Clinical and Basic Immunodermatology

Clinical and Basic Immunodermatology

Edited by

Anthony A. Gaspari, MD
Department of Dermatology
University of Maryland School of Medicine
Baltimore, MD
USA

Stephen K. Tyring, MD, PhD
Department of Dermatology
University of Texas Medical School at Houston
Houston, TX
USA

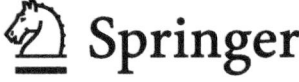 Springer

Editors
Anthony A. Gaspari, MD
University of Maryland School of Medicine
Baltimore, MD
USA

Stephen K. Tyring, MD, PhD
University of Texas Medical School at Houston
Houston, TX
USA

ISBN 978-1-84882-851-3   e-ISBN 978-1-84800-165-7
DOI 10.1007/978-1-84800-165-7
Springer Dordrecht Heidelberg London New York

British Library Cataloguing in Publication Data
A catalogue record for this book is available from the British Library

Library of Congress Control Number: 2008923739

Printed on acid-free paper

Springer is part of Springer Science+Business Media (www.springer.com)

Preface

In 1981, the first edition of *Clinical Immunodermatology* was published, with Dr. Mark Dahl as the editor and sole contributor. This textbook filled a real need for residents in training, as the focus of this textbook was immunologically mediated skin disease. It certainly was critical and highly enjoyable reading for me when I began my dermatology residency in 1982 at Emory University. Its second edition in 1985 and the third and final edition in 1996 saw further improvements in this outstanding textbook. It has been a tremendous asset for all of those interested in the immune system, and how it plays a protective and pathologic role in skin diseases. The critical features of this textbook were its concise nature, simple diagrams, and clear and direct style of delivering fundamental information about the role of the immune system and its relevance to skin diseases. All of these features made this textbook well appreciated by residents and clinicians. This textbook really was the brainchild of Dr. Mark Dahl, and reflected well his lucid approach to teaching, organizing information, and presenting a complex topic in such a high-quality product. Fortunately for our specialty, Dr. Dahl remains active in academic dermatology, teaching, patient care, and publishing.

Over the past twelve years, much has changed, stimulating Steve Tyring and I to revisit this important subject. There has been an explosion of information in the fields of cellular, molecular, innate, adaptive immunity, and immunopharmacology. In parallel, these advances have been applied to and translated to a better understanding and treatment of a number of common and less common dermatologic diseases. There are also a number of new therapeutic agents that are targeted therapies, or have an immune mechanism. All of these developments have occurred during the blossoming of the information age. Thus, we decided that it was no longer possible to present a single or even a dual authored/edited textbook. Steve Tyring and I decided to pursue the recruitment of national and international experts to author chapters on their respective areas of expertise. Hence, our approach for this important endeavor is that of a multiauthored collection of chapters that would be integrated into this book. Despite the different approach, our goal is to present the latest information related to fundamentals of the skin immune system, as well as a disease-focused textbook in the same concise, readable, and easily digested format that was initially developed by Dr. Dahl.

We thank Dr. Dahl for his vision and his original book, which has had profound influence on generations of dermatologists. We have strived to enhance the teaching of cutaneous immunology, particularly as related to skin disease, to the next generations of young dermatologists who will be caring for patients

afflicted with immune-based skin diseases. We would be delighted if our textbook triggered the kind of interest in immunology that was stimulated in Steve
and I during our training.

Anthony A. Gaspari
Stephen K. Tyring

Contents

Section II   Common Skin Diseases

Contributors

Masayuki Amagai, MD, PhD
Department of Dermatology, Keio University School of Medicine, Tokyo, Japan

John C. Ansel, MD
Department of Dermatology, University of Colorado at Denver and Health Sciences Center, Aurora, CO, USA

Jack L. Arbiser, MD, PhD
Department of Dermatology, Emory University School of Medicine, Atlanta, GA, USA

Cesar A. Arias, MD, MSc, PhD
Department of Dermatology, University of Texas Medical School at Houston, Houston, TX, USA

Cheryl A. Armstrong, MD
Department of Dermatology, University of Colorado at Denver and Health Sciences Center, Aurora, CO, USA

Anita Arora, MD
Department of Dermatology, University of Texas Health Science Center, Houston, TX, USA

Sergei P. Atamas, MD, PhD
Department of Medicine, University of Maryland School of Medicine, Baltimore, MD, USA

Brenda L. Bartlett, MD
University of Maryland School of Medicine, Baltimore, MD, USA

Donald V. Belsito, MD
Clinical Professor of Medicine (Dermatology), University of Missouri-Kansas City, Kansas City, MO, USA

Emily M. Berger, BA
Tufts University School of Medicine, Boston, MA, USA

Brian Berman, MD, PhD
Department of Dermatology and Cutaneous Surgery, Miller School of
Medicine, University of Miami, Miami, FL, USA

Thomas Bieber, MD, PhD
Department of Dermatology and Allergy, Friedrich Wilhelms University,
Bonn, Germany

Donna Bilu Martin, MD
Department of Dermatology, University of Maryland, Baltimore, MD, USA

Doerte Bittner, MD
Department of Dermatology, University Hospital Heidelberg, Heidelberg,
Germany

Andrew Blauvelt, MD
Department of Dermatology and the Department of Molecular Microbiology
and Immunology, Oregon Health and Science University and Dermatology
Service, Portland, OR, USA

Raymond E. Boissy, PhD
Department of Dermatology, University of Cincinnati College of Medicine,
Cincinnati, OH, USA

Jan D. Bos, MD, PhD, FRCP
Department of Dermatology, Academic Medical Center, University of
Amsterdam, Amsterdam, The Netherlands

Mariah R. Brown, MD
Department of Dermatology, University of Colorado at Denver and Health
Sciences Center, Aurora, CO, USA

Julie Burnett, MD
Department of Dermatology, Keck School of Medicine, University of
Southern California, Los Angeles, CA, USA

Todd V. Cartee, MD
Department of Dermatology, Emory University School of Medicine, Atlanta,
GA, USA

Mei Chen, PhD
Department of Dermatology, Keck School of Medicine, University
of Southern California, Los Angeles, CA, USA

Bernard A. Cohen, MD
Department of Dermatology, Johns Hopkins Outpatient Center, Baltimore,
MD, USA

Jennifer Z. Cooper, MD
University of Maryland School of Medicine, Baltimore, MD, USA

Edward W. Cowen, MD, MHSc
Dermatology Branch, Center for Cancer Research, National Cancer Institute,
Bethesda, MD, USA

Noah Craft, MD, PhD, DTMH
Divisions of Dermatology and Adult Infectious Diseases, David Geffen
School of Medicine at UCLA and Los Angeles Biomedical Research
Institute, Torrance, CA, USA

Ponciano D. Cruz, Jr., MD
Department of Dermatology, University of Texas Southwestern Medical
Center, Dallas, TX, USA

Luis A. Diaz, MD
Department of Dermatology, University of North Carolina School of
Medicine, Chapel Hill, NC, USA

Ilia Elenkov, MD
Institute of Neurobiology and Molecular Medicine, Rome, Italy

Alexander Enk, MD, PhD
Department of Dermatology, University Hospital Heidelberg, Heidelberg,
Germany

Clemens Esche, MD
Department of Dermatology, Johns Hopkins Outpatient Center, Baltimore,
MD, USA

David F. Fiorentino, MD, PhD
Assistant Professor of Dermatology and Medicine (Rheumatology),
Stanford University School of Medicine, Stanford, CA, USA

Levi E. Fried, BA
Department of Dermatology, Emory University School of Medicine, Atlanta,
GA, USA

Anthony A. Gaspari, MD
Department of Dermatology, University of Maryland School of Medicine,
Baltimore, MD, USA

Aron J. Gewirtzman, MD
Department of Dermatology, Center for Clinical Studies, Houston, TX, USA

Amos Gilhar, MD
Skin Research Laboratory, Technion-Israel Institute of Technology, Haifa,
Israel

Michael Girardi, MD
Department of Dermatology, Yale University School of Medicine,
New Haven, CT, USA

Laura M. Gober, MD
Division of Allergy and Clinical Immunology, Johns Hopkins University
School of Medicine, Baltimore, MD, USA

Alice B. Gottlieb, MD, PhD
Department of Dermatology, Tufts–New England Medical Center, Boston,
MA, USA

Richard D. Granstein, MD
Department of Dermatology, Joan and Sanford I. Weill Medical College of
Cornell University, New York–Presbyterian Hospital, New York, NY, USA

Gary M. Halliday, BSc (Hons), PhD, DSc
Dermatology Research Laboratories, University of Sydney, Sydney, New
South Wales, Australia

Christopher Hansen, MD
Department of Dermatology, University of Utah, Salt Lake City, UT, USA

Ulrich R. Hengge, MD, MBA
Department of Dermatology, Heinrich-Heine University, Duesseldorf,
Germany

Sherrif F. Ibrahim, MD, PhD
Department of Dermatology, University of Rochester, Rochester, NY, USA

Camille E. Introcaso, MD
Department of Dermatology, University of Pennsylvania School of Medicine,
Philadelphia, PA, USA

Nahed Ismail, MD, PhD
Department of Pathology, University of Texas Medical Branch, Galveston,
TX, USA

Heidi T. Jacobe, MD
Department of Dermatology, University of Texas Southwestern Medical
Center, Dallas, TX, USA

H. Ray Jalian, MD
Division of Dermatology, Department of Medicine, David Geffen School of
Medicine, University of California at Los Angeles, Los Angeles, CA, USA

Richard S. Kalish, MD, PhD[†]
Department of Dermatology, Stony Brook University Medical Center, Stony
Brook, NY, USA

[†] Deceased.

Ellen J. Kim, MD
Department of Dermatology, University of Pennsylvania School of Medicine, Philadelphia, PA, USA

Jenny Kim, MD, PhD
Division of Dermatology, Department of Medicine, David Geffen School of Medicine, University of California at Los Angeles, Los Angeles, CA, USA

Sidney Klaus, MD
Department of Dermatology, VA Medical Center, Dartmouth Medical School, White River Junction, VT, USA

Marcelo G. Label, MD
Department of Dermatology, Hospital Ramos Mejía, Buenos Aires, Argentina

Zelmira Lazarova, MD
Department of Dermatology, Medical College of Wisconsin, Milwaukee, WI, USA

Mark Lebwohl, MD
Department of Dermatology, Mount Sinai School of Medicine, New York, NY, USA

Erica Lee, MD
Department of Dermatology, Joan and Sanford I. Weill Medical College of Cornell University, New York–Presbyterian Hospital, New York, NY, USA

Benjamin A. Lefkove, BA
Department of Dermatology, Emory University School of Medicine, Atlanta, GA, USA

Justin J. Leitenberger, BS
Department of Dermatology, University of Texas Southwestern Medical Center, Dallas, TX, USA

I. Caroline Le Poole, PhD
Department of Pathology, Loyola University Medical Center Maywood, IL, USA

Ning Li, PhD
Department of Dermatology, University of North Carolina School of Medicine, Chapel Hill, NC, USA

Zhi Liu, PhD
Department of Dermatology, University of North Carolina School of Medicine, Chapel Hill, NC, USA

Kurt Q. Lu, MD
Department of Dermatology, University Hospitals Case Medical Center Case Western Reserve University, Cleveland, OH, USA

Thomas A. Luger, MD
Department of Dermatology, University of Münster, Münster, Germany

Irina G. Luzina, MD, PhD
Department of Medicine, University of Maryland School of Medicine,
Baltimore, MD, USA

Michael R. McGinnis, PhD, ABMM
Department of Pathology, University of Texas Medical Branch, Galveston,
TX, USA

Natalia Mendoza, MD
Department of Dermatology, Universidad El Bosque, Bogota, Colombia

Lloyd S. Miller, MD, PhD
Division of Dermatology, David Geffen School of Medicine, University of
California at Los Angeles, Los Angeles, CA, USA

Fergal J. Moloney, MD, MRCPI
Dermatology Research Laboratories, University of Sydney,
Sydney, New South Wales, Australia

Kelly Nelson, MD
Department of Dermatology, University of North Carolina School of
Medicine, Chapel Hill, NC, USA

Frank O. Nestle, MD
St. John's Institute of Dermatology, Division of Genetics and Molecular
Medicine, Kings' College London School of Medicine at Guy's Kings'
College and St. Thomas Hospitals, London, UK

James J. Nordlund, MD
Department of Dermatology, Wright State Boonshoft School of Medicine,
Dayton, OH, USA

Carlos H. Nousari, MD
Department of Dermatology, University of Miami, Miami, FL, USA

Ralf Paus, MD
Department of Dermatology, University Hospital Schleswig-Holstein,
Luebeck, Germany; Department of Cutaneous Medicine, School of
Translational Medicine, University of Manchester, Manchester, UK

Oliver A. Perez, MD
Department of Dermatology and Cutaneous Surgery, Miller School of
Medicine, University of Miami, Miami, FL, USA

Julia Prölss, MD
Department of Dermatology and Allergy, Friedrich Wilhelms University,
Bonn, Germany

Jennifer Remington, MD
Department of Dermatology, Keck School of Medicine, University of
Southern California, Los Angeles, CA, USA

Stephen K. Richardson, MD
Department of Dermatology, University of Pennsylvania School of Medicine,
Philadelphia, PA, USA

Steven Richardson, MD
Oakwood Hospital, Dearborn, MI, USA

Scott Roberts, PhD
Department of Dermatology, Yale University School of Medicine, New
Haven, CT, USA

Alain H. Rook, MD
Department of Dermatology, University of Pennsylvania School of Medicine,
Philadelphia, PA, USA

Sarbjit S. Saini, MD
Division of Allergy and Clinical Immunology, Johns Hopkins University
School of Medicine, Baltimore, MD, USA

Carolyn Senavsky, MD
Division of Dermatology, David Geffen School of Medicine, University of
California at Los Angeles, Los Angeles, CA, USA

Richard D. Sontheimer, MD
Department of Dermatology, University of Oklahoma Health Sciences
Center, Oklahoma City, OK, USA

Martin Steinhoff, MD, PhD
Department of Dermatology, University of Münster, Münster, Germany

Craig K. Svensson, PharmD, PhD
College of Pharmacy, Nursing and Health Sciences, Purdue University West
Lafayette, IN, USA

Robert A. Swerlick, MD
Department of Dermatology, Emory University School of Medicine, Atlanta,
GA, USA

Francisco A. Tausk, MD
Department of Dermatology and Psychiatry, University of Rochester School
of Medicine, Rochester, NY, USA

Marcel B.M. Teunissen, PhD
Department of Dermatology, Academic Medical Center, University of
Amsterdam, Amsterdam, The Netherlands

Anne Marie Tremaine, MD
Department of Dermatology, Center for Clinical Studies, Houston,
TX, USA

Stephen K. Tyring, MD, PhD, MBA
Department of Dermatology, University of Texas Medical School at Houston,
Houston, TX, USA

Mark C. Udey, MD, PhD
Dermatology Branch, Center for Cancer Research, National Cancer Institute,
Bethesda, MD, USA

Annemarie Uliasz, MD
Department of Dermatology, Mount Sinai School of Medicine, New York,
NY, USA

Guy F. Webster, MD, PhD
Jefferson Dermatology Associates, Philadelphia, PA, USA

Stephen E. Wolverton, MD
Department of Dermatology, Indiana University School of Medicine,
Indianapolis, IN, USA

David T. Woodley, MD
Department of Dermatology, Keck School of Medicine, University of
Southern California, Los Angeles, CA, USA

Kim B. Yancey, MD
Department of Dermatology, University of Texas Southwestern Medical
Center, Dallas, TX, USA

Section I
Concepts of Fundamental Importance for Understanding Skin Disease

1
Cytokines and Chemokines

Oliver A. Perez and Brian Berman

Key Points

- Cytokines are soluble mediators (polypeptides) that act as messengers of the immune system.
- Cytokines are critical in fundamental processes such as host defense, cell cycle control, inflammation, cancer, fibrosis, wound healing, and angiogenesis.
- Cytokines and chemokines have been implicated in the pathogenesis of a number of skin diseases, and are now being targeted by specific biologic agents produced by recombinant DNA technology.
- Chemokines are a structurally diverse collection of bioactive molecules that include lipids, peptides, and small proteins of several classes.
- Chemokines play a critical role in the pathogenesis wound healing, scarring of cell trafficking, cancer and inflammatory skin disorders.

Cytokines are soluble low-molecular weight glyco-proteins or small polypeptides that act in an auto-crine or paracrine manner between leukocytes and other cells. Cytokines have many biologic func-tions and are important for leukocyte growth and differentiation as well as activation and migration. Cytokines orchestrate defense, growth, fibrosis, angiogenesis, inflammation, and neoplasm con-trol.[1–3] They are synthesized by immunologic cells such as lymphocytes and monocytes/macrophages and by nonimmunologic cells such as keratinocytes and endothelial cells. Proinflammatory cytokines include interleukin-1 (IL-1), IL-2, interferon-γ (IFN-γ), and tumor necrosis factor-α (TNF-α), and antiinflammatory cytokines include IL-1 receptor antagonist, IL-4, IL-10, and transforming growth factor-β (TGF-β)[4,5] (Fig. 1.1). The overexpression of inflammatory cytokines or decreased levels of

antiinflammatory cytokines can lead to inflammatory cutaneous disorders.

The CD4[+] T-helper (Th) lymphocyte paradigm has also contributed to our understanding of inflam-matory cutaneous disorders. CD4[+] Th1 cells evoke cell-mediated immunity and phagocyte-depend-ent inflammation, while CD4[+] Th2 cells evoke strong antibody, or humeral, immune responses, including those of the immunoglobulin E (IgE) antibody class, and inhibit phagocytosis.[6–10] Th2 interleukins can also inhibit the development of the Th1 response.[11] A predominant Th1 cytokine pattern is characteristic in diseases such as psoria-sis and contact dermatitis, while a Th2 cytokine pattern is characteristic in diseases such as atopic dermatitis and late-stage cutaneous lymphoma[2,4] (Table 1.1).

As important as the cytokine production profiles of specific lymphocyte subsets during an immune response or disease process are the chemokines (chemotactic cytokines) released and their ulti-mate recruitment of other lymphocyte subsets. Chemokines play an important role in angio-genesis, hematopoiesis, neural development, can-cer metastasis, and infection. Chemokines belong to a structurally diverse collection of bioactive molecules that include lipids (e.g., prostaglandin D_2 and leukotrienes), peptides (e.g., chemerin nonamer), and small proteins of several classes (e.g., defensins, chemokines, and nonchemokine cytokines such as granulocyte-macrophage colony-stimulating factor (GM-CSF)). The crystal structure of all chemokines share a disordered amino terminus, a β-pleaded sheet composed of three antiparallel strands, a carboxyl-terminal α-helix, and two to

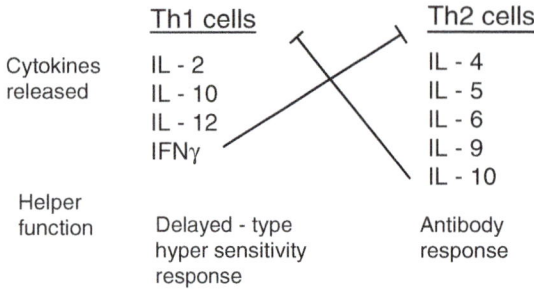

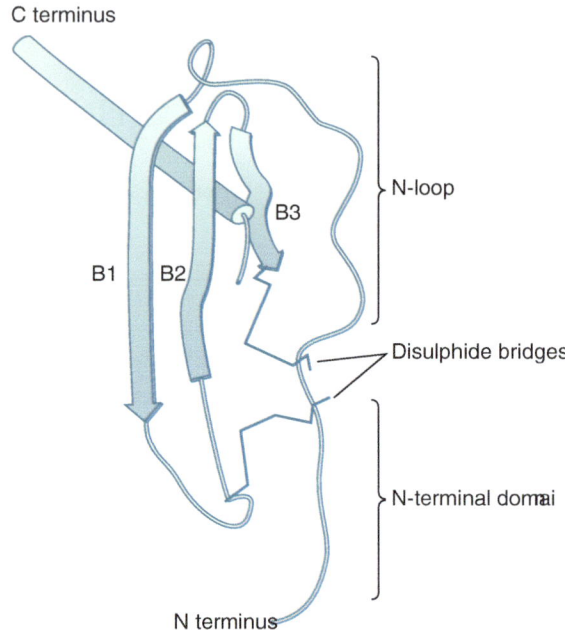

FIG. 1.1. Th1 and Th2 cytokines, their interactions and their effect on the immune response

TABLE 1.1. Cytokine production profiles of CD4[+] T-helper cell subtypes[3,6–10]

Th1	IL-2, IL-10, IL-12, IFN-γ, TNF–α/ –β, GM-CSF
Th2	IL-4, IL-5, IL-6, IL-9, IL-10, IL-13, IL-25, GM-CSF

GM-CSF – Granulocyte-macrophage Colony Stimulating Factor; IFN – Interferon; IL – Interleukin; TNF – Tumor Necrosis Factor

FIG. 1.2. Crystal structure of a chemokine. Chemokines share a disordered amino terminus, a β-pleated sheet composed of three antiparallel strands, a carboxyl-terminal α-helix and two to three disulfide bonds that stabilize the core of the protein

three disulfide bonds that stabilize the core of the protein[12] (Fig. 1.2).

During the last two decades, there has been an exponential increase in our understanding of the innate and adaptive immune systems and the role cytokine and chemokine networks play in T-cell, antigen-presenting cell (APC), and dendritic cell (DC) activation and function. Consequently, there has been a radical increase in our understanding of the pathogenesis of wound healing, scarring, skin cancer, and inflammatory dermatoses as well as improvements in their management and treatment. However, effective cures for these dermatologic conditions remain to be developed. This chapter reviews the function of cytokines and chemokines, their profiles in these common dermatologic conditions, and how present and future therapeutics are targeting known cytokine and chemokine networks.

Cytokines

Transforming Growth Factor

In the skin, TGF-β is produced by macrophages, fibroblasts, and epithelial cells, and has been shown to stimulate collagen gene expression and protein production.[13–15] It has three isoforms in humans, and TGF-β signaling involves the interaction of at least three different receptors (types I, II, and III) through a heteromeric protein kinase receptor complex. The three TGF-β receptors are serine-threonine kinases with cysteine-rich extracellular domains.[16,17] It has been shown that the expression of TGF-β receptors I and II as well as specific TGF-β isoforms are elevated in fibrotic disorders characterized by excessive accumulation of interstitial matrix material in the kidney, liver, lung, and skin.[18–23]

TGF-β1 has been identified by Northern analysis and immunohistochemistry in hypertrophic scars, and hypertrophic scar fibroblasts have been shown to produce approximately twice as much TGF-β1 as do normal skin fibroblasts.[21,24] When Smith et al.[25,26] examined the effect of exogenous TGF-β2 on keloid fibroblasts, they found increased DNA synthesis. According to their findings, TGF-β2 can induce a greater contraction of keloid fibroblasts than hypertrophic scar fibroblasts in the fibroblast-populated collagen lattice model.

The increased contraction of keloid fibroblasts was decreased with the addition of anti–TGF-β2 antibody. Other in vitro studies have also shown that TGF-β1 and −β2 stimulate fibroblasts to produce collagen and that neutralizing antibodies to TGF-β1 and −β2 inhibit scar tissue formation.[22,25–31] However, TGF-β3 prevents scarring. Fibronectin and collagen types I and III deposition in the early stages of wound healing as well as overall scarring was reduced when exogenous TGF-β3 was added to cutaneous rat wounds. By contrast, rat wounds treated with TGF-β1 and −β2 have increased extracellular matrix (ECM) deposition in the early stages of wound healing.[27,32]

In the near future, Renovo Pharmaceuticals (Manchester, UK) is planning the release of Justiva, which is derived from recombinant human (rhu) TGF-β3. Justiva has shown promise in a phase I clinical trial and two phase II clinical trials completed in the United Kingdom. In these studies, wounds treated with Justiva demonstrated a statistically significant improvement in scar appearance, with a response rate of over 70%. Safety data analysis from over 1000 subjects has revealed that Justiva is tolerable and safe in humans. Renovo Pharmaceuticals has ongoing clinical trials to study the effect of Justiva on scar improvement following surgical excision of benign head and neck nevi, bilateral breast augmentation and reduction, and varicose vein removal. Although the results of these trials are pending, Renovo Pharmaceuticals is hopeful that Justiva will soon be available on the market.[33]

Interferons

Interferons (IFNs) are naturally occurring immune response modulators produced by lymphocytes and fibroblasts. This family of cytokines demonstrates antiviral, antiproliferative, immune-enhancing, and immune-differentiating properties. The IFN family consists of type I IFN, IFN-α, and IFN-β, which are produced by leukocytes and fibroblasts, respectively, and type II IFN, or IFN-γ, which is produced by T lymphocytes (Table 1.2). These two types of IFNs bind to different high-affinity tyrosine kinase receptors from the Janus family of kinases. When activated, these kinases phosphorylate cytoplasmic signal transduction proteins that bind to cis-acting elements and subsequently regulate cellular gene transcription rates.[21,34]

Fibroblast proliferation as well as collagen, fibronectin, and glycosaminoglycan production are decreased when IFNs bind to their receptors on fibroblasts.[21,34–36] Interferon-α activates dermal fibroblast synthesis of collagenase and reduces the production of its natural inhibitor, tissue inhibitor of metalloproteinase-I (TIMP-I). In contrast, IFN-β has been shown to inhibit collagen production.[21,37] Interferon-γ inhibits fibroblast proliferation, chemotaxis, and production of ECM macromolecules, including collagen and glycosaminoglycans.[13,35–39] Interferon-γ has also been shown to decrease collagen gene expression and to downregulate collagen synthesis by reducing steady-state messenger RNA (mRNA) levels of type I, II, and III procollagen as well as to downregulate nuclear factor 1, a procollagen gene-activating transcription factor.[36,40–42]

Since IFNs have antifibrotic properties, their effect has been studied in hypertrophic and keloid scar fibroblasts. In vitro studies have shown that IFN-α-2b and IFN-γ inhibit normal and hypertrophic scar fibroblast TGF-β mRNA expression and protein production/secretion. Interferon-γ has also been demonstrated to inhibit normal fibroblast TGF-β–induced type I collagen production in vitro.[43–45] In a phase II trial by Tredget et al.[46] the effect of subcutaneous recombinant IFN-α-2b in nine subjects with severe hypertrophic scarring after thermal injury was examined. After a 3-month IFN-α-2b treatment regimen, there was a significant improvement in scar assessment in seven subjects ($p < .01$), with three of the nine subjects demonstrating a significant reduction in scar volume ($p < .05$). Before the IFN-α-2b treatment, the serum TGF-β concentrations in the nine hypertrophic scar subjects were significantly higher than control

TABLE 1.2. Classification of cytokines

Interferons (IFN)	IFN-α, -β, -γ, -δ, -ε, -κ, -τ, -ω[136]
Tumor necrosis factors (TNF)	TNF-α, -β, Lymphotoxin-β[3]
Interleukins (IL)	IL-1 to IL-33[110]
Soluble Receptors	For example, CD23, sIL1–R, sIL4–R, sIL6–R, sTNF-R[3,137]
Colony-Stimulating Factors (CSF)	G-CSF, GM-CSF, M-CSF, PDGF, erythropoietin, thrombopoietin[3]

G-CSF – Granulocyte Colony Stimulating Factor; GM-CSF – Granulocyte-macrophage Colony-Stimulating Factor; M-CSF – Macrophage Colony Stimulating Factor; PDGF – Platelet Derived Growth Factor; TNF – Tumor Necrosis Factor.

(p <.05). However, serum TGF-β levels fell significantly within 2 months of IFN-α-2b therapy and remained within the normal range 1 month after the IFN-α-2b therapy was stopped (p <.05). A later study by Tredget et al.[44] also demonstrated significantly lower TGF-β serum levels after IFN-α-2b therapy in subjects with hypertrophic scars.

Interferons have also been shown to have antineoplastic properties and to be effective in the treatment of melanoma and nonmelanoma skin cancers, Kaposi's sarcoma (KS), and cutaneous T-cell lymphoma (CTCL).[47–58] Adjuvant, high-dose IFN therapy has become the standard of care in the United States for melanomas with a high risk of recurrence. The U.S. Food and Drug Administration (FDA) has approved the use of IFN-α-2b for the treatment of patients with melanomas thicker than 4 mm and lymph node metastasis. In a study by Rusciani et al.,[59] stage II melanoma IFN-α-2b–treated subjects were compared to stage II untreated controls. The results of this study demonstrated a metastasis rate of 19.6% (10 of 51 treated subjects) vs. 60% (18 of 30 untreated controls) at 3-year follow-up, (p <.0001), and a metastasis rate of 25% (4 of 16 treated subjects) vs. 63% (12 of 19 untreated controls) at 5-year follow-up (p <.005). However, the stage I melanoma IFN-α-2b–treated subjects did not have a significantly different disease progression than the untreated stage I controls at 3- and 5-year follow-up.

Therefore, IFN-α-2b therapy appears to be more effective in patients with advanced melanoma. A recent study examined the combination of IFN-α-2b and surgery in high-risk melanoma patients. In this retrospective study of 150 patients, adjuvant high-dose IFN was an effective treatment option for patients with high-risk melanoma (stages IIC and III) after definitive surgery. The 2- and 5-year relapse-free survival were estimated at 48% and 36%, respectively.[50]

The effect of IFNs has also been studied in patients with low-risk nodular or superficial basal cell carcinoma (BCC); BCC cells have been shown to express CD95 ligand (FasL) and CD95 receptor (FasR), whereas the surrounding CD4$^+$ T cells predominantly express FasR. Thus, in IFN-treated patients, BCC may regress by FasR-FasL–mediated apoptosis.[60] Intralesional IFN-α-2b demonstrated a success rate of up to 100% when used over a 3- to 4-week period at a concentration of 1.5 million

International Units (IU).[61,62] However, when used for aggressive forms of BCC, this protocol has resulted in the cure rate of only 27% of treated patients.[63] Therefore, IFN treatment of BCCs remains an alternative only for patients with low-risk nodular or superficial BCC. Although intralesional recombinant IFN-α-2b has been shown to be effective in the treatment of squamous cell carcinoma (SCC) and actinic keratosis (AK) when administered at a dose of 1.5 million IU three times weekly for 3 weeks, its use has been limited by the pain of injections and the multiple follow-up visits necessary.[64]

The FDA has also approved the use of IFN-α-2a and -2b for the treatment of KS in patients with acquired immune deficiency syndrome (AIDS) secondary to human immunodeficiency virus (HIV). The recommended dosages for IFN-α-2a and -2b are 36 and 30 million IU subcutaneously three times per week, respectively. However, the average response rate of KS to high-dose IFN-α therapy has been approximately 30%. In many cases, tumor recurrence has been observed within 6 months after discontinuation of treatment, and response to subsequent treatments has not been reliable. This has led to indefinite IFN treatment regimens until side effects become intolerable.[65]

However, IFN-α is one of the most effective single-therapy agents for the treatment of CTCL.[66] Low-grade, non-Hodgkin's T-cell lymphomas are always associated with cutaneous involvement and include mycosis fungoides (MF) and the Sézary syndrome (SS).[67] A literature review by Bunn et al.[68] of 207 MF and SS cases treated with IFN-α-2a revealed an overall response rate of 55%, with 17% of cases being complete responders to IFN-α-2a therapy. According to this review, the optimal treatment regimen is 3 million IU of IFN-α-2a given subcutaneously three times per week to patients with early-stage disease. No therapeutic difference was observed between IFN-α-2a and -2b. Another study found that intralesional injection of MF plaques with IFN-α-2b at a dose of 1 million IU given three times per week for 4 weeks produces substantial localized clinical and histologic improvement, with 10 of 12 MF plaques demonstrating complete regression localized to the IFN-α-2b injected sites.[58]

Serendipitous findings have also supported a role for IFN in the pathogenesis of inflammatory dermatoses. Patients with psoriasis have been shown to have an immunologic response characterized by the production of Th1 CD4[+] T-cell cytokines such as IFN.[69] Topical application of imiquimod 5% cream, which upregulates the innate immune system through activation of toll-like receptors, has been shown to produce aggravation and spread of psoriasis plaques, apparently through the induction of IFN production by dendritic cell precursors.[70] Also, the treatment of cancer patients with IFN-α as well as the treatment of warts with intralesional IFN-α have produced psoriasis flares and the development of psoriasis, respectively, in a location where psoriasis had not developed previously.[71,72] The development of new psoriasis lesions has also been induced by the injection of IFN-γ into the skin of patients with psoriasis.[73,74]

Although a Th1 CD4[+] T-cell cytokine pattern predominates in diseases such as psoriasis and allergic contact dermatitis, a Th2 cytokine pattern is considered to be characteristic of acute skin lesions in patients with atopic dermatitis (AD) and late-stage CTCL.[4,75–77] Given that IFN-γ regulates the Th1–Th2 balance and favors the development of a Th1 response and downregulates IgE antibody expression, it is not surprising that IFN-γ therapy has been efficacious in the treatment of AD.[78–82] New therapies for AD are therefore targeting the reduction of the Th2 response via anti–IL-4, soluble IL-4 receptor, anti–IL-13, as well as the inhibition of chemokine action via C-C chemokine receptor-4 and cutaneous lymphocyte-associated antigen inhibition.[2,77]

Tumor Necrosis Factor

In contrast to the IFNs, the effects of TNF-α on wound healing appear to be dose dependent. Low levels of TNF-α have a profibrotic effect and may be synergistic with other growth factors, such as platelet-derived growth factor (PDGF).[83] However, high concentrations of TNF-α stimulate the production of collagenase by fibroblasts and induce the breakdown of the ECM.[53,84,85] Castagnoli et al.[86] immunostained and compared hypertrophic scar biopsies with normotrophic scar biopsies from 13 patients undergoing reconstructive plastic surgery for extensive hypertrophic scars after thermal injury. Eight percent of cells in hypertrophic scars demonstrated TNF-α immunostaining vs. 35.4% of

cells in the normotrophic scars ($p < .0155$). These findings suggest that low TNF-α levels may promote the formation of hypertrophic scars. Tumor necrosis factor-α has also been associated with keloid formation. Human keloid dermal fibroblasts are less sensitive than normal dermal fibroblasts to the inhibitory effects of TNF-α on collagen synthesis, and peripheral blood mononuclear cell fractions from patients susceptible to keloid formation have increased the levels of TNF-α when compared to controls.[87–89] The bioactivity of TNF-α overlaps with that of IL-1, and TNF-α can induce IL-1 production by several cell types.[90] Like TNF-α, IL-1 regulates collagen gene expression and protein production.[13,91]

Increased serum levels of TNF-α have also been found in patients with inflammatory dermatoses when compared to control[92,93] (Fig. 1.3). Therefore, it is not surprising that inhibition of the proinflammatory cytokine TNF-α has proven to be an effective treatment for the inflammatory dermatoses. Specifically, the soluble TNF-α receptor etanercept, which inactivates circulating TNF-α, has good efficacy in the management of psoriasis.[94,95] Chimeric mouse antihuman IgG1 monoclonal antibodies that bind to and inactivate TNF-α (e.g., adalimumab, infliximab) have also

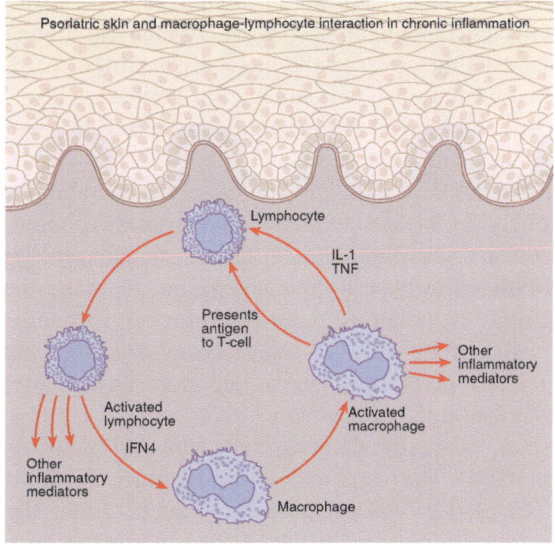

FIG. 1.3. Macrophage-lymphocyte interaction in the chronic inflammatory response of psoriatic skin. TNF, tumor necrosis factor

been demonstrated to be effective in the treatment of patients with psoriasis and marginally effective in the treatment of patients with moderate to severe AD.[96–98] The effectiveness of TNF-α inhibition in patients with psoriasis and AD has led to investigating its effectiveness in other inflammatory dermatoses. TNF-α may be efficacious in the treatment of bullous pemphigoid, subacute cutaneous lupus erythematosus, erythema annulare centrifugum, Hailey-Hailey disease, hidradenitis suppurativa, pyoderma gangrenosum, dermatomyositis, and Sweet's syndrome.[2,99–109] The effectiveness of TNF-α inhibition across a wide variety of clinical entities not only provides important information about the pathogenesis of these diseases, but also provides new directions for future research (Table 1.3).

Interleukins

An international nomenclature has been devised to standardize the names of cytokines with dominant immunoregulatory properties. These cytokines have been designated as interleukins (ILs), and newly discovered cytokines (or interleukins) are sequentially numbered. The number of interleukins is continuously growing, and it is currently up to IL-33[110] (Table 1.2). However, cytokines with immunoregulatory properties such as GM-CSF have been omitted from this nomenclature system.[5] Given the immunologic potency of interleukins and the role they play in the metabolism of the ECM, malignancy, and dermatologic inflammatory disorders, they have been targeted for the development of therapeutic applications.[4]

Interleukins not only regulate the metabolism of the ECM but also regulate fibroblast differentiation and proliferation.[111] The interleukin profiles observed in hypertrophic and keloid scars are the result of polarized specific immune responses mediated by CD4+ T-helper lymphocytes (Table 1.1). Hypertrophic and keloid scars have a predominating Th2 cytokine profile. Hypertrophic scars generally demonstrate increased numbers of CD4+ Th2 cells and a low presence of CD4+ Th1 cells.[112,113] Decreased levels of IL-2 and significantly increased levels of IL-6 ($p < .0001$) have been found in peripheral blood mononuclear cell fractions from patients susceptible to keloids when compared to controls.[88,89] Interleukin-6 has also been implicated in other fibrotic diseases such as

scleroderma and pulmonary interstitial fibrosis.[114–117] Interleukin-6 and IL-8 levels are diminished in fetal wounds, which heal without scarring, and the addition of IL-6 to fetal wounds has been shown to induce early scarring. However, IL-10 has been shown to decrease the production of IL-6 and IL-8 and to induce scarless healing when overexpressed in adult mouse wounds.[118]

Renovo Pharmaceuticals has therefore developed Prevascar, or rhu IL-10. Preclinical experiments have demonstrated that application of Prevascar to the margins of acute incisional wounds by intradermal injection decreases subsequent scarring. Renovo Pharmaceuticals is currently involved in a phase II, single-center, double-blind, placebo-controlled, randomized, clinical trial that is evaluating the antiscarring efficacy of varying doses of Prevascar in 175 subjects (1400 wounds). This trial is expected to report this year whether Prevascar is effective in preventing or reducing scarring of the skin.[33]

Interleukins have also been studied in patients with metastatic melanoma.[119] However, dose-related serious toxicities have limited IL-2 studies in melanoma patients, and low-dose IL-2 therapy has produced disappointing clinical response rates.[120] When high-dose, 100,000 units/kg, intravenous recombinant IL-2 was examined in 47 patients with metastatic malignant melanoma, up to 20% achieved objective responses; however, three patients developed myocardial infarction and one patient died during therapy.[121] Interleukin-2–based biochemotherapy (IL-2, IFN-α-2b, cisplatin, dacarbazine, and vinblastine) has shown a response rate of 48%. It appears that this combination is statistically superior to either IL-2 or chemotherapy alone.[122] Results of ongoing trials may clarify the true value of IL-2 in combination chemotherapy. Although IL-4, IL-6, and IL-7 have been evaluated for use in immunotherapy of melanoma, they have not had a significant clinical impact. However, GM-CSF has been shown to prolong both overall (37.5 months in treated patients vs. 12.2 months in matched controls) and disease-free survival when used as adjuvant therapy in patients with stage III and IV malignant melanoma ($p < .001$).[123,124]

Given that psoriasis is characterized by an overexpression of Th1 cytokines (Table 1.1) and TNF-α, the effect of rhu IL-4, a Th2 cytokine of decisive significance in regulating the Th1/Th2 balance, has been studied in an open-label trial composed

TABLE 1.3. Cytokines and their dermatologic therapeutic applications

Cytokine	Function (derived therapeutic agent)	Dermatologic application(s)
TGF		
TGF-β1,2	Stimulate fibroblast collagen gene expression and protein production	
TGF-β3	Reduces fibronectin and collagen types I and III deposition in the early stages of wound healing (rhu TGF-β3; Justiva)	Scarring[27,32,33]
IFNs		
IFN-α	T-lymphocyte and NK function enhancement, antifibrotic properties	Hypertrophic scars[44,46]
		Keloids[138]
		Malignant melanoma[50,59]
		Superficial BCC[61,62]
		AK/SCC[64]
		KS/AIDS[65]
		CTCL[58,66,68]
IFN-β	Inhibits endothelial cell migration/ neoangiogenesis	KS/AIDS[139]
IFN-γ	Promotes Th1 response	AD[78–82]
TNF-α	Promotes Th1 response, proapoptotic (chimeric TNF-α antibodies - adalimumab, infliximab)	AD[98]
		Hidradenitis suppurativa[99–101]
		PG[140–142]
		Psoriasis[94,95]
		Sarcoidosis (lupus pernio)[143,144]
	(soluble TNF-α receptor fusion protein—etanercept)	BP[109]
		Cicatricial pemphigoid[145]
		EAC[105]
		Hailey-Hailey disease[104]
		PV[146]
		PG[106]
		Psoriasis[96,97,103]
		Dermatomyositis[104]
		SCLE[104]
		Sweet's syndrome[108]
ILs		
IL-2	Stimulates T-cell activation and proliferation (rhu IL-2)	Stage IV malignant melanoma[119–122]
IL-4	Promotes Th2 response (rhu IL-4)	Psoriasis[147,148]
IL-10	Promotes Th2 response, suppresses cellular immunity and TNF-α expression, antifibrotic properties (rhu IL-10 - Prevascar)	Psoriasis[149–152]
		Scarring[33,118]
IL-12	Promotes Th1 response, proinflammatory (rhu IL-12; rhu IL-12 p40 antibody)	CTCL[126]
		Psoriasis[127]
IL-15	Stimulates T-cell activation and proliferation, upregulates angiogenesis and TNF-α expression (rhu anti-IL-15 Ab)	Psoriasis[153]
GM-CSF	Activates macrophages and stimulates peripheral blood monocytes to become cytotoxic for human melanoma cells[124]	Stage III and IV malignant melanoma[123]
CD2 fusion protein	Inhibits T-cell activation and proliferation (alefacept)	Psoriasis[154,155]
Anti-CD11a mAb	Inhibits T-cell activation (efalizumab)	Psoriasis[156,157]

AD, atopic dermatitis; AIDS, acquired immune deficiency syndrome; AK, actinic keratosis; BCC, basal cell carcinoma; BP, bullous pemphigoid; CTCL, cutaneous T-cell lymphoma; EAC, erythema annulare centrifugum; GM-CSF, granulocyte-macrophage colony-stimulating factor; IFNs, interferons; ILs, interleukins; KS, Kaposi sarcoma; NK, natural killer; PG, pyoderma gangrenosum; PV, pemphigoid vulgaris; rhu, recombinant human; SCC, squamous cell carcinoma; SCLE, subacute cutaneous lupus erythematosus; TGF, transforming growth factor; TNF, tumor necrosis factor.

of 22 subjects receiving various doses of rhu IL-4 for 6 weeks. Of the 20 subjects who completed the study, 18 had a reduction in the psoriasis area and severity index (PASI) score by 60% to 80%.[125]

Cutaneous T-cell lymphoma presents with marked defects in IL-12 production, and progression of CTCL has been associated with profound defects in cell-mediated immunity and cytokine production. A phase I dose-escalation trial examined the effect of rhu IL-12 at a concentration of 50, 100, or 300 ng/kg, given 2 times per week subcutaneously for up to 24 weeks in 10 subjects with CTCL. A complete clinical response (CR) was defined as complete disappearance of all measurable CTCL lesions for at least 1 month. A partial response (PR) was defined as at least 50% disappearance of all CTCL skin lesions for at least 1 month. Only subjects with plaque stage disease ($n = 2$) presented a CR. Two plaque stage subjects and one Sézary syndrome subject had a PR. None of the T3-stage subjects responded to the rhu IL-12 treatment. The authors announced the development of future phase II/III clinical trials based on the high response rate of plaque stage CTCL subjects to rhu IL-12.[126]

Not only has the administration of rhu IL-12 been successful in the treatment of subjects with plaque stage CTCL, but the administration of rhu IL-12 p40 antibody has also been successful in the treatment of subjects with moderate-to-severe psoriasis. A phase I, nonrandomized, open-label study evaluated the short-term safety, pharmacokinetics, and clinical response of single, ascending, intravenous doses of rhu IL-12 p40 antibody in subjects with moderate-to-severe psoriasis. Eighteen subjects with at least 3% body surface area were enrolled in an escalating dose regimen (0.1, 0.3, 1.0, and 5.0 mg/kg). The results of this study demonstrated a significant and sustained concentration-dependent improvement in psoriatic lesions in most of the subjects studied.[127]

Chemokines

There are approximately 50 human chemokines that are classified into four families based on differences in their structure and function.[128,129] The largest is the CC chemokine family. These chemokines have the first two of the four cysteine residues adjacent to each other; hence their name. These chemokines attract mononuclear cells to sites of chronic inflammation. The most widely studied CC chemokine is monocyte chemoattractant protein (MCP)-1, which is an important stimulator of monocytes, dendritic cells, and T cells. The second family of chemokines has been termed CXC, given that a single amino acid is interposed between first two of the four cysteine residues in each molecule. The most recognized

CXC chemokine is IL-8 (CXCL8), which functions to attract polymorphonuclear cells to sites of acute inflammation. The third and fourth families of chemokines only have one member each. The CX_3C is composed of fractalkine (CX_3CL1), which functions as a cell-adhesion receptor and a soluble chemoattractant when cleaved by TNF-α–converting enzyme.[130] Lymphotactin (XCL1), the only member of the fourth chemokine family, attracts T cells and natural killer cells to sites of inflammation.[131,132]

It has been a growing interest to understand chemokines and their receptor interactions in order to develop new methods to treat inflammation. However, chemokine receptors have proven difficult to antagonize. It has been hypothesized that this may be secondary to the large surface of interaction that a chemokine has with its receptor. Recent studies have shown that patients with psoriasis have an increased percentage of T cells expressing CC receptor 4 (CCR4), and the CCR4 ligands CCL17 and CCL22 may be involved in the pathogenesis of this disease.[133] The CXC receptor 3 (CXCR3)-activating chemokines CXCL9, CXCL10, and CXCL11 have also been shown to function to attract activated T-cells to areas of skin inflammation.[134] Amgen-Tularik, Inc. (Thousand Oaks, CA) has been involved in a phase 2 randomized, double-blind, placebo-controlled study to determine the safety and efficacy of T487, an oral agent that inhibits CXCR3, in subjects with moderate to severe psoriasis.[135] The results of this study will be released in the near future.

Future clinical trials on immunomodulators will continue to change the approach, management, and follow-up of patients with hypertrophic scars, keloids, skin cancer, and inflammatory dermatoses. These therapies will continue to be based on principles governing the immune system. As our current knowledge of the immune system continues to grow, the application of safe and efficacious immunomodulators to treat these common skin conditions will continue to change and shape the field of dermatology.

Conclusion

Cytokines and chemokines are critical messengers of the immune system, as well as the homeostasis of peripheral tissues such as the skin. This class of molecules has been implicated in the pathogenesis of a number of dermatologic diseases. The continued discovery of novel members of the cytokine/chemokine family will expand our understanding of the role these mediators play in health and disease, and will also lead to new therapeutic targets.

References

1. Holman DM, Kalaaji AN. Cytokines in dermatology. J Drugs Dermatol 2006;5:520–524.
2. Nickoloff BJ, Stevens SR. What have we learned in dermatology from the biologic therapies? J Am Acad Dermatol 2006;54:S143–51.
3. Trefzer U, Hofmann M, Sterry W, Asadullah K. Cytokine and anticytokine therapy in dermatology. Expert Opin Biol Ther 2003;3:733–743.
4. Asadullah K, Sterry W, Trefzer U. Cytokines: interleukin and interferon therapy in dermatology. Clin Exp Dermatol 2002;27:578–584.
5. Asadullah K, Sterry W, Trefzer U. Cytokine therapy in dermatology. Exp Dermatol 2002;11:97–106.
6. Chinen J, Shearer WT. Basic and clinical immunology. J Allergy Clin Immunol 2005;116:411–418.
7. Romagnani S. T-cell subsets (Th1 versus Th2). Ann Allergy Asthma Immunol 2000;85:9–18; quiz 18, 21.
8. Ngoc PL, Gold DR, Tzianabos AO, Weiss ST, Celedon JC. Cytokines, allergy, and asthma. Curr Opin Allergy Clin Immunol 2005;5:161–166.
9. Shibuya H, Hirohata S. Differential effects of IFN-alpha on the expression of various TH2 cytokines in human CD4+ T cells. J Allergy Clin Immunol 2005;116:205–212.
10. Dong C, Flavell RA. Th1 and Th2 cells. Curr Opin Hematol 2001;8:47–51.
11. Taylor JJ, Mohrs M, Pearce EJ. Regulatory T cell responses develop in parallel to Th responses and control the magnitude and phenotype of the Th effector population. J Immunol 2006;176:5839–5847.
12. Clark-Lewis I, Schumacher C, Baggiolini M, Moser B. Structure-activity relationships of interleukin-8 determined using chemically synthesized analogs: critical role of NH2–terminal residues and evidence for uncoupling of neutrophil chemotaxis, exocytosis, and receptor binding activities. J Biol Chem 1991;266:23128–23134.
13. Boyce DE, Ciampolini J, Ruge F, Murison MS, Harding KG. Inflammatory-cell subpopulations in keloid scars. Br J Plast Surg 2001;54:511–516.
14. Sporn MB, Roberts AB. The transforming growth factor-betas: past, present, and future. Ann N Y Acad Sci 1990;593:1–6.
15. Roberts AB, Sporn MB, Assoian RK, et al. Transforming growth factor type beta: rapid induction of fibrosis and angiogenesis in vivo and stimulation of collagen formation in vitro. Proc Natl Acad Sci U S A 1986;83:4167–4171.
16. Wrana JL, Attisano L, Carcamo J, et al. TGF beta signals through a heteromeric protein kinase receptor complex. Cell 1992;71:1003–1014.
17. Massague J, Andres J, Attisano L, et al. TGF-beta receptors. Mol Reprod Dev 1992;32:99–104.
18. Massague J. TGF-beta signal transduction. Annu Rev Biochem 1998;67:753–791.
19. Chin GS, Liu W, Peled Z, et al. Differential expression of transforming growth factor-beta receptors I and II and activation of smad 3 in keloid fibroblasts. Plast Reconstr Surg 2001;108:423–429.
20. Schmid P, Itin P, Cherry G, Bi C, Cox DA. Enhanced expression of transforming growth factor-beta type I and type II receptors in wound granulation tissue and hypertrophic scar. Am J Pathol 1998;152:485–493.
21. Tredget EE, Nedelec B, Scott PG, Ghahary A. Hypertrophic scars, keloids, and contractures. The cellular and molecular basis for therapy. Surg Clin North Am 1997;77:701–730.
22. Zhang K, Garner W, Cohen L, Rodriguez J, Phan S. Increased types I and III collagen and transforming growth factor-beta 1 mRNA and protein in hypertrophic burn scar. J Invest Dermatol 1995;104:750–754.
23. Garner WL, Karmiol S, Rodriguez JL, Smith DJ Jr, Phan SH. Phenotypic differences in cytokine responsiveness of hypertrophic scar versus normal dermal fibroblasts. J Invest Dermatol 1993;101:875–879.
24. Younai S, Venters G, Vu S, Nichter L, Nimni ME, Tuan TL. Role of growth factors in scar contraction: an in vitro analysis. Ann Plast Surg 1996;36:495–501.
25. Smith P, Mosiello G, Deluca L, Ko F, Maggi S, Robson MC. TGF-beta2 activates proliferative scar fibroblasts. J Surg Res 1999;82:319–323.
26. Smith PD, Siegler K, Wang X, Robson MC. Transforming growth factor beta 2 increases DNA synthesis and collagen production in keloid fibroblasts. Surg Forum 1998;49:617.
27. Shah M, Foreman DM, Ferguson MW. Neutralisation of TGF-beta 1 and TGF-beta 2 or exogenous addition of TGF-beta 3 to cutaneous rat wounds reduces scarring. J Cell Sci 1995;108(pt 3):985–1002.
28. Tredget EE. The molecular biology of fibroproliferative disorders of the skin: Potential cytokine therapeutics. Ann Plast Surg 1994;33:152–154.
29. Shah M, Foreman DM, Ferguson MW. Control of scarring in adult wounds by neutralising antibody to transforming growth factor beta. Lancet 1992;339:213–214.

30. Finesmith TH, Broadley KN, Davidson JM. Fibroblasts from wounds of different stages of repair vary in their ability to contract a collagen gel in response to growth factors. J Cell Physiol 1990;144:99–107.

31. Montesano R, Orci L. Transforming growth factor beta stimulates collagen-matrix contraction by fibroblasts: Implications for wound healing. Proc Natl Acad Sci U S A 1988;85:4894–4897.

32. Frank S, Madlener M, Werner S. Transforming growth factors beta1, beta2, and beta3 and their receptors are differentially regulated during normal and impaired wound healing. J Biol Chem 1996;271:10188–10193.

33. Renovo. Products in development. http://www.renovo.com.

34. Kalvakolanu DV, Borden EC. An overview of the interferon system: signal transduction and mechanisms of action. Cancer Invest 1996;14:25–53.

35. Berman B, Duncan MR. Short-term keloid treatment in vivo with human interferon alfa-2b results in a selective and persistent normalization of keloidal fibroblast collagen, glycosaminoglycan, and collagenase production in vitro. J Am Acad Dermatol 1989;21:694–702.

36. Jimenez SA, Freundlich B, Rosenbloom J. Selective inhibition of human diploid fibroblast collagen synthesis by interferons. J Clin Invest 1984;74:1112–1116.

37. Duncan MR, Berman B. Gamma interferon is the lymphokine and beta interferon the monokine responsible for inhibition of fibroblast collagen production and late but not early fibroblast proliferation. J Exp Med 1985;162:516–527.

38. Adelmann-Grill BC, Hein R, Wach F, Krieg T. Inhibition of fibroblast chemotaxis by recombinant human interferon gamma and interferon alpha. J Cell Physiol 1987;130:270–275.

39. Elias JA, Jimenez SA, Freundlich B. Recombinant gamma, alpha, and beta interferon regulation of human lung fibroblast proliferation. Am Rev Respir Dis 1987;135:62–65.

40. Jimenez SA, Hitraya E, Varga J. Pathogenesis of scleroderma. Collagen. Rheum Dis Clin North Am 1996;22:647–674.

41. Duncan MR, Hasan A, Berman B. Pentoxifylline, pentifylline, and interferons decrease type I and III procollagen mRNA levels in dermal fibroblasts: evidence for mediation by nuclear factor 1 downregulation. J Invest Dermatol 1995;104:282–286.

42. Czaja MJ, Weiner FR, Takahashi S, et al. Gamma-interferon treatment inhibits collagen deposition in murine schistosomiasis. Hepatology 1989;10:795–800.

43. Ghosh AK, Yuan W, Mori Y, Chen S, Varga J. Antagonistic regulation of type I collagen gene expression by interferon-gamma and transforming growth factor-beta. integration at the level of p300/CBP transcriptional coactivators. J Biol Chem 2001;276:11041–11048.

44. Tredget EE, Wang R, Shen Q, Scott PG, Ghahary A. Transforming growth factor-beta mRNA and protein in hypertrophic scar tissues and fibroblasts: Antagonism by IFN-alpha and IFN-gamma in vitro and in vivo. J Interferon Cytokine Res 2000;20:143–151.

45. Varga J, Olsen A, Herhal J, Constantine G, Rosenbloom J, Jimenez SA. Interferon-gamma reverses the stimulation of collagen but not fibronectin gene expression by transforming growth factor-beta in normal human fibroblasts. Eur J Clin Invest 1990;20:487–493.

46. Tredget EE, Shankowsky HA, Pannu R, et al. Transforming growth factor-beta in thermally injured patients with hypertrophic scars: effects of interferon alpha-2b. Plast Reconstr Surg 1998;102:1317–28; discussion 1329–30.

47. Vassiliadis T, Patsiaoura K, Tziomalos K, et al. Pegylated IFN-alpha 2b added to ongoing lamivudine therapy in patients with lamivudine-resistant chronic hepatitis B. World J Gastroenterol 2006;12:2417–2422.

48. Berenguer M, Palau A, Fernandez A, et al. Efficacy, predictors of response, and potential risks associated with antiviral therapy in liver transplant recipients with recurrent hepatitis C. Liver Transpl 2006;12(7):1067–1076.

49. Kreuter A, Brockmeyer NH, Weissenborn SJ, et al. 5% imiquimod suppositories decrease the DNA load of intra-anal HPV types 6 and 11 in HIV-infected men after surgical ablation of condylomata acuminata. Arch Dermatol 2006;142:243–244.

50. Fluck M, Kamanabrou D, Lippold A, Reitz M, Atzpodien J. Dose-dependent treatment benefit in high-risk melanoma patients receiving adjuvant high-dose interferon alfa-2b. Cancer Biother Radiopharm 2005;20:280–289.

51. Korman N, Moy R, Ling M, et al. Dosing with 5% imiquimod cream 3 times per week for the treatment of actinic keratosis: results of two phase 3, randomized, double-blind, parallel-group, vehicle-controlled trials. Arch Dermatol 2005;141:467–473.

52. Marchitelli C, Secco G, Perrotta M, Lugones L, Pesce R, Testa R. Treatment of bowenoid and basaloid vulvar intraepithelial neoplasia 2/3 with imiquimod 5% cream. J Reprod Med 2004;49:876–882.

53. Berman B, Villa AM, Ramirez CC. Novel opportunities in the treatment and prevention of scarring. J Cutan Med Surg 2004;8(suppl 3):32–36.

54. Smith KJ, Hamza S, Skelton H. The imidazoquinolines and their place in the therapy of cutaneous disease. Expert Opin Pharmacother 2003;4:1105–1119.

55. Bong AB, Bonnekoh B, Franke I, Schon MP, Ulrich J, Gollnick H. Imiquimod, a topical immune response modifier, in the treatment of cutaneous metastases of malignant melanoma. Dermatology 2002;205:135–138.

56. Berman B, Kaufman J. Pilot study of the effect of postoperative imiquimod 5% cream on the recurrence rate of excised keloids. J Am Acad Dermatol 2002;47:S209–11.

57. Edwards L. The interferons. Dermatol Clin 2001;19:139–46, ix.

58. Vonderheid EC, Thompson R, Smiles KA, Lattanand A. Recombinant interferon alfa-2b in plaque-phase mycosis fungoides: intralesional and low-dose intramuscular therapy. Arch Dermatol 1987;123: 757–763.

59. Rusciani L, Petraglia S, Alotto M, Calvieri S, Vezzoni G. Postsurgical adjuvant therapy for melanoma: evaluation of a 3-year randomized trial with recombinant interferon-alpha after 3 and 5 years of follow-up. Cancer 1997;79:2354–2360.

60. Buechner SA, Wernli M, Harr T, Hahn S, Itin P, Erb P. Regression of basal cell carcinoma by intralesional interferon-alpha treatment is mediated by CD95 (apo-1/Fas)-CD95 ligand-induced suicide. J Clin Invest 1997;100:2691–2696.

61. Buechner SA. Intralesional interferon alfa-2b in the treatment of basal cell carcinoma. immunohistochemical study on cellular immune reaction leading to tumor regression. J Am Acad Dermatol 1991;24:731–734.

62. Greenway HT, Cornell RC, Tanner DJ, Peets E, Bordin GM, Nagi C. Treatment of basal cell carcinoma with intralesional interferon. J Am Acad Dermatol 1986;15:437–443.

63. Stenquist B, Wennberg AM, Gisslen H, Larko O. Treatment of aggressive basal cell carcinoma with intralesional interferon: evaluation of efficacy by Mohs surgery. J Am Acad Dermatol 1992;27:65–69.

64. Edwards L, Berman B, Rapini RP, et al. Treatment of cutaneous squamous cell carcinomas by intralesional interferon alfa-2b therapy. Arch Dermatol 1992;128:1486–1489.

65. Krown SE. Interferon and other biologic agents for the treatment of Kaposi's sarcoma. Hematol Oncol Clin North Am 1991;5:311–322.

66. Apisarnthanarax N, Duvic M. Cutaneous T-cell lymphoma. new immunomodulators. Dermatol Clin 2001;19:737–748.

67. Broder S, Bunn PA Jr. Cutaneous T-cell lymphomas. Semin Oncol 1980;7:310–331.

68. Bunn PA,Jr, Hoffman SJ, Norris D, Golitz LE, Aeling JL. Systemic therapy of cutaneous T-cell lymphomas (mycosis fungoides and the Sezary syndrome). Ann Intern Med 1994;121:592–602.

69. Nickoloff BJ, Bonish B, Huang BB, Porcelli SA. Characterization of a T cell line bearing natural killer receptors and capable of creating psoriasis in a SCID mouse model system. J Dermatol Sci 2000;24:212–225.

70. Gilliet M, Conrad C, Geiges M, et al. Psoriasis triggered by toll-like receptor 7 agonist imiquimod in the presence of dermal plasmacytoid dendritic cell precursors. Arch Dermatol 2004;140:1490–1495.

71. Funk J, Langeland T, Schrumpf E, Hanssen LE. Psoriasis induced by interferon-alpha. Br J Dermatol 1991;125:463–465.

72. Shiohara T, Kobayashi M, Abe K, Nagashima M. Psoriasis occurring predominantly on warts: possible involvement of interferon alfa. Arch Dermatol 1988;124:1816–1821.

73. Fierlbeck G, Rassner G. Treatment of psoriasis and psoriatic arthritis with interferon gamma. J Invest Dermatol 1990;95:138S-141S.

74. Fierlbeck G, Rassner G, Muller C. Psoriasis induced at the injection site of recombinant interferon gamma: results of immunohistologic investigations. Arch Dermatol 1990;126:351–355.

75. Farrell AM, Antrobus P, Simpson D, Powell S, Chapel HM, Ferry BL. A rapid flow cytometric assay to detect CD4+ and CD8+ T-helper (th) 0, Th1 and Th2 cells in whole blood and its application to study cytokine levels in atopic dermatitis before and after cyclosporin therapy. Br J Dermatol 2001;144:24–33.

76. Grewe M, Walther S, Gyufko K, Czech W, Schopf E, Krutmann J. Analysis of the cytokine pattern expressed in situ in inhalant allergen patch test reactions of atopic dermatitis patients. J Invest Dermatol 1995;105:407–410.

77. Leung DY, Boguniewicz M, Howell MD, Nomura I, Hamid QA. New insights into atopic dermatitis. J Clin Invest 2004;113:651–657.

78. Kirkwood J. Cancer immunotherapy: the interferon-alpha experience. Semin Oncol 2002;29:18–26.

79. Stevens SR, Hanifin JM, Hamilton T, Tofte SJ, Cooper KD. Long-term effectiveness and safety of recombinant human interferon gamma therapy for atopic dermatitis despite unchanged serum IgE levels. Arch Dermatol 1998;134:799–804.

80. Schneider LC, Baz Z, Zarcone C, Zurakowski D. Long-term therapy with recombinant interferon-gamma (rIFN-gamma) for atopic dermatitis. Ann Allergy Asthma Immunol 1998;80:263–268.

81. Somos Z, Schneider I. Serum and secretory immunoglobulins in atopic dermatitis. Orv Hetil 1993;134:1359–1361.

82. Hanifin JM, Schneider LC, Leung DY, et al. Recombinant interferon gamma therapy for atopic dermatitis. J Am Acad Dermatol 1993;28:189–197.

83. Steenfos HH. Growth factors and wound healing. Scand J Plast Reconstr Surg Hand Surg 1994;28:95–105.

84. Rapala K. The effect of tumor necrosis factor-alpha on wound healing. an experimental study. Ann Chir Gynaecol Suppl 1996;211:1–53.

85. Duncan MR, Berman B. Differential regulation of collagen, glycosaminoglycan, fibronectin, and collagenase activity production in cultured human adult dermal fibroblasts by interleukin 1-alpha and beta and tumor necrosis factor-alpha and beta. J Invest Dermatol 1989;92:699–706.

86. Castagnoli C, Stella M, Berthod C, Magliacani G, Richiardi PM. TNF production and hypertrophic scarring. Cell Immunol 1993;147:51–63.

87. He W, Liu R, Zhong B. Response of keloid fibroblasts to the effect of tumor necrosis factor-alpha (TNF-alpha). Zhonghua Zheng Xing Wai Ke Za Zhi 2001;17:332–334.

88. O'Sullivan ST, O'Shaughnessy M, O'Connor TP. Aetiology and management of hypertrophic scars and keloids. Ann R Coll Surg Engl 1996;78:168–175.

89. McCauley RL, Chopra V, Li YY, Herndon DN, Robson MC. Altered cytokine production in black patients with keloids. J Clin Immunol 1992;12:300–308.

90. Bechtel MJ, Reinartz J, Rox JM, Inndorf S, Schaefer BM, Kramer MD. Upregulation of cell-surface-associated plasminogen activation in cultured keratinocytes by interleukin-1 beta and tumor necrosis factor-alpha. Exp Cell Res 1996;223:395–404.

91. Placik OJ, Lewis VL Jr. Immunologic associations of keloids. Surg Gynecol Obstet 1992;175:185–193.

92. Arican O, Aral M, Sasmaz S, Ciragil P. Serum levels of TNF-alpha, IFN-gamma, IL-6, IL-8, IL-12, IL-17, and IL-18 in patients with active psoriasis and correlation with disease severity. Mediators Inflamm 2005;2005:273–279.

93. Roussaki-Schulze AV, Kouskoukis C, Petinaki E, et al. Evaluation of cytokine serum levels in patients with plaque-type psoriasis. Int J Clin Pharmacol Res 2005;25:169–173.

94. Gottlieb AB, Matheson RT, Lowe N, et al. A randomized trial of etanercept as monotherapy for psoriasis. Arch Dermatol 2003;139:1627–32; discussion 1632.

95. Leonardi CL, Powers JL, Matheson RT, et al. Etanercept as monotherapy in patients with psoriasis. N Engl J Med 2003;349:2014–2022.

96. Gottlieb AB, Chaudhari U, Mulcahy LD, Li S, Dooley LT, Baker DG. Infliximab monotherapy provides rapid and sustained benefit for plaque-type psoriasis. J Am Acad Dermatol 2003;48:829–835.

97. Gottlieb AB, Evans R, Li S, et al. Infliximab induction therapy for patients with severe plaque-type psoriasis: A randomized, double-blind, placebo-controlled trial. J Am Acad Dermatol 2004;51:534–542.

98. Jacobi A, Antoni C, Manger B, Schuler G, Hertl M. Infliximab in the treatment of moderate to severe atopic dermatitis. J Am Acad Dermatol 2005;52:522–526.

99. Adams DR, Gordon KB, Devenyi AG, Ioffreda MD. Severe hidradenitis suppurativa treated with infliximab infusion. Arch Dermatol 2003;139:1540–1542.

100. Lebwohl B, Sapadin AN. Infliximab for the treatment of hidradenitis suppurativa. J Am Acad Dermatol 2003;49:S275–6.

101. Sullivan TP, Welsh E, Kerdel FA, Burdick AE, Kirsner RS. Infliximab for hidradenitis suppurativa. Br J Dermatol 2003;149:1046–1049.

102. Papp KA, Miller B, Gordon KB, et al. Efalizumab retreatment in patients with moderate to severe chronic plaque psoriasis. J Am Acad Dermatol 2006;54:S164–70.

103. Gottlieb AB, Hamilton T, Caro I, et al. Long-term continuous efalizumab therapy in patients with moderate to severe chronic plaque psoriasis: updated results from an ongoing trial. J Am Acad Dermatol 2006;54:S154–63.

104. Norman R, Greenberg RG, Jackson JM. Case reports of etanercept in inflammatory dermatoses. J Am Acad Dermatol 2006;54:S139–42.

105. Minni J, Sarro R. A novel therapeutic approach to erythema annulare centrifugum. J Am Acad Dermatol 2006;54:S134–5.

106. Roy DB, Conte ET, Cohen DJ. The treatment of pyoderma gangrenosum using etanercept. J Am Acad Dermatol 2006;54:S128–34.

107. Kress DW. Etanercept therapy improves symptoms and allows tapering of other medications in children and adolescents with moderate to severe psoriasis. J Am Acad Dermatol 2006;54:S126–8.

108. Yamauchi PS, Turner L, Lowe NJ, Gindi V, Jackson JM. Treatment of recurrent sweet's syndrome with coexisting rheumatoid arthritis with the tumor necrosis factor antagonist etanercept. J Am Acad Dermatol 2006;54:S122–6.

109. Yamauchi PS, Lowe NJ, Gindi V. Treatment of coexisting bullous pemphigoid and psoriasis with the tumor necrosis factor antagonist etanercept. J Am Acad Dermatol 2006;54:S121–2.

110. Chen Q, Carroll HP, Gadina M. The newest interleukins: recent additions to the ever-growing cytokine family. Vitam Horm 2006;74:207–228.

111. Ferrarini M, Steen V, Medsger TA,Jr, Whiteside TL. Functional and phenotypic analysis of T

lymphocytes cloned from the skin of patients with systemic sclerosis. Clin Exp Immunol 1990;79: 346–352.

112. Tredget EE, Yang L, Delehanty M, Shankowsky H, Scott PG. Polarized Th2 cytokine production in patients with hypertrophic scar following thermal injury. J Interferon Cytokine Res 2006;26:179–189.

113. Molina V, Blank M, Shoenfeld Y. Fibrotic diseases. Harefuah 2002;141:973–8, 1009.

114. Shahar I, Fireman E, Topilsky M, et al. Effect of IL-6 on alveolar fibroblast proliferation in interstitial lung diseases. Clin Immunol Immunopathol 1996;79:244–251.

115. Feghali CA, Bost KL, Boulware DW, Levy LS. Control of IL-6 expression and response in fibroblasts from patients with systemic sclerosis. Autoimmunity 1994;17:309–318.

116. Gurram M, Pahwa S, Frieri M. Augmented interleukin-6 secretion in collagen-stimulated peripheral blood mononuclear cells from patients with systemic sclerosis. Ann Allergy 1994;73:493–496.

117. Feghali CA, Bost KL, Boulware DW, Levy LS. Mechanisms of pathogenesis in scleroderma. I. Overproduction of interleukin 6 by fibroblasts cultured from affected skin sites of patients with scleroderma. J Rheumatol 1992;19:1207–1211.

118. Yang GP, Lim IJ, Phan TT, Lorenz HP, Longaker MT. From scarless fetal wounds to keloids: molecular studies in wound healing. Wound Repair Regen 2003;11:411–418.

119. Rosenberg SA, Yang JC, Topalian SL, et al. Treatment of 283 consecutive patients with metastatic melanoma or renal cell cancer using high-dose bolus interleukin 2. JAMA 1994;271:907–913.

120. Atkins MB. Interleukin-2: clinical applications. Semin Oncol 2002;29:12–17.

121. Parkinson DR, Abrams JS, Wiernik PH, et al. Interleukin-2 therapy in patients with metastatic malignant melanoma: a phase II study. J Clin Oncol 1990;8:1650–1656.

122. McDermott DF, Mier JW, Lawrence DP, et al. A phase II pilot trial of concurrent biochemotherapy with cisplatin, vinblastine, dacarbazine, interleukin 2, and interferon alpha-2B in patients with metastatic melanoma. Clin Cancer Res 2000;6:2201–2208.

123. Spitler LE, Grossbard ML, Ernstoff MS, et al. Adjuvant therapy of stage III and IV malignant melanoma using granulocyte-macrophage colony-stimulating factor. J Clin Oncol 2000;18:1614–1621.

124. Grabstein KH, Urdal DL, Tushinski RJ, et al. Induction of macrophage tumoricidal activity by granulocyte-macrophage colony-stimulating factor. Science 1986;232:506–508.

125. Thomas P. IL-4 induced immune deviation as therapy of psoriasis. Arch Dermatol Res 2001;293:39.

126. Rook AH, Wood GS, Yoo EK, et al. Interleukin-12 therapy of cutaneous T-cell lymphoma induces lesion regression and cytotoxic T-cell responses. Blood 1999;94:902–908.

127. Kauffman CL, Aria N, Toichi E, et al. A phase I study evaluating the safety, pharmacokinetics, and clinical response of a human IL-12 p40 antibody in subjects with plaque psoriasis. J Invest Dermatol 2004;123:1037–1044.

128. Rot A, von Andrian UH. Chemokines in innate and adaptive host defense: basic chemokinese grammar for immune cells. Annu Rev Immunol 2004;22:891–928.

129. Cyster JG. Chemokines, sphingosine-1–phosphate, and cell migration in secondary lymphoid organs. Annu Rev Immunol 2005;23:127–159.

130. Bazan JF, Bacon KB, Hardiman G, et al. A new class of membrane-bound chemokine with a CX3C motif. Nature 1997;385:640–644.

131. Kelner GS, Kennedy J, Bacon KB, et al. Lymphotactin: a cytokine that represents a new class of chemokine. Science 1994;266:1395–1399.

132. Charo IF, Ransohoff RM. The many roles of chemokines and chemokine receptors in inflammation. N Engl J Med 2006;354:610–621.

133. Teraki Y, Miyake A, Takebayashi R, Shiohara T. Homing receptor and chemokine receptor on intraepidermal T cells in psoriasis vulgaris. Clin Exp Dermatol 2004;29:658–663.

134. Flier J, Boorsma DM, van Beek PJ, et al. Differential expression of CXCR3 targeting chemokines CXCL10, CXCL9, and CXCL11 in different types of skin inflammation. J Pathol 2001;194:398–405.

135. Amgen-Tularik, Inc. Tularik initiates phase 2 clinical trial of T487 in psoriasis. http://wwwext.amgen.com/pdfs/tularik/TLRKT487Ph2_121003.pdf.

136. Pestka S, Krause CD, Walter MR. Interferons, interferon-like cytokines, and their receptors. Immunol Rev 2004;202:8–32.

137. Rose-John S, Scheller J, Elson G, Jones SA. Interleukin-6 biology is coordinated by membrane-bound and soluble receptors: role in inflammation and cancer. J Leukoc Biol 2006;80:227–236.

138. Davison SP, Mess S, Kauffman LC, Al-Attar A. Ineffective treatment of keloids with interferon alpha-2b. Plast Reconstr Surg 2006;117:247–252.

139. Marchisone C, Benelli R, Albini A, Santi L, Noonan DM. Inhibition of angiogenesis by type I interferons in models of Kaposi's sarcoma. Int J Biol Markers 1999;14:257–262.

140. Batres LA, Mamula P, Baldassano RN. Resolution of severe peristomal pyoderma gangrenosum with

infliximab in a child with Crohn disease. J Pediatr Gastroenterol Nutr 2002;34:558–560.

141. Jenne L, Sauter B, Thumann P, Hertl M, Schuler G. Successful treatment of therapy-resistant chronic vegetating pyoderma gangrenosum with infliximab (chimeric antitumour necrosis factor antibody). Br J Dermatol 2004;150:380–382.

142. Mimouni D, Anhalt GJ, Kouba DJ, Nousari HC. Infliximab for peristomal pyoderma gangrenosum. Br J Dermatol 2003;148:813–816.

143. Haley H, Cantrell W, Smith K. Infliximab therapy for sarcoidosis (lupus pernio). Br J Dermatol 2004;150:146–149.

144. Menon Y, Cucurull E, Reisin E, Espinoza LR. Interferon-alpha-associated sarcoidosis responsive to infliximab therapy. Am J Med Sci 2004;328:173–175.

145. Sacher C, Rubbert A, Konig C, Scharffetter-Kochanek K, Krieg T, Hunzelmann N. Treatment of recalcitrant cicatricial pemphigoid with the tumor necrosis factor alpha antagonist etanercept. J Am Acad Dermatol 2002;46:113–115.

146. Berookhim B, Fischer HD, Weinberg JM. Treatment of recalcitrant pemphigus vulgaris with the tumor necrosis factor alpha antagonist etanercept. Cutis 2004;74:245–247.

147. Ghoreschi K, Mrowietz U, Rocken M. A molecule solves psoriasis? Systemic therapies for psoriasis inducing interleukin 4 and Th2 responses. J Mol Med 2003;81:471–480.

148. Ghoreschi K, Thomas P, Breit S, et al. Interleukin-4 therapy of psoriasis induces Th2 responses and improves human autoimmune disease. Nat Med 2003;9:40–46.

149. Asadullah K, Sterry W, Stephanek K, et al. IL-10 is a key cytokine in psoriasis. Proof of principle by

IL-10 therapy: a new therapeutic approach. J Clin Invest 1998;101:783–794.

150. Asadullah K, Sabat R, Wiese A, Docke WD, Volk HD, Sterry W. Interleukin-10 in cutaneous disorders: implications for its pathophysiological importance and therapeutic use. Arch Dermatol Res 1999;291:628–636.

151. Asadullah K, Docke WD, Ebeling M, et al. Interleukin 10 treatment of psoriasis: clinical results of a phase 2 trial. Arch Dermatol 1999;135:187–192.

152. Reich K, Bruck M, Grafe A, Vente C, Neumann C, Garbe C. Treatment of psoriasis with interleukin-10. J Invest Dermatol 1998;111:1235–1236.

153. Villadsen LS, Schuurman J, Beurskens F, et al. Resolution of psoriasis upon blockade of IL-15 biological activity in a xenograft mouse model. J Clin Invest 2003;112:1571–1580.

154. Krueger GG, Papp KA, Stough DB, et al. A randomized, double-blind, placebo-controlled phase III study evaluating efficacy and tolerability of 2 courses of alefacept in patients with chronic plaque psoriasis. J Am Acad Dermatol 2002;47:821–833.

155. Lebwohl M, Christophers E, Langley R, et al. An international, randomized, double-blind, placebo-controlled phase 3 trial of intramuscular alefacept in patients with chronic plaque psoriasis. Arch Dermatol 2003;139:719–727.

156. Gottlieb AB, Krueger JG, Wittkowski K, Dedrick R, Walicke PA, Garovoy M. Psoriasis as a model for T-cell-mediated disease: immunobiologic and clinical effects of treatment with multiple doses of efalizumab, an anti-CD11a antibody. Arch Dermatol 2002;138:591–600.

157. Lebwohl M, Tyring SK, Hamilton TK, et al. A novel targeted T-cell modulator, efalizumab, for plaque psoriasis. N Engl J Med 2003;349:2004–2013.

2
Innate and Adaptive Immunity

Jan D. Bos and Marcel B.M. Teunissen

Key Points

- The skin immune system is the complex network of cells that are able to mount an immune response in the skin.
- The immune response can be divided into innate and adaptive arms. This is highly relevant to both systemic immunity, as well as immunity in the skin.
- The innate immune system responds rapidly to microbial insults, but is thought to have no memory or specificity.
- The adaptive immune system, composed of B lymphocytes and T lymphocytes, requires more time to respond to a threatening challenge to the host, but is responsible for long-lasting memory and specificity, and the development of an effector pool of lymphocytes for humoral or cell mediated immunity.
- Virtually all cells that reside in the skin play some role in the function of the skin immune system. Resident cells, such as keratinocytes, and bone marrow–derived cells, such as Langerhans' cells, monocytes, and macrophages, are critical. There are a number of cells that can migrate into the skin as well (e.g., T cells, neutrophils) that also play a critical role.
- In addition to the cellular components of the skin immune system, soluble mediators are quite important. Cytokines, chemokines, lipid mediators, and antimicrobial peptides are examples of some of the critical components of the secreted mediators that can mobilize immunocytes to migrate into skin or mediate a protective or pathogenic inflammatory response.

The beginning of immunology might have been the moment when the Russian embryologist Ilya Metchnikoff described the phagocytosis theory of host defense in the 1880s.[1] Ever since, immunology has roughly been split into two major subdivisions: cellular immunity, which comprises all different immunocompetent cells, and humoral immunity, a collection of all molecules involved in immune processes, such as cytokines, immunoglobulins, complement factors, and many others. During the infancy of immunology, the cellular approach to immune defense as chosen by Metchnikoff became a matter of vigorous debate as others advocated the humoral concept of immunity. Serum studies revealed the existence of various functional factors that were able to immobilize bacteria (immobilisins) or to precipitate bacterial components (precipitins). We now know that these factors are specific subsets of antibodies. Knowledge of both immune response–related cells and molecules expanded during many decades, and at the time immunology was recognized as a separate scientific entity, the subdivision into cellular and humoral immunity was generally accepted.

At the end of the last millennium, another subdivision of immunology into two alternative major branches emerged, which is the subject of this chapter. One branch is innate or natural immunity, which encompasses a variety of natural defense mechanisms, exemplified by phagocytosis and intracellular killing of microorganisms. That mechanism is greatly enhanced by binding of specific antibodies to surface structures of these pathogens (opsonization). The other major branch is adaptive or acquired immunity that deals with

TABLE 2.1. Cellular and humoral constituents of the skin immune system (SIS)

Cellular constituents	Humoral constituents
Keratinocytes	β-defensins, cathelicidins
(Im)mature myeloid dendritic cells (Langerhans' cells, dermal dendritic cells, IDECs, Tip-DCs)	Complement and complement regulatory proteins
Plasmacytoid dendritic cells	Mannose binding lectins
Monocytes/macrophages	Immunoglobulins
Granulocytes	Cytokines, chemokines
Mast cells	Neuropeptides
Vascular and lymphatic endothelial cells	Eicosanoids and prostaglandins
T-lymphocyte subpopulations	Free radicals

IDEC, inflammatory dendritic epidermal cell; Tip-DC, tumor necrosis factor-α (TNF-α)/inducible nitric oxide synthase (iNOS)-producing dendritic cell.
Source: Modified from Bos.[50]

specific immune responses in which specificity for antigens is represented by T-cell receptors (TCRs), B-cell receptors (BCRs), and immunoglobulins secreted by plasma cells. The division into innate and adaptive immunity is not clear-cut, however, and some overlap exists. In addition, these two branches do not operate independently but rather are able to influence each other. Both innate and adaptive immunity contain humoral and cellular elements.

Translating this idea to the organ skin, we proposed *skin immune system* (SIS) as the term for the complexity of immune-response–associated cells present in normal human skin.[2] By making a qualitative inventory of cell types present in normal human skin, it became evident that approximately half of them have immune functions and thus are part of the immune system. The concept of SIS was later extended by adding its humoral constituents.[3] Table 2.1 summarizes both the cellular and humoral constituents of SIS as we presently recognize them.

The cells that participate in SIS responses may also be subdivided based on whether they function as part of innate or of adaptive immunity, or form a bridge between these compartments. One may further divide these cells based on subcategories related to their dynamic behavior in human skin. They may be resident and an integral part of the skin's microanatomy, or they may be recruited upon request. Eosinophilic granulocytes, for example,

are a recruited cell population, being present within the skin in certain pathologic states only. Another example is the influx of neutrophilic granulocytes that is seen in infections, and after sunburn due to ultraviolet B irradiation of the skin,[4] as well as in many pathologic conditions such as in Munro's microabscesses of psoriasis. Other cellular components of SIS may be formed only from precursor cells in pathologic conditions.

Finally, the cells may be circulating, such as T cells serving a detection function of the immune system. They thereby continuously verify the presence of antigens, exogenous or endogenous, presented in the context of major histocompatibility complex (MHC) class I, class II, or CD1 molecules by antigen-presenting cells. T cells may also be involved in inflammatory responses in which they downgrade the immune response with, as a result, the prevention of excessive, collateral damage. Table 2.2 summarizes these static and dynamic cellular responses of SIS

Innate and Adaptive Compartments Linked by Dendritic Cells

Innate or natural immunity is evolutionarily old, and it is the only defense system in invertebrates. In vertebrates, an adaptive or acquired system of immune responses has developed. Innate immunity

TABLE 2.2. Innate, bridging, and adaptive cells of the skin immune system, categorized as resident, recruited, and in situ maturated and outgrown populations (substantially modified from [50])

	Resident	Recruited	Maturation, growth, malignancy
Innate	Keratinocytes		Papilloma
			Basal cell carcinoma
			Spinal cell carcinoma
		Natural killer cells	Cutaneous T-cell lymphoma
		Natural killer T cells	
		Eosinophilic granulocytes	Hypereosinophilic syndrome
		Neutrophilic granulocytes	Acute infections
			Subcorneal pustulosis
	Mast cells	Basophils	Mastocytoma
			Mastocytosis
	Macrophages	Monocytes	Epithelioid cells
			Multinucleated giant cells
	Endothelial cells	Endothelial cell precursors	Teleangiectasia
	– Vascular		Kaposi sarcoma
	– Lymphatic		
Innate and bridging	Myeloid dendritic cell subsets:	Myeloid dendritic cell subsets:	Histiocytosis X
	– Langerhans' cells	– IDECs	
	– Dermal dendritic cells	– Tip-DCs	
		Plasmacytoid dendritic cells	Cutaneous lymphoblastic lymphoma
			CD4$^+$CD56$^+$ hematodermic neoplasms
Adaptive	T lymphocytes	T lymphocytes	Cutaneous T-cell lymphoma
	– Helper T cells	– Helper T cells	
	– Cytotoxic T cells	– Cytotoxic T cells	
	– Regulatory T cells	– Regulatory T cells	
		B lymphocytes	Plasma cells
			Lymphadenosis cutis benigna
			Malignant B-cell lymphoma

IDEC, inflammatory dendritic epidermal cell; Tip-DC, tumor necrosis factor-α (TNF-α)/inducible nitric oxide synthase (iNOS)-producing dendritic cell.
Source: Modified from Bos.[50]

of the integument is represented by a number of physical, biologic, and cellular factors. Essentially, innate immunity instantly responds to microorganisms and thus serves as an instantaneous defense mechanism against invading pathogens. The adaptive subsystem, however, requires several days to develop and is primarily characterized by its specificity, which is mediated by TCRs, BCRs, and immunoglobulins.[5] In addition, both innate and adaptive compartments would include those elements that are essential in the preservation of a natural homeostasis, such as avoidance of sensitization to autoantigens in the adaptive compartment.

The highly diverse BCRs and TCRs for adaptive immunity are generated through somatic rearrangement of antigen receptor genes and subsequent clonal selection. In contrast, the pattern-recognition receptors (PRRs) of innate immunity are evolutionarily ancient and germline encoded, and they form the first natural line of defense. The PRRs recognize highly conserved molecular structures that are shared by many different pathogens. Upon ligand binding, both innate and adaptive immunoreceptors engage intracellular signaling pathways that converge on conserved core transcription factors for cell activation. One key factor for both innate and adaptive immune responses is nuclear factor (NF)-κB.[6] A precise account of the many different, interacting intracellular transcription mechanisms is beyond the scope of this chapter.

Dendritic cells, which in normal human skin are represented by epidermal Langerhans' cells and dermal dendritic cells,[7] may be seen as a bridge between the innate and adaptive immune systems. They not only recognize microbes and innocent apoptotic cells, but also are able to translate this information to T cells in the regional lymph node to induce immunity or tolerance.[8] By expression of Toll-like receptors (TLRs), they can recognize conserved molecular patterns of microbial agents and become activated, leading to the production of proinflammatory cytokines such as tumor necrosis factor-α (TNF-α). In this process, the activation of immature dermal dendritic cells or epidermal Langerhans' cells can be further enhanced by factors of the innate subsystem, such as proinflammatory cytokines TNF-α and IL-1α, which are produced by keratinocytes upon contact with pathogens.[9]

The immature skin resident dendritic cells become activated when they take up (foreign) antigens from the skin environment and they then undergo maturation as they migrate to the skin-draining lymph nodes to initiate adaptive immune responses. Maturation includes the downregulation of phagocytosis activity and the upregulation of human leukocyte antigen (HLA) expression and of co-stimulatory molecules, which are required for efficient priming of effector T lymphocytes. In particular, during activation Langerhans' cells also lose the expression of E-cadherin, a molecule used to anchor themselves to the epidermal keratinocytes. Loss of E-cadherin facilitates their exit from the epidermis. In the lymph nodes, skin-derived antigen-presenting cells prime naive T cells for the pathogens that are present in the skin and simultaneously confer skin-homing capacity to the T cells. The primed T cells subsequently migrate to the skin and mediate specific, adaptive immune responses in there.

In contrast, in normal noninflamed skin, danger signals that cause activation or maturation of dendritic cells or Langerhans' cells are absent, leading to decreased antigen presentation to T lymphocytes. It is believed that if immature dendritic cells reach the lymph node and present (auto) antigens (for example, derived from "innocent" apoptotic cells) to T lymphocytes, they will confer a more regulatory phenotype to the primed T cells rather than effector functions. This process is called peripheral tolerance, and it has an important function in maintaining homeostasis in the skin. Although most T-cell priming will likely occur in the skin-draining lymph nodes, it cannot be excluded that activated Langerhans' cells and dermal dendritic cells may also present antigens to resident T cells when passing the papillary dermis on their way from the skin to the lymph nodes.

As mentioned before, normal human skin contains two subsets of dendritic cells: the Langerhans' cells in the epidermal compartment, and the dermal dendritic cells in the dermis. However, in inflammatory conditions additional types of dendritic cells can be observed. Inflammatory dendritic epidermal cells (IDECs) represent a distinct population in the epidermis of human inflamed skin and can be discriminated from Langerhans' cells by the absence of Birbeck granules, low expression of CD1a, expression of CD1b and the mannose receptor CD206, and the bright expression of FcϵRI.[10] Although IDECs have been found in other inflammatory skin diseases, a role for IDECs in the pathogenesis of particularly atopic dermatitis has been suggested.[11]

Another distinct dendritic cell that can be found in diseased human skin is the so-called TNF/inducible nitric oxide synthase (iNOS)-producing dendritic cell (Tip-DC), which earned its name because of its very strong expression of TNF-α and of iNOS. Tip-DCs, which can be present in both epidermis and dermis, have a strong expression of CD11c and lack CD1a. A role as effector cell in psoriasis has been suggested.[12] The Langerhans' cells, dermal dendritic cells, IDECs, and Tip-DCs all are of myeloid origin.

Plasmacytoid dendritic cells arise from lymphoid precursors, and a typical feature of them is that they can produce huge amounts of IFN-α and -β in response to viruses. They can be identified by the high expression of CD123 or the specific marker BDCA2 in several inflammatory skin diseases, such as lichen planus.[13] In psoriasis, plasmacytoid dendritic cells have been suggested to initiate the development of psoriatic plaques via the release of IFN-α.[14]

Innate Immunity and the Skin Immune System

A variety of physical, humoral, and cellular elements together form the innate part of SIS. The general concept is that PRRs, which can be regarded as any receptor recognizing pathogen-associated molecular patterns (PAMPs) and capable of triggering antimicrobial function in leukocytes, are present on cell membranes or located within the cell. The PAMPs are defined as highly conserved structures of common pathogens that are essential for microbe survival and include, for example, components of bacterial cell walls such as lipopolysaccharide, peptidoglycan and lipoteichoic acid, fungal cell-wall-component zymosan, and viral double-stranded RNA.[15] Apart from the prototypic TLRs, the group of PRRs also encompasses several other gene families such as CATERPILLERs,[16] nucleotide-binding oligomerization domains (NOD) 1 and 2, and the huge family of C-type lectins that binds to unique branching and positioning of sugar residues on a given molecule and includes soluble proteins, such as the collectin mannose-binding lectin, and transmembrane proteins, such as Langerin, DC-SIGN, and Dectin-1.[17]

Binding of PAMPs to PRRs, of which variable combinations can be detected on many cells including keratinocytes[9] and dendritic cells,[18] initiates signal transduction pathways that lead to the production of antimicrobial peptides, cytokines (of which many, such as TNF-α, are proinflammatory), and chemokines.[19] Several of these cytokines upregulate adhesion molecules, and, together with chemokines, enhance recruitment of effector leukocytes.[20] Initially, these effector leukocytes may include phagocytes, such as granulocytes and macrophages, and cytotoxic cells, such as killer cells. Later, adaptive immunity-related cells such as cytotoxic T cells, memory T cells, and regulatory T cells may be recruited and lead to adaptive immune responses as well as to tapering down inflammation.

It is interesting to note that in diseases that are traditionally seen as mainly T-cell mediated, innate immune responses may be very dysfunctional. For example, innate immunity is clearly defective in atopic dermatitis,[21] while all elements of innate immunity are activated or upregulated in psoriasis.[22]

The following subsections discuss individual components of innate immunity. Humoral components of the innate immune system, especially the complement system and antimicrobial peptides, are discussed elsewhere in this volume, so the emphasis here is on the cellular elements of innate immune responses in skin.

Keratinocytes

Keratinocytes form the epithelial component of skin, and epithelia are regarded as a structural part of the innate immune system. In a process of differentiation, keratinocytes divide and gradually transform themselves into corneal cells forming the stratum corneum, which consists of protein-filled corneal envelopes (keratin, filaggrin, and others) and a lipid-rich extracellular matrix. The corneal layer forms a physical barrier that protects the body from invading pathogens, antigens, and allergens.

In addition, keratinocytes are a major source of antimicrobial peptides including cathelicidin (LL-37) and β-defensins, which are discussed in detail elsewhere in this volume. Also, keratinocytes express PRRs, including TLRs, serving as initiators of innate immune responses, which also are discussed elsewhere. Keratinocytes not only serve as a proinflammatory component of innate immune defenses, but also possess some features of the adaptive immunity branch, as they may act as antigen-presenting cells, produce downregulating factors such as interleukin-1 (IL-1) receptor antagonist (IL-Ra), and α-MSH (α-melanocyte-stimulating hormone),[23] and are able to promote type 1 T-helper cell responses in the skin through production of IL-23[24] or may steer the outcome towards a type 2 T-cell response via production of the cytokine thymic stromal lymphopoietin (TSLP).[25]

Monocytes and (Tissue) Macrophages

Normal human skin has a layer of macrophages (assumed to be monocyte-derived cells) high in the papillary layer, forming a net of phagocytes just beneath the epidermis. In addition, macrophages are also present, scattered throughout its papillary and reticular layers. They are a resident component of the innate part of SIS. Monocytes and macrophages form part of the mononuclear phagocyte system[26] that also includes epithelioid cells and multinucleated giant cells that may be encountered under pathologic conditions.

When pathogens do penetrate the epidermal barrier, for example when it is damaged by scratching or by parasitic infestation, the macrophages are there to assault them. Phagocytosis is followed by degradation of the pathogen along various pathways. Surface binding of PAMPs by

PRRs is also involved in pathogen elimination by macrophages. Upon activation, macrophages secrete a wide variety of inflammatory factors, including cytokines, chemokines, complement components, coagulation factors, growth factors, reactive metabolites, enzymes, urokinase-type plasminogen activator, and reactive lipids.[27] Many of these factors are involved in killing the pathogen, while others upregulate inflammation, enable influx of other immune-response–associated cells, such as specific memory T cells, as well as regulatory T cells that are necessary to dampen the initial inflammation in order to prevent damage that may get out of control.

Granulocytes

Neutrophilic, eosinophilic, and basophilic granulocytes are not normally present in human skin. In skin sections, they may occasionally be seen within the blood vessels, where they are circulating. But in many inflammatory diseases and particularly in infections, granulocytes are recruited from the circulation, sometimes in vast numbers. Basophils are relatively rare as infiltrating cells. Eosinophils are more common, such as in parasitic infestations and in drug hypersensitivity reactions. Neutrophils can sometimes invade the skin in such huge numbers that it becomes clinically visible as pustule formation, sterile such as in psoriasis and other idiopathic subcorneal pustuloses, or loaded with microbial agents such as in many cutaneous infections.

Neutrophils form part of the recruited compartment of innate immunity, and they can phagocytose particular matter. Eosinophils may also phagocytose and are classically known to play a role in the expulsion of parasitic infestations from the gut. Basophils have many similarities with mast cells. It may be argued that mast cells and basophils that bear Fcε receptors, and thus can bind antigen-specific immunoglobulin E (IgE),[28] have a role in acquired immunity, such as in IgE-mediated allergic inflammation and immediate (cutaneous) hypersensitivity. However, any cell that bears receptors for immunoglobulins would then be part of acquired immunity, which is not consistent with the original dichotomy of natural versus acquired immunity.

Monocytes/macrophages, neutrophils, and eosinophils share the capacity to phagocytose pathogens bound to the surface by different receptor systems including PRRs and mannose receptors. Upon phagocytosis, the phagosome fuses with the lysosome to form the intracellular phagolysosome in which the pathogen is killed by toxic substances (nitric oxide, reactive oxygen species) and degraded by various enzymes. In addition, these toxic substances are secreted to kill extracellular pathogens. Specific immunity may enhance these processes by the production of specific antibodies that opsonize pathogens, which facilitate phagocytosis via Fc receptors. Finally, antigen-specific helper T cells may activate macrophages.

Natural Killer Cells

Natural killer (NK) cells are a class of lymphocytes that respond to infection by killing cells that harbor intracellular pathogens. Approximately 10% of peripheral blood lymphocytes are NK cells. They are considered to be part of innate immunity because they do not rearrange their germline DNA to obtain specificity, as is the case with BCRs or TCRs. Instead, they rely upon a limited array of receptors with distinct specificities to become activated and to generate function. These include receptors that can sense cell stress or pathogen-specific signatures. Natural killer cells identify their targets through a set of activating or inhibitory receptors, which recognize pathogen-encoded molecules (non-self recognition), self proteins whose expression is upregulated in transformed or infected cells (stress-induced self recognition), or self proteins that are expressed by normal cells but downregulated by infected or transformed cells (missing-self recognition).[29]

Major histocompatibility complex molecules on host cells provide an inhibitory signal to NK cells, but in missing-self recognition, downregulation of MHC expression, such as occurs by many viral infections, reduces the inhibitory signal and NK cells may attack.[30] The cytolytic mechanisms then used by NK cells are the same as those used by cytolytic T cells (granzymes A and B, perforin).

Macrophages produce IL-12 when they have ingested pathogens. Interleukin-12 activates NK cells and induces them to produce interferon-γ (IFN-γ), which then activates macrophages to kill intracellular pathogens. Thus, NK cells not only eliminate infected cells themselves, but also facilitate macrophage-based innate immune mechanisms, boosting them to eradicate infestation by obligate intracellular pathogens. Isolated deficiencies of NK cells have been reported, and these patients have serious, sometimes fatal herpes virus infections (cytomegalovirus, herpes simplex virus, varicella zoster virus) or mycobacterial disease (*Mycobacterium avium-intracellulare*), all intracellular pathogens.[30]

Natural Killer T Cells

Natural killer T cells express CD3, CD56, CD161, and a limited repertoire of T-cell receptor genes, typically including Vα24 and Vβ11, which enable them to recognize glycolipid antigen in the context of the nonclassic MHC molecule CD1d. Especially this latter feature discriminates NKT cells from conventional T cells, which recognize peptide antigens. To define NKT cells as T cells that also express NK receptors (like CD161) is inadequate because many conventional T cells may upregulate NK receptors after activation, and in addition, a population of NKT cells lacking CD161 has been identified in humans. It has recently been suggested that NKT cells be categorized as type I and type II subsets. Type I or invariant NKT (iNKT) cells, also known as classic NKT cells, are the Vα24-Jα18 expressing population, and type II NKT cells are a collection of all other CD1d-dependent T cells.[31]

While there is substantial knowledge regarding the function of iNKT cells, much less is known about type II NKT cells. The iNKT cells are highly conserved both in functional and structural terms between humans and mice. Their structural hallmark is their expression of a germline TCR α-chain (Vα24-Jα18 in humans, hence the term *invariant*). The α-chain pairs with a restricted repertoire of β-chains, usually Vβ11 in humans.[32] These cells can be further subdivided into CD4$^+$ and CD4$^-$CD8$^-$ (double negative) subpopulations, having different cytokine production (type 1/type 2 phenotype and selective type 1 phenotype, respectively) and chemokine receptor expression. In addition, using CD1d tetramers loaded with the glycolipid α-galactosylceramide or dendritic cells pulsed with the same glycolipid, the existence of CD1d-dependent Vα24$^-$CD8$^+$ and Vα24$^+$CD8$^+$ NKT cells was demonstrated.[33]

Depending on the context, iNKT cells may enhance or suppress a variety of immune responses against pathogens, tumors, and auto- and alloimmune responses,[33] or mediate tolerance. The NKT cells act early in the course of an immune response, and have the remarkable ability to secrete very rapidly large amounts of immunoregulatory cytokines upon TCR engagement. Responses by NKT cells, like NK cells, are amplified by dendritic cell–derived IL-12 provoked by TLR activation by microbial products, resulting in the quick release of large quantities of IFN-γ.

The possible role of NKT cells in dermatologic diseases is just beginning to be explored. Few data on NKT cells in psoriasis are available, but NKT cells are present in psoriasis plaques in significantly increased numbers compared with nonlesional skin or normal skin,[34] while in the blood circulation of psoriasis patients, NKT cell numbers are decreased, tending to be related to disease activity.[35] Further, enhanced overexpression of CD1d by psoriatic keratinocytes and their subsequent ability to activate NKT cells to produce IFN-γ may contribute to the pathogenesis of psoriasis.[36]

Adaptive Immunity and the Skin Immune System

In vivo evidence for the presence of acquired immunity in SIS is exemplified by the concept of immunosurveillance. When acquired immunity mechanisms are inhibited, as occurs in iatrogenic immunosuppression in transplant patients and in patients with HIV-induced T-cell loss, malignancies occur more frequently. Viral and tumor escape mechanisms are enhanced by diminished immune responses, and oncogenic viruses related to tumors as well as other malignancies arise uncontrolled.

As compared to the physiology of acquired immunity responses in normal human skin, the pathology that results from ill-directed acquired immune responses in human skin is more familiar and better studied. Allergic contact dermatitis is a standard example of acquired, T-cell–mediated immunity that goes beyond its original function, leading to exaggerated responses upon hapten challenge, clinically manifesting itself in the development of localized, highly pruritic allergic contact eczema. Misdirected autoantibodies form another well-known example of cutaneous pathology induced by acquired immunity. The autoimmune bullous diseases including pemphigus, pemphigoid, linear IgA disease, and acquired epidermolysis bullosa are straightforward examples. These and many others are discussed in other chapters of this book.

B Lymphocytes

As shown in Tables 2.1 and 2.2, B cells are not a normal constituent of SIS but may be recruited during inflammatory and immune-mediated diseases. For example, B cells and plasma cells may be encountered during many infectious diseases, sometimes scattered but often lumped in the superficial and deeper layers of the dermis. Remarkably little is known as to whether or not these intracutaneous plasma cells actually produce specific antibodies directed at the infectious agent in question. B cells may also be encountered as recruited cells in primary cutaneous B-cell lymphoma and in benign lymphoproliferative skin diseases such as lymphadenosis cutis benigna.

As compared to B cells, T cells are much more common, not only in normal human skin, but especially also in many inflammatory and immune-mediated skin disorders. The basic principles of their presence, recruitment, and recirculation (percolation) warrant more detailed discussion, as follows.

T Lymphocytes: The Major Cell Population of Acquired Skin Immune Responses

The total number of T cells present in normal human skin outnumbers those in peripheral blood. Clark et al.[37] estimated a total of 2×10^{10} of T cells in the normal skin of an adult, which is approximately twice as much as in the circulation (1.2×10^{10}). This underlines the magnitude of SIS as an organ-based immune response network. Cutaneous T cells in normal skin universally display CD45RO (a marker for memory T cells) and the vast majority express CD4. Approximately 20% of the skin resident cells are central memory T cells (circulating from lymph nodes to blood to skin), as they express CCR7 and L-selectin—two receptors that control migration to the lymph nodes. Thus, the remainder and majority of the skin T cells are effector memory T cells (circulating between blood and skin). Further subdivision

of the cutaneous T cells revealed a predominance of cells that secrete T-helper-1 (Th1) cytokines IFN-γ and IL-2; less than 10% are Th2 cells, based on surface expression of Th2 markers IFN-γRβ and ST2L. Approximately 20% of normal human skin–derived T cells display the phenotype of regulatory T cells (CD4$^+$CD25^{high}CD69$^-$), which have functional regulatory activity (inhibition of CD25$^-$ T cells).

In normal human epidermis, T cells are present in very small numbers, whereas in the dermal compartment they are more regularly present. Small clusters of T cells can be detected around the postcapillary venules, in the superficial papillary dermis, but elsewhere as well, especially also around the postcapillary venules of the skin appendages.[38] The identification of cutaneous lymphocyte antigen (CLA) on a subset of circulating memory T cells, and the expression of its ligand E-selectin on endothelial cells of the dermis, gave rise to a series of studies that have further elucidated the existence of skin tissue specific T cells.[39] It is estimated that approximately 16% of the T cells in the peripheral circulation express this CLA molecule and may undergo skin tissue–specific recirculation.

The existence of tissue-specific recirculating T cells is thought to serve different purposes: increase the effectiveness of regional immune responses; decrease the possibility of tissue antigen cross-reactivity; and allow functional immune specialization of particular tissues, for example, the skin. The mechanism of cutaneous T-cell homing has been described, and it is clear that several different adhesion molecules and chemokines are involved. Murine studies have shown that the tissue microenvironment of the dendritic cell determines the T-cell trafficking to the organ of dendritic cell origin.[40] In case of dermal dendritic cells or Langerhans' cells, T cells acquire skin-homing capacity during priming, by the expression of CLA and chemokines receptors CXCR3, CCR4, and CCR10.

The subsequent process of T-cell homing is generally described in different stages. Endothelial cells express different adhesion molecules that have roles in T-cell adherence and transendothelial migration into the dermis. Tethering occurs when CLA expressed on microvilli of fast-moving T cells binds to E-selectin present on the luminal surface of endothelial cells. Subsequent rolling, arrest, and transendothelial migration occur through binding of various adhesion molecules on endothelial cells and their counterstructures on T cells (VLA-4/vascular cell adhesion molecule-1 [VCAM-1], LFA-1/intercellular adhesion molecule [ICAM], PECAM/PECAM). Migration of T cells through the connective tissue of the dermis is in part dependent on binding of T cells to counterstructures on matrix proteins.

Chemokines and their receptors have been identified as key elements of this process, adding tissue specificity to the migration of T-cell subpopulations. As mentioned before, skin-derived dendritic cells instruct T cells during priming to home to the skin, by inducing the expression of CLA and chemokine receptors CCR4, CXCR3, and CCR10. This chemokine receptor profile corresponds to many of the chemokines that are produced in human skin and especially in inflammatory conditions, and local chemokine production attracts T cells to the site where the antigen was encountered. Recognition of endothelial cell–derived chemokine TARC (CCL17) by CCR4 forms an integral part of the rolling and migration process. After arrival in the dermis, monocyte-derived chemokine MDC (CCL22) activates the migration of T cells by binding to CCR4. Finally, subsequent intraepidermal immigration is stimulated by keratinocyte-derived chemokine CTACK (CCL27) and CXCL10 (IP10) that selectively bind to CLA$^+$ T-cell chemokine receptors CCR10 and CXCR3. Especially the CCR10/CTACK (CCL27) interaction is an important feature of SIS, as CTACK seems to be exclusively produced in the skin, and not in other organs, and CCR10 expression on T cells is restricted to the CLA$^+$CD4$^+$ subset.

Skin T-cell homing is thought to be particularly necessary for immunosurveillance, serving effective acquired responses to microbial infestation and preventing the development of different cutaneous, particularly keratinocyte, malignancies. In contrast, T-cell homing is seen as disadvantageous in T-cell–mediated skin diseases, of which there are many. Knowledge of the molecular processes involved in T-cell homing may be of use in different situations. Detection of circulating adhesion molecules has been found to be correlated with disease activity in a variety of skin diseases, such as atopic dermatitis.[41] Upregulation of adhesion molecules in disease states can be used for advanced diagnostic imaging. Understanding of chemokine and adhesion molecule genetic polymorphisms might contribute to our understanding of the variability that skin diseases have in different individuals affected. Finally, adhesion molecules and chemokines might form targets of therapy.

Effector T-Helper Cells

Since the mid-1980s effector T-helper cells have been divided into type 1 (Th1) and type 2 (Th2) subsets on the basis of distinct and not overlapping cytokine secretion patterns.[42] Th1 cells produce IFN-γ, IL-2, and TNF-α, and are essential for the eradication of intracellular pathogens, whereas Th2 cells secrete IL-4, IL-5, and IL-13 and are critical for optimal antibody production and for the elimination of extracellular organisms. These polarized Th1 and Th2 cells are supposed to be responsible for orchestrating the appropriate immune response to a wide variety of pathogens, and restoration and control of a certain kind of Th1/Th2 equilibrium are important. Disturbance of the Th1/Th2 balance and inappropriate controlled polarized Th1 and Th2 responses are held responsible for chronic inflammatory disorders, autoimmune diseases, and allergy. For example, excessive Th1 responses have been associated with psoriasis, and overactive Th2 cells have been implicated in atopy.

Although this model of Th1/Th2 dichotomy has been useful for two decades, it has now become clear that another separate effector T-helper cell lineage exists. This newly identified proinflammatory T-cell subset, called Th17, is characterized by the production of a distinct profile of effector cytokines, including IL-17 (or IL-17A), IL-17F, and IL-6.[43] Interleukin-22 is also preferentially produced by Th17 cells and is an important mediator of acanthosis, that is, hyperplasia of the epidermis.[44] In addition, IL-22 in conjunction with IL-17A or IL-17F synergistically induced the expression of antimicrobial peptides, such as β-defensin.[45] Both IL-17 and IL-22 are induced by IL-23 but not by related cytokine IL-12. Remarkably, IFN-γ and IL-4, when present during the generation of Th17 cells, completely abolishes IL-17 production and moderately inhibit IL-22 production, but in fully established Th17 cells, these Th1 and Th2 cytokines did not affect the production of either IL-17 or IL-22. Because IL-17–expressing T cells have been found in lesional psoriatic skin[46] and the expression of IL-23 in the keratinocytes and antigen-presenting cells in these lesions is increased,[24] it would be interesting to study the role of Th17 cells in the pathogenesis of psoriasis.

Because the search for new factors is still going on, the list of cytokines is expected to expand. It may not be surprising if further effector T-helper-cell subtypes with distinct cytokine profiles are described in future.

Regulatory T Cells

In the early 1970s, it was suggested that a subset of T cells exists that exerts suppressive activities (hence the name suppressor T cells) and that the cells may be important in the downregulation of immune responses and immunologic self tolerance. Because at that time and in subsequent years these cells could not be convincingly characterized, the existence of this cell type was questioned or ignored. In the mid-1990s the concept of suppressor T cells was revived by the identification and characterization of suppressor T cells, which were renamed as regulatory T cells.[47]

$CD4^+CD25^+$ regulatory T cells, also called naturally occurring regulatory T cells, have been suggested to play a role in the prevention of a variety of autoimmune diseases, the regulation of allograft rejection, and in immune responses to pathogens. The regulatory T-cell subset known as Tr1, characterized by its high production of the inhibitory cytokine IL-10, controls the activation of naive and memory T cells, and suppresses Th1- and Th2-mediated immune responses to pathogens, tumors, and alloantigens. Type 3 helper T cells (Th3), producing large amounts of transforming growth factor-β (TGF-β), also suppress Th1- and Th2-mediated immune responses. To date the best marker to detect regulatory T cells is the transcription factor FoxP3, but it should be noted that it is not clear whether all regulatory T-cell subsets express this marker (Table 2.3).

Although the regulatory T cells have initially been described as subsets within the pool of CD4 T cells, it has become clear that regulatory activity can be detected in other types of T cells as well, including the CD8 population of T cells. Natural killer T cells may also have a role

TABLE 2.3. Characteristics of regulatory T cells

	Expression of FoxP3	Mechanism of suppression	In vivo functions
$CD4^+CD25^+$ Treg	++	Cell contact-dependent	Prevention of a variety of autoimmune diseases Regulation of allograft rejection Immune response to pathogens
$CD4^+CD25^-$ Treg	– ?	Cytokine mediated	Suppression of autoimmunity Control the activation of naive and memory T cells
Tr1	+ ?	IL-10	Suppress Th1- and Th2-mediated immune responses to pathogens, tumors, and alloantigens
Th3	– ?	TGF-β	Suppress Th1- and Th2-mediated immune responses
Regulatory NKT	– ?	IL-4, IL-10, TGF-β cytotoxicity	Immune regulation and T cell homeostasis Destruction of tumors and pathogens Regulations of Th1-mediated autoimmune diseases
$CD8^+$ Treg	+ ?	Cell contact-dependent cytotoxicity	Suppression of autoimmunity and regulation of peripheral TCR repertoire
$CD8^+CD28^-$ Treg	+ ?	Suppression induced via dendritic cells	Regulation of autoimmunity

IL, interleukin; NKT, natural killer T cell; TCR, T-cell receptor; TGF, transforming growth factor; Treg, regulatory T cell ;Tr1, regulatory T cell type 1; Th3, T helper cell type 3; ?, not yet clear or not yet investigated.
Source: Adapted from Zhang et al.,[29] Godfrey and Kronenberg,[33] and Beissert et al.[47]

in immune response regulation as suppressors of Th1-mediated autoimmunity.[29] In only a few years, investigations of the function of various subsets of regulatory T cells have resulted in data that are difficult to summarize (Table 2.3). In addition, not much is known about what these cell subpopulations actually do in skin diseases, for example, in the many dermatoses where immune and inflammatory mechanisms play a role. The occurrence of inflammatory skin diseases is not simply a matter of lack of suppression due to abnormalities in the numbers of regulatory T cells. There are no significant differences in frequency of FoxP3[+] cells between different inflammatory skin diseases and, remarkably, normal human skin also contains FoxP3[+] cells in the same frequency range as in diseased skin, being approximately 20%.[48] It might well be that impaired function of (subsets of) regulatory T cells is responsible for the chronicity of many inflammatory immune-mediated dermatoses, as has been demonstrated for regulatory T cells in psoriasis patients.[49]

Conclusion

From the beginning of the development of the scientific discipline of immunology, the distinction between natural and acquired immunity has been known. A major breakthrough in our understanding of acquired immunity with its clonal selection of specific receptor-bearing T and B cells was the principle of gene rearrangement in these cells, enabling the expression of millions of specificities represented by millions of different proteins, of which the corresponding DNA can never be part of the human genome. A major advance in our understanding of innate immunity was the recognition of pattern-recognition receptors (PRRs) that bind highly conserved pathogen-associated molecular patterns (PAMPs) and when activated start immediately and nonspecifically with defense responses.

All known molecular and cellular elements of innate and acquired immunity are part of the skin immune system (SIS),[50] either under physiologic circumstances, or in pathologic conditions, when they may be secreted (molecular elements) or recruited (cellular elements) in human skin. Innate and adaptive immunity overlap and influence each other and it is impossible to pinpoint a single cell type that governs the complexity of these multiple interacting processes. New subpopulations have recently been defined, and their proinflammatory or regulatory roles are just beginning to be explored. This work will provide new and highly needed insight into their possible role in the pathogenesis of a large variety of poorly understood dermatologic diseases.

Acknowledgment. Rosalie M. Luiten is gratefully acknowledged for her editorial and textual suggestions.

References

1. Tauber AI, Chernyak L. Metchnikoff and the Origins of Immunology: From Metaphor to Theory. New York: Oxford University Press, 1991.
2. Bos JD, Kapsenberg ML. The skin immune system (SIS): its cellular constituents and their interactions. Immunol Today 1986;7:235–40.
3. Bos JD, ed. Skin Immune System (SIS), 1st ed. Boca Raton, FL: CRC Press, 1990.
4. Teunissen MBM, Piskin G, di Nuzzo S, et al. Ultraviolet B radiation induces a transient appearance of IL-4+ neutrophils, which support the development of Th2 responses. J Immunol 2002;168:3732–9.
5. Janeway CA. Approaching the asymptote? Evolution and revolution in immunology. Cold Spring Harb Symp Quant Biol 1989;54:1–13.
6. Bonizzi G, Karin M. The two NF-κB activation pathways and their role in innate and adaptive immunity. Trends Immunol 2004;25:280–8.
7. Teunissen MBM. Langerhans cells and other skin dendritic cells. In: Bos JD, ed. Skin Immune System (SIS): Cutaneous Immunology and Clinical Immunodermatology, 3rd edition. Boca Raton, FL: CRC Press, 2005:123–82.
8. Banchereau J, Steinman M. Dendritic cells and the control of immunity. Nature 1998;392:245–52.
9. Lebre MC, Van der Aar AMG, Van Baarsen L, et al. Human keratinocytes express functional Toll-like receptor 3, 4, 5, and 9. J Invest Dermatol 2007;127:331–41.
10. Wollenberg A, Kraft S, Hanau D, et al. Immunological and ultrastructural characterization of Langerhans cells and a novel, inflammatory dendritic epidermal cell (IDEC) population in lesional skin of atopic eczema. J Invest Dermatol 1996;106:446–53.
11. Bieber T. FcεRI-expressing antigen-presenting cells: new players in the atopic game. Immunol Today 1997;18:311–3.

12. Lowes MA, Chamian F, Abello MV, et al. Increase in TNF-α and inducible nitric oxide synthase-expressing dendritic cells in psoriasis and reduction with efalizumab (anti-CD11a). Proc Natl Acad Sci USA 2005;102:19057–62.

13. De Vries HJC, Van Marle J, Teunissen MBM, et al. Lichen planus is associated with human herpesvirus type 7 replication and infiltration of plasmacytoid dendritic cells. Br J Dermatol 2006;154:361–4.

14. Nestle FO, Conrad C, Tun-Kyi A, et al. Plasmacytoid predendritic cells initiate psoriasis through interferon-α production. J Exp Med 2005;202:135–43.

15. Akira S, Uematsu S, Takeuchi O. Pathogen recognition and innate immunity. Cell 2006;124:783–801.

16. Ting JPY, Kastner DL, Hoffman HM. CATERPILLERs, pyrin and hereditary immunological disorders. Nat Rev Immunol 2006;6:183–95.

17. Robinson MJ, Sancho D, Slack EC, et al. Myeloid C-type lectins in innate immunity. Nat Immunol 2006;12:1258–65.

18. Van der Aar AMG, Sylva-Steenland RMR, Bos JD, et al. Cutting edge: loss of TLR2, TLR4, and TLR5 on Langerhans cells abolishes bacterial recognition. J Immunol 2007;178:1986–900.

19. Medzhitov R, Janeway CA. Innate immunity. N Engl J Med 2000;343:338–44.

20. Esche C, Stellato C, Beck LA. Chemokines: key players in innate and adaptive immunity. J Invest Dermatol 2005;125:615–28.

21. McGirt LY, Beck LA. Innate immune defects in atopic dermatitis. J Allergy Clin Immunol 2006;118:202–8.

22. Bos JD, De Rie MA, Teunissen MBM, et al. Psoriasis: activation of innate immunity. Br J Dermatol 2005;152:1098–107.

23. Chu AC, Morris JF. The keratinocyte. In: Bos JD, ed. Skin Immune System (SIS): Cutaneous Immunology and Clinical Immunodermatology, 3rd edition. Boca Raton, FL: CRC Press, 2005:77–99.

24. Piskin G, Sylva-Steenland RMR, Bos JD, et al. In vitro and in vivo expression of IL-23 by keratinocytes in healthy skin and psoriasis lesions: enhanced expression in psoriatic skin. J Immunol 2006;176:1908–15.

25. Soumelis V, Reche PA, Kanzler H, et al. Human epithelial cells trigger dendritic cell-mediated allergic inflammation by producing TSLP. Nat Immunol 2002;3:673–80.

26. Furth R van, Cohn ZA, Hirsch JG, et al. The mononuclear phagocyte system: a new classification of macrophages, monocytes and their precursor cells. Bull WHO 1972;46:845–52.

27. Lu KQ, McCormick TS, Gilliam AC, et al. Monocytes and macrophages in human skin. In: Bos JD, ed. Skin Immune System (SIS): Cutaneous Immunology and Clinical Immunodermatology, 3rd edition. Boca Raton, FL: CRC Press, 2005:183–209.

28. Knol EF, Kuijpers TW, Roos D. Neutrophils, eosinophils and basophils in the skin immune system. In: Bos JD, ed. Skin Immune System (SIS): Cutaneous Immunology and Clinical Immunodermatology, 3rd edition. Boca Raton, FL: CRC Press, 2005:263–83.

29. Zhang C, Zhang J, Tian Z. The regulatory effect of natural killer cells: do "NK-reg cells" exist? Cell Mol Immunol 2006;3:241–54.

30. Orange JS. Human natural killer cell deficiencies. Curr Opin Allergy Clin Immunol 2006;6:399–409.

31. Godfrey DI, MacDonald RH, Kronenberg M, et al. NKT cells: what's in a name? Nat Rev Immunol 2004;4:231–7.

32. Karadimitris A, Patterson S, Spanoudakis E. Natural killer T cells and haemopoiesis. Br J Haematol 2006;134:263–72.

33. Godfrey DI, Kronenberg M. Going both ways: immune regulation via CD1d-dependent NKT cells. J Clin Invest 2004;114:1379–88.

34. Cameron AL, Kirby B, Fei W, et al. Natural killer and natural killer-T cells in psoriasis. Arch Dermatol Res 2002;294:363–9.

35. Van der Vliet HJJ, Von Blomberg BME, Nishi N, et al. Circulating Vα24⁺ Vβ11⁺ NKT cell numbers are decreased in a wide variety of diseases that are characterized by autoreactive tissue damage. Clin Immunol 2001;100:144–8.

36. Bonish B, Jullien D, Dutronc Y, et al. Overexpression of CD1d by keratinocytes in psoriasis and CD1d-dependent IFN-γ production by NK-T cells. J Immunol 2000;165:4076–85.

37. Clark RA, Chong B, Mirchandani N, et al. The vast majority of CLA+ T cells are resident in normal skin. J Immunol 2006;176:4431–9.

38. Bos JD, Zonneveld I, Das PK, et al. The skin immune system (SIS): distribution and immunophenotype of lymphocyte subpopulations in normal human skin. J Invest Dermatol 1987;88:569–73.

39. Santamaria-Babi LF. CLA(+) T cells in cutaneous diseases. Eur J Dermatol 2004;14:13–8.

40. Dudda JC, Simon JC, Martin S. Dendritic cell immunization route determines CD8+ T cell trafficking to inflamed skin: role for tissue microenvironment and dendritic cells in establishment of T cell-homing subsets. J Immunol 2004;172:857–63.

41. Gutgesell C, Heise S, Seubert A, et al. Comparison of different activity parameters in atopic dermatitis: correlation with clinical scores. Br J Dermatol 2002;147:914–9.

42. Kapsenberg ML. Dendritic-cell control of pathogen-driven T-cell polarization. Nat Rev Immunol 2003;3:984–93.

43. Weaver CT, Harrington LE, Mangan PR, et al. Th17: an effector CD4 T cell lineage with regulatory T cell ties. Immunity 2006;24:677–88.

44. Zheng Y, Danilenko DM, Valdez P, et al. Interleukin-22, a TH17 cytokine, mediates IL-23–induced dermal inflammation and acanthosis. Nature 2007;445:648–51.

45. Liang SC, Tan XY, Luxenberg DP, et al. Interleukin (IL)-22 and IL-17 are coexpressed by Th17 cells and cooperatively enhance expression of antimicrobial peptides. J Exp Med 2006;203:2271–9.

46. Teunissen MBM, Koomen CW, de Waal Malefyt R, et al. Interleukin-17 and interferon-γ synergize in the enhancement of proinflammatory cytokine production by human keratinocytes. J Invest Dermatol 1998;111:645–9.

47. Beissert S, Schwarz A, Schwarz T. Regulatory T cells. J Invest Dermatol 2006;126:15–24.

48. De Boer OJ, Van der Loos CM, Teeling P, et al. Immunohistochemical analysis of regulatory T cell markers FOXP3 and GITR on CD4+CD25+ T cells in normal skin and inflammatory dermatoses. J Histochem Cytochem 2007;55:891–8.

49. Sugiyama H, Gyulai R, Toichi E, et al. Dysfunctional blood and target tissue CD4+CD25high regulatory T cells in psoriasis: mechanism underlying unrestrained pathogenic effector T cell proliferation. J Immunol 2005;174:164–73.

50. Bos JD, ed. Skin Immune System (SIS): Cutaneous Immunology and Clinical Immunodermatology, 3rd ed. Boca Raton, FL: CRC Press, 2005.

3
Neuroimmunology

Erica Lee and Richard D. Granstein

Key Points

- The skin is a complex organ system consisting of a sophisticated network of nerve fibers and specialized sensory structures.
- Cutaneous nerves release neuropeptides and neurohormones into the local milieu in response to internal and external stimuli. Many appear to serve an immunoregulatory role.
- Neuropeptides play a role in the pathophysiology of common skin diseases such as atopic dermatitis and psoriasis.
- Substance P and calcitonin gene–related peptide are among the most prevalent and multifunctional neuropeptides in the skin.

Human skin consists of a sophisticated network of nerve fibers and specialized sensory structures to transduce sensations of touch, vibration, temperature, and pain. Nerve fibers have dual functions: to transmit afferent sensory impulses to the central nervous system and to secrete mediators into the local environment. While many of these mediators are polypeptides (called neuropeptides), others are nonpeptide factors. These factors affect various biologic processes including inflammation, immunity, wound healing, and aging.

Cutaneous neurobiology is an expanding field of research with increasing clinical implications. The presence of neuropeptide receptors on epidermal and dermal cells and the close anatomic relationship of nerve fibers with immune and nonimmune cells demonstrate the direct link between the sensory nervous system and the largest organ system of the human body, the skin.

Background

The classic "triple response" of sensory nerves was demonstrated by Lewis[1] in 1927. This is seen after the skin is stroked, producing local erythema (capillary dilatation), followed by the axon-reflex flare to produce erythema (arteriolar dilatation) and a wheal (transudation of fluid). Vasodilatation has been shown to occur following dorsal nerve root stimulation and is inhibited by depleting sensory nerves of neuropeptides with capsaicin, demonstrating the role of nerves in cutaneous inflammation.[2] Furthermore, Bayliss[3] and Bruce[4] noted that patients with defective cutaneous sensory systems could not mount normal inflammatory responses to cutaneously applied inflammatory agents. Similarly, observations that patients with sensory disorders such as postherpetic neuralgia have defective responses to inflammatory stimuli suggest that the cutaneous nervous system modulates inflammation.[5]

Anatomy

Highly specialized afferent sensory and efferent autonomic nerve branches innervate the skin.[5–7] The nervous system is divided into two main divisions, the central and peripheral nervous systems. The peripheral nervous system (PNS) includes peripheral nerves, the autonomic nervous system (ANS), and the sensory nervous system. The ANS is further divided into the sympathetic, parasympathetic, and enteric nervous systems.[8]

The sensory component of the peripheral nervous system conveys mechanical and chemical activity to the central nervous system (CNS). Stimuli include external and internal physiologic and mechanical triggers. Afferent unmyelinated C or myelinated Aδ fibers from the dorsal root ganglia innervate the epidermis as fine nerve fibers with free endings that converge in the dermis.[5] Sensory receptors include encapsulated structures such as Pacini's, Ruffini's, and Meissner's corpuscles and nerve fibers with "free ends." Free nerve endings are in contact with hair follicles, pilosebaceous units, glandular structures, and the epidermis. The trunk, extremities, neck, and posterior scalp are supplied by nerves derived from the dorsal root ganglia, whereas the upper anterior neck, face, and the majority of the scalp are innervated by the trigeminal nerve.[9]

Sensory fibers are generally classified into three groups based on their size and conduction velocity. C fibers are unmyelinated, thin afferent fibers consisting of pain receptors called nociceptors and mechanoreceptors. A subpopulation termed C-polymodal nociceptors represents 70% of all cutaneous C fibers and participate in the release of neuropeptides.[10] Aδ fibers are small, myelinated fibers that innervate the skin although to a much smaller extent than C fibers. Autonomic nerves represent a minority of the cutaneous fibers. These nerves predominantly generate the neurotransmitters acetylcholine and catecholamines; however, they also produce neuropeptides such as neuropeptide Y, calcitonin gene–related peptide (CGRP), vasoactive intestinal peptide (VIP), and atrial natriuretic peptide.[2]

The skin is innervated with parasympathetic and sympathetic nerve fibers. Sweat glands are regulated by sympathetic cholinergic fibers that release acetylcholine, whereas the fibers innervating blood vessels release noradrenaline.

Neuropeptides

Neuropeptides (NPs) are a heterogeneous group of polypeptides ranging from 2 to greater than 40 amino acids in size. There are over 50 identified neuropeptides, 11 of which are found in human skin.[11] Neuropeptides are released in response to a range of stimuli from pain and temperature

to irritation in order to mediate diverse biologic processes related to injury, inflammation, infection, and wound healing. Neuropeptides are synthesized in the nerve cell bodies. The precursors are synthesized in the endoplasmic reticulum and processed and packaged in the Golgi apparatus for eventual transport to the nerve endings. The most abundant neuropeptides in the skin include substance P (SP), CGRP, neurokinin A (NKA), neurotensin, pituitary adenylate cyclase activating polypeptide (PACAP), VIP, neuropeptide Y (NPY), β-endorphin, enkephalin, somatostatin, galanin, dynorphin, atrial natriuretic peptide, α- or γ-melanocyte-stimulating hormone (MSH), parathyroid hormone–related protein, urocortin, and corticotrophin-releasing hormone.[2] Neuropeptides are released predominantly from nerve fibers; however, evidence exists that epidermal and dermal cells also produce neuropeptides and neurohormones. These cells include fibroblasts, keratinocytes, Langerhans' cells, macrophages, mast cells, melanocytes, endothelial cells, Merkel cells, and leukocytes.[2,12]

The distribution of neuropeptides varies depending on the body site. High levels of SP, NKA, and CGRP are found in areas with the greatest tactile sensation. Intermediate levels are found in the neck and face, whereas the lowest levels are present in the groin, arm, and thigh.[13] Levels of VIP and peptide histidine methionine (PHM) are also highest in axillary skin, suggesting their role in axillary eccrine sweat production. The location of neuropeptides in the layers of the skin varies as well. Substance P, NKA, and CGRP are found in nerves penetrating the epidermis, and the neuropeptides SP, CGRP, VIP, and NKA are in nerves innervating dermal structures.[9]

Neuropeptides bind to specific receptors on nerves and cells to activate intracellular signaling cascades. Neuropeptides are then inactivated by peptidases such as neutral endopeptidase or angiotensin-converting enzyme to deactivate and subsequently lead to their degradation.[14,15]

Delineating the role of neuropeptides and neurohormones has led to the emergence and explosive growth of a field investigating the intimate relationship between the nervous, immune and endocrine systems and the skin. Terms such as the *neuroimmunecutaneous system* are used to imply a relationship between immune and nonimmune cells in the skin and between the immune system and the nervous system within the skin.[16]

The skin is an ideal organ to investigate these relationships due to its location, size, and function. As the interface between the external and internal environments, the skin has a unique role in modulating and transmitting outside stimuli while maintaining homeostasis inside. As a result, there is increasing attention and focus on the skin to unravel these connections, apply them to other organ systems, and ultimately use them as a model for therapeutic interventions in several disease conditions.

This chapter highlights several neuropeptides and other neural signals, discussing their functions and role in clinical skin diseases (Table 3.1).

Receptors

There are numerous neuropeptide receptors. For example, SP has three receptors, NK_1, NK_2, NK_3. Two receptors have been identified for CGRP (1 and 2) and NPY has receptors $Y_{1,2,3,4,5}$.[17] Most cutaneous cells express several receptors; to discuss each in detail is beyond the scope of this chapter, and more comprehensive reviews are available.[9] Rather, the receptors most relevant to the skin are discussed here. These include NK-1, preferentially expressed on human keratinocytes, vasoactive intestinal polypeptide/pituitary adenylate cyclase activating polypeptide 1 receptor (VPAC-1R) on dermal endothelial cells and Langerhans' cells, VPAC-2R on keratinocytes and Langerhans' cells, and melanocortin 1 receptor (MC-1R) on melanocytes, keratinocytes, monocytes, fibroblasts, and Langerhans' cells.[2,9,18]

Substance P

Substance P is the best characterized neuropeptide. An undecapeptide, it is a member of the tachykinin family along with NKA and neurokinin B (NKB). It is released from sensory nerves that are in contact with endothelial cells, mast cells, hair follicles, and epidermal cells.[19] Its biologic effects in the skin are mediated predominantly by the NK-1 receptor. Substance P leads to the activation of phospholipase C, increase in intracellular calcium, and subsequently the activation of nuclear factor-kappa B (NF-κB).[20]

Substance P is a potent vasodilator, participating in the wheal and flare response in neurogenic inflammation. It directly acts on vascular smooth muscle and indirectly on the endothelium to enhance the production of nitric oxide, resulting in vasodilatation and increased vascular permeability.[21] In human skin, SP is also released by free nerve endings in the dermal papilla and epidermis of human fingers, in Meissner's corpuscles, and near sweat gland ducts and blood vessels.[12] Receptors for SP are on mast cells, lymphocytes, leukocytes, and macrophages. Stimulated macrophages generate prostaglandin E_2, thromboxane B_2, and superoxide ion, and SP-stimulated keratinocytes release proinflammatory cytokines interleukin (IL)-1α, IL-1β, and IL-8.[2] Furthermore, SP induces histamine release from mast cells, lymphocyte proliferation and chemotaxis, immunoglobulin production, and the release of cytokines IL-1, IL-6, and tumor necrosis factor-α (TNF-α).[22]

An increase in SP-expressing nerve fibers is seen in inflammatory skin diseases such as atopic dermatitis.[23] Substance P increases the release of proinflammatory cytokines from keratinocytes and TNF-α, histamine, leukotriene B_4, and prostaglandin D_2 from mast cells. Substance P also upregulates IL-2 production to promote T-cell proliferation and induces the expression of adhesion molecules P-selectin, intercellular adhesion molecule-1 (ICAM-1), and vascular cell adhesion molecule-1 (VCAM-1).[2,23]

Vasoactive Intestinal Peptide

Vasoactive intestinal peptide is a 28 amino acid peptide. It belongs to the glucagon-secretin family that includes PACAP and growth hormone–releasing hormone. It is localized in the deeper dermis in nerve fibers situated around eccrine sweat glands, superficial and deep vascular plexuses, and hair follicles.[21] It is a potent vasodilator contributing to the development of pruritus, erythema, and edema. Vasoactive intestinal peptide also has a role in the regulation of cutaneous blood flow, the promotion of nitric oxide synthesis, keratinocyte proliferation, and sweat production. Vasoactive intestinal polypeptide/pituitary adenylate cyclase activating polypeptide 1 receptor (VPAC-1R) is the dominant receptor on human dermal endothelial cells, whereas VPAC-2R is expressed on keratinocytes.[2]

TABLE 3.1. Neuromediators in the skin

Neuromediator	Source	Receptor	Primary function
Substance P	Sensory nerve fibers	Tachykinin (neurokinin) receptor	Mediates erythema and edema
	Meissner's corpuscles Perivascular nerves		Increases histamine and TNF-α release from mast cells
	Mast cells		Released by PAR-2 agonists
	Monocytes		Upregulates cell adhesion molecule expression in dermal endothelial cells
	Eosinophils		Stimulates release of proinflammatory cytokines from keratinocytes
VIP	Sensory nerve fibers	VPAC receptors	Vasodilation
	Sweat glands		Increases sweat secretion
	Merkel cells		Histamine release from mast cells
	PMNs		Keratinocyte proliferation and migration
			Inhibits Langerhans' cell antigen presentation
PACAP	Sensory nerve fibers	VPAC receptors	Vasodilation
	Autonomic nerves		Downregulates proinflammatory cytokines in T cells
	Lymphocytes		Modulates mast cells
	Endothelial cells		Inhibits Langerhans' cell antigen presentation
CGRP	Sensory nerve fibers	CGRP receptors	Vasodilation
	Perivascular nerves		Modulates Langerhans' cell function
	Meissner's corpuscles		Released by PAR-2 stimulation
			Keratinocyte proliferation
			Histamine release (mast cells)
POMC peptides	Keratinocytes	Melanocortin receptors	Immunomodulation (upregulates IL-10 and antagonizes effects of proinflammatory cytokines)
	Melanocytes		Inhibits NF-κB
	LCs		Melanogenesis
	Fibroblasts		Inhibit keratinocyte migration
	Mast cells		Regulate natural killer and monocyte activity
	Monocytes		Inhibit antigen presentation
	Macrophages		
	Endothelial cells		
	PMNs		
	Sensory nerves		
Catecholamines	Autonomic adrenergic nerves Keratinocytes Melanocytes	Adrenergic receptors	

CGRP, calcitonin gene-related peptide; IL, interleukin, LC, Langerhans cell; PACAP, pituitary adenylate cyclase activating polypeptide; NF-κB, nuclear factor κB; PAR-2, proteinase-activated receptor 2; PMN, polymorphonuclear cell; POMC, pro-opiomelanocortin; TNF-α, tumor necrosis factor-α; VIP, vasoactive intestinal peptide; VPAC, vasoactive intestinal polypeptide/pituitary adenylate cyclase activating polypeptide.

Source: Data from Steinhoff et al.,[2] Scholzen et al.,[10] and Kodali et al.[24,26]

Both are found on Langerhans' cells.[18] In a mouse model, VIP inhibited the ability of epidermal cells enriched for Langerhans' cell content to present antigen for elicitation of delayed-type hypersensitivity in previously immunized mice.[24] Vasoactive intestinal peptide also inhibited Langerhans' cell antigen presenting capability in in vitro assays of antigen presentation.[24]

Pituitary Adenylate Cyclase Activating Polypeptide

Pituitary adenylate cyclase activating polypeptide (PACAP) exists in two forms: PACAP-38 and a truncated form, PACAP-27.[25] It binds to two types of receptors. PAC1 binds PACAP to activate adenylate cyclase and phospholipase C, whereas the second type of receptors, VPAC1 and VPAC2, binds both PACAP and VIP to activate adenylate cyclase.[26] PACAP has the highest immunoreactivity around blood vessels, hair follicles, and sweat glands, and is shown to modulate inflammatory responses in the skin.[2] In a murine model, intradermal administration of PACAP suppresses the induction of contact hypersensitivity (CHS) at the injected site, and in vitro treatment of epidermal antigen-presenting cells inhibits their ability to present antigen for elicitation of delayed-type hypersensitivity (DTH) in previously immunized mice. PACAP also inhibits the ability of Langerhans' cells to present antigen in wholly in vitro assay systems.[26] In vitro studies suggest this may be due to PACAP-induced suppression of IL-1β release and augmentation of IL-10 production.[26]

Calcitonin Gene–Related Peptide

Calcitonin gene–related peptide (CGRP) is a 37 amino acid neuropeptide discovered in 1982.[27] There are two forms: CGRP-α or CGRP-1 and CGRP-β or CGRP-2. In human skin, CGRP is localized with SP in nerves in the dermal papillae and free nerve endings of glabrous skin; however, when co-localized with somatostatin, it is found in nerve fibers associated with the epidermis and perivascular space.[21] Calcitonin gene–related peptide is one of the most prevalent neuropeptides in the skin and is found associated with mast cells, melanocytes, keratinocytes, Langerhans' cells, and Merkel cells.[2,19]

Calcitonin gene–related peptide is a mediator of neurogenic vasodilatation and a modulator of keratinocyte proliferation and cytokine production.[2] It inhibits antigen presentation by Langerhans' cells,[28] macrophages,[29] and blood-derived dendritic cells,[30,31] and upregulates melanocyte proliferation, dendricity, and melanogenesis.[16] C fibers containing CGRP are in direct contact with the surface of epidermal Langerhans' cells, suggesting an intimate relationship.[28]

Calcitonin gene–related peptide is involved in ultraviolet radiation (UVR)-induced immunosuppression. In the low-dose model of ultraviolet B (UVB)-induced immunosuppression (sensitization to a hapten is impaired at the irradiated site), UVR releases CGRP from sensory neurons to locally impair contact hypersensitivity responses.[32] The release of CGRP after UVR may be triggering mast cells to release stored TNF-α, which in turn downregulates Langerhans' cell density and function to impair CHS induction.[33] Calcitonin gene–related peptide also contributes to the high dose or systemic model of UVR-induced immunosuppression (sensitization at a nonirradiated site is impaired) as CHS responses are suppressed when mice are pretreated with CGRP antagonists.[34]

Pro-Opiomelanocortin Peptides

The skin is a source of neuroendocrine hormones of the pro-opiomelanocortin (POMC) family termed melanocortins (MCs). The POMC hormones include α-, β-, and γ-melanocyte stimulating hormone (MSH). These are derived from POMC along with adrenocorticotropic hormone (ACTH) and endorphins. Pro-opiomelanocortin is predominantly synthesized in the pituitary gland; however, it is also present in the skin, and expressed by melanocytes, keratinocytes, Langerhans' cells, endothelial cells, mast cells, and fibroblasts.[10] The cutaneous melanocortin system is well characterized[35] with melanocortin receptor (MC-R) expression in nearly all cell types, including fibroblasts, adipocytes, endothelial cells, and mast cells.[36] MC-1R is the most prevalent among the five melanocortin receptors, with high affinity for α-MSH and ACTH.

Pro-opiomelanocortin–derived peptides influence several processes including melanogenesis and skin immunity, and are also suggested to have a role in the hair cycle, sebum, and eccrine gland function and epidermal proliferation.[36]

The known functions of melanocortins in cutaneous biology continue to expand with potential clinical applications. Human sebocytes increase lipid droplet formation in response to MCs, suggesting acne vulgaris may be affected. Evidence suggests that MCs are involved in keratinocyte proliferation and differentiation, with potential repercussions in regenerative processes.[35] In addition, although the mechanism is not completely understood, it is believed that MSH induces melanocyte prolif-eration and melanogenesis through engagement of MC1-R, serving as a substrate or promoter of the enzyme tyrosinase.[16]

Pro-opiomelanocortin messenger RNA (mRNA) and related peptides such as α-MSH and ACTH are upregulated by UVR. Ultraviolet B radiation (280 to 320 nm) upregulates ACTH, α-MSH, and MC-1R in epidermal melanocytes, and increases MC-1R expression in cultured normal and malig-nant melanocytes and keratinocytes, the latter asso-ciated with increased melanogenesis in cell culture and in vivo.[9,35] The melanogenic and dendritogenic effects of α-MSH and ACTH on the skin and fol-licular melanocytes may correlate with tanning and hair color, respectively.[35]

Pro-opiomelanocortin–derived peptides play a role in immunity and inflammation, especially α-MSH; α-MSH is antiinflammatory and may be involved in host defense. In addition, its anti-TNF and antimicrobial effects suggest it may reduce replication of the human immunodeficiency virus.[37] α-MSH also inhibits contact hypersensitivity and induces hapten-specific tolerance through IL-10 upregulation in a murine model.[38] The antiinflam-matory properties in animal models of hepatic inflammation and arthritic processes suggest that α-MSH may be an important antiinflammatory agent in the treatment of inflammatory diseases in humans.[39–41]

Catecholamines

Sympathetic fibers of the autonomic nervous system travel with sensory nerve fibers and as single fibers to innervate blood vessels, hair follicles, and sweat glands.[5] Keratinocytes also synthesize catecholamines.[9,42] Catecholamines inhibit antigen presentation in Langerhans' cells[43] through the β_2-adrenergic receptor. Interestingly, evidence exists that norepinephrine plays a role in vivo in enhancing CHS through involve-ment in the trafficking of skin dendritic cells to draining lymph nodes, possibly through effects on α-adrenergic receptors.[44] Thus, the effects of catecholamines on skin immunity may be complex, with the outcome dependent on timing exposure, the presence of other regulatory factors, and so on.

Neuropeptide Y

Neuropeptide Y (NPY) is a 36 amino acid peptide identified predominantly in periarteriolar nerve fibers in the dermal plexuses and epidermal basal cells as well as sweat glands, sebaceous glands, and hair follicles. It also appears to be produced by Langerhans' cells.[45] Neuropeptide Y causes vasoconstriction and may also play a role in eccrine sweat production.

Adenosine Triphosphate

The nucleotide adenosine triphosphate (ATP) is a ubiquitous carrier of energy involved in count-less cellular processes. Several lines of evidence suggest extracellular ATP participates in inflam-matory and regenerative responses in the skin and affects melanocyte and Langerhans' cell function.[46] Adenosine triphosphate plays a role in the nocicep-tive signaling pathways that follow cutaneous cell injury,[47] and may contribute to the pathophysiology of inflammatory skin conditions such as rosacea by augmenting the production of inflammatory media-tors by endothelial cells.[48] Purinergic agonists also appear to enhance Langerhans' cell antigen-presenting function when exposure occurs along with activa-tion by an additional signal (lipopolysaccharide).[49] The function of ATP in the neuropeptide milieu of epidermal and dermal cell types and sensory nerves in the skin remains unclear.

Neurogenic Inflammation

Cutaneous neurogenic inflammation implies the role of nerves in cutaneous inflammation. The neuropeptides secreted by sensory nerves evoke an inflammatory response referred to as neurogenic inflammation. The axon-reflex model implies that tissue injury triggers a signal to the dorsal root ganglion toward the CNS (orthodromic response) with return of the signal from branch points in the reverse direction to exert effects at the local level. The orthodromic response transmits pain, whereas the antidromic response leads to the release of neuropeptides in the innervated tissue.[12] The most prominent neuropeptides in UV-induced neuroin-flammation are SP and CGRP.

Substance P and CGRP mediate vasodilatation, and SP and NKA are responsible for plasma extravasation.[19] Substance P is well known to provoke erythema and edema by a mast cell–dependent and -independent pathway.[10] The flare is the result of the antidromic arm of the axon reflex leading to the local release of neuropeptides such as SP and CGRP.[17]

Cutaneous/Dermatologic Diseases

The relationship between neuropeptides and dermatologic diseases has been explored for over a decade. In inflammatory processes, the neuroimmuno-endocrine-cutaneous nexus participates in the trigger and maintenance of inflammation in healthy and pathologic skin. Understanding the role of neurotransmitters and their receptors may lead to the identification of novel therapeutic targets for the treatment of several common cutaneous diseases.

There are several lines of evidence suggesting a neurogenic component in dermatologic disease. Neuropeptides may induce or alleviate urticarial symptoms, hypersensitivity reactions, and rosacea, and may play a role in the pathophysiology of pruritus, psoriasis atopic dermatitis, alopecia areata, vitiligo, and nodular prurigo.[2,12] Several of these conditions are discussed below.

Urticaria

Urticaria are transient swellings or wheals due to plasma leakage. The primary effector cell in the pathogenesis of urticaria is the mast cell.[5] Neuropeptides such as SP, VIP, and somatostatin activate mast cells to secrete histamine and other mediators that induce urticaria and mediate the late-phase response.[5,50] Substance P and CGRP exert effects in cases of chronic urticaria, and ACTH is present in the cutaneous mast cells of patients with urticaria pigmentosa.[51,52] The expression of the POMC gene in mast cells suggests that α-MSH may be contributing to the cutaneous hyperpigmentation seen in patients with urticaria pigmentosa.[53] These studies suggest an interrelationship between the cutaneous nervous system and mast cells in the pathophysiology of urticaria.

Pruritus

Pruritus is one of the most common symptoms encountered in dermatology with significant potential to impact quality of life. Itch may be peripheral (dermal or neuropathic) or central (neuropathic, neurogenic, or psychogenic) in origin. Neuropathic itch originates at any point along the afferent pathway and is the result of damage to the nervous system, whereas neurogenic itch is induced centrally. In the skin, itch is induced by the stimulation of specialized C fibers by various pruritogens. This is followed by the release of neuropeptides from the cleavage of type 2 proteinase-activated receptors (PAR-2) by tryptase to release histamine, CGRP, and SP.[54]

It is important to understand the underlying mechanisms to provide effective management and treatment. Multiple cutaneous mediators such as histamine, prostanoids, cytokines, and kinins induce pruritus.[50] Pruritus-inducing mechanisms of these mediators include nerve fiber sensitization and receptor stimulation, direct pruritogenic effects, and mast cell activation.[7] Histamine is well known for its pruritic effects especially in urticaria. However, in conditions such as atopic dermatitis the inability of antihistamines to eliminate itch suggest that other mediators are involved as well. Intradermal injection of SP, VIP, and somatostatin evokes pruritus; however, CGRP does not have pruritogenic effects in humans.[50] Substance P is released from C neuron terminals by the action of mast cell tryptase on PAR-2 to directly cause itching and to induce mast cells to release histamine.

There are continuing new developments surfacing in the understanding of the pathogenesis of pruritus, including the recent identification of IL-31 and its role in inflammation and pruritus.[55]

Atopic Dermatitis

Atopic dermatitis (AD) is characterized by cutaneous hyperactivity to nonspecific stimuli leading to a cycle of pruritus, scratching, and further worsening of skin lesions.[56] There is an increased density of nerve fibers and neuropeptide levels in the various stages of skin lesions seen in atopic dermatitis.[57] The diameter of these fibers is larger than those in nonatopic control subjects, possibly due to keratinocyte-derived nerve growth factor (NGF).[58] The free nerve endings in the skin of atopics also lack a surrounding sheath of Schwann cells, suggesting an active state of excitation.[57]

Substance P is a potent pruritogenic neuropeptide in AD that is downregulated by phototherapy[59] along with CGRP.[60] An increase in nerve fibers containing SP and CGRP is observed,[61] although Fantini et al.[62] demonstrated a decrease in SP and an increase in VIP levels in chronic lesions of AD. In lesional skin of atopic dermatitis and nummular dermatitis patients, SP and CGRP but not VIP fibers in the dermis are elevated compared to nonlesional controls and are likely maintained by the increase in mast cells.[63] Intradermal SP increases nitric oxide and enhances SP-induced pruritus, while acute stress triggers skin mast cell degranulation by SP.[7] Elevated VIP was again found to be present in eczema.[64] Preliminary studies on the effects of SP and VIP on T cells indicate that there are no effects on Th1 or Th2 cytokines.[50]

Psoriasis

Psoriasis is a multifactorial disease characterized by symmetric plaque lesions. The possibility of a neurogenic component is supported by the temporal onset or exacerbation of lesions with emotional stress, the appearance of lesions at sites of injury or trauma (Koebner phenomenon, believed to be initiated by the release of proinflammatory neuropeptides in traumatized skin), and by observations that lesions resolve in areas of denervation.[50,65]

Neuropeptide levels and density of sensory nerves are increased in lesional skin[50]; however, levels of SP and VIP vary in psoriasis. Elevated levels in both SP and VIP,[66] normal SP and elevated VIP,[64] and increased SP and normal VIP levels[67] have all been demonstrated in psoriatic lesions. There are conflicting reports of CGRP expression in lesional and nonlesional skin compared to normal controls, and VIP expression is reported to be increased, yet a statistical difference is not consistently observed between lesional and normal skin.[65] Compared to psoriatic lesions, a lower level of SP is seen in lichen planus and lichen simplex chronicus, while higher levels are observed in spongiotic dermatoses.[67] Serum β-endorphin is elevated in psoriatic patients and is likely produced by inflammatory cells in the psoriatic plaques.[68] PACAP-38 is also increased in lesional psoriatic skin, and recent evidence suggests NGF is involved in the pathogenesis of psoriasis.[25,50] Keratinocyte hyperproliferation is a histologic feature in psoriasis, and NGF is suggested to induce keratinocyte proliferation and prevent apoptosis.[65] These studies demonstrate that neuropeptides play a role in psoriasis. However, further delineation of their role in the pathogenesis of the disease is needed.

Vitiligo Vulgaris

Vitiligo is a depigmenting disorder often presenting in a symmetric or segmental distribution. There are changes in neuropeptides distribution in affected skin. An increase in NPY, CGRP, and SP has been demonstrated, whereas no changes in VIP was observed, supporting the concept that neuropeptides are involved in the pathogenesis of vitiligo.[69–72]

Alopecia Areata

Alopecia areata (AA) is characterized by nonscarring patches of hair loss. The pathogenesis is complex and unclear, as immunologic, genetic, environmental, and psychological factors are implicated; however, stressful life events may trigger or exacerbate the disease.[73] The local stress response is believed to contribute to the normal hair cycle, yet its role in AA is unknown.[74] The enhanced expression of corticotropin-releasing hormone (CRH), ACTH, and α-MSH in sites of AA demonstrated by Kim et al.[74] suggest that further studies are needed.

Allergic Contact Dermatitis

In a murine model, topical application of SP, CGRP, and somatostatin reportedly enhance allergic and irritant contact dermatitis.[75] Substance P acts as an adjuvant to raise the immunogenicity of cutaneously applied haptens to promote the induction of CHS, and when it is inhibited, decreases the CHS and DTH responses in humans.[50] Furthermore, the inhibition of SP-degrading peptidases leads to an exaggerated allergic contact dermatitis (ACD) response, suggesting that SP may be capable of boosting both the sensitization and elicitation phase of ACD.[15,75] However, intradermal administration of CGRP suppresses the induction of contact hypersensitivity at the injected site.[76] Furthermore, treatment of epidermal antigen-presenting cells with CGRP in vitro inhibits their ability to present antigen for immunization of naive mice[76] or elicitation of DTH in previously sensitized mice by subcutaneous injection.[28] The difference between these results and those seen with topical application may represent concentration-dependent effects, the effects of secondary mediators induced in unknown third-party cell targets, or other factors peculiar to the route of administration. α-MSH inhibits both the induction and elicitation of CHS responses in mice.[38] Neuropeptides appear to have a modulatory role in the pathogenesis of ACD.[77]

Ultraviolet Radiation

Ultraviolet radiation produces changes in the skin such as erythema, and has immunosuppressive and carcinogenic effects as well.[5] Ultraviolet radiation acts on keratinocytes, mast cells, Langerhans' cells, dermal fibroblasts, and endothelial cells to induce the release of various cytokines, neurohormones, and growth factors.[19] Afferent sensory nerves are a source of inflammatory mediators, notably neuropeptides following UVR exposure. Ultraviolet B radiation (290 to 320 nm) induces CGRP, NKA, and SP release from cutaneous sensory nerves and NGF release from epidermal keratinocytes.[9] Langerhans' cells are also a source of nerve growth factor (NGF) that, along with NGF from keratinocytes, leads to an increase in nerve fibers in sun-exposed skin. CGRP and α-MSH appear to be immunosuppressive in the skin, at least partially through induction of IL-10 production, and SP is involved in the healing of photodamaged skin.[16] CGRP also inhibits the upregulation of IL-12 p40, IL-1β, and CD86.[78]

Ultraviolet radiation–induced immune suppression of CHS and DTH is believed to be partially mediated by IL-10, TNF-α, and the histidine metabolite cis-urocanic acid. Urocanic acid exists in the epidermis primarily as the trans isomer. UVB (and UVC) radiation induces a trans-cis isomerization and considerable evidence supports a role for cis-urocanic acid (UCA) in UVR-induced immune suppression.[79] Increasing evidence also suggests that mast cell products such as histamine are important in downstream systemic immunosuppression.

Evidence suggests that sensory C fibers and mast cells form a functional unit with bidirectional effects.[80] Cis-urocanic can activate mast cells by its effects on release of neuropeptides by afferent sensory nerves.[81] Furthermore cis-UCA induction of the release of neuropeptides such as CGRP may participate in the regulation of UVB-induced inflammation and Langerhans' cell function.[82]

Ultraviolet radiation leads to the release of both pro- and antiinflammatory mediators, and it is the balance of these factors that will determine the host response and clinical outcome. Proinflammatory neuropeptides include SP, NKA, and CGRP, whereas immunosuppressive or antiinflammatory neuropeptides include CGRP and α-MSH.[19] CGRP can be pro- or antiinflammatory, depending on the experimental system.

Wound Healing

Studies suggest the nervous system is important in wound healing and tissue repair. Patients with sensory defects due to injury or a disease process such as diabetic neuropathy, spinal cord injury, or lepromatous leprosy have nonhealing ulcers.[19] Neuropeptides participate in wound repair by initially evoking vascular responses and then influencing the proliferation and differentiation of target cells in the healing process.[50] CGRP promotes human keratinocyte and endothelial cell proliferation,[83] and, together with SP, has proliferative effects on culture fibroblasts.[50] The role of SP is further supported by the finding of elevated neutral endopeptidase expression in wounds and in the skin and ulcers of diabetics. It may contribute to deficient neuroinflammatory signaling and impaired wound healing.[84,85]

Hair Cycling

The cyclical activity of the hair follicle appears to be regulated by a "biological clock" that also affects local neuropeptide expression. The pattern of sensory innervation is also hair-cycle dependent with an increase in nerve fibers seen during growth (anagen), followed by a decrease during regression (catagen) and persistently low levels during the resting stage (telogen).[86]

The corticotropin-releasing hormone (CRH)/ POMC system may regulate the hair follicle pigmentary unit.[87] The expression and processing of POMC and its melanocortin derivatives (α-MSH, ACTH, β-endorphin) vary in the hair follicle. The POMC system appears to be most expressed during early stages of melanocyte differentiation and becomes downregulated in mature melanocytes, suggesting additional systems are involved in maintaining melanogenesis.[88]

Stress leads to premature termination or arrest of hair in telogen in an NGF and mast cell–dependent manner, suggesting that interference with neuropeptide signaling may be an effective measure in the management of stress-induced hair loss.[86]

Photoaging

Chronic, excessive exposure to the sun results in skin changes termed photoaging. Mast cell mediators participate in the dermal changes associated with photoaging,[89] and the correlation between the degree of epidermal innervation and chronic photodamage suggests a possible role of neural influences on photodamaged skin.[90] Toyoda et al.[91] demonstrated an increase in dermal nerve fibers, notably CGRP-positive fibers and increased tissue levels of SP, CGRP, and NGF in sun-exposed skin compared to sun-protected skin. Furthermore, the mast cells were intimately associated with fibroblasts and contained larger amounts of SP when compared to controls. These findings support a role for cutaneous neurogenic factors and mast cells in chronic ultraviolet injury, and suggest a potential target for future therapeutic options.

Melanoma

The role of α-MSH in experimental melanoma is controversial.[92] In the human metastatic melanoma cell lines HBL and A375SM, α-MSH inhibits invasion through a layer of human fibronectin. Furthermore, there is enhanced expression of CRH, ACTH, and α-MSH in human melanoma, squamous cell carcinoma, and basal cell carcinoma tumors demonstrated by immunohistochemical analysis. This suggests a possible role for the stress response in the pathogenesis of skin malignancies.[93] These findings suggest melanocortins, notably α-MSH, may offer new insight into the understanding of the biology of skin cancers, notably melanoma, and potential therapeutic interventions.

Melanocortin receptors are widely distributed in the human body, and of the five receptors, the MC-1 receptor (MCR1) is expressed in cutaneous cells (keratinocytes, fibroblasts melanocytes) and melanoma cells. Previous data demonstrate MCR1 variants predispose to cutaneous melanoma independent of skin type and hair color, and the Asp84Glu variant confers the highest risk.[94] *MCR1* gene variants are shown to be independent risk factors for nonmelanoma skin cancer.[95] However, recent analyses show the association of *MC1R* variants and constitutive pigmentation phenotypes is less than previously reported and has a low rather than high penetrance susceptibility locus for melanoma.[96]

Conclusion

The skin is part of an active neuroimmunoendocrine network with influence at both the local and central levels of the immune system.[36] There are complex interactions among nerve fibers, neuropeptides, target cells, and proteases that are now beginning to be understood. Research in this highly sophisticated system has significantly increased our understanding of neuropeptides and their activities in the skin. The relevance of understanding this intimate relationship is clear, as the pathogenesis of several dermatologic conditions involves the neuroimmune-endocrine network. Further understanding of these mechanisms may lead to novel approaches to the therapy of skin disorders; potential targets include neuropeptides, receptors, and proteases. Although studies are only just beginning in this area, the future is promising.[17]

References

1. Lewis T. Local Means of Producing the Triple Response in the Blood Vessels of Human Skin and Their Responses. London: Shaw & Son, 1927: 46–64.
2. Steinhoff M, Stander S, Seeliger S, et al. Modern aspects of cutaneous neurogenic inflammation. Arch Dermatol 2003;139:1479–1488.
3. Bayliss W. On the origin from the spinal cord of vasodilator fibers of the hind limb, and on the nature of these fibers. J Physiol 1901;26:173–209.

4. Bruce AN. Vasodilator axon reflexes. Q J Exp Physiol 1913;6:339–354.

5. Freedberg IM, Eisen AZ, Wolff K, et al. Fitzpatrick's Dermatology in General Medicine, 6th ed. New York: McGraw-Hill. 2003.

6. Metze D, Luger T. Nervous system in the skin: new basic science in dermatology. In: Freinkel RK, Woodley DT, eds. The Biology of the Skin. New York: Parthenon, 2001:153–165.

7. Stander S, Steinhoff M, Schmelz M, et al. Neurophysiology of pruritus. Arch Dermatol 2003; 139: 1463–1470.

8. Sternini C. Organization of the peripheral nervous system: autonomic and sensory ganglia. J Invest Dermatol Symp Proc 1997;2:1–7.

9. Slominski A, Wortsman J. Neuroendocrinology of the skin. Endocr Rev 2000;21:457–487.

10. Scholzen T, Armstrong CA, Bunnett NW, et al. Neuropeptides in the skin: interactions between the neuroendocrine and the skin immune systems. Exp Dermatol 1998;7:81.

11. Lotti T, Hautmann G, Panconesi E, Neuropeptides in skin. J Am Acad Dermatol 1995;33:482–96.

12. Zegarska B, Leinska A, Tyrakowski T. Clinical and experimental aspects of cutaneous neurogenic inflammation. Pharmacol Rep 2006;58:13–21.

13. Eedy DJ, Shaw C, Johnston CF, Buchanan KD. The regional distribution of neuropeptides in human skin as assessed by radioimmunoassay and high-performance liquid chromatography. Clin Exp Dermatol 1994;19:761–763.

14. Ansel JC, Armstrong CA, Song I, et al. Interactions of the skin and nervous system. J Invest Dermatol Symp Proc 1997;2:23–26.

15. Scholzen TE, Steinhoff M, Bonaccorshi P et al. Neutral endopeptidase terminates substance P-induced inflammation in allergic contact dermatitis. J Immunol 2001;166:1285–1291.

16. Misery L. The neuro-immuno-cutaneous system and ultraviolet radiation. Photodermatol Photoimmunol Photomed 2000;16:78–81.

17. Brain SD, Cox HM. Neuropeptides and their receptors: innovative science providing novel therapeutic targets. Br J Pharmacol 2006;147:S202–S211.

18. Torii H, Yan Z, Hosoi J, Granstein RD. Expression of neurotrophic factors and neuropeptide receptors by Langerhans cells and the Langerhans cell-like cell line XS52: further support for a functional relationship between Langerhans cells and epidermal nerves. J Invest Dermatol 1997;109:586–91.

19. Scholzen TE, Brzoska T, Kalden DH, et al. Effect of ultraviolet light on the release of neuropeptides and neuroendocrine hormones in the skin: mediators of photodermatitis and cutaneous inflammation. J Invest Dermatol Symp Proc 1999;4:55–60.

20. Koizumi H, Tanaka H, Fukaya T, Ohkawara A. Substance P induces intracellular calcium increase and translocation of protein kinase C in epidermis. Br J Dermatol 1992;127;595–9.

21. Rossi R, Johansson O. Cutaneous innervation and the role of neuronal peptides in cutaneous inflammation: a minireview. Eur J Dermatol 1998;8:299–306.

22. Seiffert K, Granstein RD. Neuropeptides and neuroendocrine hormones in ultraviolet radiation-induced immunosuppression. Methods 2002;97–103.

23. Luger TA. Neuromediators—a crucial component of the skin immune system. J Dermatol Sci 2002;30:87–93.

24. Kodali S, Ding W, Huang J, et al. Vasoactive intestinal peptide modulates langerhans cell immune function. J Immunol 2004;173:6082–6088.

25. Steinhoff M, McGregor GP, Radleff-Schlimme A, et al. Identification of pituitary adenylate cyclase activating polypeptide (PACAP) and PACAP type 1 receptor in human skin: expression of PACAP-38 is increased in patients with psoriasis. Regul Pept 1999;80:49–55.

26. Kodali S, Friedman I, Ding W, et al. Pituitary adenylate cyclase-activating polypeptide inhibits cutaneous immune function. Eur J Immunol 2003;33:3070–3079.

27. Amara SG, Jonas V, Rosenfeld MG, et al. Alternative RNA processing in calcitonin gene expression generates mRNAs encoding different polypeptide products. Nature 1982;298:240–4.

28. Hosoi J, Murphy GF, Egan CL et al. Regulation of Langerhans cell function by nerves containing calcitonin gene-related peptide. Nature 1993;363:159–63.

29. Nong YH, Titus RG, Ribeiro JM, Remold HG. Peptides encoded by the calcitonin gene inhibit macrophage function. J Immunol 1989;143:45–49.

30. Fox FE, Kubin M, Cassin M, et al. Calcitonin gene-related peptide inhibits proliferation and antigen presentation by human peripheral blood mononuclear cells: effects on B7, interleukin 10, and interleukin 12. J Invest Dermatol 1997;108:43–8.

31. Carucci JA, Ignatius R, Wei Y, et al. Calcitonin gene-related peptide decreases expression of HLA-DR and CD86 by human dendritic cells and dampens dendritic cell-driven t cell-proliferative responses via the type I calcitonin gene-related peptide receptor. J Immunol 2000;164:3494–3499.

32. Gillardon F, Moll I, Michel S, et al. Calcitonin gene-related peptide and nitric oxide are involved in ultraviolet radiation-induced immunosuppression. Eur J Pharmacol 1995;293:395–400.

33. Niizeki H, Alard P, Streilein JW. Calcitonin gene-related peptide is necessary for ultraviolet B-impaired induction of contact hypersensitivity. J Immunol 1997;159:5183–5186.

34. Garssen J, Buckley TL, Van Loveren H. A role for neuropeptides in UVB-induced systemic immuno-suppression. Photochem Photobiol 1998;68:205–10.

35. Bohm, M, Luger TA, Tobin DJ, Garcia-Borron J. Melanocortin receptor ligands: new horizons for skin biology and clinical dermatology. J Invest Dermatol 2006;126:1966–1975.

36. Brazzini B, Ghersetich I, Hercogova J, Lotti T. The neuro-immuno-cutaneous endocrine network: relationship between mind and skin. Dermatol Ther 2003;16:123–131.

37. Catania A, Airaghi L, Garofalo L, et al. The neuropeptide alpha-MSH in HIV infection and other disorders in humans. Ann NY Acad Sci 1998;840:848–56.

38. Grabbe S, Bhardwaj RS, Mahnke K, et al. Alpha-melanocyte stimulating hormone induces hapten-specific tolerance in mice. J Immunol 1996;156:473–478.

39. Catania A, Cutuli M, Garofalo L, et al. The neuropeptide α-MSH in host defense. Ann NY Acad Sci 2000;917:227–231.

40. Ceriani G, Diaz J, Murphree S, et al. The neuropeptide alpha-melanocyte-stimulating hormone inhibits experimental arthritis in rats. Neuroimmunomodulation 1994;1:28–32.

41. Chiao H, Foster S, Thomas R, et al. Alpha-melanocyte stimulation hormone reduces endotoxin-induced liver inflammation. J Clin Invest 1996;97:2038–2044.

42. Schallreuter KU, Lemke KR, Pittelkow MR, et al. Catecholamines in human keratinocyte differentia-tion. J Invest Dermatol 1995;104:953–957.

43. Seiffert K, Hosoi J, Torri, H, et al. Catecholamines inhibit the antigen-presenting capability of epidermal Langerhans cells. J Immunol 2002;168:6128:6135.

44. Maestroni GJM. Dendritic cells migration con-trolled by α1b-adrenergic receptors. J Immunol 2000;165:6743–6747.

45. Lambert RW, Campton K, Ding W, et al. Langerhans cell expression of neuropeptide Y and peptide YY. Neuropeptides 2002;36:246–251.

46. Holzer AM, Granstein RD. Role of extracellular adenosine triphosphate in human skin. J Cutan Med Surg 2004;90–96.

47. Cook SP, McCleskey EW. Cell damage excites nociceptors through release of cytosolic ATP. Pain 2002;95:41–47.

48. Seiffert K, Ding W, Wagner JA, Granstein RD. ATPγS enhances the production of inflammatory mediators by a human dermal endothelial cell line via purinergic receptor signaling. J Invest Dermatol 2006;126:1017–1027.

49. Granstein RD, Ding W, Huang J et al. Augmentation of cutaneous immune responses by ATP gamma S: purinergic agonists define a novel class of immuno-logic adjuvants. J Immunol 2005;174:7725–31.

50. Roosterman D, Goerge T, Schneider SW, et al. Neuronal control of skin function: the skin as a neuroimmunoendocrine organ. Physiol Rev 2006;86:1309–1379.

51. Borici-mazi, Kouridakis S, Kontou-Fili K. Cutaneous responses to substance P and calcitonin gene-related peptide in chronic urticaria: the effect of cetirizine and dimethindene. Allergy 1999;54:46–56.

52. Akiyama M, Watanabe Y, Nishikawa T. Immunohistochemical characterization of human cutaneous mast cells in urticaria pigmentosa (cuta-neous mastocytosis). Acta Pathol Jpn 1991;41: 344–9.

53. Artuc M, Bohm M, Grutzhau A, et al. Human mast cells in the neurohormonal network: expression of POMC, detection of precursor proteases and evi-dence for IgE-dependent secretion of alpha-MSH. J Invest Dermatol 2006;126:1976–81.

54. Twycross R, Greaves MW, Handwerker H, et al. Itch: more than scratching the surface. Q J Med 2003;96:7–26

55. Sonkoly E, Muller A, Lauerma A. IL-31: a new link between T cells and pruritus in atopic skin inflamma-tion. J Allergy Clin Immunol 2006;117:411–7.

56. Raap U, Kapp A. Neuroimmunological findings in allergic skin diseases. Curr Opin Allergy Clin Immunology 2005;5:419–424.

57. Sugiura H, Omoto M, Hirota Y, et al. Density and fine structure of peripheral nerves in various skin lesions of atopic dermatitis. Arch Dermatol Res 1997;289:125–131.

58. Pincelli C, Sevignani C, Manfredini R, et al. Expression and function of nerve growth factor and nerve growth factor receptor on cultured keratinoc-ytes. J Invest Dermatol 1994;103:13–18.

59. Staniek V, Liebich C, Vocks E, et al. Modulation of cutaneous Sp receptors in atopic dermatitis after UVA irradiation. Acta Derm Venereol 1998'78:92–94.

60. Wallengren J, Sundler F. Phototherapy reduces the number of epidermal and CGRP-positive der-mal nerve fibers. Acta Derm Venereol 2004;84: 111–115.

61. Ostlere LS, Cowen T, Rustin MH. Neuropeptides in the skin of patients with atopic dermatitis. Clin Exp Dermatol 1995;6:462–7.

62. Fantini F, Pincelli C, Romualdi P, et al. Substance P levels are decreased in lesional skin of atopic derma-titis. Exp Dermatol 1992;3:127–8.

63. Jarvikallio A, Harvima IT, Naukkarinen A. Mast cells, nerves and neuropeptides in atopic derma-titis and nummular eczema. Arch Dermatol Res 2003;295:2–7.

64. Anand A, Springall DR, Blank MA, et al. Neuropeptides in skin disease: increased VIP in eczema and psoriasis but not axillary hyperhidrosis. Br J Dermatol 1991;124:547–549.

65. Saraceno R, Kleyn CE, Terenghi G, Griffiths CEM. The role of neuropeptides in psoriasis. Br J Dermatol 2006;154:876–882.

66. Eedy DJ, Johnston CF, Shaw C, Buchanan KD. Neuropeptides in psoriasis: an immunocytochemical and radioimmunoassay study. J Invest Dermatol 1991;96:434–438.

67. Chan J, Smoller BR, Raychaudhuri SP, et al. Intraepidermal nerve fiber expression of calcitonin gene-related peptide, vasoactive intestinal peptide and substance P in psoriasis. Arch Dermatol Res 1997;289:611–616.

68. Glinska W, Brodecka H, Glinska-Ferenz M, Kowalski D. Increased concentration of beta-endorphin in sera of patients with psoriasis and other inflammatory dermatoses. Br J Dermatol 1994;131:260–4.

69. Al'Abadie MS, Senior HJ, Bleehen SS, Gawkrodger DJ. Neuropeptide and neuronal marker studies in vitiligo. Br J Dermatol 1994;131:160–5.

70. Falaballa R, Barona MI, Echeverri IC, Alzate A. Substance P may play a part during depigmentation in vitiligo. A pilot study. J Eur Acad Dermatol Venereol 2003;17:355–6.

71. Lazarova R, Hristakieva E, Lazarov N, Shani J. Vitiligo-related neuropeptides in nerve fibers of the skin. Arch Physiol Biochem 2000;108:262–267.

72. Liu PY, Bondesson L, Lontz W, Johansson O. The occurrence of cutaneous nerve endings and neuropeptides in vitiligo vulgaris: a case-control study. Arch Dermatol Res 1996;288:67–675.

73. Gulec AT, Tanriverdi N, Duru C et al. The role of psychological factors in alopecia areata and the impact of the disease on the quality of life. Int J Dermatol 2004;43:352–356.

74. Kim HS, Cho DH, Kim HJ, et al. Immunoreactivity of corticotropin-releasing hormone, adrenocorticotropic hormone and alpha-melanocyte-stimulating hormone in alopecia areata. Exp Dermatol 2006;15:515–22.

75. Gutwald J, Goebeler M, Sorg C. Neuropeptides enhance irritant and allergic contact dermatitis. J Invest Dermatol 1991;96:695–698.

76. Asahina A, Hosoi J, Beissert S, et al. Inhibition of the induction of delayed-type and contact hypersensitivity by calcitonin gene-related peptide. J Immunol 1995;154:3056.

77. Goebeler M, Henseleit U, Roth J, Sorg C. Substance P and calcitonin gene-related peptide modulate leukocyte infiltration to mouse skin during allergic contact dermatitis. Arch Dermatol Res 1994;286:341–346.

78. Torii H, Hosoi J, Beissert S, et al. Regulation of cytokine expression in macrophages and the Langerhans cell-like line XS52 by calcitonin gene-related peptide. J Leukoc Biol 1997;61:216–223.

79. Hart PH, Townley SL, Grimbaldeston MA, et al. Mast cells, neuropeptides, histamine, and prostaglandins in UV-induced systemic immunosuppression. Methods 2002;28:79–89.

80. Townley SL, Grimbaldeston MA et al. Nerve growth factor, neuropeptides and mast cells in ultraviolet-B-induced systemic suppression of contact hypersensitivity responses in mice. J Invest Dermatol 2002;396–401.

81. Noonan FP, De Fabo ED. Immunosuppression by ultraviolet B radiation: initiation by urocanic acid. Immunol Today 1992;13:250–254.

82. Khalil Z, Townley SL, Grimbaldeston MA, et al. Cis-urocanic acid stimulates neuropeptide release from peripheral sensory nerves. J Invest Dermatol 2001;117:886–891.

83. Haegerstrand A, Dalsgaard CJ, Jonzon B, et al. Calcitonin gene-related peptide stimulates proliferation of human endothelial cells. Proc Natl Acad Sci USA 1990;87:3299–303.

84. Olerud JE, Usui ML, Seckin D et al. Neutral endopeptidase expression and distribution in human skin and wounds. J Invest Dermatol 1999;112:873–81.

85. Antezana M, Sullivan S, Usui M, et al. Neutral endopeptidase activity is increased in the skin of subjects with diabetic ulcers. J Invest Dermatol 2002;119:1400–4.

86. Peters EM, Ericson ME, Hosoi J, et al. Neuropeptide control mechanisms in cutaneous biology: physiological and clinical significance. J Invest Dermatol 2006;126:1937–1947.

87. Tobin DJ, Kauser S. Hair melanocytes as neuroendocrine sensors—pigments of our imagination. Mol Cell Endocrinol 2005;243:1–11.

88. Kauser S, Thody AJ, Schallreuter KU, et al. A fully functional proopiomelanocortin/melanocortin-1 receptor system regulates the differentiation of human scalp hair follicle melanocytes. Endocrinology 2005;146:532–43.

89. Lavker RM, Kligman AM. Chronic heliodermatitis: a morphologic evaluation of chronic actinic dermal damage with emphasis on the role of mast cells. J Invest Dermatol 1998;90:325–30.

90. Toyoda M, Hara M, Bhawan J. Epidermal innervation correlates with severity of photodamage: a quantitative ultrastructural study. Exp Dermatol 1996;5:260–6.

91. Toyoda M, Nakamura M, Nakada K, et al. Characteristic alterations of cutaneous neurogenic factors in photoaged skin. Br J Dermatol 2005;153:13–22.

92. Eves PC, MacNeil S, Haycock JW. α-Melanocyte stimulating hormone, inflammation and human melanoma. Peptides 2006;27:444–452.

93. Kim MH, Cho D, Kim HJ, et al. Investigation of the corticotropin-releasing hormone-proopiomelano-cortin axis in various skin tumors. Br J Dermatol 2006;155:910–915.

94. Kennedy C, ter Huurne J, Berkhout M, et al. Melanocortin 1 receptor (MC1R) gene variants are associated with an increased risk for cutaneous melanoma which is largely independent of skin type and hair color. J Invest Dermatol 2001;117:294–300.

95. Bastiaens MT, ter Huurne JA, Kielich C, et al. Melanocortin-1 receptor gene variants determine the risk of nonmelanoma skin cancer independently of fair skin and red hair. Am J Hum Genet 2001;68:884–94.

96. Kanetsky PA, Rebbeck TR, Hummer AJ, et al. Population-based study of natural variation in the melanocortin-1 receptor gene and melanoma. Cancer Res 2006;66:9330–7.

4
Stress and Immunity

Francisco A. Tausk, Ilia Elenkov, Ralph Paus, Steven Richardson, and Marcelo Label

Key Points

- The brain and the immune system are the two major adaptive systems of the body. There is crosstalk between these two systems, which allows for maintaining homeostasis.
- There is a large body of evidence that documents the effects of stress on a variety of components of the immune response at the systemic level as well as cutaneous immunity.
- Stress can render the host more susceptible to bacterial infections and the development of cancer.
- Emotional stressors have been anecdotally linked to the development or exacerbation of a number of skin diseases (for example, acne, vitiligo, alopecia areata, lichen planus, seborrheic dermatitis, herpes infections).
- The role of stress in atopic dermatitis and psoriasis is well studied, and has established the adverse effects of stress on the clinical course of both diseases.
- There is definitely a brain–skin connection that can translate emotional stressors into biochemical mediators that can result in adverse effects on dermatologic diseases.

The association between stress and health has been extensively documented, however, the mechanisms by which it specifically influences disease susceptibility and outcome remain poorly understood. Hans Selye, the pioneer of stress research, wrote, "Stress is a scientific concept, which has suffered the mixed blessing of being too well known and too little understood." Recent evidence indicates that stress hormones affect major immune functions such as antigen presentation, lymphocyte proliferation

and traffic, secretion of cytokines and antibodies, and selection of the T-helper-1 (Th1) versus Th2 responses. Importantly, it is becoming increasingly clear that stress hormones induce inhibition or upregulation of the systemic or local pro- and antiinflammatory cytokine production, and the Th1/Th2 balance may represent a major mechanism by which stressors affect human disease.

The brain and the immune system are the two major adaptive systems of the body. During an immune response the brain and the immune system "talk" to each other, and this process is essential for maintaining *homeostasis*. Two major pathways systems are involved in this crosstalk: the hypothalamic-pituitary-adrenal (HPA) axis and the systemic/adrenomedullary sympathetic nervous system (SNS). The HPA axis and the SNS represent the peripheral limbs of the stress system,[1–3] whose activation occurs within the central nervous system (CNS) in response to distinct blood-borne, neurosensory, and limbic signals. The central components of the stress system are the corticotropin-releasing hormone (CRH) and locus ceruleus-norepinephrine (LC-NE)/autonomic (sympathetic) neurons of the hypothalamus and brainstem, which respectively regulate the peripheral activities of the HPA axis and the SNS.[2,3] The stress-induced release of hypothalamic CRH leads ultimately to systemic secretion of glucocorticoids (GCs) and catecholamines (CAs), mainly epinephrine and norepinephrine (NE), which in turn influence immune responses. Immune challenges that threaten the stability of the internal milieu can be regarded as stressors. Thus, cell products from an activated immune system, predominately the cytokines interleukin (IL)-1, tumor necrosis factor-α (TNF-α), and IL-6, stimulate CRH secretion from the hypothalamus, and hence activate both the HPA axis and the SNS.[1,3,4]

Several studies during the 1970s and 1980s revealed that stress hormones inhibit lymphocyte proliferation and cytotoxicity and the secretion of certain cytokines, such as IL-2 and interferon-γ (IFN-γ).[5] These early observations, in the context of the broad clinical use of GCs as potent antiinflammatory and immunosuppressive agents, initially led to the conclusion that stress was, in general, immunosuppressive. Recent evidence, however, indicates that stress hormones influence the immune response in a less monochromatic way: they selectively inhibit the Th1/proinflammatory but potentiate Th2/antiinflammatory cytokine production systemically, whereas locally, in certain conditions, they may exert proinflammatory effects. Through this mechanism hyperactive or hypoactive stress systems may influence the onset or course of various common human immune-related diseases. This concept, which emerged in the last decade, is briefly outlined below.

Antigen Presentation

For T cells to be optimally activated, recognition of antigen/major histocompatibility complexes (MHCs) by the T-cell receptor (TCR) must be accompanied by a second co-stimulatory signal, predominantly generated by B7.1 or B7.2 molecules, expressed on antigen-presenting cells (APCs), when engaged to their counterreceptor, CD28, present on T cells. The GCs inhibit the expression of B7.1 and B7.2 in human monocytes and dendritic cells (DCs), respectively, and downregulate MHC II expression in APCs. The downregulation of B7 and MHC II molecules may contribute to the inhibitory effects of these hormones on APC-dependent T-cell activation.[6–9] The Toll-like receptors (TLRs), which recognize conserved microbial products TLR-4 and TLR-2, mediate the host response to bacteria, leading to the activation of signaling pathways that result in the induction of inflammatory and antimicrobial innate immune responses. Recent evidence indicates that GCs induce TLR-4 in the resting condition, yet after T-cell activation they decrease TLR-4 expression.[8]

Lymphocyte Traffic and Proliferation

After a single dose of a short-acting glucocorticoid, the concentration of neutrophils increases, whereas the lymphocytes, monocytes, eosinophils, and basophils in the circulation decrease in number. The increase of neutrophils is due both to the increased influx from the bone marrow and to the demargination and impaired extravasation of neutrophils. The decreased migration of neutrophils from the blood vessels combined with diminished chemotaxis and adherence to vascular endothelium of neutrophils and monocytes results in inhibition of the accumulation of these cells at the site of inflammation. These effects underlie the potent antiinflammatory properties of GCs. The reduction in circulating lymphocytes, monocytes, eosinophils, and basophils is the result of their movement from the vascular bed to lymphoid tissue. Two phases are recognized after CA administration in humans: a quick (< 30-minute) mobilization of lymphocytes, followed by an increase of granulocytes with relative lymphopenia (maximal response at 2 to 4 hours).[9] The CAs predominantly affect natural killer (NK) cells and granulocytes circulation, whereas T- and B-cell numbers remain relatively unaffected. Infusion of both NE and epinephrine in humans results in marked increases (between 400% and 600%) of NK cell numbers (CD16$^+$CD56$^+$), most probably due to the β_2-adrenoceptor (AR)–mediated demargination of the NK pool in blood vessels. By contrast, a reduction of NK cell number is observed after 7 days of treatment with terbutaline, a β_2-AR selective agonist, changes that are identical to those seen in congestive heart failure patients.[10] Thus, in the short term, CAs acutely mobilize NK cells from depots, whereas in the long term, chronically, CAs decrease the number of lymphocytes, and particularly of NK cells in the peripheral blood.

Catecholamines inhibit the T-cell proliferation directly through stimulation of β-ARs and induction of cyclic adenosine monophosphate (cAMP) in these cells.[11–14] An additional CA-induced inhibition operates through suppression of the production of IL-2, a cytokine that is an important co-stimulatory molecule in T-cell proliferation.[15] The proliferative response of CD8$^+$ T cells is inhibited to a greater extent than CD4$^+$ T cells, presumably because

CD8[+] T cells have a higher number of β-ARs.[15] By inhibiting IL-1 production by monocytes and IL-2 and IFN-γ production by lymphocytes, GCs may also contribute for decreased lymphocyte proliferation.

Proinflammatory/Antiinflammatory Cytokine Production and the Th1/Th2 Balance

Immune responses are regulated by APCs, such as monocytes/macrophages, DCs, and other phagocytic cells that are components of innate immunity, and by the Th lymphocyte subclasses Th1 and Th2, which are components of acquired (adaptive) immunity. Homeostasis within the immune system is largely dependent on cytokines, the chemical messengers between immune cells, which play crucial roles in mediating inflammatory and immune responses. These diverse groups of proteins may be regarded as hormones of the immune system. Cytokines act in an autocrine, paracrine, or endocrine fashion to control the proliferation, differentiation, and activity of immune cells. For instance, Th1 cells primarily secrete IFN-γ, IL-2, and TNF, which promote cellular immunity, whereas Th2 cells secrete a different set of cytokines, primarily IL-4, IL-10, and IL-13, which promote humoral immunity[16–18] (Fig. 4.1). Naive CD4[+] (antigen-inexperienced) Th0 cells are bipotential and serve as precursors of Th1 and Th2 cells. Interleukin-12, produced by APCs, is the major inducer of Th1 differentiation and hence cellular immunity. It also synergizes with IL-18 to induce the production of IFN-γ by NK cells. Thus, IL-12 in concert with IL-18, IFN-α, and IFN-γ, promote the differentiation of Th0 cells toward the Th1 phenotype. Interleukin-1, IL-12, TNF-α, and IFN-γ also stimulate the functional activity of T-cytotoxic (Tc) cells, NK cells, and activated macrophages, which are the major components of cellular immunity. The type 1 cytokines IL-12, TNF-α, and IFN-γ also stimulate the synthesis of nitric oxide (NO) and other inflammatory mediators that drive chronic delayed type inflammatory responses. Because of their synergistic roles in stimulating inflammation IL-12, TNF-α and IFN-γ are considered the major

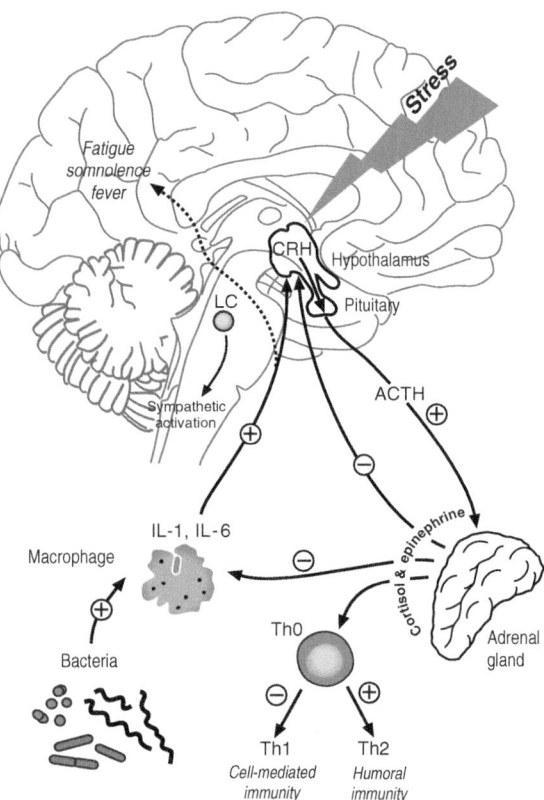

FIG. 4.1. Hypothalamic-pituitary-adrenal (HPA) axis. The "fight-flight" response is triggered by a stressor, mediating the secretion of hypothalamic corticotropin-releasing factor (CRF) and the subsequent liberation of pituitary ACTH. The latter induces the secretion of adrenal glucocorticosteroids, which act as a negative feedback, inhibiting the production of adrenocorticotropic hormone (ACTH). Cortisol stimulates the differentiation of lymphocytes toward the T-helper-2 (Th2) profile, favoring the humoral and suppressing the cellular immune response, and also inhibits macrophage cytokine production with the exception of the mostly immunosuppressing interleukin-10 (IL-10). Bacterial lipopolysaccharides bind to Toll-like receptors on these cells, favoring the secretion of IL-1, IL-6, and tumor necrosis factor (TNF) by macrophages, agents that induce liberation of hypothalamic CRF, triggering the HPA axis in a similar fashion as emotional stressors. Stress also activates the sympathetic system, with the resulting production of catecholamines and neuropeptides

proinflammatory cytokines.[16–18] Th1 and Th2 responses are mutually inhibitory. Thus, IL-12 and IFN-γ inhibit Th2, while IL-4 and IL-10 inhibit Th1 cell activities. Interleukin-4 and IL-10 promote humoral immunity by stimulating the growth and activation of mast cells and eosinophils (Eo), the differentiation of B cells into antibody-secreting B cells, and B-cell immunoglobulin (Ig) switching to IgE. Importantly, these cytokines also inhibit macrophage activation, T-cell proliferation, and the production of proinflammatory cytokines.[16–18] Therefore, the Th2 (type 2) cytokines IL-4 and IL-10 are the major antiinflammatory cytokines.

Systemic Effects of Glucocorticoids and Catecholamines

Both GCs and CAs systemically mediate a Th2 shift by suppressing APCs and Th1-cytokine production and upregulating Th2-cytokine production.[19] Thus, GCs and the two major CAs, NE and epinephrine, through stimulation of classic cytoplasmic/nuclear glucocorticoid receptors (GR) and β_2-ARs, respec-

tively, suppress the production by APCs of IL-12, the main inducer of Th1 responses.[20–23] Since IL-12 is extremely potent in enhancing IFN-γ and inhibiting IL-4 synthesis by T cells, this is also associated with decreased IFN-γ but increased production of IL-4 by T cells[21,24,25] (Fig. 4.2). The GCs also have a direct effect on Th2 cells by upregulating their IL-4, IL-10, and IL-13 production.[21,26] The GCs do not affect the production of IL-10 by monocytes,[20,27] yet lymphocyte-derived IL-10 production is upregulated by GCs.[26] This could be the result of a direct stimulatory effect of GCs on T-cell IL-10 production or a block on the restraining inputs of IL-12 and IFN-γ on lymphocyte IL-10 production. Both GCs and CAs inhibit the production of IL-1, TNF-α, and IFN-γ, while CAs inhibit the production of TNF-α by monocytes, microglial cells, and astrocytes, and suppress the production of IL-1, an effect that is mostly indirect via inhibition of TNF-α and potentiation of IL-10 production.[28–32]

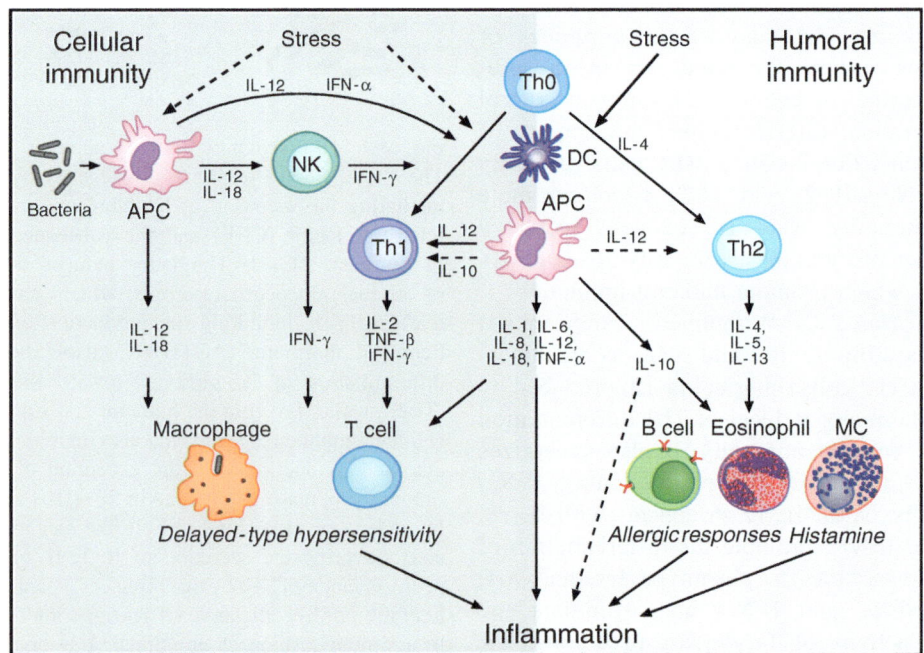

Fig. 4.2. Stress and inflammation. The stress hormones (glucocorticoids and catecholamines) modulate the maturation of naive T-helper cells (Th0) favoring the development of the Th2 profile. Pro- and antiinflammatory and Th1 and Th2 cytokines regulate cellular and humoral immunity, and inflammation. Cellular immunity provides protection against intracellular bacteria, protozoa, fungi, and several viruses, while humoral immunity provides protection against multicellular parasites, extracellular bacteria, some viruses, soluble toxins, and allergens. The cellular source of IL-4 that stimulates the Th2 differentiation is not well defined. Solid lines represent stimulation, while dashed lines inhibition. Ag, antigen; APC, antigen-presenting cell; DC, dendritic cell; IFN, interferon; IL, interleukin, Tc, T cytotoxic cell: Th, T helper cell; Th0: naive Th; TNF, tumor necrosis factor

Since β_2-ARs are expressed on Th1 cells but not on Th2 cells,[33] CAs do not affect directly the cytokine production by Th2 cells; in murine and human systems, β_2-AR agonists inhibit IFN-γ production by Th1 cells, but do not affect IL-4 production by Th2 cells.[33,34] However, CAs, through stimulation of β_2-ARs, upregulate the production of the antiinflammatory cytokine IL-10 and IL-6 by APCs.[20,35–37]

Neuropeptide Y

Sympathetic/neuropeptide Y (NPY)-positive nerve fibers predominantly supply the vasculature, where they mainly occur as perivascular plexuses, and both NE and NPY, released from these fibers, control blood flow and lymphocyte traffic. They branch off only rarely to run into the lymphoid parenchyma.[38,39] Neuropeptide Y is co-released with NE upon SNS activation. Particularly in conditions of high sympathetic activity, large dense-cored vesicles release both NPY and NE.[40] Neuropeptide Y does not usually act as a genuine cotransmitter but rather as a prejunctional or postjunctional modulator of the release or the effects of the principal transmitters, NE and adenosine triphosphate (ATP). In many tissues the major action of NPY is to enhance the postjunctional response of NE and ATP.

Neuropeptide Y inhibits IL-6 release from splenic macrophages via stimulation of the Y1 receptor. Neuropeptide Y also potentiates CA-induced inhibition and stimulation of IL-6 production by these cells through α_2- and β_2-ARs, respectively.[41] In the presence of NPY, differentiated Th1 cells produce less IFN-γ, but Th2 cells express increased IL-4 production. Additionally, administration of NPY induces inhibition of the ex vivo production of IFN-γ in antigen-specific murine lymphocytes. Thus, NPY similar to CAs might possess Th2-inducing properties.[42]

Local Versus Systemic Effects

The systemic Th2-inducing properties of stress hormones may not pertain to certain conditions or local responses in specific compartments of the body. Thus, corticosteroid treatment results in a significant increase of the number of IL-12$^+$ cells, with concurrent reduction in the number of IL-13$^+$ expressing cells in bronchial biopsy specimens of asthmatics.

Interestingly, this occurs only in steroid-sensitive but not steroid-resistant asthmatic subjects.[43] The number of IL-4$^+$ cells in the bronchial and nasal mucosa is also reduced by glucocorticoid treatment.[44,45] Furthermore, the synthesis of transforming growth factor-β (TGF-β), another cytokine with potent antiinflammatory activities, is enhanced by GCs in human T cells but suppressed in glial cells,[46] and low doses of GCs can indeed activate alveolar macrophages, leading to increased lipopolysaccharide (LPS)-induced IL-1β production.[47]

Norepinephrine, via stimulation of α_2-ARs, can augment LPS-stimulated production of TNF-α by mouse peritoneal macrophages.[48] In rodents, induction of hemorrhage, a condition associated with elevations of systemic CA concentrations or exposure of animals to mild inescapable electric shock of the foot, stress results in increased IL-1β and TNF-α production by alveolar macrophages and lung mononuclear cells.[49,50] These effects are most likely indirect; in vitro, a direct modulatory effect of CAs on LPS-induced IL-1β by alveolar macrophages was not demonstrated. Thus, stress-induced changes in alveolar macrophage activity might result from alveolar type II epithelial cell activation, leading to release of surfactant or other factors.[50]

Catecholamines also potentiate the production of IL-8 (a chemokine that promotes the recruitment of polymorphonuclear cells to an inflammatory site) by monocytes, epithelial cells of the lung and endothelial cells, indirectly, via an effect on platelets.[51–53] Furthermore, CAs (through β_2/β_3-ARs) upregulate IL-6 production by human adipocytes.[54,55] Interleukin-6 is the major inducer of C-reactive protein (CRP) production by the liver, and both GCs and CAs enhance this induction.[56] Interestingly, histamine induces the production of both IL-6 and IL-8 by coronary artery endothelial cells, whereas chronic β-AR stimulation induces myocardial, but not systemic, production of TNF-α, IL-1β, and IL-6[57,58] (Fig. 4.2).

Corticotropin-Releasing Hormone/ Substance P–Mast Cell–Histamine Interactions

Corticotropin-releasing hormone is also secreted peripherally at inflammatory sites (peripheral or immune CRH).[59] Immunoreactive CRH is identified locally in tissues from patients with rheumatoid arthritis, autoimmune thyroid diseases, and ulcerative colitis. Corticotropin-releasing hormone in early inflammation is of peripheral postganglionic sympathetic and sensory afferent nerve rather than immune-cell origin.[59,60] Peripheral CRH has vascular permeability-enhancing and vasodilatory actions. An intradermal CRH injection induces a marked increase of vascular permeability and mast cell degranulation, mediated through CRH type 1 receptors.[61] It appears that the mast cell is a major target of immune CRH. Peripheral CRH and substance P (SP), released from sensory peptidergic neurons, are two of the most potent mast cell secretagogues.[61–64] Thus, peripheral CRH and SP activate mast cells via a CRH type 1 and NK1 receptor-dependent mechanism, leading to release of histamine and other contents of the mast cell granules that cause vasodilatation, increased vascular permeability, and other manifestations of inflammation (Fig. 4.3).

Antibody Production

When B cells and Th cells are exposed to Th-cell–dependent antigens, NE, through stimulation of β_2-ARs, exerts an enhancing effect on B-cell antibody (Ab) production.[33,65] One mechanism for this enhancement may involve a CA-induced increase in the frequency of B cells differentiating into Ab-secreting cells. Moreover, Th cells activate B cells during cell-to-cell interaction, and Th2 cells provide the cytokines necessary for B-cell growth. Thus, the β_2-AR agonists salbutamol and fenoterol potentiate IL-4–induced IgE production by human peripheral blood momonuclear cells (PBMCs), while they inhibit IFN-γ production by these cells.[66] Furthermore, salbutamol induces an increase of the ex vivo release of IL-4, IL-6, and IL-10.[67] Glucocorticoid and IL-4 have synergistic effects on the triggering and differentiation of B cells into IgE-producing plasma cells. In addition,

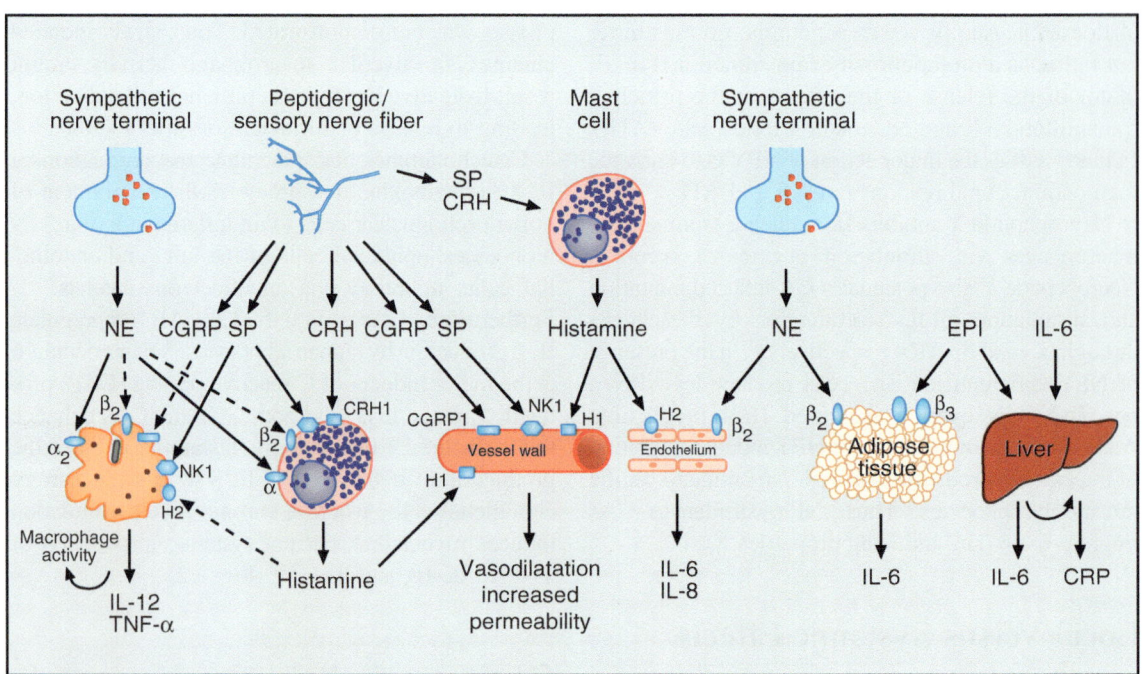

Fig. 4.3. Simplified scheme of the complex interactions among catecholamines (CAs), neuropeptides, and the CRH/SP–mast cell–histamine axis, and their pro- and antiinflammatory effects in certain local responses. Solid lines represent stimulation, while dashed lines represent inhibition. CGRP, calcitonin gene–related peptide; CRH, corticotropin-releasing hormone (peripheral); EPI, epinephrine; IL, interleukin; NE, norepinephrine; SP, substance P; TNF, tumor necrosis factor; NK1, SP receptor; H1 and H2, histamine receptors 1 and 2; CGRP1, CGRP receptor 1. (From Elenkov IJ. Neuroendocrine effects on immune system. At www.endotext.com [online endocrine source], L. DeGroot, ed., 2003.)

patients with asthma, after 7-day treatment with 40 mg of prednisone daily, experience a rise in serum IgE levels.[68,69]

Stress and Clinical Cutaneous Immunology

Seventy years ago, Selye[70] suggested that the organism has the ability to adapt to acute homeostatic challenges, but chronicity will lead to exhaustion, distress, and disease.[71] Indeed, subsequent research has shown that the nature,[72] temporality,[73] and duration[74] of the stressors are critical in determining their effect,[75] including the significant decay of general health as well as enhanced mortality.[76–79]

The response of the organism to acute stressors represents the physiologic mechanism of adaptation (fight or flight reaction), and allows the survival of the species. The effect of stress on immunity suggested that it results in an augmentation of the susceptibility to neoplasms, infections, and deficient wound healing. Dhabhar and McEwen[80,81] noted the paradox that "the suppression of immune function under all stress conditions would not be evolutionarily adaptive" for an organism that is attacked by a predator and needs protection from injuries and infections. These researchers examined the differential effects of acute or chronic stress on the cutaneous cell mediated immune response. Indeed, they found that rodents exposed to acute stressors experience changes characterized by the mobilization and redistribution of leukocytes to peripheral organs such as the skin. Delayed-type hypersensitivity (DTH) reactions were also found to be significantly enhanced, an effect that was reversed by adrenalectomy, suggesting a role played by physiologic secretion of adrenal hormones. In contrast to these findings, animals exposed to prolonged (chronic) stressors experienced a significant decrease in DTH, representing an impairment in cell-mediated immunity that would enhance their susceptibility to infections and neoplasms.

Stress and Infections

A large body of evidence links stressors to the susceptibility to infections (reviewed in Biondi and Zannino[82]) such as viral respiratory ailments during periods of psychological stress,[83] or the incidence of experimentally induced upper respiratory viral infections, which correlated with the presence of chronic stress in normal volunteers.[84,85] Similarly, studies have documented the immunosuppressive effects of chronic stressors on the evolution of cutaneous bacterial[86,87] and viral infections, such as recurrent herpetic infection precipitated by psychiatric illness, life events, and disgust.[88] As Cohen and colleagues[89] demonstrated, chronic stressors are predictive of herpes simplex recurrence, a response that is largely mediated by endogenous corticosteroids.

Stress and Cancer

For more than 50 years, research has suggested that a large variety of emotional stressors can enhance the development of malignant neoplasms[90]; similarly, studies have suggested that stress among other emotional influences can affect the evolution of neoplasms.[91–93]

A variety of psychosocial interventions such as housing conditions, differential handling, surgical procedures, and other stressors are known to favor the development of experimental tumors in laboratory animals,[94,95] suppressing lymphocyte proliferation[96] and natural killer cell activity,[97,98] an effect that could be abolished by β-adrenergic blocking agents, suggesting the role of catecholamines in this process.[99,100] Furthermore, lymphocytes from rats exposed to rotational stress expressed decreased DNA repair following irradiation.[101,102] It was only recently that we reported markedly accelerated carcinogenicity in ultraviolet B (UVB)-treated SKH mice when they were exposed to stressors.[103]

The effect of stress on the development of cancer in humans is more difficult to evaluate. Some studies appear to indicate that, for example, in the case of breast cancer, stress may have some influence over the outcome of the disease.[104–108]

Some of the evidence of psychosocial influence on neoplasia[109] stems from studies that showed that women with metastatic breast cancer who participated in weekly sessions of group therapy and hypnosis for 1 year duplicated their survival time when compared with controls.[110] Patients with metastatic melanoma were also found to have a significantly improved 6-year survival rate when they received limited sessions of psychological interventions.[111]

One possible explanation for the benefit of these interventions could be the modulatory effect of stress and stress reduction on NK cell function, presumed to represent one of the first innate lines of immune defense against foreign (including cancerous) cells.[112]

Daily life stressors and social dysfunction markers such as bereavement,[113,114] loneliness,[115] and lack of social support have been shown to suppress immune responses across a variety of different populations such as medical students,[116] divorcees,[117] married couples,[118] spouses of cancer patients,[119] caregivers of patients with Alzheimer's disease,[120–122] and normal adults.[119]

Even relatively mild forms of stress on students were associated with decreases in NK cell activity and IFN-γ production during examination periods.[115,123] Interestingly, acute stressors such as first-time parachuting appear to mediate the opposite effect of chronic aggressors; they enhance the immune response with a significant increase in NK cell numbers and function.[74,124–126] Natural killer cell activity can also be modulated by psychosocial interventions as exemplified by a study that reported increased cytotoxic function in elderly individuals following relaxation training.[127] Finally, individual variability due to personality traits appears to play an important role, as seen in the changes in NK cell activity associated with emotional stability and anxiety-stressed individuals.[128]

Acquired and Inherited Alterations of the Hypothalamic-Pituitary-Adrenal Axis Can Determine How the Individual Responds to Stressors During Adult Life

Stressors occurring early in life have a profound effect on the HPA axis; in such a manner, neonatal rodents that are not appropriately groomed by their mothers,[129] or females abused during childhood,[130] exhibit an abnormal response to stressors in adulthood, with elevated production of glucocorticosteroids over time. On the other hand, genetic hypothalamic dysfunctions can be responsible for an inappropriate secretion of corticosteroids, as reported by Sternberg, showing that very similar strains of rats, such as the Lewis and Fisher, could differ markedly in the hypothalamic response to stressors. The Lewis, but not the Fisher, would succumb to stress and artificially induced inflammation due to an inappropriate secretion of

corticosterone. Furthermore, transplanting cells of the hypothalamus from Fisher to Lewis rats corrected the defect.[131–133] These observations highlight the notion that not only the elevated production of glucocorticosteroids mediates stress induced disease, but also the inappropriate production of these hormones in response to stress can be associated with an altered homeostasis. Pediatric as well as adult patients with atopic dermatitis respond to common stressors with a significantly lower peak of cortisol, when compared to healthy controls.[134–137] This phenomenon was also seen in patients with rheumatoid arthritis[138,139] and psoriasis,[140] suggesting that these patients have inflammatory diseases that may flare when they are unable to sustain normal levels of corticosteroids when confronted with adverse stimuli.

Stress and Skin Diseases

For many years emotional stressors have been linked anecdotally to the development or evolution of a variety of cutaneous diseases, including acne,[141] vitiligo,[142,143] alopecia areata,[144] lichen planus,[145] seborrheic dermatitis, herpes simplex infections,[89] pemphigus,[146] and urticaria[147]; however, psoriasis and atopic eczema are the ones that have been most extensively studied.

Psoriasis

This is a common chronic and relapsing inflammatory skin disorder that frequently affects all aspects of quality of life, including physical, psychological, social, sexual, and occupational.[148] In addition to the genetic and immunologic basis of psoriasis, stress appears to play an important role in the variable clinical course.[149,150] These patients respond to experimental stressors with elevated blood pressure, heart rate, and epinephrine levels, and decreased plasma cortisol and dehydroepiandrosterone.[140,151]

Neurogenic inflammation also plays a significant role in the pathogenesis of psoriasis,[152–155] as suggested by the symmetrical distribution of the lesions, increased nerve density in psoriatic plaques, elevated neuropeptide expression in diseased skin,[155] and the clinical clearance of psoriatic plaques in anesthetic areas following sensory nerve injury.[156] Interestingly, in the latter case, disease recurred following reinnervation and the return of cutaneous sensitivity, suggesting a role played by these nerves.[157] The altered expression of numerous neuropeptides in psoriatic skin may contribute to the disease; for example, nerve growth factor (NGF) induces keratinocyte proliferation, mast cell migration, and degranulation; stimulates IL-2 production through T-cell proliferation; and is chemotactic for memory T cells.[152,158–160] Other neuropeptides such as calcitonin gene–related peptide (CGRP), SP, and vasoactive intestinal peptide (VIP) (discussed in Chapter 3) also play a role in this disease.

Finally, numerous reports of successful psychosocial interventions aimed at the reduction of stress in the treatment of psoriasis[161,162] highlight the deleterious role of emotional stress. Kabat Zinn's group[163,164] showed how a brief intervention such as the addition of mindfulness meditation tapes during phototherapy sessions shortened the time to complete remission by half.

Atopic Dermatitis

Atopic dermatitis (AD) (see Chapter 13) is a disease that exemplifies the delicate balance among genetic, environmental, and psychosocial factors in the maintenance of health. An increasing number of studies suggest that stress, among other psychological factors, contributes significantly (up to 70%) to exacerbations and the continuing chronic nature of AD.[165] Up to 70% of atopic patients report that significant emotional stressors predate flares of the disease.[166] However, the relationship between psychological stress and the severity of atopic dermatitis may be bidirectional. Not only is the stressor a strong predictor of worsening, but flares of atopic disease contribute significantly to a lowered stress threshold and increased levels of psychological distress.[167]

A number of studies have reported alterations in the cytokine secretion profile as well as the distribution of lymphocytes and eosinophils in these patients when exposed to experimental psychological stress.[168,169] The balance of Th lymphocytes helps us understand some aspects of the role played by stress in this disease. The presence of stressors polarize the immune status toward a Th2 response, with a predominant stimulation of humoral immunity.[170–172] Interestingly, glucocorticosteroids

appear to play a more widespread role, since they also have the ability to suppress the production of IL-4, which is an agent of differentiation toward Th2.[171,173–176] This effect tends to occur at pharmacologic levels, and explains the beneficial effect of systemic or topical application of these agents.

As discussed before, atopic patients were found to have abnormal glucocorticoid regulation, exhibiting a blunting of the HPA axis response. Compared to controls, atopic patients display an altered 24-hour cortisol profile, and children with atopic dermatitis produce lower levels of cortisol in response to psychological stress.[137,177] Furthermore, adult atopic patients injected with CRH were found to secrete attenuated levels of adrenocorticotropic hormone (ACTH) and cortisol, compared to controls [178]. The inadequate secretion of cortisol could help explain flares during taxing stressors. On the other hand, there appears to be an upregulation of glucocorticoid receptors on peripheral leukocytes in atopic patients,[178] the result of which are effector cells potentially hyperreactive to glucocorticoid stimulation. Thus in spite of a blunted HPA axis response to stress, effector cells exquisitely sensitive to systemic glucocorticoid release may respond in a hyperreactive fashion to stress cortisol, accentuating the cytokine shift from the Th1 to the Th2 constellation.

In addition to the changes in immunity patterns, stressors have been found to alter significantly the recovery kinetics of the skin barrier. Women subjected to interview stress or sleep deprivation had an altered skin barrier function, measured by recovery of transepidermal water loss.[179] This breakdown in barrier function homeostasis causes an increased susceptibility to cutaneous inoculation with environmental agents (such allergens as dust mites, dander, bacteria, and viruses). This may play an important role in the skin of atopic patients since these stimuli have all been considered as potential precipitants of acute atopic dermatitis and elicitors of atopic flares.[180]

Catecholamines and their metabolites secreted from the adrenal medulla as well as from sympathetic nerve endings during periods of stress may also contribute to disease worsening. These patients have higher concentrations of norepinephrine,[181] which may stimulate the activity of intracellular type 4 phosphodiesterases (PDE4) in mononuclear cells, which in turn have been found to be elevated in patients with atopic dermatitis,[182] leading to the secretion of IL-13 and IL-4.[183]

Finally, a number of psychosocial interventions including stress reduction, hypnosis, biofeedback, and psychotherapy[184–188] have been shown to improve significantly in patients with atopic eczema,[189] highlighting the possible role played by emotional stress in the evolution of these patients.

Stress and the Brain–Skin Connection

These increasing insights into the clinically long-appreciated close interrelatedness of psychoemotional stress and the triggering or aggravation of defined dermatoses gain even greater importance on the background of emerging, relatively recent investigations in skin biology, as follows:

1. There is increasing evidence that numerous cell populations of human skin as well as its most prominent skin appendage, the pilosebaceous unit, are direct targets for classical mediators of systemic stress responses in vitro and in vivo.
2. There is increasing evidence that the skin itself is a major source of "central" neuroendocrine stress mediators. 3. There is recognition that mammalian skin has established functionally and fully active peripheral equivalents of central stress response systems.

As we shall see, one recurrent theme in the field of brain–skin connection is that, time and again, the pilosebaceous unit has surfaced as a surprisingly productive research tool for the exploration and definition of new research frontiers in stress-related cutaneous neuroendocrinology and neuroimmunology, both in mice and humans.

The Skin and Its Appendages as a Target of Neuroendocrine Stress Mediators

While it has been recognized for decades that the pigment cells of vertebrate skin are prominent targets of neuroendocrine regulation and that, in fact, melanocortins such as α-melanocyte-stimulating hormone (α-MSH) and ACTH are key regulators of melanocyte function and melanogenesis,[190] it took much longer to recognize that many other cell populations in the skin (such as keratinocytes, sebocytes, fibroblasts, endothelial cells, mast cells, macrophages, and sensory nerve fibers innervating the skin) also are important targets of secreted neuroendocrine messengers.[191–200] Neurogenic inflammation and pruritogenic pruritus (which often occur in conjunction, as in atopic eczema and prurigo nodularis) represent particularly complex examples for multiple skin cells and structures that are targeted by stress-associated neuroendocrine mediators.[201,202]

To list but a few selected examples, it is now well recognized that CRH, the most proximal regulatory element of the HPA stress response axis, targets skin mast cells, epidermal and hair follicle keratinocytes, as well as sebocytes, and exerts surprisingly diverse functions on skin biology and skin pathophysiology. These range from skin mast cell activation via inhibition of hair follicle keratinocyte proliferation to the modulation of lipogenesis in sebocytes and the intracutaneous stimulation of pro-opiomelanocortin (POMC) gene expression.[191,198,201,203] Namely, CRH inhibits hair shaft formation and matrix keratinocyte proliferation, while it stimulates hair matrix keratinocyte apoptosis, follicular melanogenesis, POMC gene expression, melanocortin production, and melanocortin receptor expression in normal human scalp hair follicles in organ culture.[204]

The prototypic stress-associated melanocortin ACTH, whose pituitary synthesis and secretion is controlled by CRH, has long been recognized for its immunomodulatory properties relevant to skin immunity; besides its classical immunosuppressive activity (stimulation of cortisol synthesis), ACTH has mast cell–activating[194,195] and multiple lymphocyte-regulatory properties.[199] Most recently, ACTH has been reported to stimulate IL-18 expression in a human keratinocyte line on the gene and protein level, likely via the caspase-1 activation pathway.[205] The regulatory role of CRH in the release of inflammatory mediators from primary human epidermal keratinocytes in response to bacterial products (such as LPS)[206] further highlights how stress-associated neurohormones may modulate skin immune responses via direct effects on the epithelium.

However, in vivo, the effects of ACTH on the skin epithelium clearly extend beyond immunomodulation, as suggested by the hypertrichosis induced by ACTH and its potent hair cycle modulator in mice.[207,208] Moreover, the peptide content as well as the intensity of immunoreactivity and immunolocalization of ACTH in mouse all are hair cycle dependent, and ACTH exerts dose-dependent proliferation-modulatory effects on defined mouse skin compartments.[209]

Compared with CRH and ACTH, the prototypic stress-associated neuropeptide SP has both overlapping and distinct functions; SP activates skin mast cells,[193–195,210] selectively stimulates TNF-α release by mast cells,[211] and stimulates epidermal keratinocyte proliferation.[210] Depending on the cell and hair cycle status of these cells, SP either inhibits or stimulates murine keratinocyte proliferation in situ, and thus became the first neuropeptide shown to operate as a potent hair cycle modulator in vivo affecting both the growth phase as well as the regression phase in follicles.[208,212] In mice, SP also promotes hair follicle inflammation, resulting in alopecia areata.[197]

The prototypic stress-associated growth factor NGF, whose serum level rises sharply upon exposure to psychoemotional stressors, is now recognized as a major stimulator of skin mast cell survival, proliferation, and activation.[194,195,213] Moreover, NGF profoundly modulates the proliferation of murine epidermal and hair follicle keratinocytes in situ, not only in mice, but also in human epidermis and hair follicles.[213–216]

A particularly striking example for the skin and its appendages as chief targets of major stress mediators like NGF and SP has come from a murine sound stress model,[217,218] in which NGF and SP have now been documented to operate as the key mediators for executing the neurogenic perifollicular inflammation and subsequent hair growth inhibition of murine pelage hair follicles after exposure to sound stress. Upregulation of NGF expression following stressors may enhance SP synthesis and release by dorsal root ganglion sensory nerves leading to perifollicular, mast cell–dependent neurogenic inflammation, which in addition to the direct growth-inhibitory effects of NGF and SP on anagen hair follicles, results in substantial hair growth inhibition.[217–219]

Prolactin, the most prominent polypeptide product of pituitary lactotroph cells, whose pleiotropic functional properties extend beyond the control of mammary gland development and lactation and include a wide range of immunomodulatory functions, is yet another classic neuroendocrine mediator that is strongly upregulated during stress responses. Prolactin receptor–deficient mice show striking hair cycle abnormalities, while prolactin receptor expression in normal murine skin is hair cycle dependent.[220–223] Moreover, prolactin administration promotes premature hair follicle regression,[222,223] and retards anagen development,[221] while hyperprolactinemia can be associated with telogen effluvium and a hair loss pattern that imitates androgenetic alopecia.[222]

The Skin as a Source of Neuroendocrine Stress Mediators

Perhaps the most important discovery in cutaneous neuroendocrinology is that the skin itself is a potent source of major neuroendocrine stress mediators and that the pilosebaceous unit is a particularly prominent site of expression, production, and secretion of these neurohormones. Early key findings in this respect were the demonstration that murine skin transcribes, translates, and enzymatically processes the POMC gene and its products in vivo, in a hair cycle–dependent manner,[224] and that human scalp skin hair follicles in anagen are prominently immunoreactive for ACTH.[224] Another important discovery was that murine skin in vivo, namely the hair follicle epithelium and cutaneous nerve fibers, also shows hair cycle–dependent CRH immunoreactivity and CRH receptor expression.[225] Both CRH gene and protein expression now have also been documented for human scalp anagen hair follicles.[204,226] Numerous studies have now confirmed the notion that mammalian skin is a key extrahypothalamic and extrapituitary source of major stress-related neuroendocrine mediators.[203,227–233]

Human Skin Has Established Functional, Peripheral Equivalents of the Hypothalamic-Pituitary-Adrenal Stress Response Axis

The discovery that key stress mediators are expressed in mammalian skin in situ soon encouraged the hypothesis that the skin may also have established a peripheral equivalent of the central HPA stress response axis.[233] This was followed by a long series of in vitro studies with various murine and human skin cell populations that, summarily, all supported this original concept and provided evidence that mammalian skin expresses the full enzymatic repertoire even for glucocorticoid synthesis (reviewed in Slominski et al.[191]).

Definitive proof that a fully functional peripheral equivalent of the HPA stress response axis exists in normal human skin came from the documentation that the epithelium of organ-cultured human scalp hair follicles expresses CRH and responds to CRH stimulation not only by upregulating POMC gene expression and POMC product synthesis, but also by an increase in the intrafollicular synthesis of cortisol (presumably via ACTH). By demonstrating that cortisol administration downregulates intrafollicular CRH expression, these human hair follicle organ culture studies also provided evidence for the existence of regulatory feedback loops that imitate those seen in the central HPA axis,[204] suggesting the presence of novel peripheral, intracutaneous equivalents that mimic central neuroendocrine stress response systems.

It is critical to determine whether and how intracutaneous peripheral HPA axis equivalents, which appear to be fully operative in the skin epithelium, interact with the central HPA axis. This question has become even more pertinent in the face of a recent report that lesional hair follicles of patients with alopecia areata, an organ-specific form of T-cell–dependent autoimmunity long suspected to be susceptible to triggering/aggravation by psychoemotional stress in at least some patients, show an upregulation of their CRH and ACTH immunoreactivity.[234] This is supported by findings that experimental stress increases intrafollicular CRH in telogen hairs and retards anagen development.[235]

While it is likely that centrally released CRH and ACTH affect intracutaneous melanocortin and glucocorticoid synthesis, since the skin expresses functional high-affinity receptors, it remains unknown whether and to what extent skin-derived α-MSH, ACTH, β-endorphin, or cortisol actually impacts on central HPA axis functions/activity.

The challenge for understanding the pathogenesis of stress triggering or stress aggravation of skin diseases such as the ones discussed above is to apply these emerging concepts and frontiers in cutaneous neuroendocrine-immune biology to specific dermatoses.

Human scalp hair follicles and sebocytes have proven to offer very instructive, easily accessible, and clinically highly relevant discovery tools for exploring the physiology and the pathophysiology of the brain–skin connection in health and disease.[193,200,201] Further research will help us understand the role played by the pilosebaceous unit–derived neuroendocrine mediators in the multilevel responses of skin to stress as well as the molecular turning points at which physiologic cutaneous stress responses begin to promote the development/aggravation of inflammatory skin disease.

Conclusion

The challenge for understanding how stress modulates inflammation in the skin, and thus has adverse effects on chronic skin diseases, is beginning to emerge. This challenge presents opportunities to harness this information to better control skin diseases by managing stress, or the biochemical mediators that are induced by the brain–skin connection. The lessons learned from managing this connection will be of benefit to patients with skin disease, and perhaps can be applied to other organ systems such as the cardiovascular or gastrointestinal systems.

References

1. Chrousos GP. The hypothalamic-pituitary-adrenal axis and immune-mediated inflammation. N Engl J Med 1995;332(20):1351–62.
2. Besedovsky HO, del Rey A, Sorkin E. What do the immune system and the brain know about each other. Immunology Today 1983;4(12):342–6.
3. Elenkov IJ WR, Chrousos GP, Vizi ES. The sympathetic nerve—an integrative interface between two supersystems: the brain and the immune system. Pharmacol Rev 2000;52(4):595–638.
4. Besedovsky H, del Rey A, Sorkin E, Dinarello CA. Immunoregulatory feedback between interleukin-1 and glucocorticoid hormones. Science 1986;233(4764):652–4.
5. Boumpas DT, Chrousos GP, Wilder RL, Cupps TR, Balow JE. Glucocorticoid therapy for immune-mediated diseases: basic and clinical correlates. Ann Intern Med 1993;119(12):1198–208.
6. Girndt M, Sester U, Kaul H, Hunger F, Kohler H. Glucocorticoids inhibit activation-dependent expression of costimulatory molecule B7–1 in human monocytes. Transplantation 1998;66(3):370–5.

7. Pan J, Ju D, Wang Q, et al. Dexamethasone inhibits the antigen presentation of dendritic cells in MHC class II pathway. Immunol Lett 2001;76(3):153–61.

8. Galon J, Franchimont D, Hiroi N, et al. Gene profiling reveals unknown enhancing and suppressive actions of glucocorticoids on immune cells. FASEB J 2002;16(1):61–71.

9. Benschop RJ, Rodriguez-Feuerhahn M, Schedlowski M. Catecholamine-induced leukocytosis: early observations, current research, and future directions. Brain Behav Immun 1996;10(2):77–91.

10. Maisel AS, Michel MC. Beta-adrenoceptor control of immune function in congestive heart failure. Br J Clin Pharmacol 1990;30(suppl 1):49S–53S.

11. Carlson SL, Brooks WH, Roszman TL. Neurotransmitter-lymphocyte interactions: dual receptor modulation of lymphocyte proliferation and cAMP production. J Neuroimmunol 1989;24(1–2):155–62.

12. Chambers DA, Cohen RL, Perlman RL. Neuroimmune modulation: signal transduction and catecholamines. Neurochem Int 1993;22(2):95–110.

13. Elliott L, Brooks W, Roszman T. Inhibition of anti-CD3 monoclonal antibody-induced T-cell proliferation by dexamethasone, isoproterenol, or prostaglandin E2 either alone or in combination. Cell Mol Neurobiol 1992;12(5):411–27.

14. Hadden JW, Hadden EM, Middleton E Jr. Lymphocyte blast transformation. I. Demonstration of adrenergic receptors in human peripheral lymphocytes. Cell Immunol 1970;1(6):583–95.

15. Bartik MM, Bauman GP, Brooks WH, Roszman TL. Costimulatory signals modulate the antiproliferative effects of agents that elevate cAMP in T cells. Cell Immunol 1994;158(1):116–30.

16. Fearon DT, Locksley RM. The instructive role of innate immunity in the acquired immune response. Science 1996;272(5258):50–3.

17. Mosmann TR, Sad S. The expanding universe of T-cell subsets: Th1, Th2 and more. Immunol Today 1996;17(3):138–46.

18. Trinchieri G. Interleukin-12 and the regulation of innate resistance and adaptive immunity. Nature Rev 2003;3(2):133–46.

19. Elenkov IJ, Chrousos GP. Stress hormones, Th1/Th2 patterns, pro/anti-inflammatory cytokines and susceptibility to disease. Trends Endocrinol Metab 1999;10(9):359–68.

20. Elenkov IJ, Papanicolaou DA, Wilder RL, Chrousos GP. Modulatory effects of glucocorticoids and catecholamines on human interleukin-12 and interleukin-10 production: clinical implications. Proc Assoc Am Physicians 1996;108:374–81.

21. Blotta MH, DeKruyff RH, Umetsu DT. Corticosteroids inhibit IL-12 production in human monocytes and enhance their capacity to induce IL-4 synthesis in CD4+ lymphocytes. J Immunol 1997;158(12):5589–95.

22. Hasko G, Szabo C, Nemeth ZH, Salzman AL, Vizi ES. Stimulation of beta-adrenoceptors inhibits endotoxin-induced IL-12 production in normal and IL-10 deficient mice. J Neuroimmunol 1998;88(1–2):57–61.

23. Panina-Bordignon P, Mazzeo D, Lucia PD, et al. Beta2–agonists prevent Th1 development by selective inhibition of interleukin 12. J Clin Invest 1997;100(6):1513–9.

24. DeKruyff RH, Fang Y, Umetsu DT. Corticosteroids enhance the capacity of macrophages to induce Th2 cytokine synthesis in CD4+ lymphocytes by inhibiting IL-12 production. J Immunol 1998;160(5):2231–7.

25. Wu CY, Wang K, McDyer JF, Seder RA. Prostaglandin E2 and dexamethasone inhibit IL-12 receptor expression and IL-12 responsiveness. J Immunol 1998;161(6):2723–30.

26. Ramirez F, Fowell DJ, Puklavec M, Simmonds S, Mason D. Glucocorticoids promote a TH2 cytokine response by CD4+ T cells in vitro. J Immunol 1996;156(7):2406–12.

27. van der Poll T, Barber AE, Coyle SM, Lowry SF. Hypercortisolemia increases plasma interleukin-10 concentrations during human endotoxemia—a clinical research center study. J Clin Endocrinol Metab 1996;81(10):3604–6.

28. Hetier E, Ayala J, Bousseau A, Prochiantz A. Modulation of interleukin-1 and tumor necrosis factor expression by beta-adrenergic agonists in mouse ameboid microglial cells. Experimental brain research. Exp Hirnforschung 1991;86(2):407–13.

29. Koff WC, Fann AV, Dunegan MA, Lachman LB. Catecholamine-induced suppression of interleukin-1 production. Lymphokine Res 1986;5(4):239–47.

30. Nakamura A, Johns EJ, Imaizumi A, Abe T, Kohsaka T. Regulation of tumour necrosis factor and interleukin-6 gene transcription by beta2–adrenoceptor in the rat astrocytes. J Neuroimmunol 1998;88(1–2):144–53.

31. Severn A, Rapson NT, Hunter CA, Liew FY. Regulation of tumor necrosis factor production by adrenaline and beta-adrenergic agonists. J Immunol 1992;148(11):3441–5.

32. Van der Poll T, Lowry SF. Epinephrine inhibits endotoxin-induced IL-1 beta production: roles of tumor necrosis factor-alpha and IL-10. Am J Physiol 1997;273(6 pt 2):R1885–90.

33. Sanders VM, Baker RA, Ramer-Quinn DS, Kasprowicz DJ, Fuchs BA, Street NE. Differential expression of the beta2–adrenergic receptor by Th1 and Th2 clones: implications for cytokine production and B cell help. J Immunol 1997;158(9):4200–10.

34. Borger P, Hoekstra Y, Esselink MT, et al. Beta-adrenoceptor-mediated inhibition of IFN-gamma, IL-3, and GM-CSF mRNA accumulation in activated human T lymphocytes is solely mediated by the beta2–adrenoceptor subtype. Am J Respir Cell Mol Biol 1998;19(3):400–7.

35. Maimone D, Cioni C, Rosa S, Macchia G, Aloisi F, Annunziata P. Norepinephrine and vasoactive intestinal peptide induce IL-6 secretion by astrocytes: synergism with IL-1 beta and TNF alpha. J Neuroimmunol 1993;47(1):73–81.

36. Norris JG, Benveniste EN. Interleukin-6 production by astrocytes: induction by the neurotransmitter norepinephrine. J Neuroimmunol 1993;45(1–2):137–45.

37. van der Poll T, Coyle SM, Barbosa K, Braxton CC, Lowry SF. Epinephrine inhibits tumor necrosis factor-alpha and potentiates interleukin 10 production during human endotoxemia. J Clin Invest 1996;97(3):713–9.

38. Felten DL, Felten SY, Carlson SL, Olschowka JA, Livnat S. Noradrenergic and peptidergic innervation of lymphoid tissue. J Immunol 1985;135(2 suppl):755s–65s.

39. Felten SY, Felten DL, Bellinger DL, et al. Noradrenergic sympathetic innervation of lymphoid organs. Prog Allergy 1988;43:14–36.

40. Lundberg JM, Rudehill A, Sollevi A, Fried G, Wallin G. Co-release of neuropeptide Y and noradrenaline from pig spleen in vivo: importance of subcellular storage, nerve impulse frequency and pattern, feedback regulation and resupply by axonal transport. Neuroscience 1989;28(2):475–86.

41. Straub RH, Herrmann M, Frauenholz T, et al. Neuroimmune control of interleukin-6 secretion in the murine spleen. Differential beta-adrenergic effects of electrically released endogenous norepinephrine under various endotoxin conditions. J Neuroimmunol 1996;71(1–2):37–43.

42. Bedoui S, Kawamura N, Straub RH, Pabst R, Yamamura T, von Horsten S. Relevance of neuropeptide Y for the neuroimmune crosstalk. J Neuroimmunol 2003;134(1–2):1–11.

43. Naseer T, Minshall EM, Leung DY, et al. Expression of IL-12 and IL-13 mRNA in asthma and their modulation in response to steroid therapy. Am J Respir Crit Care Med 1997;155(3):845–51.

44. Bentley AM, Hamid Q, Robinson DS, et al. Prednisolone treatment in asthma. Reduction in the numbers of eosinophils, T cells, tryptase-only positive mast cells, and modulation of IL-4, IL-5, and interferon-gamma cytokine gene expression within the bronchial mucosa. Am J Respir Crit Care Med 1996;153(2):551–6.

45. Bradding P, Feather IH, Wilson S, Holgate ST, Howarth PH. Cytokine immunoreactivity in seasonal rhinitis: regulation by a topical corticosteroid. Am J Respir Crit Care Med 1995;151(6):1900–6.

46. Batuman OA, Ferrero A, Cupp C, Jimenez SA, Khalili K. Differential regulation of transforming growth factor beta-1 gene expression by glucocorticoids in human T and glial cells. J Immunol 1995;155(9):4397–405.

47. Broug-Holub E, Kraal G. Dose- and time-dependent activation of rat alveolar macrophages by glucocorticoids. Clin Exp Immunol 1996;104(2):332–6.

48. Spengler RN, Allen RM, Remick DG, Strieter RM, Kunkel SL. Stimulation of alpha-adrenergic receptor augments the production of macrophage-derived tumor necrosis factor. J Immunol 1990;145(5):1430–4.

49. Le Tulzo Y, Shenkar R, Kaneko D, et al. Hemorrhage increases cytokine expression in lung mononuclear cells in mice: involvement of catecholamines in nuclear factor-kappaB regulation and cytokine expression. J Clin Invest 1997;99(7):1516–24.

50. Broug-Holub E, Persoons JH, Schornagel K, Mastbergen SC, Kraal G. Effects of stress on alveolar macrophages: a role for the sympathetic nervous system. Am J Respir Cell Mol Biol 1998;19(5):842–8.

51. Engstad CS, Lund T, Osterud B. Epinephrine promotes IL-8 production in human leukocytes via an effect on platelets. Thromb Haemost 1999;81(1):139–45.

52. Kaplanski G, Porat R, Aiura K, Erban JK, Gelfand JA, Dinarello CA. Activated platelets induce endothelial secretion of interleukin-8 in vitro via an interleukin-1–mediated event. Blood 1993;81(10):2492–5.

53. Kavelaars A, van de Pol M, Zijlstra J, Heijnen CJ. Beta 2–adrenergic activation enhances interleukin-8 production by human monocytes. J Neuroimmunol 1997;77(2):211–6.

54. Mohamed-Ali V, Flower L, Sethi J, et al. beta-Adrenergic regulation of IL-6 release from adipose tissue: in vivo and in vitro studies. J Clin Endocrinol Metab 2001;86(12):5864–9.

55. Vicennati V, Vottero A, Friedman C, Papanicolaou DA. Hormonal regulation of interleukin-6 production in human adipocytes. Int J Obes Relat Metab Disord 2002;26(7):905–11.

56. Baumann H, Gauldie J. The acute phase response. Immunol Today 1994;15(2):74–80.

57. Li Y, Chi L, Stechschulte DJ, Dileepan KN. Histamine-induced production of interleukin-6 and interleukin-8 by human coronary artery endothelial cells is enhanced by endotoxin and tumor necrosis factor-alpha. Microvasc Res 2001;61(3):253–62.

58. Murray DR, Prabhu SD, Chandrasekar B. Chronic beta-adrenergic stimulation induces myocardial proinflammatory cytokine expression. Circulation 2000;101(20):2338–41.

59. Karalis K, Sano H, Redwine J, Listwak S, Wilder RL, Chrousos GP. Autocrine or paracrine inflammatory actions of corticotropin-releasing hormone in vivo. Science 1991;254(5030):421–3.

60. Elenkov IJ, Webster EL, Torpy DJ, Chrousos GP. Stress, corticotropin-releasing hormone, glucocorticoids, and the immune/inflammatory response: acute and chronic effects. Ann N Y Acad Sci 1999;876: 1–11; discussion 13.

61. Theoharides TC, Singh LK, Boucher W, et al. Corticotropin-releasing hormone induces skin mast cell degranulation and increased vascular permeability, a possible explanation for its proinflammatory effects. Endocrinology 1998;139(1):403–13.

62. Foreman JC. Neuropeptides and the pathogenesis of allergy. Allergy 1987;42(1):1–11.

63. Church MK, Lowman MA, Robinson C, Holgate ST, Benyon RC. Interaction of neuropeptides with human mast cells. Int Arch Allergy Appl Immunol 1989;88(1–2):70–8.

64. Theoharides TC, Spanos C, Pang X, et al. Stress-induced intracranial mast cell degranulation: a corticotropin-releasing hormone-mediated effect. Endocrinology 1995;136(12):5745–50.

65. Sanders VM, Munson AE. Norepinephrine and the antibody response. Pharmacol Rev 1985;37(3): 229–48.

66. Coqueret O, Dugas B, Mencia-Huerta JM, Braquet P. Regulation of IgE production from human mononuclear cells by beta 2-adrenoceptor agonists. Clin Exp Allergy 1995;25(4):304–11.

67. Coqueret O, Lagente V, Frere CP, Braquet P, Mencia-Huerta JM. Regulation of IgE production by beta 2–adrenoceptor agonists. Ann N Y Acad Sci 1994;725:44–9.

68. Wu CY, Sarfati M, Heusser C, et al. Glucocorticoids increase the synthesis of immunoglobulin E by interleukin 4–stimulated human lymphocytes. J Clin Invest 1991;87(3):870–7.

69. Zieg G, Lack G, Harbeck RJ, Gelfand EW, Leung DY. In vivo effects of glucocorticoids on IgE production. J Allergy Clin Immunol 1994;94(2 pt 1) :222–30.

70. Selye H. A syndrome produced by diverse nocuous agents. Nature 1936;138:32.

71. Selye H. The general adaptation syndrome and the disease of adaptation. J Clin Endocrinol 1946;6: 117–230.

72. Visintainer MA, Volpicelli JR, Seligman ME. Tumor rejection in rats after inescapable or escapable shock. Science 1982;216(4544):437–9.

73. Flint MS, Valosen JM, Johnson EA, Miller DB, Tinkle SS. Restraint stress applied prior to chemical sensitization modulates the development of allergic contact dermatitis differently than restraint prior to challenge. J Neuroimmunol 2001;113(1):72–80.

74. Schedlowski M, Jacobs R, Stratmann G, et al. Changes of natural killer cells during acute psychological stress. J Clin Immunol 1993;13(2):119–26.

75. Kiecolt-Glaser JK, McGuire L, Robles TF, Glaser R. Psychoneuroimmunology and psychosomatic medicine: back to the future. Psychosom Med 2002;64(1):15–28.

76. Stone R. Social science. Stress: the invisible hand in Eastern Europe's death rates [news]. Science 2000;288(5472):1732–3.

77. Schulz R, Beach SR. Caregiving as a risk factor for mortality: the Caregiver Health Effects Study [see comments]. JAMA 1999;282(23):2215–9.

78. Kiecolt-Glaser JK, Glaser R. Chronic stress and mortality among older adults [editorial; comment]. JAMA 1999;282(23):2259–60.

79. Kamarck TW, Everson SA, Kaplan GA, et al. Exaggerated blood pressure responses during mental stress are associated with enhanced carotid atherosclerosis in middle-aged Finnish men: findings from the Kuopio Ischemic Heart Disease Study. Circulation 1997;96(11):3842–8.

80. Dhabhar FS, McEwen BS. Acute stress enhances while chronic stress suppresses immune function in vivo: a potential role for leukocyte trafficking. Brain Behav Immun 1997;11:286–306.

81. Dhabhar FS, McEwen BS. Enhancing versus suppressive effects of stress hormones on skin immune function. Proc Natl Acad Sci U S A 1999;96(3):1059–64.

82. Biondi M, Zannino LG. Psychological stress, neuroimmunomodulation, and susceptibility to infectious diseases in animals and man: a review. Psychother Psychosom 1997;66(1):3–26.

83. Konstantinos AP SJ. Stress and influenza viral infection: modulation of proinflammatory cytokine responses in the lung. Respir Physiol 2001;128(1):71–7.

84. Cohen S, Tyrrell DA, Smith AP. Psychological stress and susceptibility to the common cold [see comments]. N Engl J Med 1991;325(9):606–12.

85. Cohen S, Line S, Manuck SB, Rabin BS, Heise ER, Kaplan JR. Chronic social stress, social status, and susceptibility to upper respiratory infections in nonhuman primates [see comments]. Psychosom Med 1997;59(3):213–21.

86. Bailey MT, Engler H, Sheridan JF. Stress induces the translocation of cutaneous and gastrointestinal microflora to secondary lymphoid organs of C57BL/6 mice. J Neuroimmunol 2006;171(1–2):29–37.

87. Rojas IG, Padgett DA, Sheridan JF, Marucha PT. Stress-induced susceptibility to bacterial infection during cutaneous wound healing. Brain Behav Immun 2002;16(1):74–84.

88. Buske-Kirschbaum A GA, Wermke C, Pirke KM, Hellhammer D. Preliminary evidence for Herpes labialis recurrence following experimentally induced disgust. Psychother Psychosom 2001;70(2):86–91.

89. Cohen F, Kemeny ME, Kearney KA, Zegans LS, Neuhaus JM, Conant MA. Persistent stress as a predictor of genital herpes recurrence. Arch Intern Med 1999;159(20):2430–6.

90. Yang EV, Glaser R. Stress-induced immunomodulation: Implications for tumorigenesis. Brain Behav Immun 2003;17(suppl 1):S37–40.

91. Reiche EM, Nunes SO, Morimoto HK. Stress, depression, the immune system, and cancer. Lancet Oncol 2004;5(10):617–25.

92. Reiche EM, Morimoto HK, Nunes SM. Stress and depression-induced immune dysfunction: implications for the development and progression of cancer. Int Rev Psychiatry (Abingdon, England) 2005;17(6):515–27.

93. Lillberg K, Verkasalo PK, Kaprio J, Teppo L, Helenius H, Koskenvuo M. Stressful life events and risk of breast cancer in 10,808 women: a cohort study. Am J Epidemiol 2003;157(5):415–23.

94. Riley V. Psychoneuroendocrine influences on immunocompetence and neoplasia. Science 1981;212(4499): 1100–9.

95. Wu W, Yamaura T, Murakami K, et al. Social isolation stress enhanced liver metastasis of murine colon 26–L5 carcinoma cells by suppressing immune responses in mice. Life Sci 2000;66(19):1827–38.

96. Laudenslager ML, Ryan SM, Drugan RC, Hyson RL, Maier SF. Coping and immunosuppression: inescapable but not escapable shock suppresses lymphocyte proliferation. Science 1983;221(4610):568–70.

97. Ben-Eliyahu S, Page GG, Yirmiya R, Shakhar G. Evidence that stress and surgical interventions promote tumor development by suppressing natural killer cell activity. Int J Cancer 1999;80(6):880–8.

98. Ben-Eliyahu S. The promotion of tumor metastasis by surgery and stress: immunological basis and implications for psychoneuroimmunology. Brain Behav Immun 2003;17(suppl 1):S27–36.

99. Bachen EA, Manuck SB, Cohen S, et al. Adrenergic blockade ameliorates cellular immune responses to mental stress in humans. Psychosom Med 1995;57(4):366–72.

100. Benschop RJ, Nieuwenhuis EE, Tromp EA, Godaert GL, Ballieux RE, van Doornen LJ. Effects of beta-adrenergic blockade on immunologic and cardiovascular changes induced by mental stress. Circulation 1994;89(2):762–9.

101. Glaser R, Thorn BE, Tarr KL, Kiecolt-Glaser JK, D'Ambrosio SM. Effects of stress on methyltransferase synthesis: an important DNA repair enzyme. Health Psychol 1985;4(5):403–12.

102. Kiecolt-Glaser JK, Stephens RE, Lipetz PD, Speicher CE, Glaser R. Distress and DNA repair in human lymphocytes. J Behav Med 1985;8(4):311–20.

103. Parker J, Klein SL, McClintock MK, et al. Chronic stress accelerates ultraviolet-induced cutaneous carcinogenesis. J Am Acad Dermatol 2004;51(6):919–22.

104. Ramirez AJ, Craig TK, Watson JP, Fentiman IS, North WR, Rubens RD. Stress and relapse of breast cancer [see comments]. BMJ 1989;298(6669):291–3.

105. Havlik RJ, Vukasin AP, Ariyan S. The impact of stress on the clinical presentation of melanoma. Plast Reconstr Surg 1992;90(1):57–61; discussion 62–64.

106. Reynolds P, Kaplan GA. Social connections and risk for cancer: prospective evidence from the Alameda County Study. Behav Med 1990;16(3):101–10.

107. Jacobs JR, Bovasso GB. Early and chronic stress and their relation to breast cancer [In Process Citation]. Psychol Med 2000;30(3):669–78.

108. Grossarth-Maticek R, Eysenck HJ, Boyle GJ, Heeb J, Costa SD, Diel IJ. Interaction of psychosocial and physical risk factors in the causation of mammary cancer, and its prevention through psychological methods of treatment. J Clin Psychol 2000;56(1):33–50.

109. Kiecolt-Glaser JK, Glaser R. Psychoneuroimmunology and cancer: fact or fiction? Eur J Cancer 1999;35(11):1603–7.

110. Spiegel D, Bloom JR, Kraemer HC, Gottheil E. Effect of psychosocial treatment on survival of patients with metastatic breast cancer [see comments]. Lancet 1989;2(8668):888–91.

111. Fawzy FI, Fawzy NW, Hyun CS, et al. Malignant melanoma. Effects of an early structured psychiatric intervention, coping, and affective state on recurrence and survival 6 years later. Arch Gen Psychiatry 1993;50(9):681–9.

112. Herberman RB, Ortaldo JR. Natural killer cells: their roles in defenses against disease. Science 1981;214:24–30.

113. Irwin M, Daniels M, Smith TL, Bloom E, Weiner H. Impaired natural killer cell activity during bereavement. Brain Behav Immun 1987;1(1):98–104.

114. Irwin M, Daniels M, Risch SC, Bloom E, Weiner H. Plasma cortisol and natural killer cell activity during bereavement. Biol Psychiatry 1988;24(2): 173–8.

115. Kiecolt-Glaser JK, Garner W, Speicher C, Penn GM, Holliday J, Glaser R. Psychosocial modifiers of immunocompetence in medical students. Psychosom Med 1984;46(1):7–14.

116. Kiecolt-Glaser JK, Speicher CE, Holliday JE, Glaser R. Stress and the transformation of lymphocytes by Epstein-Barr virus. J Behav Med 1984;7(1):1–12.

117. Kiecolt-Glaser JK, Fisher LD, Ogrocki P, Stout JC, Speicher CE, Glaser R. Marital quality, marital disruption, and immune function. Psychosom Med 1987;49(1):13–34.

118. Kiecolt-Glaser JK, Malarkey WB, Chee M, et al. Negative behavior during marital conflict is associated with immunological down-regulation [see comments]. Psychosom Med 1993;55(5):395–409.

119. Baron RS, Cutrona CE, Hicklin D, Russell DW, Lubaroff DM. Social support and immune function among spouses of cancer patients. J Pers Soc Psychol 1990;59(2):344–52.

120. Kiecolt-Glaser JK, Dyer CS, Shuttleworth EC. Upsetting social interactions and distress among Alzheimer's disease family care-givers: a replication and extension. Am J Community Psychol 1988;16(6):825–37.

121. Irwin M, Hauger R, Patterson TL, Semple S, Ziegler M, Grant I. Alzheimer caregiver stress: basal natural killer cell activity, pituitary-adrenal cortical function, and sympathetic tone. Ann Behav Med 1997;19(2):83–90.

122. Irwin M, Brown M, Patterson T, Hauger R, Mascovich A, Grant I. Neuropeptide Y and natural killer cell activity: findings in depression and Alzheimer caregiver stress. FASEB J 1991;5(15):3100–7.

123. Glaser R, Rice J, Speicher CE, Stout JC, Kiecolt-Glaser JK. Stress depresses interferon production by leukocytes concomitant with a decrease in natural killer cell activity. Behav Neurosci 1986;100(5):675–8.

124. Schedlowski M, Jacobs R, Alker J, et al. Psychophysiological, neuroendocrine and cellular immune reactions under psychological stress. Neuropsychobiology 1993;28(1–2):87–90.

125. Schedlowski M, Falk A, Rohne A, et al. Catecholamines induce alterations of distribution and activity of human natural killer (NK) cells. J Clin Immunol 1993;13(5):344–51.

126. Schedlowski M, Fluge T, Richter S, Tewes U, Schmidt RE, Wagner TO. Beta-endorphin, but not substance-P, is increased by acute stress in humans. Psychoneuroendocrinology 1995;20(1):103–10.

127. Esterling BA, Kiecolt-Glaser JK, Glaser R. Psychosocial modulation of cytokine-induced natural killer cell activity in older adults. Psychosom Med 1996;58(3):264–72.

128. Borella P, Bargellini A, Rovesti S, et al. Emotional stability, anxiety, and natural killer activity under examination stress. Psychoneuroendocrinology 1999;24(6):613–27.

129. King JA, Edwards E. Early stress and genetic influences on hypothalamic-pituitary-adrenal axis functioning in adulthood. Horm Behav 1999;36(2):79–85.

130. Heim C, Newport DJ, Heit S, et al. Pituitary-adrenal and autonomic responses to stress in women after sexual and physical abuse in childhood. JAMA 2000;284(5):592–7.

131. Aksentijevich S, Whitfield HJ Jr, Young WSd, et al. Arthritis-susceptible Lewis rats fail to emerge from the stress hyporesponsive period. Brain Res Dev Brain Res 1992;65(1):115–8.

132. Sternberg EM, Hill JM, Chrousos GP, et al. Inflammatory mediator-induced hypothalamic-pituitary-adrenal axis activation is defective in streptococcal cell wall arthritis-susceptible Lewis rats. Proc Natl Acad Sci U S A 1989;86(7):2374–8.

133. Sternberg EM, Young WSd, Bernardini R, et al. A central nervous system defect in biosynthesis of corticotropin-releasing hormone is associated with susceptibility to streptococcal cell wall-induced arthritis in Lewis rats. Proc Natl Acad Sci U S A 1989;86(12):4771–5.

134. Rupprecht M, Salzer B, Raum B, et al. Physical stress-induced secretion of adrenal and pituitary hormones in patients with atopic eczema compared with normal controls. Exp Clin Endocrinol Diabetes 1997;105(1):39–45.

135. Rupprecht M HO, Schluter D, Schafers HJ, Koch HU, Beck G, Rupprecht R. Cortisol, corticotrophin, and beta-endorphin responses to corticotrophin-releasing hormone in patients with atopic eczema. Psychoneuroendocrinology 1995;20:543–51.

136. Buske-Kirschbaum A, Jobst S, Hellhammer DH. Altered reactivity of the hypothalamus-pituitary-adrenal axis in patients with atopic dermatitis: pathologic factor or symptom? Ann N Y Acad Sci 1998;840:747–54.

137. Buske-Kirschbaum A, Jobst S, Psych D, et al. Attenuated free cortisol response to psychosocial stress in children with atopic dermatitis. Psychosom Med 1997;59(4):419–26.

138. Masi AT, Chrousos GP. Hypothalamic-pituitary-adrenal-glucocorticoid axis function in rheumatoid arthritis [editorial; comment]. J Rheumatol 1996;23(4):577–81.

139. Gudbjornsson B, Skogseid B, Oberg K, Wide L, Hallgren R. Intact adrenocorticotropic hormone secretion but impaired cortisol response in patients with active rheumatoid arthritis. Effect of glucocorticoids [see comments]. J Rheumatol 1996;23(4):596–602.

140. Richards HL, Ray DW, Kirby B, et al. Response of the hypothalamic-pituitary-adrenal axis to psychological stress in patients with psoriasis. Br J Dermatol 2005;153(6):1114–20.

141. Chiu A, Chon SY, Kimball AB. The response of skin disease to stress: changes in the severity of

acne vulgaris as affected by examination stress. Arch Dermatol 2003;139(7):897–900.

142. Papadopoulos L, Bor R, Legg C, Hawk JL. Impact of life events on the onset of vitiligo in adults: preliminary evidence for a psychological dimension in aetiology. Clin Exp Dermatol 1998;23(6):243–8.

143. Barisic-Drusko V, Rucevic I. Trigger factors in childhood psoriasis and vitiligo. Collegium Antropologicum 2004;28(1):277–85.

144. Gulec AT, Tanriverdi N, Duru C, Saray Y, Akcali C. The role of psychological factors in alopecia areata and the impact of the disease on the quality of life. Int J Dermatol 2004;43(5):352–6.

145. Chaudhary S. Psychosocial stressors in oral lichen planus. Australian dental journal 2004;49(4):192–5.

146. Goldberg I IA, Brenner S. Pemphigus vulgaris triggered by rifampin and emotional stress. Skin Med 2004;3(5):294.

147. Berrino AM, Voltolini S, Fiaschi D, et al. Chronic urticaria: importance of a medical-psychological approach. Allerg Immunologie 2006;38(5):149–52.

148. Kimball AB JC, Weiss S, Vreeland MG, Wu Y. The psychosocial burden of psoriasis. Am J Clin Dermatol 2005;6(6):383–92.

149. Fortune DG RH, Griffiths CEM, Main CJ. Psychological stress, distress and disability in patients with psoriasis: consensus and variation in the contribution of illness perceptions, coping and alexithymia. Br J Dermatol 2002;41:157–74.

150. Fortune DG RH, Griffiths CEM, Main CJ. Psychologic factors in psoriasis: consequences, mechanisms, and interventions. Dermatol Clin 2005;4:681–94.

151. Schmid-Ott G, Jacobs R, Jager B, et al. Stress induced endocrine and immunological changes in psoriasis patients and healthy controls. Psychother Psychosom 1998;67:37–42.

152. Raychaudhuri SP, Farber EM, Raychaudhuri SK. Role of nerve growth factor in RANTES expression by keratinocytes. Acta Derm Venereol 2000;80(4):247–50.

153. Nickoloff BJ, Schroder JM, von den Driesch P, et al. Is psoriasis a T-cell disease? Exp Dermatol 2000;9:357–75.

154. Farber EM, Nall L. Psoriasis: a stress-related disease. Cutis 1993;51(5):322–6.

155. Farber EM, Nickoloff BJ, Recht B, Fraki JE. Stress, symmetry, and psoriasis: possible role of neuropeptides. J Am Acad Dermatol 1986;14 (2 pt 1):305–11.

156. Farber EM, Lanigan SW, Boer J. The role of cutaneous sensory nerves in the maintenance of psoriasis. Int J Dermatol 1990;29(6):418–20.

157. Raychaudhuri SP, Farber EM. Are sensory nerves essential for the development of psoriatic lesions? J Am Acad Dermatol 1993;28(3):488–9.

158. Aloe L, Alleva E, Fiore M. Stress and nerve growth factor: findings in animal models and humans. Pharmacol Biochemi Behav 2002;73(1):159–66.

159. Raychaudhuri SP JW, Farber EM. Psoriatic keratinocytes express high levels of nerve growth factor. Acta Derm Venereol 1998;78(2):84–6.

160. Raychaudhuri SP, Jiang WY, Smoller BR, Farber EM. Nerve growth factor and its receptor system in psoriasis. Br J Dermatol 2000;143(1):198–200.

161. Ginsburg IH. Coping with psoriasis: a guide for counseling patients. Cutis 1996;57(5):323–5.

162. Tausk F, Whitmore SE. A pilot study of hypnosis in the treatment of patients with psoriasis. Psychother Psychosom 1999;68(4):221–5.

163. Benhard JD, Kristeller J, Kabat-Zinn J. Effectiveness of relaxation and visualization techniques as an adjunct to phototherapy and photochemotherapy of psoriasis. J Am Acad Dermatol 1988;19(3):572–4.

164. Kabat-Zinn J, Wheeler E, Light T, et al. Influence of a mindfulness meditation-based stress reduction intervention on rates of skin clearing in patients with moderate to severe psoriasis undergoing phototherapy (UVB) and photochemotherapy (PUVA). Psychosom Med 1998;60(5):625–32.

165. Langan SM, Bourke JF, Silcocks P, Williams HC. An exploratory prospective observational study of environmental factors exacerbating atopic eczema in children. Br J Dermatol 2006;154(5):979–80.

166. Faulstich ME, Williamson DA, Duchmann EG, Conerly SL, Brantley PJ. Psychophysiological analysis of atopic dermatitis. J Psychosom Res 1985;29(4):415–7.

167. King RM, Wilson GV. Use of a diary technique to investigate psychosomatic relations in atopic dermatitis. J Psychosom Res 1991;35(6):697–706.

168. Schmid-Ott G, Jaeger B, Adamek C, et al. Levels of circulating CD8(+) T lymphocytes, natural killer cells, and eosinophils increase upon acute psychosocial stress in patients with atopic dermatitis. J Allergy Clin Immunol 2001;107(1):171–7.

169. Schmid-Ott G, Jaeger B, Meyer S, Stephan E, Kapp A, Werfel T. Different expression of cytokine and membrane molecules by circulating lymphocytes on acute mental stress in patients with atopic dermatitis in comparison with healthy controls. J Allergy Clin Immunol 2001;108(3):455–62.

170. Kagi MK, Wutrich B, Montano E, Barandun J, Blaser K, Walker C. Differential cytokine profiles in peripheral blood lymphocyte supernatants and skin biopsies from patients with different forms of atopic dermatitis, psoriasis and normal individuals. Int Arch Allergy Immunol 1994;103(4):332–40.

171. Mori A, Yamamoto K, Dohi M, Suko M, Okudaira H. Interleukin-4 gene expression in human peripheral

blood mononuclear cells. Int Arch Allergy Appl Immunol 1991;95(2–3):282–4.

172. Tamir A, Ophir J, Brenner S. Pemphigus vulgaris triggered by emotional stress [letter]. Dermatology 1994;189(2):210.

173. Braun CM HS, Bashian GG, Kagey-Sobotka A, Lichtenstein LM, Essayan DM. Corticosteroid modulation of human, antigen-specific Th1 and Th2 responses. J Allergy Clin Immunol 1997;100(3):400–7.

174. Byron KA, Varigos G, Wootton A. Hydrocortisone inhibition of human interleukin-4. Immunology 1992;77(4):624–6.

175. Cupps TR, Gerrard TL, Falkoff RJ, Whalen G, Fauci AS. Effects of in vitro corticosteroids on B cell activation, proliferation, and differentiation. J Clin Invest 1985;75(2):754–61.

176. Schwiebert LM, Beck LA, Stellato C, et al. Glucocorticosteroid inhibition of cytokine production: relevance to antiallergic actions [published erratum appears in J Allergy Clin Immunol 1996;98(3):718]. J Allergy Clin Immunol 1996;97 (1 pt 2):143–52.

177. Buske-Kirschbaum A GA, Hollig H, Morschhauser E, Hellhammer D. Altered responsiveness of the hypothalamus-pituitary-adrenal axis and the sympathetic adrenomedullary system to stress in patients with atopic dermatitis. J Clin Endocrinol Metab 2002;87(9):4245–51.

178. Rupprecht M RR, Kornhuber J, Wodarz N, Koch HU, Riederer P, Hornstein OP. Elevated glucocorticoid receptor concentrations before and after glucocorticoid therapy in peripheral mononuclear leukocytes of patients with atopic dermatitis. Dermatologica 1991;183:100–5.

179. Altemus M, Rao B, Dhabhar FS, Ding W, Granstein RD. Stress-induced changes in skin barrier function in healthy women. J Invest Dermatol 2001;117(2):309–17.

180. Zane L. Psychoneuroendocrinimmunodermatology: pathophysiological mechanisms of stress in cutaneous disease. In: Koo JYM, CS Lee, eds. Psychocutaneous Medicine. New York: Marcel Dekker, 2003:65–95.

181. Schallreuter KU PM, Swanson NN, Beazley WD, Korner C, Ehrke C, Buttner G. Altered catecholamine synthesis and degradation in the epidermis of patients with atopic eczema. Arch Dermatol Res 1997;289:663–6.

182. Delgado M F-AM, Fuentes A. Effect of adrenaline and glucocorticoids on monocyte cAMP-specific phosphodiesterase (PDE4) in a monocyte cell line. Arch Dermatol Res 2002:190–7.

183. Chan SC BM, Willcox TM, Li SH, Stevens SR, Tara D, Hanifin JM. Abnormal IL-4 gene expression by atopic dermatitis T lymphocytes is reflected in altered nuclear protein interactions with IL-4 transcription regulatory element. J Invest Dermatol 1996;106:1131–6.

184. Cole WC, Roth HL, Sachs LB. Group psychotherapy as an aid in the medical treatment of eczema. J Am Acad Dermatol 1988;18(2 pt 1):286–91.

185. Ehlers A, Stangier U, Gieler U. Treatment of atopic dermatitis: a comparison of psychological and dermatological approaches to relapse prevention. J Consult Clin Psychol 1995;63(4):624–35.

186. Horne DJ, White AE, Varigos GA. A preliminary study of psychological therapy in the management of atopic eczema. Br J Med Psychol 1989;62(pt 3):241–8.

187. Howlett S. Emotional dysfunction, child-family relationships and childhood atopic dermatitis. Br J Dermatol 1999;140(3):381–4.

188. Stewart AC, Thomas SE. Hypnotherapy as a treatment for atopic dermatitis in adults and children. Br J Dermatol 1995;132(5):778–83.

189. Gupta MA, Gupta AK. Psychodermatology: an update. J Am Acad Dermatol 1996;34(6):1030–46.

190. Slominski A, Wortsman J, Plonka PM, Schallreuter KU, Paus R, Tobin DJ. Hair follicle pigmentation. J Invest Dermatol 2005;124(1):13–21.

191. Slominski A, Wortsman J, Luger T, Paus R, Solomon S. Corticotropin releasing hormone and proopiomelanocortin involvement in the cutaneous response to stress. Physiol Rev 2000;80(3): 979–1020.

192. Peters EM, Ericson ME, Hosoi J, et al. Neuropeptide control mechanisms in cutaneous biology: physiological and clinical significance. J Invest Dermatol 2006;126(9):1937–47.

193. Paus R, Theoharides TC, Arck PC. Neuroimmunoendocrine circuitry of the "brain-skin connection." Trends Immunol 2006;27(1):32–9.

194. Maurer M, Metz M. The status quo and quo vadis of mast cells. Exp Dermatol 2005;14(12):923–9.

195. Maurer M, Theoharides T, Granstein RD, et al. What is the physiological function of mast cells? Exp Dermatol 2003;12(6):886–910.

196. Botchkarev VA, Yaar M, Peters EM, et al. Neurotrophins in skin biology and pathology. J Invest Dermatol 2006;126(8):1719–27.

197. Siebenhaar F, Sharov AA, Peters EM, et al. Substance P as an immunomodulatory neuropeptide in a mouse model for autoimmune hair loss (alopecia areata). J Invest Dermatol 2007.

198. Zouboulis CC, Bohm M. Neuroendocrine regulation of sebocytes—a pathogenetic link between stress and acne. Exp Dermatol 2004;13(suppl 4):31–5.

199. Luger TA, Scholzen T, Brzoska T, Becher E, Slominski A, Paus R. Cutaneous immunomodulation and coordination of skin stress responses by

alpha-melanocyte-stimulating hormone. Ann N Y Acad Sci 1998;840:381–94.

200. Arck PC, Slominski A, Theoharides TC, Peters EM, Paus R. Neuroimmunology of stress: skin takes center stage. J Invest Dermatol 2006;126(8):1697–704.

201. Biro T, Ko MC, Bromm B, et al. How best to fight that nasty itch - from new insights into the neuroimmunological, neuroendocrine, and neurophysiological bases of pruritus to novel therapeutic approaches. Exp Dermatol 2005;14(3):225–40.

202. Paus R, Schmelz M, Biro T, Steinhoff M. Frontiers in pruritus research: scratching the brain for more effective itch therapy. J Clin Invest 2006;116(5):1174–86.

203. Zouboulis CC, Seltmann H, Hiroi N, et al. Corticotropin-releasing hormone: an autocrine hormone that promotes lipogenesis in human sebocytes. Proc Natl Acad Sci U S A 2002;99(10):7148–53.

204. Ito N, Ito T, Kromminga A, et al. Human hair follicles display a functional equivalent of the hypothalamic-pituitary-adrenal axis and synthesize cortisol. FASEB J 2005;19(10):1332–4.

205. Park HJ, Kim HJ, Lee JY, Cho BK, Gallo RL, Cho DH. Adrenocorticotropin hormone stimulates interleukin-18 expression in human HaCaT keratinocytes. J Invest Dermatol 2007.

206. Zbytek B, Paus R. CRH mediates inflammation induced by lipopolysaccharide in human adult epidermal keratinocytes. J Invest Dermatol 2007;127(3):730–2.

207. Paus R, Maurer M, Slominski A, Czarnetzki BM. Mast cell involvement in murine hair growth. Developmental biology 1994;163(1):230–40.

208. Maurer M, Fischer E, Handjiski B, et al. Activated skin mast cells are involved in murine hair follicle regression (catagen). Lab Invest 1997;77(4):319–32.

209. Slominski A, Botchkareva NV, Botchkarev VA, et al. Hair cycle-dependent production of ACTH in mouse skin. Biochim Biophys Acta 1998;1448(1):147–52.

210. Paus R, Heinzelmann T, Robicsek S, Czarnetzki BM, Maurer M. Substance P stimulates murine epidermal keratinocyte proliferation and dermal mast cell degranulation in situ. Arch Dermatol Res 1995;287(5):500–2.

211. Ansel JC, Brown JR, Payan DG, Brown MA. Substance P selectively activates TNF-alpha gene expression in murine mast cells. J Immunol 1993;150(10):4478–85.

212. Paus R, Heinzelmann T, Schultz KD, Furkert J, Fechner K, Czarnetzki BM. Hair growth induction by substance P. Lab Invest 1994;71(1):134–40.

213. Paus R, Luftl M, Czarnetzki BM. Nerve growth factor modulates keratinocyte proliferation in murine skin organ culture. Br J Dermatol 1994;130(2):174–80.

214. Botchkarev VA, Botchkareva NV, Albers KM, Chen LH, Welker P, Paus R. A role for p75 neurotrophin receptor in the control of apoptosis-driven hair follicle regression. FASEB J 2000;14(13):1931–42.

215. Botchkarev VA, Botchkareva NV, Peters EM, Paus R. Epithelial growth control by neurotrophins: leads and lessons from the hair follicle. Prog Brain Res 2004;146:493–513.

216. Peters EM, Stieglitz MG, Liezman C, et al. p75 Neurotrophin receptor-mediated signaling promotes human hair follicle regression (Catagen). Am J Pathol 2006;168(1):221–34.

217. Arck PC, Handjiski B, Hagen E, Joachim R, Klapp BF, Paus R. Indications for a "brain-hair follicle axis (BHA)": inhibition of keratinocyte proliferation and up-regulation of keratinocyte apoptosis in telogen hair follicles by stress and substance P. FASEB J 2001;15(13):2536–8.

218. Peters EM, Handjiski B, Kuhlmei A, et al. Neurogenic inflammation in stress-induced termination of murine hair growth is promoted by nerve growth factor. Am J Pathol 2004;165(1):259–71.

219. Arck PC, Handjiski B, Kuhlmei A, et al. Mast cell deficient and neurokinin-1 receptor knockout mice are protected from stress-induced hair growth inhibition. J Mol Med (Berlin, Germany) 2005;83(5):386–96.

220. Craven AJ, Ormandy CJ, Robertson FG, et al. Prolactin signaling influences the timing mechanism of the hair follicle: analysis of hair growth cycles in prolactin receptor knockout mice. Endocrinology 2001;142(6):2533–9.

221. Craven AJ, Nixon AJ, Ashby MG, et al. Prolactin delays hair regrowth in mice. J Endocrinol 2006;191(2):415–25.

222. Foitzik K, Krause K, Conrad F, Nakamura M, Funk W, Paus R. Human scalp hair follicles are both a target and a source of prolactin, which serves as an autocrine and/or paracrine promoter of apoptosis-driven hair follicle regression. Am J Pathol 2006;168(3):748–56.

223. Foitzik K, Krause K, Nixon AJ, et al. Prolactin and its receptor are expressed in murine hair follicle epithelium, show hair cycle-dependent expression, and induce catagen. Am J Pathol 2003;162(5):1611–21.

224. Slominski A, Wortsman J, Mazurkiewicz JE, et al. Detection of proopiomelanocortin-derived antigens in normal and pathologic human skin. J Lab Clin Med 1993;122(6):658–66.

225. Roloff B, Fechner K, Slominski A, et al. Hair cycle-dependent expression of corticotropin-releasing

factor (CRF) and CRF receptors in murine skin. FASEB J 1998;12(3):287–97.

226. Ito N, Ito T, Betterman A, Paus R. The human hair bulb is a source and target of CRH. J Invest Dermatol 2004;122(1):235–7.

227. Kauser S, Thody AJ, Schallreuter KU, Gummer CL, Tobin DJ. beta-Endorphin as a regulator of human hair follicle melanocyte biology. J Invest Dermatol 2004;123(1):184–95.

228. Kauser S, Thody AJ, Schallreuter KU, Gummer CL, Tobin DJ. A fully functional proopiomelanocortin/melanocortin-1 receptor system regulates the differentiation of human scalp hair follicle melanocytes. Endocrinology 2005;146(2):532–43.

229. Krause K, Schnitger A, Fimmel S, Glass E, Zouboulis CC. Corticotropin-releasing hormone skin signaling is receptor-mediated and is predominant in the sebaceous glands. Horm Metab Res 2007;39(2):166–70.

230. Rousseau K, Kauser S, Pritchard LE, et al. Proopiomelanocortin (POMC), the ACTH/ melano-cortin precursor, is secreted by human epidermal keratinocytes and melanocytes and stimulates melanogenesis. FASEB J 2007;21(8):1844–56.

231. Ziegler CG, Krug AW, Zouboulis CC, Bornstein SR. Corticotropin releasing hormone and its function in the skin. Horm Metab Res 2007;39(2):106–9.

232. Slominski A, Wortsman J, Tuckey RC, Paus R. Differential expression of HPA axis homolog in the skin. Mol Cell Endocrinol 2007;265–266:143–9.

233. Slominski A, Paus R, Wortsman J. On the potential role of proopiomelanocortin in skin physiology and pathology. Mol Cell Endocrinol 1993;93(1):C1–6.

234. Kim HS, Cho DH, Kim HJ, Lee JY, Cho BK, Park HJ. Immunoreactivity of corticotropin-releasing hormone, adrenocorticotropic hormone and alpha-melanocyte-stimulating hormone in alopecia areata. Exp Dermatol 2006;15(7):515–22.

235. Aoki E, Shibasaki T, Kawana S. Intermittent foot shock stress prolongs the telogen stage in the hair cycle of mice. Exp Dermatol 2003;12(4):371–7.

5
Toll-Like Receptors

Donna Bilu Martin and Anthony A. Gaspari

Key Points

- Toll-like receptors (TLRs) are part of the innate immune response.
- TLRs work through two pathways:
  - Adaptor protein myeloid differentiation factor 88 (MyD88) to activate transcription factor nuclear factor κB (NF-κB) or activating protein-1 (AP-1)
  - A lipopolysaccharide (LPS)-triggered MyD88-independent pathway that produces inflammatory cytokines
- Multiple dermatologic diseases are found to involve TLRs, including TLR-1 (psoriasis, tuberculoid leprosy), TLR2 (acne, retinoids, lepromatous leprosy, syphilis, atopic dermatitis, Lyme disease, herpes simplex virus, candidiasis), TLR4 (Kawasaki's disease, syphilis, candidiasis, melanoma), TLR5 (syphilis), and TLR9 (herpes simplex virus).
- Current and future therapies and vaccines will target TLRs.

There are two major arms of the immune system: innate immune response, and acquired, or adaptive, immune response. In the former, phagocytic cells recognize pathogens that bind to specific receptor recognition molecules or through complement fixation, and then activate pathways to contain infection.[1] Essential components of the innate immune response include neutrophils, eosinophils, natural killer cells, natural killer T cells, mast cells, cytokines, complement, and antimicrobial peptides. In the latter, T lymphocytes recognize foreign antigens presented on major compatibility complexes I and II on the cell surface of antigen-presenting cells (APCs).[1] Lymphocytes that recognize foreign antigens then clonally expand to provide an antigen-specific immune response. Table 5.1 lists the characteristics of innate versus adaptive immunity.

More recently, another key component of the innate immune response has been discovered, the Toll-like receptors (TLRs). These receptors allow the innate immune system to tailor its response depending on the stimulatory antigen and which TLR is activated. Toll-like receptors represent the innate immune mechanisms that sense danger, which triggers protective (but sometimes disease inducing) inflammation and a subsequent adaptive immune response.[2] In addition, TLRs allow the innate immune system to control activation of the adaptive response, thus helping to bridge the gap between innate and adaptive immunity.[3] The TLRs play an important role in many skin diseases (Table 5.2).

Discovery of Toll-Like Receptors in Humans

The TLRs, or so-called pathogen recognition receptors, were identified as primary sensors of the innate immune system as a result of studying the pathogenesis of sepsis.[4] Lipopolysaccharide (LPS) is a component of the cell wall of gram-negative bacteria. TLR4 was discovered as the critical transducer of the LPS signal, revealing the first of ten mammalian plasma membrane proteins with a strong homology to the receptor, Toll, present in *Drosophila melanogaster* flies.[4] In flies, Toll is a regulator of *Drosophila* embryonic

TABLE 5.1. Characteristics of innate versus adaptive immunity

Characteristics	Innate immunity	Adaptive immunity
Trigger	Pathogen-associated molecular patterns	Specific antigens
Kinetics of action	Minutes to hours	Days to weeks
Molecular receptors	Toll-like receptors	T-cell receptors, B-cell receptors
Diversity/memory	No diversity/memory	Has diversity/memory
Communication	Cytokines, chemokines	Cytokines, chemokines
Effectors	Complement, antigen presentation, phagocytosis, transdifferentiation	Complement, antigen presentation, cytotoxicity, antibody

Source: Gaspari.[3]

TABLE 5.2. Toll-like receptors (TLRs) in dermatologic disease

TLR	Disease	Comment
1	Tuberculoid leprosy	TLR1 favors Th1 phenotype; TLR1 enhances TLR2 signaling by forming heterodimers[37]
	Psoriasis	TLR1 expression increased in keratinocytes[50]
	Lyme disease	Stimulation with *B. burgdorferi* lysate increased TLR1 expression[64]
	IL-1 receptor associated kinase-4 deficiency	
		Cells from patients do not respond to ligands from TLR1–6,9[65]
2	Acne vulgaris	*P. acnes* activates TLR2 through LPS and PG[5]
	Retinoids	Antiinflammatory effects through TLR2[32]
	*Psoriasis	TLR2 expression increased in keratinocytes[50]
	Lepromatous leprosy	Polymorphism in TLR2 (mutated) favors Th2 phenotype[35]
	Syphilis	
	Meningitis	*T. pallidum* stimulates TLR2 directly[38]
	Atopic dermatitis	LPS-deficient *N. meningitidis*, porins activate TLR2[5,55, 56]
	Candidiasis	*S. aureus*, human β-defensin-2 signal through TLR2[9]; mutation in TLR2 found with increased frequency in AD patients[46]
	Plague	
	Lyme disease	
	UV-induced immunosuppression	TLR2 activated by glucan in fungal cell wall[5]
	HSV	Outer membrane protein targets TLR2 on APCs[60]
		B. burgdorferi lipoprotein mediated by TLR2[63]
		UV induces keratinocytes to secrete ligands to activate TLR2 and 4[85]
		TLR2 knockout mice have decreased response to HSV[70]
3	*SLE	snRNP Ag, an autoAb in SLE, may act via TLR3[75]
	*Melanoma	Vaccination for melanoma with poly-I:C acts via TLR3[81]
		TLR3 recognizes dsDNA (associated with viral infections like HSV)[73]
4	Acne	Distinct strains of *P. acnes* may also activate TLR4[32]
	Syphilis	*T. pallidum* stimulates TLR4 directly[38]
	Meningitis	LPS in *N. meningitidis* activates TLR4[4]
	Candidiasis	TLR4 activated by mannan in fungal cell wall[5]
	Plague	*Y. pestis* utilizes TLR4 to trigger apoptosis[61]
	*Psoriasis	HSP overexpressed in psoriasis, activate TLR4[51]
	*Melanoma	Melanoma inhibits TLR4 signaling in macrophages[79]
	*Kawasaki disease	TLR4 upregulated during acute phase[62]
	UV-induced immunosuppression	Mutated TLR4 in mice: resistant to low-dose UV immunosuppression[85]
5	Syphilis	*T. pallidum*–derived flagellin activates TLR5 and heterodimers TLR4–TLR5[39, 40]
6	Lyme disease	*B. burgdorferi* induces cooperation of TLR2 and TLR6[17]
7	Imiquimod	Synthetic TLR7 analogue, used as antiviral, antitumor[5,72]
	Loxoribine	
	Bropirimine	Synthetic TLR7 ligand, may be used as antitumor therapy in the future[5]

(continued)

TABLE 5.2. (continued)

TLR	Disease	Comment
	*Psoriasis	
	*SLE	Synthetic TLR7 ligand, used as treatment after BCG for bladder cancer[5]
	UV-induced immunosuppression	
		Imiquimod aggravates psoriatic lesions[53]
		U1 snRNP Ag stimulates TLR7[77]
		TLR7 activation on DC allows maturation despite UV exposure[86]
8	Resiquimod	Synthetic TLR8 analogue[5]
	*Psoriasis	Imiquimod aggravates psoriatic lesions[53]
	*SLE	RNA sequences in snRNP stimulate TLR8[77]
9	*SLE	snRNP Ag, an autoAb in SLE, may act via TLR9[75]
	*Melanoma	TLR9 agonist (CpG 7909) may be used as adjuvant for cancer vaccine[82]
	HSV	
		HSV activates IFN-producing cells in mice through TLR9[71]
10		
11		

*Likely, but not proven as of yet.
AD, atopic dermatitis; APC, antigen-presenting cell; DC, dendritic cell; dsDNA, double-stranded DNA; HSP, heat shock protein; HSV, herpes simplex virus; IFN, interferon; LPS, lipopolysaccharide; PG, peptidoglycan; snRNP, small nuclear ribonuclear protein.

TABLE 5.3. Historical timeline: discoveries of Toll-like receptors

	Discovery
	Toll receptor in *Drosophila* flies dictates dorsoventral patterning[88]
1996	Toll required for resistance to fungal infections in flies[6]
1989	Term *pathogen-associated molecular patterns* introduced[89]
1997	Human homologue of *Drosophila* Toll, signals activation of adaptive immunity (linking innate and adaptive immunity)[90]
1998	TLR4 is lipopolysaccharide receptor[91]
2000	TLR9 recognizes bacterial DNA[92]
2000	TLR2 can pair with TLR6 to recognize bacterial proteins[93]
2000	TLR2 can also associate with TLR1[93]
2001	TLR3 mediates response to viral double-standed RNA[73]
2001	TLR5 detects flagellate protein in whiplike tails of bacteria[94]
2001	TLR2 activation leads to tuberculosis death in macrophages[95]
2002	TLR2 triggers inflammatory response to *Propionibacterium acnes*[30]
2002	TLR2/1 heterodimers involved in response to *Borrelia burgdorferi*[96]
2002	TLR7 triggered by imiquimod, resulting in immunomodulation[15]
2003	TLR1, 2, 5 expressed in normal keratinocytes[50]
2003	TLR2, 4 expressed in normal keratinocytes[97]
2003	TLR1, 2, 3, 5, 9 expressed in normal keratinocytes[98]
2003	TLR2/1 heterodimers activated by killed *Mycobacterium leprae*[37]
2003	TLR1,2 increased and TLR5 downregulated in psoriatic keratinocytes[50]
2004	TLR8 (humans), TLR 7 (mice) recognize single-stranded RNA[99]
2004	TLR11, 12, 13 in mice discovered[100]
2005	TLR4 signaling suppressed by melanoma[79]

development, responsible for the determination of its dorsoventral axis.[5] The mutant form of Toll was found to impair antifungal defense in flies, which was the first demonstration of its role in host defense.[6] There are now 11 (and perhaps up to 13) known human pathogen recognition receptors (TLR1 to TLR11), which allow cytokine synthesis in response to various classes of microbial products and common pathogens.[7,8] For a detailed look at the history of TLRs, see Table 5.3.

Expression of Human Toll-Like Receptors

Expression of human TLRs has been detected on neutrophils, macrophages, dendritic cells, dermal endothelial cells, mucosal epithelial cells, B cells, and T cells[7] (Table 5.4). Keratinocytes constitutively express messenger RNA (mRNA) for TLRs 1, 2, 3, and 5 and potentially 4, 6, 9, and 10 as well.[9] The expression of TLR family members confers cellular responsiveness to pathogen-associated molecular patterns (PAMPs), as well as endogenous ligands (Fig. 5.1).[10] Lipopolysaccharide, viral double-stranded and single-stranded RNA, flagellin, unmethylated cytosine-phosphate-guanine (CpG)-containing DNA, peptidoglycan (PG), lipopeptides, and heat shock proteins (HSP) are several of the ligands known to activate specific TLRs. Table 5.5 provides a detailed look at the ligands that activate TLRs and the cytokines produced.[7] Thus, TLRs confer the ability to detect dangerous infections, as well as recognizing self molecules that represent a host response to such danger.

Toll-Like Receptors in Innate and Adaptive Immunity

The TLRs have a key role in host defense by linking innate and adaptive immune responses.[5] Activation of TLRs mediates the release of antimicrobial pep-

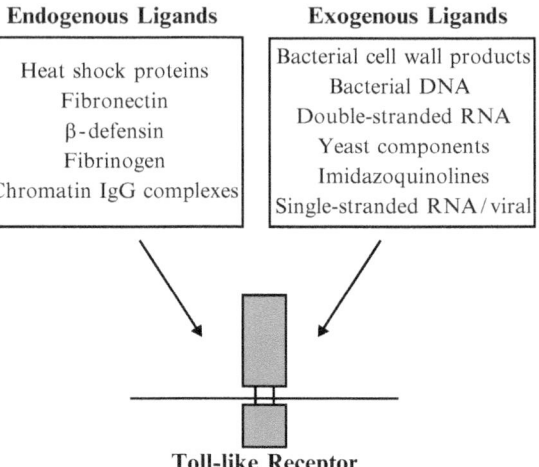

FIG. 5.1. Known activating endogenous and exogenous ligands of Toll-like receptors.

tides and chemokines that recruit phagocytic cells to the site of infection.[10]

The TLRs influence the adaptive immune response through a variety of mechanisms. TLR ligands upregulate surface expression of the major histocompatibility complex (MHC), inducing maturation of dendritic cells from phagocytic cells to potent APCs.[11] Activation of TLRs by microbial products initiates the expression of co-stimulatory molecules on both T cells and APCs.[5] If these signals are not expressed, then the T cell will not become activated to clonally expand, and a fully developed adap-

TABLE 5.4. TLR expression in different cell types

Cell type	TLR1	2	3	4	5	6	7	8	9	10	11
KC[9]	+	+	+	+	+	+			+	+	
LC[101]		+		+					+		
EC[102,103]		+	+	+	+				+		+
MC[104]		+		+							
FB*[105]	+	+	+	+	+	+	+	+	+		
DC[82, 106]	+	+	+	+	+	+	+	+	+	+	
M[106]	+	+	+	+	+	+	+	+	+		
B[106]	+	+		+		+			+		
N[106]		+	+	+		+	+		+		
BL[82,106]	+	+	+	+	+	+	+		+	+	
T$_{reg}$[106]			+		+		+	+			
NKT[106]		+	+	+	+	+		+	+		

*Murine embryonic fibroblasts: human skin fibroblasts have not been studied.

KC, keratinocyte; LC, Langerhans' cell; EC, endothelial cell; MC, mast cell; FB, fibroblast; DC, dendritic cell; M, macrophage; B, basophil; N, neutrophil; L, B lymphocyte; T$_{reg}$, T-regulatory lymphocyte; NKT, natural killer T cells.

TABLE 5.5. TLR: proposed effector function, ligands, and cytokines induced

TLR	Proposed effector function	Endogenous ligands	Exogenous ligands	Cytokines induced
1	Defense against *Mycobacteria*, organisms expressing triacylated lipoprotein	None identified	Triacylated LP, mycobacterial LP	TNF-α IL-12
2	Defense against *Mycobactera, Mycoplasma,* gram-positive bacteria (*P. acnes*), protozoa, fungi, LPS-deficient *N. meningitidis, Yersinia pestis*	HSPgp96 HSP60 HSP70	PG of gram + bacteria Triacylated LP Diacylated LP Zymosan of yeast Lipoteichoic acid GPI anchors Outer membrane protein A Phosphatidylinositol dimannoside	
	Senses oxidative stresses and cellular necrosis		Glycolipid LAM Mycobacterial LP Phenol-soluble modulin	
	Activation of respiratory burst		Measles virus hemagglutinin protein	
	Induction of antimicrobial TLR4 ligand, β-defensin-2			
	Mast cell activation and degranulation		hCMV particles	
	Induction of apoptosis		Porin protein	
3	Antiviral defense	None identified	Double-stranded RNA	IFN-β
4	Defense against gram-negative bacteria, fungi, viruses	HSPgp96	LPS	TNF-α
		HSP60 HSP70 Extra domain A of fibronectin	F protein of RSV *Escherichia Col P fimbriae* Mouse mammary tumor virus envelope protein	IFN-β IL-1 IL-6 IL-10
	Flagellum of *Treponema Pallidum*, LPS present *N. meningitidis, Y. pestis*	B-defensin-2 Fibrinogen	Taxol E5564? (LPS antagonist)	IL-13 Macrophage inflammatory protein-1α/β
	Induction of apoptosis		Glucuronoxylomannan of *Cryptococcus neoformans*	Nitric oxide Leukotrienes Prostanoids
5	Defense against flagellated bacteria, *T. pallidum*	None identified	Flagellin	TNF-α
	DC maturation			IL-1β IL-6 IL-10 IFN-γ Nitric oxide
6	Defense against bacteria, fungi, mycoplasma, protozoa	None identified	Diacylated LP Phenol-soluble modulin Zymosan of yeast GPI anchors	TNF-α
7	Antiviral and antitumor defense DC maturation Activation and migration of LCs from skin to draining lymph nodes Th1 development NK-cell activation B-cell proliferation Eosinophil activation	None identified	Imidazoquinolines Loxoribine Bropirimine Single-stranded RNA (HIV, influenza)	IFN-α IFN-γ IFN-β TNF-α IL-1 IL-6 IL-8 IL-12 IL-18 GM-CSF Superoxides

(continued)

TABLE 5.5. (continued)

TLR	Proposed effector function	Endogenous ligands	Exogenous ligands	Cytokines induced
8	Similar to TLR7	None identified	Imidazoquinolines	Similar to TLR7
			Single-stranded RNA	
9	Antibacterial and antiviral defense	Chromatin-IgG	Unmethylated Cytidine-guanine	IFN-α
	Th1 development	complexes	DNA	IFN-γ
	B-cell proliferation		Live or inactivated HSV-2	IFN-β
	DC maturation			IL-6
				IL-12
10	Unknown	None identified	None identified	Unknown
11[8]	Uropathogenic bacteria	None identified	None identified	

GM-CSF, granulocyte-macrophage colony-stimulating factor; GPI, glycosylphosphatidylinositol; hCMV, human cytomegalovirus; HSP, heat shock protein; IFN, interferon; IgG, immunoglobulin; IL, interleukin; LAM, lipoarabinomannan; LP, lipoprotein; LPS, lipopolysaccharide; MDDC, monocyte-derived dendritic cell, NO, nitric oxide; PG, peptidoglycan; TNF, tumor necrosis factor; HIV, human immunodeficiency virus

Source: Kang et al.[5]

tive immune response cannot occur. Furthermore, whether a naive T cell will differentiate toward a T-helper-1 (Th1) cell or a Th2 profile depends on the antigen and the TLR to which it binds.[5] This influences cytokine production. TLR-activated dendritic cells have been shown to secrete interleukin-6 (IL-6), which can result in the loss of suppressor activity by T-regulatory cells, allowing a more effective immune response.[5] The TLRs can also mediate B-cell proliferation and antibody production, and generate antigen-specific immune responses in naive individuals with enhancement by adjuvants.[10]

The TLRs may also mediate effects of members of the heat shock protein family of molecular chaperones, which stimulate cytokine production and APC activation.[12] Lysis of cells and HSP release may help trigger an antiviral immune response.[13] Heat shock protein has also been shown to be overexpressed by keratinocytes in psoriatic lesions and is discussed below (see Psoriasis).[3]

Pathways

There are two distinct signaling pathways that TLRs utilize. One involves the adaptor protein myeloid differentiation factor 88 and the other is independent of this protein.

The TLRs are transmembrane proteins with a series of leucine repeats in the N-terminal extracellular domain, and a cytoplasmic portion, called Toll–Interleukin 1 (IL-1) receptor (TIR) homology domain, which bears similarity to the IL-1 receptor.[5] This intracellular region is crucial to the immune response. Upon recognition of the TLR by its ligand, the TIR domain initiates a signaling cascade. It undergoes homo- or heterodimerization with another TLR and interacts with the Toll–IL-1 receptor domain of the cytoplasmic adaptor protein myeloid differentiation factor 88 (MyD88).[5,14] Interleukin-1-receptor–associated kinase (IRAK) and tumor necrosis factor (TNF) receptor–associated factor 6 (TRAF6) are then further recruited to the TLRs.[15] The pathway then diverges. One path activates transcription factor nuclear factor κB (NF-κB),[16] and the other c-Jun N-terminal kinase (JNK) and mitogen-activated protein kinase (MAPK), resulting in activation of activating protein 1 (AP-1).[15] This signaling pathway leads to the production of inflammatory cytokines (Fig. 5.2).[16]

A newly described component is Toll-interacting protein (TOLLIP), which is present in a complex with IRAK and links IRAK to IL-1R, limiting IRAK phosphorylation and NF-κB activation.[17] Overexpression of TOLLIP has been shown to inhibit TLR4– and TLR2–mediated NF-κB activation.[17] It may serve as an antiinflammatory strategy.[17]

In the LPS-triggered MyD88-independent pathway of TLR4, the biologically active portion of LPS causes upregulation of interferon (IFN)-inducible genes and activation of IFN regulatory factor (IRF)-3, which is involved in an antiviral response.[18] It also reduces proinflammatory

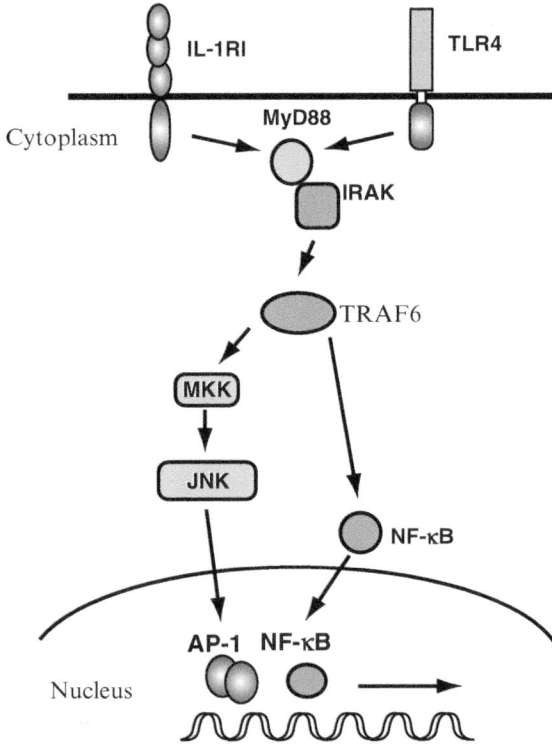

FIG. 5.2. The interleukin-1R (IL-1R)– Toll-like receptor(TLR) signaling pathway. Activated IL-1R1 or TLR4 associates with cytoplasmic adaptor molecule, MyD88, which further recruits IRAK and TRAF 6. The association activates two signaling pathways, resulting in the activation of AP-1 transcription factors through c-Jun N-terminal kinase (JNK) and mitogen-activated protein kinase (MAPK), and activation of NF-κB transcription factors in the nucleus.[16]

cytokines and cyclooxygenase induction,[19,20] suggesting that different genes were being induced. Other effects of this pathway include the upregulation of co-stimulatory molecules on DCs and activation of Kupffer cell caspase 1, leading to cleavage of endogenously stored proIL-18 into mature IL-18 to be secreted.[21,22]

Acne

Acne vulgaris is one of the most commonly seen conditions in dermatology. It is a chronic inflammatory disease of the pilosebaceous unit, characterized by comedones, inflammatory papules, pustules, nodules, cysts, and often scars. The pathogenesis of acne is multifactorial, with the principal abnormality being comedo formation resulting from hyperproliferation of keratinocytes. This leads to in follicular dilatation and disruption, resulting in the discharge of follicular contents, such as keratin, sebum, and microorganisms, namely *Propionibacterium acnes,* a gram-positive anaerobe bacteria, into the dermis.[5] It is generally accepted that inflammation in acne vulgaris may be a reaction to extracellular products of *P. acnes.*[23]

Studies have demonstrated the presence of proinflammatory cytokines in acne patients. Interleukin-1α has been demonstrated in open comedones.[24] *P. acnes* has been shown to induce monocytes to secrete IL-1β, tumor necrosis factor-α (TNF-α), and IL-8.[25] Interleukin-8 has also been produced by keratinocytes in response to *P. acnes.*[26] In addition, IL-1β, TNF-α, and IL-1α have also been demonstrated in normal sebaceous glands.[27] More recently, *P. acnes* type IA and IB isolates and LPS were found to induce human β-defensin-2 (hBD2) and proinflammatory cytokine expression, and to influence sebocyte viability in vitro.[26] hBD2 is involved in nonoxidative killing of primarily gram-negative microorganisms, but can also recruit macrophages and dendritic cells to infectious sites.[28,29] It is now known that *P. acnes* activates cytokine release through a mechanism involving pattern recognition receptors, such as the TLRs.

In 2002, it was discovered that in acne lesions, TLR2–expressing macrophages surround the pilosebaceous follicles and that *P. acnes* induced cytokine production, such as IL-6, -8, and -12, by monocytes via TLR2.[30] TLR2 forms homodimers and acts as one of the signal-transducing co-receptors for CD14.[31] *P. acnes* possesses two potential cell wall components, LPS and PG, that can serve as ligands and activate TLR2.[5] A recent study demonstrated that distinct strains of *P. acnes* induced upregulation of hBD2, and IL-8 mRNA levels in keratinocytes are both TLR2 and TLR4 dependent.[26] The authors also add that other TLRs, such as TLR1 or TLR6, in addition to other signal transduction pathways, may play a role in sensing *P. acnes.*[26] Retinoids, such as adapalene, may exert their antiinflammatory effects by decreasing local expression of TLR2 by inhibiting the expression of the gene encoding this TLR.[32] This decreased TLR2 expression, therefore, would attenuate the inflammatory response of monocytes to the *P. acnes* organism.

Leprosy

Leprosy, or Hansen's disease, caused by *Mycobacterium leprae*, is a chronic, debilitating disease that encompasses a spectrum of clinical manifestations. At one end, tuberculoid leprosy (TL) presents in patients with a strong cell-mediated immune response, resulting in high resistance to *M. leprae* and few, localized, paucibacillary lesions.[33] At the other end of the spectrum, lepromatous leprosy (LL) patients have a weak immune response, resulting in disseminated, multibacillary disease, including cutaneous and nerve involvement.[33] Other forms of the disease with unstable resistance include borderline tuberculoid, borderline, and borderline lepromatous. The former is Th1 mediated (e.g., IFN-γ, IL-12, IL-18, and granulocyte-macrophage colony-stimulating factor), whereas the latter is Th2 driven (e.g., IL-4 and IL-10).[5] Whether a patient develops one response over the other may be due, in part, to TLRs.

In 1999, it was discovered that mycobacteria activated macrophages through TLR2, resulting in production of TNF-α, an inflammatory cytokine. When a dominant negative mutation was introduced in TLR2, the receptor was unresponsive to *M. tuberculosis*.[34] Furthermore, a mutation in Arg[677]Trp in TLR2 has been associated with LL in the Korean population.[35] A more recent study confirmed that this mutation halts the ability of TLR2 to mediate a response to both *M. leprae* and *M. tuberculosis*, confirming the presence of this polymorphism.[33]

This polymorphism may play a crucial role in determining the clinical presentation of leprosy. Upon stimulation with *M. leprae*, patients with the Arg[677]Trp in TLR2 were found to have decreased production of IL-2, IL-12, IFN-γ, and TNF-α, and increased IL-10 when compared to those with the wild-type TLR2.[36] Thus, the mutated TLR2 favored a Th2 phenotype, which is consistent with what is observed in LL. The authors suggested that TLR2 plays a critical role in the alteration of cytokine profiles and determination of the type of leprosy.

TLR2-TLR1 heterodimers are also activated by *M. leprae*, and the coexpression of TLR1 has been shown to greatly enhance TLR2 activity.[37] Furthermore, TL lesions had higher TLR1 expression, and stronger TLR2 expression than LL lesions.[37] Therefore, the expression of TLR2 and TLR1 contributes to the host response. Interestingly, this study demonstrated that type 1 cytokines enhance TLR1 and TLR2 activation, whereas the Th2 cytokines inhibited activation. It was hypothesized that the cytokine pattern triggered by *M. leprae* infection both activated TLRs and modulated their expression through two distinct mechanisms. Therefore, the adaptive immune response, through cytokine release, may actually influence the innate response. This further exemplifies the role of TLRs in bridging the gap between innate and adaptive immunity.

Syphilis

Syphilis, also known as lues, is a contagious, sexually transmitted disease caused by the spirochete *Treponema pallidum*. There are three stages of syphilis. In primary syphilis, a painless genital ulcer called a chancre, appears 18 to 21 days after infection. Secondary syphilis can appear as various cutaneous eruptions—macular, papular, or polymorphous—often with lesions on the palms and soles. Tertiary syphilis often occurs 3 to 5 years after infection. Patients may develop gummas, or necrotic lesions in the skin, mucous membranes, bones, or joints. Other complications of syphilis include neurologic and cardiac involvement.

T. pallidum lacks LPS; however, it does contain many membrane lipoproteins (LPs), which are the principal proinflammatory mediators during syphilitic infection, serving to activate monocytes and macrophages.[38] In 2001, it was demonstrated that upon stimulation with *T. pallidum* or the synthetic lipopeptide, TLR2- and TLR4-expressing immature murine dendritic cells (DCs) released cytokines that favored Th1 development, including IL-12, IL-1β, TNF-α, and IL-6.[38] The DCs are a component of innate immunity. They are APCs that, upon taking up and processing foreign antigen, migrate to the lymph nodes, where they present the antigen in the context of MHC, and, with co-stimulatory molecules, activate naive T cells.[5]

Flagellin is a conserved protein monomer that makes up the flagellar filament[39] in the periplasmic space beneath the outer membrane.[5] It is an important ligand recognized by TLRs. Upon stimulation with bacterial flagellin, TLR5 expressing human monocyte–derived DCs induced maturation and chemokine production.[39] Heterodimers of TLR4-5 may be required to induce macrophage nitric oxide synthesis in response to flagellin.[40] Therefore, TLRs can recognize not only *T. pallidum* itself but also a portion of it.

It has been proposed that these three TLRs may play different, complementary roles in immunity against *T. pallidum*. TLR2 recognizes the LPs on the surface of *T. pallidum*, activating the adaptive immune system and a Th1 cytokine profile.[5] Following recognition, processing, and presentation of *T. pallidum* by DCs, flagellin would activate TLRs 4 and 5, resulting in proinflammatory cytokines and bactericidal nitric oxide synthesis.[5]

Atopic Dermatitis

Atopic dermatitis (AD) is a common, chronic, inflammatory skin condition that affects both adult and pediatric population. Patients often have asthma and seasonal allergies as well. Patients with AD often have concomitant viral, fungal, and bacterial infections, especially *Staphylococcus aureus*; 90% of patients with AD have been found to have colonization with *S. aureus* in both lesional and nonlesional skin, whereas only 5% of healthy controls exhibit colonization.[41] Up to 50% to 60% of the *S. aureus* found on patients with AD is toxin producing.[41] It is unclear why AD patients have this increased colonization; however, a defective innate immune response may play a role.

Several studies have made headway in offering explanations. Early lesions in AD have a Th2 cytokine profile, which has been shown in murine models to promote preferential skin binding to *S. aureus* over Th1 environments.[42] Furthermore, recent studies have shown that human β-defensin-2 and cathelicidin LL-37 (two endogenous antimicrobial peptides important in keratinocyte defense against pathogens, especially *S. aureus*) were significantly decreased in acute and chronic lesions of AD when compared to controls and patients with psoriasis.[43]

Both *S. aureus* and human β-defensin-2 have been found to signal though TLR2. Purified staphylococcal cell-wall components lipoteichoic acid (LTA) and peptidoglycan (PGN) are known to sig-

nal through TLR2.[9] A study involving human kidney and lung cells revealed that upon stimulation of TLR2 with synthetic bacterial LPS, human β-defensin-2 was released in a dose-dependent manner.[44] It has also been demonstrated that murine β-defensin-2 induces maturation of DCs as well as release of Th1 cytokines through TLR4.[45] Therefore, if TLR2 is defective, it may cause a decrease in human β-defensin-2, resulting in decreased killing of *S. aureus* as well as reduced activation of TLR4, amplifying a Th2 response.[5] *S. aureus* favors a Th2 environment, and would be able to multiply.[5] In 2004, it was reported that a missense mutation in the TLR2 gene *R753Q* has been found with increased frequency in patients with AD, correlating with a more severe phenotype, higher serum levels of immunoglobulin E (IgE), and greater susceptibility to *S. aureus* colonization.[46]

The loss of T-regulatory cell suppressive activity induced by toxin producing bacterial infections has been demonstrated to play a role in the flares of AD.[47] This may occur by two mechanisms: direct effects of bacterial superantigens on T-regulatory cells, and the TLR-mediated maturation of DCs that are necessary to maintain T-regulatory suppressive activity. Thus, administration of oral antibiotics may have an antiinflammatory effect by controlling DC–T-regulatory cell interaction and restoring immune tolerance.

In addition, levels of IL-1α, a known receptor of IL-1R, have been shown to be increased in skin of mice during *S. aureus* infection.[9] Interleukin-1R also uses the adaptor protein MyD88 in its pathway.[9] A recent publication demonstrated that, when exposed to *S. aureus*, both IL-1R and MyD88 knockout mice had impaired neutrophil chemotaxis, whereas a TLR2 knockout mouse did not.[48] The authors suggested a greater role for the IL-1R pathway than TLR2 in combating *S. aureus* in AD.[48] It may be that the defects mentioned above occur in all patients with AD or just a subset.[5] Regardless, exciting research is being done to better understand the mechanism.

Finally, TLR4 has been shown to be involved in allergic Th2 responses to intranasal allergen.[49] It may be that TLRs play a role in atopic patients or patients who develop IgE-mediated allergic reactions when they encounter activating polypeptides in the skin or respiratory tree.

Psoriasis

Psoriasis is a chronic, recurrent, inflammatory disease characterized by dry, scaly, circumscribed erythematous plaques predominantly located in the scalp, nails, extensor surfaces of the limbs, umbilical region, and sacrum. The pathogenesis of psoriasis, which is characterized by Th1 cytokines, involves intralesional T lymphocytes triggering primed basal stem keratinocytes to proliferate and perpetuate the disease process.[3] Advances in understanding the mechanisms involved in psoriasis and developments of new immunosuppressive and biologic treatments have occurred in the last 25 years.

Not surprisingly, TLRs have also been found to play a role in the pathogenesis of psoriasis. A study demonstrated that, in lesional epidermis from patients with psoriasis, TLR1 and TLR2 expression was increased in the suprabasal layer of keratinocytes upon comparison with normal controls.[50] Furthermore, TLR5 expression was decreased. Nuclear TLR1 staining of the epidermis of both lesional and nonlesional psoriatic skin was increased, but not in that of normal skin. The authors speculated that the upregulated TLR2 may be in response to the presence of gram-positive bacteria such as *S. aureus* on the keratin layer.[50] Interestingly, systemic and topical retinoids are used in the treatment of psoriasis, and may control inflammation through their inhibitory effects on TLR2, although this has not yet been studied.[5]

As mentioned above, heat shock protein (HSP) expression is induced by exposure to microbial pathogens and other stressful stimuli.[51] Heat shock protein 27, 60, and 70 have been shown to be overexpressed in psoriasis, and can trigger an innate immune response through TLR4 on APCs, resulting in the secretion of TNF-α, IL-12, and Th1 cytokines.[51] They also may act on the adaptive immune response by serving as autoantigens for self-reactive T cells that migrate into psoriatic lesions.[51]

Such discoveries are opening doors for novel treatments in psoriasis. Monomethyl fumarate (MMF), a bioactive metabolite of fumaric acid ester, is an immunotherapy for psoriasis that causes decreased production of Th1 cytokines and lymphocytopenia.[52] Monomethylfumarate was shown to decrease DC response to LPS and decreased IL-12p70 and IL-10 production.[52] As LPS is a potent TLR4 agonist, this may shed light on the mechanism of action of the drug in the treatment of psoriasis.[3] Furthermore, application of imiquimod, a TLR7/8 agonist, causes aggravation of psoriatic lesions, with an increase in IFN-α and infiltration of DC into lesions.[53]

Bacterial Infections

The TLRs have been implicated in the pathogenesis of multiple bacterial diseases. *Neisseria meningitidis,* a gram-negative (GN) bacteria, causes invasive meningococcal disease, severe bacterial sepsis, and the cutaneous manifestation acute infectious purpura fulminans.[5] These infarcts portend a poor outcome for patients and is evidence of tissue injury from proinflammatory cytokines, microvascular endothelial injury, and a prothrombotic state.[5] A critical component of the pathogenesis of this disease is LPS. The level of circulating LPS has been shown to directly correlate with clinical severity and risk of death from meningococcal septicemia.[54]

As previously mentioned, LPS is a component of the cell wall of gram-negative bacteria, and TLR4 is the critical transducer of the LPS.[4] In acute infectious purpura fulminans, LPS acts through TLR4 to trigger the release of cytokines TNF-α, IL-1, IL-6.[5] However, other microbial products of *N. meningitidis* play a role. Lipopolysaccharide-deficient *N. meningitidis* mutants activate TLR2 to elicit proinflammatory cytokines and induce DC maturation.[5,55] Neisserial porins, outer membrane proteins that allow diffusion of small molecules across membranes, may activate TLR2 and stimulate B cells.[56] Furthermore, the type of T-cell response (Th1 vs. Th2) appears to depend on the ligand. One study demonstrated that when LPS was the ligand for DC, greater concentrations of Th1 cytokines (IFN-γ) were produced when compared to Th2 cytokines (IL-13).[57] The reverse was shown when an LPS-deficient outer membrane vesicle stimulated the DCs.[57] Finally, LPS itself may be a potential target for treatment in patients with gram-negative septicemia. A synthetic lipodisaccharide, E5564, was found to act at the level of TLR4 to inhibit LPS and decrease production of TNF-α, IL-1β, IL-6, IL-8, and IL-10.[58] Thus, this TLR4 antagonist could be administered to patients with septicemia, thus blunting the severe systemic reaction to naturally occurring endotoxin.

Yersinia pestis is a GN bacillus that causes plague, a disease that was epidemic in Europe and killed millions of people. It was called the "Black Death." It is transmitted by the bite of the rat flea *Xenopsylla cheopis*. Clinically, painful buboes form in the axillae or groin, although other skin lesions such as vesicles, plaques, petechiae, and purpura can be seen. One mechanism by which *Yersinia* gains entry into the host's APCs is through low calcium response protein V, an outer-membrane protein.[59] It was shown that this protein targets TLR2 and CD14 on the surfaces of APCs.[60] In addition, it was also found that *Yersinia* utilizes TLR4 to trigger apoptosis.[61] These were interesting discoveries, for it revealed that *Yersinia* uses TLRs to its survival advantage.

Kawasaki disease (KD) is a syndrome seen primarily in children consisting of fever, polymorphous rash, mucous membrane involvement, and lymphadenopathy. Complications include coronary artery aneurysms. There are many suspected etiologic agents, such as *S. aureus and* other bacteria, viral, or fungal agents, but none is specifically implicated. Recently, a study in China showed that TLR4 and MyD88 were upregulated during the acute phase of KD.[62] The activation of TLR4 may initiate immune aberrance in KD.[62]

Finally, Lyme disease is a tick-borne illness caused by the spirochete *Borrelia burgdorferi*. It is loosely divided into three stages. The primary stage is characterized by constitutional symptoms and erythema chronicum migrans. The second stage occurs for 5 to 6 months after the rash resolves. In the tertiary phase, cardiac, neurologic, and rheumatologic complications can occur. In 1999, it was shown that inflammatory signaling by *B. burgdorferi* outer surface protein A lipoprotein is mediated by TLR2.[63] Later, it was found that cooperation of TLR2 and TLR6 occurred upon activation by soluble tuberculosis factor as well as *B. burgdorferi* lipoprotein.[17] Most recently, stimulation with *B. burgdorferi* lysate was found to increase the expression of TLR1 and TLR2 in all peripheral blood monocytes and human brain cells, but not neurons.[64]

Interleukin-1 Receptor-Associated Kinase 4 Deficiency

Interleukin-1 receptor-associated kinase 4 is a molecule involved in the TLR signaling cascade mentioned above.[5] Deficiency in this kinase has been shown to increase susceptibility to pyogenic infections caused mostly by *Streptococcus pneumoniae* and *S. aureus*.[65] Cells from patients with this disease did not respond to IL-1β, IL-18, or any known ligands from TLRs 1 to 6 and 9.[65] Key clinical features of this disease include early onset; recurrent pyogenic infections with minimal febrile or inflammatory responses; resistance to viral, fungal, or parasitic organisms; and neutropenia during infectious episodes.[5] The mode of inheritance is likely autosomal recessive.[5] As patients mature, their profound susceptibility to bacterial infections lessens, possibly reflecting the maturation of adaptive immunity over time.

Candidal Infections

Candida albicans is a dimorphic fungi that causes cutaneous and mucocutaneous candidiasis, which is seen in healthy patients, babies, and especially in those who are immunocompromised. It can be difficult to control and manage therapeutically. Infection by *C. albicans* triggers release of proinflammatory cytokines. Immunoreactive components of *C. albicans* include glucans, mannans, and chitin.[5] It has been demonstrated that the immune response against yeast involves TLR2, causing upregulation of TNF-α via the NF-κB pathway.[66]

Furthermore, TLR4 plays a role in mounting an immune response against *C. albicans*. Anti-CD14 and anti-TLR4 antibodies (but not anti-TLR2 antibodies) have been shown to block mannan-induced cytokine production.[67] However, when zymosan, a preparation that contains β-glucan and mannan, was used as the ligand, anti-TLR2 antibodies blocked cytokine production.[67] Thus, TLR4 is likely activated by mannan, and TLR2 is likely activated by other fungal cell components, such as glucan.[5]

In contrast to the aforementioned study, however, another study of mice with mutated TLR4 revealed lower levels of neutrophil chemokines when compared to controls, suggesting that TLR4 may induce clearing of infection through chemotaxis of neutrophils to the site of infection rather than the induction of proinflammatory cytokines.[5,68] In addition, this study revealed that anti-TLR2 antibodies decreased production of TNF and IL-1β, consistent with the previous reported findings.[68] It is likely that these TLRs work differently to foster an immune response against *C. albicans*; activation of TLR4 leads to neutrophil cytokines, whereas TLR2 partially mediated TNF and IL-1β production.[5] Finally, there is evidence that *C. albicans* resembles *Yersinia* in that it can manipulate these TLRs and host immunity to its own survival advantage.[69]

Viral Diseases

Herpes simplex virus type 1 (HSV-1) and type 2 (HSV-2) are commonly seen by dermatologists. They are double-stranded (ds) DNA viruses that produce latent yet lifelong infections by residing in immune cells and nerves. HSV-1 generally produces vesicular outbreaks at the orolabial or ocular mucosa, whereas HSV-2 typically infects genital mucosa and renders patients more susceptible to other sexually transmitted infections. However, both strains of the virus can infect either physical location.

Herpes simplex virus has been shown to be recognized by two TLRs, TLR2 and TLR9. One study revealed that TLR2 knockout mice have decreased cytokine responses to HSV, as well as an increased severity in encephalitis.[70] Herpes simplex virus has also been shown to activate interferon-producing cells in mice through TLR9.[71] However, it is likely that HSV works through other TLRs as well.[72] Furthermore, TLR polymorphisms may make certain individuals more susceptible to infection with HSV than others.[72]

In addition, dsRNA, a molecular pattern associated with viral infection, has been shown to be recognized by mammalian TLR3.[73] Upon activation, the receptor induces production of interferons through NF-κB.[73] Polyriboinosinic:polycytidylic acid complex (poly-I:C), a synthetic version of dsRNA, has been shown to trigger TLR3 pathways to elicit a strong IFN-β response, which has been associ-

ated with HSV clearance.[72] Imidazoquinolines, such as imiquimod, are recognized by TLRs 7 and 8, resulting in antiviral cytokine production and immune response.[72] Imiquimod has been used to treat HSV-2, with mixed results.[72] CpG motifs in DNA sequences activate TLR9+ dendritic cells, subsequently inducing viral Th1 cytokines.[72] These motifs have been recently used as an adjuvant in an experimental HSV-2 vaccine with promising results.[74]

Autoimmune Diseases

The autoimmune connective tissue diseases (AI-CTDs) are a group of clinical disorders that all have circulating autoantibodies (autoAbs). Such disorders include lupus erythematosus (LE), dermatomyositis, systemic sclerosis, rheumatoid arthritis, mixed connective tissue disease, Sjögren's, and more. Systemic LE (SLE) is a disease commonly seen in dermatology, in which patients may exhibit several key diagnostic signs and symptoms, including antinuclear antibody positivity, malar and discoid rashes, photosensitivity, oral ulcers, arthritis, serositis, and renal, neurologic, hematologic, and immunologic disorders.

Recently, several studies have demonstrated evidence for the role of TLR in SLE. An important target for autoAb in SLE are small nuclear ribonuclear protein particles (SnRNP) called U1 and Sm.[75] A recent study revealed that, following the engagement of TLRs, immature anti-SnRNP B cells differentiated and produced autoAb.[75] The authors postulated that snRNP Ag could act with endogenous CpG motifs or self RNA to generate stimuli for low-affinity autoreactive B-cell activation via TLR9, TLR3, and TLR7 pathways.[75] TLR9, in particular, has been shown to directly bind to single-stranded unmethylated CpG-DNA containing a phosphodiester backbone.[76] This study demonstrated that the binding of TLR9 and CpG-DNA is inhibited by chloroquine and quinacrine, suggesting a possible mechanism for the therapeutic effect seen in some autoimmune diseases, such as lupus.[76]

Furthermore, another study revealed that specific RNA sequences within snRNPs stimulate TLR7 and TLR8 as well as activate immune cells, such as plasmacytoid dendritic cells, to secrete high levels of IFN.[77] Specifically, U1 snRNP can stimulate TLR7, leading to IFN-α secretion, and TLR8, leading to TNF-α secretion from monocytes.[77]

A recent study, involving MRL[lpr/lpr] mice that spontaneously develop immune complex glomerulonephritis as part of a systemic lupus-like autoimmune syndrome, characterized the expression of TLRs 1 to 9.[78] As the mice developed nephritis, the expression of TLRs 1 to 9 increased, as measured by mRNA levels.[78] Expression of TLRs differed in specific cell types.[78] Thus, more TLR types may be involved in the pathogenesis of SLE.

Melanoma and Mycosis Fungoides

Melanoma is a tumor rising from melanocytes that has been increasing in incidence and mortality over the years. It is a common type of cancer in young adults. Melanoma, like many cancers, likely results from a combination of genetic and environmental exposures (mainly sun exposure). The body defends itself against tumor cells with an immune response, secreting cytokines and presenting antigen, and by direct tumor cytotoxicity.[79] Not surprisingly, research reveals that TLRs are likely involved in this immune response.

Peritoneal macrophages from mice transplanted with the B16 melanoma cell line have shown inhibited killing and decreases in the production of superoxide, nitric oxide, TNF-α, and NF-κB when stimulated with LPS.[79] A recent study in such mice revealed that melanoma cells inhibit TLR4 signaling in macrophages.[79] The authors suggested that the ability to avoid innate immune activation confers a selective advantage to the tumor. In addition, when melanoma cells were activated in vitro with LPS, they produced high levels of IL-8 and promoted cell adhesion. These effects were dependent on the expression of TLR4.[80] Interestingly, other tumor cell lines, such as ovarian carcinoma and neuroblastoma were not affected by LPS.[80]

Manipulation of TLRs is currently being investigated as a therapeutic option in the treatment of melanoma. Vaccination with recombinant adenovirus encoding human tyrosinase-related protein 2 (Ad-hTRP2) has previously been reported to provide protective immunity against subsequent transplantation of B16 melanoma cells.[81] However, it is not effective against established melanoma

in the skin or lungs. To increase the therapeutic efficacy, the authors added peritumoral injections of ligands CpG DNA and poly-I:C, which activate innate immunity via TLR9 and TLR3, respectively.[81] This modified regimen induced cutaneous tumor rejection in 60% of mice (18 of 30), rendering them tumor-free after 50 days.[81] Injection of the TLR ligands alone was able to significantly inhibit growth of lung metastases.[81] Such discoveries are instrumental in developing a treatment for melanoma.

Finally, CpG 7909 (PF-3512676) is an immunomodulating synthetic oligonucleotide that acts as a TLR9 agonist.[82] It is currently under development for the treatment of cancer both as monotherapy and in combination therapy, as well as an adjuvant for vaccines.[82] It acts through TLR9 receptors present on B cells and plasmacytoid dendritic cells to stimulate B-cell proliferation, IFN-α and IL-10 production, and natural killer (NK) cell activity.[82] It is currently in trials as treatment for non–small-cell lung cancer and may likely be useful in the treatment of other cancers, as well.[82]

The TLRs may also be involved in the pathogenesis and treatment of other malignancies. The most common form of cutaneous T-cell lymphoma (CTCL) is mycosis fungoides (MF).[83] Skin lesions in MF include patches, plaques, tumors, hypopigmented lesions, and erythroderma. There is no single effective treatment available currently for MF. Those utilized by dermatologist today include light therapy, retinoids, nitrogen mustard, topical steroids, and systemic interferon.[83] These treatments are not without side effects. A preliminary pilot study of six patients with patch and plaque stage MF treated with topical imiquimod, a TLR7 agonist, 5% cream three times a week for 12 weeks reported a histologic and clinical response rate of 50%.[83] The mechanism of this treatment is unclear; however, it may be in part due to the induction of local interferon production.[83]

Ultraviolet Light

Ultraviolet (UV) light has been used for decades to treat common skin diseases such as psoriasis and atopic dermatitis. In dermatology, phototherapy is done with broadband UVB, narrowband UVB, UVA-1, and UVA plus psoralen (PUVA). These treatments can be very effective. However, as with most other therapeutic interventions, they are not without side effects. UV radiation causes suppression of the immune system through Langerhans' cell (LC) depletion and inhibition of antigen presentation by LCs.[5] This UV-induced immunosuppression likely occurs as a result of IL-10 and TNF-α production.[84,85]

Studies reveal the involvement of TLRs in UV exposure. A C3H/HeJ mouse model that has a dominant-negative TLR4 exhibits impaired TNF-α production after UVB exposure and is resistant to UVB suppression of contact hypersensitivity.[85] UVB radiation likely induces keratinocytes to secrete endogenous TLR ligands, such as HSPs. These ligands activate TLRs 2 and 4, resulting in secretion of IL-10 and TNF-α.[85] Some of these ligands may also bind to TLRs on LCs, perhaps inducing the migration of these cells to regional lymph nodes.[5] This would help explain why the density of epidermal LC in UV-irradiated skin is decreased.[5]

As a result of depletion of LCs and inhibition of hapten presentation to Th1-lymphocytes, UV light exposure also results in suppression of contact hypersensitivity (CHS).[5,86] A recent study demonstrated that topical applications of imiquimod, a TLR7 agonist, to mouse skin before UV exposure prevented the loss of CHS.[86] In addition, in vitro studies utilizing XS52, a LC-like mouse line, revealed that imiquimod initiated maturation of LC despite UV exposure, and that imiquimod and UVB work synergistically to enhance IL-12 production and migration of LC in vivo, preserving CHS.[86] Thus, the authors suggest that topical imiquimod treatment may help prevent UV-induced immunosuppression by stimulation of TLR signaling.[86]

Xeroderma pigmentosum (XP) is a rare, autosomal recessive disorder characterized by photosensitivity, premature skin aging, and malignant tumor development. These patients are unable to repair DNA damaged by UV light. In 1993, it was discovered that NK cells from patients with XP failed to enhance after challenge with an IFN-inducing poly-I:C, a form of synthetic dsRNA.[87] However, when IFN-α was added exogenously, the NK cell activity was increased.[87] Thus, NK cells from XP patients had a defect in IFN production in response to poly-I:C, impairing NK cell activity.[5] It

was also discovered that poly-I:C utilizes TLR3 to activate an innate immune response.[73] A defect in TLR3 signaling could lead to decreased IL-12 and predominant IL-10 and TNF-α.[5] Furthermore, IL-12 is an activator of NK cells. Decreased activation may allow for unchecked tumor growth.[5] Thus, it may be possible that defects in TLR3 or in the TLR3 signaling pathway may prove to be partly responsible for the UV-light induced photosensitivity and tumor production in XP patients.[5]

Thus, TLRs play an integral role in countless dermatologic diseases, serving to bridge the gap between innate and adaptive immunity. It is certain that many more discoveries will be made to further characterize and understand this novel group of receptors, their role in skin diseases, as well as the potential to manipulate signaling through these TLRs to treat such diseases.

Conclusion

A key component of the innate immune response has been discovered, the Toll-Like receptors (TLRs). These receptors allow the innate immune system to tailor its response depending on the stimulatory antigen and which TLR is activated, thus helping to bridge the gap between innate and adaptive immunity. There are now 11 (and perhaps up to 13) known human pathogen recognition receptors (TLR1 to TLR11), which allow cytokine synthesis in response to various classes of microbial products and common pathogens. Keratinocytes constitutively express mRNA for TLRs 1, 2, 3, and 5 and potentially 4, 6, 9, and 10 as well. There are two distinct signaling pathways that TLRs utilize. One involves the adaptor protein myeloid differentiation factor 88, and the other is independent of this protein. There are numerous diseases in dermatology that utilize TLRs, such as atopic dermatitis.

References

1. Bilu D, Sauder D. Immunomodulatory and pharmacologic properties of imiquimod. J Am Acad Dermatol 2000;43(1 pt 2):S6–11.
2. Fuchs E, Matzinger P. Is cancer dangerous to the immune system? Semin Immunol 1996;8(5): 271–280.

3. Gaspari A. Innate and adaptive immunity and the pathophysiology of psoriasis. J Am Acad Dermatol 2006;54(3 suppl 2):S67–80.

4. Beutler B. Toll-like receptors: how they work and what they do. Curr Opin Hematol 2002;9(1):2–10.

5. Kang S, Kauls L, Gaspari A. Toll-like receptors: Applications to dermatologic disease. J Am Acad Dermatol 2006;54(6):951–983.

6. Lemaitre B, Nicolas E, Michaut L, et al. The dorsoventral regulatory gene cassette Spatze/Toll/cactus controls the potent antifungal response in Drosophila adults. Cell 1996;86(6):973–983.

7. Armant M, Fenton M. Toll-like receptors: a family of pattern-recognition receptors in mammals. Genome Biol 2002;3(8):reviews 3011.

8. Zhang D, Zhang G, Hayden M. A toll-like receptor that prevents infection by uropathogenic bacteria. Science 2004;303(5663):1522–1526.

9. McGirt L, Beck L. Innate immune defects in atopic dermatitis. J Allergy Clin Immunol 2006;118(1):202–208.

10. Sieling P, Modlin R. Toll-like receptors: mammalian "taste receptors" for a smorgasbord of microbial invaders. Curr Opin Microbiol 2002;5(1):70–75.

11. Banchereau J, Steinman R. Dendritic cells and the control of immunity. Nature 1998;392(6673):245–252.

12. Beg A. Endogenous ligands of Toll-like receptors: implications for regulating inflammatory and immune responses. Trends Immunol 2002;23(11):509–512.

13. Berwin B, Reed R, Nicchitta C. Virally induced lytic cell death elicits the release of immunogenic GRP94/gp96. J Biol Chem 2001;276(21):21083–21088.

14. Akira S. Toll-like receptors and innate immunity. Adv Immunol 2001;78:1–56.

15. Hemmi H, Kaisho T, Takeuchi O, et al. Small antiviral compounds activate immune cells via the TLR7 MyD88–dependent signaling pathway. Nat Immunol 2002;3(2):196–200.

16. Akira S, Takeda K, Kaisho T. Toll-like receptors: critical proteins linking innate and acquired immunity. Nat Immunol 2001;2(8):675–680.

17. Bulut Y, Faure E, Thomas L, et al. Cooperation of Toll-like receptor 2 and 6 for cellular activation by soluble tuberculosis factor and Borrelia burgdorferi outer surface protein A lipoprotein: role of Toll-interacting protein and IL-1 receptor signaling molecules in Toll-like receptor 2 signaling. J Immunol 2001;167(2):987–994.

18. Kawai T, Takeuchi O, Fujita T, et al. Lipopolysaccharide stimulates the MyD88–independent pathway and results in activation of IFN-regulatory factor 3 and the expression of a subset of lipopolysaccharide-inducible genes. J Immunol 2001;167(10):5887–5894.

19. Sato M, Taniguchi T, Tanaka N. The interferon system and interferon regulatory factor transcription factors: studies from gene knockout mice. Cytokine Growth Factor Rev 2001;12(2–3):133–142.

20. Taniguchi T, Takaoka A. The interferon-alpha/beta system in antiviral responses: a multimodal machinery of gene regulation by the IRF family of transcription factors. Curr Opin Immunol 2002;14(1):111–116.

21. Kaisho T, Takeuchi O, Kawai T, et al. Endotoxin induced maturation of MyD88–deficient dendritic cells. J Immunol 2001;166(9):5688–5694.

22. Seki E, Tsutsui H, Nakano H, et al. Lipopolysaccharide induced IL-18 secretion from murine Kupffer cells independently of myeloid differentiation factor 88 that is critically involved in induction of production of IL-12 and IL-1beta. J Immunol 2001;166(4):2651–2657.

23. Strauss J, Kligman A. The pathologic dynamics of acne vulgaris. Arch Dermatol 1960;82:779–791.

24. Ingham E, Eady E, Goodwin C, et al. Pro-inflammatory levels of interleukin-1–alpha-like bioactivity are present in the majority of open comedones in acne vulgaris. J Invest Dermatol 1992;98(6):895–901.

25. Vowels B, Yang S, Leyden J. Induction of proinflammatory cytokines by a soluble factor of Propionibacterium acnes: implications for chronic inflammatory acne. Infect Immun 1995;63(8):3158–3165.

26. Nagy I, Pivarcsi A, Kis K, et al. Propionibacterium acnes and lipopolysaccharide induce the expression of antimicrobial peptides and proinflammatory cytokines/chemokines in human sebocytes. Microbes Infect 2006;8(8):2195–2205.

27. Boehm K, Yun J, Strohl K, et al. Messenger RNA for the multifunctional cytokines interleukin-1alpha, interleukin-1beta, and tumor necrosis factor-alpha are present in adnexal tissues and in dermis of normal human skin. Exp Dermatol 1995;4(6):335–341.

28. Schroder J. Epithelial peptide antibiotics. Biochem Pharmacol 1999;57(2):121–134.

29. Yang D CO, Bykovskaia SN, et al. Beta-defensins: Linking innate and Adaptive immunity through dendritic and T cell CCR6. Science 1999;286:525–528.

30. Kim J, Ochoa M, Krutzik S, et al. Activation of toll-like receptor 2 in acne triggers inflammatory cytokine responses. J Immunol 2002;169(3):1535–1541.

31. Yang R, Mark M, Gurney A, et al. Signaling events induced by lipopolysaccharide-activated Toll-like receptor 2. J Immunol 1999;163(2):639–643.

32. Vega B, Ferret C, Jomard A. Regulation of Toll-Like receptor-2 expression by Adapalene: implications for the treatment of inflammatory acne. J Invest Dermatol Abstracts 2003;121:156.

33. Bochud P, Hawn T, Aderem A. Cutting edge: A Toll-Like Receptor 2 polymorphism that is associated with lepromatous leprosy is unable to mediate mycobacterial signaling. J Immunol 2003;170(7):3451–3454.

34. Underhill D, Orzinsky A, Smith K, et al. Toll-like receptor-2 mediates mycobacteria-induced proinflammatory signaling in macrophages. Proc Natl Acad Sci USA 1999;96(25):14459–14463.

35. Kang T, Chae G. Detection of Toll-like Receptor 2 (TLR2) mutation in the lepromatous leprosy patients. FEMS Immunol Med Microbiol 2001;31(1):53–58.

36. Kang T, Yeum C, Kim B, et al. Differential production of IL-10 and IL-12 in mononuclear cells from leprosy patients with a Toll-like Receptor 2 mutation. Immunol 2004;112(4):674–680.

37. Krutzik S, Ochoa M, Sieling P, et al. Activation and regulation of Toll-like receptors 2 and 1 in human leprosy. Nature Med 2003;9(5):525–532.

38. Bouis D, Popva T, Takashim A, et al. Dendritic cells phagocytose and are activated by Treponema pallidum. Infect Immun 2001;69(1):518–528.

39. Means T, Hayashi F, Smith K. The Toll-like receptor 5 stimulus bacterial flagellin induces maturation and chemokine production in human dendritic cells. J Immunol 2003;170(10):5165–5175.

40. Mizel S, Honko A, Moors M, et al. Induction of macrophage nitric oxide production by gram-negative flagellin involves signaling via heteromeric Toll-like receptor5/Toll-like receptor4 complexes. J Immunol 2003;170(12):6217–6223.

41. Leung D. Infection in atopic dermatitis. Curr Opin Pediatr 2003;15(4):399–404.

42. Cho S, Strickland I, Tomkinson A, et al. Preferential binding of Staphylococcus aureus to skin sites of Th2–mediated inflammation in a murine model. J Invest Dermatol 2001;116(5):658–663.

43. Ong P, Ohtake T, Brandt C. Endogenous antimicrobial peptides and skin infections in atopic dermatitis. N Engl J Med 2002;347(15):1151–1160.

44. Birchler T, Seibel R, Buchner K, et al. Human Toll-like receptor 2 mediates induction of the antimicrobial peptide human beta-defensin 2 in response to bacterial lipoprotein. Eur J Immunol 2001;31(11): 3131–3137.

45. Biragyn A, Ruffini P, Leifer C, et al. Toll-like receptor 4–dependent activation of dendritic cells by beta-defensin 2. Science 2002;298(5595): 1025–1029.

46. Werfel T, Heeg K, Neumaier M, et al. R753Q polymorphism defines a subgroup of patients with atopic dermatitis having severe phenotype. J Allergy Clin Immunol 2004;113(3):565–567.

47. Ou L-S, Goleva E, Hall C, et al. T regulatory cells in atopic dermatitis and subversion of their activity by superantigens. J Allergy Clin Immunol 2004;113(4):756–763.

48. Miller L, O'Connell R, Gutierrez M, et al. MyD88 mediates neutrophil recruitment initiated by IL-1R but not TLR2 activation in immunity against Staphylococcus aureus. Immunity 2006;24(1): 79–91.

49. Piggott D, Eisenbarth S, Xu L. MyD88–dependent induction of allergic Th2 responses to intranasal antigen. J Clin Invest 2005;115(2):459–467.

50. Baker B, Ovigne J-M, Powles A, et al. Normal keratinocytes express Toll-Like receptors (TLRs) 1, 2 and 5: modulation of TLR expression in chronic plaque psoriasis. Br J Dermatol 2003;148(4): 670–679.

51. Curry J, Qin J-Z, Bomish B, et al. Innate immune-related receptors in normal and psoriatic skin. Arch Pathol Lab Med 2003;127(2):178–186.

52. Litjens N, Rademaker M, Ravensbergen B, et al. Monomethylfumarate affects polarization of monocyte-derived dendritic cells resulting in down-regulated Th1 lymphocyte responses. Eur J Immunol 2004;34(2):565–575.

53. Gilliet M, Conrad C, Geiges M, et al. Psoriasis triggered by toll-like receptor 7 agonist imiquimod in the presence of dermal plasmacytoid dendritic cell precursors. Arch Dermatol 2004;140(12):1490–1495.

54. Brandtzaeg P, Kierulf P, Gaustad P, et al. Plasma endotoxin as a predictor of multiple organ failure and death in systemic meningococcal disease. J Infect 1989;159(2):195–204.

55. Ingalls R, Lien E, Golenbock D. Differential roles of TLR2 and TLR4 in the host response to gram-negative bacteria: lessons from a lipopolysaccharide-deficient mutant of Neisseria meningitidis. J Endotoxin Res 2000;6(5):411–415.

56. Massari P, Henneke P, Ho Y, et al. Cutting edge: immune stimulation by neisserial porins is Toll-like receptor 2 and MyD88 dependent. J Immunol 2002;168(4):1533–1537.

57. Al-Bader T, Christodoulides M, Heckels J, et al. Activation of human dendritic cells in modulated by components of the outer membranes of Neisseria meningitidis. Infect Immun 2003;71(10): 5590–5597.

58. Mullarkey M, Rose J, Bristol J, et al. Inhibition of endotoxin response by E5564, a novel Toll-like receptor 4–directed endotoxin antagonist. J Pharm Exp Ther 2003;304(3):1093–1102.

59. Sing A, Roggenkamp A, Geiger A, et al. Yersinia enterolitica evasion of the host innate immune response by V antigen-induced-IL-10 production of macrophages is abrogated in IL-10 deficient mice. J Immunol 2002;168(3):1315–1321.

60. Sing A, Rost D, Tvardovaskia N, et al. Yersinia V-antigen exploits Toll-Like Receptor 2 and CD14 for interleukin 10–mediated immunosuppression. J Exp Med 2002;196(8):1017–1024.

61. Haase R, Kirsching C, Sing A, et al. A dominant role of Toll-like receptor 4 in the signaling of apoptosis in bacteria-faced macrophages. J Immunol 2003;171(8):4294–4303.

62. Wang G, Li C, Zu Y, et al. The role of activation of Toll-like receptors in immunological pathogenesis of Kawasaki disease. Zhonghua Er Ke Za Zhi 2006;44(5):333–336.

63. Hirschfeld M, Kirschning C, Schwandner R, et al. Cutting edge: inflammatory signaling by Borrelia burgdorferi lipoproteins is mediated by toll-like receptor 2. J Immunol 1999;163(5):2382–2386.

64. Cassiani-Ingoni R, Cabral E, Lunemann J, et al. Borrelia burgdorferi induces TLR1 and TLR2 in human microglia and peripheral blood monocytes but differentially regulates HLA-class II expression. J Neuropathol Exp Neurol 2006;65(6):540–548.

65. Picard C, Puel A, Bonnet M. Pyogenic bacterial infections in humans with IRAK-4 deficiency. Science 2003;299(5615):2076–2079.

66. Underhill D, Ozinsky A, Hajjar A, et al. The Toll-like receptor 2 is recruited to macrophage phagosome and discriminates between pathogens. Nature 1999;401(6755):811–815.

67. Tada H, Nemoto E, Shimauchi H, et al. Saccharomyces cerevisiae- and Candida albicans- derived mannan production of tumor necrosis factor alpha by human monocytes in a CD14- and Toll-like receptor 4-dependent manner. Microbiol Immunol 2002;46(7):503–512.

68. Netea M, Van der Graaf C, Vonk A, et al. The role of Toll-like receptor (TLR 2) and TLR 4 in the host defense against disseminated candidiasis. J Infect Dis 2002;185(10):1483–1489.

69. Deva R, Shankaranarayanan P, Ciccoli R, et al. Candida albicans induces selectively transcriptional activation of cyclooxygenase-2 in HeLa cells: pivotal roles of toll-like receptors, p38 mitogen-activated protein kinases, and NF-kappaB. J Immunol 2003;171(6):3047–3055.

70. Kurt-Jones E, Chan M, Zhou S, et al. Herpes simplex virus 1 interaction with toll-like receptor 2 contributes to lethal encephalitis. Proc Natl Acad Sci USA 2004;101:1315–1320.

71. Krug A, Luker G, Barchet W. Herpes simplex virus type 1 activates murine natural interferon-producing cells through toll-like receptor 9. Blood 2004;103(4):1433–1437.

72. Herbst-Kralovetz M, Pyles R. Toll-like receptors, innate immunity and HSV pathogenesis. Herpes 2006;13(2):37–41.

73. Alexopoulou L, Holt A, Medzhitov R, et al. Recognition of double-stranded RNA and activation of NF-kappaB by Toll-like receptor 3. Nature 2001;413(6857):732–738.

74. McCluskie M, Cartier J, Patrick A, et al. Treatment of intravaginal HSV-2 infection in mice: a comparison of CpG oligodeoxynucleotides and resiquimod (R-848). Antiviral Res 2006;69(2):77–85.

75. Ding C, Wang L, Al-Ghawi H, et al. Toll-like receptor engagement stimulates anti-snRNP autoreactive T cells for activation. Eur J Immunol 2006;36(8):2013–2024.

76. Rutz M, Metzger J, Gellert T. Toll-like receptor 9 binds single-stranded CpG-DNA in a sequence- and pH- dependent manner. Eur J Immunol 2004;34(9):2541–2550.

77. Vollmer J, Tluk S, Schmitz C, et al. Immune stimulation mediated by autoantigen binding sites within small nuclear RNAs involves Toll-like receptors 7 and 8. J Exp Med 2005;202(11):1575–1585.

78. Patole P, Pawar R, Lech M, et al. Expression and regulation of Toll-like receptors in lupus-like immune complex glomerulonephritis of MRL-Fas(lpr) mice. Nephrol Dial Transplant 2006;21(11):3062–73.

79. Clarke J, Cha J, Walsh M, et al. Melanoma inhibits macrophage activation by suppressing Toll-like receptor 4 signaling. J Am Coll Surg 2005;201(3):418–425.

80. Molteni M, Marabella D, Orlandi C, et al. Melanoma cell lines are responsive in vitro to lipopolysaccharide and express TLR-4. Cancer Lett 2006;235(1):75–83.

81. Tormo D, Ferrer A, Bosch P. Therapeutic efficacy of antigen-specific vaccination and Toll-like receptor stimulation against established transplanted and autochthonous melanoma in mice. Cancer Res 2006;66(10):5427–5435.

82. Na. CpG 7909: PF 3512676, PF-3512676. Drugs in Research and Development 2006;7(5):312–316.

83. Deeths M, Chapman J, Dellavalle R. Treatment of patch and plaque stage mycosis fungoides with imiquimod 5% cream. J Am Acad Dermatol 2005;52(2):275–280.

84. Rivas J, Ullrich S. Systemic suppression of delayed-type hypersensitivity by supernatants from UV-induced keratinocytes. An essential role for keratinocyte-derived IL-10. J Immunol 1992;149(12):3865–3871.

85. Yoshikawa T, Kurimoto I, Streilein J. Tumor necrosis factor-alpha mediates ultraviolet B-enhanced expression of contact hypersensitivity. Immunology 1992;76(2):254–271.

86. Thatcher T, Luzina I, Fishelevich R, et al. Topical imiquimod treatment presents UV-light induced loss of contact hypersensitivity and immune tolerance. J Invest Dermatol 2006;126(4):821–831.

87. Gaspari A, Fleisher T, Karemer K. Impaired interferon production and natural killer cell activation in patients with the skin cancer-prone disorder, xeroderma pigmentosum. J Clin Invest 1993;92(3):1135–1142.

88. Anderson KV, Bokla L, Nusslein-Volhard C. Establishment of dorsal-ventral polarity in the Drosophila embryo: the induction of polarity by the Toll gene product. Cell 1985;42:791–798.

89. Janeway C Jr Approaching the asymptote? Evolution and revolution in immunology. Cold Spring Harbor Symp Quant Biol 1989;54(Pt 1):1–13.

90. Medzhitov R, Preston-Hurlburt P, Janeway C Jr. A human homologue of the Drosophila Toll protein signals activation of adaptive immunity. Nature 1997;388(24):394–397.

91. Beutler B, Poltorak A. The sole gateway endotoxin response: how LPS was identified as TLR 4 and its role in innate immunity. Drug Metab Dispos 2001;29(4 pt 2):474–478.

92. Hemmi H, Takeuchi O, Kawai T, et al. A Toll-like receptor recognizes bacterial DNA. Nature 2000;408(6813):740–745.

93. Ozinsky A, Underhill D, JD F, et al. The repertoire for pattern recognition of pathogens by the innate immune system is defined by cooperation between toll-like receptors. Proc Natl Acad Sci USA 2000;97:13766–13771.

94. Hayashi F, Smith K, Ozinsky A, et al. The innate immune response to bacterial flagellin is mediated by Toll-like receptor 5. Nature 2001;410(6832):1099–1103.

95. Thoma-Uszynski S, Stenger S, Takeuchi O, et al. Induction of direct antimicrobial activity through mammalian toll-like receptors. Science 2001;291(5508):1544–1547.

96. Alexopoulou L, Thomas V, Schnare M, et al. Hyporesponsiveness to vaccination with Borrelia burgdorferi OspA in humans and in TLR1– and TLR2– deficient mice. Nat Med 2002;8(8):878–884.

97. Pivarcsi A, Bodai L, Rethi B, et al. Expression and function of Toll-like receptors 2 and 4 in human keratinocytes. Int Immunol 2003;15(6):721–730.

98. Mempel M, Voelcker V, Kollisch G, et al. Toll-like receptor expression in human keratinocytes: nuclear factor kappaB controlled gene activation by Staphylococcus aureus is toll-like receptor 2 but not toll-like receptor 4 or platelet activating factor receptor dependent. J Invest Dermatol 2003;121(6):1389–1396.

99. Heil F, Hemmi H, Hochrein H, et al. Species-specific recognition of single-stranded RNA via toll-like receptor 7 and 8. Science 2003;303(5663):1526–1529.

100. Tabeta K, Georgel P, Janssen E, et al. Toll like receptors 9 and 3 as essential components of innate immune defense against mouse cytomegalovirus infection 3. Proc Natl Acad Sci USA 2004;101(10):3516–3521.

101. Mitsui H, Watanabe T, Saeki H, et al. Differential expression and function of Toll-like receptors in Langerhans cells: comparison with splenic dendritic cells. J Invest Dermatol 2004;122(1):95–102.

102. Bsibsi M, Persoon-Deen C, Verwer R, et al. Toll-like receptor 3 on adult human astrocytes triggers production of neuroprotective mediators. Glia 2006;53(7):688–695.

103. Martin-Armas M, Simon-Santamaria J, Pettersen I. Toll-like receptor 9 (TLR9) is present in murine liver sinusoidal endothelial cells (LSECs) and mediates the effect of CpG-oligonucleotides. J Hepatol 2006;44(5):939–946.

104. Supajatura V, Ushio H, Nakao A. Differential responses of mast cell Toll-like receptors 2 and 4 in allergy and innate immunity. J Clin Invest 2002;109(10):1351–1359.

105. Kurt-Jones E, Sandor F, Ortiz Y, et al. Use of murine embryonic fibroblasts to define Toll-like receptor activation and specificity. J Endotox Res 2004;10(6):419–424.

106. Majewska M, Szczepanik M. The role of Toll-like receptors (TLR) in innate and adaptive immune responses and their function in immune response regulation. Postepy Hig Med Dosw 2006;60:52–63.

6
Conventional and Unconventional T Cells

Scott Roberts and Michael Girardi

Key Points

- T lymphocytes that express an $\alpha\beta$ T cell receptor (TCR), as well as a co-receptor CD4 or CD8, are present in the peripheral blood, lymph nodes, and tissues (such as the skin), and are considered conventional T cells.
- Unconventional T cells include those lymphocytes that express a $\gamma\delta$ TCR, and may commonly reside in an epithelial environment such as the skin, gastrointestinal tract, or genitourinary tract. Their role is to recognize infections and cancer cells, and regulate inflammatory responses that arise in these tissues.
- Another subset of unconventional T cells is that of the invariant natural killer T (NKT) cell, which has phenotypic and functional capacities of a conventional T cell, as well as features of natural killer cells (cytolytic activity). NKT cells recognize glycolipids when presented in the context of CD1d, and play a role in allergy, autoimmunity, and host defense against cancer and infections.

The locally resident and infiltrating cellular components that are responsible for the coordinated immunity against various infectious organisms and environmental toxins within the skin also may manifest misdirected or overexuberant responses that underlie cutaneous inflammatory disease. As the complexities of the immune system continue to be elucidated, it has become increasingly apparent that two major types of T cells, so-called conventional and unconventional, operate in fundamentally different ways to mediate and coordinate immune responses. This terminology reflects conventional T cells as those first identified with the capacity for immunologic memory, as opposed to the subsequent elucidation of a phenotypically and functionally distinct set of unconventional T cells.[1,2] Such conventional T cells mediate a highly evolved system that centers on the ability of their collectively diverse T-cell receptors (TCRs), each composed of a heterodimeric $\alpha\beta$ chain, to recognize processed antigenic peptide presented within the grooves of major histocompatibility complex (MHC) molecules on other cells. However, there has been relatively more recent elucidation of unconventional T cells that differ from their conventional counterparts in the rapidity of their initial response, the manner in which they recognize and respond to foreign or self nonpeptide molecules, as well as their tissue distribution within the body. In contrast to the diverse repertoire of $\alpha\beta$ TCR on conventional T cells, unconventional T cells have a more limited TCR repertoire in the form of cells expressing either an alternative $\gamma\delta$ TCR (reviewed in Girardi[3]), or a nondiverse $\alpha\beta$ TCR defining a population of so-called invariant natural killer T (iNKT) cells (reviewed in Kronenberg and Engel[4]).

The multidimensionality of unconventional T cells is revealed through their relationship to cooperative arms of so-called *innate* and *adaptive* immunity (Fig. 6.1). In contrast to innate immune responses that act relatively quickly and more indiscriminately via their recognition and targeting of molecules found on a range of infectious agents, adaptive immune responses are a more evolved system whereby recognition of specific molecules (i.e., antigens) is guided by the diversity of TCRs

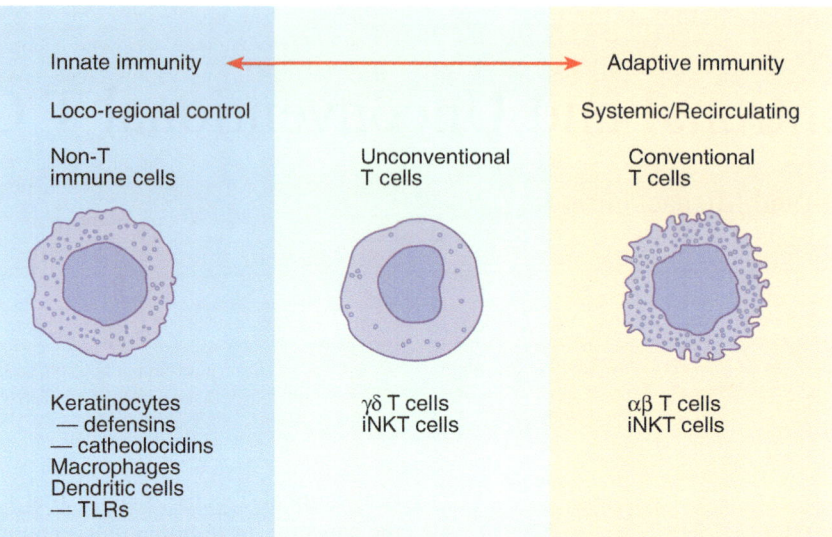

FIG. 6.1. Unconventional T cells have elements of both the innate and adaptive arms of the immune system. The innate immune system is characterized by immediate and local response to a limited set of nonpeptide molecules, while adaptive immunity responds slower and more globally to nearly any peptide antigen by virtue of the diversity present in the $\alpha\beta$ T-cell receptor (TCR) pool. Although unconventional T cells possess the ability to create a myriad of diverse TCRs, they are more often found in greater abundance in epithelia tissues with limited or nearly monomorphic sets of TCR chains. Evidence that these unconventional T cells are playing important roles in many immune functions includes their response to epithelial perturbation, clearance of pathogens, and antitumor properties. iNKT, invariant natural killer T; TLR, Toll-like receptor

expressed by conventional $\alpha\beta$ T cells (see Chapter 2). Cells and components of the innate immune system, in contrast, appear to recognize and locally respond in a rapid manner to more generic molecular components of microorganisms, or in some cases to self molecules expressed by cells under stress (see Chapter 4). Despite the fact that they express TCRs such as conventional T cells, unconventional T cells also show the following features of innate immunity: the rapidity of their response, propensity for local influences, and the fact that the nature of their response is to a less diverse set of nonpeptide (e.g., stress-induced endogenous, patterned microbial, or pharmacologic exogenous molecules). Although expression studies[1] suggest that both conventional and unconventional T cells may express similar genes—involved in, for example, the helper response to support the function of other immune cells, the cytotoxic response to target and eliminate infected or tumor cells, and the regulatory response to control immunity—the highly conserved evolution of these major subsets of T cells suggests their important and nonredundant

functions. The combination of mouse models of infection and cancer with an increasingly recognized diversity of human T cell responses to microorganisms and tumor cells has dramatically enhanced our understanding of the relative contributions of conventional and unconventional T cells to various immune responses.

Conventional T Cells

Conventional T-Cell Development, Activation, and Effector Functions

The incredible TCR diversity of conventional $\alpha\beta$ T cells, and their ability to distinguish a vast array of peptides derived from foreign versus self proteins, is endowed by an elegant process of development with the thymus (reviewed in Janeway et al.[5]). Gene rearrangements occur early during conventional T-cell differentiation and are derived from arrays of germline-encoded segments, named V (variable), D (diversity), and J (junction). Developing conventional

T cells are "educated" in the thymus, wherein the survival of T cells depends principally on the capacity of their TCR to bind processed peptide presented within MHC molecules. In general, those T cells with high-affinity binding to self-presented peptides are induced to undergo apoptosis (i.e., negative selection), while those with low-affinity specificity for self-presented peptides will survive (i.e., positive selection). This results in a conventional T-cell repertoire that binds presented self antigens with too low an affinity for activation, but will have the potential capacity to bind a vast number of foreign antigens with sufficient affinity to result in T-cell activation.

Conventional T cells generally require two major signals for activation. Signal 1 consists of binding of peptide plus the MHC complex by the TCR. Signal 2, also referred to as co-stimulation, is delivered for most conventional T cells by binding of molecules such as B7.1 (CD80) or B7.2 (CD86) on the surface of so-called professional antigen-presenting cells (APCs) (e.g., dendritic cells, macrophages) to a receptor on T cells, CD28. A T cell that receives only signal 1 results in T-cell anergy, a state of peripheral unresponsiveness. Another mechanism for limiting the magnitude of T-cell responses involves the substitution of a receptor, CTLA-4, that delivers an inhibitory suppressive signal 2 to the T cells via CD28. Only professional APCs can express both abundance amounts of MHC molecules, as well as poststimulatory molecules to provide signal 2. Resting professional APCs express co-stimulatory molecules at low levels; however, co-stimulatory molecule expression is dramatically increased on these cells when they receive a "danger signal," for example via their Toll-like receptor 4 (TLR4) (see Chapter 5). These conventional T cells that are activated will clonally expand and differentiate into effector cells and memory T cells, poised to respond more efficiently and rapidly to subsequent antigen exposure. This immunologic "memory" is a major feature of conventional T cells and is distinguished from that of unconventional T cells and their limited TCR diversity (discussed below).

Conventional T cells are generally considered to contain two major functional subsets delineated by their TCR co-receptors: CD4+ helper/inducer (Th) and CD8+ cytotoxic (T_C) (or "killer") lymphocytes. CD4-expressing T cells commonly differentiate after activation into one of two major functional subsets with characteristic cytokine profiles, although a third set of T-helper cells, termed "Th17" because of their production of interleukin-17 (IL-17),[6] has been more recently identified (Fig. 6.2). T-helper-1 (Th1)-type CD4+ cells, the major controllers of cell-mediated adaptive immunity, can greatly facilitate the effector functions against intracellular (e.g., viral, mycobacterial) pathogens or transformed cells in the skin. Their distinguishing cytokine profile (e.g., IL-2, interferon-γ [IFN-γ], IL-21) can help CD8 cytotoxic T-cell precursors to differentiate into T_C, activate macrophages to kill the pathogens that they have ingested, and boost the cytotoxic and IFN-γ production effects of natural killer (NK) cells (a major effector cell of antiviral and antitumor innate immunity).

In contrast, Th2-type CD4+ cells are specialized for the induction of "humoral immunity," critical to the response against extracellular (e.g., bacterial, fungal, certain parasitic) pathogens. For example, major Th2 cytokine effects are the stimulation of plasma cells to switch their antibody isotypes to immunoglobulins A and E (IgA and IgE), and the activation of effector cells of the innate immune system such as eosinophils, basophils, and mast cells. The distinguishing cytokines of Th2-type responses include IL-4 (a very potent B-cell activating cytokine), IL-5 (an eosinophil recruitment and key IgA class-switching factor), IL-9 (a mast cell differentiation factor), and IL-13 (important in mucus production and airway hyperactivity). The subsetting of CD4+ and CD8+ effector functions may not always be as neatly delineated as above, and in fact both CD4 and CD8 cells can be divided into functional subsets based on their cytokine profiles.[4] Many skin disorders can be classified on the basis of the predominant cytokine produced by the infiltrating T cells.[7,8] For example Th1-type cells dominate skin lesions in tuberculoid leprosy, localized leishmaniosis, allergic contact dermatitis, lichen planus, early patch/plaque cutaneous T cell lymphoma (CTCL), psoriasis, and acute graft-versus-host disease (GVHD). In contrast Th2-type cells are more prevalent in skin lesions include lepromatous leprosy, disseminated leishmaniosis, acute atopic dermatitis, advanced CTCL/Sézary syndrome, and chronic GVHD. Indeed, the T-helper cytokine profile is paramount to shaping the quality of the adaptive immune effects against

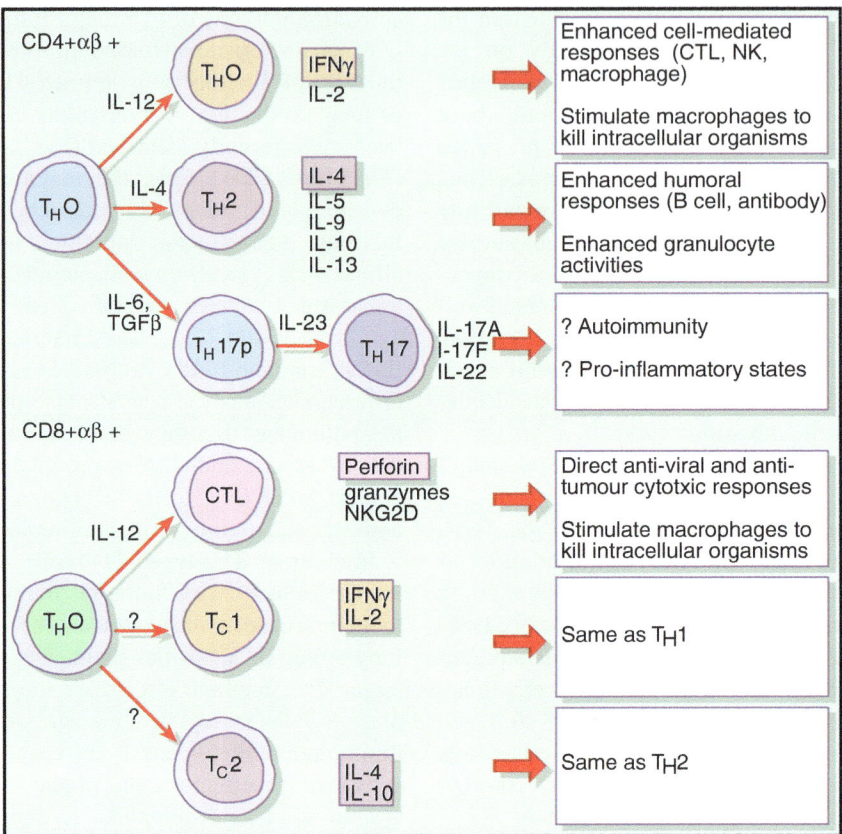

Fig. 6.2. Conventional αβ T cells are represented by two major subsets, CD4+ and CD8+ T cells. CD4 and CD8 T-cell subsets originate from precursors, Th0 and T$_C$0 cells, respectively. The various subsets are functionally defined by which cytokines they produce and the immune responses that are initiated or enhanced

cutaneous pathogens, the type of cutaneous lesions that characterize inflammatory skin diseases, and the potential influence over inflammatory disease in other organs.

Several key factors play a role in determining the differentiation of naive CD4+ T cells into Th1-type or Th2-type cells have been elucidated, and represent a major link between innate and adaptive immunity.[9–11] Dendritic cells (DCs) presenting antigen are highly influenced by the nature of antigen encountered, as well as other pathogen-associated molecular patterns (PAMPs) (e.g., bacterial lipopolysaccharide, unmethylated cytosine-phosphate-guanosine (CpG) oligonucleotides, viral double-stranded RNA), which may bind TLRs on dendritic cells or macrophages. In general, high

levels of PAMPs that bind TLRs stimulate DCs to express co-stimulatory molecules (CD80/86) as well as secrete IL-12 and other Th1-biasing cytokines (e.g., IL-23, IL-27, tumor necrosis factor-α [TNF-α], IFN-γ). Naive CD4 cells, activated in the presence of IL-12 and adequate co-stimulation, for example, differentiate into IFN-γ–producing Th1 cells under the transcription control of factor Stat4 and T-bet. Interleukin-12 can also activate NK cells to produce IFN-γ, further enhancing the Th1 polarization. In contrast, relatively lower levels of PAMPs, while still capable of inducing CD80/86 expression on DCs, are not sufficient to stimulate IL-12 production and by default may activate naive CD4 cells to differentiate into Th2 cells, an effect also influenced by the presence of IL-4.

Conventional T-Cell Trafficking to the Skin

There appears to be at least two major scenarios in which conventional T cells migrate from the circulation, through endothelial-cell–lined dermal capillaries, and into dermis.[12–14] Naive T cells are equipped to continuously course from the circulatory system via high endothelial venules (HEVs) into lymph node after lymph node within the body, migrating through the lymph node until encountering specific antigen. When naive T cells do encounter their antigen in the lymph nodes (e.g., presented by dermal dendritic cells that have migrated from the skin), the signals transmitted via TCR and co-stimulatory receptor CD28 result in not only rapidly expansion and differentiation, but also a series of newly expressed surface molecules. Key among these for enabling cutaneous homing is expression of cutaneous lymphocyte antigen (CLA), an oligosaccharide-bearing ligand for endothelial cell E-selectin that is upregulated in inflamed skin via exposure to primary cytokines (IL-1, TNF-α) and TLR engagement. In addition, chemokine receptors, including CCR4, CCR6, CCR8, and CCR10, may be induced on the activated T cells, and ligands for these can be preferentially found in the perturbed cutaneous environment. The CLA$^+$ T cell, travels through the bloodstream, attaches at sites within the skin where activated endothelium is expressing E-selectin, permitting a tethering and rolling effect that allows for interactions between chemokines and chemokine receptors as well as other adhesion molecules. The activated T cells are then induced to transmigrate through the dermal endothelial cells. Following gradients by chemokines and utilizing integrin binding, the activated T cells may further navigate within the dermis or into the epidermis. In either case, resident DC and other immunocytes (e.g., mast cells, NK cells, macrophages) may further activate and influence T-cell effector function in the cutaneous environment.

A major feature of conventional T cells is their capacity for immunologic memory. Memory T cells (e.g., those that have encountered antigen previously, markedly expanded, and have a relatively low threshold for activation) endow an individual with enhanced immunity in the face of subsequent antigen exposure. Increasingly recognized is that in addition to the rapid recruitment of cutaneous

T cells into inflamed skin described above, there is also a more homeostatic, continuous recruitment of memory T cells that take residence in noninflamed skin.[14] Low levels of constitutively expressed E-selectin, chemokines, and intercellular adhesion molecule 1 (ICAM-1) on dermal endothelial cells of noninflamed skin allow for the population with numerous memory T cells. These "resident skin cells" are not only expanded and more sensitive to activation, but are now appropriately positioned for a more likely subsequent encounter of relevant antigen via direct interactions with potential APCs also resident in the epidermis or dermis. Indeed, the adaptive immune system has evolved to greatly fortify the skin, a crucial interface with the environment, against pathogen invasion. This might in part explain why the intraepidermal population of unconventional $\gamma\delta$ T cells (discussed below) is largely conserved among mammals yet conspicuously absent in human skin.

The distinction of antigenic compartments has direct relevance to the character of the elicited adaptive immune response. For example, phagocytic dendritic cells that internalize bacteria found in the extracellular space can enzymatically cleave potential antigenic peptides and present them in MHC class II molecules on the cell surface. Since MHC-II is a co-receptor for the molecule CD4 found on a portion of T cells, then extracellular antigens are more likely to elicit a CD4$^+$ "helper" T-cell response. Similarly, intracytoplasmic antigens derived from a virally infected cell would favor presentation of viral-derived antigenic peptides within MHC-I, the co-receptor for the CD8 molecule, and elicit a CD8$^+$ "cytolytic" T-cell response aimed at killing antigen-bearing (virally infected) cells. An incompletely understood but major exception to the rule of this compartmentalization of MHC-I (cytosol-derived antigens) and MHC-II (internalized antigen) is known as "cross-presentation," whereby APC-internalized extracellular antigens (e.g., derived from internalized microbes, cancer cells, transplanted histoincompatible tissues) are readily presented not only to CD4$^+$ T cells via MHC-II but also to CD8$^+$ T cells via MHC-I.[15] Thus, professional APCs (e.g., DCs, macrophages, B cells) are the major initiators of various subsets of conventional T cells.

The capacity to distinguish between self and nonself is critical to allowing conventional

T cells to direct appropriate immunologic response (e.g., against microbial invasion) while preventing autoimmune and inflammatory damage to self tissues. Simply defined, immunologic "tolerance" is the lack of an immune response against an antigen that may come about via central (e.g., thymic "negative selection," see above) or peripheral mechanisms. In addition to the induction of anergy by DCs presenting antigen in the absence of co-stimulatory molecules to T cells (as described above), T regulatory cells (T_{reg}) are also major players mediating peripheral tolerance to provide the controls on adaptive immune responses that may cause damage to self tissues.[16] While T_{reg} are best defined functionally, several phenotypic populations have been identified. For example, naturally circulating $CD25^+CD4^+$ T_{reg} have been characterized by their expression of CTLA-4 (e.g., high affinity, negative signal-inducer through T-cell CD28) and secretion of immunosuppressive cytokines (e.g., transforming growth factor-β [TGF-β], IL-10) capable of downregulating both Th1- and Th2-type responses. More recently, T_{reg} production of IL-9 has been shown to enhance mast cell growth and function, and these cells may contribute in various ways to an immune privileged site as modeled by skin-graft rejection.[17] In addition, unconventional T cells may serve regulatory functions (Fig. 6.2).

In sum, conventional $\alpha\beta$ T cells are responsible for coordinating the adaptive immune response by virtue of their exquisite ability to respond to a vast number of potential antigens, to survey the endoreticular system for corresponding specific antigens, to serve as a home to tissues under appropriate signaling, to handle subsequent antigen exposure with a more concentrated and rapid response (i.e., immunologic memory), and to carry out and regulate a wide range of immune responses. These characteristics are all contrasted by so-called unconventional T cells, which nonetheless serve critical, complementary immune activities.

Unconventional T Cells

In contrast to conventional T cells, which are the principal controllers of adaptive immunity, unconventional T-cell subsets do not fit neatly within either arm of the innate/adaptive dichotomy

(Fig. 6.1).[1,2] The two major unconventional T cells, $\gamma\delta$ T cells and iNKT cells, both express TCRs like the conventional (predominantly $\alpha\beta$) T cells that are largely responsible for adaptive immunity, but differ from their conventional counterparts in several ways including their relatively limited TCR repertoires, the nature of the molecules that cause their activation, and their tissue distribution (Fig. 6.3). The $\gamma\delta$ T cells may be further subdivided on the basis of their particular Vγ (particularly in mice) or Vδ (particularly in humans) usage, while the majority of iNKT cells in mice use an invariant α chain paired with one of a few β chains (i.e., Vα14Jα18 paired with one of three beta chains Vβ8.2, Vβ7, or Vβ2, in mice; Vα24Jα18 paired with a variable Vβ11 chain in humans). Both $\gamma\delta$ and iNKT TCRs have antigen recognition properties fundamentally different from those of conventional $\alpha\beta$ TCRs in that they likely bind their respective antigens in a fashion similar to that of antibodies (e.g., independent of MHC presentation and in a fashion more dependent on conformational shape of intact protein or nonprotein compounds) (Fig. 6.4). Mouse models and studies in human have markedly increased our understanding of unconventional T cells and the complementary roles they play in relation to conventional T cells in infection, cancer, and inflammatory disease.

$\gamma\delta$ T Cells

The evolutionarily conserved enrichment of unconventional T cells within the intraepithelial lymphocyte (IEL) compartments (e.g., skin, intestine, genitourinary tract) has enabled further characterization of these cells through the genetic manipulation of mice, and isolation and study of these subsets (Fig. 6.3). Physiologic defense at epithelial surfaces relies on the coordinated activities of various host immune cell populations that must balance the elimination of infected, metabolically stressed, and premalignant cells, with the limitation of a potentially overexuberant response that might otherwise disrupt the epithelial barrier, enhancing cellular damage and transformation. Data derived from several laboratories collectively have shown that IELs, largely represented by $\gamma\delta$ T cells, can act relatively quickly and vigorously in response to infected or damaged epithelial cells, while also

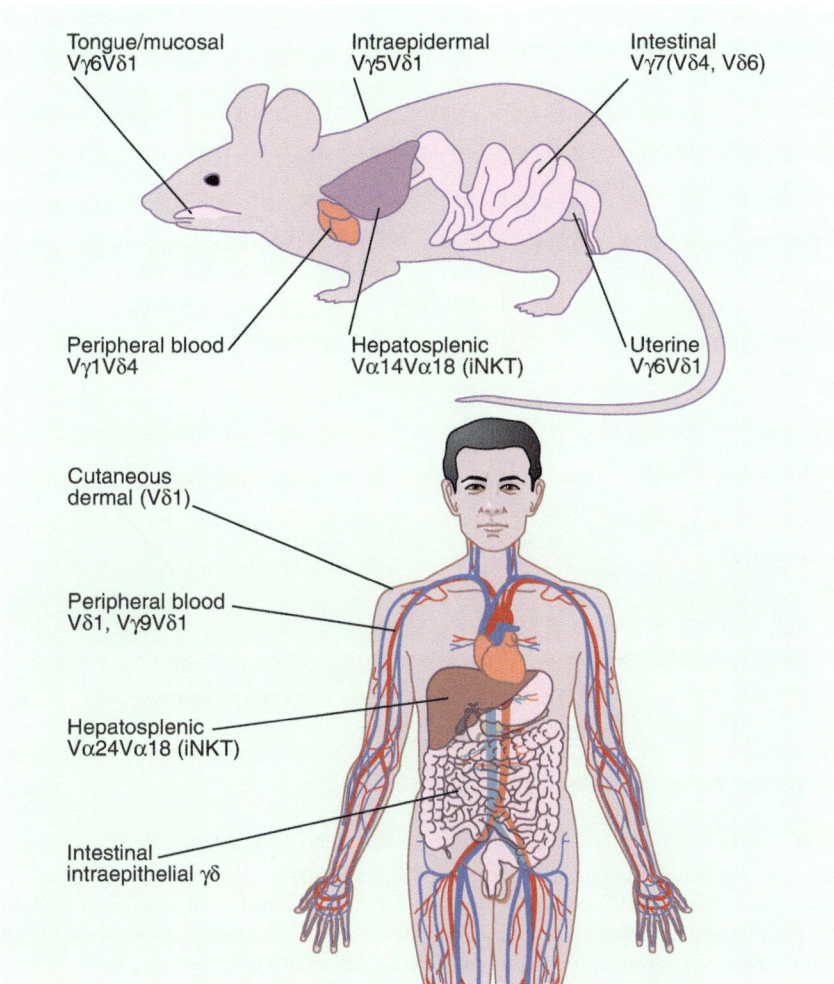

FIG. 6.3. Localization of the various subsets of unconventional T cells in mouse and humans. The γ and δ T-cell receptor chains noted are the predominant types used by γδ T cells within a given epithelium, tissue, or in the peripheral blood

providing an immunoregulatory function (reviewed in Hayday and Tigelaar[18]).

In mouse skin, TCRγδ+ cells account for almost 100% of the resident IELs and are commonly known as dendritic epidermal T cells (DETCs).[19–21] Moreover, DETCs predominantly express an identical Vγ5Vδ1 TCR, while other IEL compartments are also either monoclonal or oligoclonal, expressing distinct albeit related TCRs. Studies of fetal thymic development have shown that such subsets of γδ T cells emerge from the thymus in a series of development "waves," guided to their tissues by the loss and gain of appropriate chemokine receptors.[20,22] Thus, Vγ5Vδ1+ thymocytes are the precursors of

DETCs, and are the first mature T cells to leave the mouse fetal thymus, whereupon they take up residence in the suprabasal epidermis to form a dendritic network unique among T cells.[23]

Several studies have indicated that the particular TCR expressed by an IEL subset stabilizes its association with a particular tissue. For example, developing IEL compartments in the perineonatal period show a more diverse set of γδ TCRs than is evident at 2 to 3 weeks of age[24]; intestinal IELs ectopically expressing a transgenic γδ TCR not normally associated with the gut fail to mature properly,[25] and skin IEL repertoires from TCRδ−/− mice, that *per force* express TCRαβ, seem to decay with time.[26]

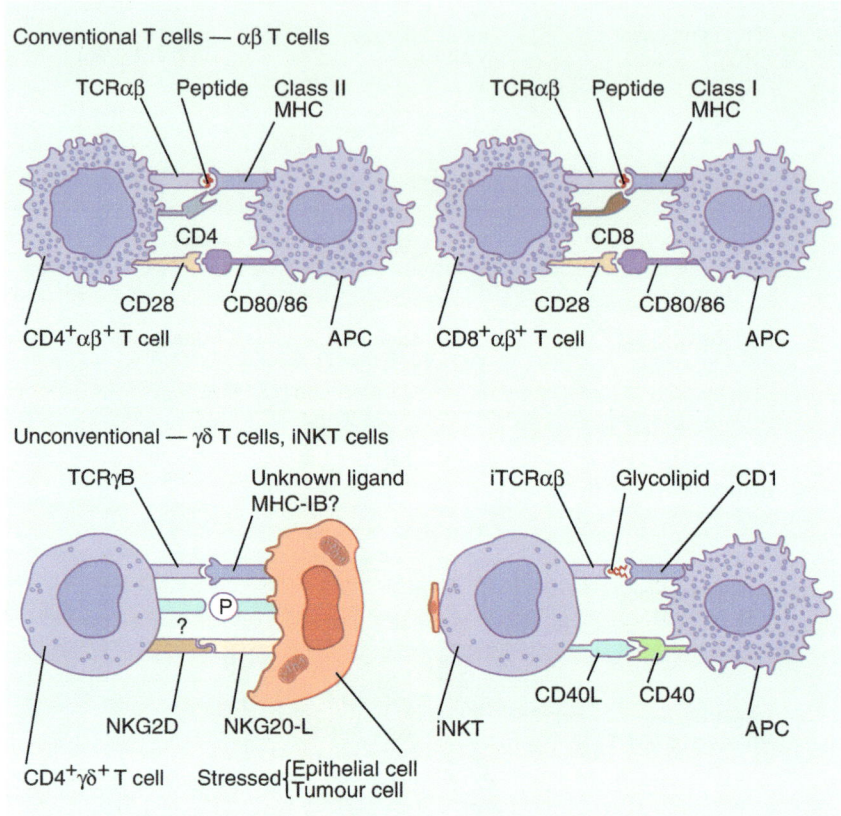

Fig. 6.4. Comparison of antigen presentation and activation signals used by conventional (CD4+ and CD8+ αβ T cells) and unconventional T cells (γδ and NKT cells). Conventional T cells recognize a diverse set of peptide antigens, while unconventional T cells recognize nonpeptide molecules, for example, glycolipids, in the case of NKT cells, and an as-yet-unclear set of intact cell-surface proteins for γδ T cells. APC, antigen-presenting cell

Such data are consistent with the hypothesis that tissue-associated γδ TCRs recognize autologous, tissue-specific ligands expressed by epithelial cells in response to cell stress. Candidates for such ligands include inducible MHC class IB gene products.[27-30] The proposed recognition of generic "stress antigens" clearly distinguishes IELs from conventional systemic T cells that are highly specific for pathogen-encoded determinants that reflect the origin of an infection. Following the recognition of "stress antigens," it has been proposed that IELs kill the stressed epithelial cells and promote wound healing, as a result of which the potentially disastrous systemic dissemination of infected or transformed cells is prevented, while the integrity of the epithelium is maintained.

γδ T Cells and Infection Control

Mice genetically deficient in γδ T cells (i.e., TCRδ[−/−]) have proven an invaluable tool for assessing the contributions of γδ T cells to host responses. However, it should be noted that not all γδ T cells reside within the IEL compartments and the TCRδ[−/−] mouse is not deficient in all IELs.[31] Nonetheless, when challenged with a variety of infectious agents (e.g., *Listeria*, vesicular stomatitis virus, malaria), TCRδ[−/−] mice show enhanced susceptibility particularly at early time points after infection, consistent with the notion that γδ T cells contribute to rapidly mounted protective responses via recognition of common, stress-induced self antigens.[27] In some instances, the contribution of γδ cells to protection is very striking. For example, TCRδ$^{-/-}$ mice infected with the lung pathogen *Nocardia asteroides* failed to mount a characteristic neutrophil attack, as a result of which there was unimpeded bacterial growth and epithelial necrosis.[32] Such data point to an important role for γδ cells in coordinating early, innate responses. This is very different from the development of antigen-specific memory that is a signature of conventional αβ T cells, a difference further highlighted by the finding that γδ cells likewise limit widespread lung damage in response to a noninfectious scenario, ozone exposure.[32] The perspective that γδ cells provide primary immunoprotection, rather than establishing antigen-specific memory, received further support from two independent studies of the responses of young mice to two related parasites, *Cryptosporidium* and the intestinal parasite *Eimeria vermiformis*.[33,34] These studies showed that the protection of young mice relies heavily on the γδ cell compartment, results that are perhaps related to the early ontogenetic development of γδ T-cell subsets.

In the human fetal thymus, γδ T cells that first emerge utilize the Vδ1 chain (paired with various Vγ chains), and these will eventually preferentially populate epithelial tissues such as in the intestine.[18] Thus, while such Vδ1$^+$ T cells comprise only a minor proportion of the γδ T cells present in human blood, these cells constitute a much larger proportion of the human IELs and have also been found enriched within various human epithelial tumors (e.g., lung, kidney, colon carcinomas) and lymphomas.[35] Vδ1 T cells appear to recognize stressed cells via presentation of self lipids presented by CD1 (like iNKT cells, discussed below) or expression of stress-induced MHC class IB molecules. In contrast, Vγ9Vδ2 T cells continually expand and take on a memory phenotype during childhood, presumably because of recurrent exposure to foreign agents, such that they eventually comprise approximately 80% of the γδ T cells of normal adult human blood. These cells recognize, markedly expand, and release cytokines in response to nonpeptide compounds found across a spectrum of microbial pathogens as well as within mammalian cells. Under this paradigm,[36] large numbers of memory Vγ9Vδ2 T cells respond within hours to common molecules produced by microbes, and highly restricted intraepithelial Vδ1 T cells respond to stressed epithelial cells bearing sentinels of danger.

A range of studies has demonstrated a marked expansion of γδ T cells in the blood of systemically infected patients, including those with leprosy, tuberculosis, malaria, tularemia, salmonellosis, brucellosis, ehrlichiosis, or bacterial meningitis due to *Haemophilus influenzae*, *Neisseria meningitidis*, or *Streptococcus pneumoniae*.[37] The broad recognition of the response may be the direct result of Vγ9Vδ2 stimulation by one of two major sets of shared nonpeptide compounds: isopentenyl pyrophosphate (IPP) and other intermediates of the mevalonate pathway; and alkylamines, nonphosphate compounds ubiquitously found in plants and bacteria.[36] In fact, the most natural stimulator of Vγ9Vδ2 T cells appears to be (e)-4-hydroxy-3- methyl-but-2-enyl diphosphate (HMB-PP), one of the precursors of IPP synthesis. Importantly, phosphoantigens are found expressed on many human tumor cells, possibly reflecting their state of raised metabolic stress, and stimulate secretion of cytotoxic molecules by Vγ9Vδ2 cells.[38] Synthetic aminobisphosphonate compounds (e.g., the drugs pamidronate and zoledronate), also stimulate Vγ9Vδ2 cells, but this is more likely due to their simulation of farnesyl diphosphate (FPP) synthetase, leading to accumulation of IPP. A complex of cell-surface apolipoprotein-A (ApoA) and adenosine triphosphatase (ATPase), derived from the mitochondria, can strongly stimulate Vγ9Vδ2 cells.[39] Studies are ongoing to use immunostimulatory phosphoantigen drugs that might be therapeutic against malignancy.[40–43]

Human peripheral Vγ9Vδ2 cells, after their exposure to foreign infectious agents or dying or metabolically stressed host cells (e.g., tumor states), may enhance other immune components as well. Through the rapid secretion of chemokines and T-helper-1 (Th1) cytokines such as IFN-γ, Vγ9Vδ2 cells may stimulate NK, NKT, and αβ T-cell functions.[44] Moreover, Brandes et al.[45] reported that Vγ9Vδ2 cells can also function as professional APCs capable of ingesting, processing, and presenting peptide antigens to stimulate both CD4$^+$ and CD8$^+$ subsets of αβ T cells. These findings collectively describe a scenario whereby Vγ9Vδ2 cells may be very early responders to states of infection or host cellular dysregulation, providing direct cytotoxic effects, altering the local cytokine/chemokine milieu to facilitate other lymphoid cells, and initiating antigen-specific αβ

T-cell immune responses through their capacity to function as APCs much like DCs.

Immunoregulatory Roles of γδ T Cells

Consistent with their contribution to immuno-protection, γδ T cells, particularly those in the IEL compartments, have been shown to be cyto-lytic[46–48]; to express various cytolytic mediators, such as granzymes and FasL[49–51]; and to be potent producers of IFN-γ.[52,53] Nonetheless, analyses of genes encoded by γδ T cells have also revealed overt expression of a spectrum of chemokines and of RNAs encoding for other putative regulatory molecules,[51,54–56] consistent with several findings that immune responses to pathogens are not prop-erly regulated in γδ T-cell deficiency. For example, adult TCRδ$^{-/-}$ mice infected with *Eimeria* showed exaggerated inflammatory responses, reflected in local hemorrhage and shedding of the intestinal epithelium. This phenomenon did not occur in ani-mals deficient in both αβ and γδ T cells, suggesting that the γδ T cells were responsible for regulating the immunoprotective but tissue-damaging αβ T-cell–driven inflammatory response.[57] Similar obser-vations were made in mice infected with *Listeria monocytogenes* where challenge in one testicle induces a contralateral inflammation that is sub-stantially exaggerated in mice lacking γδ cells.[58]

TCRδ$^{-/-}$ mice have also shown accelerated immune responses in noninfectious settings. For example, the αβ T-cell–driven, lupus-like disease of MRL/*lpr* mice was markedly worsened when the mice were rendered deficient in γδ T cells by backcrossing the TCRδ$^{-/-}$ mutation onto the sus-ceptible background; whereas ~25% of MRL/*lpr* mice die (primarily of glomerulonephritis) after 6 months, this figure rises to ~67% for TCRδ$^{-/-}$ MRL/*lpr* mice.[59] Similarly, Shiohara and col-leagues[60] observed that γδ cells would regulate αβ T-cell activity in the skin. By contrast, TCRδ$^{-/-}$ mice showed an exaggerated epidermal infiltration, and failed to develop resistance to αβ T-cell rechal-lenge.[60] Repopulation of the TCRδ$^{-/-}$ mice with γδ T cells prior to challenge restored the wild-type phenotype, revealing the capacity of γδ T cells to regulate αβ T-cell–mediated immunity in the skin. Further studies showed that the locally resident TCRγδ$^+$ DETCs, in the absence of other (e.g., sys-temic recirculating) TCRγδ$^+$ T cells, are sufficient

to protect the epidermis against exaggerated αβ T cell-mediated inflammation.[61] Essentially 100% of TCRδ$^{-/-}$ nonobese diabetic (NOD) mice show a spontaneous dermatitis, most evident in the unprotected ear skin, despite being housed under specific pathogen-free conditions. Likewise, TCRδ$^{-/-}$ FVB mice consistently show exaggerated cutaneous inflammatory responses to contact allergens and irritants. As is the case for γδ T-cell immunoregula-tion in the *Eimeria* model and the MRL/*lpr* model, the spontaneous and augmented contact responses in γδ-deficient mice on susceptible backgrounds are dependent on αβ T cells; that is, the phenotype is absent in double-knockout (TCRβ$^{-/-}$δ$^{-/-}$) mice that lack both αβ and γδ T cells.[61] These results show that γδ cells are natural physiologic regulators of cutaneous inflammation, and that their role in the mouse is nonredundant with that of other cells.

When susceptible γδ-deficient mice were injected at birth with DETC progenitors (Vγ5$^+$ thymocytes obtained from fetal thymi), their epidermis was selectively repopulated with Vγ5$^+$ DETCs, and they did not develop spontaneous or augmented induced dermatitis. The same result was not achieved when mice were repopulated with systemic γδ cells.[61] These studies unequivocally established that cutaneous immunoregulation was affected by local TCRγδ$^+$ IELs, logically suggesting that local T cells might also regulate systemic responses in other sites, for example, the intestinal epithelium, a notion consistent with reports that IEL deficiencies are associated with human inflammatory bowel disease pathologies.[62] Another clear and important finding of these studies was that the regulation of αβ T cell responses by γδ cells occurred in the effector phase of the response.[61] That is to say, the lack of γδ cells was not associated with enhanced priming and increased numbers of responding αβ T cells in the secondary lymphoid tissues, but rather was associated with an exaggerated effect of those cells in the tissue to which they migrated.

Although developing spontaneously, the derma-titis that develops in TCRδ$^{-/-}$ NOD mice can be reduced by housing mice in individually ventilated cages where humidity is low and there is less accu-mulation of chemical irritants. This strong environ-mental influence on αβ T-cell–driven dermatitis shares several properties with the human disorder atopic dermatitis (AD).[63] In addition to similar histologic features, they both show compromised barrier function, exacerbation with chemical irritants, and augmented responses to contact allergens. Moreover, they are both strikingly influenced by genetic modifiers: thus, TCRδ$^{-/-}$ C57BL/6 mice show little or no difference in cutaneous inflammation by comparison to their cage-matched TCRδ$^+$ controls. This observation may be exploited via genetic mapping to identify genes that regulate the development of dermatitis that occurs in the absence of γδ T cells; such genes may have broad implications for the local control of cutaneous inflammation and for AD.

However, an important aspect of the gene expression data that have been obtained for γδ cells is the likely pleiotropy of γδ cells. O'Briens group[64] studying the γδ cell response to enterovirus infection of mice concluded that γδ cells expressing Vγ1$^+$ TCRs were antiinflammatory while those with Vγ4$^+$ TCRs were proinflammatory.[64]

γδ$^+$ T Cells and Tumor Surveillance

A number of studies in mice have pointed to the capacity of γδ cells to regulate malignancy. Almost a decade ago, Mak's group noted that mice expressing a TCRVγδ chain transgene were spontaneously resistant to acute T-cell leukemias, although they did not reject nonhematopoietic tumors. By comparison to IELs, TCRVγδ$^+$ cells are most often found in the lymphoid organs and blood, and TCRVγδ$^+$ hybridomas isolated from the transgenic mice reacted in vitro against almost all hematopoietic tumor cell lines tested, in a fashion independent of MHC class I, MHC class II, or the transporter associated with antigen processing (TAP) peptide transporter.[65] Shortly thereafter, it was shown that *lpr* mice with mutations in the *Fas* gene rapidly and spontaneously developed massive splenic B-cell malignancies if the mice lacked both αβ T cells and γδ cells, but that this was not the case if either T-cell subset was present.[66] Both sets of data point to a capacity of γδ cells to regulate the development of hematologic malignancies, consistent with which human clinical trials are now ongoing in which the enhanced activities of γδ cells are being harnessed against non-Hodgkin's lymphoma and multiple myeloma.[67]

Tumors have been found to form more readily in TCRδ$^{-/-}$ mice following injection of squamous cell carcinoma (SCC) or melanoma tumor cell lines.[68,69]

Suggesting that γδ T cells regulate carcinogenesis more broadly, chemically induced colorectal adenocarcinoma reportedly occurs with greater frequency in γδ-deficient mice.[70] Although the mechanisms by which γδ cells exert their effects are incompletely understood, there are numerous instances in which TCRγδ$^+$ IELs have been shown to directly kill transformed or stressed epithelial cell targets, again in an MHC-independent fashion.[68,71] Additionally, their activation-induced capacity to make IFN-γ in the early stages of tumor growth appears to be important.[69] The notion that the different T-cell compartments may contribute to tumor surveillance in distinct fashions and at distinct stages of tumor growth has been further explored in a two-stage system of chemical carcinogenesis, wherein a single epicutaneous application of dimethylbenzanthracene (DMBA) is followed by repeated application of low concentrations of the tumor promoting agent (TPA).[72] The two-stage protocol permits one to measure two features of carcinogenesis: the incidence of *tumor development* via monitoring of papilloma formation, and the frequency of *tumor progression* via quantitation of the conversion of papillomas into frank SCC. In TCRδ$^{-/-}$ FVB mice, the appearance of papillomas and the progression to carcinoma were both significantly increased.[73] These data are consistent with the proposal that γδ T cells can inhibit the early stages of tumor development (see above), but that they also limit progression to carcinoma.[66] One may hypothesize that these respective effects of γδ cells may reflect their utilization of two different mechanisms.

A clue to this hypothesis was provided by the study of tumor incidence and progression in mice lacking αβ T cells.[73] In this case, there was a much less obvious increase in papilloma development. Moreover, under an intense regimen of chemical promotion, tumors were *less* likely to progress to the carcinoma stage than was the case in wild-type mice.[73] This finding highlighted a paradoxical tumor-promoting effect attributable to αβ T cells, a concept that is consistent with other experimental systems where pro-tumor contributions of αβ T cells have been reported.[74,75] Intriguingly, these results suggest that γδ cells might limit tumor progression by limiting the proinflammatory responses of αβ T cells, much as they have been described to do in several other systems (see above). More recently, the identification and characterization of a proinflammatory, tumor-promoting population of CD8[+] αβ T cells has suggested a cellular target and mechanism of γδ T-cell inhibition of carcinogenesis.[76]

In sum, as is the case in the host response to infection and to physical stress, γδ cells may exert two qualitatively distinct effects: a rapidly responsive immunoprotective effect (cytolysis, IFN-γ, etc.) and a critical immunoregulatory mechanism. Although the latter is poorly understood, it is clear from murine systems that γδ cells in some circumstances can kill or otherwise dysregulate APCs, thereby limiting the αβ T-cell response.[77,78] Moreover, γδ T-cell elimination of activated Fas[+] αβ T cells mediating Coxsackie B3 virus-induced myocarditis has been implicated as a mechanism by which γδ T cells may again limit αβ T-cell–mediated immunopathology.[79]

Within human epithelial compartments, most notably gut Vδ1[+] T cells, γδ T cells may express surface NKG2D, a molecule found on two other major subsets of cells with cytotoxic potential, namely CD8[+] αβ T cells and NK cells. NKG2D engagement by one of its several identified ligands, including MHC class I chain-related A and B (MICA and MICB) in humans[80] and retinoic acid early (Rae)-1 in mice,[81] provides a co-stimulatory function and targets cellular destruction. These molecules are upregulated under cellular stress and are expressed on a variety of tumor cells[82] including melanoma.[83] They may act as signals that target host cells for destruction by locally resident or infiltrating γδ T cells as well as other NKG2D[+] lymphoid cells.

Invariant Natural Killer Cells

Invariant natural killer (iNKT) cells, another type of unconventional T cells, have an important role in recognizing and responding to certain types of bacteria, fungi, and parasites.[84] Other activities in cancer and autoimmune disease are under active investigation. In a recent review, Kronenberg[85] has proposed that iNKT cells are defined by reactivity to tetramers of the nonclassic CD1d molecule complexed with the glycolipid α-galactosylceramide (αGalCer) (see below). This functional definition of iNKT circumvents the confusion over the expression of the natural killer cell markers (NK1.1 in mice, and CD161 in humans) that, along with TCR expression, traditionally had been used to

define the iNKT subset. In mice, almost all NK1.1 expressing T cells are specific for αGalCer, while only a small percent of CD161-expressing T cells express the iNKT receptor chains and react with αGalCer in humans.

Experiments in mice have demonstrated that iNKT cells are selected in the thymus at the double positive stage of T-cell development. Those cells that have randomly rearranged and displayed the Vα14-Jα18 alpha chain, coupled with Vβ8.2, Vβ7 or Vβ2 forming the CD1d-specific T-cell receptor of iNKT cells, are selected by the nonclassic MHC molecule CD1d.[86,87] Interestingly, the selection is mediated by double-positive thymocytes that express CD1d and not thymic epithelial cells, which are responsible for the positive and negative selection of non-NKT thymocytes. These newly selected "pre-iNKT cells" undergo numerous rounds of division and acquire memory markers. Finally, the CD8 chain is downregulated leaving mature iNKT populations that are either CD4[+] or double-negative (although in humans a percentage of CD8α[+] NKT cells has been reported).[88,89] In mice, upon exit from the thymus, the iNKT cells reside primarily in the liver (10% to 40% of murine liver lymphocytes) with spleen, thymus, blood, and bone marrow containing less than 1% iNKT cells. In sharp contrast, human liver contains less than 1% iNKT cells with other sites such as blood (0.2% circulating of circulating lymphocytes) and spleen containing percentages of NKT that are similar to or lower than those seen in mice.[90–93] iNKT cells are not common in the lymph nodes and are rarely observed in intestinal mucosa.

Given the reactivity to glycolipids that iNKT cells display, there is keen interest in iNKT cells and the immune response to bacteria, which contain glycolipids in their cell wall that could potentially be displayed on CD1d molecules and present to NKT cells.[94,95] Infection with the lipopolysaccharide (LPS)-containing gram-negative bacterium *Salmonella typhimurium*, resulted in IFN-γ production from iNKT cells. The production of IFN-γ by iNKT in this model could be induced by coculturing the iNKT with DCs supplemented with either LPS or IL-12 in the absence of *Salmonella*. Thus it was suggested that a microbial ligand (i.e., LPS) could activate the DCs to produce IL-12, which had previously been demonstrated to activate iNKT to produce IFN-γ.[95] This effect, however, required the expression of CD1d on the surface of the DCs, suggesting that the activation of the iNKT was more than merely a bystander effect. In contrast, studies of activation of iNKT cells by the LPS-negative bacteria *Sphingomonas* revealed two related glycosylceramides isolated from the CD1d molecules, strongly suggesting that these microbial derived antigens were recognized by the NKT receptor.[94,96]

Thus the iNKT cell has two distinct activation pathways, one involving a self antigen and one using exogenous antigen, to guide their response to different types of bacterial challenge. It must be noted that iNKT-intact and iNKT-deficient mice have a similar outcome when challenged with *Salmonella*. This implies that there are other mechanisms that can compensate for the loss of iNKT reactivity, but the mechanism may still be instructive for other strains of bacteria. In contrast, mice lacking iNKT cells are unable to clear *Sphingomonas* when compared to iNKT intact mice when given a low dose of bacteria. Under high-dose challenge, mice with an intact iNKT compartment show signs of sepsis and toxic shock, while those lacking iNKT cells are spared. This indicates that the response of iNKT and the resulting level of cytokine production is variable depending on the degree on iNKT activation, and as such can have substantial effects on the outcome of infection on the host.[97]

iNKT Cells and Tumor Surveillance

iNKT cells appear to also play a role in tumor immunosurveillance as seen in the methylcholanthrene (MCA)-induced sarcoma model. Initial experiments involved comparing tumor susceptibility between mice lacking iNKT cells (e.g., Jα18$^{-/-}$) and wild-type mice. Mice lacking iNKT cells were more susceptible to the MCA-induced sarcoma.[98,99] Liver-derived iNKT cells, adoptively transferred to the iNKT-deficient mice, prevented the cancers from forming.[100,101] The same investigative group also compared different NKT subsets, for example, from the thymus, spleen, and finally the CD4($^-$) versus CD4($^+$) liver derived NKT cells. Only the CD4($^-$) liver-derived subset conferred tumor protection.[102]

Using a lung metastasis model of B16F10 melanoma, it was revealed that liver-derived iNKT cells adoptively transferred into Jα18$^{-/-}$ mice, only in animals receiving αGalCer to enhance NKT responses, limited lung metastasis compared to that in thymic-derived NKT cells. However, if thymic NKT cells were taken form IL4$^{-/-}$ mice, they too could limit lung metastasis in this model. The authors argue that the thymic NKT from IL4$^{-/-}$ mice may produce IFN-γ, early production of which has been demonstrated to limit tumor formation and promote tumor rejection. Interferon-γ production was not directly demonstrated in the transferred population, so alternative explanations such as different cytokine profiles produced by the different NKT subsets could also play a key role in the outcome of the cancer progression/metastasis. iNKT subsets (thymic and liver) from wild-type mice were cocultured with liver mononuclear cells in the presence of αGalCer. There was no difference noted in the ability of each subset to promote IFN-γ production from the NK cells or the amount of CD86 upregulated on liver DCs, suggesting that the differences seen in the tumor experiments was not a result of the subsets interacting with the presenting DC cells/innate immune system (NK) in a starkly different manner.[102]

iNKT Cells in Inflammatory Disease

Work by Askenase and colleagues[103] illustrates the role iNKT may play in the initiation of contact sensitivity (CS) and delayed-type hypersensitivity (DTH). Allergic contact hypersensitivity involves sensitizing mice to an antigen, typically by topical application to the abdominal skin, followed 4 days later with a challenge application to the ears. The resultant swelling is then measured by micrometer. The reaction is antigen specific and dependent both on CD4 and CD8 T-cell populations. Mice deficient in iNKT are unable to mount a full DTH response. The hypothesized mechanism involves an immediate iNKT activation by endogenous glycolipids presented in context with CD1d. These iNKT cells then preferentially produce IL-4, which assists B-1 type B cells, a T-cell–independent antigen-specific B-cell population found in the peritoneum, which produces IgM antibodies that assist in the later recruitment of antigen-specific T cells. Of interest, the iNKT cells that produce the IL-4 in this model are located in the liver and are found there within minutes of the challenge antigen application.[104]

In numerous autoimmune conditions (e.g., diabetes, multiple sclerosis, rheumatoid arthritis, and lupus), in both human disease states and mouse models, there appears to be an overall decrease in the number of iNKT cells in both mice and humans.[105] The most widely studied autoimmune model linking iNKT activity and disease progression and prevention has been in the NOD mouse model. Mice lacking CD1d molecules had a higher penetrance and a more severe course of disease compared to mice with intact CD1d expression.[106–108] Upregulating the activity of the existing population of iNKT cells by increasing the level of CD1d ameliorates disease progression.[109] The mechanism appeared to involve a Th2 bias in the pancreas to islet autoantigens. Activation of the NKT by repeated treatments with αGalCer resulted in slower disease progression.[110–112] This protocol effected the DC population in the draining lymph nodes of the pancreas where a more tolerogenic subset of DC was observed.[113] Thus the action of NKT can be focused on downstream lymphocyte populations. This is clearly illustrated when naive T cells expressing a diabetogenic TCR are cocultured with NKT cells. The cells are not prevented from initial activation, but their ability to produce IL-2 and IFN-γ is retarded. This suppressive activity requires direct cell-to-cell contact.[114]

Experimental autoimmune encephalomyelitis (EAE) is a murine model of multiple sclerosis. It closely follows the disease course in humans in that it shows periods of disease progression followed by remission followed by relapse. In humans, and in some murine EAE models the number of iNKT cells present in diseased individuals is reduced compared to normal controls.[115–117] Treating mice with αGalCer, in some cases, ameliorates disease in a fashion similar to that seen in diabetes, in that a Th2 cytokine bias was noted.[118–120] Indeed, mice deficient in IL-10 or IL-4 were not protected from developing EAE when administered αGalCer, again suggesting that a Th2 response by NKT cells is critical to ameliorating disease.[121] However, depending on the mouse model and other variables including timing and dose of αGalCer given, the treatment may not affect the ultimate course of the disease.[122] Further studies using a truncated form of a αGalCer seems to bias responding iNKT cells more strongly to a Th2 response compared to a αGalCer, and reduced the severity of EAE in these mice.[123] Thus, in two models of autoimmune disease, NKT responses that skew Th2 are desired.

The iNKT cells, as illustrated in responses to bacteria, tumor surveillance, and contact hypersensitivity,

can contribute to a Th1-mediated response, while in autoimmune models, their role in prevention of disease progression involves biasing the immune response to Th2. This bipolar response of iNKT is reflected in its ability to produce significant quantities of either type of cytokine profile upon stimulation. How one response is favored over the other in a given immune response to either self (e.g., autoimmunity, cancer) or nonself (e.g., bacteria and other pathogens) is currently unknown. Indeed, there is growing recognition that iNKT cells may play a substantial role in cutaneous inflammatory diseases such as psoriasis.[124]

Evolving Paradigms of Unconventional T Cells

To what degree are these mouse studies relevant to the immunoprotection and immunoregulation in the skin of humans? One obstacle to direct extrapolation is the fact that there is no obvious homologue of murine (or bovine) TCRγδ DETC in the human epidermis. However, Holtmeier and colleagues[125] have provided clear evidence for human dermal γδ cells displaying a TCR repertoire that could be distinguished from that of systemic γδ cells.[125] There is likewise a human, gut-associated TCRγδ+ IEL compartment that is distinct from systemic γδ cells. Another possibility is that the crucial mechanisms exerted by murine DETCs are affected by other, non-TCRγδ+ cells in the human. A comprehensive comparison of murine gut–associated TCRγδ+ and TCRαβ+ IELs identified numerous genes expressed substantially more strongly by the latter cells, but essentially no γδ-specific genes. It was hypothesized that the TCRαβ+ population may contain within it a set of "unconventional" TCRαβ+ cells that very closely resembled TCRγδ+ cells.[1,126] In the mouse intestine, substantial numbers of CD8γδ+ TCRαβ+ IELs resemble γδ IEL in their limited TCR diversity and in their expression of strikingly similar gene profiles.[31] Moreover, Poussier and colleagues[127] showed that CD8γδ+ TCRαβ+ cells regulate systemic αβ T-cell–driven colitis. Hence, γδ cells may be mere prototypes of unconventional T cells that in different tissues in different species play important roles in the rapid response to challenge and in the regulation of systemic responses.[31,126] This perspective is consistent with the observations that the most overt phenotypes of TCRδ−/− occur in the skin, where there are few if any $\alpha\beta$ T-cell populations that might compensate for their loss. In human skin, candidates for a parallel population may be found within the aforementioned various subsets of $CD8^+$ $CCR8^+$ $\alpha\beta$ T cells, $\gamma\delta$ T cells, and iNKT cells that have been identified in normal dermis at much higher numbers than previously appreciated.

The $\gamma\delta$ T cells have features of both innate and adaptive immunity, and may serve critical roles in bridging these types of responses. The recent identification of the capacity of $V\gamma9V\delta2^+$ T cells to function as APCs[45] adds yet another layer of complexity to our understanding of $\gamma\delta$ T-cell biology. Brandes and colleagues[45] demonstrated that, comparable to dendritic cells, $V\gamma9V\delta2^+$ T cells can express co-stimulatory molecules and present conventional peptide antigens for the primary stimulation of $CD4^+$ and $CD8^+$ $\alpha\beta$ T-cell responses. Hence, $V\gamma9V\delta2^+$ T cells may provide the ultimate link of innate and adaptive immunity by rapid expansion and secretion of cytokines within hours of encountering any pathogenic organisms (e.g., through recognition of IPP and HMB-PP), and processing and presentation of foreign peptide to prime antigen-specific $\alpha\beta$ T cells and coordinate a more directed attack. In considering the potential avenues of $\gamma\delta$ T-cell immunotherapy, it may ultimately prove possible to utilize peripheral $\gamma\delta$ T cells in antitumor protocols in which such cells are activated and exposed to tumor antigen, thus potentially serving a dual role of stimulating both $\gamma\delta$ T-cell–directed antitumor activity as well as stimulation of tumor antigen-specific CD4 and CD8 $\alpha\beta$ T-cell responses. The recent identification of the importance of certain cytokines to the enhancement of cytotoxic activity of phosphoantigen stimulated $V\gamma9V\delta2^+$ T cells is a key step toward engaging these unconventional T cells in cancer immunotherapy.[128]

Conclusion

The skin and immune system are functionally integrated to provide a first line of microbial defense, and T lymphocytes are major cellular coordinators of response. The discovery of T cells and how their T-cell receptors (TCRs) recognize and respond to cells presenting peptides in the grooves of their cell-surface major histocompatibility complex (MHC) molecules gave insight into the antigen-specific responses fundamental to immunity following exposure to (or vaccination against) microbial infections, as well as the mechanisms underlying allograft rejection and autoimmunity. However, there is also a more recently appreciated set of unconventional T cells that differ from peptide-recognizing conventional T cells in several major ways. This chapter discussed how (predominantly $TCR\alpha\beta^+$) conventional T cells are complemented by a nonredundant set of unconventional T cells, specifically $TCR\gamma\delta^+$ T cells and invariant $TCR\alpha\beta^+$ natural killer T (iNKT) cells, to mediate and regulate immune responses to infectious microorganisms and to developing and established neoplasms. While conventional T cells are primarily responsible for the more antigen-specific reactivity and immunologic memory characteristics of adaptive immunity, unconventional T cells have a relatively limited TCR diversity, appear to respond to foreign or self molecules in a more generic and more rapid fashion, and have a fundamentally different tissue distribution. To explore the function of these major categories of T cells, various studies have been performed in mice, particularly those that are genetically deficient in specific T-cell subsets. In addition, studies of conventional and unconventional T cells have identified important parallels and differences between laboratory animals and humans, opening potential novel strategies to immunotherapy.

References

1. Pennington DJ, Vermijlen D, Wise EL, et al. The integration of conventional and unconventional T cells that characterizes cell-mediated responses. Adv Immunol 2005;87:27–59.
2. Kaufman SH. Gamma / delta and other unconventional T lymphocytes: what do they see and what do they do? Proc Natl Acad Sci USA 1996;93:2272–9.
3. Girardi M. Cutaneous biology of T cells. In: Advances in Dermatology, vol. 20. New York: Mosby, 2004.
4. Kronenberg M, Engel I. On the road: progress in finding the unique pathway of invariant NKT cell differentiation. Curr Opin Immunol 2007;19:186–93.
5. Janeway CA, Travers P, Walport M, et al. In: Immunobiology 5. New York: Garland, 2001.
6. Weaver CT, Hatton RD, Mangan PR, et al. IL-17 family cytokines and the expanding diversity of effector T cell lineages. Annu Rev Immunol 2007;25:821–52.

7. Modlin RL. Th1–Th2 paradigm: insights from leprosy. J Invest Dermatol 1994;102:828–32.

8. Biedermann T, Rocken M, Carballido JM. TH1 and TH2 lymphocyte development and regulation of TH cell-mediated immune responses of the skin. J Invest Dermatol Symp Proc 2004;9:5–14.

9. Heath WR, Carbone FR. Dangerous liaisons. Nature 2003;425(6957):460–1.

10. Iwasaki A, Medzhitov R. Toll-like receptor control of the adaptive immune responses. Nat Immunol 2004;5:987–95.

11. Renn CN, Sanchez DJ, Ochoa MT, et al. TLR activation of Langerhans cell-like dendritic cells triggers an antiviral immune response. J Immunol 2006;177:298–305.

12. Robert C, Kupper TS. Inflammatory skin diseases, T cells, and immune surveillance. N Engl J Med 1999;341:1817–28.

13. Kupper TS. T cells, immunosurveillance, and cutaneous immunity. J Dermatol Sci 2000;24:S41–5.

14. Clark RA, Chong B, Mirchandani N, et al. The vast majority of CLA +T cells are resident in normal skin. J Immunol 2006;176:4431–9.

15. Ackerman AL, Cresswell P. Cellular mechanisms governing cross-presentation of exogenous antigens. Nat Immunol 2004;5:678–684.

16. Beissert S, Schwarz A, Schwarz T. Regulatory T cells. J Invest Dermatol 2006;126:15–24.

17. Lu L-F, Lind EF, Gondek DC, et al. Mast cells are essential intermediaries in regulatory T-cell tolerance. Nature 2006;442:997–1002.

18. Hayday A, Tigelaar R. Immunoregulation in the tissues by gammadelta T cells. Nat Rev Immunol 2003;3:233–42.

19. Asarnow DM, Goodman T, LeFrancois L, et al. Distinct antigen receptor repertoires of two classes of murine epithelium-associated T cells. Nature 1989;341:60–2.

20. Allison JP, Havran WL. The immunobiology of T cells with invariant gamma delta antigen receptors. Annu Rev Immunol 1991;9:679–705.

21. Goodman T, Lefrancois L. Expression of the gamma-delta T-cell receptor on intestinal CD8+ intraepithelial lymphocytes. Nature 1988;333:855–8.

22. Itohara S, Farr AG, Lafaille JJ, et al. Homing of a gamma delta thymocyte subset with homogeneous T-cell receptors to mucosal epithelia. Nature 1990;343:754–7.

23. Bergstresser PR, Sullivan S, Streilein JW, et al. Origin and function of Thy-1+ dendritic epidermal cells in mice. J Invest Dermatol 1985;85:85s–90s.

24. Kyes S, Pao W, Hayday A. Influence of site of expression on the fetal gamma delta T-cell receptor repertoire. Proc Natl Acad Sci U S A 1991;88:7830–3.

25. Bonneville M, Itohara S, Krecko EG, et al. Transgenic mice demonstrate that epithelial homing of gamma/delta T cells is determined by cell lineages independent of T cell receptor specificity. J Exp Med 1990;171:1015–26.

26. Chien YH, Jores R, Crowley MP. Recognition by gamma/delta T cells. Annu Rev Immunol 1996;14:511–32.

27. Janeway CA Jr, Jones B, Hayday A. Specificity and function of T cells bearing gamma delta receptors. Immunol Today 1988;9:73–6.

28. Iwashima M, Green A, Bonyhadi M, et al. Expression of a fetal gamma delta T-cell receptor in adult mice triggers a non-MHC-linked form of selective depletion. Int Immunol 1991;3:385–93.

29. Steele CR, Oppenheim DE, Hayday AC. Gamma(delta) T cells: non-classical ligands for non-classical cells. Curr Biol 2000;10:R282–5.

30. Wu J, Groh V, Spies T. T cell antigen receptor engagement and specificity in the recognition of stress-inducible MHC class I-related chains by human epithelial gamma delta T cells. J Immunol 2002;169:1236–40.

31. Pennington DJ, Silva-Santos B, Shires J, et al. The inter-relatedness and interdependence of mouse T cell receptor gammadelta+ and alphabeta+ cells. Nat Immunol 2003;4:991–8.

32. King DP, Hyde DM, Jackson KA, et al. Cutting edge: protective response to pulmonary injury requires gamma delta T lymphocytes. J Immunol 1999;162:5033–6.

33 Waters WR, Harp JA. Cryptosporidium parvum infection in T-cell receptor (TCR)-alpha- and TCR-delta-deficient mice. Infect Immun 1996;64:1854–7.

34. Ramsburg E, Tigelaar R, Craft J, et al. Age-dependent requirement for gammadelta T cells in the primary but not secondary protective immune response against an intestinal parasite. J Exp Med 2003;198:1403–14.

35. Fisch P, Meuer E, Pende D, et al. Control of B cell lymphoma recognition via natural killer inhibitory receptors implies a role for human Vgamma9/Vdelta2 T cells in tumor immunity. Eur J Immunol 1997;27:3368–79.

36. Holtmeier W, Pfander M, Hennemann A, et al. The TCR delta repertoire in normal human skin is restricted and distinct from the TCR-delta repertoire in the peripheral blood. J Invest Dermatol 2001;116:275–80.

37. Chen ZW, Letvin NL. Vgamma2Vdelta2+ T cells and anti-microbial immune responses. Microbes Infect 2003;5:491–8.

38. Bonneville M, Fournie JJ. Sensing cell stress and transformation through Vgamma9Vdelta2 T cell-

mediated recognition of the isoprenoid pathway metabolites. Microbes Infect 2005;7:503–9.

39. Scotet E, Martinez LO, Grant E, et al. Tumor recognition following Vgamma9Vdelta2 T cell receptor interactions with a surface F1–ATPase-related structure and apolipoprotein A-I. Immunity 2005;22:71–80.

40. Wilhelm M, Kunzmann V, Eckstein S, et al. Gammadelta T cells for immune therapy of patients with lymphoid malignancies. Blood 2003;102:200–6.

41. Lozupone F, Pende D, Burgio VL, et al. Effect of human natural killer and gammadelta T cells on the growth of human autologous melanoma xenografts in SCID mice. Cancer Res 2004;64:378–85.

42. Liu Z, Guo BL, Gehrs BC, et al. Ex vivo expanded human Vgamma9Vdelta2+ gammadelta-T cells mediate innate antitumor activity against human prostate cancer cells in vitro. J Urol 2005;173:1552–6.

43. Wang L, Kamath A, Das H, et al. Antibacterial effect of human V gamma 2V delta 2 T cells in vivo. J Clin Invest 2001;108:1349–57.

44. Smith AL, Hayday AC. An alphabeta T-cell-independent immunoprotective response towards gut coccidia is supported by gammadelta cells. Immunology 2000;101:325–32.

45. Brandes M, Willimann K, Moser B. Professional antigen-presentation function by human γδT cells. Science 2005;309:264–8.

46. Kaminski MJ, Cruz PD Jr, Bergstresser PR, et al. Killing of skin-derived tumor cells by mouse dendritic epidermal T-cells. Cancer Res 1993;53:4014–9.

47. Havran WL, Poenie M, Tigelaar RE, et al. Phenotypic and functional analysis of gamma delta T cell receptor-positive murine dendritic epidermal clones. J Immunol 1989;142:1422–8.

48. Guy-Grand D, Malassis-Seris M, Briottet C, et al. Cytotoxic differentiation of mouse gut thymodependent and independent intraepithelial T lymphocytes is induced locally. Correlation between functional assays, presence of perforin and granzyme transcripts, and cytoplasmic granules. J Exp Med 1991;173:1549–52.

49. Mohamadzadeh M, McGuire MJ, Smith DJ, et al. Functional roles for granzymes in murine epidermal gamma(delta) T-cell-mediated killing of tumor targets. J Invest Dermatol 1996;107:738–42.

50. Krahenbuhl O, Gattesco S, Tschopp J. Murine Thy-1+ dendritic epidermal T cell lines express granule-associated perforin and a family of granzyme molecules. Immunobiology 1992;184:392–401.

51. Shires J, Theodoridis E, Hayday AC. Biological insights into TCRgamma delta+ and TCRalpha beta+ intraepithelial lymphocytes provided by serial analysis of gene expression (SAGE). Immunity 2001;15:419–34.

52. Huber H, Descossy P, Regier E, et al. Activation of phenotypically heterogeneous murine T cell receptor gamma delta + dendritic epidermal T cells by self-antigen(s). Int Arch Allergy Immunol 1995;107:498–507.

53. Matsue H, Cruz PD Jr, Bergstresser PR, et al. Profiles of cytokine mRNA expressed by dendritic epidermal T cells in mice. J Invest Dermatol 1993;101(4):537–42.

54. Boismenu R, Havran WL. Modulation of epithelial cell growth by intraepithelial gamma delta T cells. Science 1994;266:1253–5.

55. Boismenu R, Feng L, Xia YY, et al. Chemokine expression by intraepithelial gamma delta T cells. Implications for the recruitment of inflammatory cells to damaged epithelia. J Immunol 1996;157(3):985–92.

56. Fahrer AM, Konigshofer Y, Kerr EM, et al. Attributes of gammadelta intraepithelial lymphocytes as suggested by their transcriptional profile. Proc Natl Acad Sci USA 2001;98:10261–6.

57. Roberts SJ, Smith AL, West AB, et al. T-cell alpha beta + and gamma delta + deficient mice display abnormal but distinct phenotypes toward a natural, widespread infection of the intestinal epithelium. Proc Natl Acad Sci USA 1996;93:11774–9.

58. Mukasa A, Hiromatsu K, Matsuzaki G, et al. Bacterial infection of the testis leading to autoaggressive immunity triggers apparently opposed responses of alpha beta and gamma delta T cells. J Immunol 1995;155:2047–56.

59. Peng SL, Madaio MP, Hayday AC, et al. Propagation and regulation of systemic autoimmunity by gammadelta T cells. J Immunol 1996;157:5689–98.

60. Shiohara T, Moriya N, Hayakawa J, et al. Resistance to cutaneous graft-vs.-host disease is not induced in T cell receptor delta gene-mutant mice. J Exp Med 1996;183:1483–9.

61. Girardi M, Lewis J, Glusac E, et al. Resident skin-specific gammadelta T cells provide local, nonredundant regulation of cutaneous inflammation. J Exp Med 2002;195:855–67.

62. Van Damme N, De Keyser F, Demetter P, et al. The proportion of Th1 cells, which prevail in gut mucosa, is decreased in inflammatory bowel syndrome. Clin Exp Immunol 2001;125:383–90.

63. Beltrani VS. The clinical spectrum of atopic dermatitis. J Allergy Clin Immunol 1999;104:S87–98.

64. Huber SA, Graveline D, Newell MK, et al. gamma 1+ T cells suppress and V gamma 4+ T cells promote susceptibility to coxsackievirus B3–induced myocarditis in mice. J Immunol 2000;165:4174–81.

65. Penninger JM, Wen T, Timms E, et al. Spontaneous resistance to acute T-cell leukaemias in TCRV gamma 1.1J gamma 4C gamma 4 transgenic mice. Nature 1995;375:241–4.

66. Peng SL, Robert ME, Hayday AC, et al. A tumor-suppressor function for Fas (CD95) revealed in T cell-deficient mice. J Exp Med 1996;184(3):1149–54.

67. Wilhelm M, Kunzmann V, Eckstein S, et al. Gamma delta T cells for immune therapy of patients with lymphoid malignancies. Blood 2003;102:200–6.

68. Girardi M, Oppenheim DE, Steele CR, et al. Regulation of cutaneous malignancy by gammadelta T cells. Science 2001;294:605–9.

69. Gao Y, Yang W, Pan M, et al. Gamma delta T cells provide an early source of interferon gamma in tumor immunity. J Exp Med 2003;198:433–42.

70. Matsuda S, Kudoh S, Katayama S. Enhanced formation of azoxymethane-induced colorectal adenocarcinoma in gammadelta T lymphocyte-deficient mice. Jpn J Cancer Res 2001;92(8):880–5.

71. Havran WL, Chien YH, Allison JP. Recognition of self antigens by skin-derived T cells with invariant gamma delta antigen receptors. Science 1991;252:1430–2.

72. Owens DM, Wei S, Smart RC. A multihit, multistage model of chemical carcinogenesis. Carcinogenesis 1999;20:1837–44.

73. Girardi M, Glusac E, Filler RB, et al. The distinct contributions of murine T cell receptor (TCR)gamma delta+ and TCRalpha beta+ T cells to different stages of chemically induced skin cancer. J Exp Med 2003;198:747–55.

74. Siegel CT, Schreiber K, Meredith SC, et al. Enhanced growth of primary tumors in cancer-prone mice after immunization against the mutant region of an inherited oncoprotein. J Exp Med 2000;191:1945–56.

75. Daniel D, Meyer-Morse N, Bergsland EK, et al. Immune enhancement of skin carcinogenesis by CD4+ T cells. J Exp Med 2003;197:1017–28.

76. Roberts SJ, Ng BY, Filler RB, et al. Characterizing tumor-promoting T cells in chemically induced cutaneous carcinogenesis. Proc Natl Acad Sci USA 2007;104:6770–5.

77. Egan PJ, Carding SR. Downmodulation of the inflammatory response to bacterial infection by gammadelta T cells cytotoxic for activated macrophages. J Exp Med 2000;191:2145–58.

78. Skeen MJ, Freeman MM, Ziegler HK. Changes in peritoneal myeloid populations and their proinflammatory cytokine expression during infection with Listeria monocytogenes are altered in the absence of gamma/delta T cells. J Leukoc Biol 2004;76:104–15.

79. Huber SA, Graveline D, Born WK, et al. Cytokine production by Vgamma(+)-T-cell subsets is an important factor determining CD4(+)-Th-cell phenotype and susceptibility of BALB/c mice to coxsackievirus B3–induced myocarditis. J Virol 2001;75:5860–9.

80. Bauer S, Groh V, Wu J, et al. Activation of NK cells and T cells by NKG2D, a receptor for stress-inducible MICA. Science 1999;285:727–9.

81. Cerwenka A, Bakker AB, McClanahan T, et al. Retinoic acid early inducible genes define a ligand family for the activating NKG2D receptor in mice. Immunity 2000;12:721–7.

82. Groh V, Rhinehart R, Secrist H, et al. Broad tumor-associated expression and recognition by tumor-derived gamma delta T cells of MICA and MICB. Proc Natl Acad Sci USA 1999;96:6879–84.

83. Vetter CS, Groh V, Thor Straten P, et al. Expression of stress-induced MHC class I related chain molecules on human melanoma. J Invest Dermatol 2002;118:600–5.

84. Hansen DS, Schofield L. Regulation of immunity and pathogenesis in infectious diseases by CD1d-restricted NKT cells. Int J Parasitology 2004;34:15–25.

85. Kronenberg M. Toward an understanding of NKT cell biology: progress and paradoxes. Annu Rev Immunol 2005;23:877–900.

86. Godfrey DI, McConville MJ, Pelicci DG. Chewing the fat on natural killer T cell development. J Exp Med 2006;203:2229–32.

87. Godfrey DI, Hammond KJ, Poulton LD, et al. NKT cells: facts, functions and fallacies. Immunol Today 2000;21:573–83.

88. Gumperz JE, Miyake S, Yamamura T, et al. Functionally distinct subsets of CD1d-restricted natural killer T cells revealed by CD1d tetramer staining. J Exp Med 2002;195:625–36.

89. Takahashi T, Chiba S, Nieda M, et al. Cutting edge: analysis of human V Alpha 24+ NK T cells activated by alpha-galactosylceramide-pulsed monocyte-derived dendritic cells. J Immunol 2002;168:3140–4.

90. Prussin C, Foster B. TCR V alpha 24 and V beta 11 coexpression defines a human NK1 T cell analog containing a unique Th0 subpopulation. J Immunol 1997;159:5862–70.

91. Benlagha K, Weiss A, Beavis A, et al. In vivo identification of glycolipid antigen-specific T cells using fluorescent CD1d tetramers. J Exp Med 2000;191:1895–903.

92. Norris S, Doherty DG, Collins C, et al. Natural T cells in the human liver: cytotoxic lymphocytes with dual T cell and natural killer cell phenotype and function are phenotypically heterogenous and include Valpha24-JalphaQ and gammadelta T cell receptor bearing cells. Hum Immunol 1999;60:20–31.

93. Gadola S, Silk JD, Jeans A, et al. Impaired selection of invariant natural killer T cells in diverse mouse models of glycosphingolipid lysosomal storage diseases. J Exp Med 2006;203:2293–303.

94. Mattner J, Debord KL, Ismail N, et al. Exogenous and endogenous glycolipid antigens activate NKT cells during microbial infections. Nature 2005;434:525–9.

95. Brigl M, Bry L, Kent SC, Gumperz JE, et al. Mechanism of CD1d-restricted natural killer T cell

activation during microbial infection. Nat Immunol 2003;4:1230–7.

96. Kinjo Y, Wu D, Kim G, et al. Recognition of bacterial glycosphingolipids by natural killer T cells. Nature 2005;434:520–5.

97. Van Kaer L, Joyce S. Innate immunity: NKT cells in the spotlight. Curr Biol 2005;15:R429–31.

98. Smyth MJ, Thia KY, Street SE, et al. Differential tumor surveillance by natural killer (NK) and NKT cells. J Exp Med 2000;191:661–8.

99. Bell E. Immunotherapy: Do natural born killers specialize? Nature Rev Cancer 2005;5:914.

100. Crowe NY, Smyth MJ, Godfrey DI. A critical role for natural killer T cells in immunosurveillance of methylcholanthrene-induced sarcomas. J Exp Med 2002;196:119–27.

101. Smyth MJ, Crowe NY, Pellicci DG, et al. Sequential production of interferon-gamma by NK1.1(+) T cells and natural killer cells is essential for the antimetastatic effect of alpha-galactosylceramide. Blood 2002;99:1259–66.

102. Crowe NY, Coquet JM, Berzins SP, et al. Differential antitumor immunity mediated by NKT cell subsets in vivo. J Exp Med 2005;202:1279–88.

103. Askenase PW, Szczepanik M, Itakura A, et al. Extravascular T-cell recruitment requires initiation begun by Valpha14+ NKT cells and B-1 B cells. Trends Immunol 2004;25:441–9.

104. Campos RA, Szczepanik M, Lisbonne M, et al. Invariant NKT cells rapidly activated via immunization with diverse contact antigens collaborate in vitro with B-1 cells to initiate contact sensitivity. J Immunol 2006;177:3686–94.

105. Linsen L, Somers V, Stinissen P. Immunoregulation of autoimmunity by natural killer T cells. Hum Immunol 2005;66:1193–202.

106. Wilson SB, Delovitch TL. Janus-like role of regulatory iNKT cells in autoimmune disease and tumour immunity. Nat Rev Immunol 2003;3:211–22.

107. Wang B, Geng YB, Wang CR. CD1-restricted NK T cells protect nonobese diabetic mice from developing diabetes. J Exp Med 2001;194:313–20.

108. Shi FD, Flodstrom M, Balasa B, et al. Germ line deletion of the CD1 locus exacerbates diabetes in the NOD mouse. Proc Natl Acad Sci USA 2001;98:6777–82.

109. Falcone M, Facciotti F, Ghidoli N, et al. Upregulation of CD1d expression restores the immunoregulatory function of NKT cells and prevents autoimmune diabetes in nonobese diabetic mice. J Immunol 2004;172:5908–16.

110. Sharif S, Arreaza GA, Zucker P, et al. Activation of natural killer T cells by alpha-galactosylceramide treatment prevents the onset and recurrence of autoimmune Type 1 diabetes. Nat Med 2001;7:1057–62.

111. Hong S, Wilson MT, Serizawa I, et al. The natural killer T-cell ligand alpha-galactosylceramide prevents autoimmune diabetes in non-obese diabetic mice. Nat Med 2001;7:1052–6.

112. Naumov YN, Bahjat KS, Gausling R, et al. Activation of CD1d-restricted T cells protects NOD mice from developing diabetes by regulating dendritic cell subsets. Proc Natl Acad Sci USA 2001;98:13838–43.

113. Beaudoin L, Laloux V, Novak J, et al. NKT cells inhibit the onset of diabetes by impairing the development of pathogenic T cells specific for pancreatic beta cells. Immunity 2002;17:725–36.

114. Novak J, Beaudoin L, Griseri T, et al. Inhibition of T cell differentiation into effectors by NKT cells requires cell contacts. J Immunol 2005;174:1954–61.

115. Yoshimoto T, Bendelac A, Hu-Li J, et al. Defective IgE production by SJL mice is linked to the absence of CD4+, NK1.1+ T cells that promptly produce interleukin 4. Proc Natl Acad Sci USA 1995;92:11931–4.

116. Illes Z, Kondo T, Newcombe J, et al. Differential expression of NK T cell V alpha 24J alpha Q invariant TCR chain in the lesions of multiple sclerosis and chronic inflammatory demyelinating polyneuropathy. J Immunol 2000;164:4375–81.

117. Demoulins T, Gachelin G, Bequet D, et al. A biased Valpha24+ T-cell repertoire leads to circulating NKT-cell defects in a multiple sclerosis patient at the onset of his disease. Immunol Lett 2003;90:223–8.

118. Singh AK, Wilson MT, Hong S, et al. Natural killer T cell activation protects mice against experimental autoimmune encephalomyelitis. J Exp Med 2001;194:1801–11.

119. Pal E, Tabira T, Kawano T, et al. Costimulation-dependent modulation of experimental autoimmune encephalomyelitis by ligand stimulation of V alpha 14 NK T cells. J Immunol 2001;166:662–8.

120. Furlan R, Bergami A, Cantarella D, et al. Activation of invariant NKT cells by alphaGalCer administration protects mice from MOG35–55–induced EAE: critical roles for administration route and IFN-gamma. Eur J Immunol 2003;33:1830–8.

121. Singh AK, Wilson MT, Hong S, et al. Natural killer T cell activation protects mice against experimental autoimmune encephalomyelitis. J Exp Med 2001;194:1801–11.

122. Jahng AW, Maricic I, Pedersen B, et al. Activation of natural killer T cells potentiates or prevents experimental autoimmune encephalomyelitis. J Exp Med 2001;194:1789–99.

123. Miyamoto K, Miyake S, Yamamura T. A synthetic glycolipid prevents autoimmune encephalomyelitis by inducing TH2 bias of natural killer T cells. Nature 2001;413:531–4.

124. Nikoloff BJ, Nestle FO. Recent insights into the immunopathogenesis of psoriasis provide new therapeutic opportunities. J Clin Invest 2004;113:1664–75.

125. Holtmeier W, Pfander M, Hennemann A, et al. The TCR-delta repertoire in normal human skin is restricted and distinct from the TCR-delta repertoire in the peripheral blood. J Invest Dermatol 2001;116:275–80.

126. Hayday A, Theodoridis E, Ramsburg E, et al. Intraepithelial lymphocytes: exploring the Third Way in immunology. Nat Immunol 2001;2: 997–1003

127. Poussier P, Ning T, Banerjee D, et al. A unique subset of self-specific intraintestinal T cells maintains gut integrity. J Exp Med 2002;195: 1491–7.

128. Vermijlen D, Ellis P, Langford C, et al. Distinct cytokine-driven responses of activated blood gammadelta T cells: insights into unconventional T cell peliotropy. J Immunol 2007;178:4304–14.

7
Complement System

Kim B. Yancey and Zelmira Lazarova

Key Points

- Complement plays an important role in inflammation, opsonization of foreign materials, facilitation of phagocytosis by leukocytes, and direct cytotoxic reactions.
- The complement system is divided into three segments: initiation mechanisms, the amplification pathway, and the membrane attack complex.
- The initiation mechanisms are the classic, alternative, and lectin pathways.
- The complement system displays continuous, low-grade activation.

The complement system represents a complex group of interacting proteins and glycoproteins in blood and other body fluids (Fig. 7.1). Complement plays an important role in inflammation, opsonization of foreign materials, facilitation of phagocytosis by leukocytes, and direct cytotoxic reactions. The complement system, like the blood clotting pathways, displays continuous, low-grade activation that is subject to rapid and massive amplification based on specific and sequential cleavage of zymogen proteases. Proteases in this proinflammatory cascade can cleave many different substrate molecules (e.g., ratios of protease to substrate ranging from 1:10 to over 1:1000) to yield rapid and massive activation reactions. Accordingly, almost every step in the complement activation cascade is tightly regulated by both fluid phase and cell surface regulatory proteins. The complement system is divided into the following general segments: (1) initiation mechanisms known as the classic, alternative, and lectin pathways; (2) the amplification pathway;

and (3) the membrane attack complex (MAC). Activation of the complement system generates a number of cleavage fragments with diverse biologic activities. In many cases, such cleavage fragments bind specific plasma membrane receptors on various cells to yield responses that extend and amplify the biologic activities of the complement system.

Historical Perspectives

The first evidence for the existence of the complement system was discovered in the latter half of the 19th century.[1-4] At that time, a number of studies showed that blood contained a soluble defense system that was capable of destroying bacteria in vitro independent of the action of phagocytic cells. These studies demonstrated that the bactericidal activity of serum consisted of two basic factors. One of these factors was relatively heat stable, restricted to immune sera, and specifically reactive with a given microorganism or immunogen. This factor, specific antibody, was able to agglutinate its target but it could not cause its lysis without participation of the second factor. This second "complementing" factor was present in normal (i.e., nonimmune) as well as immune sera as a heat labile mediator. The sequential character of the interaction between specific antibody and the second factor was demonstrated by adding fresh serum to a mixture of specific antibody and bacteria, with the resultant production of bacterial lysis and death. Subsequent studies demonstrated that the second factor was composed of several subcomponent fractions that

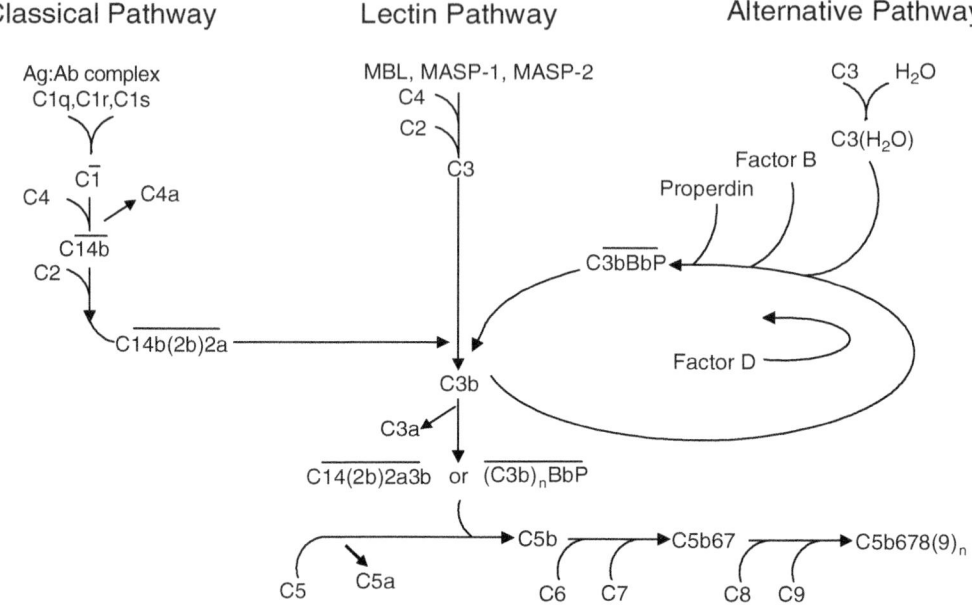

FIG. 7.1. Schematic overview of the complement system. (Modified from Goldsmith LA, ed. Physiology, Biochemistry, and Molecular Biology of the Skin, 2nd ed. New York: Oxford University Press, 1991.)

when separated were no longer active. Second factor or complement components were collectively termed alexin by Bordet and addiment or complement by Ehrlich and Morgenroth.

Biochemical Overview and Nomenclature

The human complement system consists of over 20 distinct proteins or glycoproteins that comprise approximately 3% of the total serum protein concentration (Table 7.1). The electrophoretic mobilities of these proteins range from the early γ-globulin to the albumin region. In many cases, these components are present in the circulation as inactive precursors that develop proteolytic activity upon activation. While various proteins circulate freely, some organization is afforded to this system by low-affinity, fluid-phase interactions between C1q and immunoglobulin G (IgG), C4 and C3, factor B and C3, and terminal components C5 through C9. Within the complement system, there are similar physiochemical properties among C3,

C4, and C5 as well as between C2 and factor B. Similarly, certain shared characteristics are also present between C1s and factor D as well as C6 and C7.

Traditionally, the lytic activity of complement has been used to study its functional activity. Because of its reliability and ease of use, the lysis of erythrocytes has been used as the principal in vitro functional complement assay (hence the term *hemolytic activity*). Classic assays of complement function utilize sheep erythrocytes (E) sensitized with rabbit antibody (A) and subsequently tested by the subsequent addition of serum complement components (C). This experimental paradigm is based on the high susceptibility of sheep erythrocytes to the lytic activity of complement, that such erythrocytes display the highly antigenic Forssman antigen (a target site for specific antibody binding), and that rabbits are Forssman antigen "negative" and hence a reliable source for production of specific antibody that efficiently activates complement. This combination of reagents (i.e., E + A + C) has been used to study the hemolytic activity of the classic complement pathway as well as the specific

TABLE 7.1. Complement components

	Molecular weight (daltons)	Serum concentration (μg/mL)
Classic pathway		
C1q	410,000	70
C1r	190,000	34
C1s	85,000	31
C4	206,000	600
C2	117,000	25
C3	195,000	1200
Alternative pathway		
Factor B	95,000	225
Factor D	25,000	1
Properdin	190,000	25
C3b	185,000	Derived from C3
Lectin pathway		
MBL	600,000	150
MASP-1	83,000	6
MASP-2	52,000	?
Membrane attack sequence		
C5	180,000	85
C6	128,000	60
C7	120,000	55
C8	150,000	55
C9	79,000	60
Control proteins		
C1 esterase inhibitor	105,000	180
C4 binding protein	560,000	?
Factor H (IH)	150,000	500
Factor I	90,000	34
S protein	80,000	600
Carboxypeptidase	280,000	50
CD59	20,000	?
CD46 (MCP)	45,000	?
CD55 (DAF)	70,000	?
SP-40, 40 (clusterin)	80,000	60

functional activity of individual complement components.

A commonly accepted nomenclature has been developed to designate the various components of the complement system.[1,2] The components of the classic pathway are designated by an uppercase C followed by a number (e.g., C2, C4, etc.). The components of the classic pathway react sequentially except for C4, which follows C1 and acts before C2 and C3. Alternative pathway components are designated by letter (e.g., factor B). Regulatory elements are typically designated by name (e.g., C4 binding protein), or in the case of regulatory elements closely associated with the alternative pathway, by letter (e.g., factor H). Components or complexes possessing enzymatic activity are designated with a bar over the component(s) in question; components or fragments that have been inactivated are designated by a prefix lowercase "i" (e.g., iC3b). Subunits or fragments of components are designated by a lowercase letter suffix (e.g., C3a, C3b, etc.).

The Classic Pathway

The classic pathway begins with the activation and binding of C1. Traditionally, antibody has been held responsible for C1 binding and activation. However, other materials including urate crystals, C-reactive protein, myelin basic protein, DNA, endotoxin, as well as selected bacteria and viruses have been shown to activate C1 directly in the absence of specific antibody (Table 7.2). In respect to classic pathway activation initiated by antibody-coated surfaces, immune complexes containing IgG subclasses 1 to 3 and IgM are capable of binding C1. Binding of C1 occurs via interaction of the CH_2 domain of the Fc portion of immunoglobulin.[5–8] In the case of IgG, two adjacent immunoglobulin molecules (i.e., an antibody doublet) are required to bind a single molecule of C1; conversely, one surface-bound molecule of IgM is sufficient for binding of a C1 molecule.[9]

C1 exists as a cation-dependent macromolecular complex composed of three subunits, namely C1q, C1r, and C1s. C1q, the largest of the C1 subunits, consisting of six copies of three separate chains, is the portion of the molecule that recognizes and binds immunoglobulin.[10,11] Binding of C1q to immune complexes alters the confirmation of the molecule and results in the activation of C1r and subsequently C$\overline{1s}$. Activated C1, via an active site in C$\overline{1s}$, cleaves the next two proteins in the classic pathway, C4 and C2, respectively. The rate of activation of C1 as well as its enzymatic activity is controlled in plasma by a specific regulatory protein termed the C1 inhibitor (C1-INH). C4 consists of three disulfide linked chains (i.e., α, β, and γ chains). Upon exposure to C$\overline{1s}$, the C4 molecule is cleaved into C4a, a 9-kd fragment with weak anaphylatoxin activity, and C4b.[12] While C4a is released into the fluid phase, C4b expresses a short-lived reactive site that allows it to bind

TABLE 7.2. Mechanisms of complement activation

Activators of the classic pathway
IgG (subclass 1–3) containing immune complexes
IgM containing immune complexes
C-reactive protein
Serum amyloid P
Mannose-binding lectin
Urate crystals
Endotoxin
DNA
Myelin basic protein
Activators of the alternative pathway
Bacterial polysaccharides and lipopolysaccharides
Cells infected with selected viruses
C3 tickover
Yeast cell walls (e.g., zymosan)
IgA containing immune complexes
Inulin
Amplification of classic pathway activation
Cobra venom factor
Activators of the lectin pathway
Binding of mannose-binding lectin to repeating simple sugars

TABLE 7.3. Complement control proteins

Control protein	Active site
C1 inhibitor	C1r, C1s
C4-binding protein	C4b
Factor H	C3b, C3bBb
Factor I	C3b (surface bound)
	C3b + factor H (fluid phase)
	C4b (surface bound)
	C4b + C4 binding protein
	(fluid phase)
S protein	C5b67
Serum carboxypeptidases	Carboxyl terminal arginine
	of C4a, C3a, C5a

covalently to nearby surfaces (e.g., to the inciting immune complex or to an adjacent target cell plasma membrane).[13] The interaction of C$\overline{4}$ with C1 enhances the activity of the latter with its other natural substrate, C2. In the presence of magnesium (Mg^{2+}), C2a, the major cleavage fragment of C2, binds to C4b to form the classic pathway C3 convertase (i.e., C$\overline{14b[2b]2a}$). This convertase may be formed either in the fluid phase or covalently attached to the surface of a target particle. In respect to the latter circumstance, the C4b portion of this complex remains responsible for binding the target particle while the adjacent serine protease site in the C2a molecule cleaves C3. The classic pathway C3 convertase is unstable and decays spontaneously with release of inactive C2a into the fluid phase. Interestingly, C4b remains covalently bound to its target and in the presence of C$\overline{1s}$ can accept another C2 molecule for development of additional C$\overline{14b(2b)2a}$ sites.

C3 is the complement component with the highest concentration in human serum. It plays a critical and pivotal role in the classic, alternative, and lectin pathways. C3 consists of disulfide linked α and β chains.[14,15] The α chain contains an internal thioester bond that is highly reactive, easily attacked by nucleophiles, and subject to slow hydrolysis. If C3 is hydrolyzed (i.e., C3[H$_2$O]), it

undergoes a conformational change that renders it resistant to specific cleavage.[16] Interestingly hydrolyzed C3 retains important biologic activity in the alternative pathway (see below). When the classic pathway C$\overline{3}$ convertase interacts with native C3 containing an intact internal thioester bond, two fragments are produced: C3a, a 9-kd anaphylatoxin that is released into the fluid phase, and C3b, a 185-kd molecule that contains an exposed and reactive thioester site.[17] This site may be attacked by a H$_2$O molecule to form hydrolyzed C3b, or covalently bound to an adjacent molecule or activation surface. In this manner, C3b may covalently bind to sites of complement activation in the vicinity of C$\overline{14b(2b)2a}$ leading to the formation of C$\overline{14b(2b)2a3b}$, the classic pathway C5 convertase. In this convertase, C3b presumably serves as the C5 binding site while the active site in C2a functions as the enzyme. The subsequent cleavage of C5 results in the production of C5a, the most potent anaphylatoxin produced during the activation of complement and a factor with potent chemotactic, spasmogenic, and immunomodulatory activities, and C5b, the initial component of the MAC.

Given that C3 plays a central and pivotal role in the classic, alternative, and lectin pathways, C3 inactivation represents a crucial regulatory event controlling complement activation (Table 7.3). Key to this process is further degradation of C3b. The initial cleavage of C3b is made in its α chain by factor I, with factor H serving as an essential cofactor in the fluid phase and as an accelerator for surface-associated cleavage reactions.[18,19] Such events culminate in the formation of iC3b (i.e., "inactivated" C3b). While iC3b is not easily further degraded in the fluid phase, surface bound iC3b is susceptible to another

TABLE 7.4. Complement receptors

Complement receptor	Predominant ligand	Predominant cell-type distribution
CR1 (CD35)	C3b, C4b, C1q	Erythrocytes, neutrophils, monocytes, B lymphocytes, some T lymphocytes, glomerular podocytes, mast cells, eosinophils, follicular dendritic cells, Kupffer cells
CR2 (CD21)	C3d,g, C3d, Epstein-Barr virus, CD23	Mature B lymphocytes, small subset of T lymphocytes, thymocytes, follicular dendritic cells, basophils, keratinocytes
CR3 (CD11b/CD18)	iC3b (>C3b>C3d)	Neutrophils, monocytes, NK cells, follicular dendritic cells, Kupffer cells
CR4 (CD11c/CD18)	iC3b (>C3b)	Monocytes, neutrophils
C1q receptor	C1q	Endothelial cells, fibroblasts, platelets, smooth muscle cells, selected epithelial cells, monocytes, neutrophils, B lymphocytes, small percentage of T and non-T, non-B lymphocytes
C5a receptor (CD88)	C5a	Neutrophils, monocytes, eosinophils, mast cells, T lymphocytes, hepatocytes, endothelial cells, pulmonary epithelial cells, astrocytes, selected smooth muscle cells
C3a receptor	C3a, C4a	Neutrophils, monocytes, basophils

factor I–mediated cleavage in which CR1, the C3b receptor, serves as an important cofactor.[20,21] In the presence of CR1, factor I cleaves C3b into C3c, a 145-kd molecule that is released into the fluid phase, and C3d,g, a 41-kd fragment that contains the novel thioester binding site of the original C3 molecule. Surface-bound C3d,g is susceptible to proteolysis by trypsin, elastase, or plasmin to yield C3g, a 10-kd fluid phase fragment, and C3d, a 31-kd chain remnant that contains the thioester covalent binding site of the molecule. As noted in Table 7.4 there are specific plasma membrane receptors for various C3 cleavage fragments on a wide variety of different cells.

Alternative Pathway

Fundamental differences between the alternative and classic pathways of complement activation include the following: (1) the alternative pathway does not require specific antibody for activation and thus is functional in nonimmunized hosts as part of their innate immune system; (2) the alternative pathway is activated by a wide array of substances including bacterial polysaccharides and lipopolysaccharides, viruses, inulin, yeast cell walls, IgA containing immune complexes, and other materials (Table 7.2); (3) this pathway exhibits low-grade continuous activation, in part

initiated by continuous hydrolysis of C3 that yield $C3[H_2O]$; and (4) the alternative pathway is unique in that molecules that initiate its activation (specifically, C3b or $C3[H_2O]$) can also serve as major products of this activation cascade, thus creating a powerful and positive feedback loop for both the alternative and classic pathways.[8,22] As noted above, the generation of C3b (or $C3[H_2O]$) serves as a point of entry for alternative pathway activation (so-called C3 tickover). In the presence of magnesium ions (Mg^{2+}), the binding of factor B to C3b (or $C3[H_2O]$) results in factor $\overline{D}$ mediated cleavage of factor B and the formation of the alternative pathway C3 convertase, $\overline{C3bBb}$. Properdin (P) binds to $\overline{C3bBb}$ and stabilizes this convertase by forming a complex termed $\overline{C3bBbP}$. The latter convertase complex demonstrates a reduced rate of spontaneous decay as well as a reduced rate of inactivation by factors I and H.[23] As is true for the classic pathway C3 convertase, the addition of C3b to $\overline{C3bBbP}$ confers substrate specificity for C5 upon the latter complex ($\overline{C3bBbC3bP}$). Proteolytic cleavage of C5 by the alternative pathway C5 convertase is a result of an active site within the $\overline{Bb}$ portion of the molecule.

The efficiency of $\overline{C3bBb}$ for C3 consumption is well demonstrated in patients who possess an autoantibody directed against the alternative pathway C3 convertase. This autoantibody, termed the C3 nephritic factor (C3NeF), stabilizes the alternative pathway C3 convertase and results in continuous C3 cleavage and markedly low levels of this complement component. C3NeF has been identified in patients with systemic lupus erythematosus, membranoproliferative glomerulonephritis, partial lipodystrophy, and selected other disorders.

The Lectin Pathway

The lectin pathway of complement activation is activated by the binding of mannose-binding lectin (MBL) to repeating carbohydrate moieties on the surface of various pathogens.[24] MBL is structurally similar to C1q; interestingly, MBL physically associates with two proteases, MBL-associated proteases 1 and 2 (MASP-1 and MASP-2), the latter moieties acting like C1r and C1s of the classic pathway.[25] Once MBL is bound to a target, MASP-1 and MASP-2 are activated leading to the subsequent cleavage of C4, C2, and C3. By an incompletely understood mechanism, the lectin pathway can also bypass C4 and C2 and activate C3 directly.

The Membrane Attack Complex

Cleavage of C5 by either the classic or alternative pathway C5 convertases results in identical fragmentation of the native molecule and the formation of C5a and C5b. C5a is an 11-kd cationic glycoprotein that is released into the fluid phase as the most potent anaphylatoxin produced during the activation of complement. Following its generation, C5b undergoes a conformational change that exposes a labile hydrophobic binding region that allows C5b to become noncovalently attached to an activating or exposed surface.[26,27] However, in the absence of C6, surface bound C5b rapidly loses its hemolytic activity. Alternatively, C5 cleavage in the presence of C6 results in the formation of a structurally stable C5b6 complex. C5b6 may circulate in the fluid phase, bind to unsensitized cells, and elicit the formation of the MAC by facilitating binding of other terminal complement components. C6 interacts nonenzymatically with C5b; physiochemically, C7 is quite similar to C6 and displays high-affinity binding to C5b6. The resulting C5b67 complex is capable of associating with phospholipid bilayers of plasma membranes. The addition of C8 to a surface-bound C5b67 complex allows it to enter more deeply into the lipid bilayer and disrupt the plasma membrane.[28,29] While this complex produces a sufficiently large lesion to initiate cell lysis, this process is slow and dependent on high inputs of C8.

C9, the final terminal complement component, has two interesting biologic features: (1) it is amphipathic (i.e., composed of two domains with notably different properties) in that it contains one hydrophobic and one hydrophilic domain; and (2) it has the ability to polymerize. C9 initially binds as a monomer to C5b678 in plasma membranes. Subsequently, it polymerizes to create a transmembrane tubular complex containing an internal channel and a unipolar thickened annulus.[30] Such channels allow water to enter the targeted cell and eventuate in its lysis. In this respect, C9 shares features like those seen with other pore-forming proteins such as the cytotoxic granule protein perforin. In contrast to the proteolytic activity of the early activation components, the assembly of the MAC results from conformational changes that expose new reactive sites on each subsequent complement component. The conformational and structural changes that occur in the terminal components during assembly of the MAC lead to the expression of neoantigens on the complex that are absent (or hidden) in the respective native components comprising this complex. Specific antisera against MAC neoantigens have shown that this macromolecular complex can be found in lesional skin from patients with systemic lupus erythematosus as well as in the skin of patients with bullous pemphigoid or dermatitis herpetiformis.

Anaphylatoxins

Complement activation sufficient to cleave C4, C3, and C5 results in the production of a series of low-molecular-weight fragments, C4a, C3a, and C5a, respectively, that are released into the fluid phase (Table 7.5). C4a and C3a are nonglycosylated, 77-amino-acid fragments, while C5a contains a large carbohydrate moiety and 74 amino acids. All of these peptides are regarded as anaphylatoxins because of their ability to stimulate smooth muscle contraction, enhance vascular permeability, and induce vasoactive mediator release from mast cells and basophils.[12,31]

TABLE 7.5. Biologic activities of anaphylatoxins

Target site	Biologic effects
Mast cells	Degranulation, histamine release
Leukocytes	Aggregation, adhesion, chemotaxis (C5a), degranulation, stimulation of oxidative metabolism
Smooth muscle	Contraction in selected tissues
Capillary walls	Vasopermeability
Vascular endothelial cells	Induction of leukocyte adhesion, liberation of arachidonic acid
Platelets	Aggregation, generation of arachidonic acid products

C5a, the "classic" complement anaphylatoxin, is an 11-kd peptide that contains an aspargine-linked oligosaccharide at amino acid 64 that contributes 25% of the molecular weight of this anaphylatoxin. C5a is approximately 200- and 3000-fold more potent than C3a and C4a, respectively. C5a is further distinguished from C3a and C4a by its ability to elicit directed migration of neutrophils and monocytes as well as aggregation, polarization, lysosomal enzyme release, and oxidative metabolism of the former. C5a stimulates interleukin-1 and tumor necrosis factor production by human mononuclear cells and also has been shown to augment both humoral and cell-mediated immune responses in vitro. Although the removal of the carboxyl-terminal arginine by serum carboxypeptidase N destroys or substantially reduces spasmogenic activity of all three molecules, the des Arg form of the anaphylatoxins may retain other biologic activities. Of these, C5a des Arg is clearly the most potent. C5a des Arg is approximately 10- to 100-fold less potent than C5a, but does retain numerous biologic activities.

Complement Regulatory Proteins

The complement system is tightly controlled by regulatory elements that act in various ways at a number of different sites (see Table 7.3). Such regulatory elements are found in the fluid phase, on cell membranes, and in the matrix. They can irreversibly inactivate a specific component, transiently maintain a protein in an inactive form, or dissociate proteins from multicomponent complexes. Selected regulatory elements or inactivators are briefly reviewed below.

Regulators of Complement Activation

A large number of proteins exert a controlling influence at the C3 convertase stage of complement activation. These proteins bind to fragments of C3 or C4 and either block formation of the C3 convertase or serve as a cofactor for its inactivation by factor I. This group of regulatory proteins includes C4 binding protein, factor H, decay-accelerating factor (DAF), CR1, CR2, and membrane cofactor protein (MCP, originally named gp45-70). Analysis of complementary DNA (cDNA) clones for all of these proteins has revealed a common structural motif that features multiple repeats of an approximately 60-amino-acid consensus unit. Moreover, the genes for these proteins have been localized to the long arm of human chromosome 1. These genes are regarded as a multigene family of complement regulator proteins that may have evolved from an ancestral C3-binding protein. Interestingly, this family includes both soluble as well as membrane-associated proteins.

Fluid Phase Regulatory Elements

C1 Inhibitor

C1 inhibitor (C1-INH) is a 105-kd glycoprotein that is a member of the serine proteinase inhibitor (or serpin) family. It binds active sites on C1r and C1s, thus destroying their proteinase activity.[32] It also inhibits the proteinases kallikrein, factor XIa, factor XIIa, and plasmin. A deficiency of C1-INH is seen in patients with hereditary angioedema (HAE), an autosomal dominant disorder characterized by recurrent attacks of nonpruritic, nonerythematous, and generally nonpitting edema of the face, airways, gastrointestinal tract, and extremities (see below).

Factor I

Factor I (previously known as C3b inactivator) is a 90-kd enzyme that like factor D, appears to circulate in an active state.[18] The natural substrates of factor I are C4b and C3b. C4-binding protein and factor H are obligate cofactors for the enzymatic action of factor I in fluid-phase systems. This relationship suggests that the binding proteins produce conformational changes in their substrates that expose cryptic sites susceptible to cleavage by factor I. Cleavage of C3b or C4b by factor I create specific forms of these molecules. While these degradation products can no longer act as partners of a C5 convertase, they demonstrate high affinity for specific C3 and C4 receptors.

Factor H

Factor H, previously known as β-1H, is a 150-kd, monomeric polypeptide that functions as a regulator of the "tickover" activation mechanism of the alternative pathway.[33] Factor H accelerates the decay of the alternative pathway C3 convertase by promoting the dissociation of Bb from the complex. Factor H achieves this effect by competing with both B and Bb for binding to C3b. The binding of factor H to C3b also interferes with the capacity of the latter to bind C5. Factor H also serves as an essential cofactor for the cleavage of fluid-phase C3b by factor I, and accelerates cleavage of surface-bound C3b by factor I. Although factor H lacks enzymatic activity, it regulates C3b activity in a manner analogous to that of C4 binding protein on C4. Although the combined influence of factors H and I on C3b does not abrogate all of the latter's biologic activity, it terminates C3b's capacity to participate in C3 or C5 convertases.

C4-Binding Protein

C4-binding protein is composed of seven or eight subunits linked by disulfide bridges; its molecular weight is 570 kd.[34] C4-binding protein engages in activities that parallel those of factor H (i.e., cofactor activity and decay acceleration). Interestingly, these activities are directed toward C4b and the classic activation pathway rather than C3b and the alternative activation pathway. C4-binding protein binds fluid-phase C4b and renders it susceptible to inactivation by factor I. Although C4-binding protein is not required for factor I–mediated inactivation of cell-surface bound C4b, factor I cannot interact with fluid-phase C4b in the absence of this cofactor. In binding to C4b, C4-binding protein also facilitates dissociation of C2a, thus accelerating the decay of the classic pathway convertase. C4-binding protein is also capable of binding a single molecule of the vitamin K–dependent serum protein, protein S. Subsequent to its binding to C4-binding protein, the anticoagulant function of this molecule appears to be lost.

S Protein (Vitronectin)

S protein is a glycoprotein of approximately 88 kd that is capable of forming stable, presumably hydrophobic interactions with the membrane-binding site of C5b67.[35] This interaction converts the C5b67 complex into a hydrophilic non–membrane-binding and hence inactive moiety. Although C8 and C9 can still bind to such complexes, C9 cannot polymerize.

Carboxypeptidases

Carboxypeptidases, present in normal serum in an active state, rapidly remove the carboxyl terminal arginine from C4a, C3a, and C5a, thus destroying (or substantially reducing) their activity. Such exopeptidases also display important regulatory control (either partial or complete) of kinin and fibrinolytic peptides.

Homologous Restriction Factor

Terminal component lytic efficiency is severely restricted when complement and target cells are derived from the same species (so-called homologous restriction). This activity is mediated by a 65-kd membrane protein called C8-binding protein or homologous restriction factor (HRF). The manner in which this molecule inhibits C8 and C9 lytic lesions is similar to that of CD59 (see below).

SP-40,40 (Clusterin)

SP-40,40 is a disulfide-linked heterodimer found free in normal serum as well as epithelial cells of male reproductive tissues, seminal plasma, and selected endothelial cells. In complement activated serum it associates with soluble C5b-9 complexes and exhibits regulatory activity that is similar to S protein. In this manner, clusterin is thought to interact with the hydrophobic membrane insertion domain of the nascent MAC and thus block its entry into plasma membranes.

Membrane Regulatory Elements

Decay Accelerating Factor (CD55)

Decay accelerating factor (DAF) is a 70-kd cell-surface glycoprotein that has a glycophosphatidylinositol (GPI) anchor. It acts by binding C3b or C4b on cell membranes, thus markedly increasing the spontaneous decay of both the classic and alternative pathway C3 convertases. Soluble forms of DAF have been found in a wide range of biologic fluids.

Membrane Cofactor Protein (CD46)

Membrane cofactor protein (MCP) is a widely distributed surface membrane human C3-binding protein that functions as a required cofactor for the cleavage of C3 and C4 into their hemolytically inactive forms, iC3b and iC4b. Although the role of MCP in the complement system is similar to that of DAF, the specific enzymatic activity is different and results in an inactive form of C3 protein. The expression of MCP is widespread, with the notable exception of erythrocytes, and soluble forms have been found in many biological tissues.

CD59

CD59 (MIRL, MACIF, HRF20, P18) is a widely distributed, highly disulfide-linked protein with a GPI anchor.[36] It is found on erythrocytes, monocytes, granulocytes, platelets, endothelial cells, and many cells of the nervous and reproductive tissues. A soluble form has also been found in urine, seminal plasma, serum, and amniotic fluid. CD59 can bind C8 in the C5b-8 complex and thus block the effective incorporation of C9. CD59 can also bind C9 that is already in the MAC and block its polymerization, thereby preventing the full formation of the transmembrane pore. CD59 also has non–complement-related functions (e.g., it can function as an adhesion molecule through its ability to serve as a counterreceptor for CD2).

Matrix Regulatory Elements

Decorin

In skin, bone, articular cartilage, cornea, and arterial wall adventitia, a dermatin sulfate proteoglycan, designated decorin, is expressed. Purified or recombinant decorin has been shown to bind C1q with a high affinity at physiologic strength.[37] Interestingly, decorin inhibits complement activation, presumably by binding and altering the activity of C1q. While other matrix proteins, such as fibrinogen, fibrin, fibronectin, and laminin, have also been shown to bind C1q, they have not been reported to block its activity.

Complement Receptors

A wide variety of biologic effects of complement are mediated by specific high-affinity receptors for various cleavage fragments (see Table 7.4). These effects include not only the clearance of complement-coated antigens, but also the activation of cells of the immune system. For some proteins, such as C3, different receptors exist that are relatively specific for unique activation fragments of the molecule (C3b, C3bi, C3d). By this mechanism, the immune response can be modulated with a higher degree of specificity.

Complement-activation fragments for which receptors have been well described and cloned include C1q, C5a, C3a, and cleaved forms of C3 and C4. Receptors for C4a, factor B (both Ba and Bb), factor H, and other components have been identified based on biologic activities only. Table 7.4 provides a summary overview of selected complement receptors. Readers are referred elsewhere for additional information about this topic.[4,8]

Biosynthesis and Genetics of Complement Proteins

Studies of protein polymorphism in human subjects following orthotopic liver transplants have shown that more than 90% of plasma C3, C6, C8, and factor B are synthesized in the liver.[38] However, other studies have shown that a variety of cell types such as monocytes, macrophages, fibroblasts, and epithelial cells are capable of synthesizing complement components.[39] Locally produced components may play an important role in inflammatory responses. Moreover, a variety of stimuli have been shown to modify complement component secretion.

Complement proteins demonstrate a substantial number of genetic polymorphisms. In general, these polymorphisms present as differences in charge. Polymorphic variants have been described for C2, C3, C4, C6, C7, C8, factor B, factor H, C4 binding protein, and C1-INH. The majority of these complement allotypes function normally. The most common dysfunctional variant is that of C1-INH, which may be present in antigenetically normal levels yet demonstrate no functional activity.

Complement Component Deficiencies

The incidence of inherited complement deficiency states in otherwise normal individuals is low. However, genetic deficiencies have been reported for a substantial number of complement components and complement-related proteins (Table 7.6) Individuals who lack a complement component are often at increased risk for developing infectious diseases or autoimmune syndromes. Individuals who lack a component of the classic pathway (e.g., C1, C4, C2) tend to develop systemic lupus erythematosus (SLE), SLE-like syndromes, or other autoimmune diseases. Those who lack components of the membrane attack complex or the alternate pathway tend to have recurrent pyogenic infections. Almost all genetic complement deficiency states appear to be inherited in an autosomal recessive manner. The following subsections briefly review two of the most common complement deficiency states.

TABLE 7.6. Inherited complement component deficiencies

Deficient component	Disease association
C1r, C1s, C2, C4	SLE, SLE-like syndromes, dermatomyositis, glomerulonephritis, recurrent bacterial infections
C3, factor I	Recurrent bacterial infections (esp. *Pneumococcus, Staphylococcus, Streptococcus*)
C5, C6, C7, C8	*Neisseria* infections (SLE and SLE-like syndromes also reported)
C1 inhibitor	Hereditary angioedema, SLE, DLE

DLE, disseminated lupus erythematosus; SLE, systemic lupus erythematosus.

C2 Deficiency

C2 deficiency is the most common complement component deficiency in Caucasians. It has been estimated that about 1 in 40,000 individuals is homozygous for C2 deficiency.[34] Since the gene for C2 is located in the major histocompatibility complex (MHC) (see above), it is not surprising that it is in linkage disequilibrium with certain human leukocyte antigens (HLAs). The most common disease associated with C2 deficiency is SLE, although other autoimmune diseases such as discoid lupus erythematosus, necrotizing vasculitis, and juvenile rheumatoid arthritis have been reported. Patients with SLE and C2 deficiency are not clinically different from SLE patients in general, except that their disease may have a relatively early age of onset and less severe renal involvement. Other C2-deficient patients have been reported to have an increased incidence of recurrent bacterial infections. C2 deficiency should be considered in a patient who presents with signs and symptoms of an autoimmune disease and has a hemolytic complement (CH_{50}) of zero.

C1 Inhibitor Deficiency

C1-inhibitor deficiency is the cause of HAE, an autosomal dominant disorder that has been estimated to occur in about 1 in 100,000 individuals. HAE is characterized by recurrent episodes of subcutaneous swelling of the face, extremities, upper airway, and gastrointestinal tract that last for 48 to 72 hours.[40] C1-INH binds irreversibly to activated C1r and C1s. Several types of C1-INH deficiency exist. In the most common form of HAE (type I, ~85% of patients), the individual has one normal C1-INH gene and one that does not encode protein. These patients have low levels of C1-INH (i.e., 5% to 30% of normal). In another form of HAE (type II, ~15% of patients), the individual has one normal C1-INH gene and one that encodes a molecule that is antigenically intact but functionally inactive. These patients have normal antigenic levels but markedly decreased functional activity of C1-INH due to altered structure of this molecule. A clinical syndrome resembling HAE that affects only women has been termed type III HAE. Interestingly, no abnormalities of complement or C1-INH levels have been described in these patients. The mediator responsible for the angioedema seen in patients with HAE is somewhat controversial. Increased bradykinin concentrations have been associated with clinical flares of HAE. C2 kinin, a fragment of C2b, may also contribute to the pathophysiology of this disorder. In Europe, purified C1-INH is available for treatment of acute attacks of HAE; in the United States, treatment largely consists of the use of fresh frozen plasma acutely, and androgens chronically.

Acquired angioedema (AAE) mimicking HAE is a rare syndrome. Like HAE, AAE has two distinct forms. Type I is characterized by diminished levels of C1-INH secondary to its increased catabolism. Type I AAE is associated with lymphomas, chronic lymphocytic leukemia, and other lymphoproliferative diseases. Although the exact mechanism by which these lymphoproliferative diseases lead to angioedema is not clear, the underlying cause is thought to be the formation of immune complexes that increase consumption of C1-INH. In AAE type II, while no lymphoproliferative or other underlying diseases are apparent, autoantibodies bind the reactive center of C1-INH, altering its structure and regulatory capacity.

Complement Assays

There are two basic types of complement assays—those that quantitate antigenic concentrations of various complement proteins and those that measure the functional activity of a single or group of complement components. Each of these assay methods offers certain advantages and disadvantages.[8]

Antigenic complement assays are widely available, and, in general, can be performed easily and quickly. Although antigenic assays are accurate, they are not as sensitive as functional assays and provide no information about the biologic activity of the component under study. Moreover, radial immunodiffusion assays sometimes detect fragments as well as intact components, thus providing inaccurate determinations. Commercially available assays are currently available for a variety of human complement components. In addition to radial immunodiffusion, enzyme-linked immunosorbent assay (ELISA), rocket immunoelectrophoresis, crossed immunoelectrophoresis, and nephelometry have also been used to quantitate complement component levels.

Functional complement assays are generally precise and sensitive yet not widely available. Most of these assays utilize serum samples since anticoagulants (e.g., ethylenediaminetetraacetic acid [EDTA], heparin) inhibit or interfere with complement activation. The most commonly employed functional complement assay is the CH_{50} or whole complement titer. The CH_{50} assay tests the ability of serial dilutions of test serum to lyse a standardized suspension of antibody-sensitized sheep erythrocytes. The CH_{50} titer is the reciprocal of the dilution of serum that lyses 50% of the erythrocytes. Absence or dysfunction of a classic pathway component results in a CH_{50} titer of essentially zero. Research laboratories employ similar techniques to determine the functional activity of specific complement components or regulatory molecules. Although functional test systems are relatively complex, they may detect reduced levels of certain complement components before the activated component (still reactive in some antigenic assays) is cleared from the circulation. These assays also identify nonfunctional components that are present at normal antigenic levels.

Several general caveats regarding measurement of complement components should be mentioned. First, measurements of components are static, assessing levels of these proteins at only one point in time. Because a number of complement components are synthesized and degraded at a rapid rate, static measurements should not be considered reflective of changing events in vivo. Second, plasma levels of these proteins reflect the balance between their rates of synthesis and degradation. Metabolic studies in humans have shown that normal component levels may be maintained by an increased rate of synthesis despite the presence of pronounced complement activation. Third, there is a wide range of normal values for several complement components and it is sometimes difficult to determine minor variations in a single sample. Fourth, several complement components behave as acute-phase reactants and become elevated (or normal) in various pathophysiologic alterations where some degree of complement activation is occurring.

Complement Inhibitors as Therapeutics

Because complement plays a key role in many inflammatory and autoimmune diseases, substantial effort has gone into the development of inhibitors that may attenuate the biologic activities of various complement fragments. These inhibitors have already been shown to have dramatic effects on animal models of complement-dependent inflammatory states.[41,42]

Nonrecombinant Inhibitors

Anticomplement effects have been identified in a variety of drugs. Heparin, for example, can inhibit complement activation. Because its complement inhibition appears distinct from its anticoagulant effect, there is potential for the development of a safe and specific complement inhibitor based on this drug. Other potential complement inhibitors include substituted iso-coumarines, leupeptin, peptides that mimics serine protease cleavage sites, and intravenous immunoglobulin (IVIG).

Recombinant Soluble Complement Regulatory Proteins as Complement Inhibitors

Efforts to create complement regulatory agents have focused on the development of biologically active soluble forms of CR1, CR2, DAF, MCP, and C59. Because CR1 can block activation of the alternative as well as the classic pathways, and has both decay-accelerating and cofactor activities, it is an ideal "drug" candidate. Recombinant soluble human CR1 (sCR1) has been shown to inhibit local inflammation in a number of animal models. Soluble forms of CR2, DAF, MCP, MCP-DAF fusions, and CD59 have also been created, as have cell-targeted forms of sCR1 and CD59. Finally, monoclonal antibodies directed against C5 are in human trials, and both peptide and nonpeptide inhibitors of factor D, factor B, and C3 activation are under development in preclinical studies.

Conclusion

Complement plays an important role in inflammation, opsonization of foreign materials, facilitation of phagocytosis by leukocytes, and direct cytotoxic reactions. The complement system displays continuous, low-grade activation that is subject to rapid and massive amplification based on specific and sequential cleavage of zymogen proteases. The complement system is divided into the following general segments: (1) initiation mechanisms known as the classic, alternative, and lectin pathways; (2) the amplification pathway; and (3) the membrane attack complex.

References

1. Fries L, Frank M. Molecular mechanisms of complement activation. In: Stamatoyannopoulous G, Nienhuis A, Leder P, Majerus P, eds. The Molecular Basis of Blood Diseases. Philadelphia: WB Saunders, 1987:450–98.
2. Brown E, Joiner K, Frank M. Complement. In: Paul W, ed. Fundamental Immunology. New York: Raven Press, 1984:645–68.
3. Mayer M. Complement and complement fixation. In: Kabat E, Mayer M, eds. Experimental Immunochemistry. Springfield, IL: Charles C Thomas, 1967:133–241.
4. Carroll MC. The role of complement and complement receptors in induction and regulation of immunity. Ann Rev Immunol 1998;16:545–68.
5. Metzger H. Effect of antigen binding on the properties of antibody. Adv Immunol 1974;18:169–207.
6. Yasmeen D, Ellerson JR, Dorrington KJ, Painter RH. The structure and function of immunoglobulin domains. IV. The distribution of some effector functions among the Cgamma2 and Cgamma3 homology regions of human immunoglobulin G1. J Immunol 1976;116(2):518–26.
7. Yancey KB, Lawley TJ. Circulating immune complexes: their immunochemistry, biology, and detection in selected dermatologic and systemic diseases. J Am Acad Dermatol 1984;10(5 pt 1):711–31.
8. Frank M. The complement system. In: Samster M, Talmage D, Frank M, Austen K, Claman H, eds. Immunological Diseases. Boston: Little, Brown, 1988:203–32.
9. Ziccardi RJ. Activation of the early components of the classical complement pathway under physiologic conditions. J Immunol 1981;126(5):1769–73.
10. Ziccardi RJ. The first component of human complement (C1): activation and control. Springer Semin Immunopathol 1983;6(2–3):213–30.

11. Ziccardi RJ. Nature of the metal ion requirement for assembly and function of the first component of human complement. J Biol Chem 1983;258(10):6187–92.

12. Gorski J, Hugli T, Muller-Eberhard HJ. C4a: the third anaphylatoxin of the human complement system. Proc Natl Acad Sci U S A 1979;76(10):5299–302.

13. Dodds AW, Ren XD, Willis AC, Law SK. The reaction mechanism of the internal thioester in the human complement component C4. Nature 1996;379(6561):177–9.

14. Tack BF. The beta-Cys-gamma-Glu thiolester bond in human C3, C4, and alpha 2–macroglobulin. Springer Semin Immunopathol 1983;6(4):259–82.

15. Thomas ML, Tack BF. Identification and alignment of a thiol ester site in the third component of guinea pig complement. Biochemistry 1983;22(4):942–7.

16. Isenman DE, Podack ER, Cooper NR. The interaction of C5 with C3b in free solution: a sufficient condition for cleavage by a fluid phase C3/C5 convertase. J Immunol 1980;124(1):326–31.

17. Hugli TE. Structure and function of the anaphylatoxins. Springer Semin Immunopathol 1984;7(2–3):193–219.

18. Pangburn MK, Schreiber RD, Muller-Eberhard HJ. Human complement C3b inactivator: isolation, characterization, and demonstration of an absolute requirement for the serum protein beta1H for cleavage of C3b and C4b in solution. J Exp Med 1977;146(1):257–70.

19. Gaither TA, Hammer CH, Frank MM. Studies of the molecular mechanisms of C3b inactivation and a simplified assay of beta 1H and the C3b inactivator (C3bINA). J Immunol 1979;123(3):1195–204.

20. Harrison RA, Lachmann PJ. Novel cleavage products of the third component of human complement. Mol Immunol 1980;17(2):219–28.

21. Harrison RA, Lachmann PJ. The physiological breakdown of the third component of human complement. Mol Immunol 1980;17(1):9–20.

22. Farries TC, Atkinson JP. Evolution of the complement system. Immunol Today 1991;12(9):295–300.

23. Vogt W, Dames W, Schmidt G, Dieminger L. Complement activation by the properdin system: formation of a stoichiometric. C3 cleaving complex of properdin factor B with C36. Immunochemistry 1977;14(3):201–5.

24. Muller-Eberhard HJ. Molecular organization and function of the complement system. Annu Rev Biochem 1988;57:321–47.

25. Thiel S, Vorup-Jensen T, Stover CM, et al. A second serine protease associated with mannan-binding lectin that activates complement. Nature 1997;386(6624):506–10.

26. Morgan BP. Effects of the membrane attack complex of complement on nucleated cells. Curr Top Microbiol Immunol 1992;178:115–40.

27. Koski CL, Estep AE, Sawant-Mane S, Shin ML, Highbarger L, Hansch GM. Complement regulatory molecules on human myelin and glial cells: differential expression affects the deposition of activated complement proteins. J Neurochem 1996;66(1):303–12.

28. Thompson RA, Lachmann PJ. Reactive lysis: the complement-mediated lysis of unsensitized cells. I. The characterization of the indicator factor and its identification as C7. J Exp Med 1970;131(4):629–41.

29. Lachmann PJ, Thompson RA. Reactive lysis: the complement-mediated lysis of unsensitized cells. II. The characterization of activated reactor as C56 and the participation of C8 and C9. J Exp Med 1970;131(4):643–57.

30. Podack ER, Tschopp J. Polymerization of the ninth component of complement (C9): formation of poly(C9) with a tubular ultrastructure resembling the membrane attack complex of complement. Proc Natl Acad Sci U S A 1982;79(2):574–8.

31. Yancey KB. Biological properties of human C5a: selected in vitro and in vivo studies. Clin Exp Immunol 1988;71(2):207–10.

32. Harpel PC, Cooper NR. Studies on human plasma C1 inactivator-enzyme interactions. I. Mechanisms of interaction with C1s, plasmin, and trypsin. J Clin Invest 1975;55(3):593–604.

33. Whaley K, Ruddy S. Modulation of the alternative complement pathways by beta 1 H globulin. J Exp Med 1976;144(5):1147–63.

34. Ross SC, Densen P. Complement deficiency states and infection: epidemiology, pathogenesis and consequences of neisserial and other infections in an immune deficiency. Medicine (Baltimore) 1984;63(5):243–73.

35. Podack ER, Kolb WP, Muller-Eberhard HJ. The C5b-6 complex: formation, isolation, and inhibition of its activity by lipoprotein and the S-protein of human serum. J Immunol 1978;120(6):1841–8.

36. Davies A, Wilson AB, Bramley JC, et al. Identification of MIC 11 antigen as an epitope of the CD59 molecule. Immunology 1995;85(2):220–7.

37. Ramamurthy P, Hocking AM, McQuillan DJ. Recombinant decorin glycoforms. Purification and structure. J Biol Chem 1996;271(32):19578–84.

38. Whaley K, Schwaeble W. Complement and complement deficiencies. Semin Liver Dis 1997;17(4):297–310.

39. Morgan BP, Gasque P. Extrahepatic complement biosynthesis: where, when and why? Clin Exp Immunol 1997;107(1):1–7.

40. Cooper NR, Nemerow GR, Mayes JT. Methods to detect and quantitate complement activation. Springer Semin Immunopathol 1983;6(2–3):195–212.

41. Kalli KR, Hsu P, Fearon DT. Therapeutic uses of recombinant complement protein inhibitors. Springer Semin Immunopathol 1994;15(4): 417–31.

42. Moore F. Therapeutic regulation of the complement system in acute injury states. Adv Immunol 1994;56:267–99.

8
Cutaneous Dendritic Cells in Health and Disease

Mark C. Udey

Key Points

- Specialized, bone marrow–derived antigen-presenting cells (dendritic cells, DCs) are critical in the initiation and propagation of skin-related immune reactions in both health (host defense) and disease (inflammatory skin conditions).
- These DC bridge the innate and adaptive arms of the immune system.
- Dendritic cell subsets are difficult to define and characterize from a functional perspective because of their heterogeneity and plasticity.
- All DC can act as antigen-presenting cells (APCs), and thus have the capacity to uptake and process polypeptides into antigens that are readily recognizable by the immune system. This group of cells expresses major histocompatibility complex (MHC) antigens (class I and II) and low levels of co-stimulatory molecules that are regulated. Cytokine production by DCs is also a critical feature that allows these APC to activate and educate T lymphocytes during cell–cell interactions.
- Dendritic cells can exist in tissues in an immature state, and can be activated into a mature state by microbial products (via Toll-like receptors) that results in migration from a tissue such as the skin to the local lymph node.
- Dendritic cells are present in normal and inflamed skin (Langerhans' cells in the epidermis, and dermal dendritic cells in the dermis) and may be involved in the pathogenesis of important diseases such as psoriasis and atopic dermatitis.

Specialized professional antigen-presenting cells (APCs), termed "dendritic cells" (DCs), are thought to play critical roles in the initiation and propagation of skin-centered immune and inflammatory reactions in health and disease. Although this chapter focuses almost exclusively on DCs and additionally emphasizes DCs that preferentially localize in skin, DCs are only one component of the skin immune system. The involvement of other hematopoietic cells, including lymphocytes, polymorphonuclear leukocytes, and tissue mast cells, in cutaneous inflammation is widely appreciated. Increasingly, it is apparent that skin intrinsic constituents such as keratinocytes and endothelial cells are also active participants in cutaneous inflammatory and immune reactions. Keratinocytes maintain the cutaneous barrier that excludes noxious agents, produce peptides that limit growth of microbes that breech the barrier, and release chemokines and proinflammatory cytokines that recruit and activate leukocytes. Effects on leukocyte recruitment are mediated, in part, by the actions of these epidermal-derived cytokines on microvascular endothelia that facilitate leukocyte adhesion and transmigration.

It is important to recognize that even tissue-centered immune and inflammatory reactions are organismal responses. Both innate and adaptive arms of the immune system are involved in most instances, with DCs acting as essential bridges reaching from one cell to another and between peripheral and lymphoid tissues as well. In trying to understand DC function in skin and other tissues, it is important to keep in mind that two critical drivers of evolution of immune and inflammatory mechanisms are resistance to life-threatening microbial infections and the need to avoid autoimmunity. Thus, studies of infectious and autoimmune diseases may be particularly informative when it comes to elucidating important functional aspects of cutaneous DC.

Historical Perspectives

In retrospect, studies of cutaneous DCs were ongoing for more than a century before DCs were identified as an important leukocyte subpopulation. In 1868, an Austrian medical student, Paul Langerhans, identified a distinctive cell in histologic sections of human epidermis that exhibited an unusual affinity for gold salts. Subsequently termed "Langerhans' cells" (LCs), these cells have been extensively studied by dermatologists as well as nondermatologists. Because of their dendritic morphology and lack of keratin filaments, relationships of LC to both neurons and melanocytes were conjectured. In the 1970s, Drs. Stephen Katz and Jeffrey Frelinger and their colleagues[1,2] conclusively and independently demonstrated that mouse LCs were bone marrow–derived and were therefore leukocytes. These studies led to more directed characterization of the functional activities of LCs, and it was subsequently demonstrated that they could function as APCs. Studies of patients who received allogeneic bone marrow transplants demonstrated that human LCs were also of bone marrow origin, and additional studies have confirmed that mouse and human LCs are comparable in many ways.

Dendritic cells were discovered as an identifiable leukocyte subpopulation about 30 years ago by Ralph Steinman at Rockefeller University. Working in mice, Steinman and his coworkers[3] characterized a very minor subpopulation of spleen cells that were extremely potent APCs and that were uniquely able to initiate immune responses in naive T cells. Analogous cells were subsequently described in other lymphoid tissues in relatively short order, and ultimately it was recognized that DCs populated most epithelia and solid organs as well. In 1985, more than 100 years after Paul Langerhans discovered them, another Austrian, Dr. Gerald Schuler,[4] a dermatologist, defined LCs as members of the DC family while working as a postdoctoral fellow in Dr. Steinman's laboratory, thereby definitively linking cutaneous immunophysiology and DC biology. This chapter explores this relationship and its consequences in health and disease.

Definition of Dendritic Cells

Perhaps because of their heterogeneity and plasticity, it is more difficult to identify and define DCs than other leukocyte subpopulations. Thus, we rely on a set of shared properties to clearly delineate DCs from other, in some cases related, leukocytes rather than any single characteristic (Table 8.1). Morphology is one criterion that is useful, and one that was recognized early on. Dendritic cells in tissues typically exhibit long processes ("dendrites"). This property is maintained to some extent by DCs in suspension and in culture, although in these settings cellular extensions take the form of sheets ("veils") rather than tubular projections. Because of their irregular contour, DCs have large cell surface areas with which to interface with their surroundings. Thus, although DCs are infrequently represented in their tissues of origins, comprising no more than a few percent of all cells present, a single DC may interact with many neighboring cells. Recent studies indicate that DCs actively extend and retract their cellular extensions in tissues,[5] a process that may reflect sampling activity of cells that likely function as sentinels.

All DCs can function as APCs. Minimal requirements for APCs include the ability to take up and degrade antigens into relevant peptides, cell-surface expression of MHC class I and class II antigens that can bind to appropriately processed peptides, and at least limited expression of some co-stimulatory molecules. Dendritic cells are the most potent of all APCs and can stimulate naive T cells. This latter activity of DCs likely results from their capacity to express large amounts of MHC-peptide antigen complexes, and high

TABLE 8.1. Dendritic cell characteristics

Derived from bone marrow (leukocytes)
Limited proliferation potential
Minor population in tissues
Widely distributed (epithelia, lymphoid tissues, solid organs)
Dendritic morphology
Antigen-presenting cell (APC) activity
Responsive to environmental cues (cytokines and pathogens)
Several activation/differentiation states
Can migrate from peripheral tissues to lymphoid organs
Can stimulate naive T cells
Can influence T-cell differentiation

levels of a variety of co-stimulatory molecules. The large cell surface areas with which DC can interface with responding T cells may also be a factor. The ability of many DCs to translocate in a directed fashion from peripheral tissues to lymphoid organs is another distinctive property of DCs that is integral to many of the their important functional activities.

Note that this discussion initially did not focus on cell-surface markers. B cells and T cells can be differentiated from all other leukocytes because they express immunoglobulin molecules and T-cell receptors (TCRs) for antigen, respectively, on their surfaces. Unfortunately, there is no single cell-surface antigen (or corresponding antibody) that uniquely identifies DCs. The leukocyte integrin CD11c/CD18 is perhaps the most useful single DC surface protein in this regard, being expressed by all murine and many human DCs, but CD11c is also expressed by non-DC under certain circumstances. Selected single cell-surface antigens can be used reliably to distinguish members of selected distinct DC subpopulations from each other, however (see below).

Dendritic Cell Subpopulations, Origins, and Lineages

Dendritic cells share more cell-surface markers with monocyte/macrophages than other leukocytes, a feature that was thought to indicate a lineage relationship between DCs and myeloid cells. Deciphering relationships between DCs and other leukocytes became more difficult as new DC subpopulations were described and it became increasingly apparent that DC phenotypes are influenced by their tissue environments, as well as by the degree to which DCs have been manipulated in vitro. The current consensus view is that there are three well-defined conventional DC subpopulations in both mice and humans: epidermal Langerhans' cells (LCs); interstitial DCs, as exemplified by dermal DCs (DDCs) in skin; and plasmacytoid DCs (PDCs) (Table 8.2). Two of the three subpopulations (LCs and DDCs) are represented in normal skin, and PDCs have been detected in skin in the setting of several cutaneous diseases. Recent data from studies of mice suggest that monocytes repre-

TABLE 8.2. Dendritic cells subpopulations

Conventional dendritic cells
Epidermal Langerhans' cells (LCs)
Interstitial dendritic cells (IDC), including dermal dendritic cells (DDCs)
Plasmacytoid dendritic cells (PDCs)
Unconventional dendritic cells
Dendritic cells with natural killer cell–like features (NK-DCs)
Tumor necrosis factor-α (TNF-α) and inducible nitric oxide synthase (iNOS)-producing dendritic cells (TIP-DCs)
Inflammatory dendritic epidermal cells (IDECs)

sent immediate precursors of LCs and DDCs.[6–8] The PDC lineage appears to be distinct from that of LCs and DDCs,[9] and these cells may be more closely related to lymphocytes. Elucidation of the relationships of several unconventional DCs (Table 8.2), including DCs with some features of natural killer (NK) cells,[10,11] inflammatory dendritic epidermal cells (IDECs),[12] and tumor necrosis factor-α (TNF-α)- and inducible nitric oxide synthase (iNOS)-producing DCs (TIP-DCs)[13] and conventional DCs, and the significance of these unconventional DCs in immunophysiology represents an area of active investigation (see below).

Some DCs (e.g., LCs and DDCs) localize initially in peripheral tissues (such as skin) and migrate to regional lymphoid organs in a regulated fashion, while others are found exclusively in lymphoid tissues and are derived from peripheral blood-borne precursors. When discussing tissue and lymphoid DCs that are linked in a precursor-product relationship, the convention is to refer to tissue DCs as "immature" and their lymphoid DC derivatives as "mature"[14] (Table 8.3).

Antigen Processing and Presenting Functions of Dendritic Cells

Although APC activity is a feature of all DCs, DCs are functionally distinct from other APCs (macrophages and B cells) in several important ways.[15] As already mentioned, DCs are the most potent APC known, and efficiently stimulate naive T cells. In addition, in some DCs antigen acquisition/processing and antigen presentation occur at different times and in different tissues. Highly active antigen acquisition and processing activities are characteristic of immature tissue DCs such as LCs

TABLE 8.3. Dendritic cell maturation

	Immature dendritic cells	Mature dendritic cells
Location	Periphery (e.g., skin)	Regional lymphoid tissue
Shape	Dendritic	More dendritic
Phagocytosis	Low	Absent
Macropinocytosis	High	Lower
Endocytosis	Present	Lower
Ag capture receptors	High	Low
MHC class I Ag	Present (cell surface)	High (cell surface)
MHC class II Ag	Present (intracellular)	High (cell surface)
Co-stimulatory molecules	Low (cell surface)	High (cell surface)
Migratory activity	Sessile	Motile
Cytokine production	Limited	IL-12, IL-23 and others

IL, interleukin; MHC, major histocompatibility complex.

and DDCs while they are located in skin. Immature DCs display a variety of cell-surface receptors including a number of C-type lectins (proteins that bind to microbial carbohydrates in a calcium-dependent manner),[16] Fc receptors (proteins that bind to Fc domains of immunoglobulins), complement receptors, and other proteins that enable them to physically interact with sources of antigen (e.g., microbes) and ingest them.

Ingestion of particulate antigen by DCs is accomplished by phagocytosis, while soluble antigens can be acquired via endocytosis or macropinocytosis. After ingestion, antigens are shuttled to the appropriate lysosomal enzyme containing compartments where they degraded into peptides that can bind to MHC class II antigens for presentation to CD4 T cells. Immature DCs exhibit limited phagocytic activity as compared with macrophages, but are much more active in this regard than mature dendritic cells. Immature DCs are also able to efficiently sample their extracellular environment through fluid-phase macropinocytosis. This process involves ingestion of relatively large amounts of extracellular fluid, allowing DCs to accumulate antigens that are present in low amounts in their environments.

Dendritic cells are also highly efficient stimulators of CD8 T cells. Antigenic epitopes that are recognized by CD8 T cells are displayed on the surfaces of DCs as complexes of appropriately processed peptides and polymorphic (or classic) MHC class I proteins. These complexes are assembled in the endoplasmic reticulum (ER) as MHC class I proteins are synthesized. Most peptides that are incorporated into MHC class I–containing peptides have a cytosolic origin and are generated through a process that involves proteolytic degradation by the proteosome and active transport into the ER via the transporter associated with antigen processing (TAP) protein. This pathway provides a mechanism for presentation of epitopes that are derived from self antigens or from pathogens (e.g., viruses) that infect DC to CD8 T cells.

It is at least theoretically important that DCs are also able to process and present antigenic epitopes that are derived from tumor cells or from pathogens that do not infect DCs for recognition by CD8 T cells. There is some controversy about the overall significance of this pathway, but it is clear that under some circumstances DCs can "cross-present" antigens that they do not synthesize to CD8 T cells. Although mechanistic details regarding this pathway remain to be determined, apoptotic cells comprise at least one relevant source of antigen for cross-presentation. Additionally, in the mouse, it appears that one DC subpopulation (CD8α+ lymphoid DC) is primarily responsible for cross-presentation of apoptotic cell-derived epitopes.

Finally, cutaneous DCs also express nonpolymorphic MHC class I antigens such as CD1a, CD1b, and CD1c. These cell-surface molecules are of particular interest and importance because they are involved in presentation of nonpeptide glycolipid-associated antigens, including those derived from mycobacteria such as *Mycobacterium leprae,* to T cells.

Activation and Trafficking of Cutaneous Dendritic Cells

In skin-centered immune responses, antigen acquisition occurs in the periphery (i.e., in skin), whereas antigen presentation occurs in regional lymph nodes (LNs). Thus, the ability of LCs and DDCs to translocate from one tissue to another in a directed fashion is critical. Encounters between DCs and antigen in association with one or more "danger signals" sets into motion a series of events that results in dramatic phenotypic changes, including enhanced migratory activity. Known danger signals include proinflammatory cytokines (such as interleukin-1 [IL-1] and TNF-α) and microbes. In skin, IL-1 and TNF-α can be produced by DCs and keratinocytes, and perhaps by other cells as well. Thus, DCs can respond to insults directly, or can exhibit bystander activation that is dependent on prior activation of keratinocytes or other resident skin cells. Microbes can interact with DCs via a variety of cell-surface proteins, including C-type lectins (see above)[16] and Toll-like receptors (TLRs).[17,18] Examples of cooperative interactions between selected C-type lectins and TLRs have been reported.

Interactions of immature DC with proinflammatory cytokines (via relevant receptors) and microbes (via TLRs) leads to downregulation of levels of cell-surface receptors that are involved in antigen recognition and uptake as well as decreased endocytic and macropinocytic activities. Simultaneously, activated DC express increased migratory activity, a chemokine receptor (CCR7) that facilitates directed migration to CCL21 (secondary lymphoid tissue chemokine, SLC)-expressing dermal lymphatics, increased MHC class I and class II antigens on cell surfaces, and higher levels of co-stimulatory molecules. The DDCs and LCs that have been activated in skin localize in T-cell–rich paracortical areas of regional LNs within 24 to 72 hours, where they are well positioned to activate naive T cells that are potentially reactive with antigens that were acquired in skin. Recent experiments indicate that DDCs arrive in draining LNs before LCs, and that DDCs and LCs accumulate in LNs in adjacent nonoverlapping regions.[19] The implications of these intriguing results are not yet fully understood. In the case of LCs, decreased of expression of the homotypic adhesion molecule E-cadherin (which may promote adhesion of LC to keratinocytes in vivo) also occurs as a consequence of activation.

The ability of activated DCs to express high levels of a variety of co-stimulatory molecules is, in part, responsible for their potent APC activity. Co-stimulatory molecules are cell-surface proteins that are expressed by APCs and that augment the responsiveness of T cells to ligation of T-cell receptors (TCRs) and their co-receptors CD4 and CD8 by complementary ligands on T cells. Co-stimulatory molecules are most often members of the immunoglobulin supergene family and include such proteins as CD40, CD80 (B7.1),

and CD86 (B7.2). CD40L is the T-cell co-receptor for CD40, and CD28 binds to CD80 and CD86. Although proinflammatory cytokines and TLR agonists induce comparable changes in DC surface phenotype and DCs activated by both types of stimuli cause T cells to proliferate, only DC stimulated with TLR agonists are able to efficiently induce complete T-cell differentiation and acquisition of effector function.[20] In addition to activating naive T cells, DCs influence T-cell differentiation. T-cell education is dependent on cytokines that are produced by DCs and that are present at the time of T-cell priming. DC-derived IL-12 is required for T-helper-1 (Th1) differentiation, while IL-23 promotes Th17 development (see below).

Skin-derived DCs also migrate to regional LNs in the absence of inflammatory stimuli. It has been conjectured that this baseline trafficking of skin DCs, in particular LCs, to regional LNs is a mechanism that allows for continuous presentation of self antigens to regulatory T cells that maintain peripheral tolerance.[21,22] However, all skin-derived DCs in regional LNs appear to express a mature phenotype manifested by high levels of MHC class I and II antigens and co-stimulatory molecules. Thus, it is not entirely clear how or why skin DCs would be mobilized in the absence of a danger signal or why DCs that migrated to LNs in the absence of inflammation would selectively stimulate T-regulatory lymphocytes (T$_{reg}$) to contribute to peripheral tolerance. The differential ability of TLR- and cytokine-activated DCs to promote development of T cells with effector activity indicate that there are nuances of DC function that remain to be elucidated, however.[20]

Dendritic Cell Heterogenicity and Plasticity

The heterogeneity of DCs that is encountered in vivo and in DC-like cells that are propagated in vitro is attributable to the existence of subpopulations with distinct lineages, and the influence of environment on DC phenotype. LCs, interstitial DCs, and PDCs clearly represent distinct populations, and interstitial DCs can be further subdivided based on surface phenotypes. The PDCs are functionally distinct from other DCs, but functional differences between other DC subpopulations are less well defined. Differential expression of individual C-type lectins and TLRs by different DC subpopulations suggests that DC subpopulations may have evolved to effectively recognize and respond to different microbes. As mentioned above, one subset of lymphoid DC (CD8α[+] DC) in mice is primarily responsible for ingesting apoptotic cells. Very recent experiments also suggest that, in mice, another lymphoid DC subpopulation, 33D1[+] DCs, are particularly efficient presenters of exogenous antigens to CD4 T cells.[23] It is likely that the functional significance of DC subpopulations in mice will become increasingly clear in the near future, and that results of these studies will provide important insights into functions of analogous DC subpopulations in humans.

The remarkable sensitivity of DCs to environmental influences is another feature that is undoubtedly of functional relevance. The ability of DCs to respond to proinflammatory cytokines and microbes and, in doing so, to acquire the ability to activate naive T cells has been discussed. In contrast, exposure of DCs to antiinflammatory environments, such as the IL-10–rich milieu present in some tumors, conditions DCs to preferentially induce unresponsiveness in T cells (T-cell anergy) or to activate T cells that possess negative regulatory activity. Dendritic cell plasticity is also reflected in the variety of surface phenotypes and functional activities of DCs that are propagated in vitro. Seemingly inconsequential or even imperceptible differences in culture conditions can have dramatic effects on the outcome of experimental results. This phenomenon is perhaps particularly relevant as it relates to propagation of human DCs in vitro for therapeutic purposes (as components of cancer vaccines for example), as small differences in culture conditions may lead to unanticipated differences in efficacy.

Dendritic Cells in Normal Skin

Two distinct subpopulations of conventional DCs are found in normal human and mouse skin (LCs and DDCs).[24] LCs are found in all stratified squamous epithelia and comprise 2% to 4% of all viable cells in epidermis. Cells analogous to DDCs are also identifiable in the submucosa of other epithelia and in solid organs as well. Although it has been thought that LCs

and DDCs have identical or overlapping functional activities, recent studies in mice have highlighted significant differences between these cells and provided new insights into possible functions.

A number of features distinguish LCs from DDCs and all other DCs (Table 8.4). Trilaminar racket-shaped vesicular structures termed "Birbeck granules" can be visualized in LCs via transmission electron microscopy, and have long been regarded as pathognomonic for LCs. Birbeck granules probably represent specialized endocytic vesicles, but their function is not well understood. A C-type lectin termed "langerin" (CD207) localizes to Birbeck granules and is responsible for their unusual appearance and possibly their formation. Langerin knockout mice have normal numbers of LCs and do not exhibit an obvious phenotype.[25] Thus, at this point, the importance of langerin and of Birbeck granules is not entirely clear. It is likely that, like other DC C-type lectins, langerin will ultimately be shown to play a role in microbial recognition. Indeed, some data suggest that langerin may facilitate presentation of mycobacterial-derived glycolipid antigens to CD1-restricted human T cells.

Another distinctive feature of LC is their ability to persist in unperturbed epidermis for weeks to months.[26] This property contrasts with tissue half-lives that are measured in days for all other DCs.[27–29] The ability of LCs to localize or to persist in epidermis may be related to their ability to express

TABLE 8.4. Distinctive features of conventional dendritic cells

Epidermal Langerhans' cells

Located in stratified squamous epithelia (skin, mouth, esophagus, vagina, anus)
Contain Birbeck granules (langerin-containing, Lag[+])
Express E-cadherin, CD1a
Require transforming growth factor-β1 for development

Dermal dendritic cells

Dermal (submucosal) location
No Birbeck granules (langerin and Lag[−]) or E-cadherin
Express CD1c

Plasmacytoid dendritic cells

Not found in normal skin, but present in inflamed skin
Plasmacytoid morphology (abundant rough ER, typical chromatin pattern)
Respond to TLR 7/9 agonists and produce type I interferons
Express BDCA-2

ER, endoplasmic reticulum; TLR, Toll-like receptor.

E-cadherin, a homotypic adhesion molecule that is a major component of adherens junctions in epithelial cells. Langerhans cells also selectively express the nonpolymorphic MHC class I molecule CD1a, a cell-surface protein implicated in initiation of antimycobacterial immunity, and have unique cytokine requirements for development. Although transforming growth factor β1 (TGF-β1) inhibits immune reactions, DC maturation, and the ability of DCs to activate T cells, this pleiotropic cytokine is absolutely required for LC development. TGF-β1 knockout mice are devoid of LCs, while other DC subpopulations appear to be appropriately represented. Historically, histologic stains for surface adenosine triphosphatase (ATPase) activity and S-100 protein were used to selectively identify LCs in situ, but newer reagents have largely supplanted their utility.

The first notable distinction between DDCs and LCs is their dermal location (Table 8.4). In normal dermis, a small number of DCs with LC features represent LCs that are in transit from epidermis to LNs. The DDCs can be differentiated from these LCs because they lack E-cadherin, and CD1a, and because they express another C-type lectin (DC-SIGN [CD209]) as well as CD1b and CD1c. DC-SIGN is also expressed by other interstitial DCs, and a variety of ligands have been identified. Known DC-SIGN ligands include intercellular adhesion molecule 3 (ICAM-3), selectins, viruses (including HIV and Dengue), fungi (e.g., *Aspergillus*), and parasites (*Leishmania major*). Based largely on these results, DC-SIGN has been implicated in DC trafficking, interactions between DCs and naive T cells, and microbial uptake. The significance of differential expression of CD1a and CD1c by LCs and DDCs is uncertain, but both molecules have been implicated in glycolipid antigen presentation. Differential abilities of DDCs and LCs to produce IL-12 have also been reported. The DDCs typically produce much higher levels of bioactive IL-12 p70 than LCs in response to a range of stimuli.

Cutaneous Dendritic Cell Function: Evolution of a Paradigm

Despite the distinctiveness of LC and DDC phenotypes and lineages, for technical reasons it has not been possible to assign unique functional activities to either DC population with certainty until recently. The consensus view has been that both LCs and DDCs have the capacity to initiate development of effector T-cell responses to foreign antigens that are encountered in skin. It has also been suggested that LCs, and perhaps DDCs, that travel to regional LNs in the absence of inflammatory stimuli induce and maintain peripheral tolerance by presenting self antigens to regulatory or other T cells. Several newly developed mouse models utilized in conjunction with increasingly sophisticated imaging techniques allow these concepts to be rigorously vetted, and interesting new information is accumulating.[30]

For many years, cutaneous DC function was conceptualized and studied primarily in the context of contact sensitivity reactions. However, development of a detailed understanding of the precise mechanisms involved in the initiation and propagation of immune responses to contact allergens (e.g., trinitrochlorobenzene [TNCB]) has been difficult because these substances readily penetrate skin and can therefore interact with a variety of DCs in skin and LNs directly. A second complicating factor is that the nature of the complete antigen that is recognized by contact allergen-reactive T cells is not completely defined and may be heterogeneous. New insights into DC function have come from studies of alternative mouse models including cutaneous *Leishmania* and *Herpes* virus infections, and models in which antigens are introduced into skin via gene gun immunization. The power of these approaches is increased when TCR transgenic mice, transgenic mice that are deficient in selected DC subpopulations, and bone marrow chimeric mice in which LC and DDC function can be independently manipulated are incorporated into these models.

Studies of cutaneous leishmaniasis in mice were among the first to directly implicate LCs in antigen presentation when cells containing both *Leishmania* amastigotes and Birbeck granules were detected in LNs draining *Leishmania major*–infected skin.[31,32] More recent studies indicated that *Leishmania* antigen that was available for presentation to T cells was associated with LN-resident DCs rather than cutaneous DCs that had migrated to the LN.[33] The explanation for this apparent discrepancy is not obvious at this point. Studies of mechanisms that are responsible for cutaneous gene gun immunization also implicate LCs or DDCs in T-cell priming directly.[34–36] In these experiments, complementary

DNAs (cDNAs) encoding foreign antigens of interest were coated onto subcellular-sized gold particles and introduced into skin using a biolytic nitrogen gas-driven device. Only cells that acquired beads and the associated cDNA expressed antigen. Gold beads and bead-associated antigen were detected in DCs in skin as well as in skin-derived DCs isolated from LNs after gene gun immunization. In addition, skin-derived DCs that have been isolated from LNs that drain skin genetic immunization sites can stimulate T cells that are reactive with appropriate antigens.

Inoculation of herpes simplex virus into mouse skin via scarification also results in vigorous T-cell responses involving both CD4 and CD8 cells. However, in this instance, examination of DCs from LNs draining virus-infected skin indicated that herpes antigen was exclusively associated with CD8α+ DC,[37] cells that have their origin in peripheral blood rather than skin. Recent studies indicate that although skin-derived DCs do not present herpes antigen to T cells, they do ferry it from skin to LNs.[38] Whether LCs or DDCs or cutaneous DCs participate in this process is not clear. The mechanism of virus antigen transfer from skin DCs to lymphoid DCs is not well understood. Since herpes simplex is a cytopathic virus, it is possible that skin DCs are infected in situ and migrate to LNs before they die. Subcellular fragments of virus-infected apoptotic DCs could then be efficiently ingested by CD8α+ lymphoid DCs, and these DCs might then initiate responses in T cells. Note that for activation of CD8 T cells, this scenario represents an example of cross-presentation in action.

Functional Aspects of Langerhans' Cells and Dermal Dendritic Cells

Recent insights into cutaneous DC physiology coupled with the availability of newly created transgenic mice will allow functional properties of LCs and DDCs to be delineated with more certainty in the near future. Because LCs and DDCs turn over in mouse skin at very different rates, it is possible to create bone marrow chimeric mice in which, for a period of time, LCs will be of recipient origin while virtually all other leukocytes (including DDCs and other DCs) will be derived from transplanted bone

marrow. If recipients and donors express different histocompatibility antigens, residual LCs can stimulate vigorous graft-versus-host reactions.[39]

By carefully selecting recipient/bone marrow donor pairs, it is possible to engineer mice in which some aspect of LC or DDC function is selectively impaired in the chimeric animals. For example, if one was interested in determining the relative contributions of LCs or DDCs to CD8 T-cell priming in a skin-centered immune response, one could generate chimeras using donor or recipient mice harboring β2-microglobulin (bm2) mutations that prevent expression of MHC class I molecules on cell surfaces. If bm2 bone marrow was introduced into lethally irradiated normal mice, LCs in the recipient mouse would be competent to stimulate CD8 T cells, while other DCs (including DDCs) would not. Conversely, if normal bone marrow was introduced into bm2 recipients, DDCs would be able to stimulate CD8 T cells while LCs would not.

The LCs can also be deleted in mice by selectively expressing "suicide genes" in LCs. In one strain of mice, a gene (cDNA) encoding diphtheria toxin (DT) has been expressed in LC using the langerin promoter (langerin-DT mice).[40] Because even small amounts of intracellular DT is cytotoxic, these mice never develop LC. In two other independently generated strains of mice, genes encoding the diphtheria toxin receptor (DTR) were inserted into the langerin gene locus.[19,41] In these animals, all LCs express the DTR. Because DT is not toxic to cells that lack the DTR and normal mouse cells do not express this receptor, it is possible to treat langerin-DTR mice with DT systemically and thus selectively eliminate LCs at any time without causing harm to the mice. Although LCs repopulate skin within several weeks after DT treatment, one can carry out experiments in LC-deficient animals within this window in time. Contact sensitivity reactions (CTS) have been studied in all three LC knockout mice. Although all three LC knockout mice developed CTS reactions, CTS reactions in the langerin-DT mice were enhanced approximately twofold.[40] In contrast, CTS reactions in one of the langerin-DTR mouse strains were diminished by ~50%,[41] while CTS reactions were essentially unchanged in the other langerin-DTR mouse strain.[19] It has been suggested that the results obtained in the langerin-DT mice are consistent with a negative regulatory role for LCs.

Thus, cutaneous DC may participate in skin-centered immune responses in at least three ways: (1) as APCs that acquire foreign antigen in skin, transport it to LNs, and induce effector T-cell responses; (2) as cells that transport foreign antigen to LNs but "hand it off" to lymphoid DCs for presentation to T cells; and (3) as APCs that transport self antigen to LNs and activate regulatory T cells that limit or inhibit unwanted activation of self-reactive effector T cells. We can anticipate that the relative importance of these different functional activities in normal immunophysiology and in disease states, and the degree to which LCs and DDCs contribute to the different functional activities will be clarified over the next few years.

Dendritic Cells in Selected Inflammatory Skin Diseases

Plasmacytoid DCs (PDCs) are the third clearly defined conventional DC subpopulation (Table 8.4). These DCs can be readily identified in lymphoid tissues, especially in the setting of inflammation, but they are not prominent in normal skin. The designation "plasmacytoid" refers to the abundant rough ER and mixture of hetero- and euchromatin that is detected in PDC precursors via transmission electron microscopy. Although it has been suggested that PDCs are of lymphoid origin, they do not express surface immunoglobulin or produce immunoglobulins and should not be confused with bona fide plasma cells. Appropriate stimulation of PDC results in acquisition of a dendritic morphology and the ability to activate naive T cells—two hallmarks that justify their inclusion in the DC family.[9] However, human PDCs do not express the CD11c/CD18 β_2- integrin that is characteristic of other DC.

The PDCs express several distinctive C-type lectins (BCDA-2 [CD303]), and antibodies reactive with these surface proteins can be used to identify and isolate these interesting cells. From a functional perspective, PDCs differ from other DCs and other leukocytes in that their precursors are prodigious producers of type I interferons (interferons α and β) in response to viruses and to naturally occurring or synthetic TLR 7/9 ligands (e.g., viral nucleic acids, CpG-containing oligodeoxynucleotides, and imiquimod). Consistent with a prominent role in antiviral immunity, it has also been suggested that PDCs are more effective stimulators of CD8 T cells than CD4 cells. Type I interferons and PDCs have also been implicated in both lupus erythematosus and psoriasis.[42]

Exacerbations of psoriasis in patients who were being treated with systemic interferon-α or topical imiquimod first suggested a role for PDC in this disease.[43] Subsequently, it was determined that PDC numbers were elevated in lesional psoriatic skin, and evidence of increased type I interferon production (in the form of a transcriptional type I interferon signature) was also detected. That PDC and type I interferons may have a causative role in psoriasis was suggested by mouse/human xenograft experiments in which lesional skin from psoriasis patients was grafted onto immunodeficient mice.[44] Transplanted psoriatic skin retained the psoriatic phenotype as well as the increased numbers of PDCs and the type I interferon gene expression signature that was initially detected in patients. Interestingly, inhibition of human PDC function in graft-bearing mice with an appropriate antibody led to a loss of the psoriatic phenotype. Although this result suggests that therapeutic agents that are directed against PDCs or type I interferons may be useful in patients with psoriasis, results of clinical trials have not yet been reported.

Clinical experiences with biologic therapies that inhibit TNF-α–induced signaling clearly implicate this proinflammatory cytokine in psoriasis pathogenesis in an important way. Although TNF-α can be produced by cells that are intrinsic to skin as well as a wide variety of infiltrating leukocytes, identification of increased numbers of a novel cell type in psoriatic skin point to a potentially important cellular source. These cells, termed TNF-α– and iNOS-producing DCs (TIP-DCs),[13] are analogous to a subpopulation of cells that have been identified in the spleens of mice infected with *Listeria monocytogenes*.

Dendritic cells that normally populate skin may also play a role in psoriasis pathogenesis. For a number of years, psoriasis has been viewed as an inflammatory skin disease that is characterized by overproduction of type 1 cytokines (typified by interferon-γ). Interferon-γ (IFN-γ) is produced exclusively by Th1 cells, and Th1 cell development is dependent on production of IL-12 by DCs. Thus, therapies that target IL-12 might be expected to be efficacious in psoriasis, and, indeed, clinical studies indicate that antibodies that react with one of two subunits of IL-12 (anti-p40) have considerable activity in patients.[45] Identification and characterization of a new Th subset (Th17 cells) that is distinct from Th1 and Th2 cells, and recent recognition that Th17 cells may be of critical importance in several autoimmune diseases (rheumatoid arthritis, inflammatory bowel disease, and psoriasis)[46] has led to a reinterpretation of the results of the anti-p40 trials. Although Th17 cell development does not depend on IL-12, another IL-12 family member (IL-23) that is also produced by DC is critically important.[47,48] Because the p40 subunit is common to IL-12 and IL-23, anti-p40 antibodies neutralize both cytokines. The current view is that IL-23 may be the most relevant target of anti-p40 antibodies in psoriasis. The involvement of Th17 cells and their products in psoriasis pathogenesis is an area of active investigation.

Two DC subpopulations have been detected in the established skin lesions of patients with atopic dermatitis (AD) and implicated in disease pathogenesis: LCs and inflammatory dendritic epidermal cells (IDEC).[12] Although both subsets express high levels of co-stimulatory molecules consistent with activated phenotypes, LCs and IDECs can be distinguished from each other in AD skin using several criteria. Both cells express CD1a, but CD1a levels are high on LC and low on IDEC. LCs are langerin positive and contain Birbeck granules, while IDECs lack langerin but express the macrophage mannose receptor (another C-type lectin). CD11b/CD18 (Mac 1), another leukocyte integrin, is also differentially expressed, being abundant on IDECs and absent from the surfaces of LCs. LCs and IDECs in skin of patients with atopic dermatitis also express the high affinity immunoglobulin E (IgE) Fc receptor (Fcε RI), a feature that differentiates them from DCs in normal skin and DCs in other inflammatory settings. Atopic dermatitis appears to be a mechanistically biphasic skin disease with Th2 cytokine production predominant early and Th1 cytokines predominating in chronic lesions. It has been suggested that Fcε RI–bearing LCs are particularly potent stimulators of relevant T cells by virtue of the fact that they bear antigen-reactive IgE on their surfaces and produce cytokines and chemokines that recruit IDECs into lesional skin. Stimulation of IDECs by Fcε RI cross-linking results in production of IL-12 in vitro, and it has been suggested that IDEC may be important sources of IL-12 in vivo and may lead to the Th2 to Th1 switch that is characteristic of this disease.[49] The precise relationship of IDECs to LCs or other DCs is not entirely clear at this point, and the extent to which either LCs or IDECs are involved in atopic dermatitis also remains to be conclusively demonstrated.

Challenges and Opportunities

There has been an explosion of information regarding the many ways that DCs influence immunophysiology in skin and elsewhere, but our knowledge remains incomplete in a number of critical areas (e.g., understanding of the importance of DC subpopulations). This is well illustrated in skin, where despite investigations that have been ongoing for many years, the function of LC remains largely enigmatic. Additional studies of the conditional and constitutive LC knockout mice described above will undoubtedly clarify LC function in vivo. It can be anticipated that development of analogous mice with selective defects in other DC subpopulations will allow accumulation of definitive information about these cells as well.

Better insights into the detailed mechanisms by which DCs participate in cutaneous and other diseases with inflammatory components are also required. Dendritic cells are likely to be involved in virtually every disease in which T cells are active participants. In diseases where T cells are inappropriately active, targeting DCs or their products can be reasonably expected to represent useful therapeutic strategies. The identification of DC as potentially important sources of TNF-α (TIP-DC) and IL-23 in psoriasis may provide partial explanations for the efficacy of the biologic therapeutics that modulate these important cytokines or their receptors, for example. Likewise, the suggestion that production of type I interferon by PDCs in lesional psoriatic skin is pathophysiologically relevant provides a therapeutic avenue heretofore unknown.

Conversely, in diseases where enhanced T-cell responsiveness is desired, augmentation of DC function may be a viable therapeutic option. Several years ago, considerable effort was expended to incorporate DCs that had been grown in the laboratory into cancer vaccine trials in patients. As is often the case, early clinical experience with small numbers of patients generated an inappropriately high level of optimism, and enthusiasm has subsequently diminished. Emphasis has shifted to strategies that enhance DC function in situ with adjuvants that act on DCs or that target antigens selectively to DCs in vivo, and clinical trials are ongoing. The first century of DC biology represents a period in which cellular immunology has moved from mystery to molecules, and the critical involvement of DCs in a wide variety of inflammatory processes has been delineated. Perhaps the second century will be remembered as a time when application of this fundamental information resulted in development of new therapies that had major impacts on human health.

Conclusion

Cutaneous DCs are an important component of the skin immune system and play a role in host defense, allergy, autoimmunity and cancer surveillance. Cutaneous DCs may also play a role in the maintenance of self tolerance and in the pathogenesis of a number of common skin diseases such as psoriasis and atopic dermatitis. Targeting cutaneous DCs or their products with novel biologic therapeutics may revolutionize treatment of inflammatory skin diseases.

References

1. Katz ST, Tamaki K, Sachs DH, Epidermal Langerhans cells are derived from cells originating in bone marrow. Nature 1979;282:324–6.
2. Frelinger JG, Hood L, Hill S, Frelinger JA. Mouse epidermal Ia molecules have a bone marrow origin. Nature 1979;282:321–3.
3. Steinman RM, Adams JC, Cohn ZA. Identification of a novel cell type in peripheral lymphoid organs of mice. IV. Identification and distribution in mouse spleen. J Exp Med 1975;141:804–20.
4. Schuler G, Steinman RM. Murine epidermal Langerhans cells mature into potent immunostimulatory dendritic cells in vitro. J Exp Med 1985;161:526–46.
5. Nishibu A, Ward Brant R, Jester JV, Ploegh HL, Boes M, Takashima A. Behavioral responses of epidermal Langerhans cells *in situ* to local pathological stimuli. J Invest Dermatol 2006;126:787–796.
6. Larregina AT, Morelli AE, Spencer LA, et al. Dermal-resident CD14+ cells differentiate into Langerhans cells. Nat Immunol 2001;2:1151–58.
7. Ginhoux F, Tacke F, Angeli V, et al. Langerhans cells arise from monocytes in vivo. Nat Immunol 2006;7:265–273.
8. Bogunovic M, Ginhoux F, Wagers A, et al. Identification of a radio-resistant and cycling dermal dendritic cell population in mice and men. J Exp Med 2006;203:1–12.
9. Soumelis V, Liu Y-J. From plasmacytoid to dendritic cell: morphological and functional switches during plasmacytoid pre-dendritic cell differentiation. Eur J Immunol 2006;36:2286–92.
10. Chan CW, Crafton E, Fan HN, et al. Interferon-producing killer dendritic cells provide a link between innate and adaptive immunity. Nat Med 2006;12:207–213.
11. Taieb J, Chaput N, Menard C, et al. A novel dendritic cell subset involved in tumor immunosurveillance. Nat Med 2006;12:214–219.
12. Wollenberg A, Kraft S, Hanau D, Bieber T. Immunomorphological and ultrastructural characterization of Langerhans cells and a novel, inflammatory dendritic epidermal cell (IDEC) population in lesional skin of atopic eczema. J Invest Dermatol 1996;106:446–53.
13. Lowes MA, Chamian F, Abello MV, et al. Increase in TNF-α and inducible nitric oxide synthase-expressing dendritic cells in psoriasis and reduction with efalizumab (anti-CD11a). Proc Natl Acad Sci 2005;102:19057–19062.
14. Reis e Sousa C. Dendritic cells in a mature age. Nat Rev Immunol 2006;6:476–83.
15. Steinman, RM, Hemmi H. Dendritic cells: translating innate to adaptive immunity. Curr Top Microbiol Immunol 2006;311:17–58.
16. Figdor CG, van Kooyk Y, Adema GJ. C-Type lectin receptors on dendritic cells and Langerhans cells. Nat Rev Immunol 2002;2:77–84.
17. Hemmi H, Akira S. TLR signaling and the function of dendritic cells. Chem Immunol Allergy 2005;86:120–35.
18. Reis e Sousa C. Toll-like receptors and dendritic cells: for whom the bug tolls. Semin Immunol 2004;16:27–34.
19. Kissenpfennig A, Henri S, Dubois B, et al. Dynamics and function of Langerhans cells in vivo: dermal dendritic cells colonize lymph node areas distinct from slower migrating Langerhans cells. Immunity 2005;22:643–654.
20. Sporri R, Reis e Sousa C. Inflammatory mediators are insufficient for full dendritic cell activation and promote expansion of CD4+ T cell populations lacking helper function. Nat Immunol 2005;6:163–70.

21. Steinman RM, Nussenzweig MC. Avoiding horror auto-toxicus: the importance of dendritic cells in peripheral T cell tolerance. Proc Natl Acad Sci 2002;99:351–358.

22. Steinman RM, Hawiger D, Liu K, et al. Dendritic cell function in vivo during the steady state: A role in peripheral tolerance. Ann N Y Acad Sci 2003;987:15–25.

23. Dudziak D, Kamphorst AO, Heidkamp GF, et al. Differential antigen processing by dendritic cell subsets in vivo. Science 2007;315:107–111.

24. Valladeau J, Saeland S. Cutaneous dendritic cells. Semin Immunol 2005;17:273–283.

25. Kissenpfennig A, Ait-Yahia S, Clair-Moninot V, et al. Disruption of the *langerin*/CD207 gene abolishes Birbeck granules without a marked loss of Langerhans cell function. Mol Cell Biol 2005;25:88–99.

26. Merad M, Manz MG, Karsunky H, et al. Langerhans cells renew in the skin throughout life under steady-state conditions. Nat Immunol 2002;3:1135–41.

27. Kamath AT, Pooley J, O'Keeffe MA, et al. The development, maturation, and turnover rate of mouse spleen dendritic cell populations. J Immunol 2000;165:6762–70.

28. Henri S, Vremec D, Kamath A, et al. The dendritic cell populations of mouse lymph nodes. J Immunol 2001;167:741–8.

29. Kamath AT, Henri S, Battye F, Tough DF, Shortman K. Developmental kinetics and lifespan of dendritic cells in mouse lymphoid organs. Blood 2002;100:1734–41.

30. Villadangos JA, Heath WR. Life cycle, migration and antigen presenting functions of spleen and lymph node dendritic cells: limitations of the Langerhans cells paradigm. Semin Immunol 2005;17:262–272.

31. Moll H, Flohe S, Rollinghoff M. Dendritic cells in *Leishmania major*-immune mice harbor persistent parasites and mediate an antigen-specific T cell immune response. Eur J Immunol 1995;25:693–9.

32. Baldwin T, Henri S, Curtis J, et al. Dendritic cell populations in *Leishmania major*-infected skin and draining lymph nodes. Infect Immun 2004;1991–2001.

33. Iezzi G, Frohlich A, Ernst B, et al. Lymph node resident rather than skin-derived dendritic cells initiate specific T cell responses after *Leishmania major* infection. J Immunol 2006;177:1250–1256.

34. Condon C, Watkins SC, Celluzzi CM, Thompson K, Falo LD, Jr. DNA-based immunization by *in vivo* transfection of dendritic cells. Nat Med 1996;2:1122–1128.

35. Porgador A, Irvine KR, Iwasaki A, Barber BH, Restifo NP, Germain RN. Predominant role for directly transfected dendritic cells in antigen presentation to CD8+T cells after gene gun immunization. J Exp Med 1998;188:1075–1082.

36. He Y, Zhang J, Donahue C, Falo LD Jr. Skin-derived dendritic cells induce potent CD8+ T cell immunity in recombinant lentivector-mediated genetic immunization. Immunity 2006;24:643–656.

37. Allan RS, Smith CM, Belz GT, et al. Epidermal viral immunity induced by CD8α+ dendritic cells but not by Langerhans cells. Science 2003;301:1925–28.

38. Allan RS, Waithman J, Bedoui S, et al. Migratory dendritic cells transfer antigen to a lymph node-resident dendritic cell population for efficient CTL priming. Immunity 2006;25:153–162.

39. Merad M, Hoffmann, P, Ranheim E, et al. Depletion of host Langerhans cells before transplantation of donor alloreactive T cells prevents skin graft-versus-host disease. Nat Med 2004;10:510–517.

40. Kaplan DH, Jenison MC, Saeland S, Shlomchik WD, Shlomchik MJ. Epidermal Langerhans cell-deficient mice develop enhanced contact hypersensitivity. Immunity 2005;23:611–620.

41. Bennett CL, von Rijn E, Jung S, et al. Inducible ablation of mouse Langerhans cells diminishes but fails to abrogate contact hypersensitivity. J Cell Biol 2005;169:569–576.

42. Banchereau J, Pascual V. Type 1 interferon in systemic lupus erythematosus and other autoimmune diseases. Immunity 2006;383–392.

43. Gilliet M, Conrad C, Geiges M, et al. Psoriasis triggered by toll-like receptor 7 agonist imiquimod in the presence of dermal plasmacytoid dendritic cell precursors. Arch Dermatol 2004;140:1490–1495.

44. Nestle FO, Conrad C, Tun-Kyi A, et al. Plasmacytoid predendritic cells initiate psoriasis through interferon-α production. J Exp Med 2005;202:135–143.

45. Krueger GG, Langley RG, Leonardi C, et al. A human interleukin-12/23 monoclonal antibody for the treatment of psoriasis. N Engl J Med 2007;356:580–92.

46. Lowes Michelle A, Bowcock AM, Krueger JG. Pathogenesis and therapy of psoriasis. Nature 2007;445:866–873.

47. Hunter CA. New IL-12–family members: IL-23 and IL-27, cytokines with divergent functions. Nat Rev Immunol 2005;5:521–531.

48. Weaver CT, Hatton, RD, Mangan PR, Harrington LE. IL-17 family cytokines and the expanding diversity of effector T cells lineages. Ann Rev Immunol 2007;25:821–52.

49. Novak N, Valenta R, Bohle B, et al. FcεRI engagement of Langerhans cell-like dendritic cells and inflammatory dendritic epidermal cell-like dendritic cells induces chemotactic signals and different T-cell phenotypes in vitro. J Allergy Clin Immunol 2004;113:949–57.

9
Antimicrobial Peptides

H. Ray Jalian and Jenny Kim

Key Points

- Antimicrobial peptides (AMPs) are low-molecular-weight proteins with a wide spectrum of activity against microbial pathogens.
- Antimicrobial peptides are amphipathic.
- Antimicrobial peptides include defensins, cathelicidins, granulysin, S-100 proteins, and a variety of other antimicrobial proteins.
- Antimicrobial peptides play a role in acne, wound healing, psoriasis, and atopic dermatitis.

Skin has historically been viewed as primarily a mechanical barrier to environmental insults and microbes. However, in addition to its traditional role as a physical defense mechanism, the skin also functions as a dynamic immune organ, possessing a robust immune defense mechanism to microbial invaders. Of note, antimicrobial peptides (AMP) have gained considerable attention not only for their microbicidal properties, but also for their antiinflammatory and other immune modulating effects. In 1987, Zasloff[1] described the presence of a potent antibacterial peptide present in the skin of African frog *Xenopus laevis*. Since this initial discovery, there have been numerous AMPs described in human skin, and their role in host defense has been well characterized.

Generally speaking, antimicrobial peptides are a heterogeneous group of low-molecular-weight proteins with wide-spectrum antimicrobial activity against bacteria, fungi, and viruses. These peptides are almost uniformly positively charged, and are amphipathic, having both hydrophobic and hydrophilic surfaces. The dual nature of charge allows the peptide to be soluble in an aqueous environment, while retaining its ability to bind the bacterial membrane with its hydrophobic surface. Once bound to the target membrane, the peptide can kill the organism through various mechanisms. In addition to known antimicrobial properties, there is a growing body of evidence supporting AMPs' ability to alter host immune response. This chapter focuses on the main AMPs present in human skin, and discusses the relevant dermatologic conditions in which deficiencies or overexpression of AMPs are thought to play an important etiologic role. A summary of the key antimicrobial peptides reviewed in this chapter can be found in Table 9.1.

Defensins

Defensins are a family of evolutionarily related antimicrobial peptides with a characteristic β-sheet fold and six disulfide bonds between highly conserved cysteine residues. There are two main defensin subfamilies, α- and β-defensins, differing mainly in the pairing of their cysteine residues. Members of both subfamilies consist of a triple-stranded β-sheet with a prototypic "defensin" fold (Fig. 9.1). In addition, there is a third defensin family, θ-defensins, not expressed in humans.[2] Defensins are widely distributed in cells and tissues involved in host defense, and can be found in highest concentrations within the granules of phagocytes. α-Defensins, which have disulfide bridges between cysteines 1 and 6, 2 and 4, and 3 and 5,[3] are found predominantly in neutrophils,[4] and have aptly been named human neutrophil peptides (HNPs) 1 to 4. In humans, α-defensins

TABLE 9.1. Summary of major antimicrobial peptides present in skin

	Cell source	Other properties
α-defensins	Infiltrating neutrophils	Increase tumor necrosis factor-α and interleukin-1 in *S. aureus* activated monocytes
β-defensins	Keratinocytes	Chemotaxis of T cells and Dendritic cells
Cathelicidin (LL-37)	Keratinocytes	Angiogenesis
	Ductal epithelium	Wound healing
	Eccrine glands	Chemotaxis of neutrophils, monocytes, T cells, and mast cell
	Mast cells	
Granulysin	Infiltrating T cells	Chemotaxis for T cells, monocytes, NK cells, and dendritic cells
		Cytotoxic to tumor cells
		Antiinflammatory
		Graft Rejection
Psoriasin	Keratinocytes	Chemotaxis for CD4+ lymphocytes and neutrophils
	Follicular epithelium	
	Sebocytes	
Dermcidin	Eccrine glands	Not determined
RNase 7	Keratinocytes	Not determined

are stored in azurophilic granules of neutrophils as fully processed, mature peptides. In addition, two other α-defensins, human defensin (HD)-5[5] and 6,[6] are expressed in Paneth cells of the small intestine as well as in the epithelia of the female urogenital tract.[7] α-Defensins show a wide spectrum of antimicrobial activity against bacteria and fungi. Recent evidence has shown that certain enveloped viruses, particularly adenovirus,[8] are inactivated by α-defensins. Furthermore, α-defensins have been implicated as one of the molecules that may be important in the antiviral activity seen in CD8+ T cells of HIV nonprogressors.[9] In addition, at high concentrations, defensins are toxic to mammalian cells and may be important in tissue injury and necrosis during inflammation. Finally, α-defensins contribute to the host inflammatory response by increasing the expression of tumor necrosis factor-α (TNF-α) and interleukin-1 (IL-1) in *Staphylococcus aureus*–activated monocytes.[10] The antimicrobial spectrum and regulatory mechanisms of the main AMPs expressed in the skin can be found in Table 9.2.

Human β-defensins (HBD) are also characterized by six cysteine motifs, but the distinction

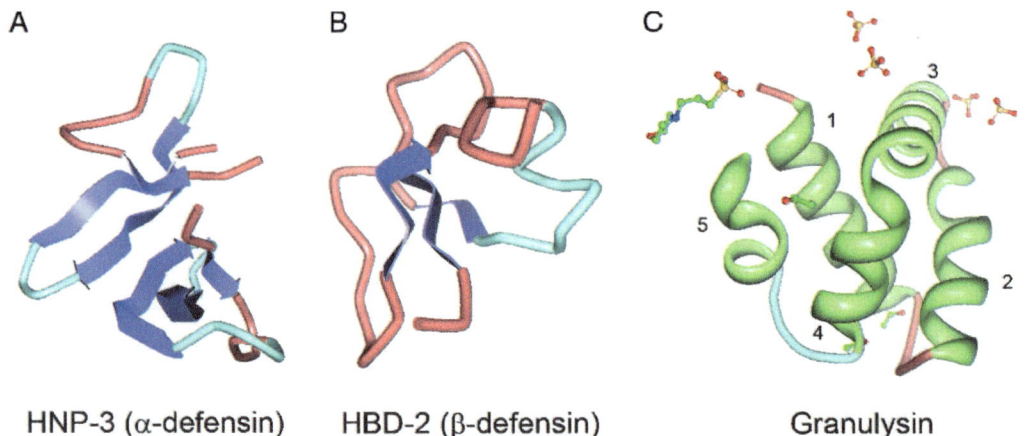

A   **B**   **C**

HNP-3 (α-defensin)   HBD-2 (β-defensin)   Granulysin

FIG. 9.1. Representative structure of defensins and granulysin. β-pleated sheets are indicated in blue arrows, α-helices indicated in green. Human neutrophil peptide 3 (HNP-3) (A), represented as a dimer, and human β-defensin (HBD-2) (B) both contain a triple stranded β-sheet as a conserved structural component. Granulysin (C) contains five α-helices important for both structure and antimicrobial activity

TABLE 9.2. Antimicrobial and immunomodulatory properties

	Antimicrobial activity			
	Gram positive	Gram negative	Fungi	Regulation
α-defensin	+	+	+	Constitutive
HBD-1	±	+	−	Constitutive
HBD-2	±	+	+	Inducible via IL-1/ NF-κB dependent mechanism Toll-like receptors
HBD-3	+	+	+	Inducible via TGF-α, and IGF-I
HBD-4	+	+	+	Via NF-κB independent pathways
Cathelicidin	+	+	+	Vitamin-D Toll-like receptors
Granulysin	+	+	+	Toll-like receptors Activator protein-1 dependent pathway
Psoriasin	±	+	−	Calcium All-trans retinoic acid Inflammatory stress
Dermcidin	+	+	+	Constitutive
RNAse 7	+	+	+	Inducible via IL-1β, IFN-γ, TNF-α Bacterial challenge

IFN, interferon; IGF, insulin-like growth factor; IL, interleukin; NF, nuclear factor; TGF, transforming growth factor; TNF, tumor necrosis factor.

of these two classes lies in their cysteine cross-bridging. The disulfide bonds of β-defensins are between cysteines 1 and 5, 2 and 4, and 3 and 6.[11] Human β-defensins 1 to 4 have been identified in many cell types, including epithelial cells, though their expression, localization, and antimicrobial specificities vary. HBD-1 is expressed predominantly in the urinary tract, but is also expressed constitutively in the skin. HBD-2, in contrast, is induced by bacteria through an IL-1/nuclear factor (NF)-κB dependent mechanism.[12] The antibacterial spectrum of HBD-2 seems to be limited predominantly to Gram-negative organisms. One study found that HBD-2 preferentially killed *Pseudomonas aeruginosa*, and was only bacteriostatic against *S. aureus*.[13] In contrast, HBD-3 is a broad-spectrum antibiotic with specificity for a wide range of both Gram-positive and Gram-negative bacteria, and fungi.[14] The induction of HBD-3 is thought to be dependent on various growth factors, including transforming growth factor-α (TGF-α), and insulin-like growth factor I (IGF-I) via transactivation of the epidermal growth factor (EGF) receptor.[15] HBD-4, also expressed in the skin, is inducible through distinct NF-κB independent pathways that have yet to be fully characterized.[16]

Both α- and β-defensins share a common antimicrobial mechanism. It is hypothesized that the permeabilization of target membranes is the critical step in defensin-mediated cytotoxicity. In experimental models using *Escherichia coli*, membrane permeabilization resulted in the subsequent inhibition of bacterial metabolism, including RNA, DNA and protein synthesis.[17] One study proposed the formation of a stable 25-Å pore, comprised of a hexamer of defensin dimers,[18] allowing for small intracellular molecules to leak out of the organism (Fig. 9.2). This mechanism, however, may only partially account for antimicrobial activity, as evidence exists for both a transient pore formation and also intracellular sites of action, which may be important in cell death.[19] In addition, some defensins have been found to bind membrane glycoproteins with high affinity, which may explain the observed antiviral activity of these peptides.[20]

Cathelicidins

Cathelicidins are a family of antimicrobial peptides that contain an N-terminal signal peptide, an evolutionary conserved cathelin domain, and a C-terminal cationic peptide.[21] Cathelicidin is first produced as a large, inactive precursor protein, which is then processed by neutrophil proteinase-3 into the cathelin domain and LL-37. From this point, further action by various cutaneous serine proteases results in multiple peptides with distinct activities.[22] The human cathelicidin family is limited to one gene whose protein product is most often referred to as LL-37 (L for two leucine residues, 37 for the number of amino present in the peptide) and also hCAP18 (human cationic AMP; 18 kD).[23] Initially, LL-37 had been identified in keratinocytes at the

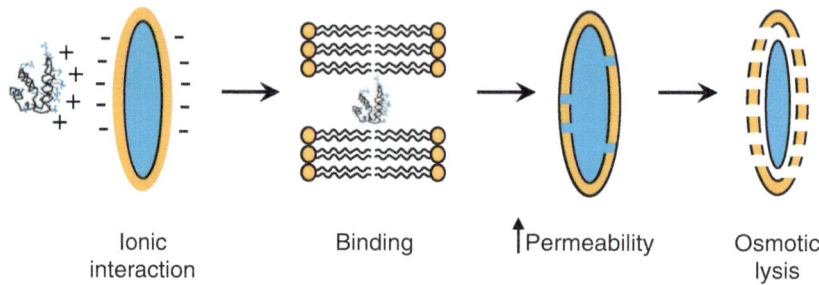

Ionic   Binding   ↑Permeability   Osmotic
interaction   lysis

Fig. 9.2. Proposed mechanism of action of antimicrobial peptides. Cationic antimicrobial peptides (AMPs) (granulysin shown) associate with the negative bacterial membrane, resulting in binding and subsequent increased permeability of the phospholipid bilayer. As a result of the increased permeability, the irreversible osmotic damage results in cell death

site of wound healing, and was found to be stored in the lamellar granules of keratinocytes.[24] It is now known that in addition to this inducible expression, constitutive expression of LL-37 occurs in certain anatomic locations, such as the nail bed and eccrine glands.[25] In addition, neonatal skin expresses LL-37 at baseline.[26]

LL-37 has a broad antibacterial spectrum, including both Gram-positive and Gram-negative organisms. In vitro evidence has shown bactericidal activity against *P. aeruginosa*, *Listeria monocytogenes*, *S. aureus*, *S. epidermidis*, *Salmonella typhimurium*, *E. coli*, and even vancomycin-resistant *Enterococci* (VRE).[27] In vivo, mice with a mutation in *CRAMP* (the gene encoding the murine homologue of LL-37) are increasingly susceptible to streptococcal infections when compared to wild-type controls.[28] In addition, LL-37 is further processed into smaller peptides, including RK-31 and KS-30, that have increasing antimicrobial activity against staphylococcal species.[29] LL-37 is also active against fungal species, most notably *Candida albicans*.[30] Recent in vitro data have also shown that LL-37 has potent activity against herpes simplex virus (HSV), and this was complemented by in vivo data showing decreased expression of LL-37 in atopic dermatitis patients with eczema herpeticum.[31]

The expression of LL-37 within human skin is both constitutive and inducible. In eccrine glands and ductal cells, LL-37 is diffusely expressed in the cytoplasm of secretory glands and also the ductal epithelium.[25] In addition, serine proteases, which are present within sweat, further cleave LL-37

into smaller peptides with enhanced antimicrobial activity against staphylococcal and candidal species.[29] LL-37 expression is induced during wound healing, and studies using a cultured keratinocyte model suggest the importance of IGF-I in this expression.[32] Recently, vitamin D has emerged as important regulator of LL-37 expression. For example, 1,25-dihydroxyvitamin D_3 can induce the expression of LL-37 in an immortalized keratinocyte cell line. In addition, the gene encoding LL-37 contains a vitamin D response element (VDRE) present in its promoter.[33] Recently, Liu and colleagues[34] found that Toll-like receptor-2 (TLR2)-dependent microbicidal activity was dependent on the vitamin-D–induced expression of LL-37.[34] This identified a novel mechanism for TLR-induced antimicrobial activity, and may represent one of the main defenses of infection from both cutaneous and systemic tuberculosis.

As with other antimicrobial peptides, LL-37 also has a role in modulating the host immune response. In addition to its direct microbicidal activity, LL-37 is chemotractant for neutrophils, monocytes, and T cells by binding of formyl-peptide-receptor-like-1 (FPRL-1). In addition, it recruits and stimulates subsequent production of LL-37 via mast cells, creating a positive feedback loop.[35]

Granulysin

Granulysin, a T-cell–derived antimicrobial peptide, belongs to a member of the larger saposin-like protein family. This family also includes other bactericidal peptides such as NK-lysin, expressed predominantly in natural killer (NK) cells.[36] Unlike defensins and cathelicidin that are expressed in the epithelial cells themselves, granulysin is found exclusively within the granules of cytotoxic T cells and NK cells recruited to sights of inflammation (e.g., skin). More specifically, granulysin colocalizes to the cytotoxic vacuole with perforin, where they act synergistically to kill intracellular bacteria.[37,38] Perforin forms pores in the cellular membrane, allowing granulysin to access the intracellular compartment in which the pathogen resides, providing a direct mechanism of intracellular pathogen targeting.

Granulysin in humans is synthesized as a 15-kD protein that is then cleaved to release the final 9-kD peptide.[39] The resultant 9-kD peptide is composed of five α-helices joined by short loops (Fig. 9.1).[40] Granulysin is effective against a wide range of Gram-positive and Gram-negative bacteria, parasites, and fungi. Notably, granulysin kills *Mycobacterium tuberculosis,*[38] and also certain fungal species such as *Cryptococcus neoformans,*[41] and parasitic species such as *Plasmodium falciparum,*[42] and *Leishmania.*[43] Granulysin also induces apoptosis in vitro of varicella-infected cells.[44] Although the structure of granulysin is significantly different from that of defensins or cathelicidin, it retains the conserved amphipathic nature. The hydrophobic surface is capable of associating closely with the target membrane, and the positively charged surface allows for association with the negatively charged bacterial membrane. In addition, studies on granulysin have shown the importance of the helix-loop-helix domain in the secondary structure. The ability of granulysin to kill *S. typhimurium* and *E. coli* has been localized to helix 2 and 3 of granulysin.[43] The amino acid residues contained within this structural component of granulysin are critical to the antimicrobial activity.[45]

Similar to other antimicrobial peptides, granulysin contains numerous immunomodulating properties. Several studies have shown that granulysin is a chemotractant for monocytes, and a subset of T cells, notably CD45Ro+ memory CD4 and CD8 T cells.[46] In addition, granulysin is also a chemotractant for cellular elements of the innate immune system, including NK cells, and monocyte-derived dendritic cells.[46] Granulysin has also been shown to be cytotoxic to tumor cells in vitro,[36] and it

has been hypothesized that granulysin plays an important role in tumor surveillance in vivo. The mechanism of cytotoxic action seems to differ from that of its antimicrobial activity. The hydrophobic surface of granulysin associates with the phospholipids of the tumor cell, altering the flux of ions[47] leading to the mitochondrial damage, liberation of cytochrome C, and activation of caspase-mediated apoptosis.[47,48] In addition, granulysin possesses antiinflammatory activity by decreasing cytokine production by monocytes stimulated with *Propionibacterium acnes.*[49]

S-100 Proteins

S-100 proteins belong to a multigene family of proteins with numerous functions including keratinocyte differentiation, epithelial defense, and wound healing. In addition, several members of the S-100 family have been implicated in direct antimicrobial activity. In general, S-100 proteins are low-molecular-weight proteins that are composed of four conserved α-helical segments, two calcium-binding regions, a central hinge, and an amino and carboxy terminal variable domain. Numerous S-100 proteins are expressed in the epidermis, and have thus been implicated in epidermal defense.

Psoriasin (S-100A7) is an antimicrobial peptide belonging to the S-100 family that is widely expressed in the human epidermis. Initially isolated from human skin on the basis of its *E. coli* bactericidal activity, psoriasin is a constitutively expressed AMP on the surface of human skin.[50] Immunohistochemical studies have shown that psoriasin is expressed focally by keratinocytes, with higher levels in areas of high bacterial colonization such as the face, axilla, and palms.[51] In addition to keratinocytes, immunohistochemical studies have also shown staining in sebocytes, indicating secretion of psoriasin into sebum.[51] In vitro studies have shown that psoriasin is preferentially active against *E. coli,* but also has some bactericidal activity for *P. aeruginosa* and *S. aureus,* albeit at much higher concentrations.[51] Although the mechanism of action is not completely known, investigators have noted that psoriasin-treated *E. coli* show no ultrastructural changes suggestive of perforation, which is the mechanism of action of most AMPs. Studies have suggested that the sequestration of

Zn^{2+} may be the mechanism of action of psoriasin, as S-100 contains two Zn^{2+} binding sites, and the antimicrobial activity is sensitive to treatment with Zn^{2+} but not other cations.[52]

In addition to its antimicrobial activity, psoriasin has immunomodulatory functions. It has also been shown to function as a chemotractant for CD4 T cells and neutrophils.[53] Although constitutive expression of S-100A7 has been reported, regulation of expression has been implicated by various exogenous agents such as all-trans retinoic acid and ultraviolet (UV) light. S-100A7 has also been shown to interact with epidermal-fatty acid binding protein, and may have some role in calcium-dependent oleic acid transport and metabolism.[54] A summary of the expression of the AMPs in the skin and their effect on the local immune system can be found in Figure 9.3

Other members of the S-100 family include S-100A8 and S-100A9, which form a heterodimer commonly referred to as calprotectin, which has some antimicrobial activity against *C. albicans*.[55,56] Increased expression of these proteins is seen in wound healing and in psoriasis. In addition, the C-terminal peptide fragment of S-100A12 (calcitermin) is capable of killing Gram-negative and fungal organisms, showing in vitro activity against *E. coli*, *L. monocytogenes*, and *C. albicans* under acidic conditions.[57] Although initially described in human airway secretions, S-100A12 is also expressed in both basal and suprabasal keratinocytes, and is seen in psoriatic skin.[58]

Other Antimicrobial Peptides

There is growing evidence to support the presence of multiple antimicrobial peptides in the human skin in addition to those discussed thus far. Discussion of all the different peptides and proteins with antimicrobial activity present within human skin is beyond the scope of this chapter. However, we highlight a few additional antimicrobial peptides found within the skin that have recently been gaining more attention. A summary of other AMPs with relevance to the skin can be found in Table 9.3.

Dermcidin, a 47-amino-acid peptide, is the primary AMP present in sweat, and is constitutively expressed by eccrine ducts.[59] It is cleaved from a 9.3-kD precursor molecule. In vitro experiments have demonstrated enhanced antibacterial activity

against a variety of organisms including, *E. coli*, *Enterococcus faecalis*, and *S. aureus*. In addition, there are also reports of activity against *C. albicans*.[60] The function of dermcidin in sweat may be to limit bacterial colonization and protect the host from infection. In addition, levels of dermcidin were measured in the sweat of patients with atopic dermatitis in comparison to matched controls. In the sweat of patients with atopic dermatitis, there is a relative deficit of dermcidin when compared to sweat from normal donors, which may in part explain the greater susceptibility of atopic dermatitis patients to cutaneous infection.[61] The tendency for superinfection in atopic dermatitis as it relates to antimicrobial peptides is further discussed below.

RNAse-7, a member of the RNAse-A family, is a 14.5-kD protein that is found within the skin.[62] It is constitutively expressed at a relatively high level in normal skin, and may be important in skin disease, as greater than a twofold level of expression is seen in psoriatic skin.[63] Structurally, RNAse-7 contains four disulfide bonds, similar to the defensin family of antimicrobial peptides. It is active against both Gram-positive organisms, such as *P. acnes* and *S. aureus*, as well as Gram-negative organisms such as *E. coli* and *P. aeruginosa*. It also has activity against the yeast *C. albicans*.[62] In addition, RNAse-7 has an extremely potent effect on VRE. Although relatively high levels of constitutive expression is seen in normal skin, the proinflammatory cytokines IL-1β, TNF-α, and interferon-γ (IFN-γ), increase messenger RNA (mRNA) transcription of the gene encoding RNAse-7 in cultured keratinocytes.[63] Other members of the RNAse-A family, in addition to their initially described function, have antimicrobial properties. For example, RNAse-3 exhibits antimicrobial activity against *S. aureus*.[64]

Psoriasis and Atopic Dermatitis

Human β-defensin-2 was initially isolated from psoriatic scale sparking numerous studies to further elucidate the role of antimicrobial peptides and host defense in human skin disease. It is well known that psoriasis is relatively resistant to bacterial superinfection. However, atopic dermatitis is often secondarily infected by streptococcal and staphylococcal species. One possible mechanism

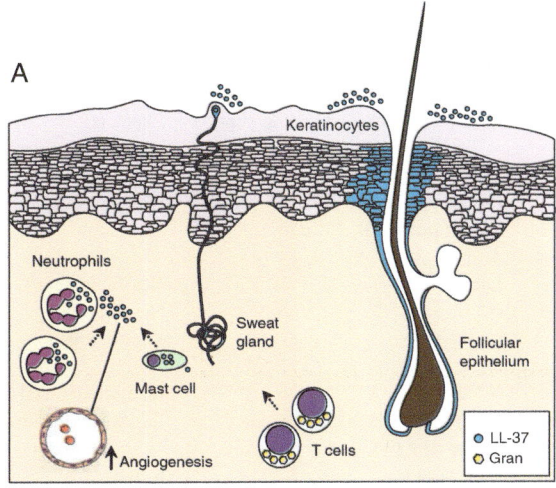

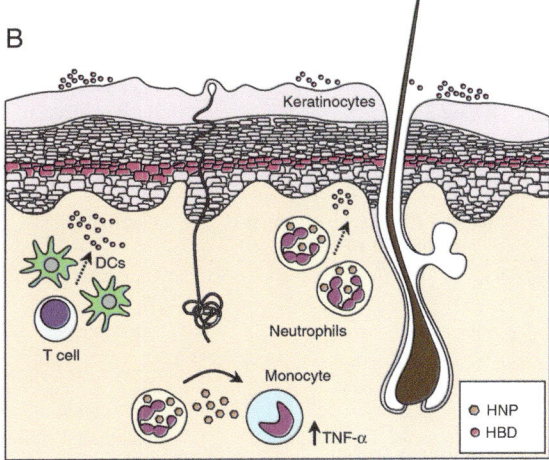

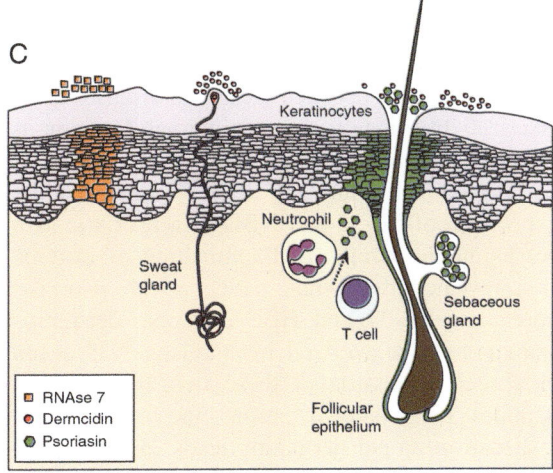

FIG. 9.3. Antimicrobial peptide expression in the skin. The expression of various AMPs by both resident cells of the skin and infiltrating inflammatory cells is demonstrated in this schematic diagram. Dashed arrows represent chemotaxis. (A) LL-37 and Granulysin. (B) HNP and HBD. (C) RNAse 7, dermcidin, and psoriasin

TABLE 9.3. Additional mammalian antimicrobial peptides with relevance to skin

	Cell type	Comments
α-melanocyte-stimulating hormone (α-MSH)	Keratinocytes	Active against *S. aureus* and *C. albicans*; inhibits HIV-1 replication
Calgranulin A/B	Keratinocytes	Inhibits growth of *C. albicans*
Connective tissue activating peptide 3 (CTAP-3)	Platelets	Microbicidal for bacteria > fungi
Elafin	Keratinocytes	Active against *P. aeruginosa*
Fibrinopeptide A (FP-A)	Platelets	Microbicidal for bacteria > fungi
Fibrinopeptide B (FP-B)		Active against Gram-negative bacteria
Lactoferrin	Keratinocytes	Decreasing IL-1, IL-2, and TNF-α
	Neutrophils	Enhancing monocyte and NK cell cytotoxicity
Lysozyme	Keratinocytes	Active against Gram-positive and some Gram-negative
Neuropeptide Y	Langerhans' cells	Broad spectrum
Neutrophil gelatinase-associated lipocalin (NGAL)	Infiltrating neutrophils	Bacteriostatic; mechanism of action based on iron sequestration
P-cystatin α	Keratinocytes	Inhibits growth of *S. aureus*
Perforin	T cells	Colocalized with granulysin
Platelet basic protein (PBP)	Platelets	Microbicidal for bacteria > fungi
Platelet factor 4 (PF-4)	Platelets	
Polypeptide YY	Langerhans' cells	Broad spectrum
RANTES	Platelets	Microbicidal for bacteria > fungi
RNase 2	Eosinophils	Antiviral activity
		Chemoattractant for dendritic cells
RNase 3	Eosinophils	Active against *S. aureus* and *E. coli*
		Antibacterial, antifungal, antiviral properties
Secretory leukocyte proteinase inhibitor (SLPI)	Keratinocytes	
	Glandular epithelium	Increased expression in psoriasis and wounds
		Active against *S. aureus*
Substance P	Macrophages	Related neuropeptides Bradykinin and neurotensin with similar, albeit weaker, antimicrobial activity
	Eosinophils	
	Endothelial cells	
Thymosin β-4 (Tβ-4)	Platelets	Microbicidal for bacteria > fungi

to explain the apparent discrepancy between rates of superinfection between these two diseases characterized by disruption in epidermal function is the disparate expression of antimicrobial peptides within lesional skin. Ong et al.[65] compared the expression of LL-37 and HBD-2 in psoriatic skin versus atopic dermatitis. Examination of lesional skin revealed that while patients with psoriasis upregulate LL-37 and HBD-2, atopic dermatitis lesions are characterized by a relatively reduced or absent expression of these two antimicrobial peptides. For unknown reasons, the inflammatory response in atopic dermatitis leads to an impairment in the upregulation of antimicrobial peptides. Several theories exist to explain the relative defi-

ciency for LL-37, including an overexpression of IL-4 and IL-13, as well as an overexpression of the antiinflammatory cytokine IL-10.[66]

A more recent study conducted by de Jongh et al.[67] compared the level of expression of keratinocyte antimicrobial peptides in psoriasis and atopic dermatitis using microarray analysis of mRNA purified from lesional skin. There was overexpression of many antimicrobial peptides in psoriatic skin when compared to atopic dermatitis lesions including HBD-1,2,3, α-defensin-4 and -6, psoriasin, calgranulin A,B,C, and LL-37. In addition, psoriatic skin has increased expression of antimicrobial signaling proteins, including TLR2, which has been implicated in HBD-2 production in other studies. Deficiency of the sweat of atopic dermatitis patients for dermcidin has also been observed when compared to normal skin.[61]

In addition to bacterial infections, patients with atopic dermatitis are at increasing risk for viral infections, particularly HSV causing eczema herpeticum and vaccinia virus (VV), leading to eczema vaccinatum. As mentioned above, LL-37 has known antimicrobial activity against both HSV and VV. The relative lack of HBD-2 and LL-37 may also account for the relatively high rates of superinfection of atopic dermatitis patients with other viruses such as HSV[31] and VV. Moreover, cathelicidin-deficient mice exhibit reduced ability to control VV replication.[68] The local deficiency of LL-37 in atopic dermatitis may in part explain not only the increased risk of bacterial superinfection but also viral infection in this patient population.

Acne

The pathogenesis of acne is multifactorial and includes follicular hyperkeratinization, increased sebum production, hormones, colonization with *Propionibacterium acnes*, and immunologic influences. Recent research has pointed to the importance of antimicrobial peptides in acne. Chronnell and colleagues[69] were among the first to suggest an important role of AMPs in acne. They analyzed both the mRNA expression and protein expression of HBD-1 and -2, via in-situ hybridization and immunohistochemistry, respectively, in the human pilosebaceous unit. High HBD-1 and -2 expression was present in the suprabasilar layers of the epidermis, as well as the distal outer root sheath, sebaceous glands, and the pilosebaceous duct in normal skin. However, HBD-2 expression in lesional and perilesional skin was further increased when compared to normal skin, suggesting a role for β-defensins in host defense in acne. A similar, albeit less dramatic, increase in HBD-1 was also observed.

New data have also implicated a role for *P. acnes* in the induction of antimicrobial peptides. Using primary human keratinocytes, one study found that distinct clinical strains of *P. acnes* could induce the expression of HBD-2, while other strains, including common laboratory strains, did not. Moreover, the expression of HBD-2 was found to be TLR2 and TLR4 dependent.[70] The selective induction of HBD-2 by different strains of *P. acnes* could in part help explain the large clinical spectrum of the disease. Individuals colonized with certain strains of *P. acnes* may produce more HBD-2, as part of host defense, and therefore have less severe clinical disease. Other studies have found that *P. acnes* induce HBD-2 production in a cultured human sebocyte cell line.[71] In vivo evidence for the importance of defensins became apparent with recently published microarray data showing that the expression of HBD-2 was significantly increased in acne lesions versus donor-matched normal skin.[72]

While there is clear evidence for the expression of AMPs in the acne, researchers are aiming to utilize antimicrobial peptides in order to treat acne. Given the increase in antibiotic-resistant *P. acnes*, the need for novel therapeutic agents is becoming increasingly urgent. Recently, McInturff et al.[49] investigated the potential role for using synthetic granulysin-derived peptides to treat acne (Fig. 9.4). Through their work they found that synthetic granulysin-derived peptides (amino acids 31 to 50) possessing a helix-loop-helix domain killed *P. acnes* in vitro. In addition, by substituting a tryptophan for the valine at amino acid 44 (peptide 31–50v44w), the authors were able to increase antimicrobial activity, presumably by increasing hydrophobicity, resulting in a stronger association with the bacterial surface. Finally, using L-type amino acids, they created a peptide that was less susceptible to degradation by proteases. In addition to the in vitro data using laboratory strains of *P. acnes*, clinical isolates of *P. acnes* from human microcomedones were also susceptible to the synthetic granulysin-derived peptides. The peptides also have potential antiinflammatory effects as they decreased *P. acnes*–induced cytokine expression.[49] Taken together, these data suggest that granulysin peptides may be useful as topical therapeutic agents, providing alternatives to current acne therapies. Due to the mechanism of action of granulysin it is less likely that bacteria can develop resistance to this potential therapy.

Mycobacterial Infections

Studies of cutaneous mycobacterial infections, such as leprosy, caused by *Mycobacterium leprae*, have provided great insight into the host innate

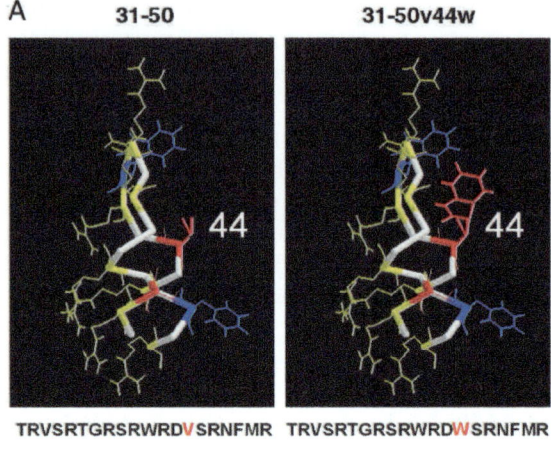

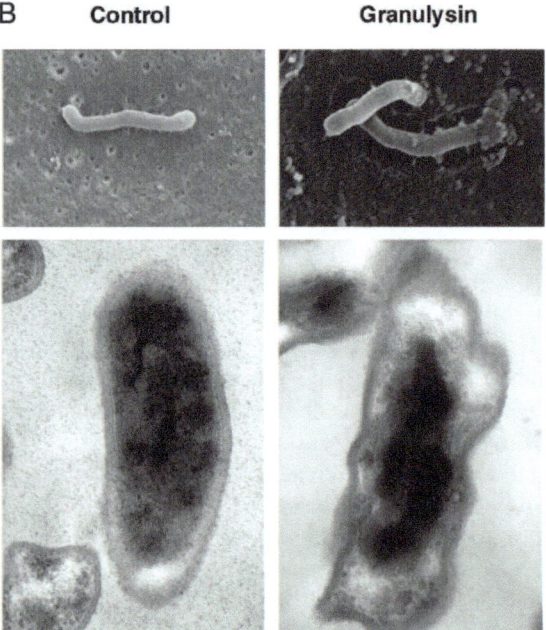

FIG. 9.4. Granulysin-derived peptides are antimicrobial. (A) Synthetic granulysin peptide containing amino acids 31 to 50 was altered by replacing the valine at position 44 with a tryptophan (31–50v44w). The resultant peptide is more hydrophobic, and has greater efficacy in killing *P. acnes*. (B) Scanning electron microscopy (top panel) revealed altered surface topography (10K magnification) of *P. acnes*, showing decreased fimbriae and a recessed and withered surface in peptide-treated samples. Transmission electron microscopy (bottom panel, 36K magnification) shows alteration in the cell wall, and a disturbance of the sharply layered surface architecture of *P. acnes* in treated samples

immune response and the role of antimicrobial peptides in skin disease. While leprosy remains a relatively rare disease in the United States, it has sparked tremendous research interest as a model for host defense and cutaneous immunity. Leprosy varies widely in its clinical presentation, which can be correlated to the host response launched against *M. leprae*. The tuberculoid form of the disease (T-lep) is characterized by localized infection, granulomas, and a cytokine milieu favoring cell-mediated immunity. The lepromatous form (L-lep), however, is a more disseminated infection, resulting in disfiguring nodules, and the expression

of cytokines favoring humoral immunity. L-lep is also characterized by a high organism load within affected tissues, and a high level of circulating antibodies that are ineffective at controlling the infection. In addition, there exist several intermediate states of disease, such as borderline forms, in which characteristics of both forms of the disease are present.

Ochoa and colleagues[73] have proposed a possible mechanism to partially explain the phenotypic expression seen in leprosy. Given that T cells are critical to cell-mediated immunity and cytolysis, the authors sought to characterize the level of granulysin expression, a T-cell–expressed antimicrobial peptide with a wide antibacterial spectrum. Granulysin-expressing T cells were detected in cutaneous T-lep lesions at a sixfold greater frequency as compared with the L-lep lesions. In contrast, perforin, a cytolytic molecule that colocalizes with granulysin in cytotoxic granules, was expressed at similar levels across the spectrum of disease. Within leprosy lesions, granulysin colocalized with CD4 T cells. Furthermore, granulysin was expressed in CD4 T-cell lines derived from skin lesions and demonstrated lysing of infected cells by the granule exocytosis pathway and reduced the viability of mycobacteria in infected cells. Thus, it appears that granulysin plays a critical role in controlling mycobacterial infection and influences the spectrum of clinical disease.

Recent evidence has implicated antimicrobial peptides in the Toll-mediated cytotoxicity pathway in humans. Although the murine model suggests a nitrous oxide–mediated mechanism for Toll-mediated cytotoxicity, evidence using primary human monocytes could not substantiate this hypothesis. However, recent studies demonstrate a role for LL-37 in the antimicrobial TLR response. Liu et al.[34] demonstrated that stimulation of human monocytes with a TLR2 ligand resulted in upregulation of the vitamin D receptor and the vitamin D-1-hydroxylase genes, leading to induction of LL-37 and killing of intracellular *M. tuberculosis*. Moreover, the effect seemed to be specific for LL-37, as increases in other antimicrobial peptides, such as HBD-2, were not observed. Finally, sera from African-American individuals, known to have increased susceptibility to tuberculosis, had low 25-hydroxyvitamin D and were inefficient in supporting cathelicidin messenger RNA induction. These data support a link between TLRs and vitamin D–mediated innate immunity, and suggest that differences in vitamin D production according to the differences in human population, including the color of skin, may contribute to susceptibility to microbial infection.

Wound Healing

A discussion of antimicrobial peptides would not be complete without a brief review of their role in wound healing. AMPs have been described in healing skin of mammals. For example, pig cathelicidin (PR-39) is found in the healing skin of pigs, and has pro–wound healing effects in fibroblasts. In particular, PR-39 increases the expression of certain extracellular matrix proteoglycans, which have been speculated to aid wound healing.[74] In agreement with the porcine data, LL-37 expression is enhanced in wounds[28] and has been shown in vitro to stimulate keratinocyte proliferation and angiogenesis. Moreover, inhibiting cathelicidins in pigs leads to increased bacterial colonization, and subsequent decreased wound healing.[75] LL-37 has also been implicated in keratinocyte migration through epidermal growth factor receptor (EGFR) transactivation.[76] In addition, LL-37 and α-defensins induce cellular proliferation, and subsequent wound closure in airway epithelium.[77,78] HNP-1 also decreases the expression of the collagen degrading enzymes, namely matrix metalloproteinase-1, while simultaneously increasing the expression of procollagen in dermal fibroblasts, suggesting one possible mechanism of action in wound healing.

In addition to LL-37 and α-defensins, a recent study has implicated the role of β-defensins in cutaneous wound healing. Niyonsaba and colleagues[79] showed that HBD-2, -3, and -4 were able to stimulate the production of various proinflammatory cytokines and chemokines in human primary keratinocytes, including IL-6, IL-10, and monocyte chemoattractant protein-1, in vitro. Moreover, they found that HBDs stimulate keratinocyte migration, and that HBDs in fact serve as chemoattractants for keratinocytes as measured by the Boyden chamber assay. An in vitro wound closure assay also showed that keratinocytes incubated with optimal doses of HBD-2, -3, and -4 migrated inwardly and covered a larger area of the wound, when compared with untreated or HBD-1–treated samples.[79] Keratinocyte-derived growth factors and antimicrobial peptides may serve as autocrine stimuli for wound healing, promoting keratinocyte migration and collagen synthesis.

In light of serious skin injuries where the structure and function of the epidermis is significantly compromised, the relative decrease in keratinocyte-derived antimicrobial peptides may be in part responsible for increased risk of infection. For example, a decrease in AMP can be used to partially explain the increased risk of *Pseudomonas* infections in burn patients. Also, deficiency in cathelicidins in mice has been reported to result in more severe and longer lasting cutaneous *S. pyogenes* infections.[13]

Conclusion

Over the past 20 years, our knowledge of the function of skin has dramatically evolved. What was once viewed as a stagnant physical barrier to the outside world, skin is now considered a dynamic immune organ, necessary and capable of mounting a specific and effective immune response. The discovery of antimicrobial peptides has greatly influenced the way we view the skin. From their initial discovery in invertebrate organisms, antimicrobial peptides have proven to be a highly conserved and important mechanism of host defense. In addition, our continuously expanding knowledge has shown the importance of overexpression, or lack of expression, of these cationic proteins in various skin conditions. Although they vary in structure and function, the mechanism of action is generally dictated by their cationic and amphipathic nature, which is a hallmark of nearly all antimicrobial peptides. Finally, with our increasing knowledge, it may be possible to develop synthetic AMPs that can be used as antibiotics and as immune modulators. Given the rapid increase in resistant bacteria, a need to add a potent antimicrobial agent to our armamentarium is imperative. With the increasing research in the field, synthetic antimicrobial peptides may hold promise in the future of antimicrobial therapy.

References

1. Zasloff M. Magainins, a class of antimicrobial peptides from Xenopus skin: isolation, characterization of two active forms, and partial cDNA sequence of a precursor. Proc Natl Acad Sci U S A 1987;84(15):5449–5453.
2. Tang YQ, Yuan J, Osapay G, et al. A cyclic antimicrobial peptide produced in primate leukocytes by the ligation of two truncated alpha-defensins. Science 1999;286(5439):498–502.
3. Selsted ME, Harwig SS. Determination of the disulfide array in the human defensin HNP-2. A covalently cyclized peptide. J Biol Chem 1989;264(7): 4003–4007.
4. Ganz T, Selsted ME, Szklarek D, et al. Defensins. Natural peptide antibiotics of human neutrophils. J Clin Invest 1985;76(4):1427–1435.
5. Jones DE, Bevins CL. Paneth cells of the human small intestine express an antimicrobial peptide gene. J Biol Chem 1992;267(32):23216–23225.
6. Jones DE, Bevins CL. Defensin-6 mRNA in human Paneth cells: implications for antimicrobial peptides in host defense of the human bowel. FEBS Lett 1993;315(2):187–192.
7. Quayle AJ, Porter EM, Nussbaum AA, et al. Gene expression, immunolocalization, and secretion of human defensin-5 in human female reproductive tract. Am J Pathol 1998;152(5):1247–1258.
8. Bastian A, Schafer H. Human alpha-defensin 1 (HNP-1) inhibits adenoviral infection in vitro. Regul Pept 2001;101(1–3):157–161.
9. Zhang L, Yu W, He T, et al. Contribution of human alpha-defensin 1, 2, and 3 to the anti-HIV-1 activity of CD8 antiviral factor. Science 2002;298(5595):995–1000.
10. Chaly YV, Paleolog EM, Kolesnikova TS, Tikhonov II, Petratchenko EV, Voitenok NN. Neutrophil alpha-defensin human neutrophil peptide modulates cytokine production in human monocytes and adhesion molecule expression in endothelial cells. Eur Cytokine Netw 2000;11(2):257–266.
11. Tang YQ, Selsted ME. Characterization of the disulfide motif in BNBD-12, an antimicrobial beta-defensin peptide from bovine neutrophils. J Biol Chem 1993;268(9):6649–6653.
12. Tsutsumi-Ishii Y, Nagaoka I. Modulation of human beta-defensin-2 transcription in pulmonary epithelial cells by lipopolysaccharide-stimulated mononuclear phagocytes via proinflammatory cytokine production. J Immunol 2003;170(8):4226–4236.
13. Nizet V, Ohtake T, Lauth X, et al. Innate antimicrobial peptide protects the skin from invasive bacterial infection. Nature 2001;414(6862):454–457.
14. Harder J, Bartels J, Christophers E, Schroder JM. Isolation and characterization of human beta-defensin-3, a novel human inducible peptide antibiotic. J Biol Chem 2001;276(8):5707–5713.
15. Sorensen OE, Thapa DR, Rosenthal A, Liu L, Roberts AA, Ganz T. Differential regulation of beta-defensin expression in human skin by microbial stimuli. J Immunol 2005;174(8):4870–4879.
16. Garcia JR, Krause A, Schulz S, et al. Human beta-defensin 4: a novel inducible peptide with a specific salt-sensitive spectrum of antimicrobial activity. FASEB J 2001;15(10):1819–1821.
17. Lehrer RI, Barton A, Daher KA, Harwig SS, Ganz T, Selsted ME. Interaction of human defensins with Escherichia coli. Mechanism of bactericidal activity. J Clin Invest 1989;84(2):553–561.
18. Wimley WC, Selsted ME, White SH. Interactions between human defensins and lipid bilayers: evidence

for formation of multimeric pores. Protein Sci 1994; 3(9):1362–1373.

19. Lichtenstein A. Mechanism of mammalian cell lysis mediated by peptide defensins. Evidence for an initial alteration of the plasma membrane. J Clin Invest 1991;88(1):93–100.

20. Wang W, Cole AM, Hong T, Waring AJ, Lehrer RI. Retrocyclin, an antiretroviral theta-defensin, is a lectin. J Immunol 2003;170(9):4708–4716.

21. Skerlavaj B, Gennaro R, Bagella L, Merluzzi L, Risso A, Zanetti M. Biological characterization of two novel cathelicidin-derived peptides and identification of structural requirements for their antimicrobial and cell lytic activities. J Biol Chem 1996;271(45):28375–28381.

22. Sorensen OE, Follin P, Johnsen AH, et al. Human cathelicidin, hCAP-18, is processed to the antimicrobial peptide LL-37 by extracellular cleavage with proteinase 3. Blood 2001;97(12):3951–3959.

23. Cowland JB, Johnsen AH, Borregaard N. hCAP-18, a cathelin/pro-bactenecin-like protein of human neutrophil specific granules. FEBS Lett 1995;368(1):173–176.

24. Braff MH, Di NA, Gallo RL. Keratinocytes store the antimicrobial peptide cathelicidin in lamellar bodies. J Invest Dermatol 2005;124(2):394–400.

25. Murakami M, Ohtake T, Dorschner RA, Schittek B, Garbe C, Gallo RL. Cathelicidin anti-microbial peptide expression in sweat, an innate defense system for the skin. J Invest Dermatol 2002;119(5):1090–1095.

26. Dorschner RA, Lin KH, Murakami M, Gallo RL. Neonatal skin in mice and humans expresses increased levels of antimicrobial peptides: innate immunity during development of the adaptive response. Pediatr Res 2003;53(4):566–572.

27. Turner J, Cho Y, Dinh NN, Waring AJ, Lehrer RI. Activities of LL-37, a cathelin-associated antimicrobial peptide of human neutrophils. Antimicrob Agents Chemother 1998;42(9):2206–2214.

28. Dorschner RA, Pestonjamasp VK, Tamakuwala S, et al. Cutaneous injury induces the release of cathelicidin anti-microbial peptides active against group A Streptococcus. J Invest Dermatol 2001;117(1):91–97.

29. Murakami M, Lopez-Garcia B, Braff M, Dorschner RA, Gallo RL. Postsecretory processing generates multiple cathelicidins for enhanced topical antimicrobial defense. J Immunol 2004;172(5):3070–3077.

30. Lopez-Garcia B, Lee PH, Yamasaki K, Gallo RL. Anti-fungal activity of cathelicidins and their potential role in Candida albicans skin infection. J Invest Dermatol 2005;125(1):108–115.

31. Howell MD, Wollenberg A, Gallo RL, et al. Cathelicidin deficiency predisposes to eczema

herpeticum. J Allergy Clin Immunol 2006;117(4): 836–841.

32. Heilborn JD, Nilsson MF, Kratz G, et al. The cathelicidin anti-microbial peptide LL-37 is involved in re-epithelialization of human skin wounds and is lacking in chronic ulcer epithelium. J Invest Dermatol 2003;120(3):379–389.

33. Gombart AF, Borregaard N, Koeffler HP. Human cathelicidin antimicrobial peptide (CAMP) gene is a direct target of the vitamin D receptor and is strongly up-regulated in myeloid cells by 1,25–dihydroxyvitamin D3. FASEB J 2005;19(9):1067–1077.

34. Liu PT, Stenger S, Li H, et al. Toll-like receptor triggering of a vitamin D-mediated human antimicrobial response. Science 2006;311(5768):1770–1773.

35. Koczulla R, von DG, Kupatt C, et al. An angiogenic role for the human peptide antibiotic LL-37/hCAP-18. J Clin Invest 2003;111(11):1665–1672.

36. Clayberger C, Krensky AM. Granulysin. Curr Opin Immunol 2003;15(5):560–565.

37. Pena SV, Krensky AM. Granulysin, a new human cytolytic granule-associated protein with possible involvement in cell-mediated cytotoxicity. Semin Immunol 1997;9(2):117–125.

38. Stenger S, Hanson DA, Teitelbaum R, et al. An antimicrobial activity of cytolytic T cells mediated by granulysin. Science 1998;282(5386):121–125.

39. Hanson DA, Kaspar AA, Poulain FR, Krensky AM. Biosynthesis of granulysin, a novel cytolytic molecule. Mol Immunol 1999;36(7):413–422.

40. Anderson DH, Sawaya MR, Cascio D, et al. Granulysin crystal structure and a structure-derived lytic mechanism. J Mol Biol 2003;325(2):355–365.

41. Ma LL, Spurrell JC, Wang JF, et al. CD8 T cell-mediated killing of Cryptococcus neoformans requires granulysin and is dependent on CD4 T cells and IL-15. J Immunol 2002;169(10):5787–5795.

42. Farouk SE, Mincheva-Nilsson L, Krensky AM, Dieli F, Troye-Blomberg M. Gamma delta T cells inhibit in vitro growth of the asexual blood stages of Plasmodium falciparum by a granule exocytosis-dependent cytotoxic pathway that requires granulysin. Eur J Immunol 2004;34(8):2248–2256.

43. Ernst WA, Thoma-Uszynski S, Teitelbaum R, et al. Granulysin, a T cell product, kills bacteria by altering membrane permeability. J Immunol 2000;165(12):7102–7108.

44. Hata A, Zerboni L, Sommer M, et al. Granulysin blocks replication of varicella-zoster virus and triggers apoptosis of infected cells. Viral Immunol 2001;14(2):125–133.

45. Wang Z, Choice E, Kaspar A, et al. Bactericidal and tumoricidal activities of synthetic peptides derived from granulysin. J Immunol 2000;165(3):1486–1490.

46. Deng A, Chen S, Li Q, Lyu SC, Clayberger C, Krensky AM. Granulysin, a cytolytic molecule, is also a chemoattractant and proinflammatory activator. J Immunol 2005;174(9):5243–5248.

47. Okada S, Li Q, Whitin JC, Clayberger C, Krensky AM. Intracellular mediators of granulysin-induced cell death. J Immunol 2003;171(5):2556–2562.

48. Kaspar AA, Okada S, Kumar J, et al. A distinct pathway of cell-mediated apoptosis initiated by granulysin. J Immunol 2001;167(1):350–356.

49. McInturff JE, Wang SJ, Machleidt T, et al. Granulysin-derived peptides demonstrate antimicrobial and anti-inflammatory effects against Propionibacterium acnes. J Invest Dermatol 2005;125(2):256–263.

50. Broome AM, Ryan D, Eckert RL. S100 protein subcellular localization during epidermal differentiation and psoriasis. J Histochem Cytochem 2003;51(5):675–685.

51. Glaser R, Harder J, Lange H, Bartels J, Christophers E, Schroder JM. Antimicrobial psoriasin (S100A7) protects human skin from Escherichia coli infection. Nat Immunol 2005;6(1):57–64.

52. Gort AS, Ferber DM, Imlay JA. The regulation and role of the periplasmic copper, zinc superoxide dismutase of Escherichia coli. Mol Microbiol 1999;32(1):179–191.

53. Jinquan T, Vorum H, Larsen CG, et al. Psoriasin: a novel chemotactic protein. J Invest Dermatol 1996;107(1):5–10.

54. Hagens G, Masouye I, Augsburger E, Hotz R, Saurat JH, Siegenthaler G. Calcium-binding protein S100A7 and epidermal-type fatty acid-binding protein are associated in the cytosol of human keratinocytes. Biochem J 1999;339(pt 2):419–427.

55. Clohessy PA, Golden BE. Calprotectin-mediated zinc chelation as a biostatic mechanism in host defence. Scand J Immunol 1995;42(5):551–556.

56. Murthy AR, Lehrer RI, Harwig SS, Miyasaki KT. In vitro candidastatic properties of the human neutrophil calprotectin complex. J Immunol 1993;151(11):6291–6301.

57. Cole AM, Kim YH, Tahk S, et al. Calcitermin, a novel antimicrobial peptide isolated from human airway secretions. FEBS Lett 2001;504(1–2):5–10.

58. Mirmohammadsadegh A, Tschakarjan E, Ljoljic A, et al. Calgranulin C is overexpressed in lesional psoriasis. J Invest Dermatol 2000;114(6):1207–1208.

59. Rieg S, Garbe C, Sauer B, Kalbacher H, Schittek B. Dermcidin is constitutively produced by eccrine sweat glands and is not induced in epidermal cells under inflammatory skin conditions. Br J Dermatol 2004;151(3):534–539.

60. Schittek B, Hipfel R, Sauer B, et al. Dermcidin: a novel human antibiotic peptide secreted by sweat glands. Nat Immunol 2001;2(12):1133–1137.

61. Rieg S, Steffen H, Seeber S, et al. Deficiency of dermcidin-derived antimicrobial peptides in sweat of patients with atopic dermatitis correlates with an impaired innate defense of human skin in vivo. J Immunol 2005;174(12):8003–8010.

62. Harder J, Schroder JM. RNase 7, a novel innate immune defense antimicrobial protein of healthy human skin. J Biol Chem 2002;277(48):46779–46784.

63. Harder J, Schroder JM. Psoriatic scales: a promising source for the isolation of human skin-derived antimicrobial proteins. J Leukoc Biol 2005;77(4):476–486.

64. Hooper LV, Stappenbeck TS, Hong CV, Gordon JI. Angiogenins: a new class of microbicidal proteins involved in innate immunity. Nat Immunol 2003;4(3):269–273.

65. Ong PY, Ohtake T, Brandt C, et al. Endogenous antimicrobial peptides and skin infections in atopic dermatitis. N Engl J Med 2002;347(15):1151–1160.

66. Howell MD, Novak N, Bieber T, et al. Interleukin-10 downregulates anti-microbial peptide expression in atopic dermatitis. J Invest Dermatol 2005;125(4):738–745.

67. de Jongh GJ, Zeeuwen PL, Kucharekova M, et al. High expression levels of keratinocyte antimicrobial proteins in psoriasis compared with atopic dermatitis. J Invest Dermatol 2005;125(6):1163–1173.

68. Howell MD, Gallo RL, Boguniewicz M, et al. Cytokine milieu of atopic dermatitis skin subverts the innate immune response to vaccinia virus. Immunity 2006;24(3):341–348.

69. Chronnell CM, Ghali LR, Ali RS, et al. Human beta defensin-1 and -2 expression in human pilosebaceous units: upregulation in acne vulgaris lesions. J Invest Dermatol 2001;117(5):1120–1125.

70. Nagy I, Pivarcsi A, Koreck A, Szell M, Urban E, Kemeny L. Distinct strains of Propionibacterium acnes induce selective human beta-defensin-2 and interleukin-8 expression in human keratinocytes through toll-like receptors. J Invest Dermatol 2005;124(5):931–938.

71. Nagy I, Pivarcsi A, Kis K, et al. Propionibacterium acnes and lipopolysaccharide induce the expression of antimicrobial peptides and proinflammatory cytokines/chemokines in human sebocytes. Microbes Infect 2006;8(8):2195–2205.

72. Trivedi NR, Gilliland KL, Zhao W, Liu W, Thiboutot DM. Gene array expression profiling in acne lesions reveals marked upregulation of genes involved

in inflammation and matrix remodeling. J Invest Dermatol 2006;126(5):1071–1079.

73. Ochoa MT, Stenger S, Sieling PA, et al. T-cell release of granulysin contributes to host defense in leprosy. Nat Med 2001;7(2):174–179.

74. Echtermeyer F, Streit M, Wilcox-Adelman S, et al. Delayed wound repair and impaired angiogenesis in mice lacking syndecan-4. J Clin Invest 2001;107(2): R9–R14.

75. Cole AM, Shi J, Ceccarelli A, Kim YH, Park A, Ganz T. Inhibition of neutrophil elastase prevents cathelicidin activation and impairs clearance of bacteria from wounds. Blood 2001;97(1):297–304.

76. Tokumaru S, Sayama K, Shirakata Y, et al. Induction of keratinocyte migration via transactivation of the epidermal growth factor receptor by the antimicrobial peptide LL-37. J Immunol 2005;175(7):4662–4668.

77. Aarbiou J, Verhoosel RM, Van WS, et al. Neutrophil defensins enhance lung epithelial wound closure and mucin gene expression in vitro. Am J Respir Cell Mol Biol 2004;30(2):193–201.

78. Shaykhiev R, Beisswenger C, Kandler K, et al. Human endogenous antibiotic LL-37 stimulates airway epithelial cell proliferation and wound closure. Am J Physiol Lung Cell Mol Physiol 2005;289(5):L842–L848.

79. Niyonsaba F, Ushio H, Nakano N, et al. Antimicrobial peptides human beta-defensins stimulate epidermal keratinocyte migration, proliferation and production of proinflammatory cytokines and chemokines. J Invest Dermatol 2007;127(3):594–604.

10
Photoimmunology

Christopher Hansen, Justin J. Leitenberger, Heidi T. Jacobe, and Ponciano D. Cruz, Jr.

Key Points

- Photoimmunology is the study of the effects of ultraviolet (UV) light between the wavelengths of 100 and 400 nm, which encompasses UVC through UVA radiation on the immune system, particularly the skin immune system.
- Ultraviolet light can serve as a therapeutic modality to treat a number of dermatologic diseases.
- Ultraviolet exposure is a major environmental risk factor for nonmelanoma skin cancer because of its mutagenic effects on epidermal cells, as well as its ability to suppress cutaneous immunosurveillance.
- Ultraviolet light is responsible for inducing or exacerbating a number of dermatologic diseases, termed photosensitivity disorders.

Photoimmunology is the study of effects of ultraviolet (UV) light/radiation (photons) on the immune system. Ultraviolet light occupies a narrow portion (100 to 400 nm) of the sun's electromagnetic radiation, which spans ionizing wavelengths (<100 nm) on one extreme and radio- and microwaves (>10,000 nm) on the other. Despite its reported diminution, our stratospheric ozone layer continues to filter solar radiation by blocking all ionizing and UVC radiation and the vast majority of UVB radiation from reaching the earth's surface. What natural exposure to sunlight provides us are some UVB, much UVA and visible light, and considerable infrared radiation (>800 nm) (Fig. 10.1).

The UV spectrum is subdivided into UVC (100 to 290 nm), UVB (290 to 320 nm), and UVA (320 to 400 nm) radiation. The ability of these wavelengths to penetrate the skin depends in great part on their absorption by different chromophores or photoreceptors (Fig. 10.2). UVC and UVB are readily absorbed by DNA within living cells, and thus almost all of these shorter wavelengths are absorbed as they pass through the epidermis, with little to none reaching the dermis. By contrast, UVA and visible light penetrate deeper into the dermis where these wavelengths are absorbed principally by aromatic amino acids on cell membrane proteins, and by collagen, elastin, and ground substance.[1]

As will be discussed later, recent development of high-energy light sources exclusively emitting 340 to 400 nm (UVA1) and its use as a therapeutic modality safer than psoralens plus UVA (PUVA) has led to discrimination between UVA2 (320 to 340 nm), which more closely resembles UVB and UVA1, which has features intermediate between UVB and visible light.

Not only are UVC and UVB absorbed by DNA, these wavelengths are also mutagenic. Indeed, UVC (germicidal) lamps are used to kill microbes, and of the solar radiation reaching the earth's surface, UVB is the most carcinogenic. It is also the most erythemogenic and is responsible for producing sunburn and immediate tanning. By contrast, UVA is considerably less erythemogenic, but more effective in producing a longer lasting tan.

Photocarcinogenesis

Human epidemiologic and laboratory animal studies overwhelmingly support the concept of UV

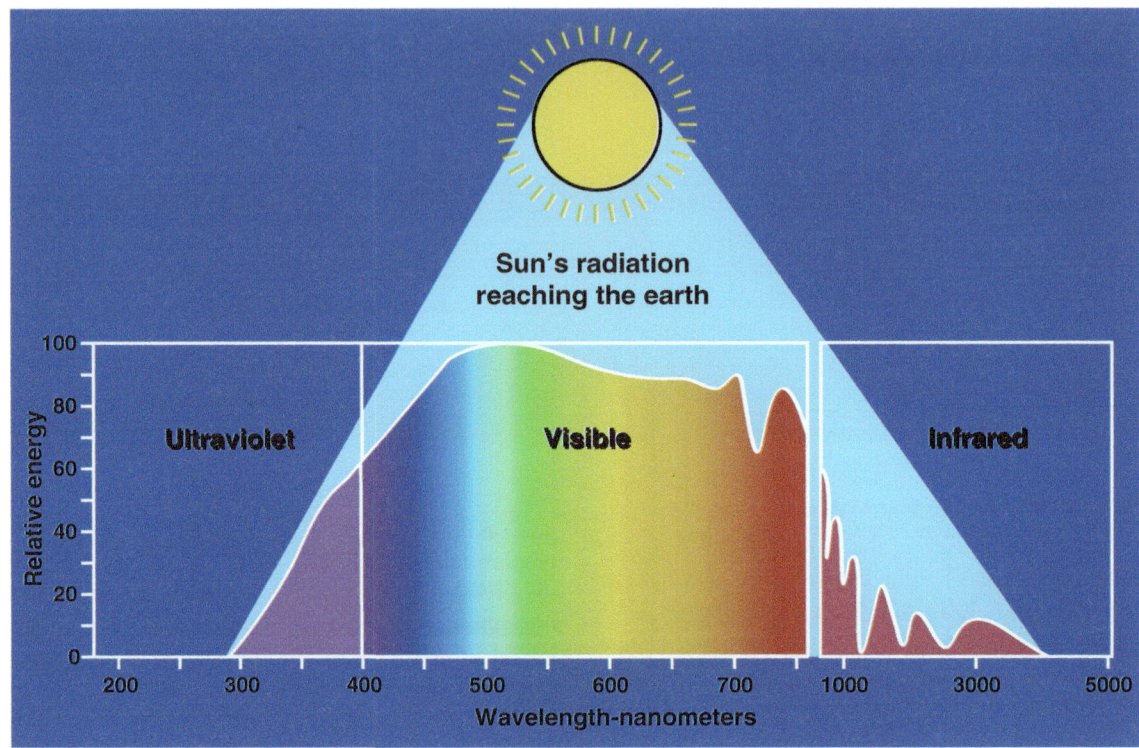

FIG. 10.1. Schematic diagram of the sun's radiation reaching the earth's surface

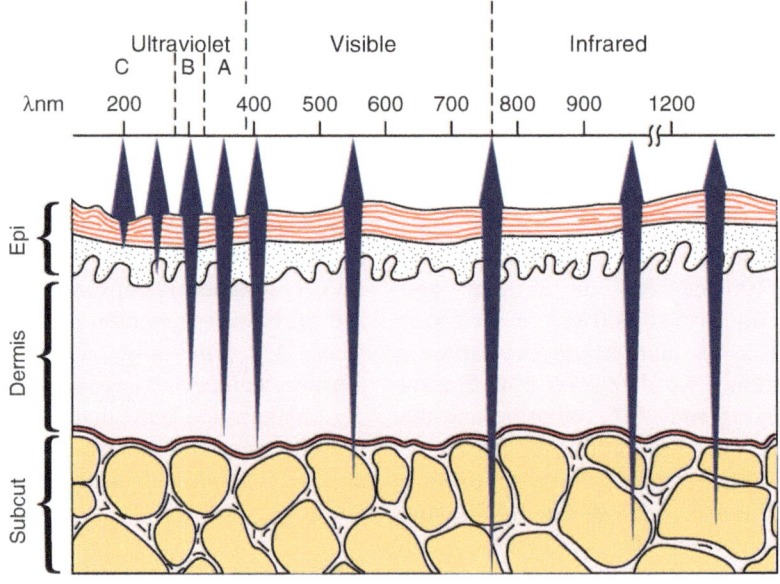

FIG. 10.2. Within 200- to 800-nm range, there is a direct relationship between wavelength and its depth of penetration into skin

exposure as the major environmental risk factor for nonmelanoma skin cancer.[2-5] In this respect and as cited previously, UVB is most carcinogenic,[6] although large doses of UVA have been shown experimentally to also cause nonmelanoma skin cancer.[7] A causative role for UV in melanoma is also supported by scientific evidence, albeit at a level less substantial than for nonmelanoma skin cancer.[8-10] Moreover, UVA rather than UVB appears may be the more relevant culprit for melanoma.[11]

Ultraviolet B causes a variety of DNA mutations, the most common of which are pyrimidine dimers. These mutations have been linked to the genesis of sunburn, tanning, and skin cancer. The biologic consequences of UVB-induced mutations depend on the ability of the host to repair DNA defects and on the specific gene mutations left unrepaired. Mutations that activate oncogenes (e.g., *ras*) or deactivate tumor suppressor genes (e.g., *p53* for squamous cell cancer; *PATCHED* for basal cell cancer), set the stage for carcinogenesis.[12] It is assumed that people with competent DNA repair mechanisms are able to correct UV-induced mutations. These protective mechanisms may deteriorate with age, allowing some mutations to escape repair, thereby leading to actinic keratoses, squamous cell cancers, and basal cell cancers. Xeroderma pigmentosa, a congenital disorder of absent or deficient DNA repair enzymes, provides a dramatic illustration of the foregoing concepts since afflicted individuals suffer from multiple skin cancers as early as childhood.

Ultraviolet B–Induced Immunosuppression

In addition to being a direct carcinogen, UVB promotes cancer growth by suppressing a second host defense mechanism—the ability of the immune system to kill UVB-induced skin cancers. Several overlapping pathways have been shown to lead to this form of immunosuppression (Fig. 10.3). Ultraviolet can induce keratinocytes to secrete soluble factors, of which tumor necrosis factor-α (TNF-α)[13,14] and interleukin-10 (IL-10)[15,16] are most critical to UVB immunosuppression; TNF-α regulates Langerhans' cells' emigration out of the epidermis into draining lymph nodes, and IL-10 shifts T-cell responses from T-helper-1 (Th1)

to Th2 phenotype.[15] Ultraviolet can also trigger lipid peroxidation on cell membranes leading to secretion of platelet aggregation factor (PAF), which in turn stimulates prostaglandin E_2 (PGE$_2$) production, which in turn prompts IL-4 secretion, which finally leads (again) to IL-10 production.[16,17] Trans-urocanic acid, a by-product of histidine metabolism, accumulates in the stratum corneum; UV nonenzymatically transforms trans-urocanic acid into the cis isomer, which contributes to immunosuppression via effects on antigen-presenting cells (APCs).[18,19] Finally, UV can directly alter the function of epidermal Langerhans' cells and other APCs; depending on the UV dose and the manner in which it is administered, UV may induce these APCs to undergo apoptosis, shift their function from stimulators of Th1 (cellular) to Th2 (humoral) responses, or cause them to activate "suppressor" T cell.[20-22]

That UVB radiation leads to suppressor T-cell activation has been demonstrated not only for UVB-induced carcinogenesis but also for UVB-induced suppression of delayed-type and contact hypersensitivity.[23,24] The immunosuppression generated is not a generalized one, but specific for the antigen to which the host is being sensitized at the time of UV exposure.[23] Until recently, the precise phenotype of the suppressor cells has eluded investigators. The current consensus is that these cells are better designated as regulatory T cells that express CD4, CD25, and CTLA-4 markers, secrete copious amounts of IL-10, and are able to bind dectin-2.[25,26]

Finally, mast cells and complement activation via the C3 pathway have been shown to participate in UVB-induced immunosuppression.[27-30]

Ultraviolet B and Vitamin D

It is well established that UVB is responsible for the nonenzymatic conversion of 7-dehydrocholesterol to cholecalciferol (vitamin D$_3$) in skin. What was discovered recently is that cholecalciferol may modulate immune responses in skin. Toll-like receptors (TLRs) activated in response to intracellular bacteria were shown to upregulate vitamin D receptors on macrophages, leading to induction of canthelicidin and intracellular killing of *Mycobacterium tuberculosis*. In addition, sera

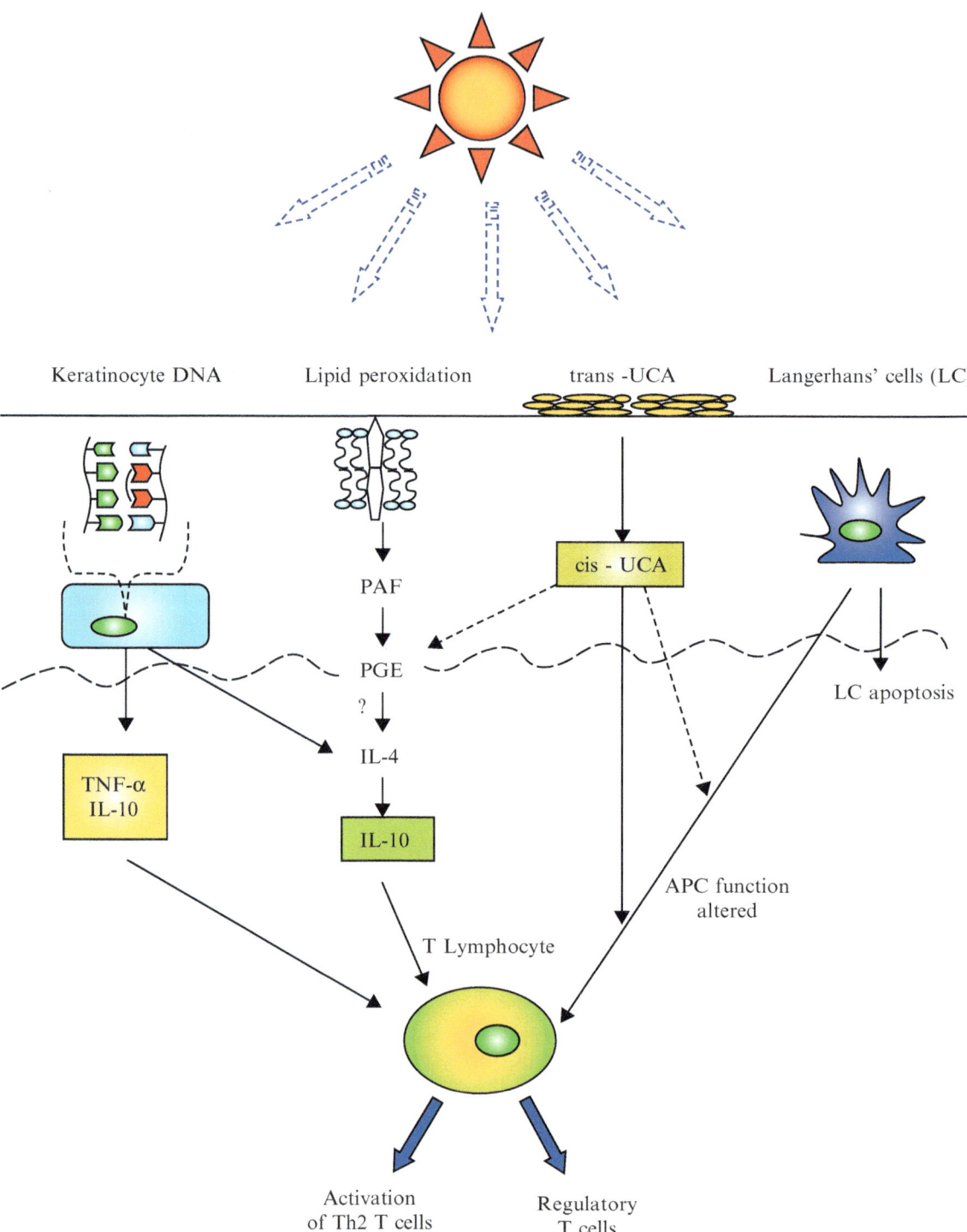

FIG. 10.3. Overlapping pathways that account for effects of ultraviolet radiation of the skin immune system. APC, antigen-presenting cell; IL, interleukin; PGE, prostaglandin E; Th, T-helper; TNF, tumor necrosis factor

from African Americans, a population known to have increased susceptibility to tuberculosis, were found to have lower levels of 25-hydroxyvitamin D compared to controls.[31]

Idiopathic (Immunologic) Photosensitivity Disorders

A useful classification of photosensitivity disorders based on presumed etiology is presented in Table 10.1. Our discussion in this chapter is limited to the "idiopathic" photosensitivity disorders for which causation remains enigmatic, although recent evidence points to immunologic underpinnings.

Polymorphic Light Eruption

Polymorphic (or polymorphous) light eruption is the most common photosensitivity disorder, with estimates as high as 20% of the general population affected.[32,33] There is greater predisposition for women, the age of onset is in the teenage and young adults years, and it more commonly affects people living in temperate climates. Recurrent outbreaks typically occur in spring, with the clinical onset occurring several hours following UV exposure. The eruption develops over sun-exposed skin, is usually pruritic, and may take several morphologic patterns (i.e., polymorphic): small to large papules, vesicles, plaques, and even ery-

thema multiforme–like eruptions.[32] The duration of the outbreaks is typically 1 to 2 weeks, and the eruption frequently improves in the summer (termed hardening). Photoprovocation studies have implicated a variety of wavelengths that span UVB, UVA, and even visible light.[34,35]

The pathogenic hypothesis is a delayed cellular hypersensitivity reaction to an endogenous cutaneous antigen possibly generated by the action of UV radiation.[36,37] Although the identity of the chromophore/antigen remains unknown, recent studies have shown patients with this condition to be deficient in generating UVB-induced suppression of the induction (but not elicitation) of contact hypersensitivity,[38] and this defect was ascribed to the inability of UVB to induce emigration of Langerhans' cells from the epidermis to draining lymph nodes.[39,40] In this model, UVB-induced immunosuppression is thought to be a natural protective mechanism that prevents autoimmunity to UV-induced autoantigens that might otherwise develop in the course of everyday exposure to solar radiation. Thus, polymorphic light eruption may represent an autoimmune disease resulting from defective UVB-induced immunosuppression.

Actinic Prurigo

Actinic prurigo is closely related to polymorphic light eruption in morphology and delayed-onset relative to sun exposure, but differs from it in several respects: actinic prurigo often starts in childhood; there is greater familial predisposition, especially among particular Native-American populations; it is linked to human leukocyte antigen (HLA) subtypes (DR4 for sporadic types; A24, Cw4, C4, and DR4 for familial types),[36] mucous membrane involvement (conjunctivitis and cheilitis) is common; and there is a tendency toward chronicity.

Solar Urticaria

Solar urticaria is a rare form of physical urticaria provoked by exposure to UV or visible light. Unlike polymorphic light eruption and actinic prurigo, solar urticaria typically develops within minutes of solar irradiation, with itching, burning, erythema, and wheals.[41] Solar urticaria represents an immediate type of photoallergic reaction mediated by immunoglobulin E (IgE) to endogenous

TABLE 10.1. Photosensitivity disorders

Idiopathic (immunologic)
Polymorphic light eruption
Actinic prurigo
Solar urticaria
Chronic actinic dermatitis
Defective DNA repair
Xeroderma pigmentosa
Trichothiodystrophy
Cockayne syndrome
Rothmund-Thomson syndrome
Autoimmune
Systemic lupus erythematosus
Dermatomyositis
Drug-induced
Phototoxic
Photoallergic
Porphyria

serum factors. The reaction can be passively transferred to normal subjects, with a positive reaction
elicited by light exposure within 2 to 6 hours after
injection of serum.

Chronic Actinic Dermatitis

Chronic actinic dermatitis is a relatively new
umbrella term that encompasses several forms of
chronic photosensitivity including photosensitive
eczema, persistent light reaction, chronic photosensitive dermatitis, and actinic reticuloid. It
often begins insidiously as nonspecific eczematous
lesions in sun-exposed areas that become more
persistent.[36] It is more common in men and tends
to occur in later adult years.[32]

Causation appears to mimic a photoallergic dermatitis in which a normal skin constituent becomes
altered and antigenic.[42] In many cases, there is a
strong association with allergic contact dermatitis,
the most common allergen being *Sesquiterpene
lactone*.[32]

Phototherapy

Along with Mohs' chemosurgery for the treatment
of skin cancer and patch testing for the diagnosis of
allergic contact dermatitis, phototherapy is among
the most quintessential of dermatologic procedures (other medical specialists rarely perform
them). Phototherapy refers to the use of artificial
UV light to treat skin disorders, a domain that for
several decades was based largely on empirical evidence. However, increasing knowledge and insight
derived from photoimmunology now provide cellular and molecular mechanisms that account for
phototherapy's beneficial effects (Table 10.2).

Both UVB and UVA1 can induce apoptosis, and
the threshold for causing programmed cell death is
much lower for lymphocytes than for other cells.

Apoptosis by UVB may be achieved via mutations or activation of death receptors (e.g., Fas/
Fas ligand, TNF receptor, TRAIL [TNF-Related
Apoptosis Inducing Ligand] receptor).[43] By contrast, apoptosis by UVA may be mediated through
reactive oxygen species, differential killing of Th1
over Th2 cells, or lysis of mast cells.[43]

As cited previously, UVB can induce secretion
of cytokines including IL-1, IL-4, IL-6, IL-8, IL-
10, and TNF-α, with the last two deemed responsible for immunosuppression.[13–17] Ultraviolet B
also generates regulatory T cells critical to this
immunosuppression.[25,26] By contrast, UVA (but not
UVB) can inhibit collagen synthesis and metalloproteinase activity, leading to changes in extracellular matrix.[43]

In general, UVB, UVA, and PUVA are useful
for treating T-cell–mediated inflammatory skin
diseases. PUVA is the most efficacious, but also
the most toxic since it is most mutagenic and is a
risk factor for both melanoma and nonmelanoma
skin cancer. Indeed, patients treated with PUVA
for more than 250 sessions remain at risk for
melanoma long after the photochemotherapy has
ceased.[44]

The commercial availability of light sources
emitting high-energy, narrower-range wavelengths
(i.e., UVA1 and narrow-band UVB) has led to phototherapy protocols that are less toxic and better
matched to treat specific skin diseases. Thus, the
older modalities of broadband UVB and PUVA
are giving way to the shorter-timed/more efficient
narrow-band UVB and the safer UVA1 treatments.

Specific therapeutic indications correlate with
depth of penetration, which in turn is based on the
nature of the absorbing chromophores (Table 10.3).
Thus, UVB is most useful for eczematous disorders

TABLE 10.2. How phototherapy works

	UVB	UVA1
Apoptosis	Yes	Yes
Cytokines	Yes	?
Regulatory T cells	Yes	?
Extracellular matrix	?	Yes

TABLE 10.3. Therapeutic indications

NB-UVB	UVA1
Psoriasis	Atopic dermatitis
Atopic dermatitis	Localized cutaneous scleroderma
Vitiligo	Urticaria pigmentosa
Patch-stage cutaneous T-cell lymphoma	Dyshidrotic eczema
Polymorphic light eruption	Disseminated granuloma annulare
Actinic prurigo	Pityriasis lichenoides
Erythropoietic porphyria	Systemic lupus erythematosus
Pityriasis lichenoides	

NB, narrow band; UV, ultraviolet.

TABLE 10.4. Risks of phototherapy

Risks	UVB	Oral PUVA
Skin aging	Yes	Yes
Skin cancer		
Nonmelanoma	Probable	Yes
Melanoma	?	Probable
Drug sensitivity	Rare	Yes
Ocular damage		
Keratitis	Yes	No
Cataracts	No	Yes
Immunosuppression	Uncertain	Uncertain
Internal malignancy	No	No

PUVA, psoralens plus UVA.

that primarily involve the epidermis and superficial dermis, such as psoriasis, atopic dermatitis, patch-stage cutaneous T-cell lymphoma, vitiligo, and pruritus due to various causes. For these diseases, narrow-band UVB is the phototherapy of choice since it approximates, if not equals, the efficacy of PUVA, while avoiding the latter's risks of greater mutagenicity/carcinogenicity and cataracts (Table 10.4). The principal limitation to UVB-based protocols is erythema, which peaks a day after exposure; this is the reason why UVB phototherapy is delivered on an every-other-day basis—to avoid causing burns. With respect to HIV infection, there is no compelling proof that UVB or PUVA leads to systemic effects in seropositive patients, although UV has been shown to activate HIV gene expression in vitro.[45,46]

Unlike UVB, UVA-based protocols allow penetration deeper into the dermis, and thus are useful for treating diseases characterized by fibrosis (e.g., scleroderma, at least during the early inflammatory phase). It has also been used for diseases for which UVB is indicated (Table 10.3). In this respect, PUVA may be more efficacious than UVA1, but the latter comes close enough to PUVA's efficacy while avoiding its toxicity. Erythema is generally not a problem with UVA1 treatment so it can be used to treat patients with erythroderma and acute flares of atopic dermatitis. The principal limitations to UVA1 are cost of the equipment and its installation (currently available in only a few centers in the United States) and hyperpigmentation.

The risks of phototherapy are dose related, so the greatest frequency of adverse events is associated with high-exposure doses of treatment. Risks are similar to those resulting from chronic exposure to sunlight and are augmented by additional exposure to sunlight. Patients should be selected appropriately and counseled on both the benefits and risks of this treatment modality.

Conclusion

Ultraviolet light is a major environmental factor that can have both acute and chronic effects on the skin. The study of the effects of UV light on the skin and its associated immune system has resulted in a better understanding of the effects of this physical modality on the skin. Ultraviolet light has an important pathogenic role in skin cancer development (photocarcinogenesis and photoimmunosuppression). However, UV light can be utilized as an effective therapy in the treatment of certain skin diseases, such as psoriasis.

References

1. Wondrak GT, Jacobson MK, Jacobson EL. Endogenous UVA-photosensitizers: mediators of skin photodamage and novel targets for skin photoprotection. Photochem Photobiol Sci 2006;5(2):215–237.
2. Black HS, deGruijl FR, Forbes PD, et al. Photocarcinogenesis: an overview. J Photochem Photobiol B 1997;40(1):29–47.
3. Sarasin A. The molecular pathways of ultraviolet-induced carcinogenesis. Mutat Res 1999;428(1–2):5–10.
4. Berneburg M, Krutmann J. Photoimmunology, DNA repair and photocarcinogenesis. J Photochem Photobiol B 2000;54(2–3):87–93.
5. Urbach F, Forbes PD, Davies RE, Berger D. Cutaneous photobiology: past, present and future. J Invest Dermatol 1976;67(1):209–224.
6. de Gruijl FR, Sterenborg HJ, Forbes PD, et al. Wavelength dependence of skin cancer induction by ultraviolet irradiation of albino hairless mice. Cancer Res 1993;53(1):53–60.
7. Sterenborg HJ, van der Leun JC. Tumorigenesis by a long wavelength UV-A source. Photochem Photobiol 1990;51(3):325–330.
8. Longstreth J. Cutaneous malignant melanoma and ultraviolet radiation: a review. Cancer Metastasis Rev 1988;7(4):321–333.
9. Armstrong BK, Kricker A. The epidemiology of UV induced skin cancer. J Photochem Photobiol B 2001;63(1–3):8–18.

10. Jhappan C, Noonan FP, Merlino G. Ultraviolet radiation and cutaneous malignant melanoma. Oncogene 2003;22(20):3099–3112.

11. Wang SQ, Setlow R, Berwick M, et al. Ultraviolet A and melanoma: a review. J Am Acad Dermatol 2001;44(5):837–846.

12. Hart RW, Setlow RB, Woodhead AD. Evidence that pyrimidine dimers in DNA can give rise to tumors. Proc Natl Acad Sci U S A 1977;74(12):5574–5578.

13. Vermeer M, Streilein JW. Ultraviolet B light-induced alterations in epidermal Langerhans cells are mediated in part by tumor necrosis factor-alpha. Photodermatol Photoimmunol Photomed 1990;7(6):258–265.

14. Yoshikawa T, Kurimoto I, Streilein JW. Tumour necrosis factor-alpha mediates ultraviolet light B-enhanced expression of contact hypersensitivity. Immunology 1992;76(2):264–271.

15. Simon JC, Cruz PD, Bergstresser PR, Tigelaar RE. Low dose ultraviolet B-irradiated Langerhans cells preferentially activate CD4+ cells of the T helper 2 subset. J Immunol 1990;145:2087–2091.

16. Shreedhar V, Giese T, Sung VW, Ullrich SE. A cytokine cascade including prostaglandin E2, IL-4, and IL-10 is responsible for UV-induced systemic immune suppression. J Immunol 1998;160(8):3783–3789.

17. Walterscheid JP, Ullrich SE, Nghiem DX. Platelet-activating factor, a molecular sensor for cellular damage, activates systemic immune suppression. J Exp Med 2002;195(2):171–179.

18. Moodycliffe AM, Kimber I, Norval M. The effect of ultraviolet B irradiation and urocanic acid isomers on dendritic cell migration. Immunology 1992;77(3):394–399.

19. El-Ghorr AA, Norval M. A monoclonal antibody to cis-urocanic acid prevents the ultraviolet-induced changes in Langerhans cells and delayed hypersensitivity responses in mice, although not preventing dendritic cell accumulation in lymph nodes draining the site of irradiation and contact hypersensitivity responses. J Invest Dermatol 1995;105(2):264–268.

20. Shreedhar VK, Pride MW, Sun Y, Kripke ML, Strickland FM. Origin and characteristics of ultraviolet-B radiation-induced suppressor T lymphocytes. J Immunol 1998;161(3):1327–1335.

21. Aberer W, Schuler G, Stingl G, Honigsmann H, Wolff K. Ultraviolet light depletes surface markers of Langerhans cells. J Invest Dermatol 1981;76(3):202–210.

22. Glass MJ, Bergstresser PR, Tigelaar RE, Streilein JW. UVB radiation and DNFB skin painting induce suppressor cells universally in mice. J Invest Dermatol 1990;94(3):273–278.

23. Schwarz A, Maeda A, Wild MK, et al. Ultraviolet radiation-induced regulatory T cells not only inhibit the induction but can suppress the effector phase of contact hypersensitivity. J Immunol 2004;172(2):1036–1043.

24. Elmets CA, Bergstresser PR, Tigelaar RE, Wood PJ, Streilein JW. Analysis of the mechanism of unresponsiveness produced by haptens painted on skin exposed to low dose ultraviolet radiation. J Exp Med 1983;158(3):781–794.

25. Aragane Y, Maeda A, Schwarz A, Tezuka T, Ariizumi K, Schwarz T. Involvement of dectin-2 in ultraviolet radiation-induced tolerance. J Immunol 2003;171(7):3801–3807.

26. Schwarz T. Regulatory T cells induced by ultraviolet radiation. Int Arch Allergy Immunol 2005;137(3):187–193.

27. Hart PH, Grimbaldeston MA, Swift GJ, Jaksic A, Noonan FP, Finlay-Jones JJ. Dermal mast cells determine susceptibility to ultraviolet B-induced systemic suppression of contact hypersensitivity responses in mice. J Exp Med 1998;187(12):2045–2053.

28. Rauterberg A, Jung EG, Rauterberg EW. Complement deposits in epidermal cells after ultraviolet B exposure. Photodermatol Photoimmunol Photomed 1993;9(4):135–143.

29. Hammerberg C, Katiyar SK, Carroll MC, Cooper KD. Activated complement component 3 (C3) is required for ultraviolet induction of immunosuppression and antigenic tolerance. J Exp Med 1998;187(7):1133–1138.

30. Yoshida Y, Kang K, Berger M, et al. Monocyte induction of IL-10 and down-regulation of IL-12 by iC3b deposited in ultraviolet-exposed human skin. J Immunol 1998;161(11):5873–5879.

31. Liu PT, Stenger S, Li H, et al. Toll-like receptor triggering of a vitamin D-mediated human antimicrobial response. Science 2006;311(5768):1770–1773.

32. Ferguson J. Diagnosis and treatment of the common idiopathic photodermatoses. Australas J Dermatol 2003;44(2):90–96.

33. Ros AM, Wennersten G. Current aspects of polymorphous light eruptions in Sweden. Photodermatol 1986;3(5):298–302.

34. Tutrone WD, Spann CT, Scheinfeld N, DeLeo VA. Polymorphic light eruption. Dermatol Ther 2003;16(1):28–39.

35. Boonstra HE, van WH, Toonstra J, van Vloten WA. Polymorphous light eruption: a clinical, photobiologic, and follow-up study of 110 patients. J Am Acad Dermatol 2000;42(2 pt 1):199–207.

36. Lecha M. Idiopathic photodermatoses: clinical, diagnostic and therapeutic aspects. J Eur Acad Dermatol Venereol 2001;15(6):499–504.

37. Norris PG, Morris J, McGibbon DM, Chu AC, Hawk JL. Polymorphic light eruption: an immunopathological study of evolving lesions. Br J Dermatol 1989;120(2):173–183.

38. Kolgen W, van WH, Den HS, et al. CD11b+ cells and ultraviolet-B-resistant CD1a+ cells in skin of patients with polymorphous light eruption. J Invest Dermatol 1999;113(1):4–10.

39. Wackernagel A, Back B, Quehenberger F, Cerroni L, Kerl H, Wolf P. Langerhans cell resistance, CD11b+ cell influx, and cytokine mRNA expression in skin after UV exposure in patients with polymorphous light eruption as compared with healthy control subjects. J Invest Dermatol 2004;122(5): 1342–1344.

40. Kolgen W, van MM, Jongsma M, et al. Differential expression of cytokines in UV-B-exposed skin of patients with polymorphous light eruption: correlation with Langerhans cell migration and immunosuppression. Arch Dermatol 2004;140(3): 295–302.

41. Horio T. Solar urticaria-idiopathic? Photodermatol Photoimmunol Photomed 2003;19(3):147–154.

42. Honigsmann H. Mechanisms of phototherapy and photochemotherapy for photodermatoses. Dermatol Ther 2003;16(1):23–27.

43. Weichenthal M, Schwarz T. Phototherapy: how does UV work? Photodermatol Photoimmunol Photomed 2005;21(5):260–266.

44. Stern RS, Nichols KT, Vakeva LH. Malignant melanoma in patients treated for psoriasis with methoxsalen (psoralen) and ultraviolet A radiation (PUVA). The PUVA Follow-Up Study. N Engl J Med 1997;336(15):1041–1045.

45. Breuer-McHam J, Simpson E, Dougherty I, et al. Activation of HIV in human skin by ultraviolet B radiation and its inhibition by NFkB blocking agents. Photochem Photobiol 2001;74:805–810.

46. McDonald H, Cruz PDJ. Phototherapy and HIV infection. In: Krutmann J, ed. Dermatological Phototherapy and Photodiagnostic Methods, 2nd ed. Heidelberg: Springer-Verlag, 2007.

11
Angiogenesis for the Clinician

Benjamin A. Lefkove, Levi E. Fried, and Jack L. Arbiser

Key Points

- Angiogenesis is the development of microvasculature in response to an infectious, neoplastic, or inflammatory agent.
- Angiogenesis contributes to the pathogenesis of many common skin disorders, such as acne, psoriasis, photoaging, common warts, and a variety of precancers and skin cancers (basal cell carcinoma, squamous cell carcinoma, actinic keratosis, and melanomas), wound healing.
- Angiogenesis in the skin is accomplished by recruitment of mesenchymal cells locally and by recruitment of the bone marrow–derived stem cells that can differentiate into endothelial cells.
- Important growth factors for endothelial cells include vascular endothelial growth factor, basic fibroblast growth factor, platelet-derived growth factor, cyclooxygenase-2, and prostaglandin E_2. There are a number of angiogenesis inhibitors, many of which are experimental. These agents have great potential as therapeutic interventions for a number of skin diseases.

Clinical Angiogenesis

Angiogenesis, the development of a microvasculature to a neoplastic, inflammatory, or infectious disease process, is a promising therapeutic target that has not been fully exploited.[1] Virtually all processes of therapy impinge on cutaneous angiogenesis, and a proper understanding of cutaneous pathophysiology with respect to angiogenesis will lead to a more effective use of current therapies

for dermatologic diseases, as well as development of novel therapies. We propose that the understanding of angiogenesis is predictable, as is the effect of current therapies on angiogenesis. With this knowledge, the clinician can make educated guesses on the effect of therapy on a process. The primary disorders of the skin are infectious, inflammatory, and neoplastic. All of these categories are capable of inducing angiogenesis through a limited and overlapping subset of mechanisms, and these mechanisms can be understood by the practicing dermatologist. This chapter discusses the primary mediators of angiogenesis and examples of common skin disorders in which they occur. Antiangiogenic therapy is also discussed. Factors that directly impact on endothelium are called direct angiogenesis stimulators or inhibitors, while factors that stimulate nonendothelial cells to make stimulators or inhibitors are called indirect angiogenesis stimulators and inhibitors (Table 11.1).

Infectious Processes

Neither acute nor chronic infections have traditionally been considered angiogenic processes, but the resolution of an acute infection and the maintenance of a chronic infection requires an intact angiogenic system. Colonization and invasion of the skin by both gram-positive and gram-negative organisms activates the innate immune system, which results in the production of antimicrobial peptides, some of which also impact on endothelial cells. While the activation of the innate immune

TABLE 11.1. Description of angiogenesis inhibitors and stimulators

Angiogenesis inhibitors

Angiostatin	Naturally occurring protein found in some animal species. Angiostatin is known to be cleaved by MMPs. Angiostatin binds to endothelial cell surface adenosine triphosphate (ATP) synthase and angiomotin.
Bevacizumab	A humanized monoclonal antibody. The first commercially available angiogenesis inhibitor. Inhibits the actions of VEGF by binding directly to VEGF-A. Used primarily for colorectal cancer. Usually used along with combination drug chemotherapy.
Celecoxib	A nonsteroidal antiinflammatory drug (NSAID). Highly selective COX-2 inhibitor. This selectivity helps reduce stomach ulcers.
Curcumin	Antiinflammatory properties are due to inhibition of eicosanoid biosynthesis. Interferes with the activity of the transcription factor NF-κB, which has been linked to a number of inflammatory diseases and tumor survival.
Epigallocatechin gallate	A flavanoid class molecule that acts as a powerful antioxidant, protects against oxidative stress and free radical damage.
Endostatin	A C-terminal fragment derived from type 18 collagen. It is a broad-spectrum angiogenesis inhibitor the interferes with the proangiogenic action of growth factors, bFGF and VEGF.
Imatinib mesylate	Acts by inhibiting particular tyrosine kinase (TK) enzymes, instead of nonspecifically inhibiting rapidly dividing cells. It occupies the TK active site, leading to a decrease in bcr-abl transformation. Imatinib mesylate is especially useful in that it is one of the few tyrosine kinase inhibitors with appropriate selectivity and limited toxicity. Studies show that imatinib may be also useful in treating small pox.[18]
Honokiol	Melanoma therapy under development. Relevant in that IFN-α, the only widely prescribed adjuvant therapy for melanoma, has marked side effects. A biphenolic ring with an ortho-allyl moiety, honokiol induced caspase-dependent cell death in B-CLL cells[18] and a variety of melanoma cell lines. Mechanism of action is likely direct inhibition of GRP78.[18]
Silymarin	Silymarin consists of a family of flavonoids commonly found in the dried fruit of the milk thistle plant. Extensive research has shown that silymarin can suppress the proliferation of a variety of tumor cells. This is accomplished by inhibition of cell-survival kinases (AKT and MAPK) and inhibition of inflammatory transcription factors (NF-κβ). It can also downregulate gene products involved in the proliferation of tumor cells (COX-2), invasion (MMP-9), angiogenesis (VEGF), and metastasis.[18]
Thalidomide	Thalidomide inhibits the release of TNF-α from monocytes and modulates other cytokine action. Thalidomide may act to heal aphthous ulcers by inhibiting angiogenesis and promoting reepithelialization.[18] Thalidomide is also useful in the treatment of multiple myelomas, autoimmune diseases, and leprosy.
Gentian violet	Occupies the chemical class of triphenylmethane dyes. Once used as a topical antiseptic, gentian violet is experiencing a reawakening as a nox4 inhibitor. Potentially useful in the treatment of melanoma, eczema, psoriasis, and verruca vulgaris.
Solenopsin[18]	Alkaloidal component of fire-ant venom. Inhibitor of phosphatidylinositol-3–kinase signaling and angiogenesis.
Rapamycin	Macrocyclic triene antibiotic, also known as sirolimus, possessing immunosuppressant and antiproliferative properties. Works through inhibition of mTOR, leading to interruption of IL-2 signaling and a cell cycle arrest at G1–S.[18] In preliminary trials for treatment of angiomyolipomas and brain tumors associated with tuberous sclerosis.[18] Used in the treatment of Kaposi's sarcoma in patients receiving renal transplants.[18]

Angiogenesis stimulators

Vascular endothelial growth factor (VEGF)	VEGF is a primary contributor to the growth of capillaries in a given network. In the presence of VEGF endothelial cells undergo angiogenesis and neovascularization. VEGF causes a large tyrosine kinase signaling cascade in endothelial cells, leading to expression of proliferation factors to be produced and these factors stimulate proliferation (survival) via bFGF, migration via MMP, and differentiation into mature blood vessels. The upregulation of VEGF is the main operator in the physiologic response during exercise. Muscle contraction increases the blood flow to the affected areas. This increased flow causes an increase in the mRNA production of VEGF receptors 1 and 2. This increase in receptors increases the signaling cascades related to angiogenesis.
Basic fibroblast growth factor (bFGF)	Basic fibroblast growth factor is a member of the fibroblast growth factor family. In normal tissue, basic fibroblast growth factor is present in basement membranes and in the subendothelial extracellular matrix of blood vessels. bFGF stays membrane-bound as long as there is no signal peptide. During both wound healing of normal tissues and tumor development, the action of heparan sulfate–degrading enzymes activates bFGF, thus mediating the formation of new blood vessels (angiogenesis).
Matrix metalloproteinase (MMP)	MMPs help degrade the proteins that keep the vessel walls solid. This proteolysis allows the endothelial cells to escape into the interstitial matrix as seen in sprouting angiogenesis. These enzymes are highly regulated during the vessel formation process because this destruction of the extracellular matrix would destroy the integrity of the microvasculature. MMP2 and MMP9 are the two proteinases linked to angiogenesis.
Cyclooxygenase-2 (COX2)–prostaglandin E_2 (PGE_2)	COX-2 inhibitors are a class of nonsteroidal antiinflammatory drugs (NSAIDs) that selectively block the COX-2 enzyme. This action impedes the production of the chemical messengers (prostaglandins) that cause the pain and swelling of arthritis inflammation. Being that COX-2 inhibitors selectively block the COX-2 enzyme and not the COX-1 enzyme, these drugs are uniquely different from traditional NSAIDs.
Platelet-derived growth factor (PDGF)	PDGF is a dimer that activates its signaling pathway by a ligand-induced receptor dimerization and autophosphorylation. PDGF has provided a market for protein receptor antagonists to treat disease. These antagonists include specific antibodies that target the molecule of interest.

system is sufficient to control and eliminate many bacterial colonizations and invasions, it is not sufficient to control high inocula of infection or particularly virulent bacterial or viral infections. Therefore, danger signals are transmitted systemically, which allow for cellular reinforcements. The arrival of cellular reinforcements requires an intact vascular system, which can respond to infection by activation of endothelial adhesions molecules (vascular cell adhesion molecule [VCAM], intercellular adhesion molecule [ICAM], E-selectin), allowing neutrophils, lymphocytes, and macrophages to proceed to the site of infection with selectivity (Fig. 11.1). One of the most graphic demonstrations of the importance of this system is the genetic deficiency of CD11, a neutrophil adhe-

sion molecule that is required for the exit of neutrophils from blood vessels. Patients lacking CD11 develop a neutrophilia due to inflammatory stimuli, but these neutrophils are unable to leave the blood vessel, leading to "cold" staphylococcal abscesses and high neutrophil counts due to the inability of these neutrophils to reach the site of infection. In the absence of bone marrow transplantations, these patients succumb to staphylococcal sepsis.

Chronic infections are usually the result of bacteria capable of intracellular colonization (treponemes, mycobacterium, *Bartonella*), viral infections that are capable of latency, or viral oncogenes (human papillomavirus [HPV], herpes virus). Bacterial infections often colonize cells of endothelial or monocyte/

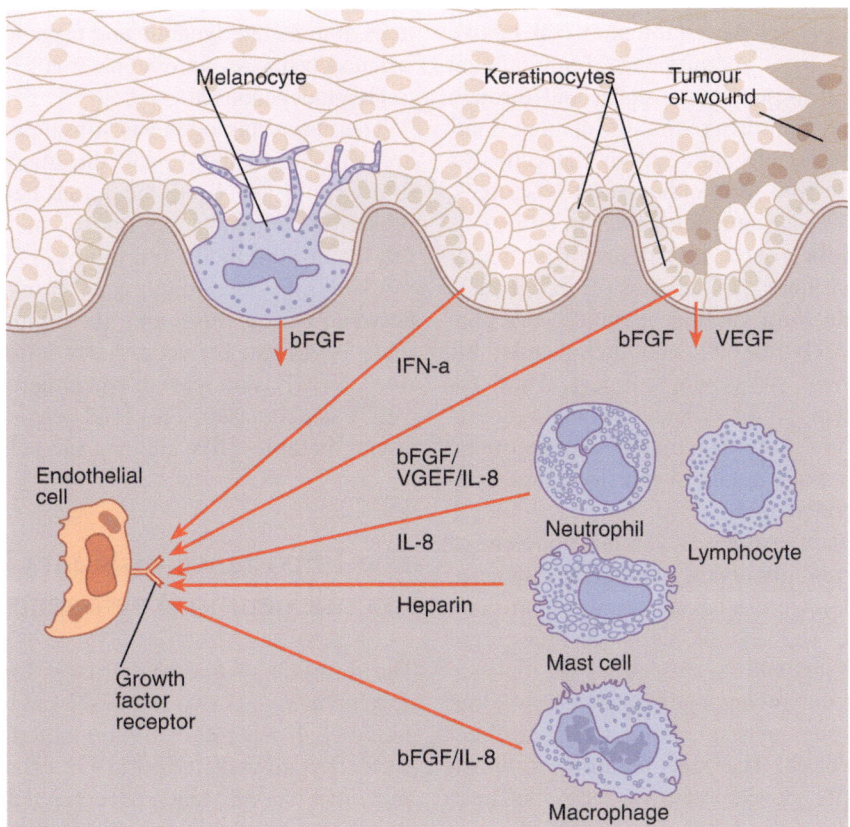

FIG. 11.1. Basement membrane-reservoir of acidic fibroblast growth factor (aFGF) and basic fibroblast growth factor (bFGF) bound to heparan sulfate proteoglycan leads to the disruption of basement membrane leads to release of growth factor. Keratinocyte-derived interferon-α (IFN-α) directly inhibits endothelial growth. Upon activation of a growth factor receptor by a growth factor, the endothelial cell is stimulated to proliferate, produce proteases that migrate toward the source of growth factors, and form tubes, the precursors of capillaries

macrophage origin, and in retrospect, this should not be surprising, since these cells share a common precursor cell in the hemangioblast. As opposed to most extracellular bacteria, chronic bacterial infections of the skin often manifest after a systemic infection, perhaps due to infection of the hemangioblast, with preferential colonization of the infected endothelial cell or monocyte in the dermis. Of note, there are two major receptors for VEGF, the major chemotactic angiogenic factor, and these are differentially expressed in the descendants of the hemangioblasts. Endothelial cells express primarily VEGFR2, while monocytes/macrophages express VEGFR1. Blockade of each of these receptors with specific antibodies impairs angiogenesis, thus demonstrating a role of both endothelial cells and hematopoietic cells in angiogenesis. This blockade likely results in the highly impaired wound healing in patients who are neutropenic.

Outside of embryonic cells, angiogenesis is affected primarily by the endothelial cell in two ways: through local recruitment of endothelial cells from local mesenchymal cells, and through recruitment and transdifferentiation of bone marrow–derived stem cells into endothelial cells. As cells may be derived from either of these sources, the efficacy of an antiangiogenic treatment is dependent on the source of cells in a particular lesion. For instance, in advanced malignancy, tumor cells can form vascular channels and phenotypically closely resemble endothelial cells; this process is known as vascular mimicry. Thus, for the development of an efficacious angiogenesis inhibitor, and for a proper understanding of the dynamic and unique nature of a lesion, angiogenesis must be understood.

One of the cornerstones in the development of angiogenesis inhibitors is the angiogenic "switch." In a given cell, there is a balance between pro- and antiangiogenic signals. As cells become more malignant, a threshold is crossed as the balance shifts toward the proangiogenic. It follows that cells produce angiogenesis stimulators and direct or indirect inhibitors. The direct inhibitors diminish endothelial cells' development of neovasculature. Indirect inhibitors block the angiogenic stimulatory pathway through inhibition of growth factors such as VEGF or the basic fibroblast growth factor (bFGF), or through blockade of releasing factors

such as the corticotropin-releasing factor. All of this functions, in the end, to impair cells' ability to promote angiogenesis.

The regulation of angiogenic growth factors is often complex, but the best elucidated is the regulatory pathways surrounding VEGF. Several stimuli regulate VEGF; on a transcriptional level there are AP1 and Sp1, and on a translational level there are hypoxia-inducible factor 2α (HIF-2α) and mitogen-activated protein kinase (MAPK) (Fig. 11.2). Though much research has focused on inhibition of HIF-1, selective HIF-2α inhibition is emerging as a more vital protein in VEGF transcription, or the inhibition thereof. The fact that HIF-deficient cells are capable of forming aggressive tumors implicates HIF-independent processes in VEGF upregulation. Though many specific and selective inhibitors of HIF, akt, and a variety of other VEGF signaling molecules are under development, it must be understood that, like many biologic systems, tumors are dynamic and capable of switching signaling pathways, for example from HIF-dependence to HIF-independence.

The major angiogenesis stimulators in the skin are VEGF and bFGF, and the major inhibitor is interferon-2 (IFN-α), the latter being a widely prescribed adjuvant therapy for melanoma. Both the major stimulants and inhibitors are produced by keratinocytes, helping to provide a barrier between vasculature and the epidermis. When there is contact between the two (barrier disruption), VEGF is increased; when there is occlusion, VEGF is decreased. This lends credence to occlusional therapies, like cautery and sclerotherapy.

The Importance of Stem Cell Recruitment in Angiogenesis

The reservoir of endothelial cells for neovascular development is of two sources: local recruitment of endothelial cells, and differentiation of quiescent mesenchymal cells. Exposure of cells to cytokines and other stimuli leads to upregulation of adhesion molecules, which bind immune effector cells; such cells can migrate to sites of infection and inflammation. Withdrawal of the stimulus will lead to apoptosis of the neovasculature. Persistent

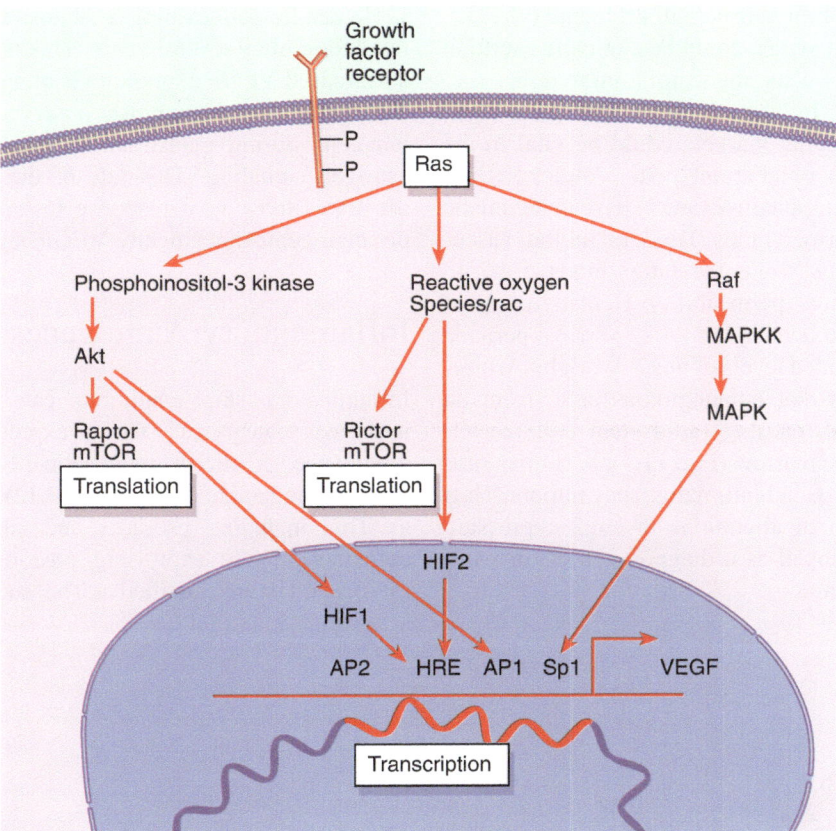

FIG. 11.2. Summary of molecular pathways that lead to vascular endothelial growth factor (VEGF) gene expression. As indicated, there are a number of signaling pathways that can activate VEGF transcriptions. HIF, hypoxia-inducible factor; MAPK, mitogen-activated protein kinase; MAPKK, mitogen-activated protein kinase kinase; mTOR, mammalian target of rapamycin; P, phosphate

endothelial stimulation, either through angiogenic growth factors, loss of endogenous factors, or mutations, will cause cells to resist physiologic apoptosis. Recall that mutations involve activation of the phosphoinositol-3-kinase (PI3K)/akt pathway; such activation accounts for neovascular formation in humans.

The recruitment of bone marrow cells is imperative for the success of vascular formation. This notion explains some observations in cancer therapy. A large group of natural products, known as chemopreventive agents, prevent cancer development but have little effect on advanced neoplasms. Xenograft models can help select for angiogenesis inhibitors

that block mesenchymal recruitment, though tumors persist in recruiting local endothelial cells. While an effective treatment may require inhibition of both pathways, recognition of the tumor's dynamic ability to switch signaling pathways may even render recruitment-inhibiting therapies ineffective.

The ligands responsible for endothelial stem cell recruitment in ischemic tissues and tumors likely start with high expression of stromal cell-derived factor 1 (SFD-1). CXCR4 (also known as fusin is a CXC chemokine receptor 4) is the SDF1 receptor, and blockade of CXCR4 is a promising new course of therapy that has been shown to block revascularization of ischemic tissue. Matrix metalloproteinase

9 (MMP-9) mobilizes the small kit ligand (sKITL). Mobilization of sKITL could be clinically useful in the treatment of acute myocardial infarction.

Recognition by the clinician and pathologist of certain signaling markers could be vital in the early detection of aberrant cells. Angiopoietin-1 (ang1) and angiopoietin-2 (ang2) have antagonistic effects: the former binds Tie-2 to inhibit vascular permeability, while the latter binds Tie-2 to stimulate vascular permeability. Hemangiomas of infancy and the hemangioma-like verruga peruana both show elevated levels of ang2. Work by Arbiser et al. suggests that hemangiomas arise from an unknown event, causing rapid stem cell recruitment from bone marrow (Fig. 11.3). A similar situation likely exists in high-malignancy tumors. Thus early detection of alterations in ang2 expression could be developed as a diagnostic tool for early detection of tumors.

Hemangiomas exhibit a characteristic natural involution after several years. This is likely due to a decreased VEGF expression leading to apoptosis. This parallels the apoptosis observed in endothelial cells during menstruation upon lessening of estrogen signaling. This fate of the hemangioma illustrates the potent response toward removal of proangiogenic, specifically VEGF, signaling.

Inflammatory Angiogenesis

Inflammatory skin conditions can be separated into two categories. Those expressing a predominance of IFN-γ, interleukin-12 (IL-12), and interferon-inducible protein 12 (IP-12) are classified as Th1, including psoriasis and allergic contact dermatitis. Those expressing predominantly IL-4, -5, -6, and -10 are classified as Th2, such as systemic

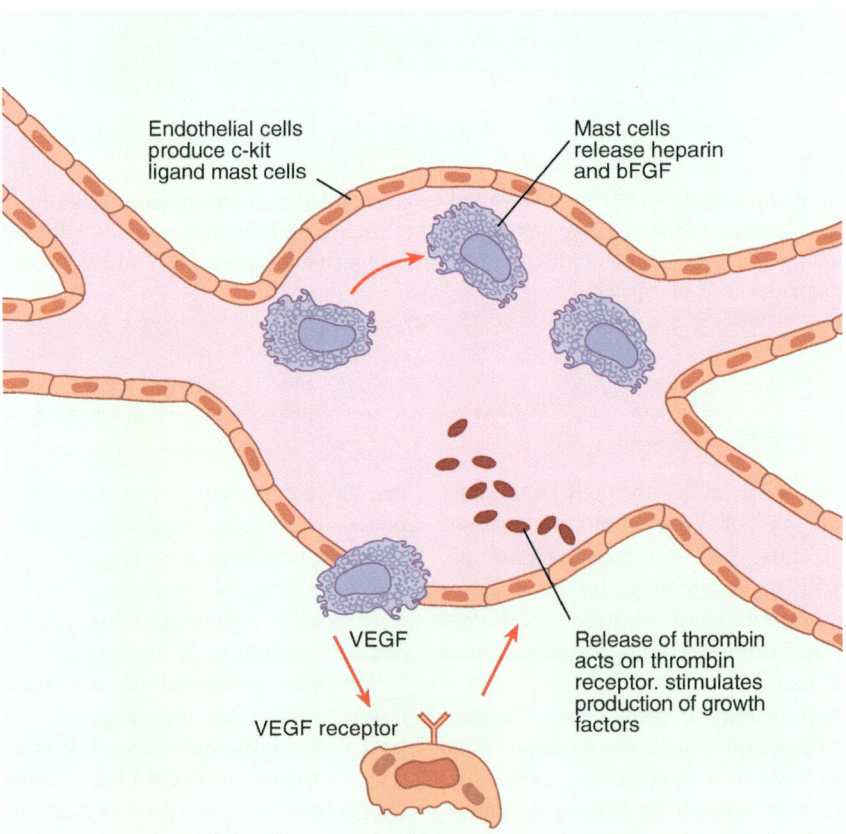

FIG. 11.3. A model for angiogenesis in hemangiomas. This model demonstrates interacting between endothelial cells. Most cells and stem cells that are recruited from bone marrow are induced to differentiate into endothelial cells

lupus erythematosus and atopic dermatitis. Both categories exhibit common features, including inflammatory infiltrates of lymphocytes, mast cells, granulocytes, and macrophages. Both conditions show excess angiogenesis (despite the presence of antiangiogenic IL-12 in Th1 disorders), showing the potential utility of angiogenesis inhibitors for treatment not merely of malignant neoplasms, but in a wide range of dermatologic disorders.

The Role of Angiogenesis in Major Skin Disorders

Acne Vulgaris

Acne is the most common cutaneous disorder in the United States. This disorder accounts for over 10% of all patient encounters with a primary care physician. While the number of cases of acne vulgaris in adolescents has remained relatively stable over the past decade, the number of cases of adult-onset acne is increasing. The majority of debilitating effects of acne are psychological, with embarrassment and anxiety being among the top reported symptoms. Scarring is not uncommon and contributes to the lifelong effects of a moderate to severe case.

The role of MMPs in acne has been somewhat unclear in recent work, though it appears that they are involved in acne progression. The source of MMPs in acne appears to be keratinocytes[2] or neutrophils.

Treatment of acne includes both topical and systemic therapies. For treatment of noninflammatory comedones, topical retinoids such as tretinoin, adapalene, and tazarotene are often prescribed. Salicylic acid also has proven comedolytic activity. The most prominent therapy, both over-the-counter and prescription-based, is topical benzoyl peroxide. Some patients experience increased inflammation due to the presence of *Propionibacterium acnes* in sebaceous follicles. Treatment of such cases usually involve topical antibiotics such as clindamycin or erythromycin. It should be noted that to lessen the opportunities for the generation of antiobiotic-resistant bacteria, treatments should be coupled with benzoyl peroxide.[3,4] In severe cases of inflammatory acne, patients can be prescribed system isotretinoin. There are prescribing restrictions for this drug that are left to the discre-tion of the physician. Blue light and laser therapy are expensive and unproven treatments for acne and should be avoided pending further data.

Psoriasis

Psoriasis is a common cutaneous disorder characterized by erythematous papules and silvery-scaled plaques. Though not entirely understood, the pathophysiology of clinical psoriasis tends to result from hyperproliferation and abnormal differentiation of epidermal keratinocytes, accompanied by inflammatory cell infiltration and vascularization. This remodeling resembles a prolonged wound response, with many reparative and remodeling processes being utilized[4] (Fig. 11.4).

To follow the wound healing analogy presented by Nickoloff, et al.,[4] tumor necrosis factor (TNF), VEGF, IL-23, and transforming growth factor (TGF) are present in high levels in psoriatic tissue. Though these cytokines are present in healthy skin, the exaggerated angiogenic response and epidermal thickening draws a definite line between healthy epidermal/dermal signaling and pathologic psoriatic skin. Genetic susceptibility plays a major role, as evidenced in the Koebner phenomenon, which describes an outbreak of psoriatic lesions on genetically susceptible patients upon mild trauma applied to the skin. Expression of TGF is a relevant early event in the formation of psoriatic lesions. Such expression leads to upregulation of VEGF, which promotes angiogenesis and changes in blood vessel morphology. In fact, elevated levels of VEGF are noted in lesional keratinocytes in psoriasis.[5] Accordingly, the angiopoietin (ang)-Tie signaling pathway is activated in psoriasis, leading to vascular remodeling, formation, and invasion. To view the whole picture, VEGF expression leads to increased vascular permeability and capillary diameter. Once this angiogenic "switch" is turned, alterations in ang1/ang2 expression allow for increased vascular proliferation. Tumor necrosis factor provides differential direct regulation of the Tie2 signaling pathway. Tumor necrosis factor and ang1/ang2 allow for vascular survival and maintenance during this proliferative phase.[6] The increased angiogenesis in the early phases of psoriasis formation allows for the proinflammatory response that will follow. It is important to note that psoriasis is not simply an epithelial hyperplasia

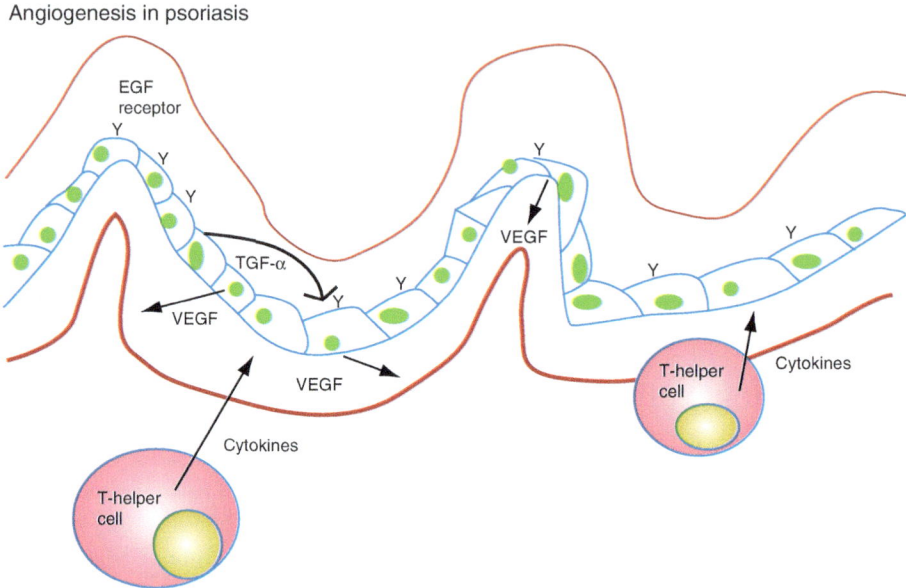

Angiogenesis in psoriasis

FIG. 11.4. Psoriasis is an example of chronic inflammation that drives excessive angiogenesis. It is a result of T cells and keratinocyte interactions, resulting in VEGF production, which then impacts endothelial cells

growth along the lines of carcinoma, but rather a metaplastic exaggerated wound response.

Treatments of psoriasis are varied, and include topical and systemic corticosteroids, immunomodulators such as cyclosporine and methotrexate, TNF blockers, and topical therapies such as calcipotriene. A long-trusted treatment has been topical coal tar treatment, and it is supposed by Arbiser that carbazole is the active ingredient in coal tar–mediated psoriasis treatment. Ultraviolet light is one of the more popular therapeutic methods. Experimental treatments include topical applications of gentian violet, a triphenylmethane dye once used as a topical antiseptic that selectively kills gram-positive bacteria.

Warts (Verruca Vulgaris)

Verrucae are a common clinical manifestation of an HPV infection of epithelial tissue. The common wart or verruca vulgaris, derived from HPV-2, is a benign proliferative lesion manifesting as a raised hyperkeratotic papillomous lesion. There are many HPV subtypes, some seemingly more site-specific than others. Though all humans are susceptible, infections are more common in children and young adults. Infection occurs through skin-to-skin contact, with macerated sites predisposing one to infection. Human papillomavirus infections from HPV-16 or HPV-18 are considered high risk as HPV-16 and HPV-18 are carcinogenic. Accordingly, there exist in all HPV infections proangiogenic signaling. There is no consensus on which cytokines actually stimulate the angiogenesis and vasodilation seen in HPV+ skin, as VEGF is commonly found in healthy uninfected human skin as well.[7] It is known that HPV-2 DNA is correlated with increases in angiogenesis,[8] but it is not confirmed whether or not VEGF is responsible for verruca angiogenesis. However, VEGF is implicated in the angiogenesis of HPV-induced cervical tumors. Though it is unconfirmed at this time, VEGF overexpression is the likely initiator of wart microvascularization in the common HPV-2 infection (Fig. 11.5).

Current therapies for cutaneous nongenital warts include debridement accompanied by freezing with liquid nitrogen, treatment with salicylic acid, bichloracetic acid, or cantharidin. Flat warts are treated with cryotherapy, 5-fluorouracil, or tretinoin,[9] while filiform warts are generally treated with

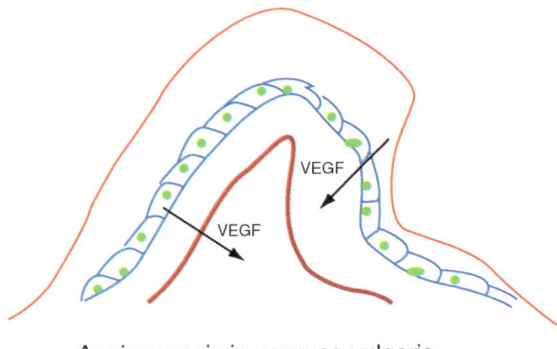

Angiogenesis in verrruca vulgaris

FIG. 11.5. Angiogenesis in common warts is the result of overproduction of VEGF by hyperproliferating epidermal keratinocytes

a snip excision. Imiquimod is a common topical treatment for anogenital warts, working through local cytokine induction (including the antiangiogenic cytokine interferon-2).

Basal Cell Carcinoma

Basal cell carcinomas (BCCs) occupy a classification of skin cancers known as the nonmelanoma skin cancers (NMSC). This classification extends to squamous cell carcinomas (SCCs) and BCCs almost exclusively. The causes of BCCs vary, but are largely attributed to overexposure to ultraviolet (UV) light, genetic predisposition (illustrated in an extreme case by xeroderma pigmentosum), and possibly HPV infection. Other risk factors include exposure to ionizing radiation, chronic immunosuppression, and long-term use of corticosteroids.[10]

The main effector of angiogenesis in BCCs appears to be the basic fibroblast growth factor (bFGF), which occupies a small family of peptides including the acidic fibroblast growth factor (aFGF) and the Kaposi fibroblast growth factor (kFGF). The fibroblast growth factors (FGFs) are small molecules, ranging from 18 to 21 kd. These molecules bind heparin and interact with a family of four receptors.[11] In mice that were irradiated with UV light, upregulation of bFGF rather than VEGF was noted. Considering that UV overexposure is considered one of the primary causes of BCCs in humans, this finding may underlie the cutaneous angiogenesis behind UV-induced

rosacea and malignancy. The regulation of bFGF is complex, as there is no signaling peptide, and any introduction of signaling peptides converts bFGF into an oncogene with the capability of malignant transformation. Basic FGF shows baseline limited expressivity in normal epidermis. However, studies have found diffuse and strong bFGF immunoreactivity in BCCs. It is known that SCCs produce a FGF-binding protein that localizes bFGF, and BCCs could work along a similar pathway.

Therapy and treatment modalities for BCCs vary, but surgical excision still remains the most reliable treatment for a primary or recurrent tumors. Among the surgeries, the most prevalent methods are cryosurgery, curettage and electrodissection, and Mohs' micrographic surgery (MMS). The latter has some marked advantages, especially in that it affords a much high confidence in a clear border. Studies have shown that MMS does not provide significantly lower rates of recurrence, but the cosmetic sensitivity of MMS often tips the scales. It is most useful on tumors of the face, neck, head, and hands. As with all surgeries, the cosmetic and practical outcome of the procedure is largely influenced by the skill of the surgeon. Adjuvant therapy for BCCs includes radiation therapy (RT), or topical treatment with imiquimod or 5-fluorouracil.

Squamous Cell Carcinoma

Squamous cell carcinomas are the second member of the class of NMSCs, and they result from malignant proliferation of keratinocytes in the epidermis. The tumors present as a hyperkeratotic nodule, papule, or plaque, closely resembling actinic keratoses. The angiogenic pathophysiology of an SCC involves dual signaling for neovascularization, blood vessel permeability, and vasodilation by both VEGF and bFGF.[12] It is theorized that the NMSCs are the result of UVB radiation, while melanomal growths result from mostly UVA radiation. It is additionally supposed by Arbiser et al. that some SCCs, such as those occurring in the mouth and throat, are the result of a p53 deficiency, while those of the epidermis are the result of direct DNA damage. Despite the fact that SCCs overexpress both VEGF and bFGF, they are predominantly only locally invasive. The most effective treatments are surgery, with reasonable effectiveness following a topical treatment with imiquimod of 5-fluorouracil. Patients must be given careful follow-up exams to ensure complete resection of all tumor tissue.

Photoaging

Photoaging is the overall process of skin aging due to UV exposure. It is characterized by wrinkle formation, blistering, and reduced recoil capacity. The cause of photoaging is likely matrix degradation or remodeling due to overexposure to UV light. The most common source of matrix degradation or remodeling in most people is chronic sun exposure. Matrix metalloproteinases secreted by dermal fibroblasts and keratinocytes are generally considered responsible for the matrix remodeling. The MMPs are zinc-dependent endopeptidases in a subclass of the metzincin superfamily of proteins. The effects of MMP can be inhibited by the tissue inhibitor of MMP (TIMP-1). Another effector of cutaneous photoaging is the serine protease granzyme B (GrB).[13] Keratinocytes irradiated with UVA simultaneously produced GrB and MMP1. The result of this finding elucidates the complementary actions of MMPs and GrB in matrix remodeling upon prolonged UV irradiation. Therapy and treatment for photoaging is limited.

Actinic Keratosis

Actinic keratosis (AK) is a premalignant lesion occurring on sun-damaged skin. Over many years AKs can progress to SCCs, exemplifying tumorigenesis through loss of tumor suppressor genes. These tumors display increased angiogenesis as the tumor progresses.[14] Angiogenesis inhibitor thrombospondin-1 (TSP-1) is strongly expressed in most AKs.[15] It has been reported that patients treated with sorafenib resulted in inflammation of AK, which in some cases progressed to invasive squamous cell carcinoma.[16] The treatment for AK is cryotherapy and in some cases a topical treatment with imiquimod of 5-fluorouracil. Physicians should be vigilant in follow-up exams, because these lesions are a risk factor for NMSC.

Ulcers

Chronic skin ulcers occur in approximately 1 million people in the United States. Little is known about the pathways leading to degeneration of tissue and ulcer formation, though common theories connect degeneration to inadequate circulation and ischemia—elements in most dermal ulcers. Collagen is the primary component of mechanical strength in most tissues. Collagen stability is dependent on adequate oxygen supply. In ischemic skin, biochemical mechanisms of tissue repair are activated, with increases in lactate, TGF-β, VEGF, collagen synthesis, and MMP-1 and -2. The upregulation of VEGF and MMP (primary angiogenesis stimulators) are known to signal increased angiogenesis to the location. In some cases unstable collagen molecules are synthesized together with upregulated MMPs, resulting in collagen denaturation, defective angiogenesis, weaker skin, and predisposition to ulceration.[17]

In chronic ulcers, slow and abnormal healing occurs due to biochemical and physiologic defects of the local tissue. The inflammatory phase may be prolonged, possibly with decreases in collagen synthesis by fibroblasts and increased levels of MMPs (Fig. 11.6). Epithelial cells and fibroblasts are senescent at the wound edges, and do not respond to growth factor signals such as platelet-derived growth factor (PDGF) or TGF-β. Nonhealing ulcers, including diabetic, venous stasis, and pressure ulcers, can be characterized by inadequate wound granulation, and thus inadequate angiogenesis. In diabetic ulcers, glucose is antiproliferative, which causes loss of angiogenic stimulators, such as PDGF-BB, TGF-β, and ang-1. In pressure ulcers, tissues compression, and vasoconstriction result in poor tissue perfusion. In venous stasis ulcers, fibrin cuffs around capillaries cause local hypoperfusion and also may sequester growth factors.

Ulcers are commonly treated through mechanical and compression therapy. Topical treatments vary, but include occlusive therapy, topical debriding agents, PDGF, and topical antibiotics. Gentian violet can be used topically to decrease inflammation in skin ulcers (Arbiser, unpublished data). In some cases, surgery (skin grafting or transposition skin) may be necessary. However, interventive care remains the best way to prevent development or exacerbation of skin ulcers.

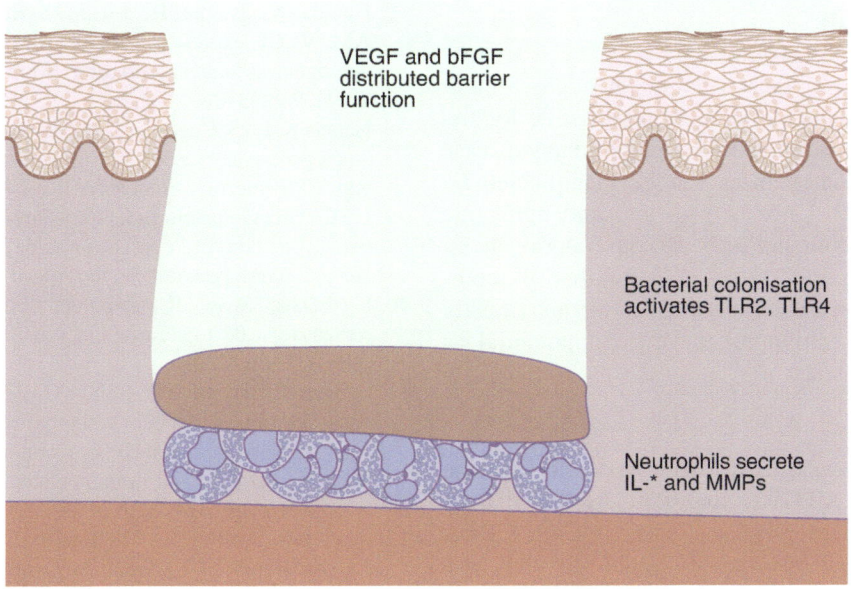

Fig. 11.6. A model for angiogenesis in venous ulcers. In chronic wounds, there is a proinflammatory process that drives angiogenesis. There is also imbalanced collagen production/degradations by fibroblasts, with the result being a chronic wound

Melanoma

Melanoma is the sixth most common cancer in the United States, with rates of occurrence increasing faster than those of any other cancer. Some risk factors for melanoma include overexposure to UVA radiation, sensitive skin type, immunosuppression, family history of melanoma, dysplastic mole syndrome, multiple common or atypical nevi, and exposure to positive mutagens.

Melanoma is infamous for its poor prognosis and resistance to treatment. Melanoma tends to metastasize via the lymphatic vessels to the areas surrounding the tumor and to draining lymph nodes. Overexpression of angiogenesis factors such as VEGF-A, FGF-2, IL-8, PDGF, and ang-2 have been observed in human melanoma. VEGFA-transfected melanomas are characterized by increased angiogenesis and tumor growth. Importantly, several receptors previously thought to be exclusively expressed on endothelial cells such as VEGFR-1, VEGFR-2, and Tie-2 are also expressed in different tumor cells. Recent experiments implicate the Tie-2 signaling pathway as an important angiogenesis modulator in melanoma. Ang1/ang2 are ligands that (de)activate the Tie-2 pathway. Dominant Ang-2 expression against ang-1 through Tie2 receptor in the presence of VEGF plays a critical role in initiating early neovascularization.[18] Akt/PI3K has emerged as a critical pathway downstream of Tie2 that is necessary for cell survival effects as well as for chemotaxis, activation of endothelial nitric oxide synthase, and perhaps for antiinflammatory effects of Tie2 activation. Mitogen-activated protein kinase (MAPK) activation has also emerged as a pathway that may be responsible for the morphogenetic effects of Tie2 on endothelial cells.

Several experimental approaches to treat melanoma using angiogenesis inhibitors have been reported. Besides the surgical modalities for the removal of melanoma, the common medical treatment modalities include adjuvant therapy with IFN. However, due to the marked side effects of IFN, many patients do not complete the full course. Cheaper, more effective, and safer methods in production include endogenous inhibitors of TSP-1, TSP-1 fragments, TRAIL, TSP-2, IL-12, angiostatin, endostatin, and other compounds such as TNP-470, thalidomide, SU6668, SR25989, solenopsin, honokiol, and batimastat. Triphenylmethane dyes are suspected to suppress Ang2 via nox4 inhibition, and are promising medical therapies for melanoma.

Conclusion

Angiogenesis, or the formation of microvasculature is a fundamental process responsible for tissue homeostasis, and is also a part of many disease processes. Angiogenesis can be manipulated by resetting the balance of pro- and antiangiogenic factors in endothelial cells. Because angiogenesis plays an important role in a number of common skin diseases, experimental agents (mostly angiogenesis inhibitors), have great potential as therapeutic agents.

Acknowledgment. J.L.A. was supported by the grants RO1 AR47901 and P30 AR42687 from the Emory Skin Disease Research Core Center of the National Institutes of Health, as well as a Veterans Administration Merit Award.

References

1. Perry BN, Arbiser JL. The duality of angiogenesis: implications for therapy for human disease. J Invest Dermatol 2006;126:2160–66.
2. Papakonstantinou E, Aletras AJ, Glass E, et al. Matrix metalloproteinases of epithelial origin in facial sebum of patients with acne and their regulation by isotretinoin. J Invest Dermatol 2005;125:673–84.
3. Eady EA, Bojar RA, Jones CE, Cove JH, Holland KT, Cunliffe WJ. The effects of acne treatment with a combination of benzoyl peroxide and erythromycin on skin carriage of erythromycin-resistant propionibacteria. Br J Dermatol 1996;134(1):107–13.
4. Nickoloff BJ, Bonish BK, Marble DJ, et al. Lessons learned from psoriatic plaques concerning mechanisms of tissue repair, remodeling, and inflammation. J Invest Dermatol Symp Proc 2006;11:16–29.
5. Detmar M, Brown LF, Claffey KP, Yeo KT, Kocher O, Jackman RW. Overexpression of vascular permeability factor/vascular endothelial growth factor and its receptors in psoriasis. J Exp Med 1994;180:1141–6.
6. Markham T, Mullan R, Golden-Mason L, et al. Resolution of endothelial activation and down-regulation of Tie2 receptor in psoriatic skin after infliximab therapy. J Am Acad Dermatol 2006; 54(6):1003–12.
7. Harada K, Baillie R, Lu S, Syrjanen S, Schor AM. VEGF expression in skin warts. Relevance to angiogenesis and vasodilation. Arch Dermatol Res 2001;293:233–38.
8. Harada K, Lu S, Chisholm DM, Syrjänen S, Schor AM. Angiogenesis and vasodilation in skin warts. Association with HPV infection. Anticancer Res 2000;20:4519–23.
9. UpToDate; Goldstein BG, Goldstein AO. http://uptodateonline.com/utd/content/topic.do?topicKey=pri_derm/8201&type=A&selectedTitle=1~5.
10. UpToDate; Shaw JC. http://uptodateonline.com/utd/content/topic.do?topicKey=skin_can/10112&type=A&selectedTitle=2~26.
11. Arbiser JL, Byers HR, Cohen C, Arbeit J. Altered basic fibroblast growth factor expression in common epidermal neoplasms: examination with in situ hybridization and immunohistochemistry. J Am Acad Dermatol 2000;42(6):973–7.
12 Perry BN, Arbiser JL. The duality of angiogenesis. J Invest Dermatol 2006;126:2160–66.
13. Hernandez-Pigeon H, Jean C, Charruyer A, et al. UVA induces granzyme B in human keratinocytes through MIF: implication in extracellular matrix remodeling. J Biol Chem 2007;16;282(11):8157–64. Epub 2007 Jan 15.
14. Klafter R, Arbiser JL. Regulation of angiogenesis and tumorigenesis by signal transduction cascades: lessons from benign and malignant endothelial tumors. J Invest Dermat Symp Proc 2000;5:79–82.
15. Burnworth B, Arendt S, Muffler S, et al. The multistep process of human skin carcinogenesis: a role for p53, cyclin D1, hTERT, p16, and TSP-1. Eur J Cell 2007;86(11–12):763–80. Epub 2007 Jan 2.
16. Lacouture ME, Desai A, Soltani K, et al. Inflammation of actinic keratoses subsequent to therapy with sorafenib, a multitargeted tyrosine-kinase inhibitor. Clin Exp Dermatol 2006;31(6):783–5.
17. Dalton SJ, Whiting CV, Bailey JR, Mitchell DC, Tarlton JF. Mechanisms of chronic skin ulceration linking lactate, transforming growth factor-β, vascular endothelial growth factor, collagen remodeling, collagen stability, and defective angiogenesis. J Invest Dermatol 2007;127(4):958–68. Epub 2007 Jan 11.
18. Zhang ZL, Liu ZS, Sun Q. Expression of angiopoietins, Tie2 and vascular endothelial growth factor in angiogenesis and progression of hepatocellular carcinoma. World J Gastroenterol 2006;12(26):4241–5.

Section II
Common Skin Diseases

12
Contact Dermatitis: Allergic and Irritant

Donald V. Belsito

Key Points

- Contact dermatitis is a common condition that affects approximately 20% of the United States population.
- Irritant and allergic contact dermatitis are the two major variants of this condition. Despite their different mechanisms, they can be difficult to distinguish at the clinical, histologic and even molecular levels.
- Allergic contact dermatitis is biphasic, with an afferent (sensitization) phase and an efferent (elicitation) phase. Cutaneous antigen-presenting cells (for example, Langerhans' cells) play a role in trafficking and presenting hapten-self complexes to T lymphocytes.
- CD8[+] T lymphocytes are thought to be the major effector cell of allergic contact dermatitis, whereas CD4[+] T lymphocytes may play a role as regulatory cells in allergic contact dermatitis.
- Patch testing plays a critical role in the management of allergic contact dermatitis, because the identification of relevant allergens enables patients to avoid the offending substance.
- Irritant contact dermatitis is a nonimmunologic response to chemicals that are damaging to the skin (surfactants, solvents, hydrocarbons, strong acids/bases, and others).

Contact dermatitis (CD) affects approximately 20% of the U.S. population.[1] Pathophysiologically, CD can be divided into allergic contact dermatitis (ACD) and irritant contact dermatitis (ICD) reactions. Despite the mechanistic differences between these two types of CD, the clinical and histopathologic findings in ACD and ICD may be quite similar.[2–6] Allergic contact dermatitis is characterized by spongiosis and a superficial lymphohistiocytic infiltrate, while ICD is marked by disruption of the stratum corneum and, occasionally, intraepidermal necrosis.[5] The exocytosis and spongiosis observed in ICD results from epidermal hyperproliferation following nonimmunologic injury.[7,8] This chapter explores the current understanding of the pathophysiology, clinical presentation, and diagnosis of these two forms of CD.

Allergic Contact Dermatitis

The Allergens

Most environmental allergens are haptens, that is, simple chemicals that must link to proteins to form a complete antigen before they can sensitize.[9] These haptens (Table 12.1) are primarily small (~500 dalton [d]), electrophilic molecules that bind to carrier proteins via covalent bonds.[11] The major exception to such covalent bonding occurs among the metallic salts (e.g., nickel and cobalt), which are thought to complex with proteins in a manner analogous to the complexing of cobalt with vitamin B_{12}.[11] Not all sensitizers penetrating the skin are complete allergens. So-called prohaptens must be metabolized in vivo to become antigenic; for example, hexavalent chromium is reduced to its trivalent form, which is the reactive form binding to cutaneous proteins.[12]

Although there are over 3700 known environmental allergens,[13] not all electrophilic, protein-binding

TABLE 12.1. The 20 most frequent allegens in the United States: 2003–2004[a,b]

Allergen	Patients tested (n)	(+) reactions (%)
Nickel sulfate	5129	18.7
Neomycin sulfate	5137	10.6
Balsam of Peru (*Myroxylon pereirae*)	5140	10.6
Fragrance mix[c]	5140	9.1
Quaternium-15	5139	8.9
Sodium gold thiosulfate	5106	8.7
Formaldehyde	5142	8.7
Cobalt	5141	8.4
Bacitracin	5143	7.9
Methyldibromoglutaronitrile/ phenoxyethanol	5140	6.1
Para-phenylenediamine	5136	4.7
Thiuram mix[d]	5141	4.6
Potassium dichromate	5142	4.3
Carba mix[e]	5142	4.0
Diazolidinyl urea	5139	3.5
Propylene glycol	5143	3.3
Imidazolidinyl urea	5139	2.9
Rosin (colophony)	5143	2.8
Tixocortol-21-pivalate	5142	2.7
Ethylenediamine dihydrochloride	5143	2.4
2-bromo-2-nitropropane-1,3-diol	5140	2.3

[a] The population studied consisted of patients with suspected ACD referred for patch testing and is therefore not necessarily representative of the general population; data from Warshaw et al.[10]
[b] Although *Toxicodendron* oleoresin in poison ivy/oak is a frequent cause of ACD, it is not listed because it was not tested in this study.
[c] Cinnamic alcohol 1%, cinnamic aldehyde 1%, hydroxycitronellal 1%, amylcinnamaldehyde 1%, geraniol 1%, eugenol 1%, isoeugenol 1%, oakmoss absolute 1%.
[d] Tetramethylthiuram disulfide 0.25%, tetramethylthiuram monosulfide 0.25%, tetraethylthiuram disulfide 0.25%, dipentamethylenethiuram disulfide 0.25%.
[e] 1.3-diphenylguanidine 1%, zinc diethyldithiocarbamate 1%, zinc dibutyl-dithiocarbamate 1%.

substances are haptens. The nature of the antigenic determinants, the type of binding that the hapten undergoes with the carrier, the final three-dimensional configuration of the conjugate, and a variety of unknown host and environmental factors undoubtedly contribute to the antigenicity of a chemical.[14] For example, in murine studies, sensitivity to dimethylbenzanthracene occurs only in strains that can metabolize this compound,[15] which suggests that the metabolic state of the host may be a key determinant in the development of reactions to at least some allergens. Of equal or greater importance is the carrier for the hapten because potent contact sensitizers, when complexed to nonimmunogenic carriers, induce tolerance rather than sensitization.[16] Class I and II molecules on the surface of the antigen-presenting cells act as the binding site (carrier) for contact allergens.[17,18]

Pathophysiology

The Afferent Phase

The antigen-presenting cells within the skin are the Langerhans' cells (LCs), which are bone marrow–derived dendritic cells situated within the suprabasilar layer of the epidermis.[19] While all epidermal cells bear class I antigens, LCs are the only cells in the epidermis that constitutively express class II human leukocyte antigens (HLA-DR). Depending on the allergen, LCs can either bind the hapten to class I or II antigens on their surface directly, or "process" the allergen internally into a complete antigen. Antigen processing by LCs may be directed toward presentation to cytotoxic CD8[+] T cells (Tc, via class I molecules) or to CD4[+] regulatory T cells (T_{reg}, class II).

Cutaneous allergens presented via class I typically undergo enzymatic digestion to yield antigenic peptides of 8 to 12 amino acids. These peptides are then transported to the endoplasmic reticulum by the transporter associated with antigen processing (TAP). The antigenic peptide is complexed to major histocompatibility complex (MHC) class I by loading from cytosolic proteins, which are rapidly destroyed by the catalytic attachment of ubiquitin (reviewed by Stingl et al.[20]). Class I molecules affixed to these peptides are released from the endoplasmic reticulum and transported to the cell surface.

In contrast, class II molecules bind peptides within endosomal or lysosomal compartments. After degradation of the allergen to peptides ranging from 15 to 22 amino acids (or longer), the antigenic peptides bind to HLA-DR, and the class II peptide complex is recycled onto the cell surface.[21–23] Adenosine triphosphatase (ATPase) on the surface of LCs, which is endocytosed with antigen, participates in this process by driving a proton pump that acidifies the environment, thus promoting degradation of allergen and the class II–associated Ii peptide (CLIP).[20,23]

Processing and presentation of the antigen are referred to as the afferent phase of cell-mediated immunity. This occurs in the paracortical (thymus-dependent) areas of the draining lymph nodes (Fig. 12.1). Upon immunologic stimulation of the epidermis, antigen-bearing LCs migrate to the lymph nodes. Migration into lymphatic vessels is evident as early as 2 to 4 hours after antigenic challenge. By 4 to 6 hours, antigen-bearing LCs are present in the T-cell–dependent, paracortical areas of the draining lymph nodes, and by 18 to 24 hours, their numbers are sufficient to transfer sensitization.[24,25]

Those factors that control the migration of LCs from the epidermis to the draining lymph nodes are now being recognized (Fig. 12.1). Within 15 minutes after application of a contact allergen, LCs synthesize interleukin-1β (IL-1β), and keratinocytes (KCs) are stimulated to produce tumor necrosis factor-α (TNF-α) and granulocyte-macrophage colony-stimulating factor (GM-CSF).[26,27] Binding of TNF-α and IL-1β to their respective receptors on LCs results in decreased expression of E-cadherin on the surface of LCs. In the epidermis, the LC and KC (which also expresses E-cadherin) are firmly associated via E-cadherin/E-cadherin junctions. Thus, the reduced expression of E-cadherin on LCs facilitates their migration away from KCs.[28] Interleukin-1β and TNF-α also inhibit the

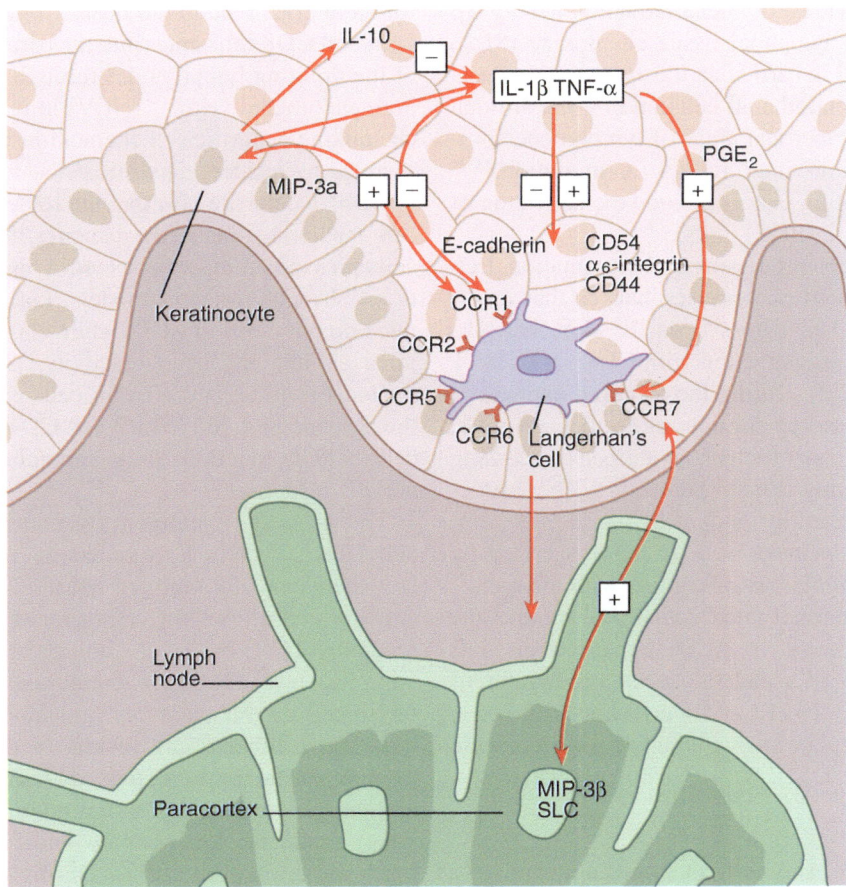

FIG. 12.1. Factors regulating Langerhans' cell (LC) trafficking between the epidermis and peripheral lymph nodes. Interleukin-1β (IL-1β) and tumor necrosis factor-α (TNF-α), secreted by LCs and keratinocytes (KCs), respectively, downregulate E-cadherin and upregulate CD54, α_6-integrin, and CD44, providing chemotactic stimuli for LC migration out of the dermis. Downregulation of CCR1, CCR2, CCR5, and CCR6 by IL-1β and TNF-α, together with upregulation of CCR7 by TNF-α and possibly prostaglandin E_2 (PGE₂), provide a chemotactic gradient toward the lymphatic endothelial cells and paracortical stromal cells due to their expression of macrophage inhibition protein 3β (MIP-3β) and secondary lymphoid tissue chemokine (SLC). IL-10, via its inhibition of IL-1β and TNF-α, can interfere with LC migration. (Courtesy of Donald V. Belsito.)

expression of a number of chemokine receptors on the LC membrane (e.g., CCR1, CCR2, CCR5, and CCR6), which recognize corresponding ligands on KCs, especially macrophage inhibition protein 3α (MIP-3α) (CCL20).[29] Finally, IL-1β and TNF-α induce the expression of adhesion molecules such as CD54, α_6-integrin, and CD44, which attract the LC to the extracellular matrix and to endothelial cells in the dermis.

To reach the dermis, LCs need to traverse the basement membrane zone, which is accomplished via secretion of matrix metalloproteinases 3 and 9 (MMP-3 and MMP-9).[30] In the dermis, upregulation of CCR7 on LCs by TNF-α and prostaglandin E_2 (PGE$_2$) provides for chemoattraction to MIP-3β and secondary lymphoid tissue chemokine (SLC) (CCL21).[29,31,32] In particular, the expression of SLC on lymphatic endothelial cells and by the stromal cells in the paracortical areas of lymph nodes provides a critical driving force for LC migration.[33–35] Other contributing factors include the activation of protein kinase C (PKC) in LCs.[36]

During antigen processing and presentation, LCs undergo profound phenotypic changes that facilitate not only their egress from the skin, but also their subsequent interaction with CD4[+] or CD8[+] T cells (Table 12.2). During the acquired expression of these accessory/adhesion molecules on LCs, they become less efficient at antigen processing and more potently antigen presenting. These processes are regulated by cytokines.

As previously mentioned, IL-1β is secreted by LCs within 15 minutes of contact with allergen.[26] Treatment of normal mice with IL-1β mimics the changes that occur in ACD: enhanced class II expression on LCs and enhanced production of IL-1α and TNF-α by KCs.[27] Interleukin-1β has been shown to upregulate intercellular adhesion molecule 1 (ICAM-1) (CD54), B7-1 (CD80), B7-2 (CD86),

CD58 (lymphocyte function–associated antigen-3 [LFA-3]), and CD40 on LCs.[40] Additionally, the interaction between CD40 and receptor activator of nuclear factor-kappa B (RANK) on LCs and their ligands (CD40-L and RANK-L) on T cells further stimulates production of ICAM-1, B7-1, and B7-2, as well as LFA-3.[41,42]

Although the accessory/adhesion molecules acquired by LCs during their "maturation" provide important secondary signals that facilitate antigen presentation via interaction with corresponding ligands on T cells (Table 12.2), antigen-bearing LCs must interact with CD4[+] T cells or CD8[+] T cells with specific receptors for the contact allergen for an allergic reaction to occur (Fig. 12.2). These CD4 and CD8 cells enter into the paracortical areas of the draining lymph nodes through postcapillary high endothelial venules (HEV) in response to the chemokine dendritic cell chemokine 1 (DC-CK-1), secreted by resident dendritic cells.[43]

CD8[+] T cells are now thought to be the principal cell mediating the ACD response,[44] while CD4[+] cells provide, in most instances, a regulatory function.[45] In experimental models, class I knockout mice do not develop ACD, while class II knockout mice exhibit enhanced reactivity.[46] Additionally, hapten-specific CD8[+] effector cells can develop in the absence of T-cell help.[46] The CD4[+], CD25[+] T$_{reg}$ cell in ACD functions to downregulate, not mediate, the response.[45]

The process of antigen presentation to CD8[+] and CD4[+] T cells is initiated by intimate contact between the antigen-bearing LCs and T cells, which allows for engagement of the T-cell receptor (TCR) on T cells and the MHC-peptide complex on LCs. This membrane interaction, facilitated by the accessory molecules previously described (Table 12.2), results in the activation of nuclear factor of activated T cells (NF-AT) and the generation of proinflammatory cytokines, which result in clonal expansion of the responding population (Fig. 12.3). During initial sensitization, "mature" antigen-primed LCs present antigen to T cells that have not been previously sensitized. These virgin T cells express L-selectin, an adhesion molecule that localizes T cells to peripheral lymph nodes,[47] hence central presentation. Appropriate presentation of antigen, in the presence of site-specific regulatory factors such as IL-6 and transforming growth factor-β

TABLE 12.2. Accessory molecules on Langerhans' cells and the corresponding ligands on T cells that enhance T-cell responses in allergic contact dermatitis (ACD)

Langerhans' cell	T cells	Reference
ICAM-1 (CD 54)	LFA-1 (CD11a/CD18)	Kuhlman et al.[37]
LFA-3 (CD58)	CD2	Prens et al.[38]
B7 (CD80, CD86)	CD28	Rattis et al.[39]

ICAM, intercellular adhesion molecule; LFA, lymphocyte function associated.

(TGF-β),[48] which are known LC products, results in the clonal expansion of antigen-specific T cells.[49] In this process, the antigen-presenting cells play a crucial role by producing IL-12,[50] which directs T-cell development toward Tc1-like memory/effector cells.[51] Thus, neutralization of IL-12 in vivo prevents the induction of ACD and induces hapten-specific tolerance.[52]

As antigen-primed LCs interact with CD4+ and CD8+ lymphocytes bearing the appropriate TCR (Fig. 12.2), LCs secrete IL-1β.[26] Interleukin-1 activates T cells to synthesize and release IL-2.[53] Interleukin-6, which is upregulated by both IL-1 and TNF-α,[54] synergizes with IL-1 in this activa-

tion of T cells. In conjunction with IL-1 and IL-6,[55] IL-2 induces one of two chains (the Tac antigen) of its own receptor (IL-2R) on T cells.[56] Expression of the high-affinity IL-2R (two chains, Tac and a 75-kd peptide) is necessary for T cells to respond optimally to the stimulating effects of IL-2.[57] The presence of B7-2[58,59] on LCs potentiate T-cell production of IL-2, which classically has been thought to be responsible for driving the clonal expansion of the responding T cells.

Although a product of the memory/effector CD8+ Tc1 cells,[60] IL-2 acts nonspecifically to stimulate T cells with and without specific antigen receptors, causing them to proliferate, to express

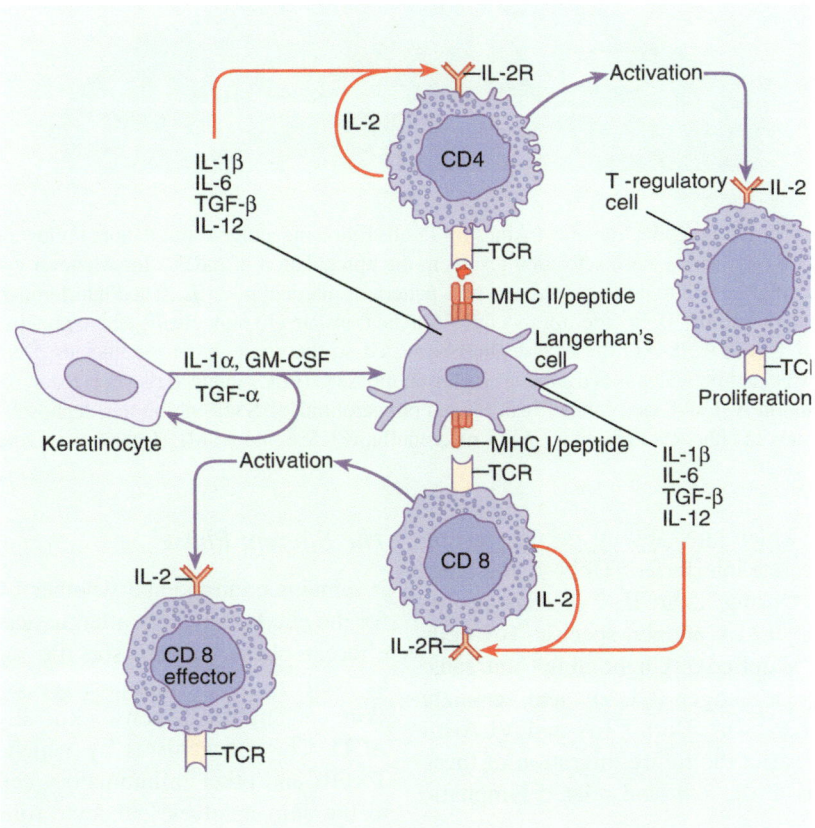

FIG. 12.2. Antigen presentation by Langerhans cells (LCs) and proliferative responses of T cells. The LCs can present antigen in association with either class I or class II molecules to T cells with the appropriate corresponding T-cell receptor (TCR). Presentation via mixed histocompatibility complex (MHC) class I results in proliferation of CD8+ cytotoxic T cells (Tc1), the effector cells for most contact allergies. Presentation via MHC class II results in proliferation of CD4+ T-regulatory (T_{reg}) cells, which act to dampen responsiveness. The keratinocyte (KC), by producing IL-1α, TNF-α, and granulocyte-macrophage colony-stimulating factor (GM-CSF), is an active participant in this process. See text for further details. (Courtesy of Donald V. Belsito.)

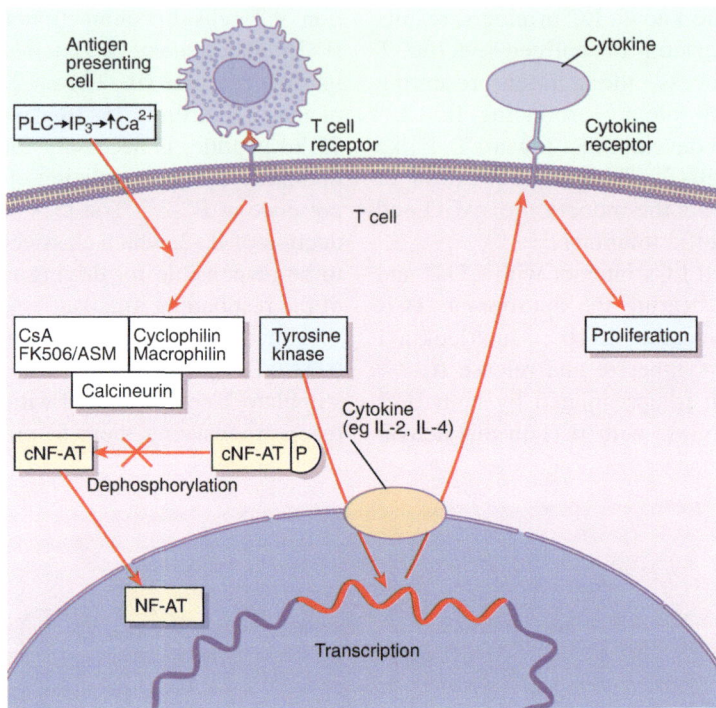

FIG. 12.3. Factors controlling production of cytokines by T cells following antigen stimulation. Following activation of the T-cell receptor (TCR), tyrosine kinase activation results in the upregulation of mRNA for whatever cytokine pattern the responding cell is programmed to produce; e.g., a type 1 pattern of interleukin-2 (IL-2) and interferon-γ (IFN-γ) or a type 2 pattern of IL-4, IL-5, and IL-10. In order for this mRNA to be translated to biologically active protein, cytosolic nuclear factor of activated T cells (cNF-AT) must be dephosphorylated so that it can enter the nucleus. Dephosphorylation is accomplished by calcineurin, which is activated via a phospholipase C (PLC)-induced rise in cytosolic calcium. The macrolactams (cyclosporin A [CsA], tacrolimus [FK506], and pimecrolimus [ASM]) inhibit this dephosphorylation by complexing calcineurin with either cyclophilin (CsA) or macrophilin (FK506 and ASM). (Courtesy of Donald V. Belsito.)

DR antigens (which are absent in the resting state), and to secrete interferon-γ (IFN-γ) and other cytokines.[61–63] During their IL-2 driven proliferation (see Fig. 12.2), antigen-specific Tc1 cells express newly acquired "skin homing" antigens: common leukocyte antigen (CLA)[49] and very late antigen α4 (VLA-α4).[64] Both CLA and VLA-α4 preferentially restrict the future migration of these memory T cells to the skin and related lymphatic beds.

As mentioned, antigen-primed Tc1 cells preferentially secrete IL-2 and IFN-γ and are the "classic" effector cells of ACD. In contrast, the CD4$^+$ T$_{reg}$, which is also CD25$^+$, preferentially secretes IL-10 and TGF-β.[60] Given their cytokine profile, it is not surprising that T$_{reg}$ cells act to downregulate ACD and are not necessary for priming of Tc1.[46,65]

The Efferent Phase

It remains controversial whether LCs are required for the elicitation of the allergic reaction.[66–70] In the efferent phase, antigen-specific memory T cells, as well as other inflammatory cells, invade the skin, causing the response clinically recognized as ACD. The mechanisms by which these memory T cells and other inflammatory cells are recruited to the skin involves leukocyte rolling, arrest, and spreading on vascular endothelium, which are mediated by the sequential activation of selectins, β_1-integrins, and β_2-integrins.[71,72]

LFA-1 (CD11a/CD18), VLA-α4, and CLA antigens (expressed on memory Tc1) and ICAM-1 (CD54), vascular cell adhesion molecule 1 (VCAM-1), and E-selectin (expressed on activated vascular

TABLE 12.3. Interaction between adhesion molecules on skin-homing; memory T cells and activated endothelial cells

T cell	Endothelial cell	Effect
CLA	E-selectin	Leukocyte rolling[73]
VLA-α4	VCAM-1	Firm adhesion[74]
LFA-1	ICAM-1	Adhesion and diapedesis[75]

CLA, common leukocyte antigen; VLA, very late antigen; VCAM, vascular cell adhesion molecule; LFA, lymphocyte function associated; ICAM, intercellular adhesion molecule.

endothelial cells) play a crucial role in homing T cells to the skin (Table 12.3). E-selectin, which is induced on vascular endothelium by IL-1 and TNF-α,[76] interacts with its corresponding ligand CLA, which memory Tc1 cells constitutively express. As a result of this molecular interaction, memory Tc1 cells circulating past activated endothelial cells are slowed in their transit and begin rolling along the endothelial cell surface.[73] After rolling, firm adhesion of leukocytes to endothelium and migration of leukocytes through the endothelial gaps are mediated by the interaction between VCAM-1 and ICAM-1 (endothelial proteins with immunoglobulin domains) and VLA-α4 (a β_1-integrin) and LFA-1 (a β_2-integrin) on lymphocytes, respectively.[74] These LFA-1+ T cells, aided by the secretion of heparanase, which degrades the heparan sulfate scaffold of the extracellular matrix,[77] migrate toward epidermal cells, which have also been induced to express ICAM-1.[78]

The induction and kinetic expression of adhesion proteins by cytokines has been well studied in vitro. Upon stimulation of endothelium with TNF-α or IL-1, E-selectin[79] and VCAM-1[80] are synthesized in, and expressed on, the endothelial cell membrane. In contrast, ICAM-1 is enhanced only after T cells have begun their adhesion to endothelial surfaces, suggesting that upregulation of ICAM-1 occurs in response to IFN-γ secreted by activated Tc1 and not to IL-1.[81]

During the course of ACD, progressively increasing amounts of ICAM-1 are expressed on epidermal cells (primarily KCs) between 48 and 96 hours after antigen challenge.[82] The strong temporal correlation between the expression of ICAM-1 on KCs and the migration of LFA-1+ T cells into the epidermis suggests that epithelial expression of ICAM-1 depends not only on epidermal cell-derived IL-1 and TNF-α, but also on T-cell–derived IFN-γ.[82] Furthermore, some allergens (e.g., urushiol[83] and

nickel[84]) may be able to directly induce ICAM-1 on KCs by activation of PKC. This may account, at least partially, for the higher frequency of reactions induced by exposure to these allergens. For most allergens, however, cytokine-coordinated expression of adhesion molecules on vascular endothelial cells and on epithelial cells more likely directs the migration of skin-homing memory Tc1s to the site of allergenic challenge.

Interleukin-1 and TNF-α are but two of the factors that contribute to homing of Tc1 effector and T_{reg} suppressor cells in ACD.[26,85] The differential recruitment of CD8+ and CD4+ cells is regulated by the expression of chemokine receptors by these T-cell subsets and by the sequential expression of chemokines in the skin during ACD. The recruitment of CD8+ effector cells seems most dependent on the interferon-inducible protein 10 (IP-10)/CXCR3 (chemokine/chemokine receptor) pathway.[86–88] In contrast, the recruitment of CD4+ T_{reg} seems to be controlled by the expression of CCL22 and CCL17 [thymus and activation-regulated chemokine (TARC)] chemokines and their receptor CCR4, which is expressed on activated CD4+ T_{reg}.[89] These latter two chemokines are upregulated in skin approximately 12 hours following antigenic challenge, the same time that mononuclear cells are observed to enter the challenged site. Finally, CTACK (CCL27) and its receptor (CCR10) also regulate the trafficking of T cells in the skin.[90,91] Of note, CTACK is constitutively expressed by KCs and is further upregulated by IL-1β and TNF-α.

While it has long been assumed that stress can exacerbate cutaneous immune responses, there is now a clearer understanding of how the nervous system regulates cutaneous responsiveness. Spurred by the observation that nerve fibers directly impinge on LCs,[92] and given the known role of neurochemicals in vascular reactivity and inflammation,[93] a number of laboratories have studied the contribution of neuropeptides, principally substance P and calcitonin gene–related peptide (CGRP), which seem to have opposing effects on ACD. Although the data are not uniformly confirmative, release of substance P from nerve fibers appears to upregulate ACD by enhancing the secretion of TNF-α from mast cells[94] and monocytes,[95] by enhancing the production of IL-1α and TNF-α by KCs,[96] and by enhancing the synthesis and secretion of IL-2, as well as expression of its receptor.[97,98] In contrast, CGRP inhibits proliferation and antigen presentation, possibly by stimulating production of IL-10, which results in decreased expression of B7-2.[99]

The end result of this exquisitely orchestrated interplay of cytokines and adhesion molecules is, for most allergens, the entrance into the skin of Tc1 cells secreting IL-2 and IFN-γ. Interferon-γ acts in a number of ways to amplify the immune response. It upregulates Fas on KCs, which renders them susceptible to apoptosis via Fas ligand, which is expressed on the infiltrating T cells or released into the microenvironment.[100] Interferon-γ also activates natural killer (NK) cells and macrophages[101] and induces IP-10 on KCs,[26] which adds to the recruitment of monocytes/macrophages.[102] Finally, the IL-1– and TNF-α–enhanced production of monocyte chemoattractant 1 (MCA-1),[103] monocyte chemotactic and activating factor (MCAF),[104] and macrophage inflammatory protein 2 (MIP-2)[26] by KCs contributes to the recruitment of monocytes/macrophages. This collection of monocytes/macrophages, proliferating T cells, and apoptotic KCs, along with their chemical mediators, is responsible for the epidermal spongiosis (intercellular edema) and dermal infiltrate that are the histologic hallmarks of ACD. Thus, the final response to a contact allergen, while induced by a specific allergen, is antigen-nonspecific.

The Resolution Phase

Data increasingly support an important role for IL-10, which is upregulated in KCs during the late phase of ACD,[105] in dampening the ongoing immune response.[106,107] Indeed, resolution of ACD has been associated with the arrival into the skin of CCR4+, CCR8+, CD4+ T$_{reg}$ cells, which produce significant amounts of IL-10, at 24 hours after antigenic challenge.[45] Other epidermal-derived cytokines may downregulate responsiveness by affecting endothelial cell expression of adhesion molecules, for example, TGF-β, also produced by T$_{reg}$.[108,109] Whether IL-4, a T-helper-2 (Th2)-type cytokine known to inhibit production of IP-10 and TNF-α by monocytes,[110] also participates in the downregulation of ACD remains controversial.[107,110]

Macrophages and CD4+ regulatory T cells may also be involved in turning off the immune response. Under stimulation by IFN-γ, macrophages produce prostaglandins (PGs), especially of the E series.[111] Both PGE$_1$ and PGE$_2$ inhibit production of IL-2 and expression of the IL-2R.[112] The E series prostaglandins also inhibit natural killer (NK) cell activation by their inhibition of IL-2.[113] Finally, different CD4+ T-cell types have been found to have downregulatory activities in murine and human models.[46,60,114,115] These subsets include Th2, Th3, and T$_{reg}$1 (CD4+/CD25+) cells.

In summary, various soluble mediators, derived from the same cells responsible for eliciting the reaction, play an active role in dampening the response. Furthermore, an expanding number of regulatory cells are being identified that suppress responses. Finally, desquamation of antigen-laden skin, cellular, or enzymatic degradation of antigen with destruction of the antigen-presenting cell and other presently unknown regulatory mechanisms contribute to the resolution of the allergic response.

Immunoregulation

Genetic Factors

Although animal studies have shown strain (presumably genetic) variation in cell-mediated immunity, the evidence for a genetic influence in humans has been slight. Skog[116] found that 5% of a defined population could not be sensitized to dinitrochlorobenzene, and suggested that this was due to inheritance. In another study, significant genetic association with the capacity to become sensitized to para-nitrosodimethylaniline was reported.[117] However, multiple attempts to correlate HLA haplotype and other factors (including T-cell receptor genes) with nickel sensitivity or other contact allergies have yielded conflicting results. Thus, definitive evidence of a genetic predisposition to ACD in humans has been meager, probably because of the diverse genetic pool and the limitations of technology.

Route of Primary Sensitization and Tolerance

The route of primary sensitization has a profound effect on the subsequent immunologic response. Sulzberger[118] demonstrated that intracardiac injection of neoarsphenamine induced tolerance rather than sensitization. Tolerance induction has also been reported after primary oral ingestion of allergens,[119] as well as after primary epicutaneous application of allergens to areas deficient in HLA-DR-positive

LCs.[120] The exact mechanism by which tolerance ensues is controversial and may depend on the route of exposure (oral, intravenous, epicutaneous, or intraperitoneal) and on the precise subset of dendritic cell responsible for antigen presentation.[121] There are data to suggest that the expression of indoleamine 2,3-dioxygenase (IDO), an intracellular heme-enzyme that catalyzes oxidative catabolism of indole rings by DCs, results in suppression of T-cell responses and promotion of tolerance.[122] In general, either induction of hapten-specific CD4+/CD25+ or Th3 suppressor T cells[120,123,124] or clonal deletion of the responding T cells[125] seems responsible for the observed tolerance. Readers interested in a better understanding of the mechanism(s) of tolerance induction are referred elsewhere.[121,123,124]

Age and Gender

Elderly individuals have been shown to have various defects in the induction and elicitation of ACD.[126] The precise reason is unknown, and many aspects of cell-mediated responses are likely involved.[127] Experiments in which contact-sensitized aged mice were injected with naive young T cells and subsequently demonstrated normal responses upon antigenic challenge suggest that a failure of T-cell amplification signals or the generation of sufficient T effector cells may be among the primary deficiencies in elderly animals.[128]

The competency of immune responses in children is also controversial.[126] In the past, it was believed that children rarely developed ACD because of an immature immune system, and that patch testing of children with standard concentrations of allergens resulted in a high percentage of irritant reactions.[129] However, other data suggest that patch testing of children with the allergens commercially available in the United States does not result in increased, and confounding, irritant responses.[130] Nonetheless, documented allergic reactions are seen mostly in older pediatric patients and are secondary to topical medications, plants, nickel, or shoe-related allergens.[131] Of note, Strauss[132] was able to sensitize 35 of 48 infants (1 to 4 days old) to *Toxicodendron (Rhus)* oleoresin, suggesting that the apparent hyporesponsiveness of children may be due to limited exposure and not to deficient immunity. Similarly, the effects of gender on the incidence of ACD seem related to the likelihood of exposure.[126,133]

Physicochemical Modulation

In experimental models and clinical practice, downregulation of ACD has been achieved with ultraviolet radiation (UVB or psoralens plus UVA [PUVA]), glucocorticoids, and calcineurin inhibitors. Each of these acts somewhat differently. UVB and PUVA significantly decrease the density of epidermal LCs, induce epidermal hyperplasia (making it more difficult for the antigen to reach any remaining epidermal antigen-presenting cells), upregulate IL-10, and induce CD4+/CD25+ T_{reg} cells.[134,135] Glucocorticoids also inhibit the type IV reaction at multiple points[134]: epidermal LCs are decreased in number; the production and function of IL-1, IL-2, and IFN-γ are inhibited; and T-cell proliferation is decreased. In contrast, cyclosporin A and other macrolactams act primarily to inhibit activation of cytosolic NF-AT (cNF-AT) via inhibition of calcineurin (Fig. 12.3). Finally, a variety of other pharmacologic agents have been reported to interfere with the induction or elicitation of ACD in murine models.[136] These include calcium channel blockers, amiloride, pentoxifylline, pentamidine, clonidine, spiperone, N-acetylcysteine, and flavonoids. Of these, only pentoxifylline has been evaluated in humans, where it was found to induce a slight reduction in responsiveness,[137] perhaps by an effect on TNF-α.

Irritant Contact Dermatitis

Irritant contact dermatitis (ICD) is a nonimmunologic response of the skin induced by a wide variety of agents, including surfactants, solvents, hydrocarbons, and strong acids or bases, among others. Like allergens, most irritants are relatively small molecules; however, unlike most allergens, irritants have the potential to disrupt membranes or interfere with metabolic processes in the epidermis or dermis. The biochemical and cellular mechanisms regulating ICD have been poorly characterized, in part because ICD encompasses a number of different clinical responses, as delineated in Table 12.4. Phototoxicity should be added to this list, as this is an irritant reaction, often acute delayed, requiring excitation by light (typically UVA) of the inducing chemical. This discussion focuses on the mechanisms underlying acute (the most well studied) and cumulative (the more common) ICD. Differences

TABLE 12.4. Subtypes of irritant contact dermatitis (ICD)[138]

Subtypes	Characteristics
Acute	Potent irritant; short lag time; burning/sting-ing with erythema, edema, vesiculobullae and/or necrosis
Acute delayed	Similar to acute but delayed in time
Irritant reaction	Subclinical resulting in either hardening or cumulative
Cumulative	Subclinical irritant; chronic exposure with long lag time; pain/itching with erythema, hyperkeratosis, lichenification and possibly fissuring,
Exsiccation eczematid	Pruritic, dry, ichthyosiform skin due to low humidity
Traumatic	Eczematous lesions, slow to heal, following acute trauma
Pustular and acneiform	Painful pustular or acneiform lesions induced by specific agents (e.g., mineral oil, tar, etc.)
Non-erythematous	Subclinical ICD in which only the corneal barrier function is disrupted (experimen-tally evident by increased transepidermal water loss [TEWL])
Subjective	Burning sensation after contact with certain agents, especially lactic acid

in the mechanism(s) inducing these two forms of ICD might exist, since acute ICD is characterized more by inflammation, while chronic ICD displays hyperproliferation and hyperkeratosis.

Pathophysiology

Following an acute insult to the epidermal barrier, messenger RNA (mRNA) and protein for several cytokines and growth factors have been found to rapidly increase, especially IL-1,[139] TNF-α,[140] and GM-CSF.[139] Repeated, subclinical, barrier insults result in epidermal hyperproliferation and dermal inflammation associated with elevated IL-1α.[141] Thus, barrier disruption, the hallmark of ICD,[142] stimulates a cytokine profile strikingly similar to that seen in the early phases of ACD (reviewed by Effendy et al.[143]). It is postulated that these proin-flammatory cytokines allow for an alternative entry into an inflammatory pathway mechanistically and clinically similar to the inflammatory cascade seen in ACD. Thus, it is not surprising that the extent of epidermal spongiosis, vesicle formation, and exocy-tosis seen in ICD may not be significantly different from that seen in ACD, although vesicle formation is more prominent in ACD and necrosis in ICD.[142]

In addition to the effects of irritants on the corneal barrier, these agents may also have direct effects on

KCs. As reviewed by Pentland,[144] some studies suggest an effect of KC-derived lipid mediators in ICD. Release of lipid peroxidation products, stimu-lation of eicosanoid production, and activation of PKC can result from oxidation or necrosis of KC cell membranes by irritants. The release of reactive oxygen species has been well demonstrated for phototoxic substances[145] and for such irritants as dithranol and sodium lauryl sulfate (SLS).[146]

The physiologic effects of these lipid mediators is myriad and could produce many of the changes seen in acute ICD. In support of this hypothesis, studies utilizing a number of different irritants (hydrochloric acid, sodium hydroxide, nonanoic acid, and sodium dodecyl sulfate) have shown activation of the PKC-related cell signal transduc-tion cascade.[147] In other experiments using gene array technology to assess the effects of different irritants (sodium lauryl sulfate, d-limonene, and m-xylene), changes in genes associated with metabo-lism, oxidative stress, and signal transduction were observed with all three irritants.[148] Of note, there was a temporal difference in irritant-induced gene expression that appeared to correlate with the pen-etration rate of the irritant.[148] Finally, the effects of ICD can be significantly reduced using peroxisome proliferating activated receptor (PPAR) agonists (e.g., linoleic acid), which have been shown to enhance barrier recovery and synthesis of lamellar bodies and neutral lipids, especially ceramides and cholesterol.[149]

Lipid mediators may also play a role in chronic cumulative ICD. However, a number of other mechanisms for this form of ICD have been pro-posed. As reviewed by Berardesca and Distante,[150] the hyperproliferation seen in chronic ICD could be due to the following: (1) production of IL-6, IL-8, and 12-hydroxyeicosatetraenoic acid (12-HETE), which can induce epidermal hyperprolifer-ation; (2) reduced cyclic adenosine monophosphate (cAMP) levels that increase cell division; and (3) stimulation of ornithine decarboxylase resulting in increased DNA synthesis and proliferation.

As with ACD, substance P has been reported to increase cutaneous irritation,[151] likely via induc-tion of proinflammatory cytokines. Substance P induces TNF-α mRNA in mast cells,[94] stimulates IL-1 production by monocytes,[152] and stimulates IL-2 production by murine lymphocytes.[153] Finally, α-melanocyte-stimulating hormone (α-MSH), most likely via induction of IL-10,[154] inhibits acute ICD.[155]

In summary, two pathways might contribute to the final picture of ICD: the direct effect of the irritant on KC membranes and the proinflammatory effects induced by barrier disruption. Both can activate the biochemical signals leading to a pathologic response not dissimilar to that in ACD. The analogy to the complement cascade, classic (antigen driven) and alternative (non-specific toxicity), should be kept in mind.

Regulatory Determinants

Subjects with sensitive skin (subjective ICD) have been demonstrated to have very dry skin with low fat content and increased penetration of water-soluble chemicals.[156] In particular, an inverse correlation has been observed for ceramide content in the skin and the proclivity to SLS-induced ICD.[157] Thus, in addition to such external factors as molecular characteristics, exposure time/chronicity, cumulative effect(s) of other irritants, and environmental conditions, endogenous differences might account for susceptibility to ICD. Those most studied are age, gender, race, anatomic site, and atopy.

Age

Using transepidermal water loss (TEWL) as a surrogate for enhanced susceptibility to irritation, many studies have shown that the skin of children and adolescents and of individuals older than 60 years is more prone to irritation (reviewed elsewhere[150,158,159]). Nonetheless, in their study comparing children 1 to 6 years of age with one of the child's parents under identical experimental conditions, Fluhr et al.[160] saw no age-related differences in TEWL, as well as in a number of other biophysical characteristics, with the exception of lower hygroscopicity, lighter color, and increased blood perfusion in the children.

Gender

No essential differences in TEWL have been shown between men and women (reviewed elsewhere[150,158,159]). Nonetheless, Agner et al.[161] did find enhanced TEWL and increased susceptibility to SLS on the first, as compared to the tenth, day of the menstrual cycle. Notwithstanding this observation, the enhanced prevalence of ICD in women would appear to be due to differences in exposure, not to innate differences between the genders.[162,163]

Race

Data regarding racial variability in the development of ICD are conflicting. As reviewed by Berardesca and Maibach,[164] the skin of African Americans exhibited higher TEWL following exposure to SLS but, nonetheless, in several clinical studies, was less easily irritated by dichloroethylsulfide, o-chlorobenzylidene, or dinitrochlorobenzene (DNCB). These results might be explained by differences in corneocyte adhesion, the thickness of the stratum corneum, and the relative lipid content of African-American skin, all of which are greater than seen in white skin. In this regard, it has been found that tape-stripped African-American skin is as susceptible to irritation by DNCB as is white skin.[165]

Anatomic Site

Percutaneous penetration varies with anatomic region, and one would predict that ICD should as well. As reviewed by Berardesca and Distante,[150] TEWL is higher on the palm, forehead, and ankle than on the back or forearm. However, significant differences in TEWL within the same area of the body make studies regarding the influence of anatomic site difficult. Indeed, the highly absorptive vulvar skin has been found to be more reactive to benzalkonium chloride,[166] but less reactive to SLS, than forearm skin.[167]

Atopic Dermatitis

Numerous studies have documented that atopics are at increased risk of developing ICD. Even atopics in apparent remission reacted more severely to SLS than controls when assessed by TEWL.[168] These findings may be explained by qualitative and quantitative differences in intercellular lipid composition, especially a reduction in ceramides associated with structural alterations in the stratum corneum that have been observed in atopic skin.[169]

Clinical Aspects

Physical Findings

The clinical appearance of ACD and ICD can vary depending on location and duration. In most instances, acute eruptions are characterized by macular erythema and papules, vesicles, or bullae, depending on the intensity of the response. In contrast, subacute to chronic ACD or ICD presents as red and scaling patches that, depending on chronicity, may be lichenified or fissured (Fig. 12.4). Thus, neither the morphology nor the histopathology of the CD is necessarily distinctive. The clinicopathologic differential diagnoses include the following dermatitides: atopic, nummular, seborrheic, dyshidrotic, and psoriatic.

At its inception, ACD usually involves the cutaneous site of principal exposure. However, as it evolves, it can spread to other more distant sites by inadvertent contact. One must be aware that the scalp, palms, and soles are relatively resistant to ACD, and that these areas may exhibit little pathology despite contact with an allergen that produces significant dermatitis in adjacent areas of the skin. In contrast, ICD, a nonimmunologic event, usually remains localized to the site of contact.

Diagnosis

A detailed history and clinical examination are crucial to the diagnosis of ACD and ICD. An underlying atopic diathesis should be sought. If an occupational cause is suspect, a description of all job-related activities, substances encountered, personal protective equipment, and cleansers must be obtained. Items encountered in the patient's avocation(s) should also be ascertained. Examination of the entire integument, rather than an examination limited to those areas identified by the patient as problematic, frequently provides vital clues not only to the offending agent(s), but

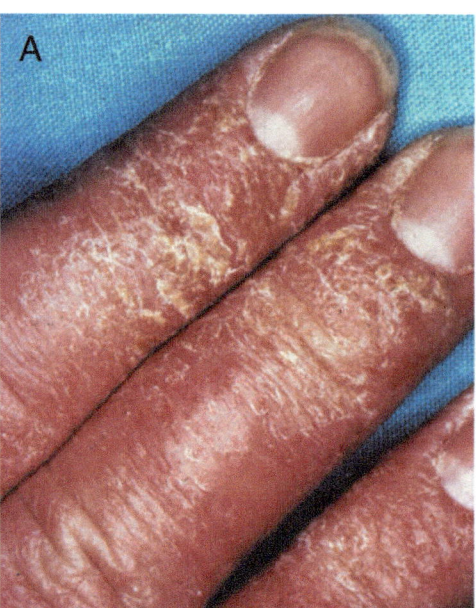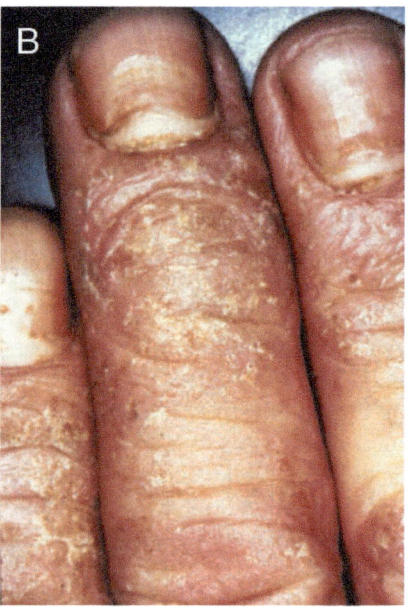

FIG. 12.4. Clinical appearance of allergic contact dermatitis (ACD) (A), and chronic cumulative irritant contact dermatitis (ICD) (B). Both patients were machinists who, as can be seen in the photographs, presented with similar-appearing rashes, except for the nail changes seen in the patient with ICD (B), which are consistent with the chronicity of the eruption. The dermatitis in A was due to ACD to 2–N-octyl-4–isothiazolin-3–one, the biocide present in his cutting oils. The dermatitis in B was due to ICD induced by the defatting action of detergents present in these oils. (Courtesy of Donald V. Belsito.)

also to the possibility of confounding endogenous (e.g., psoriasis) or exogenous (e.g., tinea) disorders.

Irritant contact dermatitis is a diagnosis of exclusion based on clinical history, physical examination, pathology (if appropriate), and, often, testing that rules out ACD. Although various laboratory tests are available to assess ACD, in vivo patch tests remain the standard.

In Vivo Tests for Allergic Contact Dermatitis

Like any in vivo assay, patch testing is subject to pitfalls, and practitioners are well advised to read Sulzberger's[170] classic review. A major issue is that, even when a chemical is found to be allergenic for a given patient, it cannot be assumed to be the cause of ACD. To determine whether an allergen is likely to be the culprit, the results of a positive patch test must always be correlated with the materials encountered by the involved areas of skin. Furthermore, even in some instances when patients are allergic to chemicals in products they are using, the allergen may be present in only minimal amounts and may not be responsible for the dermatitis.[171] In this regard, repeat open application testing (ROAT), in which the patient applies the commercial product to normal skin several times daily for 1, 2, or even 3 weeks, can be helpful.[172]

In performing patch tests, one must also be concerned with the possibility of false-positive and false-negative reactions. False-positive reactions due either to the use of allergens at irritant concentrations or to the excited skin syndrome have received much attention in the literature.[173] The false nature of these reactions can usually be resolved by repeating the patch tests individually or in lower concentrations. In contrast, false-negative reactions are more problematic and require high levels of suspicion and diligence to uncover.

One common and easily correctable cause of false-negative reactions is the failure to perform a second reading of the test sites after the initial 48-hour inspection. This second reading, sometime between 3 and 7 days after application of the patches, is particularly important for elderly patients, who take longer to mount an allergic reaction.[174] A second reading is also important in detecting positive reactions to allergens such as neomycin, more than half of which are not evident until 96 hours after application of the patch test.[175] False-negative reactions can also occur when the allergen is used in too low a concentration for patch testing, as can happen when cosmetic products are used as is. Therefore, if clinical suspicion warrants, and despite a negative patch test, additional testing such as ROAT with the suspect product can unmask the cause of ACD. Finally, with over 3700 potential allergens,[13] negative reactions may simply indicate that the responsible chemical has not been tested.

In Vitro Tests for Allergic Contact Dermatitis

Laboratory studies such as lymphocyte transformation or macrophage migration inhibition have been used as in vitro measurements of ACD in both humans and animals. However, these in vitro assays have not been reliably standardized and are therefore not clinically useful for diagnosis.[136] One of the major problems in developing in vitro systems is the lack of knowledge about what constitutes the antigenic moiety of a particular chemical. Thus, in vivo patch testing, in which the skin can process the allergen for presentation, remains the gold standard.

Treatment and Prevention

Avoidance of Allergens and Irritants

The treatment of ACD and ICD lies in correctly identifying its cause and properly instructing the patient to avoid the responsible substance(s). For certain allergens (e.g., vehicles, preservatives, stabilizers, and emulsifiers) found in topical preparations, it is important to impress upon patients the need to read labels. Patients with allergies to preservatives must be aware that these materials can be found in any water-based formulation, for example, paint. Furthermore, the name given a chemical used in a cosmetic or pharmaceutical product is frequently changed when it is used in a commercial product. For instance, the cosmetic preservative quaternium-15, when used in industry, may be referred to as Dowicil 100® or Dowicil 200®. Practitioners guiding patients through the synonymic challenges of these chemicals are advised to consult standard texts on the subject.[176]

Unfortunately for patients and their providers, the allergenic component of many materials will almost never be labeled. Rubber-related allergens, textile-related allergens, and metal-related allergens are but a few examples. In counseling patients with reactions to these materials, the patch tester must provide information about what kinds of products are likely to contain the allergen, as well as appropriate replacements. Such information can be found in standard texts.[176,177] Furthermore, some allergens are incompletely labeled. Given the proprietary nature of a fragrance's formulation, the individual fragrances that have been combined to produce the product are not listed in the U.S., although the European Union does have regulations that require labeling of 26 specific fragrance ingredients. Until the U.S. follows suit, consumers of American products with an allergic reaction to a fragrance should be advised to use fragrance-free materials, which include not only topical preparations but also a variety of other products such as toilet paper and sanitary napkins.[176,177] It is important to realize that products labeled unscented contain masking fragrances, although they are usually present in very low concentrations and are not problematic.

Because many allergens may share common antigenic moieties, one must instruct the patient not only about the known allergen, but also about possible cross-reacting allergens. For example, the patient allergic to benzocaine must be aware of the many potentially cross-reacting substances, which include agents as diverse as other aminobenzoate anesthetics (e.g., procaine), certain medications (e.g., sulfonamides), hair dyes (e.g., *para*-phenylenediamine), textile dyes (e.g., aniline dyes), some sunscreens (e.g., *para*-aminobenzoic acid), and other products.[176,177] Since cross-reactions are not always evident to the nonchemist, providers may wish to consult standard texts[176,177] when instructing their patients.

As with ACD, the primary treatment for ICD is irritant avoidance. The most common irritants are water, surfactants and solvents. However, numerous chemicals, typically found in occupational settings, can account for ICD. For guidance in the etiology of occupational ICD, the reader may want to consult relevant texts.[178]

Symptomatic Therapy

In addition to avoidance of further contact with the offending agent(s), treatment of ACD and ICD should be directed to amelioration of symptoms. Acute, vesicular, weeping eruptions benefit from drying agents such as topical aluminum sulfate/calcium acetate; chronic, lichenified eruptions are best treated with emollients. Pruritus can be controlled with topical antipruritics or oral antihistamines; topical antihistamines or anesthetics are best avoided because of the risk of inducing a secondary allergy in already dermatitic skin. Treatment with physicochemical agents that downregulate inflammation may also be required. Topical glucocorticosteroids[179] or macrolactams[1*] (Fig. 12.3)[180,181] usually suffice for most patients with ACD or ICD. However, individuals with involvement of greater than 25% of their body surface area with ACD or those exposed to certain allergens (such as *Toxicodendron (Rhus)* oleoresin, which may persist locally in the skin for weeks after exposure) may require treatment with systemic glucocorticosteroids. In those patients with ACD in whom systemic steroid therapy is not appropriate, phototherapy with UVB or PUVA can be beneficial. In addition, individuals with occupational ACD who are economically unable to discontinue working with the offending allergen and who are also unable to work with gloves or effective barrier creams may benefit from phototherapy. In these cases, chronic maintenance therapy with UVB[182] or PUVA[183] may obviate clinical manifestations of the allergy despite persistent contact.

Mechanistically, the biologics introduced for psoriasis should benefit ACD[2**]: efalizumab targeting the CD11a portion of LFA-1, alefacept binding to the CD2+ memory cells and inducing granzyme-mediated apoptosis, and the TNF-α inhibitors (etanercept, adalimumab, and infliximab) negatively affecting this crucial mediator of inflammation. Furthermore, the TNF-α inhibitors might also theoretically lessen ICD. However, the costs of these treatments make their usefulness

---

*These drugs are not currently approved for this purpose by the Food and Drug Administration.
**These drugs are not currently approved for this purpose by the Food and Drug Administration.

prohibitory in diseases such as ACD and ICD that, except in extreme cases, should be manageable by avoidance.

Physicochemical Barriers

While prevention of ACD and ICD rests with avoidance of the inducing agent, for various reasons, principally economic, this is not always possible. The hairdresser allergic to glyceryl thioglycolate (in acid-permanent solutions), which can persist in hair for months[184] and can penetrate vinyl and latex gloves,[176] may be unable to avoid daily contact with the allergen. A plastic glove made of proprietary laminate may be beneficial (4H, North Safety Products, Cranston, RI 02921; Tel. 1-800-430-4110). In clinical trials, the glove, which is only 0.07 mm thick, was impervious to more than 90% of all randomly selected organic chemicals for 4 hours at 35°C.[185] However this glove is not form-fitting and is thought by many professionals to impede the fine dexterity needed in their work.

In the future, barrier creams may be available to help patients with both ACD and ICD. Regarding ACD, barrier creams are available for only a limited number of allergens (principally poison ivy and poison oak), are effective only if the protected area is washed within several hours of contact with the allergen, and are objectionable to many patients because of their thick tack and greasy consistency. Although barrier creams may be beneficial for ICD, they must be specifically selected for the materials handled.[186,187] In general, barriers for organic solvents are less than satisfactory.[186,188] Furthermore, it is an incorrect axiom that one uses water-in-oil barriers for aqueous and oil-in-water barriers for lipophilic irritants.[186] Indeed, for "wet workers," frequent moisturization is as effective as "barrier creams" in preventing ICD.[189,190]

Conclusion

Allergic and irritant contact dermatitis is a common dermatosis in the U.S. and worldwide. The immunologic mechanisms of ACD are well defined, involving cutaneous antigen-presenting cells and T lymphocytes. For irritant contact dermatitis, there are two major pathways that trigger inflammation: direct effects of the irritant on keratinocytes, and the proinflammatory effects of barrier disruption. For both irritant and allergic contact dermatitis, effective management of these conditions involves identification of the offending agents (allergens and irritants), as these environmental exposures drive the process of contact dermatitis.

References

1. Mathias C. The cost of occupational disease. Arch Dermatol 1985;121:332–4.
2. Scheynius A, Fischer T, Forsum U, et al. Phenotypic characterization in situ of inflammatory cells in allergic and irritant contact dermatitis in vivo. Clin Exp Immunol 1984;55:81–90.
3. Scheynius A, Fischer T. Phenotypic differences between allergic and irritant patch test reactions in man. Contact Dermatitis 1986;14:297–302.
4. Willis CM, Young E, Brandon DR, et al. Immunopathological findings in human allergic and irritant contact dermatitis. Br J Dermatol 1986;115:305–16.
5. Willis CM, Stephens CJM, Wilkinson JD. Epidermal damage induced by irritants in man: a light and electron microscopic study. J Invest Dermatol 1989;93:695–99.
6. Brasch J, Burgard J, Sterry W. Common pathological pathways in allergic and irritant contact dermatitis. J Invest Dermatol 1992;98:166–70.
7. Medenica M, Rostenberg A Jr. A comparative light and electron microscopic study of primary irritant contact dermatitis and allergic. Contact Dermatitis 1971;56:259–71.
8. Le TKM, van der Valk PGM, Schwalkwijk J, et al. Changes in epidermal proliferation and differentiation in allergic and irritant contact dermatitis reactions. Br J Dermatol 1995;133:236–40.
9. Landsteiner K, Chase MW. Studies on the sensitization of animals with simple chemical compounds. IX. Skin sensitization induced by injection of conjugates. J Exp Med 1941;73:431–6.
10. Warshaw EM, Belsito DV, DeLeo VA, et al. North American Contact Dermatitis Group Patch Test Results: 2003–2004 Study Period. Dermatitis (in press).
11. Dupuis G, Benezra C. Allergic Contact Dermatitis to Simple Chemicals: A Molecular Approach. New York: Marcel Dekker, 1982.
12. Saloga J, Knop J, Kolde G. Ultrastructural cytochemical visualization of chromium in the skin of sensitized guinea pigs. Arch Dermatol Res 1988;280:214–19.

13. deGroot AC. Patch Testing: Test Concentrations and Vehicles for 3700 Chemicals. Amsterdam: Elsevier, 1994.

14. Parker D, Long PV, Turk JL. A comparison of the conjugation of DNTB and other dinitrobenzenes with free protein radicals and their ability to sensitize or tolerize. J Invest Dermatol 1983;81:198–201.

15. Anderson C, Hehr A, Robbins R, et al. Metabolic requirements for induction of contact hypersensitivity to immunotoxic polyaromatic hydrocarbons. J Immunol 1995;155:3530–7.

16. Katz DH, Davie JM, Paul WE, et al. Carrier function in anti-hapten antibody responses. IV. Experimental conditions for the induction of hapten-specific tolerance or for the stimulation of anti-hapten anamnestic responses by "non-immunogenic" hapten polypeptide conjugates. J Exp Med 1971;134:201–23.

17. Nalefski EA, Rao A:Nature of the ligand recognized by a hapten- and carrier-specific, MHC-restricted T cell receptor. J Immunol 1993;150:3806–16.

18. Martin S, Ortman B, Plugfelder U, et al. Role of hapten-anchoring peptides in defining hapten-epitopes for MHC-restricted cytotoxic T cells. Cross-reactive TNP-determinants on different peptides. J Immunol 1992;149:2569–75.

19. Katz SI, Tamaki K, Sachs DH. Epidermal Langerhans cells are derived from cells originating in bone marrow. Nature 1979;282:324–6.

20. Stingl G, Maurer D, Hauser C, et al. The Skin: an immunologic barrier. In: Freedberg IM, Eisen AZ, Wolff K, et al., eds. Fitzpatrick's Dermatology in General Medicine, 6th ed. New York: McGraw-Hill, 2003:253–73.

21. Mommaas AM, Mulder AA, Out CJ, et al. Distribution of HLA class II molecules in epidermal Langerhans cells in situ. Eur J Immunol 1995;25:520–5.

22. Sallusto F, Cella M, Danieli C, et al. Dendritic cells use macropinocytosis and the mannose receptor to concentrate macromolecules in the major histocompatibility complex class II compartment: downregulation by cytokines and bacterial products. J Exp Med 1995;182:389–400.

23. Girolomoni G, Stone DK, Bergstresser PR, et al. Vacuolar acidification and bafilomycin-sensitive proton translocating ATPase in human epidermal Langerhans cells. J Invest Dermatol 1991:96:735–41.

24. Silberberg-Sinakin I, Thorbecke GJ, Baer RL, et al. Antigen-bearing Langerhans cells in skin, dermal lymphatics and in lymph nodes. Cell Immunol 1976;25:137–51.

25. Macatonia SE, Edwards AJ, Knight SC, et al. Dendritic cells and the initiation of contact sensitivity to fluorescein isothiocyanate. Immunology 1986;59:509–14.

26. Enk AH, Katz SI. Early molecular events in the induction phase of contact sensitivity. Proc Natl Acad Sci USA 1992;89:1398–402.

27. Enk AH, Angeloni VL, Udey MC, et al. An essential role for Langerhans cell-derived IL-1 beta in the initiation of primary immune responses in skin. J Immunol 1993;150:3698–704.

28. Wang B, Kondo S, Shivji GM, et al:Tumour necrosis factor receptor II (p75) signalling is required for the migration of Langerhans' cells. Immunology 1996;88:284–8.

29. Dieu MC, Vanbervliet B, Vicari A, et al. Selective recruitment of immature and mature dendritic cells by distinct chemokines expressed in different anatomic sites. J Exp Med 1998;188:373–86.

30. Kobayashi Y, Matsumoto M, Kotani M, et al. Possible involvement of matrix metalloproteinase-9 in Langerhans cell migration and maturation. J Immunol 1999;163:5989–93.

31. Luther SA, Cyster JG. Chemokines as regulators of T cell differentiation. Nat Immunol 2001;2:102–7.

32. Scandella E, Men Y, Gillessen S, et al. Prostaglandin E2 is a key factor for CCR7 surface expression and migration of monocyte-derived dendritic cells. Blood 2002;100:1354–61.

33. Ngo VN, Korner H, Gunn MD, et al. Lymphotoxin alpha/beta and tumor necrosis factor are required for stromal cell expression of homing chemokines in B and T cell areas of the spleen. J Exp Med 1999;189:403–12.

34. Engeman TM, Gorbachev AV, Gladue RP, et al. Inhibition of functional T cell priming and contact hypersensitivity responses by treatment with antisecondary lymphoid chemokine antibody during hapten sensitization. J Immunol 2000;164:5207–14.

35. Martin-Fontecha A, Sebastiani S, Hopken UE, et al. Regulation of dendritic cell migration to the draining lymph node: impact on T lymphocyte traffic and priming. J Exp Med 2003;198:615–21.

36. Reynolds NJ, Yi JY, Fisher GJ et al. Down-regulation of Langerhans cell protein kinase C-beta isoenzyme expression in inflammatory and hyperplastic dermatoses. Br J Dermatol 1995;133:157–67.

37. Kuhlman P, Moy VT, Lollo BA, et al. The accessory function of murine intercellular adhesion molecule-1 in T lymphocyte activation: contributions of adhesion and coactivation. J Immunol 1991;146:1773–82.

38. Prens EP, Benne K, Van Joost T, et al. Differential role of lymphocyte function-associated antigens in the activation of nickel-specific peripheral blood T lymphocytes. J Invest Dermatol 1991;97:885–91.

39. Rattis FM, Péguet-Navarro J, Staquet MJ, et al. Expression and function of B7–1 (CD80) and B7–2 (CD86) on human epidermal Langerhans cells. Eur J Immunol 1996;26:449–53.

40. Ozawa H, Nakagawa S, Tagami H, et al. Interleukin-1 beta and granulocyte-macrophage colony-stimulating factor mediate Langerhans cell maturation differently. J Invest Dermatol 1996;106:441–5.

41. Péguet-Navarro J, Dalbiez-Gauthier C, Rattis FM, et al. Functional expression of CD40 antigen on human epidermal Langerhans cells. J Immunol 1995;155:4241–7.

42. Chen AI, McAdam AJ, Buhlmann JE, et al. Ox40–ligand has a critical costimulatory role in dendritic cell: T cell interactions. Immunity 1999;11:689–98.

43. Adema GJ, Hartgers F, Verstraten R, et al. A dendritic-cell-driven C-C chemokine that preferentially attracts naïve T cells. Nature 1997;387:713–7.

44. Kalish RS, Askenase PW. Molecular mechanisms of CD8+ T cell-mediated delayed hypersensitivity: implications for allergies, asthma, and autoimmunity. J Allergy Clin Immunol 1999;103:192–9.

45. Sebastiani S, Allavena P, Albanesi C. et al. Chemokine receptor expression and function in CD4+ T lymphocytes with regulatory activity. J Immunol 2001;166:996–1002.

46. Bour H, Peyron E, Gaucherand M, et al. Major histocompatibility complex class I-restricted CD8+ T cells and class II-restricted CD4+ T cells, respectively, mediate and regulate contact sensitivity to dinitrofluorobenzene. Eur J Immunol 1995;25:3006–10.

47. Bradley LM, Watson SR, Swain SL, et al. Entry of naive CD4 T cells into peripheral lymph nodes requires L-selectin. J Exp Med 1994;180:2401–6.

48. Gruschwitz MS, Hornstein OP. Expression of transforming growth factor type beta on human epidermal dendritic cells. J Invest Dermatol 1992;99:114–6.

49. Picker LJ, Treer JR, Ferguson-Darnell B, et al. Control of lymphocyte recirculation in man. J Immunol 1993;150:1105–21.

50. Kang K, Kubin M, Cooper KD, et al. IL-12 synthesis by human Langerhans cells. J Immunol 1996;156:1402–7.

51. Dilulio NA, Xu H, Fairchild RL, et al. Diversion of CD4+ T cell development from regulatory T helper to effector T helper cells alters the contact hypersensitivity response. Eur J Immunol 1996;26:2606–12.

52. Riemann H, Schwarz A, Grabbe S, et al. Neutralization of IL-12 in vivo prevents induction of contact hypersensitivity and induces hapten-specific tolerance. J Immunol 1996;156:1799–803.

53. Luqman M, Greenbaum L, Lu D, et al. Differential effect of interleukin 1 on naive and memory CD4+ T cells. Eur J Immunol 1992;22:95–100.

54. Ray A, Tatter SB, May LT, et al. Activation of the human "β_2 interferon/ hepatocyte-stimulating factor/ interleukin-6" promoter by cytokines, viruses, and second messenger agonists. Proc Natl Acad Sci USA 1988;85:6701–5.

55. Holsti MA, Raulet DH. IL-6 and IL-1 synergize to stimulate IL-2 production and proliferation of peripheral T cells. J Immunol 1989;143:2514–9.

56. Malek TR, Ashwell JD. Interleukin 2 upregulates expression of its receptor on a T cell clone. J Exp Med 1985;161:1575–80.

57. Reem GH, Yeh NH. Interleukin 2 regulates expression of its receptor and synthesis of gamma interferon by human T lymphocytes. Science 1984;225:429–30.

58. Linsley PS, Brady W, Grosmaire L, et al. Binding of the B cell activation antigen B7 to CD28 co-stimulates T cell proliferation and interleukin 2 mRNA accumulation. J Exp Med 1991;173:721–30.

59. Reiser H, Schneeberger EE. Expression and function of B7–1 and B7–2 in hapten-induced contact sensitivity. Eur J Immunol 1996;26:880–5.

60. Xu H, Dilulio NA, Fairchild RL. T cell populations primed by hapten sensitization in contact sensitivity are distinguished by polarized patterns of cytokine production: interferon-gamma producing (Tc1) effector CD8+ T cells and interleukin 4/interleukin 10 producing (Th2) negative regulatory CD4+ T cells. J Exp Med 1996;183:1001–12.

61. Chang TW, Testa D, Kung PC, et al. Cellular origin and interactions involved in gamma-interferon production induced by OKT3 monoclonal antibody. J Immunol 1982;128:585–9.

62. Ko HS, Fu SM, Winchester RJ, et al. Ia determinants on stimulated human T lymphocytes: occurrence on mitogen- and antigen-activated T cells. J Exp Med 1979;150:246–55.

63. Vilcek J, Henriksen-Destafano D, Siegel D, et al. Regulation of IFN-gamma induction in human peripheral blood cells by exogenous and endogenously produced interleukin 2. J Immunol 1985;135:1851–6.

64. Horgan KJ, Luce GE, Tanaka Y, et al. Differential expression of VLA-α4 and VLA-β_1 discriminates multiple subsets of CD4+, CD45RO+ "memory" T cells. J Immunol 1992;149:4082–7.

65. Bouloc A, Cavani A, Katz SI. Contact hypersensitivity in MHC class II-deficient mice depends on CD8 T lymphocytes primed by immunostimulating Langerhans cells. J Invest Dermatol 1998;111:44–9.

66. Krasteva M, Kehren J, Ducluzeau MT, et al. Contact dermatitis I. Pathophysiology of contact sensitivity. Eur J Dermatol 1999;9:65–77.

67. Stoitzner P, Tripp CH, Douillard P, et al. Migratory Langerhans cells in mouse lymph nodes in steady state and inflammation. J Invest Dermatol 2005;125:116–25.

68. Grabbe S, Scwarz T. Immunoregulatory mechanisms involved in elicitation of allergic contact hypersensitivity. Immunol Today 1998;19:37–44.

69. Grabbe S, Steinbrink K, Steinert M, et al. Removal of the majority of epidermal Langerhans cells by topical or systemic steroid application enhances the effector phase of murine contact hypersensitivity. J Immunol 1995;155:4207–17.

70. Baumer W, Krekeler S, DeVries VC, et al. Non-steroidal and steroidal anti-inflammatory drugs vary in their modulation of dendritic cell function in the elicitation phase of allergic contact dermatitis. Exp Dermatol 2006;15:322–9.

71. Luscinskas FW, Ding H, Lichtman AH, et al. P-selectin and VCAM-1 mediate rolling and arrest, respectively, of CD4+ T lymphocytes on TNF-α-activated vascular endothelium under flow. J Exp Med 1995;181:1179–86.

72. Luscinskas FW, Kansas GS, Ding H, et al. Monocyte rolling, arrest and spreading on IL-4–activated vascular endothelium under flow is mediated via sequential action of L-selectin, β_1 integrins, and β_2 integrins. J Cell Biol 1994;125:1417–27.

73. Lawrence MB, Springer TA. Leukocytes roll on a selectin at physiologic flow rates: distinction from and prerequisite for adhesion through integrins. Cell 1991;65:859–73.

74. Elices MJ, Osborn L, Takadq Y, et al. VCAM-1 on activated endothelium interacts with the leukocyte integrin VLA-4 at a site distinct from the VLA-4/fibronectin binding site. Cell 1990;60:577–84.

75. Dustin ML, Springer TA. Lymphocyte function-associated antigen-1 (LFA-1) interaction with intercellular adhesion molecule-1 (ICAM-1) is one of at least three mechanisms for lymphocyte adhesion to cultured endothelial cells. J Cell Biol 1988;107:321–31.

76. Bevilacqua MP. Endothelial-leukocyte adhesion molecules. Annu Rev Immunol 1993;11:767–804.

77. Lider O, Cahalon L, Gilat D, et al. A disaccharide that inhibits tumor necrosis factor-α is formed from the extracellular matrix by the enzyme heparanase. Proc Natl Acad Sci USA 1995;92:5037–41.

78. Garioch JJ, Mackie RM, Campbell I et al. Keratinocyte expression of intercellular adhesion molecule 1 (ICAM-1) correlated with infiltration of lymphocyte function associated antigen 1 (LFA-1) positive cells in evolving allergic contact dermatitis reactions. Histopathology 1991;19:351–4.

79. Bevilacqua MP, Pober JS, Mendrick DL, et al. Identification of an inducible endothelial-leukocyte adhesion molecule. Proc Natl Acad Sci USA 1987;84:9238–42.

80. Osborn L, Hession C, Tizard R, et al. Direct expression cloning of vascular cell adhesion molecule 1, a cytokine-induced endothelial protein that binds to lymphocytes. Cell 1989;59:1203–11.

81. Dustin ML, Rothlein R, Bhan AK, et al. Induction by IL1 and interferon-gamma: tissue distribution, biochemistry, and function of a natural adherence molecule (ICAM-1). J Immunol 1986;137:245–54.

82. Lewis RE, Buchsbaum M, Whitaker D, et al. Intercellular adhesion molecule expression in the evolving human cutaneous delayed hypersensitivity reaction. J Invest Dermatol 1989;93:672–7.

83. Griffiths CEM, Nickoloff BJ. Keratinocyte intercellular adhesion molecule-1 (ICAM-1) expression precedes dermal T lymphocytic infiltration in allergic contact dermatitis (Rhus dermatitis). Am J Pathol 1989;135:1045–53.

84. Guéniche A, Viac J, Lizard G, et al. Effect of nickel on the activation state of normal human keratinocytes through interleukin 1 and intercellular adhesion molecule 1 expression. Br J Dermatol 1994;131:250–6.

85. Heufler C, Topar G, Koch F et al. Cytokine gene expression in murine epidermal cell suspensions: interleukin-1β and macrophage inflammatory protein-1α are selectively expressed in Langerhans cells but are differentially regulated in culture. J Exp Med 1992;176:1221–6

86. Albanesi C, Scarponi C, Sebastiani S, et al. A cytokine-to-chemokine axis between T lymphocytes and keratinocytes can favor Th1 cell accumulation in chronic inflammatory skin diseases. J Leukoc Biol 2001;70:617–23.

87. Bonecchi R, Bianchi G, Bordignon PP, et al. Differential expressions of chemokine receptors and chemotactic responsiveness of type 1 T helper cells (Th 1s) and Th2s. J Exp Med 1998;187:129–34.

88. Flier J, Boorsma DM, Bruynzeel DP, et al. The CXCR3 activating chemokines IP-I0, Mig, and IP-9 are expressed in allergic but not in irritant patch test reactions. J Invest Dermatol 1999;113:574–8.

89. Reiss Y, Proudfoot AE, Power CA, et al. CC chemokine receptor (CCR)4 and the CCR10 ligand cutaneous T cell-attracting chemokine (CTACK) in lymphocyte trafficking to inflamed skin. J Exp Med 2001;194:1541–7.

90. Homey B, Wang W, Soto H, et al. Cutting edge: the orphan chemokine receptor G protein-coupled receptor-2 (GPR-2, CCR10) binds the skin-associated chemokine CCL27 (CTACK/ALP/ILC). J Immunol 2000;164:3465–70.

91. Homey B, Alenius H, Muller A, et al. CCL27–CCR10 interactions regulate T cell-mediated skin inflammation. Nat Med 2002;8:157–65.

92. Hosoi J, Murphy GF, Egan CL, et al. Regulation of Langerhans cell function by nerves containing calcitonin gene-related peptide. Nature 1993;363:159–63.

93. Eedy D. Neuropeptides in skin. Br J Dermatol 1993;128:597–605.

94. Ansel JC, Brown JR, Payan DG, et al. Substance P selectively activates TNF-alpha gene expression in murine mast cells. J Immunol 1993;150: 4478–85.

95. McGillis JP, Mitsuhashi M, Payan DG. Immunomodulation by tachykinin neuropeptides. Ann NY Acad Sci 1990;594:85–94.

96. Viac J, Gueniche A, Doutremepuich JD, et al. Substance P and keratinocyte activation markers: an in vitro approach. Arch Dermatol Res 1996;288:85–90.

97. Calvo CF, Chavanel G, Seni K, et al. Substance P enhances IL-2 expression in activated human T cells. J Immunol 1991;148:3498–504.

98. Calvo CF. Substance P stabilizes interleukin-2 mRNA in activated Jurkat cells. J Neuroimmunol 1995;51:85–91.

99. Fox FE, Kubin M, Cassin M, et al. Calcitonin gene-related peptide inhibits proliferation and antigen presentation by human peripheral blood mononuclear cells: effects on B7, interleukin 10, and interleukin 12. J Invest Dermatol 1997;108:43–8.

100. Trautmann A, Akdis M, Brocker EB, et al. New insights into the role of T cells in atopic dermatitis and allergic contact dermatitis. Trends Immunol 2001 22:530–2.

101. Vilcek J, Oliveira IC. Recent progress in the elucidation of interferon-gamma actions: molecular biology and biological functions. Int Arch Allergy Immunol 1994;104:311–6.

102. Taub DD, Lloyd AR, Conlon K, et al. Recombinant human interferon-inducible protein 10 is a chemoattractant for human monocytes and T lymphocytes and promotes T cell adhesion to endothelial cells. J Exp Med 1993;177:1809–14.

103. Yu X, Barnhill RL, Graves DT, et al. Expression of monocyte chemoattractant protein-1 in delayed type hypersensitivity reactions in the skin. Lab Invest 1994;71:226–35.

104. Kristensen MS, Deleuran BW, Larsen CG, et al. Expression of monocyte chemotactic and activating factor (MCAF) in skin related cells: a comparative study. Cytokine 1993;5:520–4.

105. Enk AH, Katz SI. Identification and induction of keratinocyte-derived IL-10. J Immunol 1992;149:92–5.

106. Schwarz A, Grabbe S, Riemann H, et al. In vivo effects of interleukin-10 on contact hypersensitivity and delayed-type hypersensitivity reactions. J Invest Dermatol 1994;103:211–6.

107. Berg DJ, Leach MW, Kuhn R, et al. Interleukin 10 but not interleukin 4 is a natural suppressant of cutaneous inflammatory responses. J Exp Med 1995;182:99–108.

108. Epstein SP, Baer RL, Thorbecke GJ, et al. Immunosuppressive effects of transforming growth factor beta: inhibition of the induction of Ia antigen on Langerhans cells by cytokines and of the contact hypersensitivity response. J Invest Dermatol 1991;96:832–7.

109. Gamble JR, Vadas MA. Endothelial cell adhesiveness for human T lymphocytes is inhibited by transforming growth factor-beta 1. J Immunol 1991;146:1149–54.

110. Gautam SC, Chikkala NF, Hamilton TA, et al. Anti-inflammatory action of IL-4: negative regulation of contact sensitivity to trinitrochlorobenzene. J Immunol 1992;148:1411–5.

111. Gemsa D. Stimulation of prostaglandin E release from macrophages and possible role in the immune response. In: Pick E, ed. Lymphokines. New York: Academic, 1981:335.

112. Walker C, Kristensen F, Bettens F, et al. Lymphokine regulation of activated (G1) lymphocytes: prostaglandin E_2 induced inhibition of interleukin 2 production. J Immunol 1983;130:1770–3.

113. Chun M, Krim M, Granelli-Piperno A, et al. Enhancement of cytotoxic activity of natural killer cells by interleukin 2 and antagonism between interleukin 2 and adenosine cyclic monophosphate. Scand J Immunol 1985;22:375–81.

114. Gorbachev AV, Fairchild RL. CD4+ T cells regulate CD8+ T cell-mediated cutaneous immune reactions by restricting effector T cell development through a Fas ligand-dependent mechanism. J Immunol 2004;172:2286–95.

115. Dubois B, Chapat L, Goubier A, et al. CD4+ CD25+ T cells as key regulators of immune responses. Eur J Dermatol 2003;13:111–6.

116. Skog E. The influence of pre-exposure to alkyl benzene sulphonate detergent, soap and acetone on primary irritant and allergic eczematous reactions. Acta Derm Venereol (Stockh) 1958;38:1–9.

117. Walker FB, Smith PD, Maibach HI, et al. Genetic factors in human allergic contact dermatitis. Int Arch Allergy Appl Immunol 1967;32:453–62.

118. Sulzberger MB. Hypersensitiveness to arsphenamine in guinea pigs. Arch Dermatol 1929;20: 669–73.

119. Chase MW. Inhibition of experimental drug allergy by prior feeding of the sensitizing agent. Proc Soc Exp Biol Med 1946;61:257–63.

120. Elmets CA, Bergstresser PR, Tigelaar RE, et al. Analysis of the mechanism of unresponsiveness produced by haptens painted on skin exposed to low dose ultraviolet radiation. J Exp Med 1983;158:781–94.

121. Akbari O, Umetsu DT. Role of regulatory dendritic cells in allergy and asthma. Curr Allergy Asthma Rep 2005;5:56–61.

122. Mellor AL, Munn DH. IDO expression by dendritic cells: tolerance and tryptophan catabolism. Nat Rev Immunol 2004;4:762–74.

123. Girolomoni G, Gisondi P, Ottaviani C, et al Immunoregulation of allergic contact dermatitis. J Dermatol 2004;31:264–70.

124. Cavani A. Breaking tolerance to nickel. Toxicology 2005;209:119–21.

125. Nossal GJ. Molecular and cellular aspects of immunologic tolerance. Eur J Biochem 1991;202: 729–37.

126. Kwangsukstith C, Maibach HI. Effect of age and sex on the induction and elicitation of allergic contact dermatitis. Contact Dermatitis 1995;33: 289–98.

127. Belsito DV, Dersarkissian RM, Thorbecke RJ, et al. Reversal by lymphokines of the age-related hyporesponsiveness to contact sensitization and reduced Ia expression on Langerhans cells. Arch Dermatol Res 1987;279:S76–80.

128. Belsito DV, Possick LE. Age-related changes in allergic contact hypersensitivity: functional T cell deficiencies are primarily responsible. J Invest Dermatol 1988;90:546.

129. Marcussen PV. Primary irritant patch-test reactions in children. Arch Dermatol 1963;87:378–82.

130. Rietschel RL, Rosenthal LE, Adams RM, et al. Standard patch test screening series used diagnostically in young and elderly patients. Am J Contact Dermatitis 1990;1:53–55.

131. Gonçalo S, Gonçalo M, Azenha A, et al. Allergic contact dermatitis in children: a multicenter study of the Portuguese Contact Dermatitis Group (GPEDC). Contact Dermatitis 1992;26:112–5.

132. Strauss HW. Artificial sensitization of infants to poison ivy. J Allergy 1931;2:137–46.

133. Schubert H, Berova N, Czernielewski A, et al. Epidemiology of nickel allergy. Contact Dermatitis 1987;16:122–8.

134. Belsito DV. The pathophysiology of allergic contact hypersensitivity. Clin Rev Allergy 1989;7:347–79.

135. Aubin F, Mousson C. Ultraviolet light-induced regulatory (suppressor) T cells: an approach for promoting induction of operational allograft tolerance? Transplantation 2004;77:S29–31.

136. Belsito DV. Patch-testing: after 100 years, still the gold standard in diagnosing cutaneous delayed-type hypersensitivity. In: Kurth R, ed. Regulatory Control and Standardization of Allergenic Extracts: The Eighth International Paul Ehrlich Seminar. Stuttgart: Gustav Fischer, 1997:195–202.

137. Balato N, Patruno C, Lembo G, et al. Effect of pentoxifylline on patch test response. Contact Dermatitis 1996;35:128–30.

138. Elsner PL. Clinical irritant contact dermatitis syndromes. Am J Contact Dermat 1997;8:81–82.

139. Wood LC, Jackson SM, Elias PM, et al. Cutaneous barrier perturbation stimulates cytokine production in the epidermis of mice. J Clin Invest 1992;90: 482–7.

140. Tsai J-C, Feingold KR, Crumrine D, et al. Permeability barrier disruption alters the localization and expression of TNF-alpha protein in the epidermis. Arch Dermatol Res 1994;286:242–8.

141. Denda M, Wood LC, Emami S, et al. The epidermal hyperplasia associated with repeated barrier disruption by acetone treatment or tape stripping cannot be attributed to increased water loss. Arch Dermatol Res 1996;288:230–8.

142. Astner S, González E, Cheung AC, et al. Non-invasive evaluation of the kinetics of allergic and irritant contact dermatitis. J Invest Dermatol 2005;124:351–9.

143. Effendy I, Löffler H, Maibach HI. Epidermal cytokines in murine cutaneous irritant responses. J Appl Toxicol 2000;20:335–41.

144. Pentland AP. The role of prostaglandins and other lipid mediators in irritant contact dermatitis. Am J Contact Dermatol 1994;8:98.

145. Onoue S, Tsuda Y. Analytical studies on the prediction of photosensitive/phototoxic potential of pharmaceutical substances. Pharm Res 2006;23:156–64.

146. Willis CM, Reiche L, Wilkinson JD. Immunocytochemical demonstration of reduced Cu,Zn-superoxide dismutase levels following topical application of dithranol and sodium lauryl sulphate: an indication of the role of oxidative stress in acute irritant contact dermatitis. Eur J Dermatol 1998;8:8–12.

147. Li L-F, Fiedler VC, Kumar R. Down-regulation of protein kinase C isoforms in irritant contact dermatitis. Contact Dermatitis 1998;38:319–24.

148. Rogers JV, Garrett CM, McDougal JN. Gene expression in rat skin induced by irritating chemicals. J Biochem Mol Toxicol 2003;17:123–37.

149. Schürer NY. Implementation of fatty acid carriers to skin irritation and the epidermal barrier. Contact Dermatitis. 2002;47:199–205.

150. Berardesca E, Distante F. The modulation of skin irritation. Contact Dermatitis 1994;31:281–7.

151. Gutwald J, Goebeler M, Sorg C. Neuropeptides enhance irritant and allergic contact dermatitis. J Invest Dermatol 1991;96:695–8.

152. Laurenzi MA, Persson MA, Dalsgaard CJ, et al. The neuropeptide substance P stimulates production of interleukin 1 in human blood monocytes: activated cells are preferentially influenced by the neuropeptide. Scand J Immunol 1990;31:529–33.

153. Rameshwar P, Gascon P, Ganea D. Stimulation of IL-2 production in murine lymphocytes by

substance P and related tachykinins. J Immunol 1993;151:2484–96.

154. Ceriani G, Macaluso A, Catania A, et al. Central neurogenic antiinflammatory action of alpha-MSH: modulation of peripheral inflammation induced by cytokines and other mediators of inflammation. Neuroendocrinology 1994;59:138–43.

155. Luger TA, Scholzen TE, Brzoska T, et al. New insights into the function of alpha-MSH and related peptides in the immune system. Ann NY Acad Sci 2003;994:133–40.

156. Roussaki-Schulze AV, Zafiriou E, Nikoulis D, et al. Objective biophysical findings in patients with sensitive skin. Drugs Exp Clin Res 2005;31(suppl): 17–24.

157. DiNardo A, Sugino K, Wertz P, et al. Sodium lauryl sulfate induced irritant contact dermatitis: a correlation study between ceramides and in vivo parameters of irritation. Contact Dermatitis 1996;33:86–91.

158. Patil S, Maibach HI. Effect of age and sex on the elicitation of irritant contact dermatitis. Contact Dermatitis 1994;30:257–64.

159. Lee CH, Maibach HI. The sodium lauryl sulfate model: an overview. Contact Dermatitis 1995;33: 1–7.

160. Fluhr JW, Pfisterer S, Gloor M. Direct comparison of skin physiology in children and adults with bioengineering methods. Pediatr Dermatol 2000;17:436–9.

161. Agner T, Damm P, Skouby SO. Menstrual cycle and skin reactivity. J Am Acad Dermatol 1991;24: 566–70.

162. Lantinga H, Nater JP, Coenraads PJ. Prevalence, incidence and course of eczema on the hands and forearms in a sample of the general population. Contact Dermatitis 1984;10:135–9.

163. Meding B, Swanbeck G. Prevalence of hand dermatitis in an industrial city. Br J Dermatol 1987;116:627–34.

164. Berardesca E, Maibach H. Racial differences in skin pathophysiology. J Am Acad Dermatol 1996;34:667–72.

165. Weigand DA, Gaylor JR. Irritant reaction in Negro and Caucasian skin. South Med J 1974;67:548–51.

166. Britz MB, Maibach HI. Human cutaneous vulvar reactivity to irritants. Contact Dermatitis 1979;5:375–7.

167. Elsner P, Wilhelm D, Maibach HI. Effects of low concentration sodium lauryl sulfate on human vulvar and forearm skin. J Reprod Med 1991;36:77–81.

168. Tupker RA, Pinnagoda J, Coenraads PJ, et al. Susceptibility to irritants: role of barrier function, skin dryness, and history of atopic dermatitis. Br J Dermatol 1990;123:199–205.

169. Imokawa, G, Abe A, Jin K, et al. Decreased level of ceramides in stratum corneum of atopic dermatitis: an etiologic factor in atopic dry skin? J Invest Dermatol 1991;96:523–6.

170. Sulzberger MB. The patch test: who should and should not use it and why. Contact Dermatitis 1975;1:117–9.

171. Marks JG Jr, Moss JH, Parno JR, et al. Methylchl oroisothiazolinone/ methylisothiazolinone (Kathon CG) Biocide-United States multicenter study of human skin sensitization. Am J Contact Dermatitis 1990;1:157–61.

172. Epstein WL. The use test for contact hypersensitivity. Arch Dermatol Res 1982;272:279–81.

173. Mitchell JC. Multiple concomitant positive patch test reactions. Contact Dermatitis 1975;3:315–20.

174. Przybilla B, Burg G, Thieme C. Evaluation of the immune status in vivo by the 2,4–dinitro-1–chlorobenzene contact allergy time (DNCB-CAT). Dermatologica 1983;167:1–5.

175. Belsito DV, Storrs FJ, Taylor JS, et al. Reproducibility of patch tests: a U.S. multicenter study. Am J Contact Dermatitis 1992;3:193–200.

176. Rietschel RL, Fowler JF Jr. Fisher's Contact Dermatitis, 5th ed. Baltimore: Williams & Wilkins, 2001.

177. Guin JD. Practical Contact Dermatitis. New York: McGraw-Hill, 1995.

178. Kanerva L, Elsner P, Wahlberg JE, et al., eds. Handbook of Occupational Dermatology. Heidelberg: Springer-Verlag, 2000.

179. Ramsing DW, Agner T. Efficacy of topical corticosteroids on irritant skin reactions. Contact Dermatitis 1995;32:293–7.

180. Belsito, DV, Fowler J, Marks J, et al. A potential new treatment for chronic hand dermatitis. Cutis 2004;73:31–8.

181. Belsito DV, Wilson DC, Warshaw E, et al. A prospective randomized clinical trial of 0.1% tacrolimus ointment in a model of chronic allergic contact dermatitis. J Am Acad Dermatol 2006;55:40–6.

182. Mork NJ, Austad J. Short wave ultraviolet light (UVB) treatment of allergic contact dermatitis of the hands. Acta Derm Venereol (Stockh) 1982;63:87–9.

183. Bruynzeel DP, Boon WJ, Van Ketel WG, Oral psoralen photo-chemotherapy of allergic contact dermatitis of the hands. Dermatosen Beruf Umwelt 1982;30:16–20.

184. Warshawshki L, Mitchell JC, Storrs FJ. Allergic contact dermatitis from glyceryl monothioglycolate in hair dressers. Contact Dermatitis 1981;7:351–2.

185. Henriksen HR. Beskyttelsesklaeder mod Kemikalier, Oplosnings-parametre og Taethed. Lyngby, Denmark: Instituttet for Kemiindustri, 1986.

186. Frosch PJ, Kurte A. Efficacy of skin barrier creams (IV): the repetitive irritation test (RIT) with a

set of 4 standard irritants. Contact Dermatitis 1994;31:161–8.

187. Wigger-Alberti W, Elsner P. Do barrier creams and gloves prevent or provoke contact dermatitis? Am J Contact Dermat 1998;9:100–6.

188. Frosch PJ, Schulze-Dirks A, Hoffmann M, et al. Efficacy of skin barrier creams (I): the repetitive irritation test (RIT) in the guinea pig. Contact Dermatitis 1993;28:94–100.

189. McCormick RD, Buchman TL, Maki DG. Double blind, randomized trial of scheduled use of a novel barrier cream and an oil-containing lotion for protecting the hands of health care workers. Am J Infect Control 2000;28:302–10.

190. Perrenoud D, Gallezot D, vanMelle G. The efficacy of a protective cream in a real world apprentice hairdresser environment. Contact Dermatitis 2001;45:134–8.

13
Atopic Dermatitis

Thomas Bieber and Julia Prölss

Key Points

- Atopic dermatitis is a very common skin condition, estimated to affect 15% to 30% of children and 2% to 10% of adults. There are distinct morphologic variants of atopic dermatitis that evolve during the maturation of an individual with atopic dermatitis.
- This is a complex disease process that involves polygenic inheritance as well as gene–environment interactions.
- Because this condition is so common in industrialized nations, it has been hypothesized that the avoidance of common childhood diseases (because of hygienic conditions and vaccination) interferes with the normal development of the immune system.
- A variety of factors play a role in atopic dermatitis: abnormal barrier function, neuroimmune-psychiatric factors, impaired innate immunity, and abnormal acquired immunity.
- Bacterial products, and the aberrant immune response to such products, are important pathogenic flare factors for eczema.
- Treatment involves management of flare factors, topical and systemic glucocorticosteroids, topical calcineurin inhibitors, topical and oral antibiotics, oral antihistamines, and, in severe cases, phototherapy, cytotoxic drugs, and cyclosporine.

Among the various chronic inflammatory skin diseases, atopic dermatitis (AD) (also called eczema in some countries) has a singular place since it is considered the most common itchy and relapsing inflammatory skin condition. Its increasing prevalence is well documented and represents a major public health problem,

mostly in industrialized countries. Much progress has been made in the understanding of its genetic background and pathophysiology. Recent studies in genetics, epidemiology, and immunology have provided new important pieces of the complex puzzle and have dramatically changed our view on the mechanisms, its natural history, and future ways to control the disease in the context of the so-called atopic march.

Atopy

Recently the World Allergy Organization (WAO) has launched a revised terminology for atopy and atopic diseases, defining atopy only in association with immunoglobulin E (IgE)-sensitization, that is, atopic diseases due to IgE-mediated pathophysiology. Hence, the term *atopy* should be used in combination with documented specific IgE antibodies in serum or with a positive skin prick test.[1] This terminology is aimed at replacing the term *extrinsic AD* and includes only patients with proven IgE-mediated sensitizations. For the subgroup of patients (20% to 30%) who show the clinical phenotype of AD but lack any IgE sensitization,[2] the term *nonatopic eczema/dermatitis* is now proposed, replacing the previous term *intrinsic AD*. However, in this chapter, the term *AD* is used to define the classic clinical phenotype.

Epidemiology

The lifetime prevalence of AD is estimated to be 15% to 30% in children and 2% to 10% in adults, while the incidence of AD has increased by two- to threefold during the past three decades in industrialized countries. The 12-month prevalence in 11-year-old children has been shown to vary from 1% to 20%, with the highest prevalence typically found in Northern Europe (International Study of Asthma and Allergies in Childhood, ISAAC).[3] In children, the onset of AD occurs in 45% during the first 6 months of life, 60% during the first year, and 85% are affected before the age of 5.

The prevalence of AD in rural areas and in non-affluent countries is significantly lower, emphasizing the importance of lifestyle and environment in the mechanisms of atopic disease, which may be explained by the hygiene hypothesis,[4] a concept that is still debated.[5]

Pathomechanisms

Atopic dermatitis is a paradigmatic genetic complex disease developing on the background of gene–gene and gene–environment interactions. Much progress has been achieved in the recent years in unraveling genetic predisposition, immunologic abnormalities, and environmental factors.

Genetics

The role of genetic factors in AD (Online Mendelian Inheritance in Man [OMIM] number *603165) is clearly demonstrated by twin studies, which consistently showed a higher concordance rate (0.77) in monozygotic (MZ) twins compared to dizygotic (DZ) twins (0.15).[6] The importance of genetic factors in AD is further underlined by the finding that a positive parental history is the strongest risk factor for AD; the incidence rate is doubled if AD is present in one parent, and tripled if both parents are affected.

In the modern era of genomics, two main strategies have been developed to chase the responsible genes operating in complex diseases: the linkage analysis and the candidate gene approach[7] (Fig. 13.1).

Up to now, four linkage analyses (genome-wide scans) have been published, identifying several possible gene loci on chromosomes 1q21, 3q21, 17q25, and 20p.[8,9] Interestingly, some of these regions correspond to those found in patients with psoriasis, suggesting some common genetic aspects between both psoriasis and AD, which are otherwise almost mutually exclusive chronic skin diseases.

Candidate gene studies have investigated the role of genetic variants or polymorphisms (caused

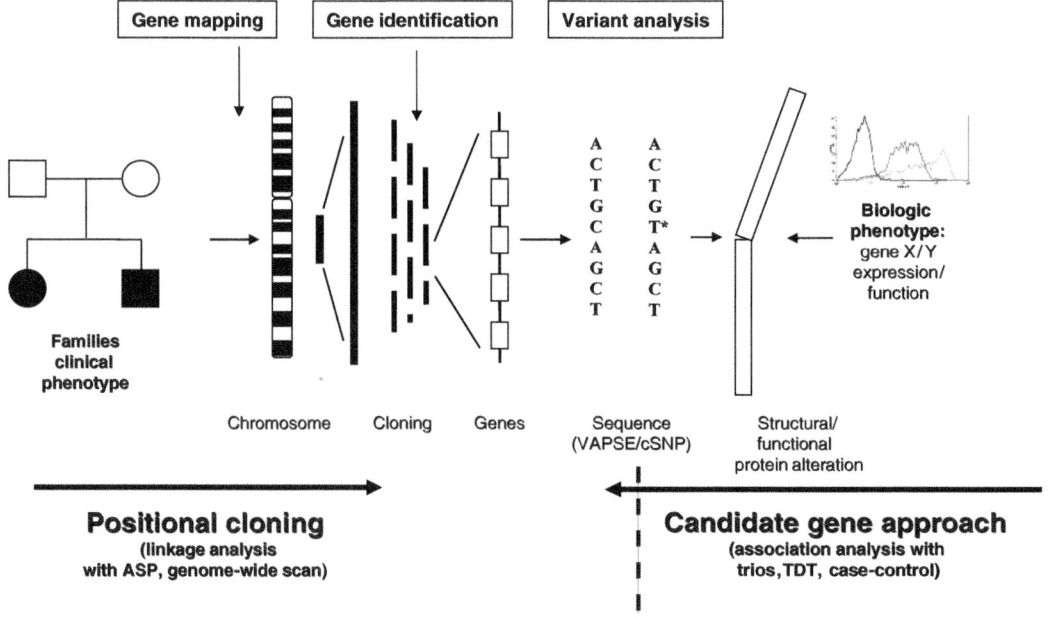

FIG. 13.1. The two approaches to determining the genes responsible for atopic dermatitis: the linkage analysis and the candidate gene approach. ASP, affected-sib-pair method; TDT; transmission disequilibrium test; VAPSE, variant affecting protein structure or expression; cSNP, coding single nucleotide polymorphisms

by the exchange of single base pairs; *single nucleotide polymorphisms* [SNPs]) in genes assumed to be of pathophysiologic relevance, most of them being genes involved in immunologic mechanisms. For example, on chromosome 5q31-33, the locus containing genes for the T-helper-2 (Th2) cytokines interleukin-3 (IL-3), IL-4, IL-5, IL-13, and granulocyte-macrophage colony-stimulation factor (GM-CSF)[10] has been suggested. Further studies identified variants of the IL-13 encoding region, functional mutations of the promoter region of the chemokine RANTES (regulated on activation, normal T cell expressed and secreted) (17q11) and gain-of-function polymorphisms in the α-subunit of the IL-4 receptor (16q12).[11] This could be linked to the incidence of nonatopic (formerly *intrinsic*) eczema, which occurs without any IgE sensitization.[12] The unbalance between Th1- and Th2-immune responses in AD may be elucidated by the detection of polymorphisms of the IL-18 gene, resulting in Th2 predominance.[13]

The recent demonstration of loss-of-function mutations of the profilaggrin/filaggrin gene, a key protein in terminal differentiation of the epidermis, can be considered as a breakthrough.[14–19] Indeed, these variations may be important risk factors for AD (with IgE) and in combination with sensitization and asthma, since they seem to be more associated with the true atopic (extrinsic) dermatitis form. It is expected that other yet-to-be-defined genetic variants from epidermal structures such as those localized in the epidermal differential complex (EDC) on chromosome 1q21, for example, stratum corneum chymotryptic enzyme (SCCE),[20] may also play a role in these phenomena. These genetic findings provide an important support for the well-known impairment of the epidermal barrier observed in AD, and could also deliver further clues to the natural history of the disease, that is, the transition of a nonatopic eczema to an atopic eczema due to a facilitated penetration of and sensitization to aeroallergens during chronic inflammation.

Environmental Factors and Hygiene Hypothesis

In 1989, Strachan[4] first coined the term *hygiene hypothesis* when he postulated that infections during early childhood are important for the prevention of allergic diseases. Environmental factors such as increased air pollution, indoor exposure to house dust mite (HDM) antigens or to pets, the use of antibiotics, infections, and dietary changes have been suggested to have an impact in the development of allergic diseases. The exposure to bacteria-derived toxins such as lipopolysaccharide (LPS) and others during early childhood, such as observed in a farming environment, seems to be important for the development and maturation of immunity. It has been postulated that Th1 immune response is enforced by some bacterial and viral inflammation. However, whether this concept applies also for AD is still not clear.[5,21]

Neuroimmunologic Factors

Neuropeptides and neurotropins mediate different actions such as vasodilatation, edema, itch and pain, or sweat gland secretion, and have a minor ability to regulate T-cell activation.[22] They can be detected in blood and within the epidermal nerve fibers in close association with mast cells or epidermal Langerhans' cells, suggesting a tight link between the immune system and the nervous system.[23] Recent studies have documented increased levels of nerve growth factor (NGF) and substance P (SP) in plasma of AD patients, which correlated positively with disease activity.[24] Brain-derived growth factor (BDGF), detected recently in sera and plasma of patients with AD, enhances the survival of eosinophils while increasing their chemotactic response in vitro.[25]

Skin Barrier Dysfunction

One of the major hallmarks of AD is xerosis, which affects lesional and nonlesional skin areas as witnessed by increased transepidermal water loss. It may favor the penetration of high-molecular-weight structures such as allergens, bacteria, and viruses.[26] Several mechanisms have been postulated: (1) a decrease in skin ceramides, serving as the major water-retaining molecules in the extracellular space[27]; (2) alterations of the stratum corneum pH[28]; (3) overexpression of the chymotryptic enzyme (chymase); and (4) defect in Filaggrin as well as molecules of the EDC such as SCCE or the S-100 protein family (see above).

Immunologic Mechanisms

The immune system has been classified into two branches: innate and adaptive/acquired immunity.

Adaptive immunity relies on antigen-presenting cells to capture and present antigen to T and B cells and is therefore the backbone of cellular and humoral immune response. Innate immunity is characterized by an immediate response to pathogens through genetically encoded and evolutionary conserved receptors and antimicrobial proteins.

Innate Immunity

The innate immune system of the epidermis presents the first-line defense against cutaneous infections. Once the epidermis is invaded by microorganisms, antimicrobial peptides are activated and form part of the defense system.[29] Up to now, three antimicrobial peptides are known in human skin: the human β-defensins 2 and 3 (HBD-2 and HBD-3), as well as the cathelicidin hCAP18/LL-37. All of them show different spectra of activity: HBD-2 is effective against gram-negative organisms such as *Escherichia coli, Pseudomonas aeruginosa,* and yeasts. HBD-3 and cathelicidin are more potent, broad-spectrum antibiotics that kill both gram-positive and gram-negative organisms as well as *Candida albicans.* Atopic dermatitis skin is characterized by a significant decrease in expression of antimicrobial peptides, explaining the susceptibility of AD patients to bacterial infections.[30–32] The innate skin defense system of patients with AD may be further reduced by the deficiency of dermcidin-derived antimicrobial peptides in sweat, which correlates with infectious complications.[33]

Acquired Immunity

T Cells

T cells represent an important component of the inflammatory infiltrate in AD and carry the allergen specificity observed in each individual patient.[34] In animal models of AD, eczematous rashes do not occur in the absence of T cells,[35] and treatment with specific T-cell–mediated medication such as calcineurin inhibitors significantly reduces eczema. Furthermore, it has been shown that Th1 and Th2 cytokines play an important role in the skin's inflammatory response.[36]

However, AD is not a classic Th2 disease; it represents biphasic inflammatory reaction starting with Th2 and switching to a Th1/Th0 profile[37](see below). Recently, most interest has been focused on the role regulatory T (T_{reg}) cells in the control of the adaptive immune response.[38,39] This family of cells has the ability to suppress T-cell response, irrespective of their profile (Th1 and Th2). Depending on the type of T_{reg}, they are characterized by some few surface markers (CD4/CD25/CD103) as well as the expression of the nuclear transcription factor FOXP3.[39] Mutations in FOXP3 result in hyper-IgE, food allergy, and eczema, which is subsumed as the immunodysregulation polyendocrinopathy enteropathy X-linked (IPEX) syndrome.[40] In addition, several studies document an association between atopy and the loss of T_{reg} function.[41,42] With regard to the hygiene hypothesis, a loss of T_{reg} cells may be the result of a limited exposure to infectious pathogens during infancy and could explain the rapid increase in the prevalence of allergies in developed countries.[43]

Cytokines and Chemokines

Inflammatory reaction in AD is the result of a distinct microenvironment provided by a series of cytokines and chemokines.[44] A predominant Th2 unbalance with increased IgE levels and eosinophilia is widely accepted in the pathogenesis of AD.[45,46] The production of Th2-mediated cytokines, notably IL-4, IL-5, and IL-13, can be detected in lesional and nonlesional skin during the acute phase of disease. Interleukin-4 and IL-13 are implicated in the initial phase of tissue inflammation and may mediate an isotype switching to IgE synthesis and upregulation expression of adhesion molecules on endothelial cells.[47] Interleukin-5 increases the survival of eosinophils, and a systemic eosinophilia with an increase of the eosinophilic cationic protein (ECP) correlates to disease severity.[48,49]

Although Th2-mediated cytokines seem to be predominant in the acute phase of AD, they are less important during its chronic course. In chronic AD skin, interferon-γ (IFN-γ) and IL-12 are dominant, as well as IL-5 and GM-CSF, being characteristic for a Th1/Th0 profile.[37] The maintenance of chronic AD further involves the production of the Th1-like cytokines IL-12 and IL-18, as well as several remodeling-associated cytokines such as IL-11, IL-17, and transforming growth factor β1 (TGF-β1).[50]

Different chemokines have gained interest in the pathology of AD. Great amounts of chemokines like MIP-4/CCL18, TARC/CCL17, PARC/CCL18, MDC/CCL22, and CCL1 seem instrumental in the development of acute and chronic lesions.[44] C-C chemokines (monocyte chemoattractant protein 4 [MCP-4], RANTES, and eotaxin) contribute to the infiltration of macrophages, eosinophils, and T cells into acute and chronic AD skin lesions. However, macrophage inhibition protein 3a (MIP-3a), which also has some antiviral activity, seems to be deficient in AD due to the particular inflammatory microenvironment.[51]

Thymic stromal lymphopoietin (TSLP) is an IL-7–like cytokine[52] expressed primarily by epithelial cells, including keratinocytes. It is associated with the activation and migration of DC within the dermis of AD. It is thought to prime naive CD4[+] T cells to differentiate into Th2 cells, which ultimately contribute to the induction of allergic inflammation. The TSLP-activated cutaneous DCs prime Th cells to produce the proallergic cytokines IL-4, IL-5, IL-13, and TNF-α. However, expression of the antiinflammatory cytokine IL-10 and the Th1 cytokine IFN-γ are inhibited. These features suggested that TSLP represents a critical mediator in uncontrolled allergic inflammation.[53]

Gene profiling experiments using microarray technology currently provides profound knowledge about the complex cytokine and chemokine microenvironment in AD,[31,54] but their exact value in the pathogenesis is still not fully resolved.

Dendritic Cells

Dendritic cells (DCs) represents a complex family of highly professional antigen-presenting cells.[55] They have been classically divided in myeloid (mDC) and plasmacytoid dendritic cells (pDC). In the epidermis of AD patients, besides Langerhans' cells (LCs), which express the high-affinity receptor for IgE (FcεRI) in the atopic but not in the nonatopic form,[56,57] another population of newly migrated DC has been reported: the so-called inflammatory dendritic epidermal cells (IDECs).[58] The IDECs belong to the group of mDC and highly express FcεRI in AD. While LCs play a dominant role in the initiation of the allergic immune response and prime naive T cells into T cells of Th2 type,[59] they do not display a strong proinflammatory profile.

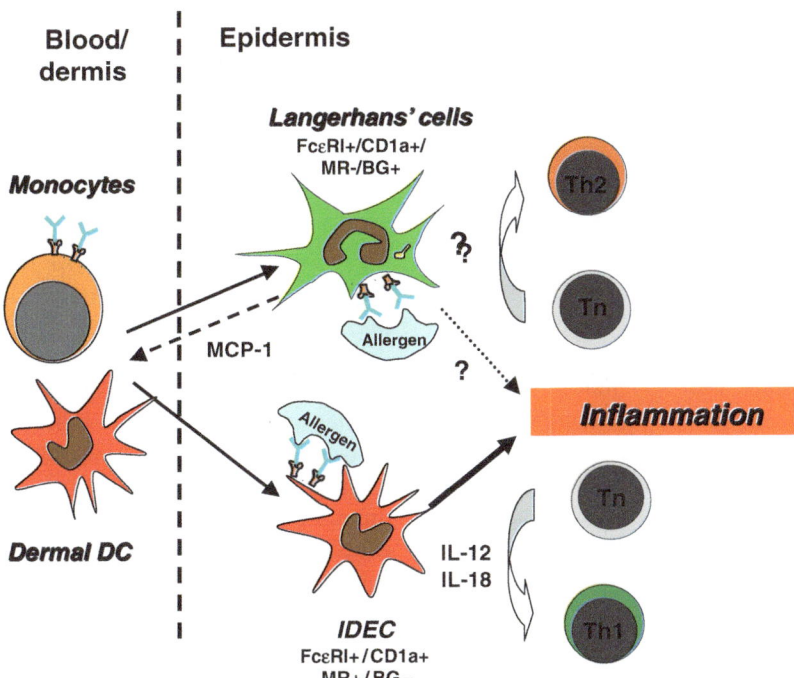

FIG. 13.2. Different roles of FcεRI+ Langerhans' cells (LCs), and inflammatory dendritic epidermal cells (IDECs) in the generation of skin inflammation. While LCs are able to induce a Th2 response, they are less proinflammatory but produce monocyte recruiting chemokines such as monocyte chemoattractant protein 1 (MCP-1). These chemokines contribute to the migration of IDEC precursors into the skin. In contrast to LCs, IDECs produce large amounts of proinflammatory mediators and drive the T cells into a Th1 profile

In contrast, FcεRI+ IDECs produce high amounts of proinflammatory cytokines and thereby contribute to the amplification of the allergic immune response (Fig. 13.2). Moreover, IDECs produce IL-12 and IL-18, contributing to the Th2-Th1 switch observed in the transition from acute to chronic lesions.[60]

Plasmacytoid dendritic cells (pDCs) are known to play a major role in the defense against viral infections by producing type 1 interferons (i.e., IFN-α and IFN-ß). They are virtually absent in AD lesions[61] but are increased in peripheral blood.[62] In the blood, pDCs express high amounts of FcεRI, the activation of which leads to an altered surface expression of major histocompatibility complex (MHC) molecules, an enhanced apoptosis of pDCs, but most importantly to a reduced secretion of type 1 interferons.[59] Overall, together with the decrease in antimicrobial peptide (AMP) production in AD, these phenomena may contribute to the susceptibility of patients for viral skin infections such as herpes simplex–induced eczema herpeticum.

Microbial Agents

Lesional and normal skin of patients with AD is highly colonized with toxins-producing *Staphylococcus aureus*.[63] This colonization is due to the decreased production of antimicrobial peptides, which are downregulated by the particular inflammatory micromilieu in AD.[32,64] Infections often provoke exacerbation or aggravation of lesional skin, particularly in children. Interestingly, *S. aureus* enterotoxins A (SEA), B (SEB), C (SEC), and D (SED) gained increasing importance in the pathogenesis of AD since they (1) induce a specific IgE sensitization, (2) act as superantigens,[65] and (3) alter the function of T_{reg}. Specific IgE antibodies directed against staphylococcal superantigens correlate with their skin disease severity.[66] Additionally, it has been shown that (1) binding of *S. aureus* to the skin is significantly enhanced by AD skin inflammation; (2) scratching may enhance *S. aureus* binding by disturbing the skin barrier; and (3) isolated *S. aureus* was detected to possess an increased activity of ceramidase, thereby aggravating the skin barrier dysfunction. Therefore, the overgrowth of these bacteria should be one of the objectives in the management of AD.

Evidence of IgE-Mediated Autoimmunity in Atopic Dermatitis

There is some evidence that autoimmune response may play a role in AD. Indeed, patients with severe AD display IgE response to so-called autoallergens.[67] These structures represent an increasing group of proteins to which the immune systems produces IgE autoantibodies due to their homology with environmental allergens. Up to now, several autoallergens have been detected, including the transcription factor LEDGF/DSF70[19], the atopy-related autoantigens (ARA) Hom S1–S5 produced by keratinocytes,[68] and the manganese superoxide dismutase (MnSOD) to which patients with AD produce specific IgE. This sensitization is induced by skin colonization with *Malassezia sympodialis*, which causes, due to its high homology, a sensitization against the human MnSOD.[69] This cross-sensitization is predominantly seen in patients with eczema of the head and neck (head and neck dermatitis). There is good evidence that IgE-related autoimmunity develops during the first years of life.[70] However, their relevance of the clinical course and the natural history of the disease remain unclear.

Clinical Aspects of Atopic Dermatitis

The clinical phenotype of AD varies with age and may differ during the course of disease.[71] The eczematous lesions may present with acute (oozing, crusted, eroded vesicles or papules on erythematous plaques), subacute (thick and excoriated plaques), and chronic (lichenified, slightly pigmented, excoriated plaques) forms. Furthermore, xerosis and a lowered threshold for itching are usual hallmarks of AD. Pruritus attacks can occur throughout the day and worsen during the night, causing insomnia and exhaustion, and overall they substantially impair quality of life. Three different stages can be distinguished clinically: infancy, childhood, and adolescent/adulthood.

Clinical Features in Infants

In the second of third month of life, the first signs of AD usually emerge with eczematous, papulovesicular and patchy lesions on the cheeks. Scratching due to itching occurs mostly a few weeks later and leads to crusty erosions. Perioral and paranasal areas are usually spared in the beginning. The term *milk crust* or *milk scurf* refers to the occurrence of yellowish crusts on the scalp that resemble scaled milk. This stage is clinical quite similar to seborrheic dermatitis. Persisting pruritus leads the infant to become restless and agitated during sleep.

Later the inner and outer parts of the arms and legs also may be affected while the diaper area is usually spared. In about 20% to 30% of the cases, lesions heal by the end of the second year of life but the atopic carrier may continue with the first signs of asthma provoked by viral infection. Interestingly, in about 50% of the AD cases at this age, there is no evidence yet for IgE-mediated sensitization; that is, these patients should be classified as having nonatopic eczema.

Clinical Features in Childhood

At this stage, eczematous lesions typically involve flexural areas (antecubital fossae, neck, wrists, and ankles) and the nape of the neck, dorsum of the feet, and hands. These lesions can either arise de novo or develop from the preceding phase. Postinflammatory hypopigmentation may occur when chronic inflammation has resolved. About 60% of the childhood eczema forms will disappear completely, but the stigmata may remain, xerosis being the most important one.

Clinical Features of Adolescents and Adults

When eczema lesions persist from childhood to adolescence and adulthood, or the disease starts de novo at adulthood, flexural areas as well as the head (forehead, periorbital and perioral region) and neck are typically involved with mostly lichenified plaques. Dry skin continues to be a persistent problem, especially in the winter months.

Complications

The most important complications of AD are due to secondary bacterial and viral infections most probably due to the above-mentioned reduced cell-mediated immunity and the deficiency in antimicrobial peptides. Staphylococci frequently provoke an impetiginization of lesions in children, leading to yellow, impetigo-like crusting. Patients with AD are at increased risk for fulminant herpes simplex virus infections (eczema herpeticum).[72] The course of this complication may be severe, with high fever and widespread eruptions. Clinically numerous vesicles in the same stage of development are a characteristic sign. It is unclear whether viral warts or mollusca contagiosa are more prevalent in AD.

Diagnosis of Atopic Dermatitis

Diagnosis of AD relies primarily on the patient's and family's history as well as on clinical findings. The clinical diagnosis of AD is based on the clinical phenotype according to the morphology and distribution of the lesions at the different stages (see above). In 1980, Hanifin and Rajka[73] proposed major and minor diagnostic criteria based on clinical symptoms of AD. A revision of the diagnostic criteria was accomplished by Williams et al.[74]

The severity of AD can be evaluated by different scoring systems such as the Score in Atopic Dermatitis (SCORAD),[75] the Eczema Area and Severity Index (EASI),[76] and others. These scoring systems can be of help in the daily praxis but are mandatory in clinical trials.

Skin tests and laboratory investigations (specific IgE) may be of help in the search for provocation factors such as food or environmental allergens. Provocation tests are additionally performed to determine the clinical significance of positive laboratory tests since skin tests and in vitro testing should complement one another yet do not always have to be concordant. The atopy patch test (APT)[77] may be helpful in the search of AD-relevant allergen. While the sensitivity of APT is average, its specificity is high for the individual context of a given patient.[78] Most importantly, laboratory results always have to be interpreted in the context of the patient's history and skin tests.

For the differential diagnosis, several rare syndromes have to be taken into account such as phenylketonuria, Wiskott-Aldrich syndrome, hyper-IgE syndrome, Netherton's syndrome, DiGeorge's syndrome, and ataxia telangiectasias syndrome.

Management

Besides allergologic diagnostics, management of AD remains a clinical challenge where the primary goals are to control inflammation and microbial colonization and to correct the barrier dysfunction (Fig. 13.3). Education of the patient or the parents of an affected child is as important as other strategies.

Topical Treatment

Skin Care

A key feature of AD is xerosis due to the epidermal barrier dysfunction as witnessed by increased transepidermal water loss. Individually adapted emollients containing urea (4% in children; up to 10% in adults) should be used to support the skin barrier function and allow hydration of the skin. The patient should be educated adequately to avoid specific provocation factors.[79]

Antiinflammatory Approach

Topical Glucocorticosteroids

Most topical glucocorticosteroids (GCSs) present a safe and effective medication when used properly.[80] This is particularly the case for GCSs with double esters and a favorable therapeutic index, that is, high efficiency with low side effects. Besides their antiinflammatory activity, GCSs contribute to a reduction of skin colonization with *S. aureus*.[81] Only mild to moderately potent preparations should be used on genital, facial, or intertriginous skin areas. Less potent topical steroids such as hydrocortisone can also be used on children younger than 1 year old. Different therapeutic schemes have been established: initial treatment should be with moderately to highly potent steroids followed by a dose reduction or a switch to a lower potency preparation.[82] Combined therapy with emollients should be routine during the course of treatment. It is advised to continue an intermittent antiinflammatory treatment over a longer period

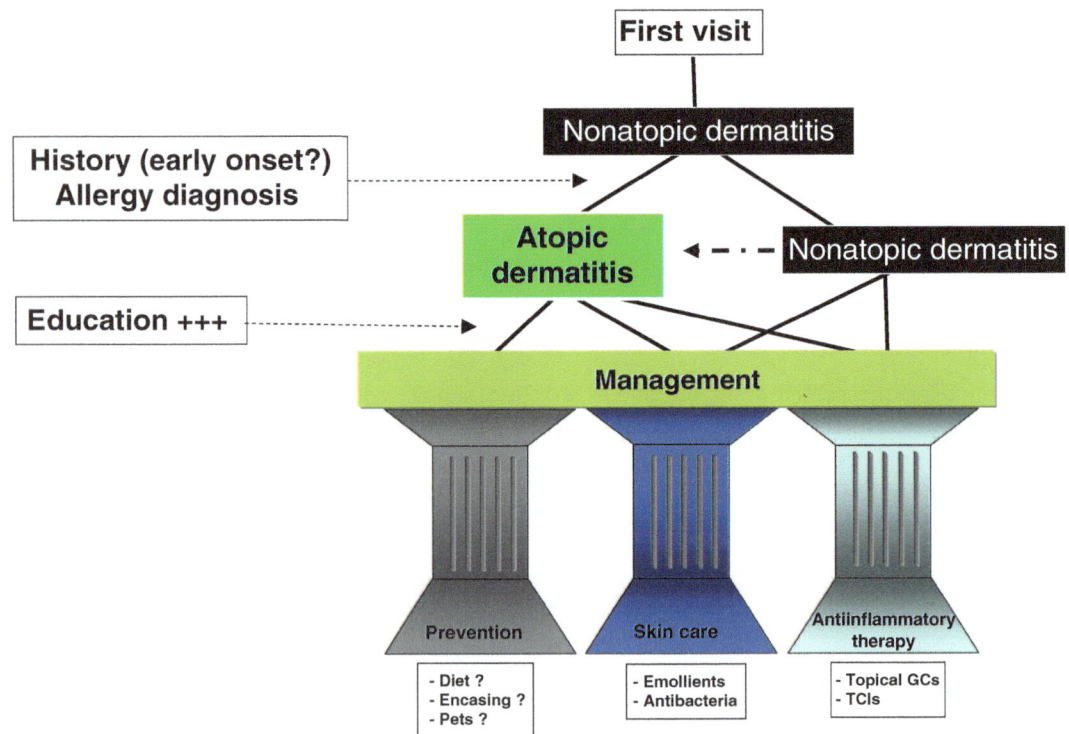

FIG. 13.3. A practical approach to the management of atopic dermatitis

of time (3 to 6 months) in order to better control the subclinical inflammation and the occurrence of flares.[83,84]

Topical Calcineurin Inhibitors

Pimecrolimus and tacrolimus are topical medications that inhibit the calcium-activated phosphatase called calcineurin. They suppress the early phase of T-cell activation and multiple cytokines involved in cellular immunity, and affect IDECs but not LCs in AD lesions. Their antiinflammatory potency is similar to that of GCSs of mild to moderate potency and have an important role in the antiinflammatory management of AD.[85,86] Side effects include a transient burning sensation of the skin. While using calcineurin inhibitors, excessive exposure to natural or artificial sunlight (tanning beds or UVA/B treatment) should be avoided. Long-term safety studies analyzing the evidence of a causal link of cancer and calcineurin inhibitors as well as an increased incidence of viral infections are ongoing. Despite the accepted favorable safety profile,[87] a black boxed warning has been released by the Food and Drug Administration (FDA), and a "red-hand letter" from the European Medicine Agency (EMEA) emphasizes the use of these products as second-line therapy.

Topical Antimicrobial Therapy

Topical antiseptics such as triclosan and chlorhexidine have a low sensitizing potential and show low resistance rates.[88] They can be used in emollients or syndets (synthetic detergents) or as part of an additional "wet wrap" dressing. Short-term fusidic acid is preferentially used in the treatment of bacterial infections with *S. aureus* because of its low minimal inhibitory concentration and good tissue penetration.[89] Intranasal eradication of methicillin-resistant *S. aureus,* frequently found in AD patients, can be achieved by the topical use of mupirocin. In the case of widespread bacterial secondary infection seen mainly in children (primarily *S. aureus*), systemic antibiotic treatment is indicated. Prophylactic treatment only increases resistance rates and has no benefit on the course of disease. The use of silver-coated textiles and silk fabric with a durable antimicrobial finish is still under investigation, but seems to be promising, especially for children.[90]

Systemic Treatment

Antihistamines

There is no specific antipruritic treatment except local applications of antiinflammatory preparations and emollients. H_1-receptor antagonists (alimemazine and promethazine) are predominantly used for their sedative effect and should be given 1 hour before bedtime. Most studies conclude that nonsedating antihistamines seem to have little or no value in the treatment of AD.[91]

Systemic Corticosteroids

Oral corticosteroids have a limited but definite role in the treatment of severe exacerbations of AD. A brief course may be used to control severe disease, and ongoing use of systemic corticosteroids leads to significant adverse effects. After discontinuation of the medication, severe relapses have been noted. Data from randomized clinical trials are lacking.

Cyclosporin A

The ongoing treatment with cyclosporin (CyA) should be reserved for very severe cases of disease that are not responding to other measures.[92,93] Multiple studies have shown a positive effect for children and adults. Treatment should be performed following body-weight–dependent dosing with 3 to 5 mg/kg/day as a high-dose regimen or 2.5 mg/kg/day as a low-dose treatment. The lowest dose for minimal side effects should be applied. Despite its effectiveness, side effects, especially concerning renal toxicity with hypertension and renal impairment, are of particular concern. A close monitoring of creatinine, blood pressure, and CyA serum levels is important.

Azathioprine

Azathioprine is an immunosuppressant drug that has been reported to be effective in severe AD.[94,95] It affects the purine nucleotide synthesis and metabolism and has antiinflammatory and antiproliferative effects. Controlled trials are lacking so far; side effects are high, including myelosuppression, hepatotoxicity, gastrointestinal disturbances, increased susceptibility for infections, and possible development of skin cancer. As azathioprine is metabolized by the thiopurine methyltransferase (TPMT); a deficiency of this enzyme should be excluded before starting an oral immunosuppression with azathioprine.

Biologics

Anti-IgE strategy (omalizumab), which is approved for asthma, has been tried with variable results in AD.[96,97] Since these patients usually display very high levels of IgE, neutralizing these levels would require extremely high amounts of this biologic. Nevertheless, some recent case reports have suggested the successful use of omalizumab in selected patients. Efalizumab (anti-CD11a) has been introduced as a promising alternative to current immunosuppressive therapies, although further double-blind placebo-controlled studies are needed to test its efficacy and safety.[98] Infliximab (anti–TNF-α) has been also reported to be successful in a some reports.[99,100] However, one has to keep in mind that side effects of biologics may be serious and need further evaluation.

Phototherapy

Atopic dermatitis patients usually report benefit from natural sun exposition. Therefore, different spectra of UV light—UVB (280 to 320 nm), narrow-band UVB (311 to 313 nm), UVA (320 to 400 nm), medium and high-dose UVA$_1$ (340 to 400 nm), PUVA, and Balneo-PUVA—have undergone trials for the treatment of AD. Clearly, UVA$_1$ irradiation seems to be superior to conventional UVA-UVB phototherapy in patients with severe AD.[101,102] Narrow-band UVB alone is also effective, and its activity seems to be partially due to a decrease in the microbial colonization.[103] In children UV-therapy should be restricted since data about long-term side effects of UV-therapy are still not available.

Immunotherapy

It is well accepted that allergen-specific immunotherapy, which has been reported since 1911 in the management of allergic diseases, represents the only causative therapeutic approach. Unfortunately, with regard to AD, only limited and often contradictory information is available. A recently published study, reexamining the efficacy of a subcutaneous immunotherapy (SCIT) in atopic patients sensitized to house dust mites (HDMs), demonstrated effectiveness in reducing eczema and allergic sensitization to

HDMs.[104] The improvement of eczema was accompanied by a reduction of topical corticosteroids needed to treat eczema. Interestingly, because of its limited side effects, sublingual immunotherapy (SLIT) may represent an alternative to SCIT. Further studies to verify the benefit of SCIT and SLIT are currently ongoing and we may experience a revival of immunotherapy in AD in the near future.[105]

Education

As mentioned above, education of especially young patients and their parents emphasizing the knowledge about the disease and its management will lead to a higher compliance rate as well as psychological stability.[106] Patient's education also significantly contributes to improvement in quality of life. Adequate educational programs are of great value when offered in interdisciplinary cooperation with dermatologists as well as pediatricians, dietitians, psychologists, and nursing staff, with patients and their families.

Future Perspectives

Combining data from epidemiology, genetics, skin physiology, immunology, and allergy provides new areas of research that will certainly provide us new perspectives and new concepts in the pathophysiology and management of this disease. The role of innate immunity, which has been underestimated for years, is now the subject of numerous projects, and functional genomics will help us to better understand the consequences of so many genetic variants in candidate genes and could potentially deliver future prognostic tools for this disease, its prevention, and its therapeutic response.

Conclusion

The understanding of the pathophysiology of atopic dermatitis is still evolving. Central to the pathogenesis of this disease is the abnormal barrier function of the epidermis, impaired innate immunity, and host–pathogen interactions and environmental allergens that promote aberrant immune response to perpetuate the cutaneous inflammatory response. A better understanding of what drives this process will result in targeted therapies, and perhaps halt the progression of what has been termed the "atopic march."

References

1. Johansson SG, Bieber T, Dahl R, et al. Revised nomenclature for allergy for global use: Report of the Nomenclature Review Committee of the World Allergy Organization, October 2003. J Allergy Clin Immunol 2004;113(5):832–6.
2. Novak N, Bieber T. Allergic and nonallergic forms of atopic diseases. J Allergy Clin Immunol 2003;112(2):252–62.
3. Asher MI, Montefort S, Bjorksten B, et al. Worldwide time trends in the prevalence of symptoms of asthma, allergic rhinoconjunctivitis, and eczema in childhood: ISAAC Phases One and Three repeat multicountry cross-sectional surveys. Lancet 2006;368(9537):733–43.
4. Strachan DP. Hay fever, hygiene, and household size. BMJ 1989;299(6710):1259–60.
5. Williams H, Flohr C. How epidemiology has challenged 3 prevailing concepts about atopic dermatitis. J Allergy Clin Immunol 2006;118(1):209–13.
6. Schultz Larsen FV, Holm NV. Atopic dermatitis in a population based twin series. Concordance rates and heritability estimation. Acta Derm Venereol Suppl (Stockh) 1985;114:159.
7. Cookson WO, Ubhi B, Lawrence R, et al. Genetic linkage of childhood atopic dermatitis to psoriasis susceptibility loci. Nat Genet 2001;27(4):372–3.
8. Bradley M, Soderhall C, Luthman H, Wahlgren CF, Kockum I, Nordenskjold M. Susceptibility loci for atopic dermatitis on chromosomes 3, 13, 15, 17 and 18 in a Swedish population. Hum Mol Genet 2002;11(13):1539–48.
9. Lee YA, Wahn U, Kehrt R, et al. A major susceptibility locus for atopic dermatitis maps to chromosome 3q21. Nat Genet 2000;26(4):470–3.
10. Forrest S, Dunn K, Elliott K, et al. Identifying genes predisposing to atopic eczema. J Allergy Clin Immunol 1999;104(5):1066–70.
11. Hershey GK, Friedrich MF, Esswein LA, Thomas ML, Chatila TA. The association of atopy with a gain-of-function mutation in the alpha subunit of the interleukin-4 receptor. N Engl J Med 1997;337(24):1720–5.
12. Novak N, Kruse S, Kraft S, et al. Dichotomic nature of atopic dermatitis reflected by combined analysis of monocyte immunophenotyping and single nucleotide polymorphisms of the interleukin-4/interleukin-13 receptor gene: the dichotomy of extrinsic and intrinsic atopic dermatitis. J Invest Dermatol 2002;119(4):870–5.
13. Novak N, Kruse S, Potreck J, et al. Single nucleotide polymorphisms of the IL18 gene are associated with atopic eczema. J Allergy Clin Immunol 2005;115(4):828–33.
14. Palmer CN, Irvine AD, Terron-Kwiatkowski A, et al. Common loss-of-function variants of the epidermal barrier protein filaggrin are a major predisposing factor for atopic dermatitis. Nat Genet 2006;38(4):441–6.
15. Weidinger S, Illig T, Baurecht H, et al. Loss-of-function variations within the filaggrin gene predispose for atopic dermatitis with allergic sensitizations. J Allergy Clin Immunol 2006;118(1):214–9.
16. Morar N, Cookson WO, Harper JI, Moffatt MF. Filaggrin mutations in children with severe atopic dermatitis. J Invest Dermatol 2007.
17. Barker JN, Palmer CN, Zhao Y, et al. Null mutations in the filaggrin gene (FLG) determine major susceptibility to early-onset atopic dermatitis that persists into adulthood. J Invest Dermatol 2007;127(3):564–7.
18. Marenholz I, Nickel R, Ruschendorf F, et al. Filaggrin loss-of-function mutations predispose to phenotypes involved in the atopic march. J Allergy Clin Immunol 2006;118(4):866–71.
19. Nomura T, Sandilands A, Akiyama M, et al. Unique mutations in the filaggrin gene in Japanese patients with ichthyosis vulgaris and atopic dermatitis. J Allergy Clin Immunol 2007;119(2):434–40.
20. Vasilopoulos Y, Cork MJ, Murphy R, et al. Genetic association between an AACC insertion in the 3′UTR of the stratum corneum chymotryptic enzyme gene and atopic dermatitis. J Invest Dermatol 2004;123(1):62–6.
21. Zutavern A, Hirsch T, Leupold W, Weiland S, Keil U, von Mutius E. Atopic dermatitis, extrinsic atopic dermatitis and the hygiene hypothesis: results from a cross-sectional study. Clin Exp Allergy 2005;35(10):1301–8.
22. Peters EM, Raap U, Welker P, et al. Neurotrophins act as neuroendocrine regulators of skin homeostasis in health and disease. Horm Metab Res 2007;39(2):110–24.
23. Hosoi J, Murphy GF, Egan CL, et al. Regulation of Langerhans cell function by nerves containing calcitonin gene-related peptide. Nature 1993;363(6425):159–63.
24. Toyoda M, Nakamura M, Makino T, Hino T, Kagoura M, Morohashi M. Nerve growth factor and substance P are useful plasma markers of disease activity in atopic dermatitis. Br J Dermatol 2002;147(1):71–9.
25. Raap U, Kapp A. Neuroimmunological findings in allergic skin diseases. Curr Opin Allergy Clin Immunol 2005;5(5):419–24.

26. Proksch E, Folster-Holst R, Jensen JM. Skin barrier function, epidermal proliferation and differentiation in eczema. J Dermatol Sci 2006;43(3):159–69.

27. Sator PG, Schmidt JB, Honigsmann H. Comparison of epidermal hydration and skin surface lipids in healthy individuals and in patients with atopic dermatitis. J Am Acad Dermatol 2003;48(3):352–8.

28. Rippke F, Schreiner V, Doering T, Maibach HI. Stratum corneum pH in atopic dermatitis: impact on skin barrier function and colonization with Staphylococcus aureus. Am J Clin Dermatol 2004;5(4):217–23.

29. Izadpanah A, Gallo RL. Antimicrobial peptides. J Am Acad Dermatol 2005;52(3 pt 1):381–90; quiz 391–2.

30. McGirt LY, Beck LA. Innate immune defects in atopic dermatitis. J Allergy Clin Immunol 2006;118(1):202–8.

31. Nomura I, Goleva E, Howell MD, et al. Cytokine milieu of atopic dermatitis, as compared to psoriasis, skin prevents induction of innate immune response genes. J Immunol 2003;171(6):3262–9.

32. Ong PY, Ohtake T, Brandt C, et al. Endogenous antimicrobial peptides and skin infections in atopic dermatitis. N Engl J Med 2002;347(15):1151–60.

33. Rieg S, Steffen H, Seeber S, et al. Deficiency of dermcidin-derived antimicrobial peptides in sweat of patients with atopic dermatitis correlates with an impaired innate defense of human skin in vivo. J Immunol 2005;174(12):8003–10.

34. Santamaria-Babi LF. Skin-homing T cells in cutaneous allergic inflammation. Chem Immunol Allergy 2006;91:87–97.

35. Spergel JM, Mizoguchi E, Oettgen H, Bhan AK, Geha RS. Roles of TH1 and TH2 cytokines in a murine model of allergic dermatitis. J Clin Invest 1999;103(8):1103–11.

36. Reinhold U, Kukel S, Goeden B, Neumann U, Kreysel HW. Functional characterization of skin-infiltrating lymphocytes in atopic dermatitis. Clin Exp Immunol 1991;86(3):444–8.

37. Grewe M, Bruijnzeel-Koomen CA, Schopf E, et al. A role for Th1 and Th2 cells in the immunopathogenesis of atopic dermatitis. Immunol Today 1998;19(8):359–61.

38. Beissert S, Schwarz A, Schwarz T. Regulatory T cells. J Invest Dermatol 2006;126(1):15–24.

39. Ziegler SF. FOXP3: of mice and men. Annu Rev Immunol 2006;24:209–26.

40. Ochs HD, Ziegler SF, Torgerson TR. FOXP3 acts as a rheostat of the immune response. Immunol Rev 2005;203:156–64.

41. Verhagen J, Akdis M, Traidl-Hoffmann C, et al. Absence of T-regulatory cell expression and function in atopic dermatitis skin. J Allergy Clin Immunol 2006;117(1):176–83.

42. Ou LS, Goleva E, Hall C, Leung DY. T regulatory cells in atopic dermatitis and subversion of their activity by superantigens. J Allergy Clin Immunol 2004;113(4):756–63.

43. Bach JF. Infections and autoimmune diseases. J Autoimmun 2005;25(suppl):74–80.

44. Homey B, Steinhoff M, Ruzicka T, Leung DY. Cytokines and chemokines orchestrate atopic skin inflammation. J Allergy Clin Immunol 2006;118(1):178–89.

45. Biedermann T, Rocken M, Carballido JM. TH1 and TH2 lymphocyte development and regulation of TH cell-mediated immune responses of the skin. J Invest Dermatol Symp Proc 2004;9(1):5–14.

46. Fiset PO, Leung DY, Hamid Q. Immunopathology of atopic dermatitis. J Allergy Clin Immunol 2006;118(1):287–90.

47. Hamid Q, Boguniewicz M, Leung DY. Differential in situ cytokine gene expression in acute versus chronic atopic dermatitis. J Clin Invest 1994;94(2):870–6.

48. Kimura M, Tsuruta S, Yoshida T. Correlation of house dust mite-specific lymphocyte proliferation with IL-5 production, eosinophilia, and the severity of symptoms in infants with atopic dermatitis. J Allergy Clin Immunol 1998;101(1 Pt 1):84–9.

49. Park JH, Choi YL, Namkung JH, et al. Characteristics of extrinsic vs. intrinsic atopic dermatitis in infancy: correlations with laboratory variables. Br J Dermatol 2006;155(4):778–83.

50. Toda M, Leung DY, Molet S, et al. Polarized in vivo expression of IL-11 and IL-17 between acute and chronic skin lesions. J Allergy Clin Immunol 2003;111(4):875–81.

51. Kim BE, Leung DY, Streib JE, Boguniewicz M, Hamid QA, Howell MD. Macrophage inflammatory protein 3alpha deficiency in atopic dermatitis skin and role in innate immune response to vaccinia virus. J Allergy Clin Immunol 2007;119(2):457–63.

52. Soumelis V, Reche PA, Kanzler H, et al. Human epithelial cells trigger dendritic cell mediated allergic inflammation by producing TSLP. Nat Immunol 2002;3(7):673–80.

53. Liu YJ. Thymic stromal lymphopoietin: master switch for allergic inflammation. J Exp Med 2006;20:203(2):269–73.

54. Neis MM, Peters B, Dreuw A, et al. Enhanced expression levels of IL-31 correlate with IL-4 and IL-13 in atopic and allergic contact dermatitis. J Allergy Clin Immunol 2006;118(4):930–7.

55. Shortman K, Naik SH. Steady-state and inflammatory dendritic-cell development. Nat Rev Immunol 2007;7(1):19–30.

56. Bieber T, de la Salle H, Wollenberg A, et al. Human epidermal Langerhans cells express the high affinity

receptor for immunoglobulin E (Fc epsilon RI). J Exp Med 1992;175(5):1285–90.

57. Wollenberg A, Wen SP, Bieber T. Langerhans cell phenotyping—a new tool for differential-diagnosis of inflammatory diseases. Lancet 1995;346(8990):1626–7.

58. Wollenberg A, Kraft S, Hanau D, Bieber T. Immunomorphological and ultrastructural characterization of Langerhans cells and a novel, inflammatory dendritic epidermal cell (IDEC) population in lesional skin of atopic eczema. J Invest Dermatol 1996;106(3):446–53.

59. Novak N, Valenta R, Bohle B, et al. FcεRI engagement of Langerhans cell-like dendritic cells and inflammatory dendritic epidermal cell-like dendritic cells induces chemotactic signals and different T-cell phenotypes in vitro. J Allergy Clin Immunol 2004;113(5):949–57.

60. Novak N, Bieber T. The role of dendritic cell subtypes in the pathophysiology of atopic dermatitis. J Am Acad Dermatol 2005;53(2 Suppl 2):S171–6.

61. Wollenberg A, Wagner M, Gunther S, et al. Plasmacytoid dendritic cells: a new cutaneous dendritic cell subset with distinct role in inflammatory skin diseases. J Invest Dermatol 2002;119(5):1096–102.

62. Hashizume H, Horibe T, Yagi H, Seo N, Takigawa M. Compartmental imbalance and aberrant immune function of blood CD123+ (plasmacytoid) and CD11c+ (myeloid) dendritic cells in atopic dermatitis. J Immunol 2005;174(4):2396–403.

63. Cardona ID, Cho SH, Leung DY. Role of bacterial superantigens in atopic dermatitis : implications for future therapeutic strategies. Am J Clin Dermatol 2006;7(5):273–9.

64. Howell MD, Gallo RL, Boguniewicz M, et al. Cytokine milieu of atopic dermatitis skin subverts the innate immune response to vaccinia virus. Immunity 2006;24(3):341–8.

65. Strickland I, Hauk PJ, Trumble AE, Picker LJ, Leung DY. Evidence for superantigen involvement in skin homing of T cells in atopic dermatitis. J Invest Dermatol 1999;112(2):249–53.

66. Leung DY, Harbeck R, Bina P, et al. Presence of IgE antibodies to staphylococcal exotoxins on the skin of patients with atopic dermatitis. Evidence for a new group of allergens. J Clin Invest 1993;92(3):1374–80.

67. Mittermann I, Aichberger KJ, Bunder R, Mothes N, Renz H, Valenta R. Autoimmunity and atopic dermatitis. Curr Opin Allergy Clin Immunol 2004;4(5):367–71.

68. Valenta R, Natter S, Seiberler S, et al. Molecular characterization of an autoallergen, Hom s 1, identified by serum IgE from atopic dermatitis patients. J Invest Dermatol 1998;111(6):1178–83.

69. Schmid-Grendelmeier P, Fluckiger S, Disch R, et al. IgE-mediated and T cell-mediated autoimmunity against manganese superoxide dismutase

in atopic dermatitis. J Allergy Clin Immunol 2005;115(5):1068–75.

70. Mothes N, Niggemann B, Jenneck C, et al. The cradle of IgE autoreactivity in atopic eczema lies in early infancy. J Allergy Clin Immunol 2005;116(3):706–9.

71. Williams HC. Clinical practice. Atopic dermatitis. N Engl J Med 2005;352(22):2314–24.

72. Wollenberg A, Wetzel S, Burgdorf WH, Haas J. Viral infections in atopic dermatitis: pathogenic aspects and clinical management. J Allergy Clin Immunol 2003;112(4):667–74.

73. Hanifin J, Rajka G. Diagnostic features of atopic eczema. Acta Derm Venereol 1980;92:44–7.

74. Williams HC, Burney PG, Hay RJ, et al. The U.K. Working Party's diagnostic criteria for atopic dermatitis. I. Derivation of a minimum set of discriminators for atopic dermatitis. Br J Dermatol 1994;131(3):383–96.

75. Severity scoring of atopic dermatitis: the SCORAD index. Consensus Report of the European Task Force on Atopic Dermatitis. Dermatology 1993;186(1):23–31.

76. Housman TS, Patel MJ, Camacho F, Feldman SR, Fleischer AB Jr, Balkrishnan R. Use of the Self-Administered Eczema Area and Severity Index by parent caregivers: results of a validation study. Br J Dermatol 2002;147(6):1192–8.

77. Ring J, Bieber T, Vieluf D, Kunz B, Przybilla B. Atopic eczema, Langerhans cells and allergy. Int Arch Allergy Appl Immunol 1991;94(1–4):194–201.

78. Darsow U, Vieluf D, Ring J. Atopy patch test with different vehicles and allergen concentrations: an approach to standardization. J Allergy Clin Immunol 1995;95(3):677–84.

79. Morren MA, Przybilla B, Bamelis M, Heykants B, Reynaers A, Degreef H. Atopic dermatitis: triggering factors. J Am Acad Dermatol 1994;31 (3 pt 1):467–73.

80. Callen J, Chamlin S, Eichenfield LF, et al. A systematic review of the safety of topical therapies for atopic dermatitis. Br J Dermatol 2007;156(2):203–21.

81. Stalder JF, Fleury M, Sourisse M, Rostin M, Pheline F, Litoux P. Local steroid therapy and bacterial skin flora in atopic dermatitis. Br J Dermatol 1994;131(4):536–40.

82. Thomas KS, Armstrong S, Avery A, et al. Randomised controlled trial of short bursts of a potent topical corticosteroid versus prolonged use of a mild preparation for children with mild or moderate atopic eczema. BMJ 2002;324(7340):768.

83. Berth-Jones J, Damstra RJ, Golsch S, et al. Twice weekly fluticasone propionate added to emollient maintenance treatment to reduce risk of relapse in

atopic dermatitis: randomised, double blind, parallel group study. BMJ 2003;326(7403):1367.

84. Bieber T, Vick K, Folster-Holst R, et al. Efficacy and safety of methylprednisolone aceponate ointment 0.1% compared to tacrolimus 0.03% in children and adolescents with an acute flare of severe atopic dermatitis. Allergy 2007;62(2):184–9.

85. Alomar A, Berth-Jones J, Bos JD, et al. The role of topical calcineurin inhibitors in atopic dermatitis. Br J Dermatol 2004;151(suppl 70):3–27.

86. Breuer K, Werfel T, Kapp A. Safety and efficacy of topical calcineurin inhibitors in the treatment of childhood atopic dermatitis. Am J Clin Dermatol 2005;6(2):65–77.

87. Bieber T, Cork M, Ellis C, et al. Consensus statement on the safety profile of topical calcineurin inhibitors. Dermatology 2005;211(2):77–8.

88. Wohlrab J, Jost G, Abeck D. Antiseptic efficacy of a low-dosed topical triclosan/chlorhexidine combination therapy in atopic dermatitis. Skin Pharmacol Physiol 2006;20(2):71–6.

89. Wilkinson JD. Fusidic acid in dermatology. Br J Dermatol 1998;139(suppl 53):37–40.

90. Juenger M, Ladwig A, Staecker S, et al. Efficacy and safety of silver textile in the treatment of atopic dermatitis (AD). Curr Med Res Opin 2006;22(4):739–50.

91. Wahlgren CF, Hagermark O, Bergstrom R. The antipruritic effect of a sedative and a non-sedative antihistamine in atopic dermatitis. Br J Dermatol 1990;122(4):545–51.

92. Griffiths CE, Katsambas A, Dijkmans BA, et al. Update on the use of cyclosporin in immune-mediated dermatoses. Br J Dermatol 2006;155 (suppl 2):1–16.

93. Hijnen DJ, ten Berge O, Timmer-de Mik L, Bruijnzeel-Koomen CA, de Bruin-Weller MS. Efficacy and safety of long-term treatment with cyclosporin A for atopic dermatitis. J Eur Acad Dermatol Venereol 2007;21(1):85–9.

94. Meggitt SJ, Gray JC, Reynolds NJ. Azathioprine dosed by thiopurine methyltransferase activity for moderate-to-severe atopic eczema: a double-blind, randomised controlled trial. Lancet 2006;367(9513):839–46.

95. Meggitt SJ, Reynolds NJ. Azathioprine for atopic dermatitis. Clin Exp Dermatol 2001;26(5):369–75.

96. Krathen RA, Hsu S. Failure of omalizumab for treatment of severe adult atopic dermatitis. J Am Acad Dermatol 2005;53(2):338–40.

97. Lane JE, Cheyney JM, Lane TN, Kent DE, Cohen DJ. Treatment of recalcitrant atopic dermatitis with omalizumab. J Am Acad Dermatol 2006;54(1):68–72.

98. Takiguchi R, Tofte S, Simpson B, et al. Efalizumab for severe atopic dermatitis: a pilot study in adults. J Am Acad Dermatol 2007;56(2):222–7.

99. Cassano N, Loconsole F, Coviello C, Vena GA. Infliximab in recalcitrant severe atopic eczema associated with contact allergy. Int J Immunopathol Pharmacol 2006;19(1):237–40.

100. Jacobi A, Antoni C, Manger B, Schuler G, Hertl M. Infliximab in the treatment of moderate to severe atopic dermatitis. J Am Acad Dermatol 2005;52(3 pt 1):522–6.

101. Dawe RS. Ultraviolet A1 phototherapy. Br J Dermatol 2003;148(4):626–37.

102. Tzaneva S, Seeber A, Schwaiger M, Honigsmann H, Tanew A. High-dose versus medium-dose UVA1 phototherapy for patients with severe generalized atopic dermatitis. J Am Acad Dermatol 2001;45(4):503–7.

103. Silva SH, Guedes AC, Gontijo B, et al. Influence of narrow-band UVB phototherapy on cutaneous microbiota of children with atopic dermatitis. J Eur Acad Dermatol Venereol 2006;20(9):1114–20.

104. Werfel T, Breuer K, Rueff F, et al. Usefulness of specific immunotherapy in patients with atopic dermatitis and allergic sensitization to house dust mites: a multi-centre, randomized, dose-response study. Allergy 2006;61(2):202–5.

105. Bussmann C, Bockenhoff A, Henke H, Werfel T, Novak N. Does allergen-specific immunotherapy represent a therapeutic option for patients with atopic dermatitis? J Allergy Clin Immunol 2006;118(6):1292–8.

106. Staab D, Diepgen TL, Fartasch M, et al. Age related, structured educational programmes for the management of atopic dermatitis in children and adolescents: multicentre, randomised controlled trial. BMJ 2006;332(7547):933–8.

14
Psoriasis

Frank O. Nestle

Key Points

- Psoriasis is a common, immune-mediated inflammatory papulosquamous skin disease that results in recurring scaly, erythematous plaques, typically in a symmetrical distribution.
- There is strong evidence that psoriasis is determined by genetic predisposition. It is thought that there is not a single disease gene, but rather a complex set of gene variants that results in an abnormal response to environmental factors.
- Psoriasis is now considered to be a disease caused by the infiltration of effector immunocytes in the epidermis and dermis.
- Important effector cells are CD4 and CD8 conventional T-lymphocytes, as well as natural killer (NK) T cells, plasmacytoid dendritic cells (PDCs), TIP-DCs.
- Other cell types that participate in this pathologic process include keratinocytes, endothelial cells, fibroblasts, monocytes/macrophages, and neutrophils.
- Pathologic cytokines include inflammatory cytokines such as tumor necrosis factor-α (TNF-α), interferon-α (IFN-α), T-helper-1 (Th1) cytokines such as IFN-γ, Th17 cytokines such as interleukin-17 (IL-17) and IL-22, and antigen-presenting cell (APC)-derived cytokines such as IL-12 and IL-23.
- Biologic agents have emerged as effective treatments for psoriasis. They include anti–T-cell agents (efalizumab and alefecept), and anti–TNF-α agents (etanercept, infliximab, and adalimumab).

Psoriasis is a chronic inflammatory skin disease that results from polygenic predisposition.[1] It is characterized by recurring erythematous, scaly plaques in often symmetric configuration. Disease recognition and classification is very much based on the descriptive pathology of the 19th century. While scaly erythematous lesions were described as early as the Hippocratic school (460–377 BC), it was only in the 19th century that Willan gave an accurate description of psoriasis and Hebra[2] defined it as a clinical entity distinct from lepra. While we have made some progress in our understanding of the pathogenesis of psoriasis, especially with regard to its immunologic basis, disease classification is still very much based on distinctive morphology of skin lesions. Ongoing progress in the dissection of the molecular events leading to psoriasis is only beginning to have some impact on disease classifications.

The prevalence of psoriasis is around 2% with variations from 0.4% to 0.7% in African and Asian populations, to 4% in the United States and Canada. Typical peaks of first appearance are at ages 20 to 30 and 50 to 60. Psoriasis is classically responsive to trigger factors that might induce psoriasis de novo or exacerbate skin lesions. Trigger factors range from nonspecific triggers such as skin trauma to more specific triggers such as pathogens (e.g., streptococci) or drugs (e.g., lithium, interferon-α). The investigation of these trigger factors is important since they might lead to a better understanding of critical starting events of the disease. One of the omissions in the field is based on the fact that most studies are performed on established inflammatory lesions where the "noise" of unspecific inflammatory events might obscure psoriasis-specific processes. Thus in the past and still continuing, nearly every novel immunologic cell or mediator has been (re-)discovered in fully established psoriasis lesions. The real challenge with these purely observational data is to add some functional significance, which is only possible in the context of relevant disease models or proof-of-principle studies in patients.

Psoriasis is associated with a significant decrease in quality of life and prominent psychosocial morbidity. Suffering is comparable to that of patients with other major chronic illnesses such as cancer, heart disease, and diabetes.[3] Economic impacts such as treatment costs and loss of work hours are associated with decreased quality of life and psoriasis severity.

Psoriasis patients have an increased risk of diabetes, obesity, and myocardial infarction.[4–6] There is an association with symptoms of metabolic syndrome,[7] a complex disorder that includes hypertension, dyslipidemia, obesity, and impaired glucose tolerance. Some of these systemic comorbidities might be explained by shared inflammatory pathways including a major role for the cytokine tumor necrosis factor-α (TNF-α). Therapies targeting such pathways might not only improve psoriasis but also alleviate other associated comorbidities including cardiovascular events.

Genomics and the Immune System

There is strong evidence that psoriasis is a multifactorial disorder based on the combined influence of predisposing gene variants, genetic modifiers, and environmental factors. In contrast to mendelian disorders where a single gene defect is causing disease, psoriasis belongs to the group of complex genetic disorders where multiple gene variants in response to environmental factors contribute to disease risk. The predisposing gene variants may often confer only small risks (e.g., relative risks of less than 3), but in their combined impact are important in setting the genetic stage for the development of psoriasis.

The strong influence of genes in psoriasis is supported by a high concordance rate in monozygotic twins of up to 72% (vs. a concordance rate of approximately 15% to 23% in dizygotic twins).[8] Psoriasis is thus concordant about three times as often in identical twins compared to fraternal

twins with lower concordance rates in Australia vs. Northern Europe. Estimates have placed the heritability of psoriasis in the range of 60% to 90%, among the highest of the complex genetic disorders.[9]

In recent years, multiple genetic genome scans have been performed in psoriasis patients, resulting in a catalogue of at least 19 genetic susceptibility loci, but replication of single loci has been provided for only a few of those. The most prominent genetic risk region in psoriasis patients is confined to an approximately 160-kilobase (kb) stretch of DNA on the short arm of chromosome 6 (termed PSORS1) encompassing genes including human leukocyte antigen *HLA-Cw6* as a potential immunologic candidate gene, and corneodesmosin as a potential epidermal structure candidate gene.[10] Gene candidate approaches are currently underway to determine the role of these genes in the pathogenesis of psoriasis.

While previous linkage or association studies were done with rather low resolution genetic mapping tools, recent progress has led to the performance of whole genome scans using between 300 K and 500 K single nucleotide polymorphism (SNP) markers, providing exciting insights into the genetic variation underlying complex genetic inflammatory disorders at a very high resolution. The first of these scans are beginning to be published and have already resulted in interesting findings related to novel genes involved in critical immune pathways of complex genetic disorders.[11] One gene variant identified in such scans is a protective nonsynonymous SNP in the IL-23R on chromosome 1p31, leading to an exchange of a glutamine for an arginine at position 381 of the IL-23R intracellular signaling chain and has a putative functional role in the responsiveness of psoriasis patients to the important cytokine IL-23.[12,13] It is noteworthy that four psoriasis susceptibility loci, namely PSORS2, PSORS4, PSORS5, and the chromosome 20p locus, overlap susceptibility regions for atopic dermatitis, potentially indicating shared biochemical pathways between psoriasis and another major inflammatory skin disease.[14] Whole genome analysis of genes is mirrored by analysis of gene transcripts in psoriasis. A recent study has identified 1338 genes differentially expressed in psoriatic skin, the majority of them involved in immune response and proliferation.[15] A significant

TABLE 14.1. Arguments for a role of the immune system in psoriasis

Presence of immune cells in psoriasis lesions
Clonal expansion of T cells in lesions over time
Bone marrow transplantation transfers/cures the disease
Therapeutic activity of drugs targeting the immune system
Essential role of T cells/cytokines in humanized mouse models
Genetic association with human leukocyte antigen (HLA) locus

part of the psoriasis-specific transcriptome derives from dendritic cells, specialized antigen-presenting sentinel cells of the immune system (J. Krueger, Rockefeller University, personal communication). The challenge of future investigations will be to combine the massive amount of data coming out of gene variant and gene transcript analyses into a meaningful pathogenic framework.

Both at the gene and transcriptome level, alterations in genes that are affecting the immune system are abundantly present in psoriasis, furthering the case of psoriasis being an immune-mediated disease (Table 14.1).

Immune Effector Cells and Cytokines

Given the striking morphologic and functional alterations in psoriatic epidermis, it is quite understandable why the prevailing view of psoriasis pathogenesis prior to the 1980s has focused on the biology of the epidermis and its main constituents the keratinocytes. This view was challenged by a serendipitous observation of rheumatologists, who described dramatic improvement of psoriatic arthritis patients treated with cyclosporine A not only in their joints but also in their skin.[16] Other investigators confirmed this initial observation about the efficacy of a potent immunosuppressive drug for skin lesions in psoriasis patients and provided thus the first solid framework in terms of thinking about psoriasis as an immune-mediated disease.[17,18] The arguments in favor of an important role of the immune system, especially T cells, in psoriasis include (1) expansion of clonal T cells in lesions over time[19]; (2) therapeutic activity of drugs targeting the immune system[17,20–22]; (3) transfer or cure of psoriasis after bone marrow transplantation, depending on the transplanted marrow and the

recipient[23,24]; (4) essential role of T cells/cytokines in humanized mouse models[25]; and (5) possible genetic association with *HLA-Cw6* (Table 14.1).[10]

There are numerous immune cells present in psoriasis lesions that could contribute to disease pathogenesis, including T cells, monocytes/macrophages, and dendritic cells.[26–28] While CD4 helper T cells are mainly located in the dermis with a preference for the upper stratum papillare, CD8 T cells are mainly positioned in the epidermis in close contact with keratinocytes and Langerhans' cells. Substantial evidence points to an important role of epidermal T cells including clonality of T-cell receptors[29] and association of reduced numbers of epidermal T cells with therapeutic response.[20] The majority of T cells are activated expressing the CD25 chain of the interleukin receptor[30] and secrete predominantly interferon-γ, classifying psoriatic T cells as T helper-1 (Th1) or T1 cells.[31–33] Recent interest has focused on T cells producing interleukin-17 (IL-17) and IL-22, but their functional role in psoriasis awaits further experimental evidence.[34]

There is also spectrum of so-called unconventional T cells that recognize lipid antigens in the context of the nonpolymorphic major histocompatibility complex (MHC) class I like protein CD1d. These natural killer T cells (NKT cells) as well as CD1d expressing keratinocytes and dendritic cells are present in psoriasis lesions and potentially contribute to the inflammatory process.[35,36] There is considerable interest in the understanding of immunosuppressive effector pathways in autoimmunity. Immunosuppressive regulatory T cells (T_reg) act either through cytokine production or cell–cell contact to suppress inflammation. While T_reg numbers are not altered in psoriasis, there seems to be a defect in their suppressive activity.[37] T cells are primed and activated by interaction with antigen-presenting dendritic cells (DCs). Dermal DCs are increased in psoriasis lesions.[33] Dermal DCs were isolated, extensively characterized, and shown to induce autoproliferation of T cells and Th1 cytokine production in psoriasis patients.[33] It has been further demonstrated that a subset of CD1 α-DR+ dendritic cells induce increased autologous T-cell proliferation.[38] The role of DCs in psoriasis is further substantiated by the fact that cyclosporin A (CsA) treatment affects dendritic cell numbers[39] and that biologics such as alefacept decrease

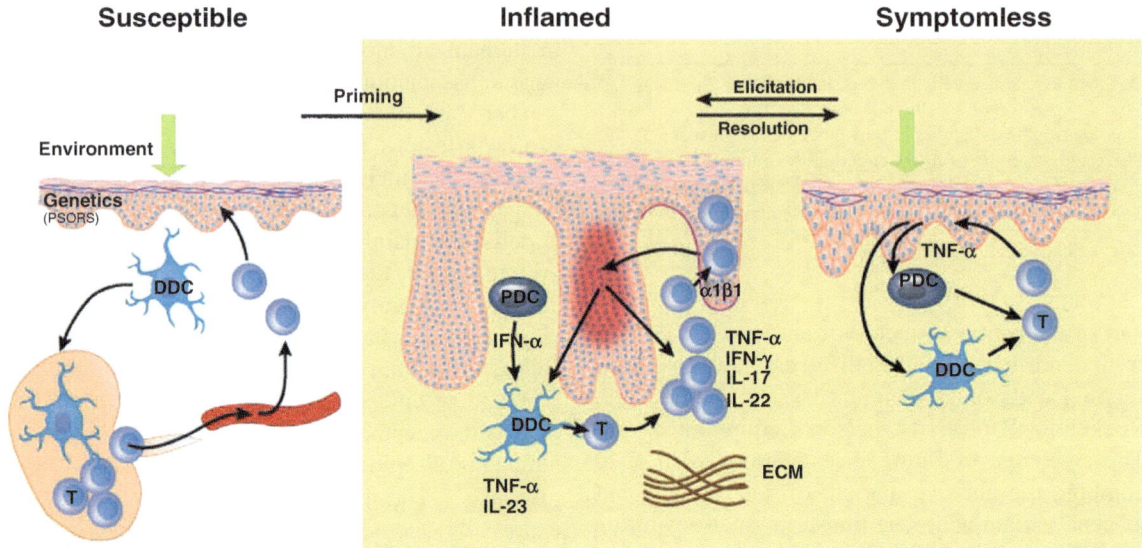

FIG. 14.1. Proposed immunopathogenesis of psoriasis. Environmental factors (infection, physical trauma, cytokines, drugs) trigger a first manifestation of psoriasis in a healthy individual with genetically determined susceptibility (psoriasis susceptibility loci PSORS) (priming). This process is proposed to require stimulation of dermal dendritic cells (DDCs), which migrate to the local lymph node and lead to the proliferation and priming of (auto)antigen-specific T cells (T). These T cells then migrate to the skin, where they are crucial for the formation of a psoriasis lesion in concert with PDCs, DDCs, a network of cytokines, and the extracellular matrix (ECM). Key check points in the inflammatory process include activation of PDCs, DDCs, the activation and proliferation of T cells, their transmigration into the epidermis controlled by the integrin α1β1 and the production of cytokines including IFN-α, IL-23, TNF-α, IFN-γ, IL-17, and IL-22. This "inflamed" state can resolve spontaneously or through therapeutic intervention (resolution). Once an individual has experienced psoriasis lesion(s), it is proposed that normal-appearing symptomless skin has a lower activation threshold owing to the strategic positioning of PDCs, DDCs, and T cells. Thus, a normally innocuous trigger can activate local skin-resident immune cells (elicitation) leading to an inflamed lesion, without the requirement for recirculation or recruitment of other cells. DDC, dermal dendritic cell; ECM, extracellular matrix; IFN, interferon; IL, interleukin; PDC, plasmacytoid dendritic cell; TNF, tumor necrosis factor. (Adapted from Boyman et al.,[62] with permission.)

lesional DC numbers.[40] The DCs can be subdivided into myeloid DCs such as dermal DC or plasmacytoid dendritic cells (PDCs). Interferon-α–producing PDCs are increased in psoriasis lesions and functionally relevant in the inflammatory psoriatic cascade as proximal producers of IFN-α.[79] Thus, there is substantial scientific evidence that various subsets of DC are key activators of psoriatic T cells and potential therapeutic targets.

Other immune cells with potential relevance in psoriasis include monocyte/macrophages, neutrophils, and mast cells with a possible contribution from immunologically active endothelial cells, fibroblasts, and especially keratinocytes.[41–43] Two publications using transgenic mouse models of psoriasis have demonstrated the key role of macrophages in the disease process; these studies await conformation from functional investigation of human psoriasis.[44–46] Immune cells communicate with each other by hormone-like secreted molecules, so-called cytokines. The cytokine network hypothesis in psoriasis predicted a key role for proinflammatory cytokines such as TNF-α and IL-8 based on extensive laboratory investigations.[47] The substantial therapeutic success of anti–TNF-α therapy in the treatment of psoriasis (see below) has validated the cytokine network hypothesis and revives interest in the definition of key effector cytokines in psoriasis. IFN-γ and IFN-γ–induced gene products are key features of the psoriatic cytokines milieu; however, blockade of IFN-γ has yet to demonstrate its efficacy in psoriasis.

The cytokine network hypothesis has been recently revisited to include novel cytokines such as IL-23 and IL-17 in this framework.[48] Interleukin-23 belongs to the IL-12 family of cytokines and is increased in psoriatic lesions with a major contribution from IL-23 producing dendritic cells.[49] Blocking IL-12 cytokine family members including IL-23 has recently shown therapeutic benefit[50]; however, due to the absence of an IL-23–specific monoclonal antibody used in functional studies, the functional role of IL-23 independent from IL-12 awaits further clarifications. Interleukin-23 stimulates IL-17, producing Th17 cells, which are also characterized by the production of IL-22. Interleukin-22 induces epidermal hyperplasia and therefore provides a potential link among IL-23 production, Th17 cells, and epidermal hyperplasia. However, this sequence of pathologic events is only hypothetical and still far from being proven in the case of psoriasis (Fig. 14.1).

Is There a Psoriasis-Specific Antigen?

Evidence for a potential antigen-driven expansion of T cells in psoriasis comes from molecular studies of T-cell receptor clonality. The usage of certain T-cell receptor motives in psoriasis seems to be highly restricted, and the same T-cell receptor clone could be followed over time in evolving lesions and was present in lesions of identical twins.[19,51] The best defined antigenic trigger for psoriasis is β-hemolytic streptococci as part of a streptococcal tonsillitis. While incidence rates of streptococcal infections preceding psoriasis have been reported as ranging from 60% to 97%,[52,53] the percentage of patients in whom streptococci can be cultured from tonsillar swaps is quite low.[54] It has been proposed that psoriasis is as autoimmune disease induced by streptococcal superantigens[55]; however, psoriasis does not resemble the transitory skin rash of streptococcal superantigen-induced scarlet fever and is generally not responsive to antibiotic treatment. An alternative scenario is related to the concept of molecular mimicry, which is based on the recognition of an infectious agent and a self antigen by the same T-cell clone. In the case of streptococci, it has been proposed the T cells reactive to streptococcal M proteins cross-react with keratins in human epidermis and thus lead to a sustained sterile (but originally antibacterial) inflammation.[56] A convincing molecular link is provided by the finding of identical T-cell receptor (TCR) clonality in streptococcal angina and skin lesions of patients with psoriasis.[57] Thus, accumulating evidence suggests the involvement of specific antigens in the pathogenesis of psoriasis.

Challenges to an Immunologic View of Psoriasis

There are also challenges to the view that the immune system is the principal driver of the psoriatic disease process. Overexpression of genes such as the transcription factor STAT3 or deletion of members of the nuclear factor κB (NF-κB) family or the AP-1 family of proteins in the epidermis of mice leads to skin lesions resembling psoriasis.[45,58,59] In some of these disease models inflammatory lesions are independent of T cells,[45,59] while in others T cells are necessary.[58] These models are of interest and stimulate thinking about a key initiating role of transcription factor dysregulation in keratinocytes in psoriasis. A recent challenge was also provided by the fact that the other major inflammatory skin disease, atopic dermatitis, is to a large extent based on a gene defect of the epidermal structural protein filaggrin. Thus in a revised scenario of the pathogenesis of atopic dermatitis, a genetic defect in a keratinocyte structural protein potentially leads to an altered epidermal barrier, increased exposure of the immune system to transepidermal challenges such as novel antigens, as well as skin irritation. It thus provides the basis for a self-perpetuating inflammatory process. Even the case for genetic linkage to *HLA-Cw6* in psoriasis is not a perfect one. There is still a reasonable scenario that in fact other genes in the PSORS1 complex close to *HLA-Cw6,* such as intronic regulatory regions or indeed other genes such as the structural epidermal gene corneodesmosin, play a key role in the genetic risk conferred by the PSORS1 locus.

Thus, the current view that epidermal hyperplasia is based on a reaction to immunologic injury has still some reasonable opposing viewpoints that need to be clarified in future research.[60]

What, then, is the potential relationship between the epithelium and the activated immune system in psoriasis? Studies of early psoriasis indicate that infiltrating immune cells are the earliest sign of psoriasis.[61] A humanized mouse model of psoriasis also demonstrates expansion of T cells before epidermal hyperplasia takes place.[62] What are the potential factors activating keratinocytes in psoriasis? The production of IFN-γ has been proposed as a key link between activated T cells and activated keratinocytes.[30] Supernatants of T-cell clones from psoriasis patients are mitogenic for keratinocytes, and IFN-γ has been identified as a key factor mediating this effect.[63] Furthermore, injection of IFN-γ (as well as IL-2) in patients with a history of psoriasis induces inflammatory lesions resembling psoriasis.[64,65] Other candidates potentially involved in feedback of immune cells to epidermal cells include keratinocyte growth factor (KGF), insulin-like growth factor I (IGF-I), amphiregulin, oncostatin M (OSM), and the IL-20 family of cytokines such as IL-22. On the other hand, keratinocytes are "cytokine factories" producing numerous immune effector molecules and thus amplifying the inflammatory vicious circle.[66]

Immunointervention

While most therapeutic strategies for psoriasis were found by serendipity, recent progress in the understanding of the immunopathogenesis of psoriasis has resulted in a variety of new treatment approaches that are based on the blockade of an immunologically relevant molecules using an antibody or a receptor fusion protein. Current approaches can be broadly divided in therapies targeting T cells or blocking cytokines.

T-cell targeted therapies include targets such as CD11a (anti-CD11a moAb efalizumab) or leukocyte function–associated antigen-3 (LFA-3; the fusion protein alefacept) targeting CD2/LFA-3 interactions.

Efalizumab is a humanized antibody directed against CD11a, the α-subunit of LFA-1 and inhibits its interaction with CD54 (intercellular adhesion molecule 1 [ICAM-1]). Its potential mechanism of action ranges from blocking T-cell/dendritic-cell interaction in the skin to blocking entrance of immune cells into skin and a possible blockade of T-cell/dendritic-cell interaction in skin draining lymph nodes. Efalizumab is injected weekly through the subcutaneous route typically over 12 weeks with a reduced starting dose to

prevent an initial flu-like syndrome. It has a reasonable clinical efficacy with a psoriasis area-and-severity index (PASI) 75% response rate (often corresponding to a physician global assessment of clear to almost clear) of about 22%,[67] which might be increasing over prolonged treatment periods. Long-term treatment over 27 months has demonstrated efficacy and safety in an open label study.[68] Efalizumab is generally well tolerated. Side effects include initial transitory flu-like syndrome, transient papular eruptions, and rare cases of thrombocytopenia.

Alefacept is an LFA-3 fusion protein that blocks engagement of LFA-3 with its ligand CD2, for example, on memory T cells. An additional mechanism of action relates to the killing of alefacept-binding targets through antibody-dependent cell-mediated cytotoxicity (ADCC). After a 12-week course of intramuscular alefacept (15 mg weekly), 33% of patients achieved at least a PASI 75 response at any time.[69] Alefacept depletes circulating memory T cells,[70] but primary and secondary humoral immune responses are maintained.[71]

The dominant target in anticytokine therapy is TNF-α, mostly based on the success story of this type of treatment in rheumatoid disease.[72] Multiple antibodies and fusion proteins are currently on the market or are on their way to the market aiming at the blockade of TNF-α in the treatment of psoriasis.[73]

Treatment of psoriasis patients with *infliximab*, a monoclonal antibody targeting TNF-α, was one of the first investigator-initiated proof-of-concept studies of the activity of biologics in psoriasis.[74] Infliximab has multiple potential mechanisms of action including (1) neutralization of circulating trimeric TNF-α, (2) binding to cell-surface–bound TNF-α or to TNF-α to TNF receptors, and (3) generation of high molecular anti-TNF/TNF complexes with potential activity through Fc receptors and complement receptors. It has one of the highest clinical efficacies of current systemic antipsoriatic treatments with a PASI 75 response rate of 80% at week 10 and prolonged treatment response until week 50.[75] Potential side effects include immediate and delayed-type hypersensitivity infusion reactions, infections (including serious infections such as tuberculosis, listeriosis, or histoplasmosis), hepatitis, and, in very rare cases, potentially fatal hepatosplenic T-cell lymphoma (mostly young adults with concomitant immunosuppression).

Etanercept is a p75 TNF receptor fusion protein that binds to soluble and membrane-bound TNF and lymphotoxin. Etanercept is injected twice weekly through the subcutaneous route. Efficacy is dose related, with 34% and 49% of patients receiving 25 mg and 50 mg twice weekly, respectively, achieving >75% improvement in PASI 75 response after 12 weeks of treatment.[76] Safety concerns reflect the overall immunosuppressive profile of anti-TNF agents and includes few cases with demyelination.

A novel anticytokine approach targets the members of the IL-12 superfamily (i.e., IL-12 and IL-23), heterodimeric cytokines that share a common p40 chain. An antibody targeting the common chain of IL-12 and IL-23 p40 has demonstrated efficacy in a phase II trial with at least 75% improvement in the PASI at week 12 in 52% of patients who received a single 45-mg dose and in 59% of those who received a single 90-mg dose, compared with 2% of those who received placebo.[50] This impressive clinical efficacy after a single dose needs confirmation in future phase III trials as well as safety data in a higher number of patients.

The new age of biologics has brought long-sought pathogenesis-based and effective systemic therapies to patients with psoriasis.[77] One potential concern is long-term safety issues with these novel immunosuppressive biologic interventions. The first data coming out of well-controlled registries for rheumatologic diseases do not show major new safety signals compared to other systemic treatment approaches.[78]

Future Perspectives

The increased insights related to the pathogenesis of psoriasis are accumulating at an unprecedented rate, in part due to the proof-of-principle studies that targeted immunointervention using biologic agents that have a major impact on the disease. Future trends might include (1) a focus on the skin-specific tissue environment; (2) the role of skin-resident immune effector cells and their interaction with the epithelium and the connective tissue[62]; (3) a focus on the systemic inflammatory components of psoriasis, with impacts on other organ systems including the cardiovascular system[5,7]; and (4) a focus on very early initiating of events in the pathogenesis of psoriasis,[79] and a synergistic view between advances in our genomic and immunologic understanding of the disease.[8]

Conclusion

Psoriasis is a genetically determined chronic inflammatory skin condition with typical clinical presentation. Accumulating evidence suggests an important role of the immune system in the initiation and maintenance of the disease. Fueled by the successful introduction of novel biologic therapies targeting key immunologic pathways, both the understanding of the immune system and its potential therapeutic application is becoming a central issue for dermatologists and investigative skin scientists. Recent successes in the translation of insights from the immunologic bench to the dermatologic bedside predict exciting future advances in both our immunologic understanding and immunologic therapies in psoriasis.

References

1. Lowes MA, Bowcock AM, Krueger JG. Pathogenesis and therapy of psoriasis. Nature 2007;445:866–873.
2. von Hebra F. Acute Exantheme und Hautkrankheiten. In: von Virchow, ed. Handbuch der Speciellen Pathologie und Therapie. Erlangen: Verlag von Ferdinand Enk, 1860.
3. Choi J, Koo JY. Quality of life issues in psoriasis. J Am Acad Dermatol 2003;49:S57–61.
4. Henseler T, Christophers E. Disease concomitance in psoriasis. J Am Acad Dermatol 1995;32:982–986.
5. Gelfand JM, Neimann AL, Shin DB, Wang X, Margolis DJ, Troxel AB. Risk of myocardial infarction in patients with psoriasis. JAMA 2006;296:1735–1741.
6. Neimann AL, Shin DB, Wang X, Margolis DJ, Troxel AB, Gelfand JM. Prevalence of cardiovascular risk factors in patients with psoriasis. J Am Acad Dermatol 2006;55:829–835.
7. Sommer DM, Jenisch S, Suchan M, Christophers E, Weichenthal M. Increased prevalence of the metabolic syndrome in patients with moderate to severe psoriasis. Arch Dermatol Res 2006;298:321–328.
8. Bowcock AM, Krueger JG. Getting under the skin: the immunogenetics of psoriasis. Nat Rev Immunol 2005;5:699–711.

9. Elder JT, Nair RP, Henseler T, et al. The genetics of psoriasis 2001: the odyssey continues. Arch Dermatol 2001;137:1447–1454.

10. Capon F, Munro M, Barker J, Trembath R. Searching for the major histocompatibility complex psoriasis susceptibility gene. J Invest Dermatol 2002;118: 745–751.

11. Duerr RH, Taylor KD, Brant SR, et al. A genome-wide association study identifies IL23R as an inflammatory bowel disease gene. Science 2006;314: 1461–1463.

12. Cargill M, Schrodi SJ, Chang M, et al. A large-scale genetic association study confirms IL12B and leads to the identification of IL23R as psoriasis-risk genes. Am J Hum Genet 2007;80:273–290.

13. Nestle F, Capon F, Tonel G, et al. Genetic and functional evidence for a role of the interleukin-23 pathway in the pathogenesis of psoriasis. J Invest Dermatol 2007;127:13.

14. Cookson WO, Ubhi B, Lawrence R, et al. Genetic linkage of childhood atopic dermatitis to psoriasis susceptibility loci. Nat Genet 2001;27:372–373.

15. Zhou X, Krueger JG, Kao MC, et al. Novel mechanisms of T-cell and dendritic cell activation revealed by profiling of psoriasis on the 63,100–element oligonucleotide array. Physiol Genomics 2003;13:69–78.

16. Mueller W, Herrmann B. Cyclosporin A for psoriasis. N Engl J Med 1979;301:555.

17. Ellis CN, Gorsulowsky DC, Hamilton TA, et al. Cyclosporine improves psoriasis in a double-blind study. JAMA 1986;256:3110–3116.

18. Griffiths CE, Powles AV, Leonard JN, Fry L, Baker BS, Valdimarsson H. Clearance of psoriasis with low dose cyclosporin. Br Med J (Clin Res Ed) 1986;293:731–732.

19. Menssen A, Trommler P, Vollmer S, et al. Evidence for an antigen-specific cellular immune response in skin lesions of patients with psoriasis vulgaris. J Immunol 1995;155:4078–4083.

20. Gottlieb SL, Gilleaudeau P, Johnson R, et al. Response of psoriasis to a lymphocyte-selective toxin (DAB389IL-2) suggests a primary immune, but not keratinocyte, pathogenic basis. Nat Med 1995;1:442–447.

21. Prinz J, Braun-Falco O, Meurer M, et al. Chimaeric CD4 monoclonal antibody in treatment of generalised pustular psoriasis. Lancet 1991;338:320–321.

22. Bachelez H, Flageul B, Dubertret L, et al. Treatment of recalcitrant plaque psoriasis with a humanized non-depleting antibody to CD4. J Autoimmun 1998;11:53–62.

23. Eedy DJ, Burrows D, Bridges JM, Jones FG. Clearance of severe psoriasis after allogenic bone marrow transplantation. BMJ 1990;300:908.

24. Gardembas-Pain M, Ifrah N, Foussard C, Boasson M, Saint Andre JP, Verret JL. Psoriasis after allogeneic bone marrow transplantation. Arch Dermatol 1990;126:1523.

25. Nestle FO, Nickoloff BJ. From classical mouse models of psoriasis to a spontaneous xenograft model featuring use of AGR mice. Ernst Schering Res Found Workshop 2005;203–212.

26. Braun-Falco O, Burg G. [Inflammatory infiltrate in psoriasis vulgaris. A cytochemical study]. Arch Klin Exp Dermatol 1970;236:297–314.

27. Bos JD, Hulsebosch HJ, Krieg SR, Bakker PM, Cormane RH. Immunocompetent cells in psoriasis. In situ immunophenotyping by monoclonal antibodies. Arch Dermatol Res 1983;275:181–189.

28. Baker BS, Swain AF, Fry L, Valdimarsson H. Epidermal T lymphocytes and HLA-DR expression in psoriasis. Br J Dermatol 1984;110:555–564.

29. Chang JC, Smith LR, Froning KJ, et al. CD8+ T cells in psoriatic lesions preferentially use T-cell receptor V beta 3 and/or V beta 13.1 genes. Proc Natl Acad Sci U S A 1994;91:9282–9286.

30. Gottlieb AB, Lifshitz B, Fu SM, Staiano-Coico L, Wang CY, Carter DM. Expression of HLA-DR molecules by keratinocytes, and presence of Langerhans cells in the dermal infiltrate of active psoriatic plaques. J Exp Med 1986;164:1013–1028.

31. Uyemura K, Yamamura M, Fivenson DF, Modlin RL, Nickoloff BJ. The cytokine network in lesional and lesion-free psoriatic skin is characterized by a T-helper type 1 cell-mediated response. J Invest Dermatol 1993;101:701–705.

32. Schlaak JF, Buslau M, Jochum W, et al. T cells involved in psoriasis vulgaris belong to the Th1 subset. J Invest Dermatol 1994;102:145–149.

33. Nestle FO, Turka LA, Nickoloff BJ. Characterization of dermal dendritic cells in psoriasis. Autostimulation of T lymphocytes and induction of Th1 type cytokines. J Clin Invest 1994;94:202–209.

34. Zheng Y, Danilenko DM, Valdez P, et al. Interleukin-22, a T(H)17 cytokine, mediates IL-23–induced dermal inflammation and acanthosis. Nature 2007; 445:648–651.

35. Bonish B, Jullien D, Dutronc Y, et al. Overexpression of CD1d by keratinocytes in psoriasis and CD1d-dependent IFN-gamma production by NK-T cells. J Immunol 2000;165:4076–4085.

36. Gerlini G, Hefti HP, Kleinhans M, Nickoloff BJ, Burg G, Nestle FO. Cd1d is expressed on dermal dendritic cells and monocyte-derived dendritic cells. J Invest Dermatol 2001;117:576–582.

37. Sugiyama H, Gyulai R, Toichi E, et al. Dysfunctional blood and target tissue CD4+CD25 high regulatory T cells in psoriasis: mechanism underlying unre-

strained pathogenic effector T cell proliferation. J Immunol 2005;174:164–173.

38. Baadsgaard O, Gupta AK, Taylor RS, Ellis CN, Voorhees JJ, Cooper KD. Psoriatic epidermal cells demonstrate increased numbers and function of non-Langerhans antigen-presenting cells. J Invest Dermatol 1989;92:190–195.

39. Baker BS, Griffiths CE, Lambert S, et al. The effects of cyclosporin A on T lymphocyte and dendritic cell sub-populations in psoriasis. Br J Dermatol 1987;116:503–510.

40. Chamian F, Lowes MA, Lin SL, et al. Alefacept reduces infiltrating T cells, activated dendritic cells, and inflammatory genes in psoriasis vulgaris. Proc Natl Acad Sci U S A 2005;102: 2075–2080.

41. Nickoloff BJ, Mitra RS, Green J, et al. Accessory cell function of keratinocytes for superantigens. Dependence on lymphocyte function-associated antigen-1/intercellular adhesion molecule-1 interaction. J Immunol 1993;150:2148–2159.

42. Pober JS, Kluger MS, Schechner JS. Human endothelial cell presentation of antigen and the homing of memory/effector T cells to skin. Ann N Y Acad Sci 2001;941:12–25.

43. Filer A, Raza K, Salmon M, Buckley CD. Targeting stromal cells in chronic inflammation. Discov Med 2007;7:20–26.

44. Wang H, Peters T, Kess D, et al. Activated macrophages are essential in a murine model for T cell-mediated chronic psoriasiform skin inflammation. J Clin Invest 2006;116:2105–2114.

45. Stratis A, Pasparakis M, Rupec RA, et al. Pathogenic role for skin macrophages in a mouse model of keratinocyte-induced psoriasis-like skin inflammation. J Clin Invest 2006;116:2094–2104.

46. Clark RA, Kupper TS. Misbehaving macrophages in the pathogenesis of psoriasis. J Clin Invest 2006;116:2084–2087.

47. Nickoloff BJ. The cytokine network in psoriasis. Arch Dermatol 1991;127:871–884.

48. Nickoloff BJ. Cracking the cytokine code in psoriasis. Nat Med 2007;13:242–244.

49. Lee E, Trepicchio WL, Oestreicher JL, et al. Increased expression of interleukin 23 p19 and p40 in lesional skin of patients with psoriasis vulgaris. J Exp Med 2004;199:125–130.

50. Krueger GG, Langley RG, Leonardi C, et al. A human interleukin-12/23 monoclonal antibody for the treatment of psoriasis. N Engl J Med 2007;356: 580–592.

51. Prinz JC, Vollmer S, Boehncke WH, Menssen A, Laisney I, Trommler P. Selection of conserved TCR VDJ rearrangements in chronic psoriatic plaques indicates a common antigen in psoriasis vulgaris. Eur J Immunol 1999;29:3360–3368.

52. Whyte HJ, Baughman RD. Acute guttate psoriasis and streptococcal infection. Arch Dermatol 1964;89:350–356.

53. Prinz J. Psoriasis. In: Bos J, ed. Skin Immune System. Boca Raton, FL: CRC Press, 2004;615–626.

54. Gudjonsson JE, Thorarinsson AM, Sigurgeirsson B, Kristinsson KG, Valdimarsson H. Streptococcal throat infections and exacerbation of chronic plaque psoriasis: a prospective study. Br J Dermatol 2003;149:530–534.

55. Valdimarsson H, Baker BS, Jonsdottir I, Powles A, Fry L. Psoriasis: a T-cell-mediated autoimmune disease induced by streptococcal superantigens? Immunol Today 1995;16:145–149.

56. Gudmundsdottir AS, Sigmundsdottir H, Sigurgeirsson B, Good MF, Valdimarsson H, Jonsdottir I. Is an epitope on keratin 17 a major target for autoreactive T lymphocytes in psoriasis? Clin Exp Immunol 1999;117:580–586.

57. Diluvio L, Vollmer S, Besgen P, Ellwart JW, Chimenti S, Prinz JC. Identical TCR beta-chain rearrangements in streptococcal angina and skin lesions of patients with psoriasis vulgaris. J Immunol 2006;176:7104–7111.

58. Sano S, Chan KS, Carbajal S, et al. Stat3 links activated keratinocytes and immunocytes required for development of psoriasis in a novel transgenic mouse model. Nat Med 2005;11:43–49.

59. Zenz R, Eferl R, Kenner L, et al. Psoriasis-like skin disease and arthritis caused by inducible epidermal deletion of Jun proteins. Nature 2005;437: 369–375.

60. Gaspari AA. Innate and adaptive immunity and the pathophysiology of psoriasis. J Am Acad Dermatol 2006;54:S67–80.

61. Christophers E, Parzefall R, Braun-Falco O. Initial events in psoriasis: quantitative assessment. Br J Dermatol 1973;89:327–334.

62. Boyman O, Conrad C, Tonel G, Gilliet M, Nestle FO. The pathogenic role of tissue-resident immune cells in psoriasis. Trends Immunol 2007;28: 51–57.

63. Bata-Csorgo Z, Hammerberg C, Voorhees JJ, Cooper KD. Flow cytometric identification of proliferative subpopulations within normal human epidermis and the localization of the primary hyperproliferative population in psoriasis. J Exp Med 1993;178: 1271–1281.

64. Fierlbeck G, Rassner G, Muller C. Psoriasis induced at the injection site of recombinant interferon gamma. Results of immunohistologic investigations. Arch Dermatol 1990;126:351–355.

65. Lee RE, Gaspari AA, Lotze MT, Chang AE, Rosenberg SA. Interleukin 2 and psoriasis. Arch Dermatol 1988;124:1811–1815.

66. Albanesi C, Scarponi C, Giustizieri ML, Girolomoni G. Keratinocytes in inflammatory skin diseases. Curr Drug Targets Inflamm Allergy 2005;4:329–334.

67. Lebwohl M, Tyring SK, Hamilton TK, et al. A novel targeted T-cell modulator, efalizumab, for plaque psoriasis. N Engl J Med 2003;349:2004–2013.

68. Gottlieb AB, Hamilton T, Caro I, Kwon P, Compton PG, Leonardi CL. Long-term continuous efalizumab therapy in patients with moderate to severe chronic plaque psoriasis: updated results from an ongoing trial. J Am Acad Dermatol 2006;54: S154–163.

69. Lebwohl M, Christophers E, Langley R, Ortonne JP, Roberts J, Griffiths CE. An international, randomized, double-blind, placebo-controlled phase 3 trial of intramuscular alefacept in patients with chronic plaque psoriasis. Arch Dermatol 2003;139:719–727.

70. Ellis CN, Krueger GG. Treatment of chronic plaque psoriasis by selective targeting of memory effector T lymphocytes. N Engl J Med 2001;345:248–255.

71. Gottlieb AB, Casale TB, Frankel E, et al. CD4+ T-cell-directed antibody responses are maintained in patients with psoriasis receiving alefacept: results of a randomized study. J Am Acad Dermatol 2003;49:816–825.

72. Feldmann M, Maini RN. Anti-TNF alpha therapy of rheumatoid arthritis: what have we learned? Annu Rev Immunol 2001;19:163–196.

73. LaDuca JR, Gaspari AA. Targeting tumor necrosis factor alpha. New drugs used to modulate inflammatory diseases. Dermatol Clin 2001;19:617–635.

74. Chaudhari U, Romano P, Mulcahy LD, Dooley LT, Baker DG, Gottlieb AB. Efficacy and safety of infliximab monotherapy for plaque-type psoriasis: a randomised trial. Lancet 2001;357:1842–1847.

75. Reich K, Nestle FO, Papp K, et al. Infliximab induction and maintenance therapy for moderate-to-severe psoriasis: a phase III, multicentre, double-blind trial. Lancet 2005;366:1367–1374.

76. Leonardi CL, Powers JL, Matheson RT, et al. Etanercept as monotherapy in patients with psoriasis. N Engl J Med 2003;349:2014–2022.

77. Smith CH, Barker JN. Psoriasis and its management. BMJ 2006;333:380–384.

78. Dixon WG, Watson K, Lunt M, Hyrich KL, Silman AJ, Symmons DP. Rates of serious infection, including site-specific and bacterial intracellular infection, in rheumatoid arthritis patients receiving anti-tumor necrosis factor therapy: results from the British Society for Rheumatology Biologics Register. Arthritis Rheum 2006;54:2368–2376.

79. Nestle FO, Conrad C, Tun-Kyi A, et al. Plasmacytoid predendritic cells initiate psoriasis through interferon-alpha production. J Exp Med 2005;202:135–143.

15
The Immunology of Acne

Guy F. Webster and Jenny Kim

Key Points

- Acne is a complex disease with multiple pathogenic factors.
- *Propionibacterium acnes* is the trigger for inflammatory acne.
- There is no suitable animal model for acne.

Acne is a complex disease with multiple pathogenic factors that act together to produce disease.[1] Dystrophic keratinization is involved in the formation of the plug in the follicle (comedo or microcomedo) that is the central lesion of acne. Hormonal stimulation of the sebaceous gland occurs at puberty, which causes production of sebum, a complex mixture of lipids that is about 50% triglycerides. Triglycerides are a rich carbon source for lipase producing bacteria and are a powerful determinant of the skin microflora.[2] *Propionibacterium acnes*, an anaerobic diphtheroid, dominates the follicular microflora after puberty and is the trigger for inflammatory acne. The study of acne pathogenesis has been hampered by the lack of a suitable animal model. Although animals can be induced to have keratinous impactions in the follicles, they cannot be induced to have inflammatory lesions since animal sebum lacks triglycerides and *P. acnes* will not colonize the follicle.[3]

Early attempts to explain inflammation in acne were based on studies of sebum composition in acne patients. Free fatty acids were found to be elevated in skin surface lipid from patients with inflammatory acne. These were derived from lipolysis of triglycerides and were suggested to be a trigger for inflammation in acne. In addition, therapy that reduced "pimples," such as tetracy-cline, reduced the free fatty acids to normal levels, apparent confirmation that the fatty acids were central to acne inflammation. Later work showed that the lipid fraction of microcomedones was not inflammatory and that only the *P. acnes*–containing fractions induced inflammation when injected intradermally. Free fatty acids were found to be the result of *P. acnes*' metabolism and to be present in proportion to the bacterial population rather than being a facet of aberrant sebaceous gland function, and more attention began to be paid to the role of the organism itself in acne. This was not a new thought; Unna, Sabouraud, and Fleming all speculated on the possibility that the "acne bacillus" was involved in acne. Fleming went so far as to demonstrate increased agglutination of the organism by sera from acne patients, but the idea lapsed until the mid-1970s, when investigative techniques caught up with researchers' needs (reviewed by Webster[4]).

Propionibacterium Acnes and Acne

Propionibacterium acnes is the predominant organism living on sebaceous regions of the skin. An aerotolerant anaerobe, *P. acnes* grows in the sebaceous follicle and is carried onto the skin surface by the flow of sebum. It lives from metabolizing the triglyceride fraction of sebum and hence is absent or low in children, but rises rapidly at puberty when androgens stimulate the start of sebum secretion acne.[5]

Puhvel and Sakamoto[6] studied the contents of comedones in vitro and found that comedonal material attracted human neutrophils. The attractant was water soluble and of low molecular weight. A similar factor was detected in the supernatant of *P. acnes* cultures. Lee et al.[7] found that *P. acnes* also produced higher molecular weight chemotactic factors, one of which was the lipase molecule itself. Subsequent studies found that *P. acnes* may simultaneously produce both high- and low-molecular-weight chemoattractants, and that the majority of neutrophil chemotactic activity in *P. acnes* culture supernatant was less than 2 kd. The amount of chemotactic material produced was proportional to the *P. acnes* population and is of a molecular weight that might conceivably diffuse from an intact follicle.[8] The comedo may also contain other inflammatory factors. Allaker et al.[9] showed that *P. acnes* produces compounds that have histamine-like activity, and Hellgren and Vincent[10] demonstrated prostaglandin like activity in *P. acnes* culture supernatants. Ingham et al.[11] found significant levels of interleukin (IL)-1 like activity and tumor necrosis factor (TNF)-like molecules in a majority of open comedones.

Once neutrophils arrive at the comedo, gross rupture of follicular epithelium may be caused by enzymatic digestion of the follicular wall by neutrophil lysosomal hydrolytic enzymes. In vitro studies have shown that neutrophils readily secrete their degradative enzymes extracellularly when exposed to *P. acnes* that has been opsonized by C3b or immunoglobulin. Release of hydrolases is greatest when the anti–*P. acnes* antibody titer is elevated.[12] These degradative lysosomal enzymes are capable of digesting tissue and may promote further comedonal rupture. Finally, *P. acnes* itself also elaborates proteases and other degradative enzymes, which may also play some part in comedonal rupture.

After exposure of comedonal contents to the immune system, a clinically detectable inflammation may result. The magnitude of the response is variable. Small, superficial papulopustules or deep nodules may develop. Complement deposition has been demonstrated in both early and late acne lesions, suggesting at least one means by which inflammation may be promoted. *P. acnes* is thought to be the cause of this deposition because the organism is a potent activator of both the classic and alternative complement pathways. The alternative pathway is triggered by *P. acnes* cell wall carbohydrate and the classic pathway by *P. acnes*-antibody complexes, and is activated in proportion to the antibody titer.[13,14] Crude comedonal material also activates complement by the classic and alternative pathways, and this activation is also stimulated by anti–*P. acnes* antibody.[15] Finally, *P. acnes* is a persistent stimulus, being only degraded and removed over many weeks.[16]

Propionibacterium acnes can also induce inflammatory response by activating other innate immune cells, such as monocytes/macrophages. Volwels et al. demonstrated that *P. acnes* induces proinflammatory cytokine production in monocytes, although the exact mechanism by which this occurs was not known.[16] Recently, with the discovery of the Toll-like receptors (TLRs), we have a better understanding of how innate immune cells respond to microbes and how this leads to immune response.

The innate immune response in the skin is composed of both the physical barriers provided by skin and mucosa as well as rapid cellular responses provided by epithelial cells, dendritic cells, monocytes, natural killer cells, and granulocytes. These cells express pattern recognition receptors (PRRs), such as the human TLRs, which are transmembrane proteins capable of mediating responses to pathogen-associated molecular patterns (PAMPs) conserved among microorganisms. The extracellular portion of TLRs is composed of leucine-rich repeats while the intracellular portion shares homology with the cytoplasmic domain of the IL-1 receptor. When TLRs are activated by exposure to microbial ligands, the intracellular domain of the TLR may trigger a MyD88-dependent pathway involving factors such as IL-1 receptor-associated kinase (IRAK) and tumor necrosis factor receptor-activated factor 6 (TRAF6) that ultimately lead to the nuclear translocation of the transcription nuclear factor κB (NF-κB); NF-κB then modulates expression of many immune response genes.[17-19] In some microbial activation of TLR, MyD88-independent pathways may be triggered.

Currently, 10 TLRs have been identified in humans. The microbial ligands for many of these receptors have been identified and include bacterial cell wall components and genetic material. More specifically, TLR2 mediates host responses to peptidoglycan from gram-positive bacteria, TLR4 mediates responses to bacterial lipopolysaccharide (LPS) from gram-negative bacteria, TLR5 is activated by bacterial flagellin,[20–22] and TLR9 mediates the response to the unmethylated Cytosine Guanine dinucleotide (CpG) DNA comprising bacterial genomes. Viral products such as double-stranded RNA activate TLR3.[23,24] In addition, imiquimod, an immunomodulatory agent commonly used in dermatology, has been shown to activate TLR7.[24]

Kim et al.[25] demonstrated that *P. acnes* contains a TLR2 ligand and that *P. acnes* activates human monocytes to secrete proinflammatory cytokines, including IL-12 and IL-8 via a TLR2-dependent mechanism. The TLR2-dependent production of IL-8 may be important in the pathogenesis of acne, as it is a known neutrophil chemoattractant, and neutrophils contribute to the formation of inflammatory lesions. The production of IL-12, a key regulator of adaptive immune response, may be important in generating a cell-mediated immune response to *P. acnes*. The importance of TLR-mediated immune response in the pathogenesis of acne was further supported by the in vivo finding that TLR2-expressing cells were present in increased numbers in inflammatory acne lesions.[25] In addition, recent studies have suggested that matrix metalloproteinases (MMPs) play a role in inducing inflammation and scar formation in acne.[26,27] *P. acnes* induces MMP-1 and MMP-9, and MMP-9 production in human monocytes was shown to be through a TLR2-dependent mechanism (R. Jalian et al., American Academy of Dermatology poster presentation, 2007). Furthermore, it was shown that the addition of all-*trans* retinoic acid (ATRA), a commonly used agent for the treatment of acne, inhibits MMP production and upregulates MMP regulators and tissue inhibitors of metalloproteinases (TIMPs), thus shifting from a tissue-degrading phenotype to tissue-preserving phenotype.

Another outcome of TLR activation is the triggering of direct antimicrobial pathways, inducing release of nonspecific antibacterial molecules such as antimicrobial peptides. Studies have shown upregulation of human β-defensin-1 and -2 in acne lesions compared to controls to suggest that β-defensins may be part of the host defense in acne.[28,29] Recent data suggest that the production of antimicrobial peptides induced by *P. acnes* in innate cells appears to be TLR2-dependent.[30] Since antimicrobial peptides are known to

have immunomodulatory effects, including both antiinflammatory and proinflammatory responses, whether the antimicrobial peptides modulate the inflammatory response found in acne in addition to eliciting a direct antimicrobial effect against *P. acnes* remains to be determined.

Interestingly, there is evidence that the same mechanism that bacteria utilize to induce inflammation and contribute to the disease state is also used in host defense. *P. acnes* activation of TLR2 appears to induce peripheral monocytes to differentiate into at least two different subsets of cells including CD1b+ dendritic cells and CD209+ macrophages. Although both cells induce cytokine production in response to *P. acnes*, it was shown that CD209+ macrophages efficiently take up the bacteria and induce the killing of *P. acnes;* thus CD209+ innate cells directly regulate the growth of pathogens.[31] Furthermore, the addition of ATRA directly induced differentiation of monocytes into CD209+ macrophages, and enhanced the *P. acnes*–mediated differentiation of the CD209+ subset. These data imply that ATRA can enhance the innate immune response, by expanding the CD209+ cell population that has the ability to phagocytose and inhibit the growth of microbial pathogens.

Explaining the Variation in Acne Severity

After puberty, most individuals have stable *P. acnes* populations, some degree of microcomedo formation and significant sebum secretion, yet only some have inflammatory acne, and only a proportion of those have severe disease. In fact, when specific factors (e.g., sebum secretion, fatty acid concentration, or *P. acnes* populations) are compared in patients with and without acne, clear differences may be difficult to detect. In each category the acne population as a group is higher than the normal group, but great overlap exists in the range of values in each cohort (e.g., some persons have minimal or no acne, but high sebum production and some with acne have lower values), which suggests that each of these important factors is involved in, but is not the determining cause of inflammatory acne (reviewed by Webster[32]).

A second observation to be accounted for is that in severe inflammatory acne almost all lesions arise from microcomedones, whereas larger comedones in patients with noninflammatory acne become clinically inflamed only rarely yet show histologic evidence of previous subclinical inflammatory episodes.[1] Likewise, clinically uninflamed microcomedones from persons with no apparent acne contain neutrophil markers suggesting earlier, limited inflammatory episodes that were not sufficiently severe to produce a clinical lesion.[33]

Finally, the familial association of severe acne must be explained. The observation that severe acne is familial has been made by most clinicians, but there are few studies. Conglobate acne and hidradenitis may have autosomal dominant single-gene inheritance, and several reports have been published of acne of similar severity in monozygotic twins.[34–37] Thus factors favoring the development of severe acne may be genetically determined.

An explanation that accounts for all these observations centers on differing individual reactivity to P. acnes. There is support for this concept. In vitro studies found P. acnes to generate greater complement activation and lysosomal enzyme release in the presence of anti–P. acnes antibodies.[38] Patients with acne have elevated precipitating, agglutinating, and complement-fixing antibody titers to P. acnes but not to other organisms.[39–42] The antibody titers increase in proportion to the severity of acne inflammation, with little or no overlap between the normal and most severe acne groups.

Some studies have addressed the identity of the P. acnes antigens potentially relevant to acne. One study found that the anti–P. acnes antibody response in a group of patients with severe nodular acne was apparently uniform, directed against a carbohydrate structure in the cell wall.[39] Of all the potential protein and carbohydrate antigens present in the P. acnes to which they were exposed, these patients appeared to hyperrespond to a single antigen. This reactivity was not detected in patients with less severe acne, and the mechanism by which it occurs has not been elucidated. Ingham et al.[43] have made a complementary observation.

Cell-mediated immunity to P. acnes is also increased in proportion to acne severity. P. acnes–stimulated lymphocyte transformation is elevated in mononuclear cells from inflammatory acne patients, and skin test reactivity to P. acnes is elevated in proportion to the severity of acne inflammation.[44,45] Wilcox et al.[46] recently studied the cellular responses in acne lesions from patients prone to scarring and those not likely to scar. They found that nonscarring patients had a greater initial influx of lymphocytes than the scarring patients, but the scarring patients had a much greater proportion of memory-effector cells, implying that the more severe acne patient has an immunologic predisposition to severity.

Conclusion

Acne is a complex disease with multiple pathogenic factors. The trigger for inflammation is P. acnes. Although there is no suitable animal model for acne, understanding of the immunology of acne has advanced from clinical studies and in vitro investigations.

References

1. Kligman AM. An overview of acne. J Invest Dermatol 1974;62:268–287.
2. McGinley KJ, Webster GF, Ruggieri MR, Leyden JJ. Regional variations of cutaneous propionibacteria, correlation of Propionibacterium acnes populations with sebaceous secretion. J Clin Microbiol 1980;12:672–675.
3. Webster GF, Ruggieri MR, McGinley KJ. Correlation of Propionibacterium acnes populations with the presence of triglycerides on non-human skin. Appl Environ Microbiol 1981;41:1269–1270.
4. Webster GF. Acne. Curr Prob Dermatol 1996;8: 240–262.
5. Marples RR, McGinley KJ. Corynebacterium acnes and other anaerobic diphtheroids from human skin. J Med Microbiol 1974;7:349–61.
6. Puhvel SM, Sakamoto M, Cytotaxin production by comedonal bacteria. J Invest Dermatol 1978;71: 324–329.
7. Lee WL, Shalita AR, Sunthralingam K. Neutrophil chemotaxis to P. acnes lipase and its inhibition. Infect Immun 1982;35:71–78.
8. Webster GF, Leyden JJ, Tsai C-C. Characterization of serum independent polymorphonuclear leukocyte chemotactic factors produced by Propionibacterium acnes. Inflammation 1980;4:261–271.
9. Allaker RP, Greenman J, Osborne RH. The production of inflammatory compounds by Propionibacterium

acnes and other skin organisms. Br J Dermatol 1987;117(2):175–83.

10. Hellgren L, Vincent J. New group of prostaglandin-like compounds in P. acnes. Gen Pharmacol 1983;14(1):207–8.

11. Ingham E, Eady EA, Goodwin CE, Cove JH, Cunliffe WJ. Pro-inflammatory levels of interleukin-1 alpha-like bioactivity are present in the majority of open comedones in acne vulgaris. J Invest Dermatol 1992;98(6):895–901.

12. Webster GF, Leyden JJ, Tsai CC, Baehni P, McArthur WP. Polymorphonuclear leukocyte lysosomal release in response to Propionibacterium acnes in vitro and its enhancement by sera from inflammatory acne patients. J Invest Dermatol 1980;74(6):398–401.

13. Webster GF, Nilsson UR, McArthur WR, Activation of the alternative pathway of complement by *Propionibacterium acnes* cell fractions. Inflammation 1981;5:165–176.

14. Webster GF, McArthur WR. Activation of components of the alternative pathway of complement by *Propionibacterium acnes* cell wall carbohydrate. J Invest Dermatol 1982;79:137–140.

15. Webster GF, Leyden JJ, Musson RA, Douglas SD. Susceptibility of *Propionibacterium acnes* to killing and degradation by human monocytes and neutrophils in vitro. Infect Immun 1985;49:116–121,

16. Vowels BR, Yang S, Leyden JJ. Induction of proinflammatory cytokines by a soluble factor of Propionibacterium acnes: implications for chronic inflammatory acne. Infect Immun 1995;63:3158–3165.

17. Suzuki S, Duncan GS, et al. Severe impairment of interleukin-1 and Toll-like receptor signalling in mice lacking IRAK-4. Nature 2002;416:750–756.

18. Takeda K, Kaisho T, Akira S. Toll-like receptors. Annu Rev Immunol 2003;21:335–376.

19. Poltorak A, He X, Smirnova I, et al. Defective LPS signaling in C3H/HeJ and C57BL/10ScCr mice: mutations in Tlr4 gene. Science 1998;282:2085–2088.

20. Yoshimura A, Lien E, Ingalls RR, et al. Recognition of Gram-positive bacterial cell wall components by the innate immune system occurs via Toll-like receptor 2. J Immunol 1999;163:1–5.

21. Hayashi F, Smith KD, Ozinsky A, et al. The innate immune response to bacterial flagellin is mediated by Toll-like receptor 5. Nature 2001;410:1099–1103.

22. Hemmi H, Takeuchi O, Kawai T, et al. A Toll-like receptor that recognizes bacterial DNA. Nature 2000;408:740–745.

23. Alexopoulou L, Holt AC, Medzhitov R, et al. Recognition of double-stranded RNA and activation of NF-kappaB by Toll-like receptor 3. Nature 2001;413:732–738.

24. Hemmi H, Kaisho T, Takeuchi O, et al. Small anti-viral compounds activate immune cells via the TLR7 MyD88–dependent signaling pathway. Nature Immunol 2002;3:196–200.

25. Kim J, Ochoa MT, Krutzik SR, et al. Activation of toll-like receptor 2 in acne triggers inflammatory cytokine responses. J Immunol 2002;169:1535–1541.

26. Trivedi NR, Gilliland KL, Zhao W, et al. Gene array expression profiling in acne lesions reveals marked upregulation of genes involved in inflammation and matrix remodeling. J Invest Dermatol 2006;126:1071–1079.

27. Kang S, Chung JH, Hammerberg C, et al. Inflammation and extracellular matrix degradation mediated by activated transcription factors nuclear factor-kappaB and activator protein-1 in inflammatory acne lesions in vivo. Am J Pathol 2005;166:1691–1699.

28. Philpott MP. Defensins and acne. Mol Immunol 2003;40:457–462.

29. Scott MG, Davidson DJ, Gold MR, et al. The human antimicrobial peptide LL-37 is a multifunctional modulator of innate immune responses. J Immunol 2002;169:3883–3891.

30. Phan J, Liu P Krutzik SR, et al. *Propionibacterium acnes* differentiates monocytes into CD209+ monocytes and CD1b+ dendritic cells. J Invest Dermatol 2006;126:124.

31. Liu PT, Phan J, Tang D, Kanchanapoomi M, Hall B, Krutzik SR, Kim J. CD209(+) macrophages mediate host defense against Propionibacterium aches. J Immunol 2008;180(7):4919–23.

32. Webster GF. Inflammation in acne vulgaris. J Am Acad Dermatol 1995;33(2 pt 1):247–53.

33. Webster GF, Kligman AM. A method for the assay of inflammatory mediators in follicular casts. J Invest Dermatol 1979;73(4):266–8.

34. Tosti A, Guerra L, Bettoli V, et al. Solid facial edema as a complication of acne in twins. J Am Acad Dermatol 1987;17:843–844.

35. Fitzsimmins JS, Guilbert PR. A family study of hidradinitis suppurativa. J Med Gen 1985;22:367–373.

36. Fitzsimmons JS, Fitzsimmons EM, Gilbert G. Familial hidradenitis suppurativa: evidence in favour of single gene transmission. J Med Genet 1984;21(4):281–5.

37. Quintal D, Jackson R. Aggressive squamous cell carcinoma arising in familial acne conglobata. J Am Acad Dermatol 1986;14:207–214.

38. Webster GF, Leyden JJ, Norman ME, Nilsson UR. Complement activation in acne vulgaris: in vitro studies with Propionibacterium acnes and Propionibacterium granulosum. Infect Immun 1978;22(2):523–9.

39. Webster GF, Indrisano JP, Leyden JJ. Antibody titers to Propionibacterium acnes cell wall carbohydrate

in nodulocystic acne patients. J Invest Dermatol 1985;84(6):496–500.

40. Puhvel SM, Hoffman IK, Sternberg TH. Corynebacterium acnes. Presence of complement fixing antibodies to Corynebacterium acnes in the sera of patients with acne vulgaris. Arch Dermatol 1966;93(3):364–6.

41. Puhvel SM, Barfatani M, Warnick M, Sternberg TH. Study of antibody levels to C. acnes in the serum of acne patients. Arch Dermatol 1964;90:421–7.

42. Ashbee HR, Muir SR, Cunliffe WJ, Ingham E. IgG subclasses specific to Staphylococcus epidermidis and Propionibacterium acnes in patients with acne vulgaris. Br J Dermatol 1997;136(5):730–3.

43. Ingham E, Gowland G, Ward RM, Holland KT, Cunliffe WJ. Antibodies to P. acnes and P. acnes exocellular enzymes in the normal population at various ages and in patients with acne vulgaris. Br J Dermatol 1987;116(6):805–12.

44. Puhvel SM, Amirian D, Weintraub J, Reisner RM. Lymphocyte transformation in subjects with nodulocystic acne. Br J Dermatol 1977;97(2):205–11.

45. Puhvel SM, Hoffman IK, Reisner RM, Sternberg TH. Dermal hypersensitivity of patients with acne vulgaris to Corynebacterium acnes. J Invest Dermatol 1967;49(2):154–8.

46. Wilcox HE, Farrar MD, Cunliffe WJ, Holland KT, Ingham E. Resolution of inflammatory acne vulgaris may involve regulation of CD4+ T-cell responses to Propionibacterium acnes. Br J Dermatol 2007;156(3):460–5.

16
Nonmelanoma Skin Cancer

Fergal J. Moloney and Gary M. Halliday

Key Points

- Nonmelanoma skin cancers (NMSCs) usually include basal cell carcinoma and squamous cell carcinoma, but can also include rare cancers such as Merkel cell carcinoma.
- Sunlight (and other sources of ultraviolet light) is the primary risk factor for NMSC.
- Immunosuppression increases the risk of NMSC.
- Human papillomaviruses are a major cause of NMSC in the anogenital area and may play a role elsewhere on the skin.
- Cell-mediated immunity helps protect against NMSC.
- Therapy of NMSC usually involves surgery, but can also include photodynamic therapy and immune response modifiers (e.g., imiquimod).
- The optimal management of NMSC should always start with prevention.

Nonmelanoma skin cancer (NMSC), basal cell carcinoma (BCC), and squamous cell carcinoma (SCC) are malignant proliferations of the same cell type, the keratinocyte. Most occur on sun-damaged skin, indicating the causal relationship with exposure to ultraviolet radiation (UVR). The BCCs arise de novo from cells in the basal layer of the epidermis or follicular structures; however, SCCs can arise from noninvasive precursor lesions of Bowen's disease and actinic keratosis (AK). While an aberrant sonic hedgehog pathway is strongly associated with BCC development, the genotypic associations with SCC are more complex with incremental levels of genomic instability related to clinicopathological stage.[1,2] This chapter outlines the role of the immune system in the pathogenesis, prevention, and treatment of NMSC, and examines how tumor development and progression is enhanced when normal immunosurveillance is compromised.

Types of Nonmelanoma Skin Cancer

Basal Cell Carcinoma

Basal cell carcinoma occurs more commonly than SCC, with a number of clinical presentations including nodular, cystic, ulcerated, superficial (Fig. 16.1), morpheic (sclerosing), keratotic, and pigmented variants. Clinical subtypes correlate well with histologic findings, which aid classification of subtypes as low or high risk. The high-risk subtype is characterized by an increased probability of subclinical extension, incomplete excision, aggressive local invasive behavior, or local recurrence.[3] Nodular BCC is the main low-risk subtype. High-risk BCCs include infiltrative, morpheic, and micronodular subtypes. Basal cell carcinomas can invade local structures but rarely metastasize. Basal cell carcinoma tumor cells typically have large oval darkly staining nuclei and little cytoplasm. Tumor cells aggregate into nests of varying size, aligning more densely at the edges to produce the characteristic peripheral palisading. The presence of mitotic figures is associated with a more aggressive course.

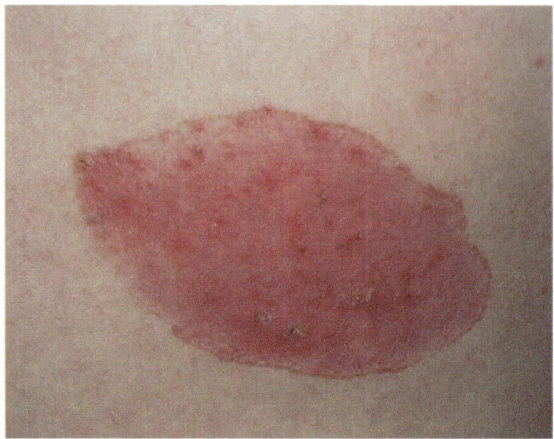

FIG. 16.1. Superficial basal cell carcinoma on the back of a 40-year-old man. The diagnosis, suggested by the slightly raised pearled margin, was confirmed histologically

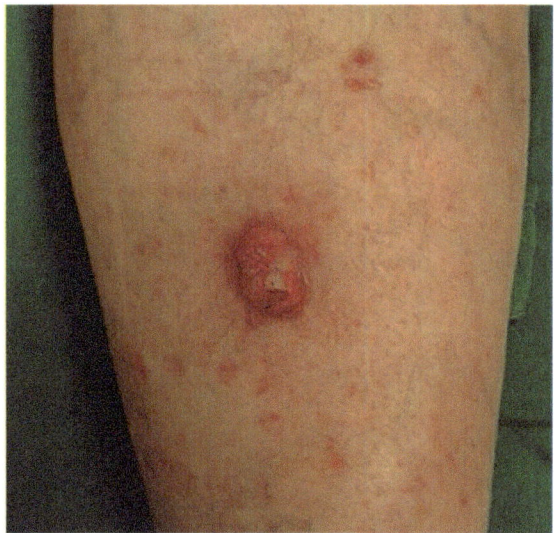

FIG. 16.2. Squamous cell carcinoma. Keratotic indurated nodule on the anterior shin of a 62-year-old woman

Squamous Cell Carcinoma

Squamous cell carcinoma presentation varies from an indurated keratotic papule or nodule (Fig. 16.2), to a crusted tumor that may ulcerate, to an ulcer without evidence of keratinization. Squamous cell carcinoma invades locally with the potential to metastasize to other organs of the body. The diagnosis is established histologically by demonstrating the extension of atypical keratinocytes beyond the dermoepidermal junction into the dermis. The grading of SCC is based on the degree of cellular differentiation; however, other variables that influence recurrence and metastatic potential include site and size of the tumor, perineural involvement, other precipitating factors such as chronic arsenic ingestion, and host immunosuppression.[4] Actinic keratosis and invasive SCC share histopathologic features and genetic tumor markers.[5] Nearly all SCCs contain histopathologic changes of AK at the periphery or within the confines of the SCC. The percentage of AKs that progress to invasive SCC and the percentage that regress spontaneously or with prolonged photoprotection remain poorly defined.[6]

Merkel Cell Carcinoma/Kaposi's Sarcoma

While a detailed discussion of other skin malignancies is beyond the scope of this chapter, we briefly consider two other less common skin cancers in which the immune system plays an important role. Kaposi's sarcoma (KS) is a spindle-cell tumor thought to be derived from endothelial cell lineage that develops in the presence of human herpesvirus 8 (HHV-8), the incidence of KS paralleling HHV-8 seroprevalence.[7] Merkel cell carcinoma is an uncommon tumor of the skin. It displays neuroendocrine features shared by normal epidermal Merkel cells and is diagnosed mostly on histologic examination. The relative risk of both tumors is markedly increased in the setting of immunosuppression secondary to HIV infection or organ transplantation. Merkel cell carcinoma behaves aggressively with a high metastatic potential particularly in an immunosuppressed setting where wide resection with nodal dissections is often required.[8] Changing the immune environment either by reducing immunosuppression therapy or changing to newer agents with potential antineoplastic properties can result in regression of Kaposi's sarcoma in immunocompromised transplant recipients.[9]

Sunlight and Nonmelanoma Skin Cancer

Sunlight is the main cause of skin cancer in humans.[10] Ultraviolet radiation is most likely the region within sunlight responsible for skin carcinogenesis, as these wavebands are able to cause both gene mutations and immunosuppression, which are the important biologic events that lead to skin cancer. However, a role for the longer visible wavelengths cannot be discounted. Ultraviolet radiation that reaches the surface of the earth from the sun is divided into two wavebands, UVB (290–320 nm) and UVA (320–400 nm), with visible light being at longer wavelengths. The shorter wavelength UVC does not reach the surface of the earth as it is absorbed or reflected by the ozone layer and the atmosphere.

Shorter wavelengths have higher energy levels per photon, and therefore UVB contains more energy than UVA. However, the amount of damage to the skin is also dependent on intensity within sunlight, penetration of the skin, and the chromophores for that particular wavelength. As UVR penetrates the skin, UVB is attenuated more than UVA with increasing depth, so that UVA penetrates deeper than UVB into the skin[11] where it can reach chromophores too deep for UVB to affect. As it is five times more likely that UVA than UVB will penetrate the epidermis to the dermis, and UVA is about 20 times more abundant in sunlight than UVB (depending on time of day and latitude), it has been estimated that 100 times more UVA than UVB photons reach the deeper regions of the skin.[12] Also, while the chromophore, or molecule that directly absorbs UVB, is accepted as being DNA, the chromophore for UVA is unknown. The chromophore not only absorbs the UVR, but also may pass the energy to other cellular molecules; it is therefore the first step in the damage process. Depth of the chromophores within the skin, and associations with other molecules are important issues with regard to the damage caused. Considering all of these issues, the relative roles of UVA and UVB in human skin carcinogenesis cannot be predicted and is an important issue when devising preventative strategies. Small animal models, which have thinner skin than humans, and may lack important chromophores or contain different levels or localization of protective mechanisms also, cannot be used to determine whether UVA or UVB causes human skin carcinogenesis. Hence, at present, while we can be convinced that sunlight causes skin cancer, the responsible wavebands are not yet known.

Ultraviolet radiation can cause gene mutations. Skin cancer, like other cancers, is fundamentally a disease resulting from deregulation of cell cycle control or differentiation, and this is largely due to mutations or epigenetic changes in genes that control these functions in cells. Ultraviolet B is directly absorbed by DNA, forming photolesions. These are essentially damaged DNA and are frequently repaired by a range of enzymes. If a cell divides prior to DNA repair, then the damaged nucleotides are not correctly recognized by the cell's replicative machinery, so that an incorrect nucleotide is incorporated into the newly synthesised DNA. This is a mutation. Alternatively UVB can result in misincorporation of an additional nucleotide, or deletion, or strand breaks. All of these forms of DNA damage, if they occur in a gene that is important for regulation of keratinocyte growth or differentiation, can be a step toward forming an NMSC.

Ultraviolet B absorbed by two adjacent cytosine (C) residues in DNA causes the formation of cyclobutane pyrimidine dimers (CPDs), which results in GC to AT mutations.[13,14] It has been widely thought that these only occur in response to UVB; however, recently it has been demonstrated that UVA can also cause this type of photolesion.[15] The major damage to DNA induced by UVA is the oxidation of guanine.[16,17] However, UVR can also cause a wide range of different mutations.[18]

In a recent study of microdissected human AK and SCC, it was shown that both of these NMSCs contain mutations in the *p53* gene. Based on the pattern of the mutations, it appears that UVA and UVB make similar contributions toward the level of mutational burden in these tumors.[19,20] However, the UVA-associated mutations were deeper in the tumors than the UVB-associated mutations, indicating that the issues raised above such as chromophore localization, depth of UV penetration, and probably localization of repair systems are important in the type and localization of mutations within human NMSC. Ultraviolet A has also been shown to cause malignant transformation of a human keratinocyte cell line.[21] Therefore, both wavebands are able to cause the essential features of skin cancer development. A more direct indication that UVA and UVB make similar contributions to the formation of NMSC in humans came from a study of human skin grafted into immunodeficient mice. Actinic keratosis developed on 10% of grafts exposed to UVB and 18% of grafts exposed to

UVB and UVA,[22] suggesting that UVA and UVB make approximately equal contributions to formation of human NMSC.

Both UVB and UVA are also immunosuppressive in humans. Irradiation with approximately half the amount of UVA present in a minimum erythema dose (MED) of sunlight suppresses recall immunity to nickel in humans.[23] An MED is the amount of sunlight required to cause barely perceptible sunburn. Another study found UVA, like UVB, to suppress memory immunity to the multitest kit Merieux, which is a delayed-type hypersensitivity (DTH) test to seven antigens to which humans are commonly exposed.[24,25] It has also been shown that a UV spectrum designed to mimic sunlight induced a greater level of immunosuppression than that provoked by UVB or UVA.[23,26] Therefore, interactions between UVB and UVA make sunlight more suppressive than either waveband alone.

While it is clear that both UVB and UVA are immunosuppressive in humans, direct evidence that this is important for NMSC induction and progression can only come from animal studies. Ultraviolet radiation immunosuppression enhances the outgrowth of primary skin cancer. Lymphocytes from UV-irradiated mice transferred into unirradiated mice enable the development of primary skin cancers on UV-irradiated skin grafts.[27] Ultraviolet immunosuppression also enables the growth of transplanted skin tumor lines, including SCC, that would be immunologically rejected in immunocompetent, unirradiated mice.[28,29]

Considering all of these issues, it appears likely that both UVB and UVA wavebands within sunlight cause NMSC in humans, by inducing genetic modifications, cellular transformation, and immunosuppression. It is therefore important to protect from both UVB and UVA.

Induction of Immunity to Skin Cancer

Cell-mediated immunity in the skin begins with skin localized dendritic cells (DCs). Like other cells of the immune system, they are produced in the bone marrow, and from here they populate other organs, including the skin, as immature DCs. When they localize to the epidermis, they are called Langerhans' cells (LCs), named after Paul

Langerhans, who was the first to observe them in the epidermis. Dendritic cells that localize to the dermis are called dermal DCs. They usually sit in the skin and only cycle slowly to the draining lymph nodes. Under conditions of stress or damage to the skin, such as wounding or death of neighboring cells, or the recognition by the DCs of a range of different factors commonly produced by invading pathogens, the DCs migrate from the skin to draining lymph nodes (Fig. 16.3). During this process they differentiate into mature DCs. They then present any antigen they encountered in the skin to T lymphocytes within the draining lymph node, resulting in their activation. This antigen presentation is likely to be a complex issue, involving the recruitment of lymph node DCs to which antigen is passed, and interactions with multiple T-cell types.[30,31]

During this process of T-cell activation, the lymph node undergoes shutdown, whereby cells are unable to leave the lymph node but are still allowed to enter. This leads to an accumulation of T cells in this lymph node in order to increase the number of antigen-reactive lymphocytes at this location. There is then a complex interplay between different populations of T cells, including CD4 and CD8 T cells, resulting in massive clonal expansion and activation of antigen-specific T cells. These effector T cells then migrate into the skin, where they will attempt to destroy the tumor cells expressing the antigen to which they have been activated. Activated T cells will also migrate to other lymph nodes to disseminate the immune response throughout the body, or differentiate into memory lymphocytes that can react more rapidly to further encounters with the same antigen.[32–34]

Risk Factors for Nonmelanoma Skin Cancer

Analysis of known risk factors for NMSC further demonstrates the role of UVR and immune status in skin cancer pathogenesis. Both SCC and BCC are strongly associated with increasing age; however, SCC incidence increases more rapidly with age than does BCC incidence.[35] The higher risk of skin cancer with age is contributed to by a number of factors: increased cumulative UVR exposure,[36] an accumulation of cell clones with cancer predisposing muta-

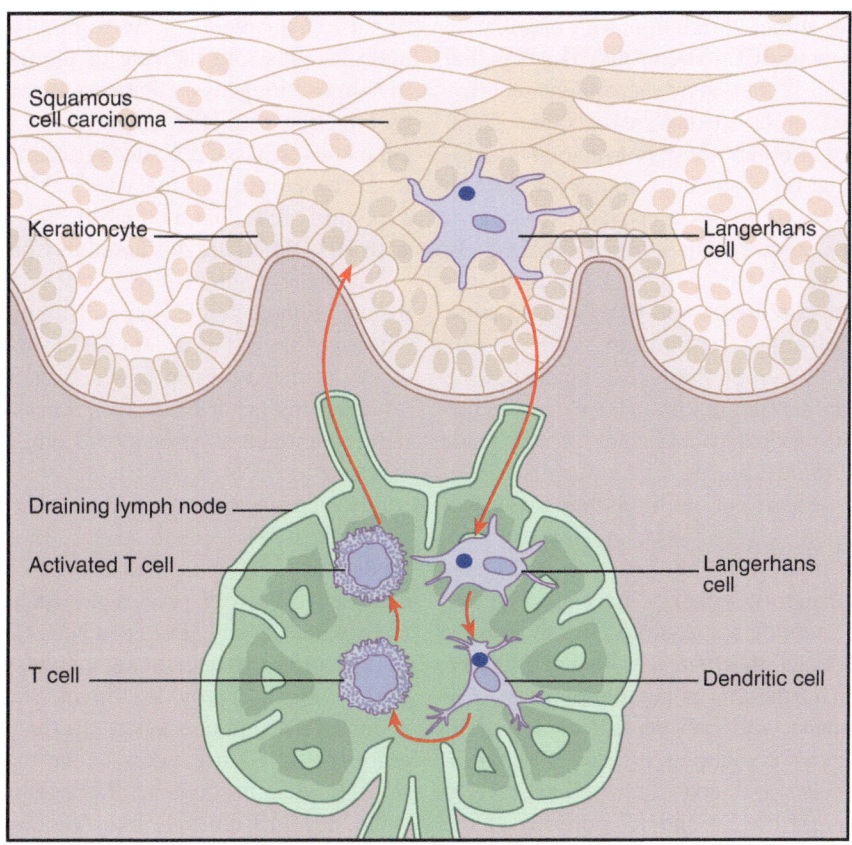

No apostrophe on Langerhans as he had an 's' on the end

Fig. 16.3. The induction of immunity to skin tumors. The epidermis consists primarily of keratinocytes (K), with basal keratinocytes sitting on the basement membrane (brown line). Keratinocytes may transform into a skin tumor such as a squamous cell carcinoma (SCC). Langerhans' cells (LCs) within the epidermis, or infiltrating the SCC, are phagocytic and they sample neighboring material, including segments of SCC (blue circle within LC). Upon activation, LCs, with phagocytosed antigen, migrate from the skin or tumor, to draining lymph nodes via dermal lymphatics. During migration they mature and present the antigen on their surface in association with major histocompatibility complex (MHC) I and II molecules. Antigen may also be passed to lymph node resident dendritic cells (DCs). These dendritic cells then interact with T lymphocytes (T), leading to their activation (T_{act}). Activated T cells then migrate to the tumor, which they attempt to kill

tions, reduced DNA repair capacity, and decreased expression of DNA-repair proteins.[37] The number of epidermal Langerhans' cells[38] and their capacity to stimulate an immune response also decline with age,[39] as does T-cell–mediated immunity.[40] It is probable that decreased immunosurveillance with age further contributes to skin cancer development.

Fairer skin types that burn easily have also been established as an independent risk factor for skin cancer.[41] In contrast, skin cancer other than human-papilloma–related anogenital cancer is rare in black-skinned individuals.[42] There is some evidence that UV radiation induces less immunosuppression in darker skin types.[43]

Ultraviolet radiation exposure also correlates with the anatomic distribution of skin cancer.[44] Although the body site incidence rates for NMSC differ in magnitude between the sexes, with a higher incidence in males, the distribution on the body is similar, except for the ears and scalp in females, which are largely spared.[45] While both SCC and BCC are more common on sun-exposed sites, BCC does not demonstrate the direct correlation with cumulative UV dose seen with SCC. The orbit and nasolabial fold where BCC is particularly prevalent receives only one fifth the UV exposure of other facial areas.[45] Studies in organ transplant recipients demonstrate a similar body-site distribution for NMSC; however, the increase in posttransplant NMSC risk relative to the general population is approximately three times greater on the scalp, neck and the upper limbs when compared with non–UV-exposed areas such as the trunk and lower limbs.[46]

Infection with certain high-risk mucosotropic types of human papilloma virus (HPV) is a major risk factor for cervical cancer and for skin cancers in epidermodysplasia verruciformis (EV), an autosomal recessive condition that results in extensive sheeted velvety warts, maximal in UV-exposed sites, that are highly prone to malignant conversion.[47] Patients with EV have a defective cell-mediated immune response to HPV infection; however, the exact mechanisms involved in the malignant transformation of keratinocytes in skin lesions of patients with EV are still unclear. EV-associated tumors contain high-risk HPV types, such as HPV types 5, 8, and 47, which selectively retain and express the E6 and E7 portions of the viral genome. Both E6 and E7 are multifunctional proteins that promote cell growth.[48]

The role of HPV in non–EV-associated skin cancer pathogenesis remains controversial. The HPV antibodies occur more frequently in SCC patients (odds ratio of 1.6) but not BCC patients when compared with control subjects.[49] Normal skin, however, also harbors multiple different HPV subtypes, mostly of the low-risk subtype, particularly in hair bulbs and sun-exposed sites. Such HPV subtypes can commonly persist for many years on healthy skin in both immunosuppressed and immunocompetent populations.[50] These findings correlate with work by Harwood et al.[51] demonstrating an association between NMSC status and EV-associated HPV DNA but not cutaneous HPV DNA. Recent work has also pointed to associations between skin cancer development and HPV38, which is known to promote keratinocyte immortality in vitro.[52]

High-Risk Populations

Skin cancers occurring in patients with HIV infection, a long history of phototherapy and in particular organ transplantation, offer a number of pathogenetic insights into the role of the immune system in skin carcinogenesis. Patients immunosuppressed by infection with HIV can develop rapidly growing cutaneous SCCs at a young age, with a high risk of local recurrence and metastasis.[53] The progressive depletion and dysfunction of T-cells associated with HIV/AIDS are discussed in Chapter 21.

Psoralens combined with UVA (PUVA) phototherapy is both mutagenic and immunosuppressive and may thus act as a complete carcinogen. Recent work has demonstrated how activation of the platelet-activating factor pathway is necessary for PUVA-induced immune suppression.[54] Long-term high-dose exposure to PUVA is consistently observed to significantly increase the risk of SCC.[55] Ultraviolet B and narrowband UVB phototherapy are safer treatment modalities, although population-based studies with extended follow-up periods are required to definitively calculate any associated NMSC risk.[56,57]

It is organ transplant recipients (OTRs), however, who have provided direct evidence of how a depressed immune system influences skin carcinogenesis. Skin cancers occur more frequently in OTRs than in the general population. The OTRs often develop multiple skin cancers (Fig. 16.4), with a higher rate of local recurrence and a greater propensity to invade locally and metastasize. The Israel Penn International Transplant Tumor Registry reported the aggressive nature and the significant mortality associated with posttransplant SCCs alone or in combination with BCCs. The registry demonstrated a 9% incidence of nodal or secondary site involvement affecting the cervix, perineum, or lung among transplant recipients with SCC.[58] Transplant recipients are at a particularly high risk of SCC with up to a 100-fold increase in the relative risk when compared with age-matched immunocompetent individuals.[46] This compares with a 10- to 16-fold increase in BCC for renal transplant recipients. The net result is a reversal of the usual ratio of BCC/SCC when compared with the nontransplanted population. A ratio of 3:1 (SCC/BCC) has been demonstrated in Australian, Irish, and Scandinavian transplant populations but not in studies from Spain and Italy where BCC remained the most common skin cancer posttransplant. This difference may reflect the effect of genetic background and skin type on UVR-induced immunosuppression.

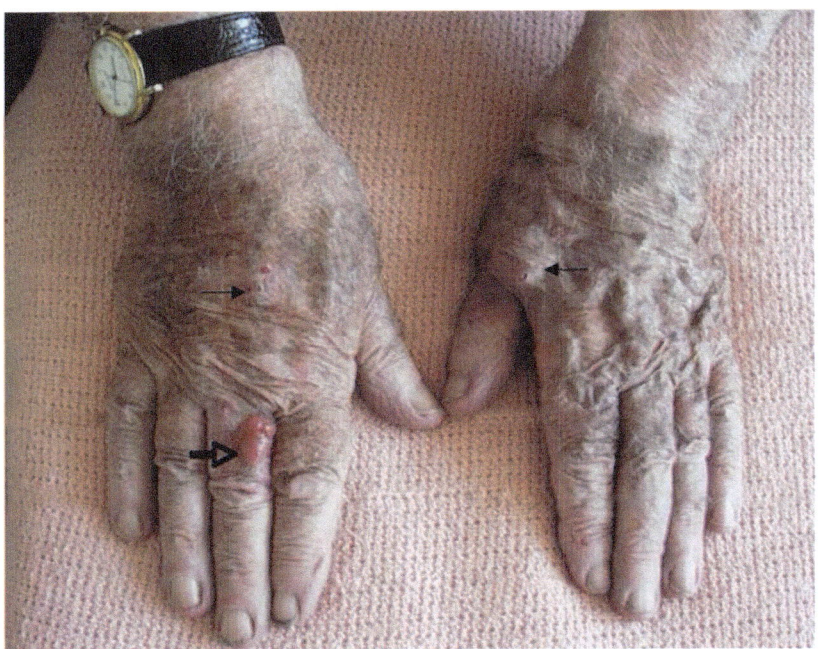

Fig. 16.4. The hands of a 72-year-renal transplant recipient. Diffuse actinic damage, multiple actinic keratoses (small arrows), and a large squamous cell carcinoma (large arrow) are displayed

Immunosuppressive Drugs and Skin Cancer

A recent study directly calculated skin cancer risk relative to duration of immunosuppression for individual renal transplant recipients compared with an age-matched immunocompetent population.[46] The relative risk of NMSC, in patients older than 50, increased rapidly as early as 2 years posttransplant, peaking by year 6. For transplant recipients younger than 50, there was a very minor increase in the relative risk of NMSC until the sixth year of immunosuppression but then a rapid increase. This peaked from 8 to 12 years after transplant, at 200 times the relative skin cancer risk of a group of similar age in the general population.[46] The majority of tumor precursor cells are detected and removed by the immune system. However, the observations in older transplant patients suggest that a percentage of the malignant clones are not eliminated, but held in check by a normal functioning immune system and grow rapidly once this surveillance is lifted. This may be due to the normal decline in cell-mediated immunity with age, compounded by immunosuppressing drugs.

Restoring immunosurveillance, by reducing or stopping immunosuppressive therapy, has been shown to lower the risk of skin cancer development in high-risk transplant recipients and may lead to deceleration of cutaneous carcinogenesis in those with skin cancers.[59] Reduction of immunosuppression has traditionally been the first-line approach in the management of Kaposi's sarcoma and posttransplant lymphoproliferative disorder. There is also evidence to support the reduction of immunosuppression as part of a treatment strategy for aggressive NMSC with a high metastatic potential.[60,61] Similarly, newer immunosuppressants with both antigraft rejection and antineoplastic properties have been developed and introduced in the posttransplant clinical setting. Work by Luan et al.[62] suggested that rapamycin in conjunction with cyclosporine may reduce the risk of cyclosporine-induced posttransplant malignancy, possibly as a result of rapamycin-induced E-cadherin expression. A study at 2 years posttransplant suggests that malignancy rates are lower for patients receiving rapamycin-based therapy without cyclosporine or for patients on rapamycin maintenance therapy after early cyclosporine withdrawal.[63]

The mechanisms whereby immunosuppressive drugs promote NMSC development are still being elucidated. Immunosuppressive therapies result in a profound suppression of T-cell activation and a decrease in the number and function of Langerhans' cells.[64] This model has been extended based on studies demonstrating how individual immunosuppressive agents can also have direct carcinogenic effects. Hojo et al.[65] identified a cell-autonomous and host-immunity–independent mechanism for cyclosporine-associated tumor progression. They found in mice that lack both T cells and natural killer cells that cyclosporine increases the number of metastases resulting from injection of adenocarcinoma cells. The increase in metastases was prevented by the use of monoclonal antibodies blocking transforming growth factor-β (TGF-β) receptors. This suggested that cyclosporine might alter cells and promote tumor progression directly by inducing the synthesis of TGF-β. Further studies showed tacrolimus to have a similar effect on tumor progression and TGF-β expression.[66] A recent study also showed that cyclosporine causes local inhibition of DNA repair and UVB-induced apoptosis in the skin.[67] Azathioprine, another commonly used immunosuppressive agent, causes the accumulation of 6-thioguanine (6-TG), the active metabolite of azathioprine, in the DNA of patients' skin cells. O'Donovan et al.[68] demonstrated that on exposure to UVA in sunlight, 6-TG is converted in an oxygen-dependent reaction into mutagenic guanine-6-sulfonate (G-6-SO$_3$) and reactive oxygen species. The increased reactive oxygen species causes oxidative stress, which indirectly leads to deletions and point mutations in DNA. This again demonstrates a further potential mechanism where an immunosuppressive agent, in conjunction with UV, can directly contribute to skin carcinogenesis. Whether these drugs enhance photocarcinogenesis solely due to their immunosuppressive effects and to what extent these secondary mechanisms contribute remain to be established.

Mechanisms of Immunity to Skin Cancer

There is conclusive evidence that the immune system is able to destroy skin cancers or at least inhibit their growth. Cell-mediated immunity, rather than humoral immunity, is the main arm of the immune system responsible for rejection of skin cancers.

In order for the immune response to kill NMSC, the tumor cells need to express an antigen capable of activating T cells. Transplantation experiments in mice show that UVR-induced NMSC do express antigens that enable the tumors to be targeted and destroyed by the immune system.[28,69] Spontaneous regression is the partial, or on occasion complete, disappearance of a tumor in the absence of any treatment capable of inducing regression. Clinical longitudinal studies indicate that AKs frequently undergo spontaneous regression.[70] Complete or partial regression is often observed in BCC both clinically and histologically. Curson and Weedon[71] identified spontaneous partial regression in 20% of excised primary BCCs, while Hunt et al.[72] reported active or prior regression in two thirds of nonulcerated, primary BCCs. Observations in humans that NMSC can spontaneously regress due to activation of the immune system[73] implies that human NMSCs also express tumor rejection antigens. While such antigens have been well characterized in melanoma, and are used in immunotherapy trials in humans,[74,75] tumor rejection antigens for NMSC have been poorly defined. Analysis of T-cell antigen binding receptor usage in patients with SCC and BCC has indicated selective T-cell receptor expression that is supportive of T-cell responses to a defined antigen in at least some patients.[76,77] The SCCs also express some of the tumor rejection antigens that have been defined for melanoma.[78] An SCC antigen (SCCA) has been described that is a member of the serpin superfamily; however, this antigen is not specifically expressed within tumor tissue[79–81] and appears to protect the tumor cells from apoptosis.[82] Therefore, while sufficient evidence exists that NMSCs express tumor rejection antigens, further work is required for their identification.

In vivo depletion of T-cell subsets from mice with a transplanted UVR-induced SCC found that immune rejection of the tumor was mediated mainly by CD8 T lymphocytes, with minor involvement of CD4 T cells.[83] T cells but not B cells or natural killer (NK) cells are found infiltrating human BCC and SCC, with a lower number of T cells in more aggressive tumors.[84–87] It is therefore likely that T lymphocytes are important for killing NMSC in humans. The predominant T cell infiltrating NMSC, including SCC, BCC, and AK, has been found to be CD4 T cells and a large proportion of these express activation markers,[88,89] markers of effector or memory lymphocytes, and the cutaneous lymphocyte-associated antigen that directs the migration of effector T cells into the skin.[85] Comparisons of spontaneously regressing human BCC with nonregressing BCC have found increased numbers of activated CD4 T cells within the regressing tumors, and these were adjacent to areas of apoptotic tumor cells.[72,73] Regressing human BCC also express higher levels of T-helper type 1 (Th1) cytokines such as interferon-γ (IFN-γ), which support cell-mediated immunity.[90] As spontaneous regression occurs when the immune response is able to effectively cause tumor destruction, it appears that CD4 T cells are of major importance in immune destruction of human NMSC. However, a role for CD8 T cells cannot be excluded.

CD4 T cells may either directly kill the tumor cells themselves, or may provide help to the CD8 T cell that causes the ultimate tumor cell death (Fig. 16.5). CD4 T cells are only able to recognize and directly kill major histocompatibility complex (MHC) class II expressing tumor cells, while CD8 T cells recognize tumor cells via MHC class I antigens. MHC I is expressed on all cells, including tumor cells, while MHC II is expressed only under conditions of activation such as in the presence of IFN-γ. However, a central role for CD4 T cells in tumor immunity is recognized.[91]

T cells may kill the NMSC via a variety of mechanisms, including perforin/granzyme, Fas/FasL, or secretion of effector cytokines such as IFN-γ.[92] Perforin secreted by cytotoxic lymphocytes punches holes in the membrane of target tumor cells, enabling the entry of granzyme, which triggers the mitochondrial apoptosis pathway, leading to death of the tumor cell.[93] Perforin expressing T cells are present within human BCC, suggesting that perforin-mediated T-cell cytotoxicity may be one mechanism by which the immune system controls growth of BCC.[94] Fas ligand (CD95L) is a member of the tumor necrosis factor (TNF) family, and is expressed on activated T cells. It binds to and trimerizes surface Fas antigen (CD95) expressed by target tumor cells that subsequently undergo apoptosis.[95] Mutations in the *Fas* gene in BCC and SCC have been described,[96] suggesting that this pathway is important for NMSC development. About 50% of T cells infiltrating SCC express FasL, suggesting that they may use this mechanism to kill tumor cells.[97] Cytokines can activate CD4 T cells to become cytotoxic by mechanisms such as TNF-

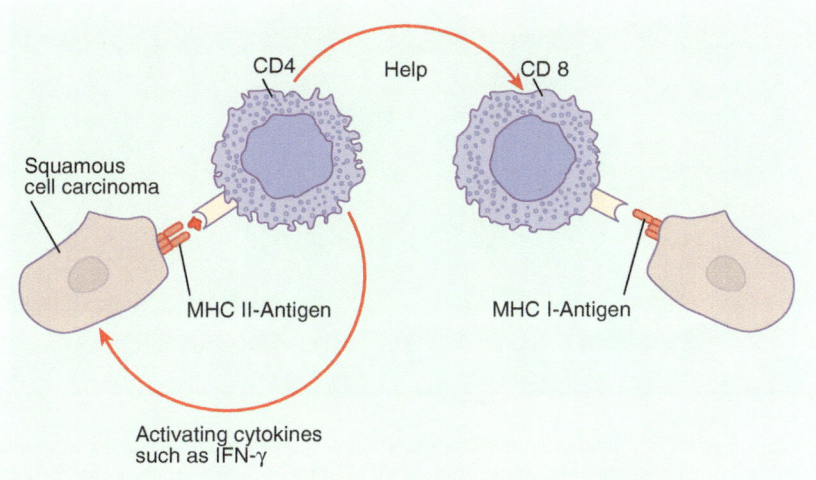

FIG. 16.5. Role of CD4 T cells in antitumor immunity. Tumor cells such as squamous cell carcinoma (SCC) may be killed by CD4 or CD8 T cells, although CD4 T cell numbers appear crucial. CD4 T cells may secrete activating cytokines such as interferon-γ (IFN-γ) that induce expression of MHC II on the tumor cells. MHC II can then present the tumor antigen (Ag) on the surface of the SCC in a manner that enables the tumor to be recognized and killed by the CD4 T cell. Alternatively, the CD4 T cell may provide help, either by direct cell contact or production of activating cytokines, to CD8 T cells. CD8 T cells recognize tumor antigen presented by MHC I. T cells can then kill the tumor cells by the mechanisms described in the text (Fas/FasL, perforin/granzyme)

related apoptosis-inducing ligand (TRAIL) expression.[98] The relative importance of these mechanisms of immune destruction of NMSC remains to be determined. It is likely that all of them play some role.

Mast cells may also regulate immunity to NMSC, as it has been shown that patients with a history of BCC have a higher number of mast cells in sun-protected skin than subjects without a history of BCC.[99] Mast cells are able to regulate skin immunity as they produce high levels of a large array of immunomodulators including the cytokines interleukin-4 (IL-4) and TNF. It is possible that they inhibit immunity to NMSC.

Nonmelanoma Skin Cancer Evasion of Immunity

Despite effective immunity to NMSC, many skin tumors grow progressively. This is because they establish effective processes for evading or inhibiting the immune system (Fig. 16.6).

A study of 34 patients with a previous history of multiple skin cancers (29 with BCC only, two with BCC and melanoma, and three with BCC and SCC) found that they had impaired cell-mediated immunity. This was characterized by reduced cuta-

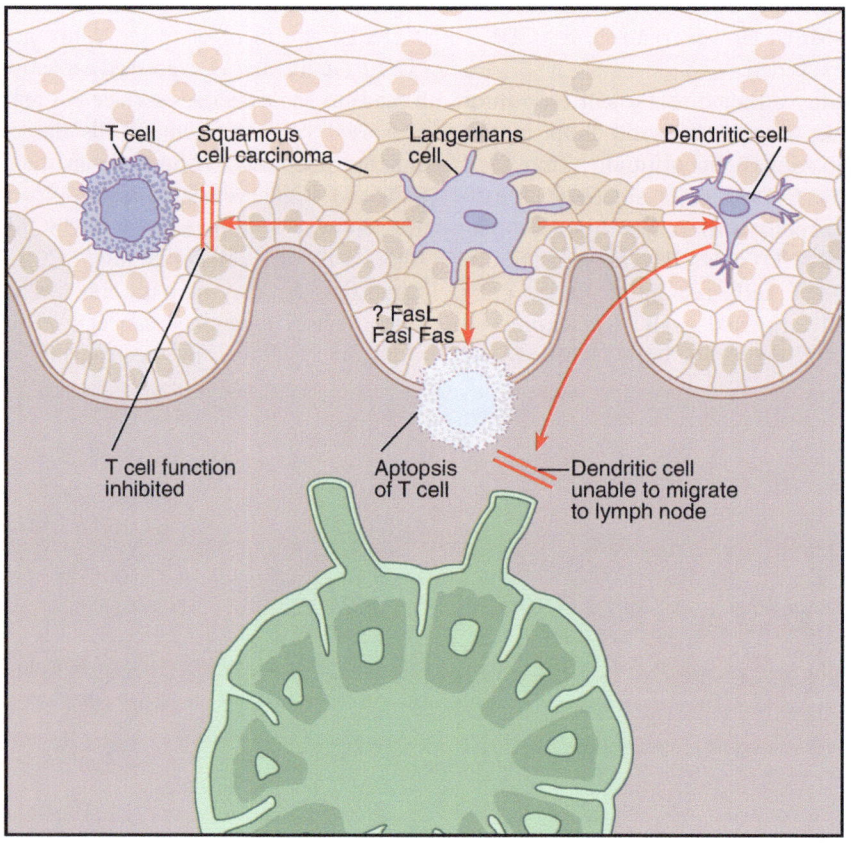

FIG. 16.6. Tumor evasion of the immune system. Skin tumor cells, such as squamous cell carcinoma (SCC), develop mechanisms to avoid destruction by the immune system. They produce cytokines such as interleukin-4 (IL-4) and IL-10, that inhibit the function of T lymphocytes (T). They also produce transforming growth factor-β (TGF-β), which inhibits migration of Langerhans' cells (LCs) from the tumor to draining lymph nodes, thereby preventing the induction of immunity to the tumor. They subvert the FasL mechanism used by T cells to kill targets. By downregulating expression of Fas (?), T cells are unable to engage Fas on the tumor cells with their FasL, and therefore are unable to induce apoptosis of the tumor cell. Additionally, skin tumor cells aberrantly express FasL, which can trigger Fas on the surface of T cells, leading to apoptosis of the T cells. Therefore, subversion of this T-cell killing mechanism results in apoptosis of the T cell rather than the tumor cell

neous reactions to recall antigens and lymphocyte counts.[100] This could have been due to the skin cancers' inhibiting immunity, even after the skin cancers were removed, or to skin cancers' being more prevalent in patients with a lower level of cell-mediated immunity. While two of the patients had melanoma, the majority of the skin cancer patients had NMSC only.

In a comparison of BCC to seborrheic keratosis, a benign epidermal growth, BCC were found to express messenger RNA (mRNA) for the Th2-type cytokines IL-4, IL-5, IL-10, and granulocyte-macrophage colony-stimulating factor (GM-CSF). This cytokine pattern usually inhibits Th1, or cell-mediated immunity.[101] Another study also found increased expression of IL-4 and IL-10 in BCC and SCC compared to peripheral blood mononuclear cells. Interleukin-10 was found to be produced by the tumor cells, not by the infiltrating lymphocytes.[102] Therefore, production of IL-10 by the tumor cells may inhibit T-cell immunity to NMSC, thereby contributing to tumor cell evasion of immunity.

Another mechanism by which NMSC escapes the immune system is by expression of FasL (CD95L) and downregulation of Fas antigen (CD95). Most cells in the body express Fas antigen. When FasL (usually on the surface of T lymphocytes) engages Fas on the surface of target cells, the Fas antigen expressing target cell dies by apoptosis. As discussed earlier in this chapter, this is a mechanism used by T cells to kill their target cell. However, in contrast to normal keratinocytes and most other types of normal cells, BCCs express FasL but fail to express Fas antigen. This not only makes BCC refractory to T-cell–mediated killing via this mechanism but also enables the BCC cells to kill infiltrating T cells. BCC expression of FasL is associated with apoptotic T cells.[103] Using double-label immunohistochemistry to differentiate Fas and FasL expression on tumor cells from T cells infiltrating AK and SCC, it was found that FasL was expressed in nine of 18 SCCs, compared with only one of 20 AKs. The expression of Fas was lower on SCC tumor cells compared with AK.[97] Progressor SCCs that evade immune destruction, but not regressor SCCs that are immunologically destroyed, express high levels of FasL.[104] This shows that SCC and AK tumor cells evade immune destruction by reducing Fas antigen and express-

ing FasL, making the tumor cells insensitive to T-cell killing, and giving them the ability to attack infiltrating T cells. This subversion of the Fas/FasL mechanism of T-cell–mediated cytotoxicity becomes more accentuated as AKs develop into SCC.

Dendritic cells within skin tumors are also defective. The DCs infiltrating BCC have a reduced expression of the co-stimulatory molecules CD80 and CD86 that are important for stimulation of T cells and display defective ability to activate T cells.[105] While DCs appear to be the major phagocytic cell in regressor tumors that do not escape immune destruction, macrophages expressing high levels of MHC II are the major phagocyte in progressor SCCs.[106] Thus a change in the main antigen-presenting cell from a DC to a macrophage may also be a mechanism by which NMSC evade immune destruction. The SCCs also interfere with DC migration from the tumor to local lymph nodes, thereby inhibiting the activation of antitumor immunity. Transforming growth factor-β (TGF-β) inhibits DC migration from progressing, but not regressing SCC, to draining lymph nodes.[107,108] Thus production of TGF-β by SCCs inhibits DC migration to draining lymph nodes, preventing the induction of immunity and therefore tumor regression.

Protection from Skin Cancer and Immunosuppression

The most effective way to prevent skin cancer is to avoid sun exposure by the use of clothing, a hat, and sunglasses, and by staying in the shade. This is not always practical due to work or recreational activities, and therefore additional procedures for sun protection are required. However, a small level of sun exposure is likely to be beneficial. Ultraviolet exposure is involved in the production of vitamin D, which is crucial for bone and muscle function, and it has been recommended that humans receive about one third of the MED of UV to about 15% of their body surface on most days.[109] It is a difficult issue to determine a beneficial level of sun exposure before the damage outweighs the health benefits. Even these low levels of sun exposure recommended for vitamin D production can damage the immune system.

Vitamin D has also been shown to reduce the levels of UVR-induced damage to DNA, probably by enhancing DNA repair,[110,111] and epidemiologic data have indicated that sunlight may be beneficial for some cancers, including melanoma survival, possibly via a vitamin D–related mechanism.[112] Therefore, UV-induced vitamin D is likely to be photoprotective.

Sunscreens containing chemical filters or reflectors to reduce the amount of UVR available to cause damage to the skin are widely used to prevent sunburn. There is evidence that sunscreen use for 4.5 years reduces the incidence of SCC but not BCC.[113] Sunburn is largely caused by UVB,[114] while, as discussed above, UVR-induced immunosuppression and gene mutations can be caused by both UVB and UVA. Therefore, it would not be expected that sunscreens designed to protect from sunburn would show the same efficacy in preventing skin carcinogenesis. It has been shown that the ability of a sunscreen to prevent immunosuppression in humans is related to the UVA protective capacity of the sunscreen,[115] and a number of studies have confirmed that sunscreens with a high level of UVA protection are required to provide substantial immunoprotection to humans.[24,116–120] This is consistent with studies described earlier in this chapter showing that UVA is immunosuppressive, and indicates the importance of UVA protection for preventing sunlight-induced skin damage.

Melanin can protect from skin cancer, and studies using congenic mice that differ only in their capacity to produce melanin in response to UVR exposure have shown that sunlight-induced tanning reduces skin carcinogenesis.[121] However, the UVR exposure required for tanning is damaging. Synthetic melanotrophins have been shown to induce tanning in humans in the absence of sun exposure, and this increased melanin density reduces DNA damage resulting from UVR exposure.[122] DNA oligonucleotides have also been found to increase both melanization and DNA repair, thereby reducing UVR-induced DNA damage.[123] Therefore, melanin can be photoprotective in humans, and if melanin induction can be induced safely by practical means in humans, this may help reduce the incidence of skin cancer in the future.

Other strategies that interfere with the biologic processes of sun damage can also reduce skin cancer formation and prevent UVR-induced immunosuppression. Topical application of the enzyme T4 endonuclease V encapsulated in liposomes protects the immune system of mice and humans from UVR.[124,125] This enzyme initiates repair of the UVR-induced photolesion cyclobutane pyrimidine dimers, and has been shown to reduce the incidence of new skin cancer formation in patients with xeroderma pigmentosum.[126] Therefore, topical agents that enhance DNA repair can be photoprotective. Topical antioxidants can also reduce immunosuppression and skin carcinogenesis.[127–129] A number of botanically derived products have also been shown to be photoprotective to the immune system in humans, such as topical isoflavonoids,[130] polysaccharides from tamarind,[131] and green tea extracts.[132] Another potential means of protecting from skin cancer is photoadaption, whereby skin protective mechanisms are upregulated so that subsequent UVR exposure is less damaging.[133]

Treatment of Nonmelanoma Skin Cancer

Surgical and Ablative Therapies

Guidelines for the treatment of NMSC identify the goal of treatment as complete (preferably histologically confirmed) removal or destruction of the primary tumor while recognizing the paucity of randomized controlled trials for all treatments of both primary cutaneous SCC and BCC.[3,134] The BCCs can be divided into relatively low- and high-risk categories based on histologic growth patterns and to a lesser extent on histologic differentiation. Similarly, malignant behavior varies significantly in tumors that fall within the histologic diagnostic category of primary cutaneous SCC. Choosing the best treatment for an individual patient requires a thorough assessment of both tumor and patient, and discussion of the different treatment modalities available with all concerned.

Where feasible, surgical excision, including Mohs' micrographic surgery (MMS) where appropriate, should be regarded as the treatment of first choice for cutaneous SCC and high-risk BCC, particularly at difficult sites.[134] Mohs' micrographic surgery is a surgical technique that allows precise definition of marginal clearance by examining horizontal frozen sections of the excised tissue. Not all BCCs require treatment; aggressive treatment might be inappropriate for patients of advanced age or poor general health, especially for asymptomatic low-risk lesions that are unlikely to cause significant morbidity. The use of curettage and cautery/electrodesiccation, cryotherapy, and nonsurgical techniques require the careful selection of low-risk lesions (small, well-defined primary lesions with nonaggressive histology) in order to achieve high cure rates.[135] Curettage and cautery involve the shave excision of the superficial component of a tumor with destruction of the base, while cryotherapy induces tissue necrosis, which results from the freezing and thawing of cells. Such approaches do not necessarily provide histologic characterization of the tumor or enable histologic examination of margins of excised tissue. The outcome of such techniques also in part depends on the experience of the physician and the compliance of the patient.

Radiotherapy has been used to treat both BCC and SCC, especially in difficult head and neck sites and for elderly patients with large tumors. Again, the absence of histologic confirmation of adequacy of treatment and poor cosmetic outcomes has resulted in a decline in radiotherapy for NMSC.

Immune-Mediated Therapies

Other options for treating both BCC and SCC include therapies aimed at upregulating the host immune response to the developing skin cancer. Immune-mediated regression of NMSC can occur spontaneously or as part of the wound-healing process following a partial biopsy of the lesion.[136] Similarly, induction of contact dermatitis with topical sensitizing agents was shown some decades ago to cause regression of established skin cancers.[137] This concept of harnessing the body's innate immune response to target and destroy skin cancers is the basis of a number of different licensed and investigational approaches to immunotherapy.

Interferon

Interferon (IFN)-α-2b is used as adjuvant high-dose therapy for the treatment of patients with thick melanomas metastasizing to lymph nodes and as systemic therapy for AIDS-associated Kaposi's sarcoma. The ability of IFN-α to represses the clinical tumorigenic phenotype in certain malignancies is an example of how focal cytokine production can enable activation of tumor-infiltrating lymphocytes, which in turn can set in place a cascade of events leading to tumor regression.[138] Intralesional injections of IFN-α-2b, while expensive and time-consuming, have been investigated in the treatment of nodular or superficial BCC, the largest series demonstrating an 81% clearance rate with a 19% recurrence rate at 1 year.[139] A marked increase in dermal CD4 T cells surrounding BCC nests has been observed after intralesional IFN-α therapy.[140] Buechner et al.[141] postulated that this subset of T cells expresses cytolytic activity against tumor cells, by inducing apoptosis. They demonstrated that apoptosis induced by Fas-FasL interaction is the major mechanism of tumor cell death in regressing BCC after intralesional IFN-α treatment.

Photodynamic Therapy

Photodynamic therapy (PDT) involves applying a photosensitizer (a porphyrin chemical) to a target region prior to activation with a visible light source. The preferential absorbance of photosensitizer by hyperproliferative tissue allows for targeted treatment of NMSC while minimizing damage to surrounding healthy skin. Photodynamic therapy is effective in the treatment of AK, Bowen's disease, and superficial BCC. Nonsuperficial BCC and SCC are intuitively not treated with PDT due to limited depth of penetration of the photosensitizer. Interestingly, two reports have indicated that responses to aminolevulinic acid–PDT treatment are less effective in immunocompromised populations when compared with immunocompetent individuals.[142,143] This correlates with a new broader understanding of how PDT impacts on tumorigenesis. In addition to causing a shutdown of the microcirculation to the tumor and a direct killing of tumor cells by apoptosis and necrosis, PDT also induces a rapid inflammatory response with cytokine-induced migration of neutrophils into the treated tumor.[144] This induction of host responses is an important contributor to short- and long-term suppression of tumor growth.[145] There is also murine evidence that PDT enhances the host antitumor immune response and generates tumor-specific vaccines, which in turn induce a cytotoxic T-cell response.[146]

Topical Therapies and Immune-Response Modifiers

Increasingly, topical therapies are being used, in carefully selected patients and carefully selected skin cancers, prior to or in place of definitive surgical procedures. Meta-analysis demonstrates that topical therapies such as imiquimod and 5-fluorouracil effectively treat actinic keratosis.[147] While long-term follow-up and randomized controlled trials are lacking, efficacy has also been shown for superficial BCCs.[148,149] A number of small case series also report successful use of 5% imiquimod in the treatment of in-situ and invasive SCC.[150,151] Imiquimod is a topical immune response modifier that binds to Toll-like receptor-7 and -8 predominately expressed on DC and monocytes, inducing IFN-α. Its use is associated with activity of both the adaptive and the innate immune response and the induction of apoptosis. Imiquimod induces an early influx of DC and CD4 T cells into the tumor, followed by a later wave of CD8 T cells after the tumor has been destroyed, suggesting that it activates similar cell-mediated immune responses as those responsible for spontaneous regression.[152] This modulation of immune response by imiquimod is also in part mediated by enhanced migration of LCs from the treated skin to draining lymph nodes,[153] which may enhance the activation of cell-mediated immunity.

Future Strategies

Work continues on potential future immunologic strategies to fight NMSC. In DC-based immunotherapy, tumor antigens are presented by DCs harvested from a patient. The activated DCs are placed back into the patient, which activates a cytotoxic response targeted against these antigens on cancerous cells. Studies to date have failed to show an effective antitumor response in murine cutaneous SCC.[154] Another theoretical approach to harnessing the immune system to fight skin cancers is T-cell–based adoptive immunotherapy. This involves the in vitro expansion of tumor infiltrating lymphocytes, which are then transferred back into the patient in conjunction with exogenous administration of IL-2. A recent study has also demonstrated how DNAzymes (synthetic nucleic acid–based drugs that can be engineered to target and cleave mRNA) can block c-Jun protein expression in SCC cells, thereby inhibiting SCC tumor growth and tumor angiogenesis.[155]

Conclusion

Nonmelanoma skin cancers are a group of skin cancers mainly derived from malignantly transformed keratinocytes, although Merkel cell and endothelial cell tumors are also classified in this group. Keratinocyte-derived NMSCs are categorized as SCC or BCC based on their clinical diagnosis and histopathology. Actinic keratosis and Bowen's disease (SCC in situ) can develop into the more aggressive and malignant SCC with the potential to invade and metastasize. Basal cell carcinoma is rarely metastatic. The major risk factor for NMSC is cumulative exposure to sunlight, and the risk increases with age and is higher in people with fairer skin. Human papilloma virus may also be a risk factor; however, this is less well established. Immunosuppression, including psoralens combined with UVA and pharmacologic immunosuppression to inhibit transplant rejection, greatly increases the risk of NMSC, in particular SCC.

The immune response is a crucial factor in NMSC development and plays an important role in both its induction and its development. The immune system is able to inhibit the outgrowth of new tumors in humans, and UVR-induced immunosuppression and pharmacologically induced immunosuppression greatly increases the incidence of skin cancer. The immune system also controls development of skin tumors, as immunosuppressed patients tend to develop more aggressive skin tumors, while reducing or stopping immunosuppression can reduce skin cancer risk. Further evidence for a role of the immune system in controlling growth of a developed NMSC is spontaneous regression. In the absence of causative therapy it is common for NMSC to undergo partial regression. Complete regression can also occur, although not so frequently. This is due to the immune system gaining control over tumor growth so that it is able to destroy cancer cells faster than they can grow. Therefore, there is clinical evidence that the immune system is involved in restraining skin cancers at all stages of their development: initial outgrowth, progression toward malignancy, and growth once established.

How the immune response recognizes and kills NMSC cells is not known. This area of knowledge is much more advanced for melanoma than for NMSC, and considerably more research attention is required. The tumor rejection antigens that enable the immune system to kill the tumor cells are not defined. Evidence based on cytokine patterns and cell types infiltrating skin tumors indicates that cell-mediated immunity, rather than humoral immunity, is responsible for destruction of NMSC. Investigations of spontaneously regressing NMSC, as well as other studies, highlight the importance of CD4 T cells in immunity to NMSC. CD4 T cells can be directly cytotoxic, but only for MHC class II–positive tumor cells. Therefore, it is unclear whether they are directly responsible for tumor cell destruction or whether they provide help to CD8 T cells, which then kill the tumor cells. A variety of mechanisms could be involved in T-cell killing of NMSC, including FasL, perforin, granzyme, or cytokines that switch on cytotoxic mechanisms such as TRAIL or induce MHC class II expression, enabling CD4 T cells to kill the tumors. However, NMSCs develop strategies to avoid killing by the immune system, including inhibition of DC migration from the tumor to inhibit the activation of immunity in draining lymph nodes, production of IL-10 to inhibit cell mediated immunity, and tumor cell expression of FasL so that the tumor cells can kill tumor-infiltrating T cells. The tumor rejection antigen, mechanisms of killing, and immune evasion probably have a dynamic relationship whereby as the immune system is able to cause regression by one mechanism, the tumor evolves ways of evading that particular mechanism, or loses expression of that antigen.

Efficacy of treatment and low recurrence rates remain the primary determinants when treating NMSC. In this regard, surgical excision remains the most common therapy for NMSC. Due consideration must also be given to cosmetic outcome and patient preference. There is an emerging trend for less invasive interventions such as photody-namic therapy and topical immune-response modifiers such as imiquimod in the treatment of AK, Bowen's disease, and superficial BCC. While such treatments are attractive to patients, comparative studies with other treatment modalities and further long-term follow-up studies are required.

Ultraviolet radiation from sunlight is the major cause of NMSC. In humans, both the UVA and UVB wavebands cause immunosuppression and gene mutations, and therefore both UVA and UVB are likely to contribute to induction and development of NMSC in humans. The best way to prevent skin cancer is to avoid sun exposure. However, this is not possible, as humans cannot function without sun exposure for work or recreation, and sunlight is also required for the formation of vitamin D, which has essential health benefits. It is a difficult and unresolved health issue to determine a level of sun exposure that is optimal for human health while avoiding the damaging events that lead to skin cancer. This is particularly difficult as immunosuppression occurs in response to low levels of sunlight exposure. Therefore, protective measures that prevent immunosuppression but not vitamin D production need to be developed. Protective measures could include artificial melanization in the absence of UVR exposure, and the use of antioxidants, botanicals, or photoadaption. While all of these have been shown to protect the immune system from sunlight, it is not known whether they spare vitamin D production.

Nonmelanoma skin cancer is a considerable medical health problem. Research into the causes and mechanisms underling the immunology and genetics of this disease will enable the development of more effective preventative and therapeutic strategies.

References

1. Boukamp P. Non-melanoma skin cancer: what drives tumor development and progression? Carcinogenesis 2005;26(10):1657–67.
2. Rehman I, Quinn AG, Healy E, Rees JL. High frequency of loss of heterozygosity in actinic keratoses, a usually benign disease. Lancet 1994;344(8925): 788–9.
3. Telfer NR, Colver GB, Bowers PW. Guidelines for the management of basal cell carcinoma. British

Association of Dermatologists. Br J Dermatol 1999;141(3):415–23.

4. Rowe DE, Carroll RJ, Day CL Jr. Prognostic factors for local recurrence, metastasis, and survival rates in squamous cell carcinoma of the skin, ear, and lip. Implications for treatment modality selection. J Am Acad Dermatol 1992;26(6):976–90.

5. Ackerman AB, Mones JM. Solar (actinic) keratosis is squamous cell carcinoma. Br J Dermatol 2006;155(1):9–22.

6. Thompson SC, Jolley D, Marks R. Reduction of solar keratoses by regular sunscreen use. N Engl J Med 1993;329(16):1147–51.

7. Brown EE, Whitby D, Vitale F, et al. Virologic, hematologic, and immunologic risk factors for classic Kaposi sarcoma. Cancer 2006;107(9):2282–90.

8. Buell JF, Trofe J, Hanaway MJ, et al. Immunosuppression and Merkel cell cancer. Transplant Proc 2002;34(5):1780–1.

9. Stallone G, Schena A, Infante B, et al. Sirolimus for Kaposi's sarcoma in renal-transplant recipients. N Engl J Med 2005;352(13):1317–23.

10. Armstrong BK, Kricker A. The epidemiology of UV induced skin cancer. J Photochem Photobiol B Biol 2001;63(1–3):8–18.

11. Bruls WA, Slaper H, van der Leun JC, Berrens L. Transmission of human epidermis and stratum corneum as a function of thickness in the ultraviolet and visible wavelengths. Photochem Photobiol 1984;40(4):485–94.

12. Lim HW, Naylor M, Honigsmann H, et al. American Academy of Dermatology Consensus Conference on UVA protection of sunscreens: Summary and recommendations. J Am Acad Dermatol 2001;44(3):505–8.

13. Setlow RB. Shedding light on proteins, nucleic acids, cells, humans and fish. Mutat Res 2002;511(1):1–14.

14. Wikonkal NM, Brash DE. Ultraviolet radiation induced signature mutations in photocarcinogenesis. J Invest Dermatol Symp Proc 1999;4(1):6–10.

15. Mouret S, Baudouin C, Charveron M, Favier A, Cadet J, Douki T. Cyclobutane pyrimidine dimers are predominant DNA lesions in whole human skin exposed to UVA radiation. Proc Natl Acad Sci USA 2006;103(37):13765–70.

16. Kawanishi S, Hiraku Y, Oikawa S. Mechanism of guanine-specific DNA damage by oxidative stress and its role in carcinogenesis and aging. Mutat Res 2001;488(1):65–76.

17. Halliday GM. Inflammation, gene mutation and photoimmunosuppression in response to UVR-induced oxidative damage contributes to photocarcinogenesis. Mutat Res 2005;571(1–2):107–20.

18. Pattison DI, Davies MJ. Actions of ultraviolet light on cellular structures. In: Cancer: Cell Structures,

19. Agar NS, Halliday GM, Barnetson RS, Ananthaswamy HN, Wheeler M, Jones AM. The basal layer in human squamous tumors harbors more UVA than UVB fingerprint mutations: A role for UVA in human skin carcinogenesis. Proc Natl Acad Sci USA 2004;101(14):4954–9.

20. Halliday GM, Agar NS, Barnetson RSC, Ananthaswamy HN, Jones AM. UV-A fingerprint mutations in human skin cancer. Photochem Photobiol 2005;81(1):3–8.

21. He YY, Pi J, Huang JL, Diwan BA, Waalkes MP, Chignell CF. Chronic UVA irradiation of human HaCaT keratinocytes induces malignant transformation associated with acquired apoptotic resistance. Oncogene 2006;25(26):3680–8.

22. Berking C, Takemoto R, Binder RL, et al. Photocarcinogenesis in human adult skin grafts. Carcinogenesis 2002;23(1):181–7.

23. Damian DL, Barnetson RS, Halliday GM. Low-dose UVA and UVB have different time courses for suppression of contact hypersensitivity to a recall antigen in humans. J Invest Dermatol 1999;112(6):939–44.

24. Fourtanier A, Moyal D, Maccario J, et al. Measurement of sunscreen immune protection factors in humans: a consensus paper. J Invest Dermatol 2005;125(3):403–9.

25. Moyal DD, Fourtanier AM. Broad-spectrum sunscreens provide better protection from the suppression of the elicitation phase of delayed-type hypersensitivity response in humans. J Invest Dermatol 2001;117(5):1186–92.

26. Poon TSC, Barnetson RSC, Halliday GM. Sunlight-induced immunosuppression in humans is initially because of UVB, then UVA, followed by interactive effects. J Invest Dermatol 2005;125(4):840–6.

27. Fisher MS, Kripke ML. Suppressor T lymphocytes control the development of primary skin cancers in ultraviolet-irradiated mice. Science 1982;216:1133–4.

28. Kripke ML. Immunologic unresponsiveness induced by UV radiation. Immunol Rev 1984;80:87–102.

29. Sluyter R, Halliday GM. Enhanced tumor growth in UV-irradiated skin is associated with an influx of inflammatory cells into the epidermis. Carcinogenesis 2000;21(10):1801–7.

30. Byrne SN, Halliday GM. Dendritic cells: Making progress with tumour regression? Immunol Cell Biol 2002;80(6):520–30.

31. Shortman K, Naik SH. Steady-state and inflammatory dendritic-cell development. Nature Rev Immunol 2007;7(1):19–30.

32. Halliday GM. Skin immunity and melanoma development. In: Thompson JF, Morton DL, Kroon BBR,

Carcinogens and Genomic Instability. Basel: Birkhauser Verlag AG, 2006:131–57.

eds. Textbook of melanoma. London: Martin Dunitz, 2004:25–42.

33. Weninger W, Crowley MA, Manjunath N, von Andrian UH. Migratory properties of naive, effector, and memory CD8(+) T cells. J Exp Med 2001;194(7):953–66.

34. von Andrian UH, Mackay CR. Advances in immunology: T-cell function and migration—two sides of the same coin [Review]. N Engl J Med 2000;343(14):1020–33.

35. Miller DL, Weinstock MA. Nonmelanoma skin cancer in the United States: incidence. J Am Acad Dermatol 1994;30(5 pt 1):774–8.

36. Vitaliano PP. The use of logistic regression for modelling risk factors: with application to non-melanoma skin cancer. Am J Epidemiol 1978;108(5):402–14.

37. Wei Q, Matanoski GM, Farmer ER, Hedayati MA, Grossman L. DNA repair and aging in basal cell carcinoma: a molecular epidemiology study. Proc Natl Acad Sci USA 1993;90(4):1614–8.

38. Bergfelt L. UV-related skin conditions and Langerhans' cell populations in human skin. Acta Derm Venereol 1993;73(3):194–6.

39. Grewe M. Chronological ageing and photoageing of dendritic cells. Clin Exp Dermatol 2001;26(7):608–12.

40. Thivolet J, Nicolas JF. Skin ageing and immune competence. Br J Dermatol 1990;122 Suppl 35:77–81.

41. Lejeune FJ. Epidemiology and etiology of malignant melanoma. Biomed Pharmacother 1986;40(3):91–9.

42. Rees JL. The melanocortin 1 receptor (MC1R): more than just red hair. Pigment Cell Res 2000;13(3):135–40.

43. Kelly DA, Young AR, McGregor JM, Seed PT, Potten CS, Walker SL. Sensitivity to sunburn is associated with susceptibility to ultraviolet radiation-induced suppression of cutaneous cell-mediated immunity. J Exp Med 2000;191(3):561–6.

44. Franceschi S, Levi F, Randimbison L, La Vecchia C. Site distribution of different types of skin cancer: new aetiological clues. Int J Cancer 1996;67(1):24–8.

45. Raasch B, Maclennan R, Wronski I, Robertson I. Body site specific incidence of basal and squamous cell carcinoma in an exposed population, Townsville, Australia. Mutat Res 1998;422(1):101–6.

46. Moloney FJ, Comber H, O'Lorcain P, O'Kelly P, Conlon PJ, Murphy GM. A population-based study of skin cancer incidence and prevalence in renal transplant recipients. Br J Dermatol 2006;154(3):498–504.

47. Jablonska S, Majewski S. Epidermodysplasia verruciformis: immunological and clinical aspects. Curr Top Microbiol Immunol 1994;186:157–75.

48. Boxman IL, Mulder LH, Noya F, et al. Transduction of the E6 and E7 genes of epidermodysplasia-verruciformis-associated human papillomaviruses alters human keratinocyte growth and differentiation in organotypic cultures. J Invest Dermatol 2001;117(6):1397–404.

49. Karagas MR, Nelson HH, Sehr P, et al. Human papillomavirus infection and incidence of squamous cell and basal cell carcinomas of the skin. J Natl Cancer Inst 2006;98(6):389–95.

50. Hazard K, Karlsson A, Andersson K, Ekberg H, Dillner J, Forslund O. Cutaneous human papillomaviruses persist on healthy skin. J Invest Dermatol 2006.

51. Harwood CA, Surentheran T, Sasieni P, et al. Increased risk of skin cancer associated with the presence of epidermodysplasia verruciformis human papillomavirus types in normal skin. Br J Dermatol 2004;150(5):949–57.

52. Caldeira S, Zehbe I, Accardi R, et al. The E6 and E7 proteins of the cutaneous human papillomavirus type 38 display transforming properties. J Virol 2003;77(3):2195–206.

53. Nguyen P, Vin-Christian K, Ming ME, Berger T. Aggressive squamous cell carcinomas in persons infected with the human immunodeficiency virus. Arch Dermatol 2002;138(6):758–63.

54. Wolf P, Nghiem DX, Walterscheid JP, et al. Platelet-activating factor is crucial in psoralen and ultraviolet A-induced immune suppression, inflammation, and apoptosis. Am J Pathol 2006;169(3):795–805.

55. Stern RS, Lunder EJ. Risk of squamous cell carcinoma and methoxsalen (psoralen) and UV-A radiation (PUVA). A meta-analysis. Arch Dermatol 1998;134(12):1582–5.

56. Lee E, Koo J, Berger T. UVB phototherapy and skin cancer risk: a review of the literature. Int J Dermatol 2005;44(5):355–60.

57. Man I, Crombie IK, Dawe RS, Ibbotson SH, Ferguson J. The photocarcinogenic risk of narrowband UVB (TL-01) phototherapy: early follow-up data. Br J Dermatol 2005;152(4):755–7.

58. Buell JF, Hanaway MJ, Thomas M, Alloway RR, Woodle ES. Skin cancer following transplantation: the Israel Penn International Transplant Tumor Registry experience. Transplant Proc 2005;37(2):962–3.

59. Otley CC, Coldiron BM, Stasko T, Goldman GD. Decreased skin cancer after cessation of therapy with transplant-associated immunosuppressants. Arch Dermatol 2001;137(4):459–63.

60. Otley CC, Maragh SL. Reduction of immunosuppression for transplant-associated skin cancer: rationale and evidence of efficacy. Dermatol Surg 2005;31(2):163–8.

61. Moloney FJ, Kelly PO, Kay EW, Conlon P, Murphy GM. Maintenance versus reduction of immunosuppression in renal transplant recipients with aggressive

squamous cell carcinoma. Dermatol Surg 2004;30(4 pt 2):674–8.

62. Luan FL, Hojo M, Maluccio M, Yamaji K, Suthanthiran M. Rapamycin blocks tumor progression: unlinking immunosuppression from antitumor efficacy. Transplantation 2002;73(10):1565–72.

63. Mathew T, Kreis H, Friend P. Two-year incidence of malignancy in sirolimus-treated renal transplant recipients: results from five multicenter studies. Clin Transplant 2004;18(4):446–9.

64. Bergfelt L. Langerhans cells, immunomodulation and skin lesions. A quantitative, morphological and clinical study. Acta Derm Venereol Suppl (Stockh) 1993;180:1–37.

65. Hojo M, Morimoto T, Maluccio M, et al. Cyclosporine induces cancer progression by a cell-autonomous mechanism. Nature 1999;397(6719):530–4.

66. Maluccio M, Sharma V, Lagman M, et al. Tacrolimus enhances transforming growth factor-beta1 expression and promotes tumor progression. Transplantation 2003;76(3):597–602.

67. Yarosh DB, Pena AV, Nay SL, Canning MT, Brown DA. Calcineurin inhibitors decrease DNA repair and apoptosis in human keratinocytes following ultraviolet B irradiation. J Invest Dermatol 2005;125(5):1020–5.

68. O'Donovan P, Perrett CM, Zhang X, et al. Azathioprine and UVA light generate mutagenic oxidative DNA damage. Science 2005;309(5742):1871–4.

69. Kripke ML. Antigenicity of murine skin tumors induced by ultraviolet light. J Natl Cancer Inst 1974;53:1333–6.

70. Marks R, Foley P, Goodman G, Hage BH, Selwood TS. Spontaneous remission of solar keratoses: the case for conservative management. Br J Dermatol 1986;115(6):649–55.

71. Curson C, Weedon D. Spontaneous regression in basal cell carcinomas. J Cutan Pathol 1979;6(5):432–7.

72. Hunt MJ, Halliday GM, Weedon D, Cooke BE, Barnetson RS. Regression in basal cell carcinoma: an immunohistochemical analysis. Br J Dermatol 1994;130(1):1–8.

73. Halliday GM, Patel A, Hunt MJ, Tefany FJ, Barnetson RSC. Spontaneous regression of human melanoma/ non-melanoma skin cancer: association with infiltrating CD4+ T cells. World J Surg 1995;19(3):352–8.

74. Romero P, Cerottini JC, Speiser DE. Monitoring tumor antigen specific T-cell responses in cancer patients and phase I clinical trials of peptide-based vaccination. Cancer Immunol Immunother 2004;53(3):249–55.

75. Speiser DE, Pittet MJ, Rimoldi D, et al. Evaluation of melanoma vaccines with molecularly defined antigens by ex vivo monitoring of tumor-specific T cells. Semin Cancer Biol 2003;13(6):461–72.

76. Caignard A, Dietrich PY, Morand V, et al. Evidence for T-cell clonal expansion in a patient with squamous cell carcinoma of the head and neck. Cancer Res 1994;54(5):1292–7.

77. Ohmen JD, Moy RL, Zovich D, et al. Selective accumulation of T cells according to T-cell receptor V beta gene usage in skin cancer. J Invest Dermatol 1994;103(6):751–7.

78. Gaugler B, Vandeneynde B, Vanderbruggen P, et al. Human gene Mage-3 codes for an antigen recognized on a melanoma by autologous cytolytic T lymphocytes. J Exp Med 1994;179(3):921–30.

79. Kato H. Expression and function of squamous cell carcinoma antigen. Anticancer Res 1996;16(4B): 2149–53.

80. Torre GC. SCC antigen in malignant and nonmalignant squamous lesions. Tumor Biol 1998;19(6):517–26.

81. Cataltepe S, Gornstein ER, Schick C, et al. Co-expression of the squamous cell carcinoma antigens 1 and 2 in normal adult human tissues and squamous cell carcinomas. J Histochem Cytochem 2000;48(1):113–22.

82. Suminami Y, Nagashima S, Vujanovic NL, Hirabayashi K, Kato H, Whiteside TL. Inhibition of apoptosis in human tumour cells by the tumour-associated serpin, SCC antigen-1. Br J Cancer 2000;82(4):981–9.

83. Cavanagh LL, Halliday GM. Dendritic epidermal T cells in ultraviolet-irradiated skin enhance skin tumor growth by inhibiting Cd4(+) T-cell-mediated immunity. Cancer Res 1996;56(11):2607–15.

84. Deng JS, Brod BA, Saito R, Tharp MD. Immune-associated cells in basal cell carcinomas of skin. J Cutan Pathol 1996;23(2):140–6.

85. Gelb AB, Smoller BR, Warnke RA, Picker LJ. Lymphocytes infiltrating primary cutaneous neoplasms selectively express the cutaneous lymphocyte-associated antigen (CLA). Am J Pathol 1993;142(5):1556–64.

86. Garciaplata D, Mozos E, Carrasco L, Solana R. HLA molecule expression in cutaneous squamous cell carcinomas—an immunopathological study and clinical-immunohistopathological correlations. Histol Histopathol 1993;8(2):219–26.

87. Patel A, Halliday GM, Cooke BE, Barnetson RS. Evidence that regression in keratoacanthoma is immunologically mediated: a comparison with squamous cell carcinoma. Br J Dermatol 1994;131(6):789–98.

88. Markey AC, Churchill LJ, Allen MH, MacDonald DM. Activation and inducer subset phenotype of the lymphocytic infiltrate around epidermally derived tumors. J Am Acad Dermatol 1990;23(2 pt 1):214–20.

89. Myskowski PL, Safai B. The immunology of basal cell carcinoma. Int J Dermatol 1988;27(9):601–7.

90. Wong DA, Bishop GA, Lowes MA, Cooke B, Barnetson RS, Halliday GM. Cytokine profiles in spontaneously regressing basal cell carcinomas. Br J Dermatol 2000;143(1):91–8.

91. Pardoll DM, Topalian SL. The role of CD4+ T cell responses in antitumor immunity. Curr Opin Immunol 1998;10(5):588–94.

92. Smyth MJ, Godfrey DI, Trapani JA. A fresh look at tumor immunosurveillance and immunotherapy. Nature Immunol 2001;2(4):293–9.

93. Sutton VR, Davis JE, Cancilla M, et al. Initiation of apoptosis by granzyme B requires direct cleavage of Bid, but not direct granzyme B-mediated caspase activation. J Exp Med 2000;192(10):1403–13.

94. Deng JS, Falo LD, Kim B, Abell E. Cytotoxic T cells in basal cell carcinomas of skin. Am J Dermatopathol 1998;20(2):143–6.

95. Melnikova VO, Ananthaswamy HN. Cellular and molecular events leading to the development of skin cancer. Mutat Res 2005;571(1–2):91–106.

96. Boldrini L, Loggini B, Gisfredi S, et al. Mutations of Fas (APO-1/CD95) and p53 genes in nonmelanoma skin cancer. J Cutan Med Surg 2003;7(2):112–8.

97. Satchell AC, Barnetson RS, Halliday GM. Increased Fas ligand expression by T cells and tumour cells in the progression of actinic keratosis to squamous cell carcinoma. Br J Dermatol 2004;151(1):42–9.

98. Dorothee G, Vergnon I, Menez J, et al. Tumor-infiltrating CD4(+) T lymphocytes express APO2 ligand (APO2L)/TRAIL upon specific stimulation with autologous lung carcinoma cells: role of IFN-alpha on APO2L/TRAIL expression and -mediated cytotoxicity. J Immunol 2002;169(2):809–17.

99. Grimbaldeston MA, Skov L, Finlay-Jones JJ, Hart PH. Increased dermal mast cell prevalence and susceptibility to development of basal cell carcinoma in humans. Methods 2002;28(1):90–6.

100. Czarnecki D, Zalcberg J, Kulinskaya E, Kay T. Impaired cell-mediated immunity of apparently normal patients who had multiple skin cancers. Cancer 1995;76(2):228–31.

101. Yamamura M, Modlin RL, Ohmen JD, Moy RL. Local Expression of Antiinflammatory Cytokines in Cancer. J Clin Invest 1993;91(3):1005–10.

102. Kim J, Modlin RL, Moy RL, et al. IL-10 production in cutaneous basal and squamous cell carcinomas. A mechanism for evading the local T cell immune response. J Immunol 1995;155:2240–7.

103. Gutierrezsteil C, Wronesmith T, Sun XM, Krueger JG, Coven T, Nickoloff BJ. Sunlight-induced basal cell carcinoma tumor cells and ultraviolet-b-irradiated psoriatic plaques express Fas ligand (Cd95l). J Clin Invest 1998;101(1):33–9.

104. Byrne SN, Halliday GM. High levels of Fas ligand and MHC class II in the absence of CD80 or CD86 expression and a decreased CD4(+) T cell infiltration, enables murine skin tumours to progress. Cancer Immunol Immunother 2003;52:396–402.

105. Nestle FO, Burg G, Fah J, Wronesmith T, Nickoloff BJ. Human sunlight-induced basal-cell-carcinoma-associated dendritic cells are deficient in T cell co-stimulatory molecules and are impaired as antigen-presenting cells. Am J Pathol 1997;150(2):641–51.

106. Byrne SN, Halliday GM. Phagocytosis by dendritic cells rather than MHC II high macrophages is associated with skin tumour regression. Int J Cancer 2003;106(5):736–44.

107. Halliday GM, Le S. Transforming growth factor-beta produced by progressor tumors inhibits, while IL-10 produced by regressor tumors enhances, Langerhans cell migration from skin. Int Immunol 2001;13(9):1147–54.

108. Weber F, Byrne SN, Le S, et al. Transforming growth factor-beta(1) immobilises dendritic cells within skin tumours and facilitates tumour escape from the immune system. Cancer Immunol Immunother 2005;54(9):898–906.

109. Diamond TH, Eisman JA, Mason RS, et al. Vitamin D and adult bone health in Australia and New Zealand: a position statement. Med J Aust 2005;182(6):281–5.

110. Wong G, Gupta R, Dixon KM, et al. 1,25-dihydroxyvitamin D and three low-calcemic analogs decrease UV-induced DNA damage via the rapid response pathway. J Steroid Biochem Mol Biol 2004;89–90(1–5):567–70.

111. Dixon KM, Deo SS, Wong G, et al. Skin cancer prevention: a possible role of 1,25dihydroxyvitamin D3 and its analogs. J Steroid Biochem Mol Biol 2005;97(1–2):137–43.

112. Kricker A, Armstrong B. Does sunlight have a beneficial influence on certain cancers? Prog Biophys Mol Biol 2006;92(1):132–9.

113. Green A, Williams G, Neale R, et al. Daily sunscreen application and betacarotene supplementation in prevention of basal-cell and squamous-cell carcinomas of the skin: a randomised controlled trial. Lancet 1999;354(9180):723–9.

114. Anders A, Altheide HJ, Knalmann M, Tronnier H. Action spectrum for erythema in humans investigated with dye lasers. Photochem Photobiol 1995;61(2):200–5.

115. Poon TSC, Barnetson RS, Halliday GM. Prevention of immunosuppression by sunscreens in humans is unrelated to protection from erythema and dependent on protection from ultraviolet A in the face of

constant ultraviolet B protection. J Invest Dermatol 2003;121(1):184–90.

116. Damian DL, Halliday GM, Barnetson RS. Broadspectrum sunscreens provide greater protection against ultraviolet-radiation-induced suppression of contact hypersensitivity to a recall antigen in humans. J Invest Dermatol 1997;109(2):146–51.

117. Fourtanier A, Gueniche A, Compan D, Walker SL, Young AR. Improved protection against solar-simulated radiation-induced immunosuppression by a sunscreen with enhanced ultraviolet A protection. J Invest Dermatol 2000;114(4):620–7.

118. Wolf P, Hoffmann C, Quehenberger F, Grinschgl S, Kerl H. Immune protection factors of chemical sunscreens measured in the local contact hypersensitivity model in humans. J Invest Dermatol 2003;121(5):1080–7.

119. Kelly DA, Seed PT, Young AR, Walker SL. A commercial sunscreen's protection against ultraviolet radiation-induced immunosuppression is more than 50% lower than protection against sunburn in humans. J Invest Dermatol 2003;120(1):65–71.

120. Baron ED, Fourtanier A, Compan D, Medaisko C, Cooper KD, Stevens SR. High ultraviolet A protection affords greater immune protection confirming that ultraviolet A contributes to photoimmunosuppression in humans. J Invest Dermatol 2003;121(4):869–75;.

121. Halliday GM, Robertson BO, Barnetson RS. Topical retinoic acid enhances, and a dark tan protects, from subedemal solar-simulated photocarcinogenesis. J Invest Dermatol 2000;114(5):923–7.

122. Barnetson RS, Ooi TKT, Zhuang LQ, et al. Nle(4)-D-Phe(7) -alpha-melanocyte-stimulating hormone significantly increased pigmentation and decreased UV damage in fair-skinned Caucasian volunteers. J Invest Dermatol 2006;126(8):1869–78.

123. Arad S, Konnikov N, Goukassian DA, Gilchrest BA. T-oligos augment UV-induced protective responses in human skin. FASEB J 2006;20(11):U95–U105.

124. Kripke ML, Cox PA, Alas LG, Yarosh DB. Pyrimidine dimers in DNA initiate systemic immunosuppression in UV-irradiated mice. Proc Natl Acad Sci USA 1992;89(16):7516–20.

125. Kuchel JM, Barnetson RS, Halliday GM. Cyclobutane pyrimidine dimer formation is a molecular trigger for solar-simulated ultraviolet radiation-induced suppression of memory immunity in humans. Photochem Photobiol Sci 2005;4(8):577–82.

126. Yarosh D, Klein J, O'Connor A, Hawk J, Rafal E, Wolf P. Effect of topically applied T4 endonuclease V in liposomes on skin cancer in xeroderma pigmentosum: a randomised study. Lancet 2001;357(9260):926–9.

127. Russo PAJ, Halliday GM. Inhibition of nitric oxide and reactive oxygen species production improves the ability of a sunscreen to protect from sunburn, immunosuppression and photocarcinogenesis. Br J Dermatol 2006;155(2):408–15.

128. Kuchel JM, Barnetson RS, Halliday GM. Nitric oxide appears to be a mediator of solar-simulated ultraviolet radiation-induced immunosuppression in humans. J Invest Dermatol 2003;121(3):587–93.

129. Yuen KS, Halliday GM. Alpha-tocopherol, an inhibitor of epidermal lipid peroxidation, prevents ultraviolet radiation from suppressing the skin immune system. Photochem Photobiol 1997;65(3):587–92.

130. Friedmann AC, Halliday GM, Barnetson RS, et al. The topical isoflavonoid NV-07 alpha reduces solar-simulated UV-induced suppression of Mantoux reactions in humans. Photochem Photobiol 2004;80(3):416–21.

131. Kuchel JM, Barnetson RSC, Zhuang L, Strickland FM, Pelley RP, Halliday GM. Tamarind inhibits solar-simulated ultraviolet radiation-induced suppression of recall responses in humans. Letters in Drug Design and Discovery 2005;2:165–71.

132. Elmets CA, Singh D, Tubesing K, Matsui M, Katiyar S, Mukhtar H. Cutaneous photoprotection from ultraviolet injury by green tea polyphenols. J Am Acad Dermatol 2001;44(3):425–32.

133. Decraene D, Smaers K, Maes D, Matsui M, Declercq L, Garmyn M. A low UVB dose, with the potential to trigger a protective p53–dependent gene program, increases the resilience of keratinocytes against future UVB insults. J Invest Dermatol 2005;125(5):1026–31.

134. Motley R, Kersey P, Lawrence C. Multiprofessional guidelines for the management of the patient with primary cutaneous squamous cell carcinoma. Br J Plast Surg 2003;56(2):85–91.

135. Salasche SJ. Status of curettage and desiccation in the treatment of primary basal cell carcinoma. J Am Acad Dermatol 1984;10(2 Pt 1):285–7.

136. Swetter SM, Boldrick JC, Pierre P, Wong P, Egbert BM. Effects of biopsy-induced wound healing on residual basal cell and squamous cell carcinomas: rate of tumor regression in excisional specimens. J Cutan Pathol 2003;30(2):139–46.

137. Klein E. Immunotherapeutic approaches to skin cancer. Hosp Pract 1976;11(11):107–16.

138. Gutterman JU. Cytokine therapeutics: lessons from interferon alpha. Proc Natl Acad Sci USA 1994;91(4):1198–205.

139. Cornell RC, Greenway HT, Tucker SB, et al. Intralesional interferon therapy for basal cell carcinoma. J Am Acad Dermatol 1990;23(4 pt 1):694–700.

140. Mozzanica N, Cattaneo A, Boneschi V, Brambilla L, Melotti E, Finzi AF. Immunohistological evaluation

of basal cell carcinoma immunoinfiltrate during intralesional treatment with alpha 2–interferon. Arch Dermatol Res 1990;282(5):311–7.

141. Buechner SA, Wernli M, Harr T, Hahn S, Itin P, Erb P. Regression of basal cell carcinoma by intralesional interferon-alpha treatment is mediated by CD95 (Apo-1/Fas)-CD95 ligand-induced suicide. J Clin Invest 1997;100(11):2691–6.

142. de Graaf YG, Kennedy C, Wolterbeek R, Collen AF, Willemze R, Bouwes Bavinck JN. Photodynamic therapy does not prevent cutaneous squamous-cell carcinoma in organ-transplant recipients: results of a randomized-controlled trial. J Invest Dermatol 2006;126(3):569–74.

143. Dragieva G, Hafner J, Dummer R, et al. Topical photodynamic therapy in the treatment of actinic keratoses and Bowen's disease in transplant recipients. Transplantation 2004;77(1):115–21.

144. Gollnick SO, Evans SS, Baumann H, et al. Role of cytokines in photodynamic therapy-induced local and systemic inflammation. Br J Cancer 2003;88(11):1772–9.

145. Oseroff A. PDT as a cytotoxic agent and biological response modifier: Implications for cancer prevention and treatment in immunosuppressed and immunocompetent patients. J Invest Dermatol 2006;126(3):542–4.

146. Gollnick SO, Vaughan L, Henderson BW. Generation of effective antitumor vaccines using photodynamic therapy. Cancer Res 2002;62(6):1604–8.

147. Gupta AK, Davey V, McPhail H. Evaluation of the effectiveness of imiquimod and 5–fluorouracil for the treatment of actinic keratosis: Critical review and meta-analysis of efficacy studies. J Cutan Med Surg 2005;9(5):209–14.

148. Geisse J, Caro I, Lindholm J, Golitz L, Stampone P, Owens M. Imiquimod 5% cream for the treatment of superficial basal cell carcinoma: results from two phase III, randomized, vehicle-controlled studies. J Am Acad Dermatol 2004;50(5):722–33.

149. Epstein E. Fluorouracil paste treatment of thin basal cell carcinomas. Arch Dermatol 1985;121(2):207–13.

150. Peris K, Micantonio T, Fargnoli MC, Lozzi GP, Chimenti S. Imiquimod 5% cream in the treatment of Bowen's disease and invasive squamous cell carcinoma. J Am Acad Dermatol 2006;55(2):324–7.

151. Hengge UR, Schaller J. Successful treatment of invasive squamous cell carcinoma using topical imiquimod. Arch Dermatol 2004;140(4):404–6.

152. Ooi T, Barnetson RS, Zhuang L, et al. Imiquimod-induced regression of actinic keratosis is associated with infiltration by T lymphocytes and dendritic cells: a randomized controlled trial. Br J Dermatol 2006;154(1):72–8.

153. Suzuki H, Wang B, Shivji GM, et al. Imiquimod, a topical immune response modifier, induces migration of Langerhans cells. J Invest Dermatol 2000;114(1):135–41.

154. O'Sullivan I, Kim TS, Chopra A, Cohen EP. Therapeutic properties of DNA-based fibroblast and dendritic cell vaccines in mice with squamous carcinoma. Anticancer Res 2006;26(2A):873–84.

155. Zhang G, Luo X, Sumithran E, et al. Squamous cell carcinoma growth in mice and in culture is regulated by c-Jun and its control of matrix metalloproteinase-2 and -9 expression. Oncogene 2006;25(55):7260–6.

17
Immunobiology and Immune-Based Therapies of Melanoma

Mariah R. Brown, John C. Ansel, and Cheryl A. Armstrong

Key Points

- Human regulatory T cells (T_{reg}s) play an important role in suppressing antitumor immune responses.
- Melanoma-derived factors may convert dendritic cells into tolerance-inducing, antigen-presenting cells.
- Adhesion molecules such as integrins, cadherins, and intercellular adhesion molecule 1 (ICAM-1) have been implicated in progression of melanoma.
- Melanoma cells produce a variety of cytokines that allow tumor progression.
- Surgery, chemotherapy, and immunotherapy (e.g., interferon-α and interleukin-2) are used in the treatment of melanoma.
- A variety of vaccines are being studied for therapy of melanoma.

Cutaneous malignant melanoma originates from melanocytes, the neural crest–derived pigment cells residing in the basal layer of the epidermis. The transition of melanocytes into neoplastic melanoma cells that initially grow in the skin and later metastasize to distant sites involves complex host–tumor cell interactions. Our understanding of these interactions has progressed rapidly in recent decades. However, translating these basic science developments into effective clinical advancements for the treatment of melanoma has proved more difficult. Melanoma remains an important health issue, with an estimated 59,940 new cases of malignant melanoma diagnosed in 2007, making it the fifth most common cancer in both women and men.[1]

Our current understanding of melanoma development involves a stepwise progression through stages of growth, including atypia, radial growth, vertical growth, and the development of metastases[2] (Fig. 17.1). This model corresponds to the American Joint Commission on Cancer (AJCC) staging classification of melanoma that categorizes primary cutaneous melanoma as stage I or stage II disease, lymph node metastases as stage III disease, and distant metastases as stage IV disease.[3] Standard treatment modalities including chemotherapy have been utilized for the treatment of metastatic melanoma, with overall disappointing results.[4] As a result, the need to discover new effective treatment modalities for melanoma has become a pressing issue. Insights into our understanding of the host immune response to malignant melanoma continue to stimulate the development of new approaches to melanoma therapy.

Melanoma Immunology

It is widely accepted that melanoma cells are capable of triggering host immunologic responses, and melanoma has long been a model for immunogenic tumors. Depigmentation and regression of primary melanomas provides supporting evidence that host immune surveillance to this tumor can occur.[5,6] Additionally, systemic immune suppression is associated with increased rates and more aggressive behavior of malignant melanoma, in particular in patients with HIV disease.[7–9] Finally, different types of immune cells have been noted infiltrating tumor sites in malignant melanoma, and increased numbers of immune cells have been associated with an improved prognosis, even in

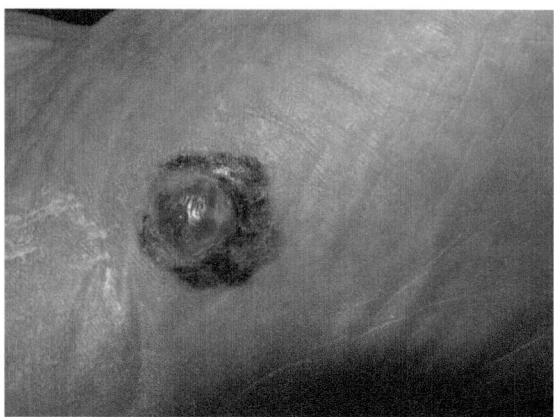

FIG. 17.1. Cutaneous melanoma. The clinical appearance of this cutaneous melanoma on the sole of a foot exhibits both radial growth (dark brown pigmentation) and vertical growth (amelanotic nodule) of neoplastic cells

more advanced disease.[10] As a result, understanding and then modulating the immune system for the treatment of malignant melanoma has been an active area of research for many years. To date these studies have yielded mixed results.

Because different components of the immune system are activated in response to melanoma cells, basic investigations of these immune responses are critical to the development of immune-based therapeutic approaches to melanoma. Numerous studies have shown that T lymphocytes play a major role in melanoma immunology and immunotherapy. T cells have been observed to accumulate in melanoma lesions and specifically lyse autologous tumor cells in vitro as well as causing tumor regression when transferred in vivo in 30% of melanoma patients.[11] Cytotoxic T cells (principally CD8+ cells) respond primarily to target cells with specific antigens associated with major histocompatibility complex (MHC) class I proteins. Activation of the cytotoxic T cells results in destruction of target cells that have altered MHC class I antigen expression. Helper T cells (CD4+ cells) respond primarily to self MHC class II proteins and the associated antigen on antigen-presenting cells. Activated CD8+ cytotoxic T lymphocytes and CD4+ T helper lymphocytes produce a variety of cytokines that function to amplify and modify the immune response to the growing tumor.[12,13] The role of B cells and humoral immunologic responses

to melanoma cells remains to be defined. Natural killer cells also appear to play a role in melanoma immune surveillance and destruction of neoplastic cells with reduced MHC expression.[14,15]

T-cell–mediated immunity to melanoma can be seen in early tumors, but also in late-stage metastatic disease. Techniques such as vaccination with tumor cells and tumor antigens can increase the T-cell–mediated immune response against melanoma tumor cells. However, like many types of tumors, melanoma cells have mechanisms to avoid host immune surveillance and defense, as demonstrated by the fact that brisk immune activation in clinical trials is rarely reflected in successful clinical responses.[16] Tumor cells evade the immune response by a number of mechanisms including antigen loss, downregulation of MHC expression, and reduction of the T-helper-1 (Th1) arm of the immune response.[17] In addition, a subpopulation of human regulatory T cells (T_{reg}s), characterized as CD4+CD25+ T cells, has recently been described that function to suppress self-reactive T cells.[18] There is evidence that T_{reg}s play an important role in suppressing antitumor immune responses, including those observed in animal models of melanoma.[19] Patients with metastatic melanoma have increased numbers of these CD4+CD25+ T cells that may influence responses to various immune modulating therapies.[20]

Dendritic cells also participate in the host immune response to melanoma. Dendritic cells are bone marrow–derived leukocytes that are potent antigen-presenting cells and play a critical role in initiation of T-cell immune responses.[21] Dendritic cells express high levels of both MHC class I and class II molecules as well as T-cell co-stimulatory molecules [i.e., CD40, CD80 (B7-1), CD86 (B7-2)].[22] Dendritic cells are capable of secreting a variety of cytokines, such as interleukin-1 (IL-1) and IL-12, which serve as accessory factors for T-cell activation. Activated dendritic cells are mobile, monocyte-derived cells that travel to lymphoid organs to present foreign or tumor cell antigens to specific populations of T cells, which results in the activation of antigen-specific effector T cells.[23] Even though it has been documented that dendritic cells infiltrate melanomas, their specific role in host immune responses to melanoma needs to be defined.[24] Previous studies have suggested that melanoma-derived factors may convert dendritic cells from potent immune response inducers into tolerance-inducing antigen-presenting cells,[21] which may be problematic in the development of dendritic cell melanoma immunotherapies.

Adhesion Molecules

A number of distinct cellular adhesion molecules and cytokines have been implicated in the local growth and metastatic progression of melanoma cells. Tumor progression and the development of metastatic disease are often associated with loss of normal cellular controls. The alteration of tumor cellular adhesion molecule expression and function allows neoplastic cells to separate from the primary tumor mass to establish metastatic lesions. With separation of the metastatic cells from the primary tumor mass, neoplastic cells are free of local cell contact inhibitory mechanisms. Altered expression of adhesion molecules in neoplastic cells can improve their ability to adhere to vascular endothelium, facilitating metastases to distant sites. Many different tumor-associated cell adhesion molecules have been implicated in the progression of melanoma from radial growth, to vertical growth, to metastases. These key adhesion molecules include integrins, cadherins and immunoglobulins such as intercellular adhesion molecule 1 (ICAM-1).[25] In vitro and in vivo studies have shown that melanoma cells alter their cell surface adhesion molecules as they progress through different stages of growth, and that expression of certain cell surface molecules by melanoma can yield prognostic information.[25,26]

One example of a cell adhesion molecule associated with melanoma pathogenesis is MUC18/ MCAM/CD146, a cell surface glycoprotein that mediates adhesion to different cell types. MUC18 is expressed on both vascular endothelia and activated T lymphocytes, facilitating the extravasation or homing of activated T cells.[27,28] The expression of MUC18 on melanoma cells is associated with tumor progression and increased metastatic potential in both humans and mice.[29,30] The level of expression of MUC18 on primary melanoma tumors increases as tumors increase in thickness and develop metastatic potential.[29,31] Indeed, the ability of human melanoma cell lines to form metastases in mice has been correlated with the

level of expression of MUC18.[32] In light of these findings, a human monoclonal antibody against MUC18, ABX-MA1, has demonstrated therapeutic promise in mouse models of melanoma.[33]

Cytokines

Melanoma cells are capable of producing a variety of cytokines, which not only can modulate the growth of melanoma cells, but also may either promote or inhibit the host antitumor inflammatory and immune response.[34] These melanoma-derived cytokines have different biologic activities and can act as autocrine growth factors, growth inhibitors, growth promoters, or immunosuppressive factors. Some of these cytokines allow the melanoma cells to grow independently of exogenous growth factors.

Basic fibroblast growth factor (bFGF), IL-6, and chemokines such as IL-8 are capable of acting as melanoma autocrine growth factors. Basic FGF is expressed by melanoma cells, but not by melanocytes and appears to provide a growth advantage to tumor cells.[35,36] Some melanoma cell lines produce IL-6, which is a major immune and inflammatory mediator that appears to have conflicting roles in regulating melanoma growth and progression.[37–39] Previous studies indicate that IL-6 may be both a growth inhibitor and an autocrine growth stimulant for melanoma cells depending on the stage of tumor progression.[40] In vitro studies also demonstrate the ability of IL-8 to function as an autocrine growth factor for melanoma cells.[41] A positive correlation between melanoma IL-8 production and tumor thickness in primary cutaneous melanoma has been reported.[42] Additionally, IL-8 production has been reported to correlate with melanoma metastatic potential in nude mice[43] and with the induction of migration by melanoma cells.

Tumor-derived transforming growth factor-β (TGF-β) and colony-stimulating factors (CSFs) may also modulate the growth and progression of melanoma. The TGF-βs are potent regulators of the immune response, cellular proliferation, differentiation, and extracellular matrix synthesis and deposition.[44] The proliferation of most melanoma cell lines is inhibited by TGF-β.[35,45] However, some melanoma cell lines established from metastatic tumors have been shown to become resistant to the growth inhibitory effects of TGF-β, and this cytokine may even act as a growth stimulator in certain of these advanced melanoma cell lines.[46] Since TGF-β has potent immunosuppressive activities, the production of this cytokine by melanoma cells may inhibit the host immune responses to this neoplasm. Some melanoma cells are capable of producing a number of CSFs including granulocyte colony-stimulating factor (G-CSF), granulocyte-macrophage colony-stimulating factor (GM-CSF), stem cell factor/mast cell growth factor, and monocyte colony-stimulating factor.[38,47] Host antimelanoma effects have been most clearly demonstrated with GM-CSF. Studies have shown that GM-CSF produced by melanoma cells can induce monocyte TNF-α production that could contribute to host antitumor responses.[48] GM-CSF gene transfection

into melanoma cells results in significant inhibition of melanoma progression by activating host immune responses[49,50] (Fig. 17.2). In human pathologic specimens, it has also been reported that melanoma tumor thickness inversely correlates with GM-CSF melanoma cell production, suggesting that GM-CSF may have an antimelanoma role in early primary lesions.[42]

Interleukin-10 (IL-10), which has a number of immunosuppressive properties, is another cytokine produced by some melanoma cells. Other studies have also demonstrated that in some circumstances, IL-10 appears to act as a growth factor for melanoma cells in vitro and can downregulate the expression of human leukocyte antigen I (HLA-I), HLA-II, as well as ICAM-I.[51] Patients with advanced metastatic melanoma have been found to have elevated serum IL-10 levels, which are

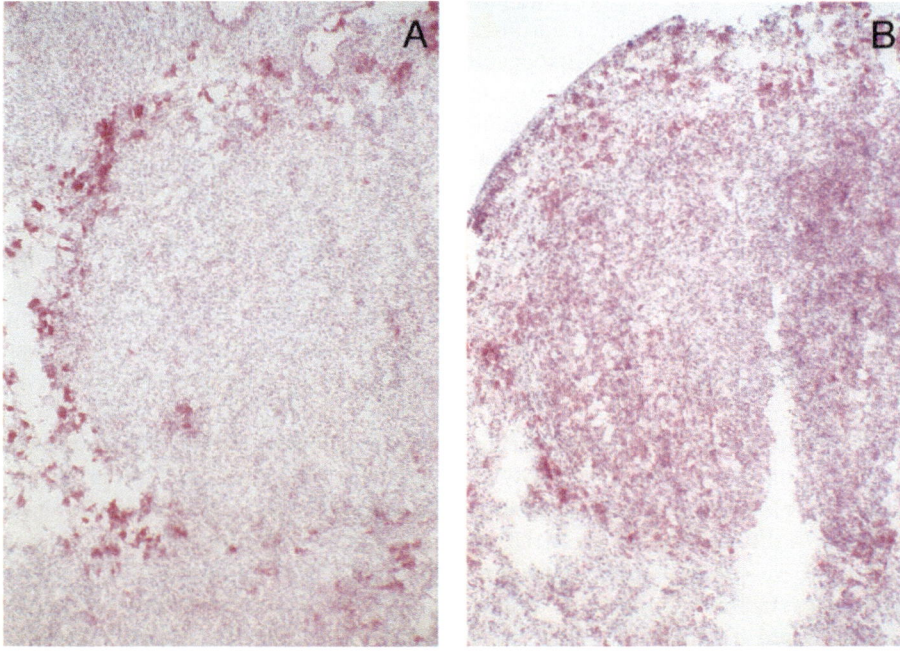

Fig. 17.2. Granulocyte-macrophage colony-stimulating factor (GM-CSF) facilitates dendritic cell infiltration in pulmonary melanoma metastases in a preclinical model. Experimental murine melanoma metastases were generated in immunocompetent mice using murine melanoma cells that did not produce GM-CSF (A) or that were transfected with the murine GM-CSF gene to produce significant amounts of GM-CSF (B). Lung tissue at the study end point was stained with a monoclonal antimurine dendritic cell antibody. Without GM-CSF, dendritic cells are localized only at the periphery of the melanoma nodules (A). In contrast, there are large numbers of dendritic cells within the GM-CSF–producing melanoma nodule (B), suggesting a potential mechanism for the antimelanoma effect of GM-CSF observed in this preclinical model system

rarely observed in healthy patients.[52] Thus, IL-10 predominantly has immunosuppressive activities, but in some cases may activate certain immune responses.[53]

Melanoma-Associated Antigens

A number of antigens located on the cell surface of melanomas have been referred to as melanoma-associated antigens (MAAs). These antigens can be divided into two major categories: HLA-associated antigens that are recognized by T cells, and cell surface antigens such as gangliosides that do not directly activate T cells.[17,54] Unlike gangliosides, melanoma associated antigens recognized by T cells are derived from proteins that do not normally reside on the surface of normal cells and thus can evoke an immune response in association with particular MHC molecules on the cell surface. These peptide-based antigens can be grouped into three different categories: antigens expressed only on cells of melanocytic lineage (e.g., tyrosinase, TRP-1, TRP-2, Melan-A/MART-1, and gp100), antigens expressed in different kinds of tumor cells but not in normal adult tissues outside of the gonads (e.g., MAGE, BAGE, GAGE, NY-ESO-1, and PRAME), and unique antigens found only on some tumor cells.[17] Interest in MAAs focuses on potential immunotherapies for melanoma, particularly vaccine therapy.

Cytotoxic T-cell clones that have been identified and expanded from melanoma patients may recognize specific antigens expressed on both melanoma cells and normal melanocytes.[55] Melanoma-associated cytotoxic T-cell antigens include tyrosinase, tyrosinase-related protein 2, tyrosinase-related protein 1/gp75, silver/gp100 protein, Melan-A/MART-1, and the Lerk proteins (lerk-1/protein B61 and Lerk-5/Eplg5/Elf2/HTK-L). Tyrosinase is an enzyme that converts tyrosine into dihydroxyphenylalanine (DOPA), the precursor of melanin. The gene that codes for tyrosinase is found in all melanoma cells as well as normal melanocytes, but is not expressed in other cell types. The silver/gp100 protein (also referred to as Pmel[56]) is a melanosomal matrix protein that acts as a solid-phase substrate for the accumulation of melanin.[57] The gp100 peptide is a melanocyte differentiation antigen that is recognized by HLA-A2 restricted

T lymphocytes.[58] Another gene that is expressed only in cells of melanocytic origin is Melan-A.[59] The antigen encoded by Melan-A is called MART-1 and is found only on normal melanocytes, melanoma cells, and retinal cells.[60] MART-1 is presented by HLA-A2 and is capable of causing a strong T-cell immune response.[61]

Antigens that are expressed almost exclusively on tumor cells and extensively on melanoma cells include products of the MAGE gene family. MAGE genes are all located on the long arm of the X chromosome and are only found on the testis in normal adult tissue. The MAGE proteins are commonly expressed on melanoma cells and less frequently on the surface of other tumor cells. The genes MAGE-1, −2, −3, −4, −6, and −12 are expressed in different tumors such as breast carcinomas, non–small-cell lung carcinomas, head and neck tumors, sarcomas, and ovarian carcinomas.[62–65] The products of MAGE-1 and MAGE-3 have been found to produce proteins that bind the different MHC class I molecules expressed on melanoma tumor cells. Products of MAGE-1 have been reported to be expressed on 48% of metastatic melanomas, while products of MAGE-3 are expressed in >90% of metastatic melanomas.[66,67] Even though some proteins produced from MAGE genes have been characterized and found to be expressed on the surface of certain tumor cells, their function is unknown.

Melanoma Gangliosides

Melanoma cells also express a number of gangliosides on their cell surfaces. Gangliosides are glycolipids that are characteristically found in neural crest–derived tissues.[12] Gangliosides regulate cell growth by altering growth factor signals and are involved in cell adhesion and cell matrix interactions.[68] The monosialoganglioside GM3 makes up 90% of the gangliosides found on normal melanocyte cell surfaces, while the disialoganglioside GD3 comprises only 5%.[68] It has been shown that quantitative and qualitative changes occur in the expression of gangliosides during oncogenic transformation.[69] The predominant gangliosides in melanoma are GM3 and GD3. GM3 is found on virtually all melanoma cells. GD3 is found on few normal melanocytes and at lower levels than melanoma cells. The minor gangliosides are expressed on most melanoma cells but less often in normal tissues. These minor gangliosides include GM2, GD2, GT3, and 9-O-Ac-GD3.[70] Melanoma gangliosides are therefore a possible target for immunotherapy against melanoma, and recent work has focused on several of these molecules in vaccine therapy.

Treatment Strategies for Melanoma

When detected early, melanoma responds well to treatment. However, it remains a difficult cancer to treat once it extends outside of the skin. About 8000 individuals are estimated to die from malignant melanoma in 2007, and the incidence of the disease continues to increase yearly.[1] Surgical removal of thin primary cutaneous melanomas is associated with 5-year survival rates of greater than 90% if the lesion is 1 mm or less in thickness.[71] However, in patients with thick cutaneous primary melanomas (>4 mm), ulcerated melanomas >1 mm, or melanomas with positive lymph nodes, survival declines dramatically.[71] Five-year survival for metastatic disease outside of the skin is less than 15%.[1] In spite of intensive experimental efforts, there is no current effective therapy that has significantly altered the poor prognosis associated with thicker, more invasive melanomas and metastatic disease. Recent advances in our understanding of the immunobiology of malignant melanoma offer the potential for new and more effective approaches for disease management.

Nonimmunologic Treatments

Surgical Treatment

As noted above, melanoma has an excellent prognosis when detected early and treated with surgical intervention. The depth of the tumor determines the local surgical margins and, for most thin tumors, surgery is curative.[72] However, the presence of local lymph node metastases (stage III disease) is a strong predictor of a poor clinical outcome.[73] The technique of sentinel lymph node dissection (SLND) has been developed as a way to identify patients with lymph node metastases without subjecting them to the morbidity of elective lymph node dissection. The technique involves the injection of a vital blue dye or radiolabeled agent into the area of the primary lesion to identify the sentinel node and the primary lymphatic drainage area from a cutaneous melanoma prior to wide local excision.[74] The sentinel lymph node is removed and a regional lymphadenectomy is performed if metastatic disease is detected histologically. Studies have shown that if the sentinel node is negative, there is less than a 1% chance of positive nodes elsewhere in the lymph node basin.[74] This technique has been studied in melanomas at high risk for metastatic disease, but still amenable to early intervention.[75]

Data from recent studies indicate that SLND yields valuable prognostic information.[75] In those patients who underwent SLND, the 5-year survival rate of those with positive sentinel nodes is 72%, versus 90% for those patients with a negative sentinel node.[75] Sentinel node biopsy can help identify patients who would benefit from adjuvant therapies. As a result of these studies, SLND is now considered the gold standard for management of melanoma of intermediate depths (1.2 to 3.5 mm).[76] However, in spite of significant optimism for this technique as an aid in melanoma therapy, clinical trials have not been able to show an overall survival benefit from SLND, and, as a result, the technique remains a subject of much debate.[77]

Chemotherapy

Dacarbazine (DTIC) is the only chemotherapeutic agent approved for the treatment of advanced melanoma by the Food and Drug Administration (FDA). Clinical trials demonstrate that approximately 10% to 20% of patients with metastatic melanoma have a measurable clinical response to the drug, but fewer than 5% achieve complete responses.[78] Innumerable combinations of different chemotherapeutics have been tried in the treatment of metastatic melanoma.[79] In spite of this effort, a recent meta-analysis failed to show a benefit in several different multidrug chemotherapy regimens when compared to DTIC alone.[79] Recently, interest has shifted to the drug temozolomide, an oral formulation of DTIC. The drug has been shown to have equal efficacy to DTIC,[80] with an increase in central nervous system (CNS) penetration that may increase activity against brain metastases.[81]

Immunologic Therapies

Overview

Immunotherapeutic approaches to melanoma can be classified as those designed as adjuvant therapy after treatment of the primary lesion to prevent subsequent metastatic disease, and those designed as immunotherapy for clinically apparent metastatic tumors. Adjuvant therapy is administered to patients at high risk for the development of metastatic disease but who have no detectable disease at the time of surgical resection of the primary neoplasms or after surgical resection of limited metastatic lesions such as to regional lymph nodes. High-risk melanoma patients include those with thick primary lesions in the skin, those with ulcerated melanomas or those in which tumor cells are detected in regional lymph nodes. Current melanoma adjuvant treatment options beyond surgery are limited and, for the most part, ineffective.

Previous therapeutic approaches for high-risk cutaneous melanoma have included clinical trials with interferons, specific and nonspecific immunotherapy, adjuvant chemotherapy and biochemotherapy, isolated limb perfusion, adjuvant radiation therapy, adjuvant hormonal therapy, and adjuvant retinoid therapy.[82–84] The development of active specific immunotherapy has resulted in therapeutic melanoma vaccines employing purified gangliosides, shed tumor antigens, specific isolated tumor peptides, mechanical or viral melanoma cell lysates, antigen-primed dendritic cells, and allogeneic or autologous whole tumor cell preparations that have been used as postoperative treatments for prevention and regression of cutaneous melanoma.[88,86] To date, although some positive results have been noted in some of these cutaneous melanoma studies, for the most part these approaches have shown little survival advantage over surgical therapy alone.

Research in tumor immune-based therapy has focused not only on the adjuvant setting after treatment of primary cutaneous melanoma, but also on the treatment of advanced metastatic melanoma.[72,87] These patients are a significant therapeutic challenge because they are often immunosuppressed and debilitated. A number of clinical immunotherapeutic trials for metastatic melanoma are currently in progress for patients with stage IV disease. Many of the same approaches that are under investigation as adjuvant therapies have been utilized in patients with detectable metastatic disease. The role of various cytokines as immunotherapy for cancer treatment remains an active area of investigation,[88] as well as the use of tumor vaccines and techniques such as adoptive immunotherapy.[86,89]

Immunotherapeutic Agents

Cytokines

The role of cytokines in immunotherapeutic approaches to cancer treatment remains an active area of investigation. Much of the data dealing with the role of melanoma-derived cytokines in the immunology of melanoma has been obtained by transfecting immunomodulating cytokine genes into neoplastic cells and observing the biologic response in murine model systems. This approach has also been useful to evaluate the in vivo consequences of tumor cell cytokine production in an animal host in a number of different tumor systems.[90–94] The in vivo consequences of tumor cell cytokine production have been evaluated for a number of cytokines including IL-2, IL-4, IL-18, IL-12, G-CSF, GM-CSF, M-CSF, interferon-γ (IFN-γ), IL-6, and IL-10.[49,50,90–98] Although IL-2 and IFN-α are the only FDA-approved cytokines for the treatment of melanoma, several other molecules in this family have also entered phase I and phase II clinical trials. Interleukin-12 has shown promise in early studies,[99] and phase II studies are ongoing to evaluate iboctadekin (rhIL-18) for the treatment of metastatic melanoma.[100]

Interleukin-2

Currently, one of the few FDA-approved treatments for metastatic melanoma is IL-2. High-dose IL-2 has been shown to induce a clinical response in 16% of patients with metastatic melanoma, with 10% of patients achieving partial response and 6% achieving complete response.[101] While response rates to IL-2 are low, recent studies demonstrate that the treatment appears able to induce durable responses in a small percentage of patients.[102] Follow-up data at 5 years indicates that, of the patients with metastatic melanoma who responded longer than 30 months to IL-2 therapy, none have had disease progression.[88] Attempts have been made to identify clinical, genetic, or immune characteristics of melanoma patients who have a vigorous response to IL-2 in order to determine which patients might benefit most from the treatment.[103,104] Targeting patients who would most likely respond to IL-2 would be beneficial, as IL-2 does not have a favorable toxicity and side effect profile. Most significantly, treatment results in a septic shock profile with hypotension in 64% of patients, limiting both the patients who can receive the medication and the medical centers eligible to administer this therapy.[102]

The role of high-dose IL-2 has been recently investigated in the context of regulatory T-cell (T_{reg}) induction. In patients with metastatic melanoma, treatment with standard high-dose IL-2 caused an increase in $CD4^+CD25^+$ T cells,[20,105] but high-dose IL-2 resulted in a significant decrease in T_{reg}s in those patients who achieved an objective clinical response.[20] Further investigation of genetic and molecular features of T_{reg}s in responding patients as well as mechanisms to eliminate T_{reg}s prior to IL-2 therapy are under investigation.

Interferon

The FDA approved high-dose IFN-α-2b as an adjuvant treatment for thick melanoma lesions or positive nodal disease in 1995. The approval stemmed from a phase III trial demonstrating an improvement in disease-free survival from 1.1 to 1.7 years and overall survival from 2.8 to 3.8 years with interferon treatment after surgical excision.[106] However, subsequent trials have not supported these results,[107] with a recent meta-analysis concluding that interferon is associated with an increase in disease-free survival, but not an improvement in overall survival.[108] Additionally, attempts to modify the dosing of interferon in order to decrease toxicity and improve efficacy have not been successful. Trials with both intermediate and low dose levels of interferon have also failed to show an improvement in survival.[109–111] As a result, the role of interferon as an adjuvant treatment in melanoma remains controversial.

Granulocyte-Macrophage Colony-Stimulating Factor

Granulocyte-macrophage colony-stimulating factor (GM-CSF) is a growth factor that functions as a potent inhibitor of the growth and progression of melanoma.[49,50] This effect is mediated by the host immunologic system and appears to involve activation of dendritic cells.[112] The antimelanoma effects of GM-CSF have been evaluated in patients with high-risk stage III and stage IV disease, demonstrating an increase in disease-free and overall survival in a phase II study of 48 patients.[113] The control arm of this trial consisted of historical patient data, and thus studies are under way to confirm this result.[114] Other studies have looked at GM-CSF as an adjuvant immunotherapy[115] and in perilesional injection of melanoma sites.[116,117] Most current work is focusing on the use of GM-CSF as an adjuvant therapy to increase immune response in vaccine trials.[118]

Biochemotherapy

Researchers have attempted to combine immunotherapy with other treatment modalities in an attempt to increase response rates. Several groups have combined IL-2 and IFN with chemotherapy for "biochemotherapy." Although some initial results were promising, larger trials have failed to show that the combinations selected result in longer survival times.[119–122] Pooled trial data have indicated increased response rates with biochemotherapy, but this comes at the cost of decreased quality of life and increased treatment related toxicity for patients receiving chemotherapy and immunotherapy concurrently.[122]

Cytotoxic T-Lymphocyte Antigen 4

Cytotoxic T-lymphocyte antigen 4 (CTLA-4) is a T-cell surface glycoprotein that functions as an inhibitor to T-cell activation, working in opposition to CD28.[123] As a result, CTLA-4 functions to prevent the breaking of self-tolerance by the immune system. Initial studies demonstrated in murine models that antibody inhibition of CTLA-4 could enhance the destruction of certain tumors, particularly those that were more immunogenic.[124] In vitro studies in humans sought to demonstrate whether inhibition of CTLA-4 could enhance the immune cell response against self antigens, such as gp100 and MART-1, which are expressed by melanoma cells.[125–127] Overall response rates appear around 15%, for an antibody to CTLA-4 administered alone or with other agents, such as vaccines against tumor antigens. As expected, response rates appear to correlate with the development of autoimmunity.[128,129]

However, the autoimmune side effects induced by anti–CTLA-4 are severe, including uveitis, gastroenteritis, dermatitis, and hypophysitis,[130] which may inhibit the usefulness of CTLA-4 as an agent for melanoma treatment.

Adoptive Immunotherapy

Adoptive immunity against melanoma antigens is achieved by the isolation of immunocompetent lymphocytes from patients, in vitro expansion of specific subsets of these cells, and then reinfusion of these T cells back into patients. The source of infused lymphocytes can be derived from the tumor itself, which yields tumor-infiltrating lymphocytes, from lymph nodes draining the site of the primary lesion, or from the peripheral blood. Several different clinical trials have investigated various types of adoptive immunotherapy as treatment for metastatic melanoma,[131–133] as well as a possible adjuvant therapy for less advanced disease.[134] Early studies demonstrated that while tumor-specific cytotoxic T cells harvested from lymph nodes draining areas of melanoma showed little or no tumor-specific cytotoxic activity, culture of these cells with irradiated autologous tumor cells in the presence of IL-2 rendered them cytotoxic to autologous tumor.[135] Treatment regimens for melanoma have included intravenous infusion of tumor-infiltrating lymphocytes with IL-2[136,137] and intralesional injection of IL-2–cultured lymphoid cells.[138] One primary limitation of adoptive cell transfer has been the inability to generate a sustained level of tumor infiltrating lymphocytes, a significant setback given that persistence of tumor infiltrating lymphocytes has been correlated with clinical response for in vitro trials.[139] A recent study has demonstrated that lymphodepleting chemotherapy prior to cell transfer results in more sustained responses in metastatic melanoma, possibly by decreasing the numbers of regulator T cells and by modifying the immune environment.[89] As a result, increasing myeloabation prior to T-cell transfer is being considered as a possible future direction for the field.[140]

Specific Immunotherapy

Specific immunotherapy agents stimulate the host immune system to recognize and destroy neoplastic cells bearing tumor-associated antigens. Also referred to as active specific immunotherapy, this approach often involves vaccination with modified melanoma cells or melanoma-derived antigens. Melanoma vaccines are currently under investigation for the treatment of advanced metastatic melanoma (stage IV) and as an adjuvant treatment of patients at high risk for metastatic disease after surgical treatment (stages II and III). Multiple trials with melanoma vaccines have been completed in the past decade, although there has been minimal overall success in phase III clinical trials.

Autologous Vaccines

One approach to generate a specific host immune response is to vaccinate patients with their own tumor cells or cellular lysates made from their own tumor cells, known as autologous vaccination. For this procedure the tumor cells are harvested from the patient, processed in vitro, often in combination with an immunostimulatory agent, and injected subcutaneously back into the patient as an autologous vaccine. The theoretical advantage of this technique is that it targets the specific antigens of a patient's tumor cells. Some of the major limitations to this approach are the limited number of tumor cells required for vaccine preparation and the labor-intensive and technically challenging nature of culturing and expanding the patient's melanoma cells.

Early randomized trials with autologous whole tumor cells plus BCG (bacille Calmette-Guérin) failed to demonstrate improvement in overall outcome.[141–143] Recent work has focused on modulating a patient's tumor cells to increase the immune response. Haptenation of tumor cells with dinitrofluorobenzene (DNFB), administered after sensitizing to DNFB, appears to increase immune response and potentially survival in patients who develop cell-mediated immunity to tumor antigens.[144,145] Additional work has focused on extraction of a patient's heat shock proteins from melanoma cells to create an autologous vaccine.[146] The vaccine, known as Oncophage, consists of autologous tumor-derived heat shock protein gp96 and has been tested in a phase II trial. This study demonstrated that 50% of patients develop HLA-restricted T cells in response to the vaccine, and further trials are under way.[147] Finally, a third technique takes advantage of the antitumor properties of GM-CSF by transfecting autologous melanoma cells with the gene for this molecule.[148,149] Using retrovirus-mediated gene transfer for transfection, investigators, have been able to create an autologous vaccine that in early studies increases tumor necrosis and invasion by immune cells.[148,149]

Allogeneic Vaccines

An alternative approach to autologous melanoma vaccines is the use of tumor vaccines derived from allogeneic melanoma cells. The goal of this approach is to stimulate the host immune system with a variety of tumor antigens associated with an allogeneic MHC background. In addition to making a vaccine that would be widely available to many patients, the foreign MHC expression on the surface of these tumor cells further augments the patient's antitumor immune response. Multiple investigators have initiated clinical trials utilizing allogeneic vaccines as monotherapy for metastatic disease, as well as adjuvant therapy after surgical excision of the tumor. Improvement in time to disease progression was shown in a double-blind, placebo-controlled trial of a polyvalent shed antigen vaccine. This small trial of 38 patients demonstrated a 2.5 times increase in time to disease progression, from 0.6 years to 1.5 years, in the vaccine group.[150] Results with other vaccines in larger trials have been less promising. Melacine, a vaccine derived from two melanoma cell line lysates administered with a detoxified end toxin adjuvant, has been studied in phase III clinical trials, with no improvement in outcomes in advanced disease as compared to chemotherapy.[151] In a large trial studying this vaccine as adjuvant therapy in stage II disease, no improvement was noted in relapse-free survival,[152] although statistically significant improvement was seen in patients expressing HLA-A2 or HLA-C3.[153] Canavaxin, an allogeneic vaccine derived from three melanoma cells lines mixed with BCG, also failed to show success in phase III trials.[154]

Viral Oncolysates

Administration of viral oncolysates is another form of specific immunotherapy that has shown significant potential in stimulating a clinical antimelanoma response when used as adjuvant therapy.[155] Viral oncolysates are produced by infecting cultured melanoma cells with virus to generate a mixture of lysed cells plus virion that can be administered as vaccines. Vaccinia virus melanoma cell oncolysates have shown promise in phase I/phase II studies in patients with stage I and stage II melanoma but not in a phase III study with stage III melanoma patients,[156] although a subsequent retrospective subset analysis showed a subset of men with one to five positive nodes between the ages of 44 and 57 years with a survival advantage when treated with vaccinia melanoma oncolysate.[157] Previous studies have demonstrated that patients with stage III metastatic melanoma with palpable lymph node disease have shown a remarkable response to postsurgical vaccination with Newcastle disease virus (NDV) melanoma cell oncolysate.[158,159] We have further reported that this group of patients treated with allogeneic melanoma cell oncolysates produced by the 73T NDV strain had a 55% survival rate at 15-year follow-up as compared to historical controls with 6% to 33% 10-year survival rates.[160] We have also detected alterations in the peripheral blood CD8 T-cell populations in NDV oncolysate patients, consistent with activation by a chronic immune stimulus.[160] The antitumor mechanisms of action triggered by NDV oncolysate are unknown, although some studies indicate that it may act in part through the induction of certain cytokines with antitumor properties.[161]

Peptide Vaccines

The identification of genes encoding melanoma-specific antigens has led to their use in specific immunotherapy. As previously discussed, these are antigens that are expressed on cells of melanocytic lineage or melanoma cells that have been shown to play a role in tumor immunology. Multiple clinical trials have studied the effect of immunization against melanoma peptides such as gp100,[162] MAGE,[163] MART,[164] and tyrosinase in patients with advanced melanoma.[165] To increase HLA binding, peptides can be modified by changing amino acids to form "heteroclytic" peptides, which enhance the immune response against the native peptide.[86] Overall, positive clinical outcomes with peptide vaccines have been few, as obstacles such as tumor escape, preexisting neutralizing antibodies, and antigen loss variants hamper vaccine success.[17] However, continued advances in heteroclytic peptides, coadministration with immune adjuvants and cytokines, and altered dosing schedules may yet provide a role for these vaccines in melanoma treatment.[166]

Ganglioside Vaccines

Other investigators have focused on melanoma gangliosides as melanoma antigen targets. Although expressed in all tissues, gangliosides are often overexpressed in melanoma cells. The minor ganglioside antigen GM2 has been used as a melanoma vaccine administered in conjunction with BCG,[167] or conjugated with keyhole limpet hemocyanin[168] due to its role as the most immunogenic ganglioside.[86] The conjugated form of the vaccine has been studied in a phase III trial against interferon for adjuvant therapy of high-risk melanomas with disappointing results.[169] The vaccine did not show superiority to interferon and indeed showed a poorer patient survival at a median follow-up at 16 months, leading to discontinuation of the study. The major ganglioside antigens GD2 and GD3 have also sparked interest as possible vaccine targets, although both molecules are less immunogenic than GM3. As a result, investigations have focused on methods to increase the antibody response to these molecules[170] or to use antiidiotypic monoclonal antibody vaccines.[171–173]

Dendritic Cell Vaccines

Dendritic cell–based melanoma vaccines are also under investigation as yet another type of specific immunotherapy for the treatment of advanced melanoma.[174] The rationale behind this strategy is that dendritic cells modified to present specific melanoma antigens will more effectively stimulate naïve T cells to generate an antimelanoma response. Numerous preclinical studies have demonstrated that various types of dendritic cells can be loaded ex vivo with tumor antigens and administered to tumor-bearing hosts to elicit T-cell–mediated tumor destruction.[175,176] An initial study with advanced melanoma patients utilized professional antigen-presenting cells pulsed ex vivo with purified melanoma peptides or tumor lysates, which were delivered by direct injection into the inguinal lymph nodes of patients.[177] This study paved the way for other clinical trials using dendritic cells exposed to multiple melanoma peptides[178,179] or autologous tumor lysates.[180,181] Although it is difficult to compare trials given the use of different antigens and different dendritic cell lineages, it appears that dendritic cell vaccines induce tumor responses in about 9.5% of patients.[174] Thus, the use of dendritic cells in melanoma immunotherapy offers another approach to the treatment of patients with advanced melanoma.

Conclusion

Recent advances in our understanding of the immunobiology of melanoma have triggered the development of novel immunotherapeutic approaches that are undergoing evaluation in preclinical studies and clinical trials. Because clinical response rates and cure rates remain low in studies utilizing single immunomodulatory agents, new approaches, refinements of current approaches, and improved patient selection criteria are imperative to the achievement of significant cure rates and to overcome a number of logistical, technical, and toxicity problems. Immunotherapy continues to hold significant promise for the treatment of patients at risk for the development of metastatic melanoma and those with advanced disease.

References

1. Jemal A, Siegel R, Ward E, et al. Cancer statistics, 2007. CA Cancer J Clin 2007;57:43–66.
2. Clark WH Jr, Elder DE, Guerry DT, et al. A study of tumor progression: the precursor lesions of superficial spreading and nodular melanoma. Hum Pathol 1984;15:1147–65.
3. Balch CM, Soong SJ, Atkins MB, et al. An evidence-based staging system for cutaneous melanoma. CA Cancer J Clin 2004;54(3):131–49.
4. Bajetta E, Del Vecchio M, Bernard-Marty C, et al. Metastatic melanoma: chemotherapy. Semin Oncol 2002;29:427–45.
5. Wagner SN, Schultewolter T, Wagner C, et al. Immune response against human primary malignant melanoma: a distinct cytokine mRNA profile associated with spontaneous regression. Lab Invest 1998;78:541–50.
6. Armstrong CA, Ansel JC. Immunology of malignant melanoma. Photochem Photobiol 1996;63:418–20.
7. Wilkins K, Turner R, Dolev JC, et al. Cutaneous malignancy and human immunodeficiency virus disease. J Am Acad Dermatol 2006;54:189–206; quiz 207–10.

8. Rodrigues LK, Klencke BJ, Vin-Christian K, et al. Altered clinical course of malignant melanoma in HIV-positive patients. Arch Dermatol 2002;138:765–70.

9. Burgi A, Brodine S, Wegner S, et al. Incidence and risk factors for the occurrence of non-AIDS-defining cancers among human immunodeficiency virus-infected individuals. Cancer 2005;104:1505–11.

10. Mihm MC Jr, Clemente CG, Cascinelli N. Tumor infiltrating lymphocytes in lymph node melanoma metastases: a histopathologic prognostic indicator and an expression of local immune response. Lab Invest 1996;74:43–7.

11. Kawakami Y, Zakut R, Topalian SL, et al. Shared human melanoma antigens. Recognition by tumor-infiltrating lymphocytes in HLA-A2.1–transfected melanomas. J Immunol 1992;148:638–43.

12. Cebon J, MacGregor D, Scott A, et al. Immunotherapy of melanoma: targeting defined antigens. Australas J Dermatol 1997;38(suppl 1):S66–72.

13. Topalian SL, Rivoltini L, Mancini M, et al. Human CD4+ T cells specifically recognize a shared melanoma-associated antigen encoded by the tyrosinase gene. Proc Natl Acad Sci USA 1994;91:9461–5.

14. Hill LL, Perussia B, McCue PA, et al. Effect of human natural killer cells on the metastatic growth of human melanoma xenografts in mice with severe combined immunodeficiency. Cancer Res 1994;54:763–70.

15. Rouas-Freiss N, Bruel S, Menier C, et al. Switch of HLA-G alternative splicing in a melanoma cell line causes loss of HLA-G1 expression and sensitivity to NK lysis. Int J Cancer 2005;117:114–22.

16. Anichini A, Vegetti C, Mortarini R. The paradox of T-cell-mediated antitumor immunity in spite of poor clinical outcome in human melanoma. Cancer Immunol Immunother 2004;53:855–64.

17. Komenaka I, Hoerig H, Kaufman HL. Immunotherapy for melanoma. Clin Dermatol 2004;22:251–65.

18. Shevach EM. Regulatory T cells in autoimmmunity. Annu Rev Immunol 2000;18:423–49.

19. Antony PA, Restifo NP. CD4+CD25+ T regulatory cells, immunotherapy of cancer, and interleukin-2. J Immunother 2005;28:120–8.

20. Cesana GC, DeRaffele G, Cohen S, et al. Characterization of CD4+CD25+ regulatory T cells in patients treated with high-dose interleukin-2 for metastatic melanoma or renal cell carcinoma. J Clin Oncol 2006;24:1169–77.

21. Enk AH, Jonuleit H, Saloga J, et al. Dendritic cells as mediators of tumor-induced tolerance in metastatic melanoma. Int J Cancer 1997;73:309–16.

22. Liu Y, Janeway CA, Jr. Cells that present both specific ligand and costimulatory activity are the most efficient inducers of clonal expansion of normal CD4 T cells. Proc Natl Acad Sci USA 1992;89:3845–9.

23. Steinman RM. The dendritic cell system and its role in immunogenicity. Annu Rev Immunol 1991;9:271–96.

24. Becker Y. Dendritic cell activity against primary tumors: an overview. In Vivo 1993;7:187–91.

25. Haass NK, Smalley KS, Li L, et al. Adhesion, migration and communication in melanocytes and melanoma. Pigment Cell Res 2005;18:150–9.

26. Johnson JP. Cell adhesion molecules in the development and progression of malignant melanoma. Cancer Metastasis Rev 1999;18:345–57.

27. Sers C, Riethmuller G, Johnson JP. MUC18, a melanoma-progression associated molecule, and its potential role in tumor vascularization and hematogenous spread. Cancer Res 1994;54:5689–94.

28. Shih IM, Elder DE, Speicher D, et al. Isolation and functional characterization of the A32 melanoma-associated antigen. Cancer Res 1994;54:2514–20.

29. Lehmann JM, Holzmann B, Breitbart EW, et al. Discrimination between benign and malignant cells of melanocytic lineage by two novel antigens, a glycoprotein with a molecular weight of 113,000 and a protein with a molecular weight of 76,000. Cancer Res 1987;47:841–5.

30. Yang H, Wang S, Liu Z, et al. Isolation and characterization of mouse MUC18 cDNA gene, and correlation of MUC18 expression in mouse melanoma cell lines with metastatic ability. Gene 2001;265:133–45.

31. Brocker EB, Suter L, Bruggen J, et al. Phenotypic dynamics of tumor progression in human malignant melanoma. Int J Cancer 1985;36:29–35.

32. Luca M, Hunt B, Bucana CD, et al. Direct correlation between MUC18 expression and metastatic potential of human melanoma cells. Melanoma Res 1993;3:35–41.

33. Melnikova VO, Bar-Eli M. Bioimmunotherapy for melanoma using fully human antibodies targeting MCAM/MUC18 and IL-8. Pigment Cell Res 2006;19:395–405.

34. Armstrong C, Luger T, Ansel J. Cytokines and malignant melanoma. In: Mukhtar H, ed. Skin Cancer: Mechanisms and Human Relevance. Boca Raton, FL: CRC Press, 1995:273–80.

35. Rodeck U, Melber K, Kath R, et al. Constitutive expression of multiple growth factor genes by melanoma cells but not normal melanocytes. J Invest Dermatol 1991;97:20–6.

36. Halaban R, Langdon R, Birchall N, et al. Basic fibroblast growth factor from human keratinocytes is a natural mitogen for melanocytes. J Cell Biol 1988;107:1611–9.

37. Colombo MP, Maccalli C, Mattei S, et al. Expression of cytokine genes, including IL-6, in human malignant melanoma cell lines. Melanoma Res 1992;2:181–9.

38. Armstrong CA, Tara DC, Hart CE, et al. Heterogeneity of cytokine production by human malignant melanoma cells. Exp Dermatol 1992;1:37–45.

39. Lazar-Molnar E, Hegyesi H, Toth S, et al. Autocrine and paracrine regulation by cytokines and growth factors in melanoma. Cytokine 2000;12:547–54.

40. Lu C, Kerbel RS. Interleukin-6 undergoes transition from paracrine growth inhibitor to autocrine stimulator during human melanoma progression. J Cell Biol 1993;120:1281–8.

41. Schadendorf D, Moller A, Algermissen B, et al. IL-8 produced by human malignant melanoma cells in vitro is an essential autocrine growth factor. J Immunol 1993;151:2667–75.

42. Hensley C, Spitzler S, McAlpine BE, et al. In vivo human melanoma cytokine production: inverse correlation of GM-CSF production with tumor depth. Exp Dermatol 1998;7:335–41.

43. Singh RK, Gutman M, Radinsky R, et al. Expression of interleukin 8 correlates with the metastatic potential of human melanoma cells in nude mice. Cancer Res 1994;54:3242–7.

44. Wahl S. Regulation of tissue inflammation, repair, and fibrosis by transforming growth factor beta. In: Luger TA, Schwarz T, eds. Epidermal Growth Factors and Cytokines. New York: Marcel Dekker, 1994:241–52.

45. Pittelkow MR, Shipley GD. Serum-free culture of normal human melanocytes: growth kinetics and growth factor requirements. J Cell Physiol 1989;140:565–76.

46. Rodeck U, Bossler A, Graeven U, et al. Transforming growth factor beta production and responsiveness in normal human melanocytes and melanoma cells. Cancer Res 1994;54:575–81.

47. Mattei S, Colombo MP, Melani C, et al. Expression of cytokine/growth factors and their receptors in human melanoma and melanocytes. Int J Cancer 1994;56:853–7.

48. Sabatini M, Chavez J, Mundy GR, et al. Stimulation of tumor necrosis factor release from monocytic cells by the A375 human melanoma via granulocyte macrophage colony-stimulating factor. Cancer Res 1990;50:2673–8.

49. Armstrong CA, Botella R, Galloway TH, et al. Antitumor effects of granulocyte-macrophage colony-stimulating factor production by melanoma cells. Cancer Res 1996;56:2191–8.

50. Dranoff G, Jaffee E, Lazenby A, et al. Vaccination with irradiated tumor cells engineered to secrete murine granulocyte-macrophage colony-stimulating factor stimulates potent, specific, and long-lasting anti-tumor immunity. Proc Natl Acad Sci USA 1993;90:3539–43.

51. Yue FY, Dummer R, Geertsen R, et al. Interleukin-10 is a growth factor for human melanoma cells and down-regulates HLA class-I, HLA class-II and ICAM-1 molecules. Int J Cancer 1997;71:630–7.

52. Dummer W, Becker JC, Schwaaf A, et al. Elevated serum levels of interleukin-10 in patients with metastatic malignant melanoma. Melanoma Res 1995;5:67–8.

53. Chen WF, Zlotnik A. IL-10: a novel cytotoxic T cell differentiation factor. J Immunol 1991;147:528–34.

54. Kirkin AF, Dzhandzhugazyan K, Zeuthen J. The immunogenic properties of melanoma-associated antigens recognized by cytotoxic T lymphocytes. Exp Clin Immunogenet 1998;15:19–32.

55. Anichini A, Maccalli C, Mortarini R, et al. Melanoma cells and normal melanocytes share antigens recognized by HLA-A2–restricted cytotoxic T cell clones from melanoma patients. J Exp Med 1993;177: 989–98.

56. Theos AC, Truschel ST, Raposo G, et al. The Silver locus product Pmel17/gp100/Silv/ME20: controversial in name and in function. Pigment Cell Res 2005;18:322–36.

57. Sakai C, Kawakami Y, Law LW, et al. Melanosomal proteins as melanoma-specific immune targets. Melanoma Res 1997;7:83–95.

58. Zhai Y, Yang JC, Spiess P, et al. Cloning and characterization of the genes encoding the murine homologues of the human melanoma antigens MART1 and gp100. J Immunother 1997;20:15–25.

59. Coulie PG, Brichard V, Van Pel A, et al. A new gene coding for a differentiation antigen recognized by autologous cytolytic T lymphocytes on HLA-A2 melanomas. J Exp Med 1994;180:35–42.

60. Kawakami Y, Eliyahu S, Delgado CH, et al. Cloning of the gene coding for a shared human melanoma antigen recognized by autologous T cells infiltrating into tumor. Proc Natl Acad Sci USA 1994;91: 3515–9.

61. Romero P, Valmori D, Pittet MJ, et al. Antigenicity and immunogenicity of Melan-A/MART-1 derived peptides as targets for tumor reactive CTL in human melanoma. Immunol Rev 2002;188:81–96.

62. Chambost H, Brasseur F, Coulie P, et al. A tumour-associated antigen expression in human haematological malignancies. Br J Haematol 1993;84:524–6.

63. Rimoldi D, Romero P, Carrel S. The human melanoma antigen-encoding gene, MAGE-1, is expressed by other tumour cells of neuroectodermal origin such as glioblastomas and neuroblastomas. Int J Cancer 1993;54:527–8.

64. De Smet C, Lurquin C, van der Bruggen P, et al. Sequence and expression pattern of the human MAGE2 gene. Immunogenetics 1994;39:121–9.

65. Brasseur F, Marchand M, Vanwijck R, et al. Human gene MAGE-1, which codes for a tumor-rejection antigen, is expressed by some breast tumors. Int J Cancer 1992;52:839–41.

66. Brasseur F, Rimoldi D, Lienard D, et al. Expression of MAGE genes in primary and metastatic cutaneous melanoma. Int J Cancer 1995;63:375–80.

67. Roeder C, Schuler-Thurner B, Berchtold S, et al. MAGE-A3 is a frequent tumor antigen of metastasized melanoma. Arch Dermatol Res 2005;296: 314–9.

68. Mukerjee S, Nasoff M, McKnight M, Glassy M. Characterization of human IgG1 monoclonal antibody against gangliosides expressed on tumor cells. Hybridoma 1998;17:133–42.

69. Hakomori S. Aberrant glycosylation in cancer cell membranes as focused on glycolipids: overview and perspectives. Cancer Res 1985;45:2405–14.

70. Hamilton WB, Helling F, Lloyd KO, et al. Ganglioside expression on human malignant melanoma assessed by quantitative immune thin-layer chromatography. Int J Cancer 1993;53:566–73.

71. Balch CM, Buzaid AC, Soong SJ, et al. Final version of the American Joint Committee on Cancer staging system for cutaneous melanoma. J Clin Oncol 2001;19:3635–48.

72. Jack A, Boyes C, Aydin N, et al. The treatment of melanoma with an emphasis on immunotherapeutic strategies. Surg Oncol 2006;15:13–24.

73. Morton DL, Wanek L, Nizze JA, et al. Improved long-term survival after lymphadenectomy of melanoma metastatic to regional nodes. Analysis of prognostic factors in 1134 patients from the John Wayne Cancer Clinic. Ann Surg 1991;214:491–9; discussion 499–501.

74. Morton DL, Wen DR, Wong JH, et al. Technical details of intraoperative lymphatic mapping for early stage melanoma. Arch Surg 1992;127:392–9.

75. Morton DL, Thompson JF, Cochran AJ, et al. Sentinel-node biopsy or nodal observation in melanoma. N Engl J Med 2006;355:1307–17.

76. Balch CM, Cascinelli N. Sentinel-node biopsy in melanoma. N Engl J Med 2006;355:1370–1.

77. Johnson TM, Sondak VK, Bichakjian CK, et al. The role of sentinel lymph node biopsy for melanoma: evidence assessment. J Am Acad Dermatol 2006;54: 19–27.

78. Houghton AN, Legha S, Bajorin DF. Chemotherapy for Metastatic Melanoma, 2nd ed. Philadelphia: 1994.

79. Huncharek M, Caubet JF, McGarry R. Single-agent DTIC versus combination chemotherapy with or without immunotherapy in metastatic melanoma: a meta-analysis of 3273 patients from 20 randomized trials. Melanoma Res 2001;11:75–81.

80. Middleton MR, Grob JJ, Aaronson N, et al. Randomized phase III study of temozolomide versus dacarbazine in the treatment of patients with advanced metastatic malignant melanoma. J Clin Oncol 2000;18:158–66.

81. Agarwala SS, Kirkwood JM. Temozolomide, a novel alkylating agent with activity in the central nervous system, may improve the treatment of advanced metastatic melanoma. Oncologist 2000;5:144–51.

82. Barth A, Morton DL. The role of adjuvant therapy in melanoma management. Cancer 1995;75(2 suppl):726–34.

83. Molife R, Hancock BW. Adjuvant therapy of malignant melanoma. Crit Rev Oncol Hematol 2002;44: 81–102.

84. Verma S, Quirt I, McCready D, et al. Systematic review of systemic adjuvant therapy for patients at high risk for recurrent melanoma. Cancer 2006;106:1431–42.

85. Pardoll DM. Cancer vaccines. Nat Med 1998;4(5 suppl):525–31.

86. Perales MA, Chapman PB. Immunizing against partially defined antigen mixtures, gangliosides, or peptides to induce antibody, T cell, and clinical responses. Cancer Chemother Biol Response Modif 2005;22:749–60.

87. Rietschel P, Chapman PB. Immunotherapy of melanoma. Hematol Oncol Clin North Am 2006;20:751–66.

88. Atkins MB. Cytokine-based therapy and biochemotherapy for advanced melanoma. Clin Cancer Res 2006;12:2353s–8s.

89. Dudley ME, Wunderlich JR, Yang JC, et al. Adoptive cell transfer therapy following non-myeloablative but lymphodepleting chemotherapy for the treatment of patients with refractory metastatic melanoma. J Clin Oncol 2005;23:2346–57.

90. Tepper RI, Pattengale PK, Leder P. Murine interleukin-4 displays potent anti-tumor activity in vivo. Cell 1989;57:503–12.

91. Colombo MP, Ferrari G, Stoppacciaro A, et al. Granulocyte colony-stimulating factor gene transfer suppresses tumorigenicity of a murine adenocarcinoma in vivo. J Exp Med 1991;173:889–97.

92. Gansbacher B, Zier K, Daniels B, et al. Interleukin 2 gene transfer into tumor cells abrogates tumorigenicity and induces protective immunity. J Exp Med 1990;172:1217–24.

93. Golumbek PT, Lazenby AJ, Levitsky HI, et al. Treatment of established renal cancer by tumor cells engineered to secrete interleukin-4. Science 1991;254:713–6.

94. Fearon ER, Pardoll DM, Itaya T, et al. Interleukin-2 production by tumor cells bypasses T helper

function in the generation of an antitumor response. Cell 1990;60:397–403.

95. Armstrong CA, Murray N, Kennedy M, et al. Melanoma-derived interleukin 6 inhibits in vivo melanoma growth. J Invest Dermatol 1994;102:278–84.

96. Tepper RI, Mule JJ. Experimental and clinical studies of cytokine gene-modified tumor cells. Hum Gene Ther 1994;5:153–64.

97. Simons JW, Mikhak B. Ex-vivo gene therapy using cytokine-transduced tumor vaccines: molecular and clinical pharmacology. Semin Oncol 1998;25:661–76.

98. Gansbacher B, Bannerji R, Daniels B, et al. Retroviral vector-mediated gamma-interferon gene transfer into tumor cells generates potent and long lasting antitumor immunity. Cancer Res 1990;50:7820–5.

99. Atkins MB, Robertson MJ, Gordon M, et al. Phase I evaluation of intravenous recombinant human interleukin 12 in patients with advanced malignancies. Clin Cancer Res 1997;3:409–17.

100. Kirkwood J, Kefford, R, Logan, T, et al. Phase II trial of iboctadekin (rhIL-18) on a daily X 5 schedule in metastatic melanoma (MM). J Clin Oncol 2006 ASCO Annual Meeting Proceedings Part I 2006;24(18S):10043.

101. Atkins MB, Lotze MT, Dutcher JP, et al. High-dose recombinant interleukin 2 therapy for patients with metastatic melanoma: analysis of 270 patients treated between 1985 and 1993. J Clin Oncol 1999;17:2105–16.

102. Atkins MB, Kunkel L, Sznol M, et al. High-dose recombinant interleukin-2 therapy in patients with metastatic melanoma: long-term survival update. Cancer J Sci Am 2000;6(suppl 1):S11–4.

103. Phan GQ, Attia P, Steinberg SM, et al. Factors associated with response to high-dose interleukin-2 in patients with metastatic melanoma. J Clin Oncol 2001;19:3477–82.

104. Boasberg PD, Hoon DS, Piro LD, et al. Enhanced survival associated with vitiligo expression during maintenance biotherapy for metastatic melanoma. J Invest Dermatol 2006;126:2658–63.

105. Ahmadzadeh M, Rosenberg SA. IL-2 administration increases CD4+ CD25(hi) Foxp3+ regulatory T cells in cancer patients. Blood 2006;107:2409–14.

106. Kirkwood JM, Strawderman MH, Ernstoff MS, et al. Interferon alfa-2b adjuvant therapy of high-risk resected cutaneous melanoma: the Eastern Cooperative Oncology Group Trial EST 1684. J Clin Oncol 1996;14:7–17.

107. Kirkwood JM, Ibrahim JG, Sondak VK, et al. High- and low-dose interferon alfa-2b in high-risk melanoma: first analysis of intergroup trial E1690/S9111/C9190. J Clin Oncol 2000;18:2444–58.

108. Kirkwood JM, Manola J, Ibrahim J, et al. A pooled analysis of eastern cooperative oncology group and intergroup trials of adjuvant high-dose interferon for melanoma. Clin Cancer Res 2004;10:1670–7.

109. Eggermont AM, Suciu S, MacKie R, et al. Post-surgery adjuvant therapy with intermediate doses of interferon alfa 2b versus observation in patients with stage IIb/III melanoma (EORTC 18952): randomised controlled trial. Lancet 2005;366(9492):1189–96.

110. Kleeberg UR, Suciu S, Brocker EB, et al. Final results of the EORTC 18871/DKG 80-1 randomised phase III trial. rIFN-alpha2b versus rIFN-gamma versus ISCADOR M versus observation after surgery in melanoma patients with either high-risk primary (thickness >3 mm) or regional lymph node metastasis. Eur J Cancer 2004;40:390–402.

111. Hancock BW, Wheatley K, Harris S, et al. Adjuvant interferon in high-risk melanoma: the AIM HIGH Study—United Kingdom Coordinating Committee on Cancer Research randomized study of adjuvant low-dose extended-duration interferon Alfa-2a in high-risk resected malignant melanoma. J Clin Oncol 2004;22:53–61.

112. Avigan D. Dendritic cells: development, function and potential use for cancer immunotherapy. Blood Rev 1999;13:51–64.

113. Spitler LE, Grossbard ML, Ernstoff MS, et al. Adjuvant therapy of stage III and IV malignant melanoma using granulocyte-macrophage colony-stimulating factor. J Clin Oncol 2000;18:1614–21.

114. Kirkwood JM, Moschos S, Wang W. Strategies for the development of more effective adjuvant therapy of melanoma: current and future explorations of antibodies, cytokines, vaccines, and combinations. Clin Cancer Res 2006;12:2331s–6s.

115. de Gast GC, Klumpen HJ, Vyth-Dreese FA, et al. Phase I trial of combined immunotherapy with subcutaneous granulocyte macrophage colony-stimulating factor, low-dose interleukin 2, and interferon alpha in progressive metastatic melanoma and renal cell carcinoma. Clin Cancer Res 2000;6:1267–72.

116. Hoeller C, Jansen B, Heere-Ress E, et al. Perilesional injection of r-GM-CSF in patients with cutaneous melanoma metastases. J Invest Dermatol 2001;117:371–4.

117. Si Z, Hersey P, Coates AS. Clinical responses and lymphoid infiltrates in metastatic melanoma following treatment with intralesional GM-CSF. Melanoma Res 1996;6:247–55.

118. Luiten RM, Kueter EW, Mooi W, et al. Immunogenicity, including vitiligo, and feasibility of vaccination with autologous GM-CSF-transduced

tumor cells in metastatic melanoma patients. J Clin Oncol 2005;23:8978–91.

119. Rosenberg SA, Yang JC, Schwartzentruber DJ, et al. Prospective randomized trial of the treatment of patients with metastatic melanoma using chemotherapy with cisplatin, dacarbazine, and tamoxifen alone or in combination with interleukin-2 and interferon alfa-2b. J Clin Oncol 1999;17:968–75.

120. Keilholz U, Goey SH, Punt CJ, et al. Interferon alfa-2a and interleukin-2 with or without cisplatin in metastatic melanoma: a randomized trial of the European Organization for Research and Treatment of Cancer Melanoma Cooperative Group. J Clin Oncol 1997;15:2579–88.

121. Atkins MB, Flaherty LE, Sosman JA, et al. prospective randomized phase III trial of concurrent biochemotherapy (BCT) with cisplatin, vinblastine, dacarbazine (CVD), IL-2 and interferon alpha-2b (IFN) versus CVD alone in patients with metastatic melanoma (E3695): an ECOG-coordinated intergroup trial (abstr 2847). Proc Am Soc Clin Oncol 2003;22.

122. Sasse A, Sasse E, Clark L, et al. Chemoimmunotherapy versus chemotherapy for metastatic malignant melanoma. Cochrane Database Syst Rev 2007: CD005413.

123. Krummel MF, Allison JP. CD28 and CTLA-4 have opposing effects on the response of T cells to stimulation. J Exp Med 1995;182:459–65.

124. Leach DR, Krummel MF, Allison JP. Enhancement of antitumor immunity by CTLA-4 blockade. Science 1996;271:1734–6.

125. Maker AV, Yang JC, Sherry RM, et al. Intrapatient dose escalation of anti-CTLA-4 antibody in patients with metastatic melanoma. J Immunother 2006;29:455–63.

126. Reuben JM, Lee BN, Li C, et al. Biologic and immunomodulatory events after CTLA-4 blockade with ticilimumab in patients with advanced malignant melanoma. Cancer 2006;106:2437–44.

127. Hodi FS, Mihm MC, Soiffer RJ, et al. Biologic activity of cytotoxic T lymphocyte-associated antigen 4 antibody blockade in previously vaccinated metastatic melanoma and ovarian carcinoma patients. Proc Natl Acad Sci USA 2003;100:4712–7.

128. Phan GQ, Yang JC, Sherry RM, et al. Cancer regression and autoimmunity induced by cytotoxic T lymphocyte-associated antigen 4 blockade in patients with metastatic melanoma. Proc Natl Acad Sci USA 2003;100:8372–7.

129. Attia P, Phan GQ, Maker AV, et al. Autoimmunity correlates with tumor regression in patients with metastatic melanoma treated with anti-cytotoxic T-lymphocyte antigen-4. J Clin Oncol 2005;23:6043–53.

130. Blansfield JA, Beck KE, Tran K, et al. Cytotoxic T-lymphocyte-associated antigen-4 blockage can induce autoimmune hypophysitis in patients with metastatic melanoma and renal cancer. J Immunother 2005;28:593–8.

131. Yee C, Thompson JA, Byrd D, et al. Adoptive T cell therapy using antigen-specific CD8+ T cell clones for the treatment of patients with metastatic melanoma: in vivo persistence, migration, and antitumor effect of transferred T cells. Proc Natl Acad Sci USA 2002;99:16168–73.

132. Meidenbauer N, Marienhagen J, Laumer M, et al. Survival and tumor localization of adoptively transferred Melan-A-specific T cells in melanoma patients. J Immunol 2003;170:2161–9.

133. Dudley ME, Wunderlich JR, Robbins PF, et al. Cancer regression and autoimmunity in patients after clonal repopulation with antitumor lymphocytes. Science 2002;298:850–4.

134. Ridolfi L, Ridolfi R, Riccobon A, et al. Adjuvant immunotherapy with tumor infiltrating lymphocytes and interleukin-2 in patients with resected stage III and IV melanoma. J Immunother 2003;26:156–62.

135. Darrow TL, Slingluff CL, Seigler HF. Autologous lymph node cell-derived tumor-specific cytotoxic T-cells for use in adoptive immunotherapy of human melanoma. Cancer 1988;62:84–91.

136. Rosenberg SA, Yannelli JR, Yang JC, et al. Treatment of patients with metastatic melanoma with autologous tumor-infiltrating lymphocytes and interleukin 2. J Natl Cancer Inst 1994;86:1159–66.

137. Arienti F, Belli F, Rivoltini L, et al. Adoptive immunotherapy of advanced melanoma patients with interleukin-2 (IL-2) and tumor-infiltrating lymphocytes selected in vitro with low doses of IL-2. Cancer Immunol Immunother 1993;36:315–22.

138. Adler A, Stein JA, Kedar E, et al. Intralesional injection of interleukin-2–expanded autologous lymphocytes in melanoma and breast cancer patients: a pilot study. J Biol Response Mod 1984;3:491–500.

139. Robbins PF, Dudley ME, Wunderlich J, et al. Cutting edge: persistence of transferred lymphocyte clonotypes correlates with cancer regression in patients receiving cell transfer therapy. J Immunol 2004;173:7125–30.

140. Muranski P, Boni A, Wrzesinski C, et al. Increased intensity lymphodepletion and adoptive immunotherapy–how far can we go? Nat Clin Pract Oncol 2006;3:668–81.

141. McIllmurray MB, Embleton MJ, Reeves WG, et al. Controlled trial of active immunotherapy in management of stage IIB malignant melanoma. Br Med J 1977;1:540–2.

142. McIllmurray MB, Reeves WG, Langman MJ, et al. Active immunotherapy in malignant melanoma. Br Med J 1978;1:579.

143. Aranha GV, McKhann CF, Grage TB, et al. Adjuvant immunotherapy of malignant melanoma. Cancer 1979;43:1297–303.

144. Berd D, Sato T, Cohn H, et al. Treatment of metastatic melanoma with autologous, hapten-modified melanoma vaccine: regression of pulmonary metastases. Int J Cancer 2001;94:531–9.

145. Berd D, Sato T, Maguire HC Jr, et al. Immunopharmacologic analysis of an autologous, hapten-modified human melanoma vaccine. J Clin Oncol 2004;22:403–15.

146. Belli F, Testori A, Rivoltini L, et al. Vaccination of metastatic melanoma patients with autologous tumor-derived heat shock protein gp96–peptide complexes: clinical and immunologic findings. J Clin Oncol 2002;20:4169–80.

147. Lee KP, Raez LE, Podack ER. Heat shock protein-based cancer vaccines. Hematol Oncol Clin North Am 2006;20:637–59.

148. Soiffer R, Hodi FS, Haluska F, et al. Vaccination with irradiated, autologous melanoma cells engineered to secrete granulocyte-macrophage colony-stimulating factor by adenoviral-mediated gene transfer augments antitumor immunity in patients with metastatic melanoma. J Clin Oncol 2003;21:3343–50.

149. Soiffer R, Lynch T, Mihm M, et al. Vaccination with irradiated autologous melanoma cells engineered to secrete human granulocyte-macrophage colony-stimulating factor generates potent antitumor immunity in patients with metastatic melanoma. Proc Natl Acad Sci USA 1998;95:13141–6.

150. Bystryn JC, Zeleniuch-Jacquotte A, Oratz R, et al. Double-blind trial of a polyvalent, shed-antigen, melanoma vaccine. Clin Cancer Res 2001;7:1882–7.

151. Mitchell MS. Perspective on allogeneic melanoma lysates in active specific immunotherapy. Semin Oncol 1998;25:623–35.

152. Sondak VK, Liu PY, Tuthill RJ, et al. Adjuvant immunotherapy of resected, intermediate-thickness, node-negative melanoma with an allogeneic tumor vaccine: overall results of a randomized trial of the Southwest Oncology Group. J Clin Oncol 2002;20:2058–66.

153. Sosman JA, Unger JM, Liu PY, et al. Adjuvant immunotherapy of resected, intermediate-thickness, node-negative melanoma with an allogeneic tumor vaccine: impact of HLA class I antigen expression on outcome. J Clin Oncol 2002;20:2067–75.

154. Faries MB, Morton DL. Therapeutic vaccines for melanoma: current status. BioDrugs 2005;19:247–60.

155. Sinkovics J, Horvath J. New developments in the virus therapy of cancer: a historical review. Intervirology 1993;36:193–214.

156. Wallack MK, Sivanandham M, Balch CM, et al. A phase III randomized, double-blind multiinstitutional trial of vaccinia melanoma oncolysate-active specific immunotherapy for patients with stage II melanoma. Cancer 1995;75:34–42.

157. Wallack MK, Sivanandham M, Balch CM, et al. Surgical adjuvant active specific immunotherapy for patients with stage III melanoma: the final analysis of data from a phase III, randomized, double-blind, multicenter vaccinia melanoma oncolysate trial. J Am Coll Surg 1998;187:69–77.

158. Cassel WA, Murray DR, Phillips HS. A phase II study on the postsurgical management of Stage II malignant melanoma with a Newcastle disease virus oncolysate. Cancer 1983;52:856–60.

159. Cassel WA, Murray DR. A ten-year follow-up on stage II malignant melanoma patients treated postsurgically with Newcastle disease virus oncolysate. Med Oncol Tumor Pharmacother 1992;9:169–71.

160. Batliwalla FM, Bateman BA, Serrano D, et al. A 15-year follow-up of AJCC stage III malignant melanoma patients treated postsurgically with Newcastle disease virus (NDV) oncolysate and determination of alterations in the CD8 T cell repertoire. Mol Med 1998;4:783–94.

161. von Hoegen P, Zawatzky R, Schirrmacher V. Modification of tumor cells by a low dose of Newcastle disease virus. III. Potentiation of tumor-specific cytolytic T cell activity via induction of interferon-alpha/beta. Cell Immunol 1990;126:80–90.

162. Rosenberg SA, Yang JC, Schwartzentruber DJ, et al. Immunologic and therapeutic evaluation of a synthetic peptide vaccine for the treatment of patients with metastatic melanoma. Nat Med 1998;4:321–7.

163. Marchand M, van Baren N, Weynants P, et al. Tumor regressions observed in patients with metastatic melanoma treated with an antigenic peptide encoded by gene MAGE-3 and presented by HLA-A1. Int J Cancer 1999;80:219–30.

164. Cormier JN, Salgaller ML, Prevette T, et al. Enhancement of cellular immunity in melanoma patients immunized with a peptide from MART-1/Melan A. Cancer J Sci Am 1997;3:37–44.

165. Scheibenbogen C, Schmittel A, Keilholz U, et al. Phase 2 trial of vaccination with tyrosinase peptides and granulocyte-macrophage colony-stimulating factor in patients with metastatic melanoma. J Immunother 2000;23:275–81.

166. Talebi T, Weber JS. Peptide vaccine trials for melanoma: preclinical background and clinical results. Semin Cancer Biol 2003;13:431–8.

167. Livingston PO, Wong GY, Adluri S, et al. Improved survival in stage III melanoma patients with GM2 antibodies: a randomized trial of adjuvant vaccination with GM2 ganglioside. J Clin Oncol 1994;12:1036–44.

168. Chapman PB, Morrissey DM, Panageas KS, et al. Induction of antibodies against GM2 ganglioside by immunizing melanoma patients using GM2–keyhole limpet hemocyanin + QS21 vaccine: a dose-response study. Clin Cancer Res 2000;6:874–9.

169. Kirkwood JM, Ibrahim JG, Sosman JA, et al. High-dose interferon alfa-2b significantly prolongs relapse-free and overall survival compared with the GM2–KLH/QS-21 vaccine in patients with resected stage IIB-III melanoma: results of intergroup trial E1694/S9512/C509801. J Clin Oncol 2001;19:2370–80.

170. Ragupathi G, Meyers M, Adluri S, et al. Induction of antibodies against GD3 ganglioside in melanoma patients by vaccination with GD3–lactone-KLH conjugate plus immunological adjuvant QS-21. Int J Cancer 2000;85:659–66.

171. Chapman PB. Vaccinating against GD3 ganglioside using BEC2 anti-idiotypic monoclonal antibody. Curr Opin Invest Drugs 2003;4:710–5.

172. Foon KA, Lutzky J, Baral RN, et al. Clinical and immune responses in advanced melanoma patients immunized with an anti-idiotype antibody mimicking disialoganglioside GD2. J Clin Oncol 2000;18:376–84.

173. Alfonso M, Diaz A, Hernandez AM, et al. An anti-idiotype vaccine elicits a specific response to N-glycolyl sialic acid residues of glycoconjugates in melanoma patients. J Immunol 2002;168:2523–9.

174. Saito H, Frleta D, Dubsky P, Palucka AK. Dendritic cell-based vaccination against cancer. Hematol Oncol Clin North Am 2006;20:689–710.

175. Campton K, Ding W, Yan Z, et al. Tumor antigen presentation by dermal antigen-presenting cells. J Invest Dermatol 2000;115:57–61.

176. Klein C, Bueler H, Mulligan RC. Comparative analysis of genetically modified dendritic cells and tumor cells as therapeutic cancer vaccines. J Exp Med 2000;191:1699–708.

177. Nestle FO, Alijagic S, Gilliet M, et al. Vaccination of melanoma patients with peptide- or tumor lysate-pulsed dendritic cells. Nat Med 1998;4:328–32.

178. Schuler-Thurner B, Schultz ES, Berger TG, et al. Rapid induction of tumor-specific type 1 T helper cells in metastatic melanoma patients by vaccination with mature, cryopreserved, peptide-loaded monocyte-derived dendritic cells. J Exp Med 2002;195:1279–88.

179. Banchereau J, Palucka AK, Dhodapkar M, et al. Immune and clinical responses in patients with metastatic melanoma to CD34(+) progenitor-derived dendritic cell vaccine. Cancer Res 2001;61:6451–8.

180. O'Rourke MG, Johnson M, Lanagan C, et al. Durable complete clinical responses in a phase I/II trial using an autologous melanoma cell/dendritic cell vaccine. Cancer Immunol Immunother 2003;52:387–95.

181. Chang AE, Redman BG, Whitfield JR, et al. A phase I trial of tumor lysate-pulsed dendritic cells in the treatment of advanced cancer. Clin Cancer Res 2002;8:1021–32.

18
Drug Eruptions

Craig K. Svensson

Key Points

- Drug eruptions are common adverse reactions to systemically administered medications, with clinical manifestations ranging from local skin changes such as the fixed drug eruption to life-threatening diseases such as toxic epidermal necrolysis.
- Such drug eruptions, in most cases, have been demonstrated to be mediated by immunologic mechanisms, and can involve type I (immunoglobulin E [IgE]-mediated), type II (cytotoxic), type III (immune complex), type IV (cell-mediated immunity), or a combination of multiple mechanisms.
- Certain drugs may be linked to specific types of drug eruptions (for instance, anticonvulsants are notorious for causing severe cutaneous reactions).
- There are predisposing factors that place a patient at increased risk for drug eruptions (viral infections, past history of medicament allergies, polymorphisms in human leukocyte antigen).
- There is a systematic approach to determining whether a medicament is triggering a drug eruption.

Clinicians are commonly faced with the problem of a patient presenting with a skin rash of unknown origin. Could it be due to a drug the patient is receiving? If so, which one? Does the rash necessitate the withdrawal of drug therapy, or can the agent be safely continued? If the rash is serious in nature, what can be done to prevent its progression? These and related questions have no simple answers. Determining the proper course of action requires clinical skill and an understanding of the pathophysiology of drug eruptions.

Epidemiology of Drug Eruptions

An accurate assessment of the true incidence of drug eruptions is complicated by many factors, including underreporting of events, uncertainty of diagnosis, and the limited sample size of most studies. Nevertheless, it is clear that drug eruptions are among the most common adverse drug reactions (ADRs). Studies report that between 10% and 30% of all ADRs involve the skin.[1–4] The incidence of drug eruptions in hospitalized patients is estimated to be between 1% and 3%.[1,5,6] Recent data suggest that dermatologic ADRs comprise over 26% of ADRs that result in an emergency room visit.[7] In an assessment of published rates for drug eruptions, Bigby[8] found that the female-to-male ratio increased with age, with a 35% higher incidence in adult females. Numerous factors that predispose subjects to drug eruptions increase the incidence in certain subgroups of patients substantially (see Predisposing Factors for Drug Eruptions).

Since approximately 90% of drug eruptions are relatively benign,[9] of greatest interest to the clinician is the incidence of severe cutaneous adverse reactions (SCARs). A SCAR is a reaction that may result in hospitalization, persistent disability, or death. While based on spontaneous reports, it has been estimated that the percent of drug eruptions that are SCARs is 17%[3]; other investigators have suggested that only 2% of all drug eruptions represent severe reactions.[10] The incidence of

Stevens-Johnson syndrome (SJS) is estimated to be 1 to 6 per million person-years, while that for toxic epidermal necrolysis (TEN) is estimated as 0.4 to 1.2 per million person-years.[10] This low incidence means that most clinicians have little experience in the diagnosis and management of the most severe forms of drug eruptions.

Evidence that Drug Eruptions are Immune-Mediated

The heterogeneity of skin eruptions associated with drug ingestion suggests that a single mechanistic scheme is unlikely to explain these phenomena. However, while some cutaneous manifestations of ADRs are most likely direct toxic effects (e.g., hyperpigmentation and phototoxicity), substantial evidence suggests that most skin reactions to drugs are immune-mediated (Table 18.1). Among the evidence that supports this assumption is the need for prior sensitization before eliciting a reaction to the drug. This is consistent with the need to create immunologic memory in order to mount an immune response to an antigen. In addition, the delayed development of most drug eruptions parallels the expected development of an immunologic response.[11] Immunohistochemical analysis of drug eruptions demonstrates the infiltration of immune cells to the affected site in drug-induced skin eruptions (Table 18.2).

Perhaps the strongest evidence for a role of the immune system in provoking cutaneous eruptions after drug administration is the demonstration of drug-reactive T cells in patients with a history of such eruptions. Exposure of mixed T cells from patients with a history of drug eruption to the suspected causative agent (including sulfamethoxazole,

Table 18.1. Evidence that drug eruptions are immune mediated

- Necessity for prior sensitization
- Delayed nature of their development
- Quicker onset upon re-challenge
- Association with drug fever
- Infiltration of immune cells at affected site
- Isolation of reactive drug-specific T-cell clones from patients with history of drug eruption
- Association with human leukocyte antigen (HLA) genotype

lidocaine, phenytoin, and carbamazepine) has been shown to result in the proliferation of T cells, from which drug-specific clones can be isolated.[12–14]

Recent studies demonstrating an association with serious drug eruptions and human leukocyte antigen (HLA) genotype with a limited number of agents (discussed further in Predisposing Factors for Drug Eruptions) provide significant evidence for involvement of the immune system in these reactions.[15–19] These genotype associations suggest presentation of drug-derived antigen is a key determinant of which patients will experience serious reactions to these drugs.

Taken together, these lines of evidence provide strong support for many drug eruptions in humans as immune-mediated events. In addition, recently the first animal model for a drug eruption has been reported, with compelling evidence for an immune mechanism in the pathogenesis.[20]

Classification of Drug Eruptions

Drug administration is associated with a variety of skin eruptions. Indeed, a single drug may be associated with numerous forms of skin eruption. For example, sulfonamides have been reported to be associated with morbilliform and urticarial rashes, erythema multiforme, erythema nodosum, SJS, and TEN, as well as photosensitivity. Drug eruptions may be classified in terms of both their clinical morphology and the presumed mechanism of action.[11]

Morphologic Classification

Accurate diagnosis of drug eruptions necessitates a careful assessment of the clinical manifestations associated with a given drug eruption. Specific diagnosis is aided by differences in presentation, time course, associated signs and symptoms, and histologic features (Tables 18.2 to 18.4).

Exanthemas

Morbilliform or maculopapular exanthemas are the most frequently observed drug eruptions (~90% of all eruptions) and have been reported with a wide range of medicines. Usually appearing first on the trunk, exanthemas appear as erythematous

TABLE 18.2. Immunohistologic features of drug eruptions

Reaction	Histologic features of affected skin
Exanthema	Presence of dyskeratotic and necrotic keratinocytes (KC) at dermal-epidermal junction; infiltration of eosinophils, CLA+ T cells; upregulation of ICAM-1; TNF-α, IL-5, IL-6 induction[22,81–85]
Urticaria	Sparse interstitial and perivascular mononuclear cell infiltrate along with eosinophils and dermal edema[23, 83]
Fixed drug eruptions	Acutely affected skin shows scattered KC along with infiltration of lymphocytes, neutrophils, and eosinophils at the dermal-epidermal junction; chronic biopsies show acanthosis, hyperkeratosis, hypergranulosis, and infiltration of melanophages in dermis[23, 83]
Erythema multiforme/SJS and TEN	Infiltration of inflammatory cells at the dermal region along with discrete regions of epidermal necrosis; SJS and TEN show widespread epidermal necrosis, reduction in Langerhans' cells, KC expression of HLA-DR[23, 86]

Source: Khan et al.,[28] with permission.

TABLE 18.3. Comparison of the characteristics of drug eruptions

Characteristic	Exanthema	Urticarial	FDE	AGEP	EMM/SJS/TEN
Time of onset	4–14 days	Within 36 hours	4–48 hours	48 hours	1–3 weeks
Duration	1 week	Single lesions <24 hours	<5 days	<1 week	1–3 weeks
Fever	Yes	No	Yes	Yes	Yes
Pustules	No	No	Yes	Yes	Yes
Angioedema	No	Yes	No	Yes	No
Pruritus	Yes	Yes			No
Mortality	~0%	2% when associated with anaphylaxis	~0%	5%	10–30%

AGEP, acute generalized exanthematous pustulosis; EMM, erythematous multiforme majus; FDE, fixed drug eruption; SJS, Stevens-Johnson syndrome; TEN, toxic epidermal necrolysis.

TABLE 18.4. Diagnostic criteria for severe cutaneous adverse reactions

Classification	Pattern of lesions	Distribution	Extent of blisters/ % detachment
Erythema multiforme majus (EMM)	Typical targets, raised atypical targets	Localized	<10
Stevens-Johnson syndrome (SJS)	Blisters to macules, flat atypical targets	Widespread	<10
Overlap SJS-TEN	Blisters to macules, flat atypical targets	Widespread	10–29
Toxic epidermal necrolysis (TEN) with spots	Blisters to macules, flat atypical targets	Widespread	≥30
TEN without "spots"	No discrete lesions, large erythematous areas	Widespread	≥10

Source: Auquier-Dunant et al.,[24] with permission.

macules or papules, and are commonly associated with a mild fever. Symmetrical spreading of the exanthema to the extremities often occurs. The onset of exanthemas after initiation of drug therapy is generally reported to be between 4 and 14 days, though a later onset may occur.[21,22]

Urticarial Eruptions

Urticarial eruptions associated with drug therapy appear to be the second most common form of drug eruption, comprising approximately 5% of reactions across a series of studies.[8] These eruptions may occur in the first few hours after drug ingestion and appear as raised, pink wheals associated with intense itching. Individual eruptions generally resolve within 24 hours, though new eruptions may be manifested. The angioedema that can be associated with these eruptions may persist for days and, on occasion, occur in the absence of urticarial eruptions. When associated with anaphylaxis, urticarial eruptions represent a life-threatening ADR.

Fixed Drug Eruptions

Fixed drug eruptions (FDEs) generally appear more rapidly than the more common exanthemas, most often within 2 days of initiation of drug therapy.[21] With these eruptions, few lesions occur, sometimes limited to a single eruption. Appearing as well-demarcated lesions with significant edema, these eruptions are usually associated with itching and burning at the site. Upon reexposure to the offending agent, lesions associated with FDE commonly recur at the same location on the skin, though new lesions in different areas may also occur.[23] Interestingly, characteristic patterns of the affected anatomic site for FDE appear to occur with specific agents.

Acute Generalized Exanthematous Pustulosis

Acute generalized exanthematous pustulosis (AGEP) is characterized by a substantial number of small pustules occurring on an erythematous region of skin. These eruptions are associated with fever and occur most commonly on the trunk, upper extremities, and manifold regions (e.g., neck, groin, axillae). Common with FDE, AGEP usually develops within the first 2 days of therapy. The eruptions themselves last several days and give rise to a superficial desquamation.

Erythema Multiforme, Stevens-Johnson Syndrome, and Toxic Epidermal Necrolysis

Historically, erythema multiforme, SJS, and TEN have been viewed by some as a spectrum of the same disease. Work by the international SCAR study group[24] has provided important insight into the distinct nature and causes of these syndromes, as well as the development of clear diagnostic criteria (Table 18.4). Indeed, an assessment of 552 patients with a tentative diagnosis of SCAR

revealed that in most cases of erythema multiforme drugs did not appear to be the etiologic factor.[24] Stevens-Johnson syndrome and TEN represent life-threatening conditions that must be recognized rapidly. Commonly, skin eruptions associated with these syndromes are preceded by 1 to 3 days of fever and other constitutional symptoms. Eruptions begin with a symmetrical distribution on the upper trunk of the body and the face. Pain or a burning sensation associated with these lesions are viewed by many as an early sign of a severe reaction. As outlined in Table 18.4, the degree of blistering or skin detachment is the primary criteria for differentiating SJS, SJS/TEN, and TEN.

Mechanistic Classification

While classification of drug eruptions by clinical morphology is an essential component of the diagnosis of these drug-induced diseases, classification by presumed mechanism provides insight into anticipated time course of development, likely risk upon reexposure, laboratory tests that may aid in diagnosis, and potential therapeutic interventions to prevent or attenuate these reactions.[11]

Immediate-Type Immune-Mediated Drug Eruptions

Immediate-type immune-mediated drug eruptions have been the most carefully studied reactions. Also known as type I hypersensitivity, these drug eruptions are mediated by immunoglobulin E (IgE). As with all IgE-mediated immune responses, prior sensitization to the drug or a chemically related compound must occur in order to provoke a drug eruption upon exposure to the agent. Importantly, this sensitization may occur as a result of a previous exposure to the drug or during the initial phase of treatment with a multiple dose regimen. Obviously, sensitization due to prior drug exposure may result in an extremely rapid drug eruption upon subsequent exposure, whereas if sensitization occurs during the initial phase of treatment, the drug eruption will not occur until several doses have been administered.

As described later in this text, elicitation of an immediate-type immune-mediated reaction requires cross-linking between the antigen and adjacent preformed IgE on mast cells. The degranulation that results from this binding releases toxic mediators (e.g., histamine, cytokines, leukotrienes, platelet-activating factor), which may occur within seconds of exposure to the drug. When initiated by a local intradermal injection (via allergy testing), the result is a localized wheal-and-flare reaction. Immunoglobulin E–mediated responses arising in response to systemic exposure result in urticaria (e.g., hives)—skin eruptions that are large, erythematous, and itchy welts. If disseminated mast cell activation occurs, a marked increase in vascular permeability, constriction of airways, swelling of the epiglottis, and vascular collapse may occur. This life-threatening condition is known as *anaphylactic shock* and, without immediate intervention, may result in death.

Recognizing a reaction as being of the immune-mediated immediate-type provides important insight into laboratory tests that may aid in the diagnosis. First, where available, measurement of antigen-specific IgE provides confirmation of sensitization to the offending agent.[25] Second, the use of skin tests may prove quite useful in identifying the offending agent.[26] In addition, recognizing the mediators that are responsible for the inflammatory reaction resulting in a drug eruption provides important insight into potential therapeutic interventions. As histamine and inflammatory mediators are key signals for these reactions, the use of antihistamines and antiinflammatory agents (e.g., corticosteroids) provides a rational approach to the treatment of skin eruptions associated with immediate-type immune-mediated reactions.

Delayed-Type Immune-Mediated Drug Eruptions

Delayed-type immune-mediated drug eruptions are characterized by their delayed onset after initiation of therapy, primarily occurring 7 to 10 days after initiation of a drug regimen. As with other delayed-type hypersensitivity reactions, drug eruptions that are of the delayed-type appear to be mediated by T cells.[27] While the mechanisms by which cutaneous eruptions are provoked after epicutaneous application have been fairly well elucidated, the mechanism by which systemically administered drugs elicit such eruptions is less clear.[28] Nevertheless, numerous studies have demonstrated the presence of drug-

specific reactive T cells from patients with a history of such reactions.[12–14] Moreover, it has been demonstrated that patients with a history of such reactions exhibit circulating drug-reactive T cells for as long as 12 years after the event.[29]

As described in earlier chapters, T-cell activation requires multiple signals.[11] The first signal is derived from interaction of the antigen in the context of major histocompatability complex (MHC) and the T-cell receptor. Antigen presentation in the context of MHC occurs via interaction of the T cell with antigen-presenting cells (APCs). In isolation, however, this interaction results in immune tolerance. A second signal is required in conjunction with antigen presentation in order to provoke T-cell activation. A variety of molecules (e.g., inflammatory cytokines, uric acid, and heat shock protein) have been suggested as being capable of upregulating the expression of secondary signals on APCs.[30,31] Release of such regulatory molecules may explain the predisposition of patients with viral infections to drug eruptions.[32,33]

Based on the presumed role for T cells in delayed-type immune-mediated drug eruptions, it was proposed that determination of the ability of drug to provoke proliferation of isolated lymphocytes could be used as a diagnostic tool in efforts to identify the agent responsible for a drug eruption.[34] While several investigators have provided evidence for the utility of such tests, their complexity and expense make them relatively impractical for routine clinical use.[35] Further refinement of the methodology may open the door for more widespread application of this diagnostic tool in the future.

As contact sensitivity to environmental and occupational chemicals is known to be mediated by T cells,[36,37] it seemed likely that skin testing may provide a useful diagnostic tool for drug eruptions after systemic administration that are consistent with a delayed-type immune-mediated response. While skin testing has been shown to be useful in the identification of the causative agent for such reactions, early negative responses must be followed to determine the occurrence of a delayed positive response to skin tests.[26]

Treatment of such reactions remains largely empirical and supportive at present. While withdrawal of the drug would appear to be the first step, continued treatment in mild reactions has been relatively common in certain patient groups (i.e., AIDS patients). However, it appears that the death rate is lower in SCAR among patients in whom drug therapy with the suspected drug is stopped upon the first appearance of cutaneous eruptions.[38] Based on the presumed mechanism of action, agents that modulate T-cell activation and T-cell–mediated killing would appear to be logical targets for attenuating the severe forms of these reactions (e.g., SJS and TEN). In addition, modulation of inflammatory cytokine release or action represents a reasonable approach to preventing or treating SCARs. However, initial studies in this direction using thalidomide to inhibit tumor necrosis factor-α action found a higher death rate with this treatment modality.[39] As the cell surface death receptor Fas (CD95) on keratinocytes may mediate the massive cell death observed in TEN, the use of intravenous immunoglobulin (which contains natural anti-Fas antibodies) has been evaluated in patients with TEN. While uncontrolled studies suggest potential benefit, a prospective controlled clinical trial is needed to assess the validity of this treatment modality.[40]

Challenges in the Diagnosis of Drug Eruptions

Attribution of causation of skin pathology to a specific drug represents a complex challenge for clinicians. For example, in one French referral center for SCAR, in only two thirds of patients referred was the diagnosis of drug-induced severe cutaneous drug eruption confirmed.[10] It is likely that the accuracy of diagnosis of less severe forms of reaction is lower, since these mild reactions may be mediated by many nondrug factors. As many skin eruptions have numerous sources of causation, a careful differential diagnosis is an essential element in the assessment. A component of this assessment must be a careful drug history, including the temporal relationship between drug ingestion and the appearance of the skin eruption. As patient recall of drug ingestion is often limited, specific probing questions (e.g., Did you take anything for a headache over the last few days?) may be necessary to elicit a complete drug history. Graphing the time course of drug ingestion and clinical manifestations (including body temperature, lab abnormalities, etc.) may prove insightful for the clinician seeking to identify the likely cause of a skin eruption in a patient receiving multiple agents. This can be a helpful step in preventing a diagnosis based solely on guilt by association—attributing a skin eruption to a drug simply because it has been previously reported to be associated with ingestion of the drug.

Since diagnosing a patient as having experienced a drug-induced skin eruption generally results in future avoidance of that and chemically related drugs in the patient, precise assessment of the level of certainty of diagnosis (and communication of that to the patient and in the medical record) is an important but often neglected step. Edwards and Aronson[41] have provided helpful criteria for causality assessment of drug-induced disease (Table 18.5). Frequently, the most definitive level a clinician can achieve with the information available is that a skin eruption is "likely" to have been caused

TABLE 18.5. Causality assessment for suspected drug eruptions

Certain

- A skin eruption that occurs in a plausible time relation to drug administration, and which cannot be explained by concurrent disease or other drugs or chemicals
- The response to withdrawal of the drug (de-challenge) should be clinically plausible
- The events must be definitive pharmacologically or phenomenologically, using a satisfactory re-challenge procedure if necessary

Probable/likely

- A skin eruption with a reasonable time relation to administration of the drug, unlikely to be attributed to concurrent disease or other drugs or chemicals, and which follows a clinically reasonable response on withdrawal (de-challenge)
- Re-challenge information is not required to fulfill this definition

Possible

- A skin eruption with a reasonable time relation to administration of the drug, but which could also be explained by concurrent disease or other drugs or chemicals
- Information on drug withdrawal are lacking or unclear

Unlikely

- A skin eruption with a temporal relation to administration of the drug that makes a causal relation improbable, and in which other drugs, chemicals, or underlying disease provide plausible explanations

Source: Adapted from Edwards and Aronson.[41]

by a specific drug. Clear communication of this level of certainty can provide important guidance for future management of the patient in weighing the cost-benefit ratio of rechallenge if therapy with the suspected or chemically related agent is deemed optimal therapy for an ailment.

Therapeutic Agents Commonly Associated with Drug Eruptions

A careful search of the literature reveals that most drugs have been reported to be associated with drug eruptions. The confidence of such associations varies widely. However, for a number of important therapeutic agents, there is significant evidence of causation for these eruptions. As a class, antimicrobial agents appear to have the highest incidence of drug eruptions, with reaction rates as high as 20 to 50 per 1000 recipients.[6] Of the many antimicrobial agents approved for human use, sulfonamides exhibit the highest frequency of skin eruptions, followed by the fluoroquinolones.[3,42]

Of greatest concern for clinicians are those agents associated with SCAR. As shown in Table 18.6, a wide variety of therapeutic agents have been associated with the development of SJS or TEN. Among the highest incidence of SCAR are those associated with sulfonamides, with an incidence estimated to be 1:1000 to 1:100,000.[43,44] The most frequent reports are associated with ingestion of trimethoprim-sulfamethoxazole, though this may reflect prescribing frequency. In one case-control study, this combination product was responsible for almost 70% of cases of SCAR reported.[45]

Several anticonvulsant agents have been associated with SCAR, as well as a syndrome frequently

Table 18.6. Drugs frequently associated with severe cutaneous adverse reactions (SCAR)

Allopurinol
Aminopenicillins
Antiretrovirals
Carbamazepine
Cephalosporins
Lamotrigine
Nonsteroidal antiinflammatory drugs (NSAIDs)
Phenobarbital
Phenytoin
Sulfonamides

referred to as anticonvulsant hypersensitivity syndrome (AHS). This syndrome is manifested by fever, widespread drug eruption, lymphadenopathy, and liver injury.[46] The relative risk of SCAR appears to be similar with carbamazepine, phenobarbital, and phenytoin.[44] The newer anticonvulsant lamotrigine has also been associated with SCAR, with incidence as high as 1 in 300 reported in clinical trials.[45] Slower escalation of initiating doses substantially reduces the rate of such reactions for this drug.

The association of nonsteroidal antiinflammatory drugs (NSAIDs) with SCAR must be recognized, as these agents are widely available without a prescription. Indeed, of all over-the-counter medications, it would appear that these agents pose the highest risk for SCAR. However, it is the oxicam NSAIDs (e.g., piroxicam and tenoxicam) that pose the most significant risk for these reactions,[45] and these remain available by prescription only in most countries.

Antiretroviral agents represent another important class of drugs associated with SCAR. As management of HIV infection is characterized by multidrug therapy, identification of causation for SCAR that occur in this population is problematic. Nevertheless, there is significant evidence that nevirapine in particular is a causative agent for these reactions.[47]

How Do Systemically Administered Drugs Mediate Drug Eruptions?

As substantial evidence exists that most drug eruptions are immune-mediated events, elucidation of the mechanism of these reactions will require determination of the means by which systemically administered drugs provoke an immune response in the skin. Studies in animal models of cutaneous hypersensitivity have yielded critical insight into the dynamic interaction of the skin immune system and antigens applied epicutaneously (Fig. 18.1).

After passage through the stratum corneum, antigen may be taken up by either epidermal keratinocytes or Langerhans' cells (LCs). Epidermal keratinocytes serve as an important source of cytokines, and perhaps other danger signals, that mediate activation of LCs.[48,49] This activation results in downregulation of E-cadherin expressed on the surface of LCs, resulting in detachment from epidermal

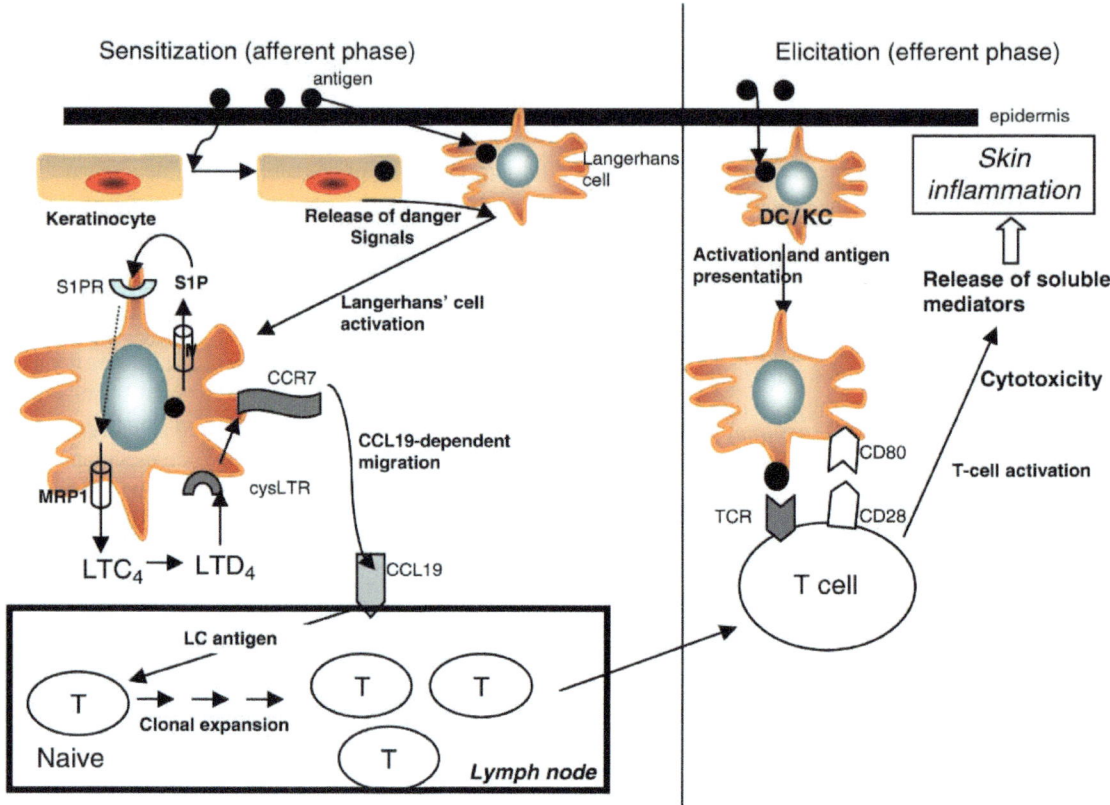

FIG. 18.1. Events associated with the provocation of an immune response in the skin. CCR7-CC, chemokine receptor 7; CCL-19-CC, chemokine ligand-19; cysLTR, cysteinyl leukotriene receptor; DC, dendritic cell; KC, keratinocyte; LC, Langerhans' cell; LT, leukotriene; MDR1, multidrug resistance transporter 1; MRP1, multidrug resistance associated protein 1; S1P, sphingosine-1-phosphate; S1PR, sphingosine-1-phosphate receptor; TCR, T-cell receptor. (Slide drawn using objects from ScienceSlides, VisiScience Corp. From Khan et al.,[28] with permission.)

keratinocytes.[50,51] Release of matrix metallopro-teinases enhances the migration of LCs through the epidermis.[52,53] During this activation process, there is an upregulation of CC chemokine recep-tor 7 (CCR7) on the LC surface.[54] Studies in skin explant models suggest that this upregulation involves the sequential engagement of two adenos-ine triphosphate (ATP)-binding cassette membrane transporters (ABCB1 and ABCC1), the latter of which mediates the efflux of leukotriene C_4 and the upregulation of CCR7.[55,56] CCR7 upregulation in LCs provides the platform for chemokine (CCL19)-guided migration to regional lymph nodes.[55,57]

Upon arrival at the regional lymph node, migrated LCs present antigenic peptides in the context of MHC, resulting in a clonal expansion of antigen-reactive T cells. These T cells are released into

the peripheral circulation and express skin-homing receptors, such as cutaneous lymphocyte antigen. The expression of such receptors permits the cap-ture of cells by E-selectin expressing endothelial cells, which appears to mediate the extrusion of T cells into the skin.[58]

T-cell–mediated cytotoxicity appears to be an essential component of the local inflamma-tory reaction observed in contact sensitivity.[59] Targeting of cells for killing by these recruited T cells necessitates the further expression of antigen in the context of MHC I or II (Fig. 18.2). While keratinocytes constitutively express MHC I, expression of MHC II may be induced in these cells by inflammatory cytokines, whose release is presumably prompted by the con-tact sensitizer.[60,61] T-cell release of granzyme

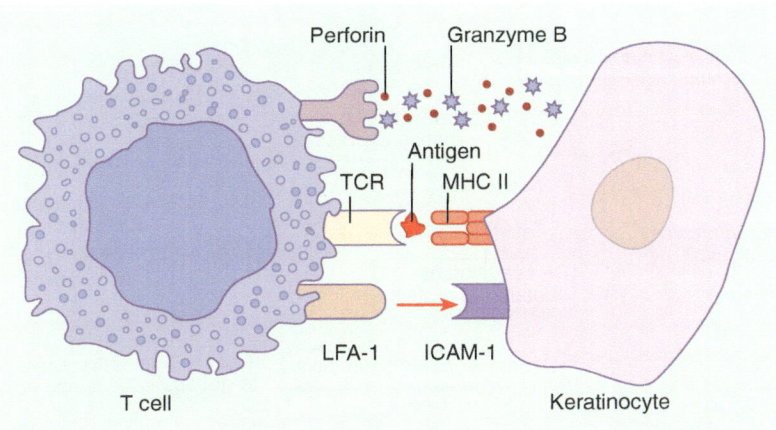

FIG. 18.2. Schematic representation of events associated with T-cell–mediated keratinocyte cell killing. ICAM-1, intercellular adhesion molecule 1; LFA-1, leukocyte function-related antigen 1; MHC, major histocompatability complex; TCR, T-cell receptor. (Adapted from Pichler.[27])

or perforin mediates keratinocytes cell death, which prompts an inflammatory response in the skin.

Recognizing the outlined mechanism for skin inflammatory responses to chemicals applied epicutaneously, how might systemically administered drugs provoke such reactions? It would appear that a systemically administered drug either provokes a systemic response that prompts migration of effector cells to the skin, or drug distributes to the skin and provokes an eruption by initiating events locally. Experimental evidence suggests the latter is most likely. For example, intradermal administration of prehaptenated dendritic cells sensitizes mice for a cutaneous reactions, whereas administration of such cells via the intraperitoneal or intravenous route does not.[62,63] This observation suggests haptenation of dendritic cells must occur in the cutaneous environment to provoke a drug eruption.

As outlined in Figure 18.3, we have proposed a model wherein bioactivation of drug in keratinocytes or localization to the skin of reactive metabolite formed in the liver serves as a key initiating event for drug eruptions.[64] In addition to resulting in protein haptenation, these reactive metabolites may result in oxidative stress and provoke the release of key secondary signals necessary for dendritic and T-cell activation. While numerous in vitro studies provide support for this hypothesis, in vivo evaluation of the hypothesis remains a necessary step prior to acceptance of the proposed mechanism.

Predisposing Factors for Drug Eruptions

The idiosyncratic nature of drug eruptions has prompted investigations into potential factors that may predispose patients to such reactions. Based on the foregoing discussion, it would seem logical that differences in drug metabolism may serve as an important predisposing factor. Indeed, early studies suggested that patients with the slow acetylator phenotype were at increased risk for the development of cutaneous reactions to sulfonamides.[65,66] Subsequent studies, however, have not found a significant association between acetylator phenotype or genotype and cutaneous reactions to these drugs.[67] Moreover, genetic variation in other drug metabolizing enzymes does not appear to correlate with risk for skin eruptions during therapy with sulfonamides.[68,69] Assessment of the potential role for variation in enzymes that mediate the bioactivation of other drugs (e.g., carbamazepine) have also not been fruitful in identifying allelic variants of such enzymes that significantly impact that risk of drug eruptions.[70] Hence, it does not appear that genetic variation in drug metabolizing enzymes is able to explain the idiosyncratic nature of these reactions. This suggests that the level of reactive metabolite formed and the rate of

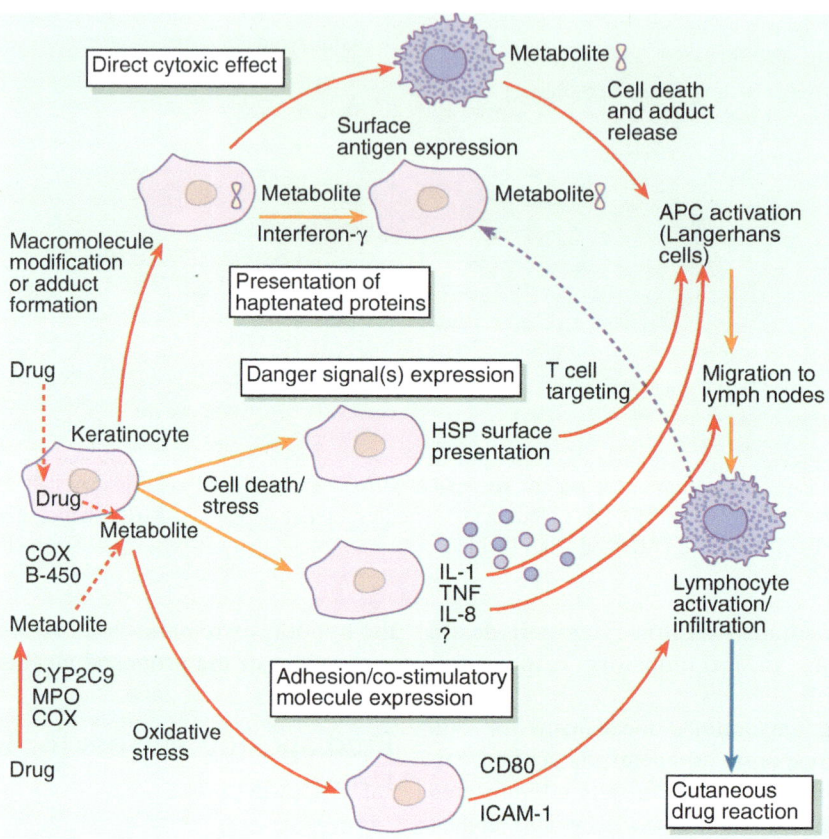

FIG. 18.3. Working hypothesis for the mechanism of cutaneous drug reactions to sulfonamides. APC, antigen-presenting cell; CD80, B7.1 co-stimulatory molecule; COX, cyclooxygenase; P-450, cytochrome P-450; HSP, heat shock protein; ICAM-1 intercellular adhesion molecule 1; IL-1, interleukin-1; IL-8, interleukin-8; TNF, tumor necrosis factor. (Adapted from Reilly et al.[64])

its detoxification is unlikely to make the difference between who exhibits an immune-mediated adverse reaction and who does not.

More fruitful investigations have arisen from probing the role of allelic variants of key immune molecules as predisposing factors for the development of drug-induced skin eruptions. For example, therapy with abacavir in patients with HIV infection is associated with hypersensitivity reactions in 5% of patients. Studies found that patients with the HLA-B[*]5701 genotype have a markedly increased incidence of hypersensitivity reactions.[16,17,71,72] As a consequence of these observations, some centers have implemented pre-prescription pharmacogenetic testing prior to initiating therapy with abacavir, a strategy that has recently been demonstrated to be cost-effective in a Caucasian population.[73] Interestingly, this association was not confirmed in a population of black patients.[17]

Striking associations between HLA genotype and severe cutaneous reactions have recently been reported for two drugs. In a Han Chinese population, 100% of patients with carbamazepine-induced SJS possessed the HLA-B[*]1502 genotype, whereas only 3% of patients receiving the drug without SJS exhibited this genotype.[15] In addition, this same group of investigators reported that 100% of patients with SCAR to allopurinol had the HLA B[*]5801 genotype, which was present in 15% of tolerant patients.[18] While ongoing studies are aimed at determining the presence of similar associations for these drugs in other ethnic populations, these results provide compelling evidence for the potential to identify at-risk patients through genotype analysis of HLA.

In addition to genetic predisposition, the presence of a viral infection appears to markedly increase the incidence of cutaneous eruptions associated with some drugs. For example, almost all patients with active infectious mononucleosis who are administered ampicillin exhibit a skin eruption.[74–77] Re-challenge with the drug after the infection has cleared results in a rash frequency of only 5%. In addition, prior to the introduction of highly active antiretroviral therapy for HIV infection, the frequency of skin eruptions during therapy with sulfonamides was about 10 times that observed in non–HIV-infected patients.[78–80] The frequency of such reactions in AIDS patients appears to have decreased with the advent of therapies that yield improved health such patients, as well as a substantial decrease in the use of sulfonamides in their management.

The mechanism by which viral infection increases the risk of developing a skin eruption is unclear.[32,33] As viral infections may provoke the release of inflammatory cytokines, which may result in the upregulation of secondary molecules on dendritic cells, such infections may predispose patients by provoking dendritic activation.

Conclusion

Drug eruptions are unfortunately common, involve immune mechanisms, and can range from mild localized or generalized rashes to life-threatening conditions. Early recognition of such adverse reactions are critical, and familiarity with the drugs and associated conditions is critical in the recognition of this reaction. In most cases, discontinuation of the offending agents results in resolution of signs and symptoms. However, severe cutaneous reactions may require supportive therapy, as well as the administration of antiinflammatory drugs or biologic agents such as intravenous immunoglobulin (IVIG).

References

1. Stewart R, May F, Cullen S. Dermatologic adverse drug reactions in hospitalized patients. Am J Hosp Pharm 1979;36:609–12.
2. Faich G, Knapp D, Dreis M, Turner W. National adverse drug reaction surveillance. JAMA 1987;257:2068–70.
3. Naldi L, Conforti A, Venegoni M, et al. Cutaneous reactions to drugs. An analysis of spontaneous reports in four Italian regions. Br J Clin Pharmacol 1999;48:839–46.
4. Suh DC, Woodall BS, Shin SK, Hermes-DesSantis ER. Clinical and economic impact of adverse drug reactions in hospitalized patients. Ann Pharmacother 2000;34:1373–9.
5. Arndt KA, Jick H. Rates of cutaneous reactions to drugs. A report from the Boston Collaborative Drug Surveillance Program. JAMA 1976;235:918–22.
6. Bigby M, Jick S, Jick H, Arndt K. Drug-induced cutaneous reactions. JAMA 1986;256:3358–63.
7. Budnitz DS, Pollock DA, Weidenbach KN, Mendelsohn AB, Schroeder TJ, Annest JL. National surveillance of emergency department visits for outpatient adverse drug events. JAMA 2006;296:1858–66.
8. Bigby M. Rates of cutaneous reactions to drugs. Arch Dermatol 2001;137:765–70.
9. Hunziker T, Kunzi UP, Braunschweig S, Zehnder D, Hoignw R. Comprehensive hospital drug monitoring (CHDM): adverse skin reactions, a 20-year survey. Allergy 1997;52:388–93.
10. Bachot N, Roujeau JC. Differential diagnosis of severe cutaneous drug eruptions. Am J Clin Dermatol 2003;4:561–72.
11. Svensson CK, Cowen EW, Gaspari AA. Cutaneous drug reactions. Pharmacol Rev 2001;53:357–79.
12. Mauri-Hellweg D, Bettens F, Mauri D, Brander C, Hunziker T, Pichler WJ. Activation of drug-specific CD4+ and CD8+ T cells in individuals allergic to sulfonamides, phenytoin, and carbamazepine. J Immunol 1995;155:462–72.
13. Naisbitt DJ, Farrell J, Wong G, et al. Characterization of drug-specific T cells in lamotrigine hypersensitivity. J Allergy Clin Immunol 2003;111:1393–403.
14. Zanni M, Mauri-Hellweg D, Brander C, et al. Characterization of lidocaine-specific T cells. J Immunol 1997;158:1139–48.
15. Chung WH, Hung SI, Hong HS, et al. A marker for Stevens-Johnson syndrome. Nature 2004;428:486.
16. Hettherington S, Hughes AR, Mosteller M, et al. Genetic variations in HLA-B region and hypersensitivity reactions to abacavir. Lancet 2002;359:1121–2.
17. Hughes AR, Mosteller M, Bansal AT, et al. Association of genetic variations in HLA-B region with hypersensitivity to abacavir in some, but not all, populations. Pharmacogenomics 2004;5:203–11.
18. Hung SI, Chung WH, Liou LB, et al. HLA-B*5801 allele as a genetic marker for severe cutaneous adverse reactions caused by allopurinol. Proc Natl Acad Sci USA 2005;102:4134–9.
19. Hung S-I, Chung W-H, Jee S-H, et al. Genetic susceptibility to carbamazepine-induced cutaneous adverse drug reactions. Pharmacogenet Genomics 2006;16:297–306.
20. Uetrecht JP. Role of animal models in drug-induced hypersensitivity reactions. AAPS J 2005;7(4):E914–E21.

21. Roujeau JC. Clinical heterogeneity of drug hypersensitivity. Toxicology 2005;209:123–9.
22. Yawalkar N. Drug-induced exanthemas. Toxicology 2005;209:131–4.
23. Crowson AN, Brown TJ, Margo CM. Progress in the understanding of the pathology and pathogenesis of cutaneous drug eruptions. Am J Clin Dermatol 2003;4:407–28.
24. Auquier-Dunant A, Mockenhaupt M, Naldi L, Correia O, Schroder W, Roujeau JC. Correlations between clinical patterns and causes of erythema multiforme majus, Stevens-Johnson syndrome, and toxic epidermal necrolysis: results of an international prospective study. Arch Dermatol 2002;138:1019–24.
25. Vervloet D, Durham S. Adverse reactions to drugs. Br Med J 2006;316:1511–4.
26. Barbaud AM, Goncalo M, Bruynzeel D, Bircher A. Guidelines for performing skin tests with drugs in the investigation of cutaneous adverse drug reactions. Contact Dermatitis 2001;45:321–8.
27. Pichler WJ. Delayed drug hypersensitivity reactions. Ann Intern Med 2003;139:683–93.
28. Khan FD, Roychowdhury S, Gaspari AA, Svensson CK. Immune response to xenobiotics in the skin: from contact sensitivity to drug allergy. Expert Opin Drug Metab Toxicol 2006;2:261–72.
29. Beeler A, Engler OB, Gerber BO, Pichler WJ. Long-lasting reactivity and high frequency of drug-specific T cells after severe systemic drug hypersensitivity reactions. J Allergy Clin Immunol 2006;117:455–62.
30. Gallucci S, Matzinger P. Danger signals: SOS to the immune system. Curr Opin Immunol 2001;13:114–9.
31. Gruchalla R. Drug metabolism, danger signals, and drug-induced hypersensitivity. J Allergy Clin Immunol 2001;108:475–88.
32. Haverkos H, Amsel Z, Drotman D. Adverse virus-drug reactions. Rev Infect Dis 1991;13:697–704.
33. Levy M. Role of viral infections in the induction of adverse drug reactions. Drug Safety 1997;16:1–8.
34. Warrington R, Sauder P, McPhillips S. Lymphocyte transformation studies in suspected hypersensitivity to trimethoprim-sulphamethoxazole. Clin Allergy 1983;13:235–40.
35. Pichler WJ, Tilch J. The lymphocyte transformation test in the diagnosis of drug hypersensitivity. Allergy 2004;59:809–20.
36. Enk A, Katz S. Early molecular events in the induction phase of contact sensitivity. Proc Natl Acad Sci USA 1992;89:1398–402.
37. Grabbe S, Schwarz T. Immunoregulatory mechanisms involved in elicitation of allergic contact hypersensitivity. Immunol Today 1998;19:37–44.
38. Garcia-Doval I, LeCleach L, Bocquet H, Otero XL, Roujeau JC. Toxic epidermal necrolysis and Stevens-Johnson syndrome—does early withdrawal of causative drugs decrease the risk of death? Arch Dermatol 2001;136:323–7.
39. Wolkenstein P, Latarjet J, Roujeau JC, et al. Randomized comparison of thalidomide versus placebo in toxic epidermal necrolysis. Lancet 1998;352:1586–9.
40. French LE, Trent JT, Kerdel FA. Use of intravenous immunoglobulin in toxic epidermal necrolysis and Stevens-Johnson syndrome: our current understanding. Int Immunopharmacol 2006;6:543–9.
41. Edwards I, Aronson J. Adverse drug reactions: definitions, diagnosis, and management. Lancet 2000;356:1255–9.
42. van der Linden P, van der Lei J, Vlug A, Stricker B. Skin reactions to antibacterial agents in general practice. J Clin Epidemiol 1998;51:703–8.
43. Chan H-L, Stern R, Arndt K, et al. The incidence of erythema multiforme, Stevens-Johnson syndrome, and toxic epidermal necrolysis. A population-based study with particular reference to reactions caused by drugs among outpatients. Arch Dermatol 1990;126:43–7.
44. Roujeau JC, Stern RS. Severe adverse cutaneous reactions to drugs. N Engl J Med 1994;331:1272–85.
45. Roujeau JC, Kelly JP, Naldi L, et al. Medication use and the risk of Stevens-Johnson syndrome or toxic epidermal necrolysis. N Engl J Med 1995;333:1600–7.
46. Knowles SR, Shapiro LE, Shear NH. Anticonvulsant hypersensitivity syndrome: incidence, prevention and management. Drug Safety 1999;21:489–501.
47. Fagot JP, Mockenhaupt M, Bouwes-Bavinck JN, Naldi L, Viboud C, Roujeau JC. Nevirapine and the risk of Stevens-Johnson syndrome or toxic epidermal necrolysis. AIDS 2001;15:1843–8.
48. Gaspari A. The role of keratinocytes in the pathophysiology of contact dermatitis. Immunol Allergy Clin North Am 1997;17:377–405.
49. Grone A. Keratinocytes and cytokines. Vet Immunol Immunopathol 2002;88:1–12.
50. Schwarzenberger K, Udey MC. Contact allergens and epidermal proinflammatory cytokines modulate Langerhans cell E-cadherin expression in situ. J Invest Dermatol 1996;106:553–8.
51. Jakob T, Udey MC. Regulation of E-cadherin-mediated adhesion in Langerhans cell-like dendritic cells by inflammatory mediators that mobilize Langerhans cells in vivo. J Immunol 1998;160:4067–73.
52. Jakob T, Ring J, Udey MC. Multistep navigation of Langerhans/dendritic cells in and out of the skin. J Allergy Clin Immunol 2001;108:688–96.
53. Lebre M, Kalinski P, Das P, Everts V. Inhibition of contact sensitizer-induced migration of human Langerhans cells by matrix metalloproteinase inhibitors. Arch Dermatol Res 1999;291:447–52.

54. Yanagihara S, Komura E, Nagafune J, Watarai H, Yamaguchi Y. EB11/CCR7 is a new member of dendritic cell chemokine receptor that is up-regulated upon maturation. J Immunol 1998;161:3096–102.

55. Robbiani D, Finch R, Jager D, Muller W, Sartorelli A, Randolph G. The leukotriene C_4 transporter MRP1 regulates CCL19 (MIB-3b, ELC)-dependent mobilization of dendritic cells to lymph nodes. Cell 2000;103:757–68.

56. Randolph G. Dendritic cell migration to lymph nodes: cytokines, chemokines, and lipid mediators. Semin Immunol 2001;13:267–74.

57. Randolph GJ, Angeli V, Swartz MA. Dendritic-cell trafficking to lymph nodes through lymphatic vessels. Nat Rev Immunol 2005;5:617–28.

58. Santamaria LF, Perez-Soler MT, Hauser C, Blasker K. Allergen specificity and endothelial transmigration of T cells in allergic contact dermatitic and atopic dermatitis are associated with the cutaneous lymphocyte antigen. Int Arch Allergy Appl Immunol 1995;107:359–62.

59. Kehren J, Desvignes C, Krasteva M, et al. Cytotoxicity is mandatory for CD8+ T cell-mediated contact hypersensitivity. J Exp Med 1999;189:779–86.

60. Albanesi C, Cavani A, Girolomoni G. Interferon-g-stimulated human keratinocytes express the genes necessary for the production of peptide-loaded MHC class II molecules. J Invest Dermatol 1998;110:138–42.

61. Basham T, Nickoloff B, Merigan T, Morhenn V. Recombinant gamma interferon induces HLA-DR expression on cultured human keratinocytes. J Invest Dermatol 1984;83:88–90.

62. Dudda JC, Lembo A, Bachtanian E, et al. Dendritic cells govern induction and reprogramming of polarized tissue-selective homing receptor patterns of T cells: important roles for soluble factors and tissue microenvironments. Eur J Immunol 2005;35:1056–65.

63. Dudda JC, Simon JC, Martin S. Dendritic cell immunization route determines CD8+ T cell trafficking to inflamed skin: Role for tissue microenvironment and dendritic cells in establishment of T cell-homing subsets. J Immunol 2004;172:857–63.

64. Reilly TP, Lash LH, Doll MA, Hein DW, Woster PM, Svensson CK. A role for bioactivation and covalent binding within epidermal keratinocytes in sulfonamide-induced cutaneous drug reactions. J Invest Dermatol 2000;114:1164–73.

65. Rieder MJ, Shear NH, Kanee A, Tang BK, Spielberg SP. Prominence of slow acetylator phenotype among patients with sulfonamide hypersensitivity reactions. Clin Pharmacol Ther 1991;49:13–7.

66. Shear NH, Spielberg SP, Grant DM, Tang BK, Kalow W. Differences in metabolism of sulfonamides predisposing to idiosyncratic toxicity. Ann Intern Med 1986;105:179–84.

67. Svensson CK. Do arylhydroxylamine metabolites mediate the idiosyncratic reactions associated with sulfonamides and sulfones? Chem Res Toxicol 2003;16:1034–43.

68. Pirmohamed M, Alfirevic A, Vilar J, et al. Association analysis of drug metabolizing enzyme gene polymorphisms in HIV-positive patients with co-trimoxazole hypersensitivity. Pharmacogenetics 2000;10:705–13.

69. Alfirevic A, Stalford AC, Vilar FJ, Wilkins EGL, Park BK, Pirmohamed M. Slow acetylator phenotype and genotype in HIV-positive patients with sulphamethoxazole hypersensitivity. Br J Clin Pharmacol 2003;55:158–65.

70. Pirmohamed M. Genetic factors in the predisposition to drug-induced hypersensitivity reactions. AAPS J 2005;8(1):E20–E6.

71. Mallal S, Nolan D, Witt C, et al. Association between presence of *HLA-B*5701*, *HLA-DR7*, and *HLA-DQ3* and hypersensitivity to HIV-1 reverse-transcriptase inhibitor abacavir. Lancet 2002;359:727–32.

72. Martin AM, Nolan D, Gaudieri S, et al. Predisposition to abacavir hypersensitivity conferred by *HLA-B*5701* and a haplotypic *Hsp70–Hom* variant. Proc Natl Acad Sci USA 2004;101:4180–5.

73. Hughes DA, Vilar FJ, Ward CC, Alfirevic A, Park BK, Pirmohamed M. Cost-effectiveness analysis of HLA B*5701 genotyping in preventing abacavir hypersensitivity. Pharmacogenetics 2004;14:335–42.

74. Klemola E. Hypersensitivity reactions to ampicillin in cytomegalovirus mononucleosis. Scand J Infect Dis 1970;2:29–31.

75. Nazareth I, Mortimer P, McKendrick GD. Ampicillin sensitivity in infectious mononucleosis - temporary or permanent? Scand J Infect Dis 1972;4:229–30.

76. Patel BM. Skin rash with infectious mononucleosis and ampicillin. Pediatrics 1967;40:910–1.

77. Pullen H, Wright N, Murdoch JM. Hypersensitivity reactions to antibacterial drugs in infectious mononucleosis. Lancet 1967;2:1176–8.

78. Gordin FM, Simon GL, Wofsy CB, Mills J. Adverse reactions to trimethoprim-sulfamethoxazole in patients with the acquired immunodeficiency syndrome. Ann Intern Med 1984;100:495–9.

79. Jaffe HS, Abrams DL, Ammann AJ, Lewis BJ, Golden JA. Complications of co-trimoxazole in treatment of AIDS-associated *Pneumocystis carinii* pneumonia in homosexual men. Lancet 1984;2:1009–11.

80. Roudier C, Caumes E, Rogeaux O, Bricaire F, Gentilini M. Adverse cutaneous reactions to trimethoprim-sulfamethoxazole in patients with the acquired immunodeficiency syndrome and *Pneumocystis carinii* pneumonia. Arch Dermatol 1994;130:1383–6.

81. Yawalkar N, Shrikhande M, Hari Y, Nievergelt H, Braathen LR, Pichler WJ. Evidence for a role for IL-5

and eotaxin in activating and recruiting eosinophils in drug-induced cutaneous eruptions. J Allergy Clin Immunol 2000;106:1171–6.

82. Yawalkar N, Egli F, Hari Y, Nievergelt H, Braathen LR, Pichler WJ. Infiltration of cytotoxic T cells in drug-induced cutaneous eruptions. Clin Exp Allergy 2000;30:847–55.

83. Crowson AN, Margo CM. Recent advances in the pathology of cutaneous drug eruptions. Dermatol Clin 1999;17:537–60.

84. Blanca M, Posadas S, Torres MJ, et al. Expression of the skin-homing receptor in peripheral blood lymphocytes from subjects with non-immediate cutaneous allergic drug reactions. Allergy 2000;55:998–1004.

85. Posadas SJ, Torres MJ, Mayorga C, Juarez C, Blanca M. Gene expression levels of cytokine profile and cytotoxic markers in non-immediate reactions to drugs. Blood Cells Mol Dis 2002;29:179–89.

86. Villada G, Roujeau JC, Clerici T, Bourgault I, Revuz J. Immunopathology of toxic epidermal necrolysis. Keratinocytes, HLA-DR Expression, Langerhans Cells, and mononuclear cells: An immunopathologic study of five cases. Arch Dermatol 1992;128:50–3.

19
Cutaneous Vasculitis

Sherrif F. Ibrahim and Carlos H. Nousari

Key Points

- Vasculitis can be caused by many different mechanisms.
- Skin biopsies for hematoxylin and eosin (H&E) and direct immunofluorescence (DIF) are the cornerstones of diagnosing vasculitis
- Serology, histories, and physical examinations can help determine the type of vasculitis.
- Treatments can include corticosteroids, cyclophosphamide, azathioprine, methotrexate, colchicine, dapsone, mycophenolate mofetil, thalidomide, or intravenous immunoglobulin.

Vasculitis is defined as inflammation of blood vessel walls. With inflammation of the vasculature, there is resultant wall destruction and increased permeability, which can lead to aneurysm formation, extravasation of blood cells, and stenosis. Clinically, these processes present as hemorrhage, tissue ischemia, or infarction of the affected organ. Depending on the organs and caliber of blood vessels involved, vasculitis can manifest with a wide spectrum of clinical findings—from a benign, self-limiting course, to death. Vasculitis of any organ can be a primary process (idiopathic) or a secondary manifestation of other triggers such as trauma, infection, malignancy, systemic inflammatory conditions, connective tissue disease, and drug hypersensitivity.

The skin in particular is among the most common organs affected by vasculitis due to its rich vascular supply, exposure to cold temperatures and trauma, and predisposing hemodynamic conditions (e.g., venous hypertension, stasis in the lower extremities).

Because lesions of the skin are readily visible to the clinician, often they are the first indication of potentially life-threatening vasculitic processes occurring elsewhere in the body. As such, it is critical to develop a systematic and thorough approach to the patient with suspected vasculitis. Cutaneous signs are varied and are primarily a reflection of the size of the affected vessels. Involvement of small, superficial vessels results in erythema and purpuric macules, whereas deeper involvement of larger vessels presents with increasingly severe lesions including livedo, palpable purpura, vesicles, ulcers, urticaria, subcutaneous nodules, distal gangrene, and necrosis. In this regard, the morphology of lesions can be a clue to the underlying vasculitic process; however, multiple lesion types are often present, as a range of blood vessel sizes may be involved. While the majority of cases of vasculitis restricted to the skin are self-limited, the physiologic response to inflammation from blood vessels results in the release of chemical mediators that may give rise to a variety of systemic findings, such as malaise, fever, weight loss, arthralgias, arthritis, myalgia, night sweats, and laboratory abnormalities.[1–3] Therefore, a complete history, physical exam, review of systems, and laboratory workup are necessary to further classify suspected vasculitis and identify extracutaneous involvement. In all cases, biopsy and clinical-histologic correlation provide the gold standard for diagnosis. This chapter discusses features common to most, if not all, variants of cutaneous vasculitis, including workup, common etiologies, and specific presentations.

Cutaneous Vasculitides

Cutaneous vasculitis most often manifests as palpable purpura in dependent areas[4] and under tight-fitting clothing. These lesions may be asymptomatic, tender, or pruritic,[5] and, depending on the disease process and the size of the affected vessels, there may be varying degrees of involvement of other organs such as the kidneys, gastrointestinal (GI) tract, or lungs. While accompanying signs and symptoms may give hints to systemic disease, there are no pathognomonic indicators of extracutaneous involvement, although tools have been proposed that may identify patients with more extensive disease.[6,7] Furthermore, because different vasculitic processes can present with the same skin findings, and because many conditions can mimic vasculitis, prognosis cannot be determined from physical examination alone.[9–12]

The annual incidence of biopsy-confirmed cutaneous vasculitis has been reported from 40 to 60 cases per million.[13,16,18] Approximately 30% to 60% of vasculitides limited to the skin are idiopathic without evidence of extracutaneous involvement and with no obvious trigger.[4,23,24] These cases are typically solitary, self-limited episodes, although as many as 10% of these patients may have recurrent or chronic disease.[25,26] Of the remaining patients, 20% are attributable to adverse drug reactions, 22% to infection, 12% to connective tissue disease (CTD), 10% to Henoch-Schönlein purpura (HSP), and less than 5% each to malignancy, systemic vasculitis, or other systemic disease[24] (Table 19.1). There is a slight predilection in women over men, and all ages can be affected (mean adult onset = 47 years, mean pediatric onset = 7 years), with 90% of pediatric cases represented by HSP.[23]

TABLE 19.1. Causes of cutaneous vasculitis.[14,23–26]

Idiopathic	30–60%
90% self-limited	
10% recurrent	
Drug reaction	20%
Infection	22%
Connective tissue disease	12%
Malignancy	<5%
Systemic vasculitis	<5%
Other systemic disease	<5%

Initial Workup of Cutaneous Vasculitis

In cases of suspected vasculitis, the laboratory results and the histologic workup provide invaluable information beyond the history and the physical examination in both determining the degree of systemic involvement and uncovering underlying causes for the vasculitic process, with biopsy providing the gold standard for diagnosis. While physical findings can afford initial clues as to the types of vessels involved, the diagnosis of vasculitis can only be confirmed histologically, keeping in mind that the verification of the diagnosis does not lend information regarding the degree of extracutaneous involvement; palpable purpura may represent vasculitis limited to the skin, or a harbinger of life-threatening systemic disease.[1,8] Table 19.2 lists the appropriate initial laboratory workup for all patients and other tests that should be considered on a case-by-case basis. Taken together, these data ultimately contribute to decisions regarding prognosis and treatment modalities. For example, serum complement is a known mediator of vascular inflammation, and low levels indicate excessive consumption, sug-

TABLE 19.2. Suggested laboratory workup for suspected vasculitis.

Standard workup
Complete blood count w/differential
Complete metabolic panel (including creatinine)
Urinalysis with microscopic evaluation
Biopsy for hematoxylin and eosin staining
Biopsy for direct immunofluorescence
Infectious serologies (blood, urine, swabs)
Rheumatoid factor
C-reactive protein
Antinuclear antibody
Antineutrophil cytoplasmic antibody
Cryoglobulins
Complement (C3, C4, CH_{50})
Hepatitis panel
Stool guaiac
Chest x-ray
HIV
Serum protein electrophoresis/urine protein electrophoresis

Other tests to consider based on the individual case
Renal biopsy
Nerve conduction studies
Hypercoagulability panel
Echocardiogram

gesting more extensive or systemic involvement.[29] An elevated erythrocyte sedimentation rate (ESR) has been described in up to 50% of patients with limited cutaneous vasculitis; however, significant elevations (up to 60 mm/h) have been associated with higher rates of systemic involvement.[25]

Skin biopsies sent for both routine hematoxylin and eosin (H&E) staining as well as direct immunofluorescence (DIF) are the cornerstones in determining whether physical findings represent true vasculitis or other conditions that can clinically mimic vasculitis. Decisions as to which lesions should be biopsied have direct impact on the diagnostic information elicited. Tissue should be acquired from lesions between 24 and 48 hours after their appearance, as sampling before or after this time range may result in false-negative results. Biopsies with thrombosis or perivascular lymphocytic inflammation are characteristic of older lesions. In cases where suspicion of vasculitis is high but histology does not correlate with clinical findings, biopsy should be repeated. Likewise, if a medium-vessel vasculitis such as polyarteritis nodosa (PAN) is suspected, the biopsy must be of sufficient depth to include the subcutaneous tissue where these vessels are found. In general, ulcerated lesions should be avoided.[1]

The diagnosis of vasculitis is confirmed unequivocally by the presence of an inflammatory infiltrate around and within the walls of vasculature with fibrin deposition. These areas of fibrinoid necrosis are accompanied by swelling and necrosis of endothelial cells, as well as secondary changes such as erythrocyte extravasation and necrosis leading to purpura and infarction, respectively.[1,23] Apoptotic cells are seen frequently as well as overlying ulceration. Determination of vessel size, type of cellular infiltrate, depth, and degree of involvement on H&E stains helps in classification and generation of differential diagnoses (Fig. 19.1).

The pathogenic features of vasculitis in the skin are related to vessel wall injury, which can be toxin mediated, immune mediated, or from direct infection, and all three mechanisms can result in the histologic pattern of fibrinoid necrosis mentioned above. It is critical to identify those patients in which pathogenesis is caused by antibody-mediated toxicity and immune complex formation, as they are more likely to have extracutaneous involvement.[1] Deposition of immune complexes leads to complement activation, further recruitment of

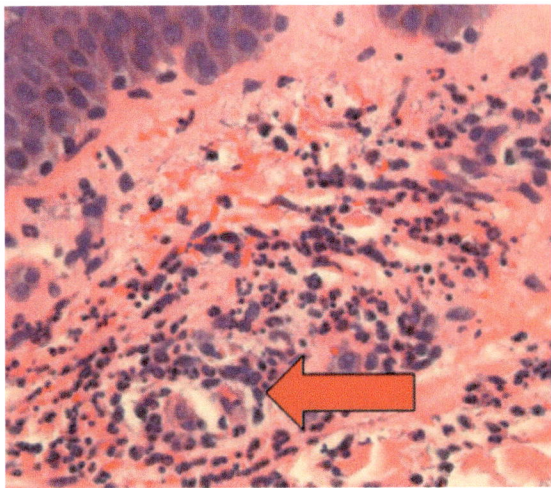

Fig. 19.1. Hematoxylin and eosin (H&E) staining of skin biopsy from a patient with cutaneous small-vessel vasculitis (CSVV). This is a leukocytoclastic vasculitis involving small, superficial vessels, rich in neutrophils (arrow)

inflammatory cells and cytokines, and expression of adhesion molecules such as E-selectin, P-selectin, and intercellular adhesion molecule 1 (ICAM-1). With endothelial cell retraction, there is vascular deposition of immune complexes, neutrophil infiltration, edema, hemorrhage, and thrombosis.[2]

Immunofluorescence is an essential diagnostic tool in the evaluation of cutaneous vasculitis, especially in the small-vessel group. This technique consists of the detection of immunoglobulins (Igs) and complement deposited within tissue. Deposition of IgA, IgG, IgM, and C3 in or around vessels identified by DIF characterizes antibody- and immune complex–mediated vasculitis, and the patterns of deposition further classify disease. Lesion age is critical to evaluation, as up to 30% of immune-mediated vasculitides are negative on DIF by 72 hours and only C3 is detected after this point.[28] Tissue samples are transported in Michell's medium and stored at 4°C prior to processing at specialized laboratories. Samples are washed, flash frozen, sectioned, and then stained to detect antibodies and complement in and around blood vessels. Certain diagnoses cannot be made without characteristic DIF patterns, which will be discussed with their associated conditions below.

Serologic testing has become routine in evaluation of vasculitis. In particular, antineutrophil cytoplasmic antibodies (ANCAs) have established clinical utility in dermatology.[31] Initially described in patients with rheumatoid arthritis, ANCA-associated vasculitides include small and medium-sized involvement such as Wegener's granulomatosis, microscopic polyangiitis, Churg-Strauss syndrome, and many drug-induced cases of vasculitis, as well as systemic inflammatory conditions and connective tissue diseases.[32] It is believed that vasculitides associated with ANCAs have a distinct mode of pathogenesis.[5] Antibodies can be directed against cytoplasmic (c-ANCA) and perinuclear (p-ANCA) neutrophil-derived products. C-ANCA antibodies are directed against proteinase 3 (PR3) and ANCA antibodies are directed toward myeloperoxidase (MPO) and elastase. Inflammatory cytokines are believed to induce the translocation of these targets to the surface of neutrophils, allowing binding of ANCAs and adherence to endothelial cells, ultimately causing damage to vessel walls.[33] Titers may predict clinical relapse or disease activity,[34] and serial testing is recommended, as transient elevations in ANCAs can be seen with acute infections.[35] Because c-ANCA is represented by only one antigen (PR3), enzyme-linked immunosorbent assay (ELISA) is a more sensitive and specific assay. Since several antigens are responsible for the p-ANCA pattern, immunofluorescence is preferred.

Drug–Induced Vasculitis

Medications from virtually every pharmacologic class (including herbal supplements) have been linked to drug-induced vasculitis, resulting in a range of clinical presentations[36–38] (Table 19.3). The onset of findings after exposure to the causative agent is typically 5 to 20 days,[1] and while withdrawal is often sufficient to reverse the vasculitic process, there have been cases of fatal drug-induced allergic vasculitis in previously healthy patients.[62] There have also been reports of cutaneous vasculitis stemming from vaccines,[63] foods,[64] and alcohol.[65] Ironically, many of the medications used for the treatment of systemic inflammatory conditions have also been linked to the development of cutaneous vasculitis.[66,67] One recent report linked the appearance of cutaneous vasculitis as a marker for therapeutic response in chemotherapy for non-Hodgkin's lymphoma.[68] Although the precise pathogenic mechanisms are varied, there appears

TABLE 19.3. Partial list of commonly used medications reported to cause vasculitis; essentially any drug in any class is capable of acting as a trigger for vasculitis.

Metformin[47]
Olanzapine[48]
Leukotriene receptor antagonists[49]
Famciclovir[50]
Bosentan[51]
Cyclooxygenase inhibitors[52]
Sirolimus[53]
Nonsteroidal antiinflammatory drugs[54]
Vancomycin[56]
Paroxetine[59]
Oxacillin[61]
Hepatitis B vaccine[63]
Alcohol[65]
Infliximab[66]
Etanercept[67]

to be a combination of cell-mediated and humoral immune responses contributing to the development of the observed vasculitis. As such, a thorough medication history is critical in the initial evaluation of the patient with suspected vasculitis, and all recently added medications should be discontinued. In those patients with both p-ANCA and c-ANCA, as well as eosinophilic infiltrates, the notion of drug-induced vasculitis should be entertained.[69,70] Finally, one should keep in mind that the vast majority of drug-induced small-vessel vasculitis falls into the category of cutaneous leukocytoclastic vasculitis (hypersensitivity vasculitis) or IgA vasculitis (Henoch-Schönlein purpura).

Vasculitis Associated with Systemic Conditions

Cutaneous vasculitis may result from a number of infectious, inflammatory, autoimmune, and malignant diseases, as well as pregnancy.[71–77] Essentially any of the above conditions can result in vasculitides of varying severity, and the workup of patients often points to a specific underlying condition. Vasculitis can present prodromally or at any time during the disease. Table 19.4 lists the potential underlying systemic triggers for vasculitis. Among malignant diseases associated with vasculitis, hematologic cancers are seen most frequently. In a recent study of 95 hospitalized patients with hematologic malignancies, 23 (24%) had biopsy proven

TABLE 19.4. Immunoglobulin A vs. non–immunoglobulin A vasculitides.

Immunoglobulin A (IgA) predominance seen on direct immunofluorescence?
IgA vasculitis
Henoch-Schönlein purpura
No IgA or IgG/IgM predominance?
Non-IgA vasculitis
Cryoglobulinemia II/III
Hypocomplimentemic urticarial vasculitis syndrome
Rheumatoid vasculitis
Connective tissue disease
Wegener's granulmatosis
Churg-Strauss syndrome
Microscopic polyangiitis
Behçet's syndrome

cutaneous vasculitis. Skin findings developed before (26%), during (39%), and after (35%) the diagnosis of malignancy.[78] Once again, thorough history, physical, and laboratory workup often point to the underlying disease processes, and in cases where there is failure to respond to treatment, investigation for occult malignancy should be considered.

Treatment

If systemic conditions are excluded and potentially causative agents discontinued, treatment for vasculitis is driven by the severity of symptoms and extent of extracutaneous involvement. The majority of cases are isolated occurrences and can be managed supportively with rest, warming, compression, elevation of affected lower extremities, and symptomatic treatment for pain control, inflammation (nonsteroidal antiinflammatory drugs [NSAIDs]), and pruritus (antihistamines). For recalcitrant disease or with evidence of systemic involvement, more aggressive therapy, including immunosuppressive agents, is necessary. Therapeutic decisions are based on the experience of the clinician and the details of the specific patient. Corticosteroids, cyclophosphamide, azathioprine, methotrexate, colchicine, dapsone, mycophenolate mofetil, thalidomide, and intravenous immunoglobulin (IVIG) have all been reported[5] and are discussed in further detail below. More recently, there have been reports of effective treatment with tumor necrosis factor-α (TNF-α) inhibitors[79,80] and anti-CD20 antibodies.[81,82] Newer

therapies targeted toward neutrophil chemotaxis, activation, and adhesion are certain to appear in the near future.[5]

Clinical Mimickers of Cutaneous Vasculitis

A variety of conditions are capable of clinically simulating cutaneous vasculitis and have been termed pseudovasculitides.[83] Many of these conditions can be excluded by biopsy, and are typically associated with conditions that cause hemorrhage or vessel occlusion, and should always be in the differential diagnosis for vasculitis. Vessel wall dysfunction or incompetence from infiltrative processes, nutritional deficits such as scurvy,[84] infection, embolism, vasospasm, and trauma can all present with varying degrees of purpura, petechia, ecchymoses, ulcers, and necrosis. Likewise, hypercoagulable states such as antiphospholipid syndrome and factor V Leiden can lead to similar clinical pictures and need to be excluded.[9]

Classification of Cutaneous Vasculitis

Classification of vasculitis in the skin is typically based on the size of predominantly affected blood vessels and type of inflammatory response, which when interpreted with DIF examination and laboratory workup, correlate with disease etiology and affect the treatment decisions. Vessels of varying sizes are frequently involved, however, as vasculitic processes do not always recognize arbitrary boundaries of vessel size. Most texts refer to the classification schemes outlined by the Chapel Hill Consensus Criteria or the American College of Rheumatology, although it is often difficult to characterize individual patient variations.[85–87]

Small blood vessels are ubiquitous in the skin. They include arterioles, capillaries, and postcapillary venules. They are typically 50 µm or less in diameter, and may not have a fully developed muscular layer. Clinical lesions of cutaneous small-vessel vasculitis (CSVV) are most commonly nonblanchable and purpuric, and are found in dependent areas (buttocks, back, lower extremities).

When urticarial lesions are present, they are less pruritic, short-lived (<24 hours), and can occur anywhere on the body. They include Wegener's granulomatosis, Churg-Strauss syndrome, microscopic polyangiitis, Henoch-Schönlein purpura, essential cryoglobulinemic vasculitis, and cutaneous leukocytoclastic angiitis.

Medium-sized blood vessels are larger than 50μm, have fully developed muscular layers, and are located deeper within the dermis or subcutaneous fat. Clinically, these processes present with livedo, nodules, ulcerations, or digital infarcts. Wedge biopsy is typically needed for sufficient diagnostic yield, and biopsy of necrotic or ulcerated areas is of low yield. Included among this group are polyarteritis nodosa and Kawasaki disease. Vasculitis of these vessels is commonly referred to as necrotizing vasculitis, reflecting the hyalinization, coagulative necrosis, and degeneration of muscular layers, where it is more readily visible. Occasionally nerve or muscle biopsy can provide additional diagnostic information if histology is inconclusive.

Large-vessel vasculitides rarely have cutaneous manifestations and include giant cell (temporal) arteritis and Takayasu's arteritis, and will be mentioned only briefly.

Cutaneous Leukocytoclastic Angiitis

As defined by the Chapel Hill Criteria, *cutaneous leukocytoclastic angiitis* (CLA) is the term applied to patients with hypersensitivity vasculitis. Exogenous chemicals, infectious agents, cytokines, and circulating immune entities that do not strongly activate complement can cause CLA by inducing an inflammatory cascade in endothelium of CSVV. Most commonly triggered by infections or drugs, the onset is acute with both palpable and nonpalpable purpuric and urticarial lesions on the lower extremities appearing 5 to 20 days after initial exposure, and 2 to 4 days after repeat exposures.[88] These cases tend to be single episodes, and relapsing cycles can result from systemic inflammatory conditions, infection, and malignancy. Extracutaneous involvement is rare, with the exception of constitutional symptoms caused by mediators of inflammation released locally.[100] Serum sickness resulting from the injection of nonhuman serum can present with a similar picture, but is rarely seen in modern practice.[1]

Routine laboratory tests are usually normal, as extracutaneous disease is rare. The ESR is elevated in up to 50% of cases, while complement levels and urinalysis are normal. There are no specific serologic markers for CLA, making it largely a diagnosis of exclusion, and normocomplementemic urticarial vasculitis is likely to be a clinical variant of this condition.[97]

On histology, there is a neutrophil predominant vasculitis of superficial vessels with varying numbers of surrounding eosinophils (Fig. 19.2). Direct immunofluorescence is positive in roughly half of these biopsies, displaying mild to moderately intense granular IgM deposits with weak or absent C3. The lack of complement involvement may correlate with the relatively benign course of this condition and low level of systemic involvement. Although DIF is frequently negative, it is a key factor in discriminating CLA from IgA vasculitis, which shares the same triggers and clinical presentation.[96,98]

Up to half of the cases of CLA are idiopathic and resolve spontaneously. In cases with a known trigger, treatment consists of removal of the offending agent or resolution of underlying sys-

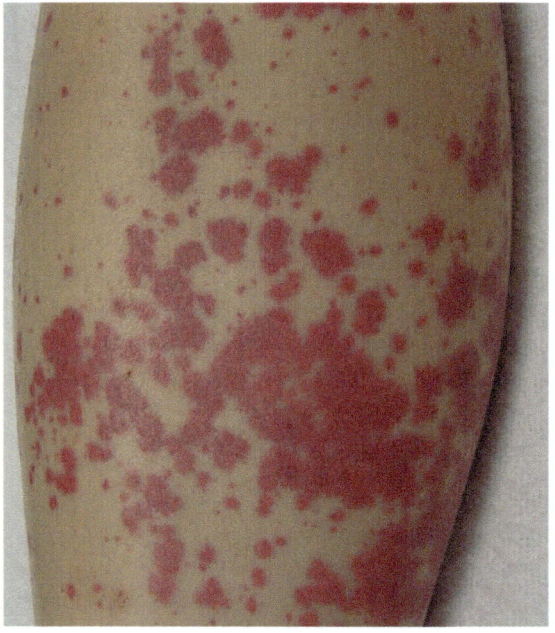

FIG. 19.2. Acute palpable purpura of cutaneous leukocytoclastic angiitis (hypersensitivity vasculitis)

temic condition. Immunosuppressive treatment is largely unnecessary in CLA, with the exception of the most severe cases, and is aimed at reducing constitutional symptoms and synovitis. Moderately dosed corticosteroids (0.5mg/kg/day) are a reasonable option until symptoms resolve. Recalcitrant cases warrant more extensive investigation.

Henoch-Schönlein Purpura

Henoch-Schönlein purpura (HSP) is defined as an IgA-mediated syndrome presenting with a tetrad of purpura, abdominal pain, arthralgias, and hematuria.[91] It is most commonly seen in children, but there have been increasing reports of HSP in adults.[94] As with CLA, HSP is often preceded by medications or infection—most commonly upper respiratory, gastrointestinal (GI), and genitourinary (GU). When associated with GI and GU infections, it can be difficult to discern findings related to infection from those caused by the vasculitic process itself. Approximately 50% of those affected develop systemic involvement such as nephritis, neuropathy, and GI symptoms.[92] Skin lesions are seen in all patients and are typically palpable purpura or urticaria of the lower extremities and buttocks that turn into purpura with annular configuration (Fig. 19.3). Koebnerization is known to occur in HSP. A subset of patients displays only urticarial lesions, and lesions above the waist have been associated with renal disease, as are elevated ESR, fever, and adult onset.[137] Women have an increased risk for the development of proteinuria or preeclampsia in future pregnancies.[138,139] Ulcerative lesions have been reported in HIV-positive patients.[130]

Extracutaneous involvement can appear in any organ, with the kidneys, GI tract, and joints being most common. Renal failure secondary to glomerulonephritis is the most serious complication of HSP, with some degree of renal involvement occurring in up to 40% of adult patients. Patients with fibronectin-rich IgA1 complexes or with abnormal glycosylation of the hinge region of IgA1 have higher rates of renal involvement. Renal disease typically manifests within the first 3 months of HSP, and 5% of patients progress to chronic renal failure. Children with renal involvement have a higher incidence of hypertension and renal failure as adults, and 15% of children on hemodialysis

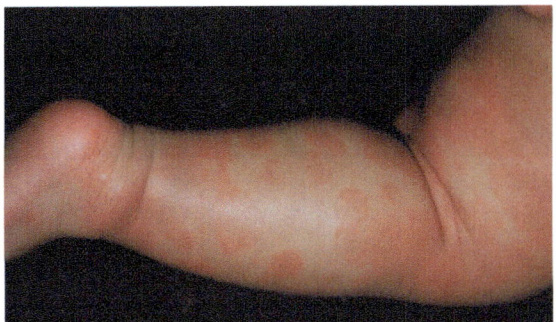

a

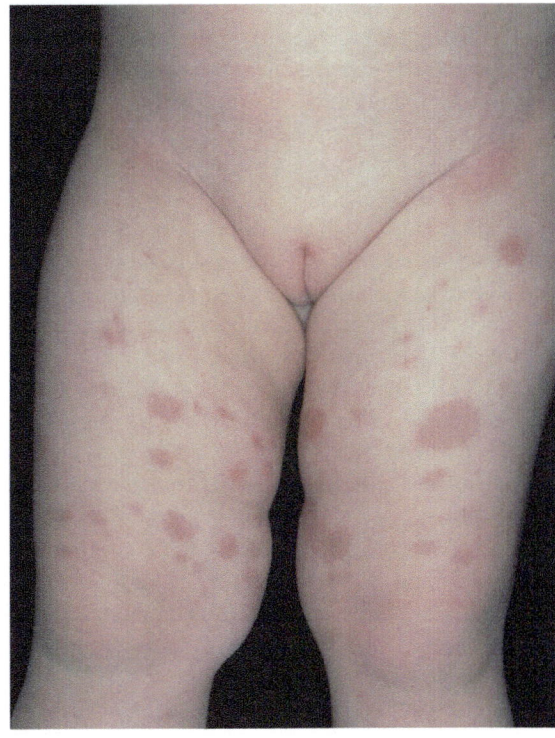

b

FIG. 19.3. (A,B) Infants with typical lesions of Henoch-Schönlein purpura (HSP). Lesions above the waistline are associated with a worse prognosis. (Courtesy of Dr. M. Mercurio.)

have renal failure secondary to HSP.[140] Urinalysis is an absolute requirement for the patient with suspected HSP, with hematuria providing the most sensitive measurement for renal involvement. Gastrointestinal involvement can range from pain to hemorrhage and necrosis of the bowel from mesenteric vasculitis, and pulmonary hemorrhage has also been reported.[90] Once again, however, it is difficult to determine if involvement of these organs is the result of a prodromal infection or from the vasculitic process itself.

There is mounting evidence that acute hemorrhagic edema of infancy (AHEI) is a variant of HSP, although in contrast with HSP, extracutaneous involvement is rare and IgA deposition is rarely seen with DIF.[93] AHEI is frequently seen after bacterial infection, and lesions appear on the face and extremities.

There are no specific serology associations with HSP, although up to 40% of adult patients demonstrate some degree of IgA gammopathy.[137] When appropriate, additional workup should include serum and urine protein electrophoresis (SPEP and UPEP), total immunoglobulin quantitation, and immunofixation.

Routine H&E staining reveals a neutrophil-rich small-vessel vasculitis of the superficial dermis with leukocytoclasia and few eosinophils. DIF provides the gold standard for diagnosis, with IgA deposits in small, superficial vessels found in virtually all biopsies. Granular deposits of other Ig classes are occasionally seen, with IgA being the most prominent.[86]

As with any of the vasculitides, treatment decisions hinge on the degree of involvement and constitutional symptoms. While the cutaneous findings are largely refractory to therapy, synovitis and GI symptoms are quite responsive to moderate doses of oral corticosteroids. Skin lesions frequently have an initial response to steroids, followed by rapid relapse upon completion of treatment. Antimetabolites such as azathioprine and mycophenolate mofetil, as well as alkylating agents can be effective for treating glomerulonephritis. There is growing evidence for a role of TNF-α in pathogenesis in HSP, and the utility of TNF-α antagonists is currently under investigation.[79]

Urticarial Vasculitis

Urticarial vasculitis presents clinically as urticaria of the trunk and proximal extremities, and histologically as vasculitis (Fig. 19.4). It occurs in two forms differentiated by serum complement levels. The normocomplementemic variant is a subset of CLA, while the hypocomplementemic type (HUVS) is a subset of systemic lupus erythematosus

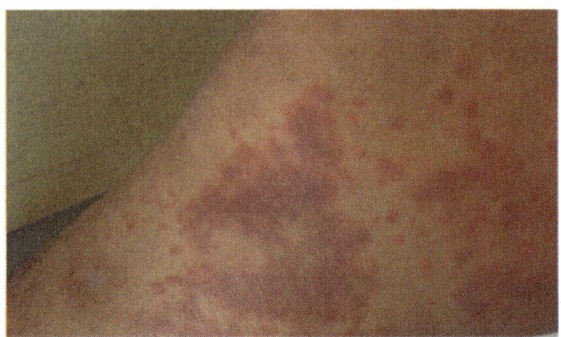

Fig. 19.4. Urticarial vasculitis. These lesions are difficult to distinguish clinically from traditional urticaria and can occur on the face and upper extremities. (Courtesy of Dr. F. Tausk.)

(SLE).[95,97] Patients with low levels of C3, C4, and total serum hemolytic complement (CH_{50}) have dramatically increased rates of complement consumption. CH_{50} is a more sensitive predictor of HUVS since C3 and C4 are acute-phase reactants and may be normal in mild disease or early-stage disease. Thorough workup of patients with urticarial vasculitis should include the quantitation of C3a, C5a, and C3bi when available.[97,98]

Ninety percent of normocomplementemic urticarial vasculitis (NUV) are triggered by infection or medications, and are self-limited without indication of systemic involvement.[96] The clinical differential includes urticarial HSP, neutrophilic urticaria, Schnitzler's syndrome, and urticarial cryoglobulinemia II and III.

Neutrophilic urticaria, also known as polymorphonuclear predominant urticaria (PPU) is a subset of chronic urticaria.[103] Lesions are typically pruritic, and mild constitutional symptoms can be present. Histologic features of PPU can be confused with NUV, as perivascular neutrophilic infiltrates can be dense, with occasional karyorrhexis; however, there is no definite disruption of vasculature and DIF is consistently negative in PPU. Chronicity and no obvious underlying cause argue against NUV. Treatment consists of antihistamines, leukotriene antagonists, dapsone, or colchicine. In cases of PPU it is important to rule out Schnitzler's syndrome, which is characterized by NUV, fever, lymphadenopathy, hepatosplenomegaly, peripheral neuropathy, bone pain, and monoclonal IgM gammopathy.[99]

In contrast to patients with NUV, the hypocomplementemic variant of urticarial vasculitis presents as a chronic, relapsing syndrome (HUVS) with signs and symptoms typically seen with SLE, including fever, arthralgias, and myalgias.[95,96] In contrast to lesions of NUV, HUVS lesions tend to have a purpuric component upon careful examination. Synovitis, GI involvement, scleritis, and synovitis are not uncommon associated findings. A subset of HUVS patients with more overt symptoms of SLE will display angioedema, thought to be mediated by a high rate of consumption of C1 esterase caused by autoantibodies to C1q. In both variants of urticarial vasculitis, histology reveals a dense neutrophilic infiltrate in and around the walls of small vessels that disrupts normal architecture. In HUVS, dermal edema and neutrophils extend to the dermal-epidermal junction (DEJ), resulting in vacuolar changes and clefting of the basement membrane zone (BMZ). The only serologic marker associated with NUV is an elevation in ESR in up to 70% of patients, while essentially all patients with HUVS have high ESR and an antinuclear antibody (ANA) titer greater than 1:320 at some point in their disease course.[1]

As with CLA, 50% of patients with NUV have immune deposition within and around blood vessel walls seen with DIF. IgM is seen more frequently than IgG, and C3, if present, is weak and patchy. In contrast, essentially all patients with HUVS show significant IgG and C3 intravascularly and perivascularly within superficial dermal vessels extending to the BMZ (Fig. 19.5). It has been reported that

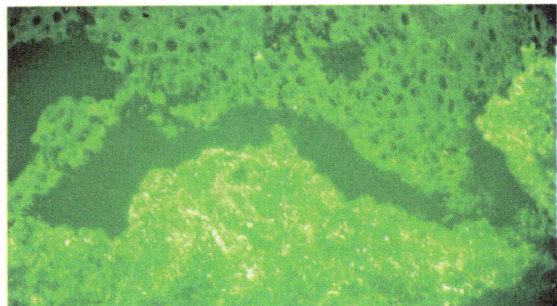

FIG. 19.5. Direct immunofluorescence of biopsy from a patient with hypocomplimentemic urticarial vasculitis syndrome (HUVS) revealing granular immunoglobulin G (IgG) in and around superficial vessels

this latter finding resembles the lupus band test, further linking HUVS with SLE.[98,108]

Treatment of NUV is similar to that for CLA—conservative and directive toward alleviation of mild symptoms. HUVS, however, frequently requires systemic immunosuppressive therapy such as corticosteroids, azathioprine (3 to 4 mg/kg/day), or mycophenolate mofetil (40 to 50 mg/kg/day); these medications are usually sufficient. Antiinflammatory agents such as dapsone, colchicine, methotrexate, and calcineurin inhibitors are not typically effective, as they have no effect on the production of immune complexes or anti-C1q synthesis.

Cryoglobulinemia

Cryoglobulinemic vasculitis affects both small and medium-sized skin blood vessels. Cryoglobulins are antibodies that precipitate with cold, and three types of cryoglobulinemia exist as defined by the type of antibodies present. Type I is a monoclonal gammopathy that commonly presents as a hyperviscosity syndrome and thrombotic events in the context of myeloproliferative disorders, and does not represent true vasculitis. Type II is mixed, with an IgM monoclonal component (usually an IgM rheumatoid factor) in conjunction with polyclonal gammopathy. Type III consists of polyclonal cryoglobulins. Because types II and III readily form immune complexes, they are more likely to cause vasculitis, as opposed to the thrombotic vasculopathy seen with type I cryoglobulins.[1,104–107] Cryoglobulinemia type II has antibodies that form immune complexes with much higher avidity and levels of complement fixation, resulting in more significant clinical syndromes. Hepatitis C is by far the most common cause of type II cryoglobulinemia, representing essentially all cases previously labeled as essential mixed cryoglobulinemia (Fig. 19.6).[104,105] It is felt that the virus stimulates the immune system chronically, causing B-cell expansion and production of autoantibodies. Other associated infections include endocarditis, hepatitis B, and HIV. Connective tissue disease, other autoimmune conditions, and malignancy have been associated with both types II and III cryoglobulinemic vasculitis.[109]

Clinically, skin lesions associated with cryoglobulinemia type I are indistinguishable from

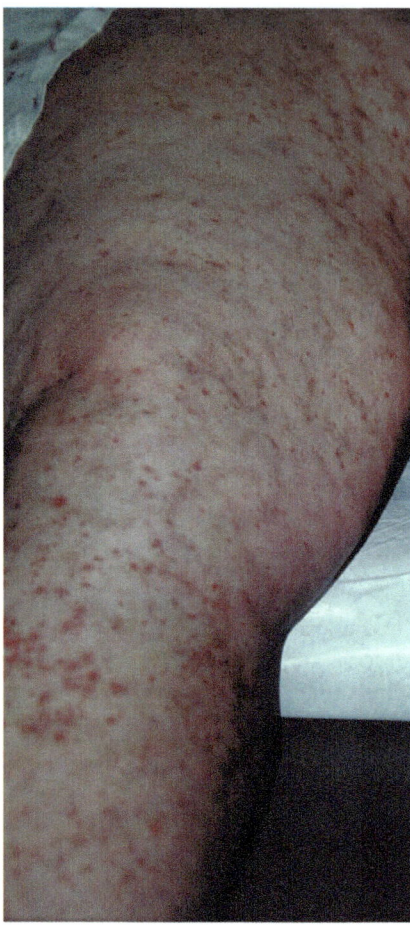

FIG. 19.6. Clinical image of patient with known hepatitis C presenting with the CSVV (purpura) and medium-sized vessel vasculitis (MSVV) (livedo) lesions associated with cryoglobulinemia type II

those seen with type II, and resemble the palpable purpura and urticarial findings seen with any CSVV. As with most vasculitides other than urticarial vasculitis, lesions most commonly appear on the lower extremities. Cryoglobulin-associated nonpalpable purpura can also present as the capillaritic eruption seen in Schamberg's disease. The benign hypergammaglobulinemic purpura seen in Waldenström's (lymphocytic vasculitis) is clinically, serologically, and histologically indistinguishable from that seen with cryoglobulinemia type III, and, as such, is generally believed to belong to the same spectrum of disease.[109] Pigmented purpura above the waistline or involving the soles

of the feet favor cryoglobulinemic vasculitis over Schamberg's, as do lesions seen at different stages of evolution, ulcerative lesions, and constitutional symptoms. Ulceration signals the involvement of medium-sized vessels and can help differentiate from other CSVV. As mentioned, medium-sized vessels can also be seen with cryoglobulinemia. These patients also tend to have systemic symptoms such as nephropathy, neuropathy, arthralgias, and gastrointestinal involvement.[1,110]

Serologically, cryoglobulin type II patients demonstrate monoclonal IgM rheumatoid factor (RF) and polyclonal IgG. All patients have an RF greater than 1:320, and over 90% have decreased C4 but essentially normal C3. Therefore, a negative cryoglobulin assay and negative RF in the setting of low C4 virtually excludes cryoglobulinemia type II, whereas a low titer cryoglobulinemia in the absence of vasculitis is common after many infections. A positive cryoglobulinemia with negative RF activity likely represents an incidental finding and not vasculitis. Cryoglobulinemia type III demonstrates a polyclonal gammopathy without any specific monoclonal spike, and low levels of both C3 and C4.[1]

Histology demonstrates findings consistent with CSVV or both CSVV and medium-sized vessel vasculitis (MSVV), but not MSVV alone. Some texts report the deposition of a nonspecific, homogeneous intravascular infiltrate associated with cryoglobulinemic vasculitis; however, this likely represents thrombotic vasculopathy seen with type I cryoglobulinemia and not true vasculitis.[109]

Direct immunofluorescence in cryoglobulinemia type II usually reveals significant granular IgM and C3 deposition in and around small and medium-sized vessels, while type III has both IgG and IgM in addition to C3. In practice, it is often difficult to distinguish between types II and III cryoglobulinemia by DIF.

Because types II and III cryoglobulinemias are difficult to distinguish histologically and clinically, treatment decisions should hinge on the serologic workup and be directed toward the underlying etiology (e.g., hepatitis C) as well as the vasculitis. Treatment of the latter is similar to that of other vasculitides and is based on combinations of steroids and steroid-sparing agents that are used in an effort to target antibody and immune complex–mediated inflammation. Differences do exist, however, when treating the underlying condition in type II as opposed to type III cryoglobulinemia. For instance, in the setting of hepatitis C–induced type II cryoglobulinemia with high titers of cryoglobulins and RF and low complement, antiviral treatment with interferon-γ could potentially result in massive formation of immune complexes, exacerbation of vasculitis, and multiorgan failure.[110] This group of patients should be treated with immunosuppressive agents of low hepatotoxicity for at least 6 months prior to antiviral therapy.[106]

An additional difference in the management of type II versus type III cryoglobulinemia is with plasmapheresis aimed at removing pathogenic immunoglobulins. Because antibodies in type II cryoglobulinemia are intravascular as opposed to the intra- and extravascular deposition seen in type III cryoglobulinemia, plasmapheresis is much more effective in the prior condition, as extravascular antibodies are not affected by plasmapheresis.

Antineutrophil Cytoplasmic Antibody–Positive Vasculitis

As described earlier, ANCAs are antineutrophil cytoplasmic antibodies and are found in varied autoimmune disorders. In the setting of vasculitis, they are associated with three conditions: Wegener's granulomatosis (WG), microscopic polyangiitis (MPA), and Churg-Strauss syndrome (CSS). Skin findings of these three conditions are those of CSVV or cutaneous medium-vessel vasculitis (CMVV), with palpable purpura being most common.[112,113] Papules and nodules are occasionally seen on extensor surfaces and can be ulcerated or necrotic, occasionally with overhanging borders as seen with pyoderma gangrenosum.[114,116] However, primary cutaneous disease in these conditions is essentially nonexistent, as all patients with WG, MPA, and CSS have varying degrees of extracutaneous involvement. Wegener's granulomatosis has significant associated extracutaneous involvement including upper and lower respiratory, renal, and nervous system manifestations, and almost all of these patients are c-ANCA positive. Churg-Strauss syndrome is hard to distinguish from WG except for the presence of significant tissue and blood eosinophilia, higher levels of p-ANCA, and associated atopy in CSS.[117] The diagnosis of CSS requires eosinophil predominance in a mixed

infiltrate. Some patients with CSS describe pruritus as a symptom preceding the development of vasculitic lesions, and this is thought to be related to the high number of eosinophils. Microscopic polyangiitis is the most common cause of vasculitis associated with pulmonary-renal syndrome, and almost all of these patients are p-ANCA positive.[100,102]

Histologically, lesions from the ANCA-associated vasculitides demonstrate classic findings of vasculitis or Churg-Strauss (cutaneous extravascular necrotizing) granulomas. (CENG).[114,118] The latter is a misnomer, as the blood vessels in these infiltrates demonstrate clear evidence of vasculitis. Originally observed in CSS, but later seen in several vasculitides, CENG lesions contain four components: (1) a central area of degenerated extracellular substance surrounded by (2) a palisaded mononuclear infiltrate; (3) variable polymorphonuclear interstitial infiltrate; and (4) variable degrees of vasculitis or vasculopathy of small or medium-sized vessels.[116,118,119] This fact helps differentiate CENG seen in systemic vasculitides from the palisaded granulomas of rheumatoid nodules. Both the histologic and clinical appearances are similar to those of rheumatoid nodules. Oscillating titers of pathogenic antibodies cause sustained damage to the endothelial lining, leading to slow death and degeneration of the extracellular matrix, resulting in a palisading inflammatory reaction. Because extensor surfaces of the extremities are prone to trauma and injury, they tend to be a common site for their location. Whether typical vasculitis or CENG is present, marked levels of eosinophils seen on biopsy (>60%) are pathognomonic for CSS. Direct immunofluorescence in all types of ANCA vasculitis is positive in approximately 80% of cases for IgG and IgM deposition, but not C3. Cutaneous extravascular necrotizing granuloma is also referred to as CSG, Winkelmann's granuloma, interstitial granuloma, palisaded neutrophilic and granulomatous dermatitis of connective tissue disease, superficial ulcerating rheumatoid necrobiosis, and rheumatoid papule.[1,117,118]

Because ANCA-associated vasculitis occurs in the setting of extracutaneous disease, treatment of the primary vasculitis treats the cutaneous findings. Standard management involves combinations of steroids and steroid-sparing immunosuppressive agents.[32–34]

Connective Tissue Disease–Associated Vasculitis

Essentially any cutaneous vasculitic syndrome can be triggered by connective tissue disease (CTD). Furthermore, these patients are more prone to infections and drug exposure, resulting in higher rates of CLA or IgA-mediated vasculitides. Three vasculitic entities in particular are associated with CTD: CTD-associated vasculitis, HUVS (discussed above), and lymphocytic vasculitis (LV).[120] Connective tissue disease–associated vasculitis is most frequently seen with SLE, but can also happen with other CTDs such as Sjögren's syndrome, dermatomyositis, systemic sclerosis, and mixed connective tissue disease.[120,121]

Clinically, these diseases can present as CSVV of the lower extremities. Although they may resemble the lesions of cryoglobulinemia, CTD vasculitides may present as a pure CMVV without small-vessel involvement, whereas small vessels will always be involved in cryoglobulinemia. Systemic involvement is present in essentially all patients, with the kidneys being the most affected organ. Central and peripheral neuropathies and GI and cardiac involvement can also occur at varying rates.

Serologically, high titers of antinuclear antibodies (ANAs) and low complement are present. Different combinations of ANA are commonly seen including anti–double-stranded DNA (anti-dsDNA, ribonucleoprotein (RNP), Ro, and Sm), further increasing the chance for vasculitis.

Histologically, CTD-associated vasculitis shows CSVV or CMVV without any distinguishing features. Lymphocytic vasculitis is rare and more commonly seen in SS and SLE; however, it can occur in association with other CTDs as well. Lymphocytic vasculitis is also known as benign hypergammaglobulinemic purpura (BHP) of Waldenström. Most experts believe that both LV and BHP of Waldenström are type III cryoglobulins associated with CTDs.[120,121]

As opposed to cryoglobulinemia, however, DIF reveals IgG in and around small and medium-sized vessels as the predominant immunoglobulin. C3 is usually very strongly deposited. Interestingly, in vivo ANA is very commonly present. This reflects the high titer of ANA, especially RNP in keratinocytes and dermal cells in these patients.[1]

As the development of vasculitis in CTD is often associated with an ominous prognosis, aggressive treatment of the underlying CTD is mandatory. Combinations of corticosteroids, with high doses of antimetabolites or alkylating agents and occasionally plasmapheresis, are necessary to control the progression of this disease.

Rheumatoid Vasculitis

Rheumatoid vasculitis (RV) is a rare but severe complication in patients with advanced, usually otherwise quiescent seropositive rheumatoid arthritis (RA).[122] It can affect virtually any sized vessel, with palpable purpura being the most common presenting sign, but ulcerations, livedo reticularis, digital infarcts, or cutaneous nodules can also be seen. Isolated, fluctuating periungual splinter hemorrhages, known as Bywater's lesions, are caused by digital small-vessel vasculitis. Cutaneous medium-vessel vasculitis involvement typically presents as deep geographic ulcers at the malleoli. As with cryoglobulinemia, these patients frequently have accompanying mononeuritis multiplex.[108,110]

Serologically, high titers of RF often with low levels of both C3 and C4 are characteristic of RV. This often helps in distinguishing RV from cryoglobulinemia since RF is elevated in both, and, even in RA patients with higher titers of RF, low levels of cryoglobulins are not uncommon. Thorough exclusion of other causes of CMVV in RA patients with cryoglobulins is mandatory (e.g., viral hepatitis, lymphoma, HIV).[122–124]

Histologic findings in RV are indistinguishable from those in other CSVVs and CMVVs.

Direct immunofluorescence is indistinguishable from cryoglobulinemia, with heavy granular IgM and variable degrees of C3 in and around small and medium vessels.[122]

The aim of therapy in RV is to reduce IgM immunocomplexes with combinations of corticosteroids with antimetabolites or alkylating agents. Methotrexate is effective for the synovitis and T-cell–mediated symptoms of RA, but is not effective for RV. Because of the IgM RF, plasmapheresis in combination with steroids and alkylating agents is a good choice in patients with life-threatening disease (as with cryoglobulinemia type II).[124] Bywaters lesions alone do not necessitate aggressive systemic therapy.

Polyarteritis Nodosa

Polyarteritis nodosa (PAN) is the prototype of a pure medium-sized vessel vasculitis (Fig. 19.7), often presenting as a systemic illness with multiorgan involvement. It is a diagnosis of exclusion when other causes of CMVV such as RV, ANCA vasculitis, and cryoglobulinemia have been ruled out. The most common presentation is with painful cutaneous nodules and ulcerations with a predilection for the malleoli,[125] but since PAN is a pure CMVV, other lesions can include nodules, ulcers, livedo (Fig. 19.8), and digital infarcts (Fig. 19.9), and less frequently papulonecrotic lesions on extensor surfaces (CENG).[126] Ulcerations heal with stellate, atrophic, ivory-colored scars or hyperpigmentation, designated as atrophie blanche or livedoid vasculitis in the past, or even Degos' like lesions. They are often accompanied by neuropathic pain resulting from involvement of the vasa nervorum. Focal synovitis and

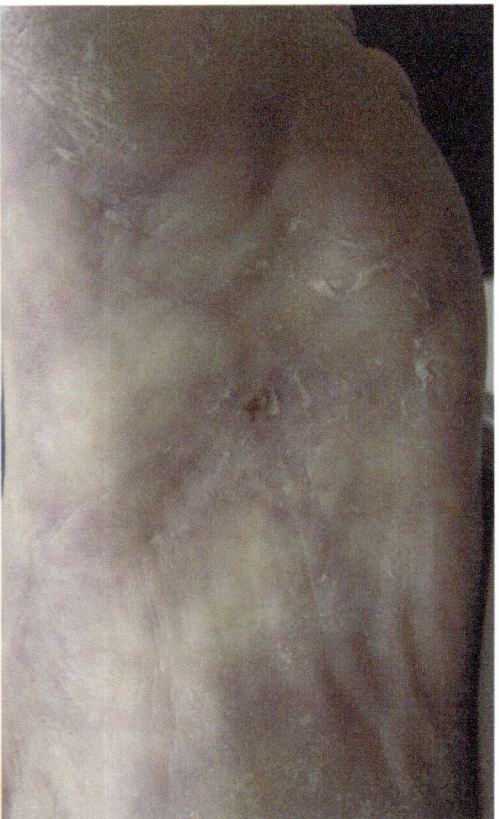

FIG. 19.8. Livedo reticularis in a patient with PAN

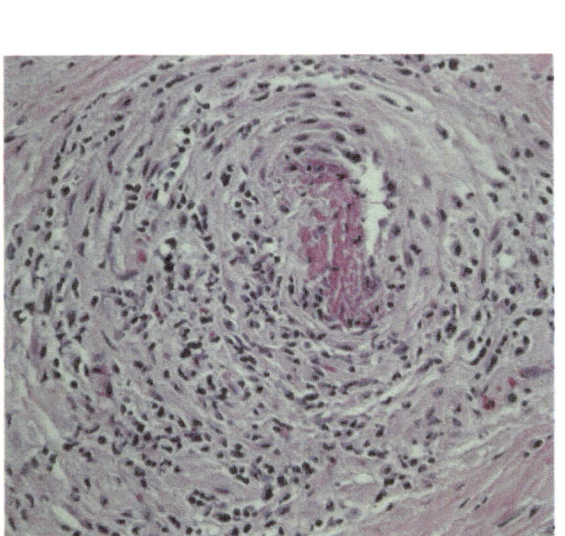

FIG. 19.7. H&E staining of a skin biopsy from patient with polyarteritis nodosa (PAN). Note involvement of medium-sized vessel

arthralgia may be present in the joints close to areas of cutaneous involvement, particularly the ankle, as opposed to erythema nodosum, where generalized arthralgias may be present. Disease limited to the skin occurs in less than 10% of those affected, and PAN can occur in children after streptococcal infection.[133]

Differential diagnosis for nodular lesions includes erythema nodosum, nodular vasculitis, and erythema induratum.[127–129] The latter two are most likely variants of this disorder, with a prominent component of panniculitis present. Infectious causes of ulceration, pyoderma gangrenosum, calciphylaxis, and other causes of medium-sized vessel vasculitis must be included in the differential. Patients with nodules limited to around the ankles may have cutaneous PAN, and even these patients require close and long-term follow-up for progression to systemic disease.[131,132] Systemic disease is present in virtually all patients with extensive

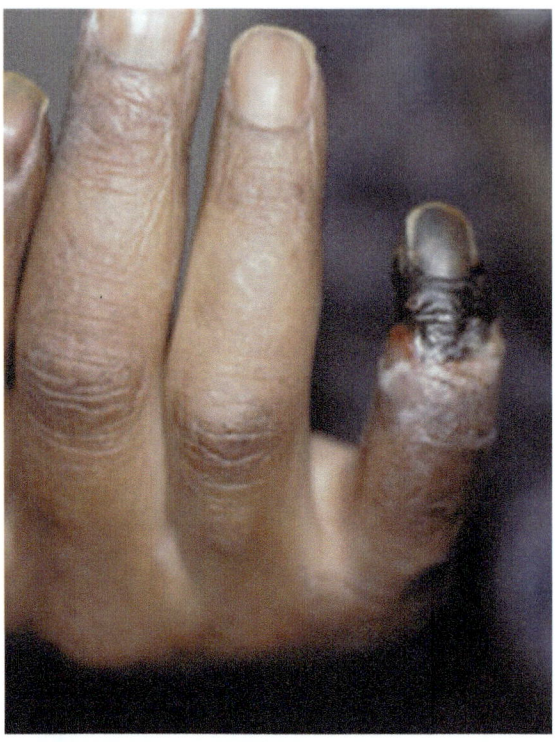

Fig. 19.9. Digital infarct in a patient with PAN

nodulo-ulcerative disease. Synovitis, hypertension, and mononeuritis multiplex are the most common systemic findings.

Kawasaki's disease is an equivalent of PAN in children with a predilection for the coronary arteries, leading to coronary aneurysms and myocardial infarction.[131–135]

Serologic testing may reveal elevated ESR with hypocomplementemia. Antineutrophil cytoplasmic antibody, ANA, and RF are typically negative, but may be present at insignificant titers.

By definition, small-vessel involvement should rule out the diagnosis of PAN. Because PAN is a pure CMVV, shallow biopsies that do not sample deeper skin vessels will lead to frequent misdiagnosis. Therefore, multiple, deep biopsies are recommended. The diagnostic yield in PAN is the following: nodules (90% to 100%), ulcers (50% to 80%), livedo (0% to 20%), and digital infarcts (0% to 5%). Direct immunofluorescence shows granular IgM in and around medium-sized vessels and weak C3 in approximately 60% of cases.[1]

Corticosteroids alone may be sufficient for mild nodular disease, while ulcerative disease without significant systemic involvement may respond to prednisone in combination with azathioprine. Severe cutaneous disease with digital infarcts and systemic involvement should be treated with corticosteroids and alkylating agents. Plasmapheresis is not effective in PAN since IgM immune complexes and RF do not play a prominent role in this disease in contrast to the high titers of these factors seen in RV and cryoglobulinemia.[126]

Cutaneous Large-Vessel Vasculitis

Cutaneous large-vessel vasculitis (CLVV) is rare, as there simply are not large vessels found in the skin. These disorders typically targeted the great vessels of the body such as the aorta and its major branches and include giant cell (temporal) arteritis and Takayasu's arteritis. Giant cell arteritis is more likely in Caucasian patients over 50 years, with a predilection for the extracranial branches of the carotid artery, while Takayasu's arteritis is more common in persons of Far Eastern descent under age 50, affecting the thoracic aorta and branches supplying the upper extremities.[2] Involvement of large vessels can occasional manifest as lesions of the scalp and tongue.[136]

Conclusion

Vasculitis, or inflammation of the vasculature, can be caused by many different mechanisms that ultimately result in varying degrees of vessel wall destruction, hemorrhage, ischemia, or infarction of affected organs. Any sized vessel in any organ can be affected and will determine the clinical and pathologic findings, with fibrinoid necrosis being the pathognomonic feature. The patient with vasculitis can present initially to dermatologists, rheumatologists, or primary medical service, as a wide range of initial presenting signs occur. Because even mild cutaneous disease does not rule out severe and significant systemic involvement, thorough workup including history and physical, serology, histology, and immunofluorescence is mandatory for these patients.

References

1. Rencic A, Rivadeneira A, Cummins D, Nousari CH. Cutaneous vasculitides. In: Kerdel F, ed. Dermatology: Just the Facts. McGraw-Hill, New York: pp. 45–57.
2. Suresh E. Diagnostic approach to patients with suspected vasculitis. Postgrad Med J 2006;82(970):483–8.
3. Carlson JA, Chen KR. Cutaneous vasculitis update: neutrophilic muscular vessel and eosinophilic, granulomatous, and lymphocytic vasculitis syndromes. Am J Dermatopathol 2007;29(1):32–43.
4. Russell JP, Gibson LE. Primary cutaneous small vessel vasculitis: approach to diagnosis and treatment. Int J Dermatol 2006;45(1):3–13.
5. Grzeszkiewicz TM, Fiorentino DF. Update on cutaneous vasculitis. Semin Cutan Med Surg 2006;25(4):221–5.
6. Flossmann O, Bacon P, de Groot K, et al. Development of comprehensive disease assessment in systemic vasculitis. Ann Rheum Dis 2007;66(3):283–92.
7. Quinet RJ, Zakem JM, McCain M. Localized versus systemic vasculitis: diagnosis and management. Curr Rheumatol Rep 2003;5(2):93–9.
8. Leshem E, Davidovitz Y, Meltzer E, et al. Fulminant vasculitis: a rare fatal complication of lymphoma. Acta Haematol 2006;115(1–2):117–22.
9. Carlson JA, Chen KR. Cutaneous pseudovasculitis. Am J Dermatopathol 2007;29(1):44–55.
10. Kao NL, Broy S, Tillawi I. Malignant angioendotheliomatosis mimicking systemic necrotizing vasculitis. J Rheumatol 19(7):1133–5, 1992.
11. Thomas R, Vuitch F, Lakhanpal S. Angiocentric T cell lymphoma masquerading as cutaneous vasculitis. J Rheumatol 21(4):760–2, 1994.
12. Walker UA, Herbst EW, Ansorge O, Peter HH. Intravascular lymphoma simulating vasculitis. Rheumatol Int 1994;14(3):131–3.
13. Watts RA, Jolliffe VA, Grattan CE, et al. Cutaneous vasculitis in a defined population—clinical and epidemiological associations. J Rheumatol 1998;25(5):920–4.
14. Lapraik C, Watts R, Scott DG. Modern management of primary systemic vasculitis. Clin Med 2007;7(1):43–7.
15. Watts R, Lane S, Hanslik T, Hauser T, et al. Development and validation of a consensus methodology for the classification of the ANCA-associated vasculitides and polyarteritis nodosa for epidemiological studies. Ann Rheum Dis 2007;66(2):222–7.
16. Watts RA, Scott DG. Epidemiology of the vasculitides. Semin Respir Crit Care Med 2004;25(5):455–64.
17. Sunderkotter C, Sindrilaru A. Clinical classification of vasculitis. Eur J Dermatol 2006;16(2):114–24.
18. Watts RA, Scott DG. Epidemiology of the vasculitides. Curr Opin Rheumatol 2003;15(1):11–6.
19. Watts RA, Lane S, Scott DG. What is known about the epidemiology of the vasculitides? Best Pract Res Clin Rheumatol 2005;19(2):191–207.
20. Lane SE, Watts RA, Shepstone L, Scott DG. Primary systemic vasculitis: clinical features and mortality. Q J Med 2005;98(2):97–111.
21. Stavropoulos PG, Boubouka DC, Anyfantakis NV, et al. Cutaneous small vessel vasculitis and pulmonary tuberculosis: an unusual association. Int J Dermatol 2006;45(8):996–8.
22. Chen CH, Chen YK, Chou CT, Chao YC. A large ulcer and cutaneous small-vessel vasculitis associated with syphilis infection. J Rheumatol 2006;35(2):147–51.
23. Carlson JA, Ng BT, Chen KR. Cutaneous vasculitis update: diagnostic criteria, classification, epidemiology, etiology, pathogenesis, evaluation and prognosis. Am J Dermatopathol 2005;27(6):504–28.
24. Carlson JA, Cavaliere LF, Grant-Kels JM. Cutaneous vasculitis: diagnosis and management. Clin Dermatol 2006;24(5):414–29.
25. Sais G, Vidaller A, Jucgla A, et al. Prognostic factors in leukocytoclastic vasculitis: a clinicopathologic study of 160 patients. Arch Dermatol 1998;134(3):309–15.
26. Cupps TR, Springer RM, Fauci AS. Chronic, recurrent small-vessel cutaneous vasculitis. Clinical experience in 13 patients. JAMA 1982;247(14):1994–8.
27. Ioannidou DJ, Krasagakis K, Daphnis EK, et al. Cutaneous small vessel vasculitis: an entity with frequent renal involvement. Arch Dermatol 2002;138(3):412–4.
28. Kulthanan K, Pinkaew S, Jiamton S, Mahaisavariya P, Suthipinittharm P. Cutaneous leukocytoclastic vasculitis: the yield of direct immunofluorescence study. J Med Assoc Thai 2004;87(5):531–5.
29. Blanco R, Martinez-Taboada VM, Rodriguez-Valverde V, Garcia-Fuentes M. Cutaneous vasculitis in children and adults. Associated diseases and etiologic factors in 303 patients. Medicine (Baltimore) 1998;77(6):403–18.
30. Davis MD, Daoud MS, Kirby B, Gibson LE, Rogers RS 3rd. Clinicopathologic correlation of hypocomplementemic and normocomplementemic urticarial vasculitis. J Am Acad Dermatol 1998;38(6 pt 1):899–905.
31. Gibson LE, Specks U, Homburger H. Clinical utility of ANCA tests for the dermatologist. Int J Dermatol 2003;42(11):859–69.
32. Preston GA, Yang JJ, Xiao H, Falk RJ. Understanding the pathogenesis of ANCA: where are we today? Cleve Clin J Med 2002;69(suppl 2):SII51–4.
33. Heeringa P, Huugen D, Tervaert JW. Anti-neutrophil cytoplasmic autoantibodies and leukocyte-endothelial interactions: a sticky connection? Trends Immunol 2005;26(11):561–4.

34. Birck R, Schmitt WH, Kaelsch IA, van der Woude FJ. Serial ANCA determinations for monitoring disease activity in patients with ANCA-associated vasculitis: systematic review. Am J Kidney Dis 2006;47(1):15–23.

35. Hermann J, Demel U, Stunzner D, Daghofer E, Tilz G, Graninger W. Clinical interpretation of antineutrophil cytoplasmic antibodies: parvovirus B19 infection as a pitfall. Ann Rheum Dis 2005;64(4):641–3. Epub 2004 Oct 14.

36. Doyle MK, Cuellar ML. Drug-induced vasculitis. Expert Opin Drug Saf 2003;2(4):401–9.

37. Cuellar ML. Drug-induced vasculitis. Curr Rheumatol Rep 2002;4(1):55–9.

38. Ingraffea A, Donohue K, Wilkel C, Falanga V. Cutaneous vasculitis in two patients taking an herbal supplement containing black cohosh. J Am Acad Dermatol 2007;56(5 suppl):S124–6.

39. Yaghoubian B, Ngo B, Mak M, et al. Warfarin-induced leukocytoclastic vasculitis. Cutis 2005;75(6): 329–38.

40. Lillicrap MS, Merry P. Cutaneous vasculitis associated with rofecoxib. Rheumatology (Oxford) 2003;42(10):1267–8.

41. Scheinfeld N. Impact of phenytoin therapy on the skin and skin disease. Expert Opin Drug Saf 2004;3(6):655–65.

42. Chamberlain AJ, Poon E. Cutaneous reactions to interferon and ribavirin. Intern Med J 2004;34(8):519.

43. Poon DY, Law NM. A case of cutaneous leukocytoclastic vasculitis associated with gabapentin. Singapore Med J 2003;44(1):42–4.

44. Flores-Suarez LF, Vega-Memije ME, Chanussot-Deprez C. Cutaneous vasculitis during selective serotonin reuptake inhibitor therapy. Am J Med 2006;119(10):e1–3.

45. Abad S, Kambouchner M, Nejjari M, Dhote R. Additional case of minocycline-induced cutaneous polyarteritis nodosa. Arthritis Rheum 2006;55(5):831.

46. Storsley L, Geldenhuys L. Ciprofloxacin-induced ANCA-negative cutaneous and renal vasculitis— resolution with drug withdrawal. Nephrol Dial Transplant 2007;22(2):660–1.

47. Salem C, Hmouda H, Slim R, Denguezli M, Belajouza C, Bouraoui K. Rare case of metformin-induced leukocytoclastic vasculitis. Ann Pharmacother 2006;40(9): 1685–7.

48. Papaioannides D, Sinapidis D, Korantzopoulos P, Charalabopoulos K. A case of cutaneous vasculitis associated with olanzapine. Int J Low Extrem Wounds 2006;5(2):116–7.

49. Ng J, Savage R, McQueen F. Churg-Strauss vasculitis syndrome and leukotriene receptor antagonists. Ann Rheum Dis 2005;64(9):1382.

50. Ali SO, McCarty RD, Davis BM. Case reports: cutaneous small vessel vasculitis due to famciclovir therapy. J Drugs Dermatol 2005;4(4):486–9.

51. Gasser S, Kuhn M, Speich R. Severe necrotising leucocytoclastic vasculitis in a patient taking bosentan. BMJ 2004;329(7463):430.

52. Gupta S, Gandhi NM, Ferguson J, et al. Cutaneous vasculitis secondary to ramipril. Cutaneous vasculitis induced by cyclo-oxygenase-2 selective inhibitors. J Am Acad Dermatol 2004;51(6):1029–30.

53. Hardinger KL, Cornelius LA, Trulock EP 3rd, Brennan DC. Sirolimus-induced leukocytoclastic vasculitis. Transplantation 2002;74(5):739–43.

54. Friedman ES, LaNatra N, Stiller MJ, et al. NSAIDs in dermatologic therapy: review and preview. J Cutan Med Surg 2002;6(5):449–59.

55. Meziani F, Chartier C, Alt M, Jaeger A. Fatal allergic vasculitis associated with celecoxib. Lancet 2002;359(9309):852–3.

56. Rocha JL, Kondo W, Baptista MI, Da Cunha CA, Martins LT. Uncommon vancomycin-induced side effects. Braz J Infect Dis 2002;6(4):196–200.

57. Gal AA, Morris RJ, Pine JR, Spraker MK. Cutaneous lesions of Churg-Strauss syndrome associated with montelukast therapy. Br J Dermatol 2002;147(3): 618–9.

58. Gonzalez-Gay MA, Garcia-Porrua C, Lueiro M, Fernandez ML. Orlistat-induced cutaneous leukocytoclastic vasculitis. Arthritis Rheum 2002;47(5):567.

59. Margolese HC, Chouinard G, Beauclair L, Rubino M. Cutaneous vasculitis induced by paroxetine. Am J Psychiatry 2001;158(3):497.

60. Holm EA, Balslev E, Jemec GB. Vasculitis occurring during leflunomide therapy. Dermatology 2001;203(3):258–9.

61. Koutkia P, Mylonakis E, Rounds S, Erickson A. Cutaneous leucocytoclastic vasculitis associated with oxacillin. Diagn Microbiol Infect Dis 2001;39(3):191–4.

62. Schneider F, Meziani F, Chartier C, Alt M, Jaeger A. Fatal allergic vasculitis associated with celecoxib. Lancet 2002;359(9309):852–3.

63. Chave T, Neal C, Camp R. Henoch-Schonlein purpura following hepatitis B vaccination. J Dermatol Treat 2003;14(3):179–81.

64. Businco L, Falconieri P, Bellioni-Businco B, Bahna SL. Severe food-induced vasculitis in two children. Pediatr Allergy Immunol 2002;13(1):68–71.

65. Chua IC, Aldridge CR, Finlay AY, Williams PE. Cutaneous IgA-associated vasculitis induced by alcohol. Br J Dermatol 2005;153(5):1037–40.

66. Anandacoomarasamy A, Kannangara S, Barnsley L. Cutaneous vasculitis associated with infliximab in

the treatment of rheumatoid arthritis. Intern Med J 2005;35(10):638–40.
67. Lee A, Kasama R, Evangelisto A, Elfenbein B, Falasca G. Henoch-Schonlein purpura after etanercept therapy for psoriasis. J Clin Rheumatol 2006;12(5):249–51.
68. Gerecitano J, Goy A, Wright J, et al. Drug-induced cutaneous vasculitis in patients with non-Hodgkin lymphoma treated with the novel proteasome inhibitor bortezomib: a possible surrogate marker of response? Br J Haematol 2006;134(4):391–8.
69. Bahrami S, Malone JC, Webb KG, Callen JP. Tissue eosinophilia as an indicator of drug-induced cutaneous small-vessel vasculitis. Arch Dermatol 2006;142(2):155–61.
70. Merkel PA. Drug-induced vasculitis. Rheum Dis Clin North Am 2001;27(4):849–62.
71. Jaing TH, Hsueh C, Chiu CH, et al. Cutaneous lymphocytic vasculitis as the presenting feature of acute lymphoblastic leukemia. J Pediatr Hematol Oncol 2002;24(7):555–7.
72. Kembre PS, Mahajan S, Kharkar V, Khopkar U. Cutaneous vasculitis as a presenting feature of multiple myeloma: a report of 2 cases. Indian J Dermatol Venereol Leprol 2006;72(6):437–9.
73. Koulaouzidis A, Campbell S, Bharati A, et al. Primary biliary cirrhosis associated pustular vasculitis. Ann Hepatol 2006;5(3):177–8.
74. Ferrero P, Orzan F, Marchisio F, Trevi G. Vasculitis mimicking bacterial endocarditis. Ital Heart J 2003;4(11):816–8.
75. Golden MP, Hammer SM, Wanke CA, et al. Cytomegalovirus vasculitis. Case reports and review of the literature. Medicine (Baltimore) 1994;73(5):246–55.
76. Lee YS, Lee SW, Lee JR, Lee SC. Erythema induratum with pulmonary tuberculosis: histopathologic features resembling true vasculitis. Int J Dermatol 2001;40(3):193–6.
77. Feldmann R, Rieger W, Sator PG, Gschnait F, Breier F. Schonlein-Henoch purpura during pregnancy with successful outcome for mother and newborn. BMC Dermatol 2002;2:1.
78. Bachmeyer C, Wetterwald E, Aractingi S. Cutaneous vasculitis in the course of hematologic malignancies. Dermatology 2005;210(1):8–14.
79. Raza K, Carruthers DM, Stevens R, Filer AD, Townend JN, Bacon PA. Infliximab leads to a rapid but transient improvement in endothelial function in patients with primary systemic vasculitis. Ann Rheum Dis 2006;65(7):946–8.
80. van der Bijl AE, Allaart CF, Van Vugt J, Van Duinen S, Breedveld FC. Rheumatoid vasculitis treated with infliximab. J Rheumatol 2005;32(8):1607–9.
81. Chung L, Funke AA, Chakravarty EF, Callen JP, Fiorentino DF. Successful use of rituximab for cutaneous vasculitis. Arch Dermatol 2006;142(11):1407–10.
82. Eriksson P. Nine patients with anti-neutrophil cytoplasmic antibody-positive vasculitis successfully treated with rituximab. J Intern Med 2005;257(6):540–8.
83. Carlson JA, Chen KR. Cutaneous vasculitis update: small vessel neutrophilic vasculitis syndromes. Am J Dermatopathol 2006;28(6):486–506.
84. Francescone MA, Levitt J. Scurvy masquerading as leukocytoclastic vasculitis: a case report and review of the literature. Cutis 2005;76(4):261–6.
85. Jennette JC, Falk RJ, Andrassy K, et al. Nomenclature of systemic vasculitides. Proposal of an international consensus conference. Arthritis Rheum 1994;37(2):187–92.
86. Rao JK, Allen NB, Pincus T. Limitations of the 1990 American College of Rheumatology classification criteria in the diagnosis of vasculitis. Ann Intern Med 1998;129(5):345–52.
87. Sorensen SF, Slot O, Tvede N, Petersen J. A prospective study of vasculitis patients collected in a five year period: evaluation of the Chapel Hill nomenclature. Ann Rheum Dis 2000;59(6):478–82.
88. Koutkia P, Mylonakis E, Rounds S, Erickson A. Leucocytoclastic vasculitis: an update for the clinician. Scand J Rheumatol 2001;30(6):315–22.
89. Saulsbury FT. Henoch-Schonlein purpura. Curr Opin Rheumatol 2001;13(1):35–40.
90. Besbas N, Duzova A, Topaloglu R, et al. Pulmonary haemorrhage in a 6-year-old boy with Henoch-Schonlein purpura. Clin Rheumatol 2001;20(4):293–6.
91. Callen JP. A clinical approach to the vasculitis patient in the dermatologic office. Clin Dermatol 1999;17(5):549–53.
92. Garcia-Porrua C, Gonzalez-Louzao C, Llorca J, et al. Predictive factors for renal sequelae in adults with Henoch-Schonlein purpura. J Rheumatol 2001;28(5):1019–24.
93. Paradisi M, Annessi G, Corrado A. Infantile acute hemorrhagic edema of the skin. Cutis 2001;68(2):127–9.
94. Zurada JM, Ward KM, Grossman ME. Henoch-Schonlein purpura associated with malignancy in adults. J Am Acad Dermatol 2006;55(5 Suppl):S65–70.
95. Chang S, Carr W. Urticarial vasculitis. Allergy Asthma Proc 2007;28(1):97–100.
96. Venzor J, Lee WL, Huston DP. Urticarial vasculitis. Clin Rev Allergy Immunol 2002;23(2):201–16.
97. Davis MD, Daoud MS, Kirby B, et al. Clinicopathologic correlation of hypocomplementemic and normocomplementemic urticarial vasculitis J Am Acad Dermatol 1998;38(6 pt 1):899–905.

98. Mehregan DR, Hall MJ, Gibson LE. Urticarial vasculitis: a histopathologic and clinical review of 72 cases. J Am Acad Dermatol 1992;26(3 pt 2): 441–8.

99. Nousari HC, Kimyai-Asadi A, Stone JH. Annular leukocytoclastic vasculitis associated with monoclonal gammopathy of unknown significance. J Am Acad Dermatol 2000;43(5 pt 2):955–7.

100. Fiorentino DF. Cutaneous vasculitis. J Am Acad Dermatol 2003;48(3):311–40.

101. Gibson LE. Cutaneous vasculitis update. Dermatol Clin 2001;19(4):603–15.

102. Alexander B, Rameshkumar K, Jayaseelan E. Cutaneous vasculitis—a dynamic process posing diagnostic challenge. J Assoc Physicians India 2003;51:574–7.

103. McGirt LY, Vasagar K, Gober LM, Saini SS, Beck LA. Successful treatment of recalcitrant chronic idiopathic urticaria with sulfasalazine. Arch Dermatol 2006;142(10):1337–42.

104. Karlsberg PL, Lee WM, Casey DL, et al. Cutaneous vasculitis and rheumatoid factor positivity as presenting signs of hepatitis C virus-induced mixed cryoglobulinemia. Arch Dermatol 1995;131(10):1119–23.

105. Mendez P, Saeian K, Reddy KR, et al. Hepatitis C, cryoglobulinemia, and cutaneous vasculitis associated with unusual and serious manifestations. Am J Gastroenterol 2001;96(8):2489–93.

106. Pawlotsky JM, Dhumeaux D, Bagot M. Hepatitis C virus in dermatology. A review. Arch Dermatol 1995;131(10):1185–93.

107. Ramos-Casals M, Cervera R, Yague J, et al. Cryoglobulinemia in primary Sjogren's syndrome: prevalence and clinical characteristics in a series of 115 patients. Semin Arthritis Rheum 1998;28(3):200–5.

108. Tseng MT, Hsieh SC, Shun CT, Lee KL, et al. Skin denervation and cutaneous vasculitis in systemic lupus erythematosus. Brain 2006;129(pt 4):977–85.

109. Braun GS, Horster S, Wagner KS, et al. Cryoglobulinaemic vasculitis: classification and clinical and therapeutic aspects. Postgrad Med J 2007;83(976):87–94.

110. Scelsa SN, Herskovitz S, Reichler B. Treatment of mononeuropathy multiplex in hepatitis C virus and cryoglobulinemia. Muscle Nerve 1998;21(11):1526–9.

111. Stone JH, Nousari HC. "Essential" cutaneous vasculitis: what every rheumatologist should know about vasculitis of the skin. Curr Opin Rheumatol 2001;13(1):23–34.

112. Lauque D, Cadranel J, Lazor R, et al. Microscopic polyangiitis with alveolar hemorrhage. A study of 29 cases and review of the literature. Groupe d'Etudes et de Recherche sur les Maladies "Orphelines" Pulmonaires (GERM"O"P). Medicine (Baltimore) 2000;79(4):222–33.

113. Mangold MC, Callen JP. Cutaneous leukocytoclastic vasculitis associated with active Wegener's granulomatosis. J Am Acad Dermatol 1992;26(4):579–84.

114. Daoud MS, Gibson LE, DeRemee RA, et al. Cutaneous Wegener's granulomatosis: clinical, histopathologic, and immunopathologic features of thirty patients. J Am Acad Dermatol 1994;31(4):605–12.

115. Raustia AM, Autio-Harmainen HI, Knuuttila ML, Raustia JM. Ultrastructural findings and clinical follow-up of 'strawberry gums' in Wegener's granulomatosis. J Oral Pathol 1985;14(7):581–7.

116. Gibson LE, Daoud MS, Muller SA, Perry HO. Malignant pyodermas revisited. Mayo Clin Proc 1997;72(8):734–6.

117. Guillevin L, Cohen P, Gayraud M, et al. Churg-Strauss syndrome. Clinical study and long-term follow-up of 96 patients. Medicine (Baltimore) 1999;78(1):26–37.

118. Chen KR, Sakamoto M, Ikemoto K, Abe R, Shimizu H. Granulomatous arteritis in cutaneous lesions of Churg-Strauss syndrome. J Cutan Pathol 2007;34(4):330–7.

119. Chu P, Connolly MK, LeBoit PE. The histopathologic spectrum of palisaded neutrophilic and granulomatous dermatitis in patients with collagen vascular disease. Arch Dermatol 1994;130(10):1278–83.

120. Tsokos M, Lazarou SA, Moutsopoulos HM Vasculitis in primary Sjogren's syndrome. Histologic classification and clinical presentation. Am J Clin Pathol 1987;88(1):26–31.

121. Ramos-Casals M, Anaya JM, Garcia-Carrasco M, et al. Cutaneous vasculitis in primary Sjogren syndrome: classification and clinical significance of 52 patients. Medicine (Baltimore) 2004;83(2): 96–106.

122. Schneider HA, Yonker RA, Katz P, et al. Rheumatoid vasculitis: experience with 13 patients and review of the literature. Semin Arthritis Rheum 1985;14(4):280–6.

123. Nousari HC, Kimyai-Asadi A, Stebbing J, Stone JH. Purple toes in a patient with end-stage rheumatoid arthritis. Arch Dermatol 1999;135(6):648–50.

124. Winkelstein A, Starz TW, Agarwal A. Efficacy of combined therapy with plasmapheresis and immunosuppressants in rheumatoid vasculitis. J Rheumatol 1984;11(2):162–6.

125. Maillard H, Szczesniak S, Martin L, et al. Cutaneous periarteritis nodosa: diagnostic and therapeutic aspects of 9 cases. Ann Dermatol Venereol 1999;126(2):125–9.

126. Daoud MS, Hutton KP, Gibson LE. Cutaneous periarteritis nodosa: a clinicopathological study of 79 cases. Br J Dermatol 1997;136(5):706–13.

127. Martin JI, Dronda F, Chaves F. Erythema elevatum diutinum, a clinical entity to be considered in patients infected with HIV-1. Clin Exp Dermatol 2001;26(8):725–6.

128. Gibson LE, el-Azhary RA. Erythema elevatum diutinum. Clin Dermatol 2000;18(3):295–9.

129. Nguyen VU. Study of erythema nodosum leprosum. Ann Dermatol Venereol 1994;121(2):194–6.

130. Birchmore D, Sweeney C, Choudhury D, et al. IgA multiple myeloma presenting as Henoch-Schonlein purpura/polyarteritis nodosa overlap syndrome. Arthritis Rheum 1999;39(4): 698–703.

131. Kumar L, Thapa BR, Sarkar B, et al. Benign cutaneous polyarteritis nodosa in children below 10 years of age—a clinical experience. Ann Rheum Dis 1995;54(2):134–6.

132. Siberry GK, Cohen BA, Johnson B. Cutaneous polyarteritis nodosa. Reports of two cases in children and review of the literature. Arch Dermatol 1994;130(7):884–9.

133. Fathalla BM, Miller L, Brady S, Schaller JG. Cutaneous polyarteritis nodosa in children. J Am Acad Dermatol 2005;53(4):724–8.

134. Royle J, Burgner D, Curtis N. The diagnosis and management of Kawasaki disease. J Paediatr Child Health 2005;41(3):87–93.

135. Dillon MJ, Ozen S. A new international classification of childhood vasculitis. Pediatr Nephrol 2006;21(9):1219–22.

136. Dourmishev AL, Serafimova DK, Vassileva SG, et al. Segmental ulcerative vasculitis: a cutaneous manifestation of Takayasu's arteritis. Int Wound J 2005;2(4):340–5.

137. Tancrede-Bohin E, Ochonisky S, Vignon-Pennamen MD, Flageul B, Morel P, Rybojad M. Schonlein-Henoch purpura in adult patients. Predictive factors for IgA glomerulonephritis in a retrospective study of 57 cases. Arch Dermatol 1997;133(4):438–42.

138. Ronkainen J, Koskimies O, Ala-Houhala M, et al. Early prednisone therapy in Henoch-Schonlein purpura: a randomized, double-blind, placebo-controlled trial. J Pediatr 2006;149(2):241–7.

139. Ronkainen J, Nuutinen M, Koskimies O. The adult kidney 24 years after childhood Henoch-Schonlein purpura: a retrospective cohort study. Lancet 2002;360(9334):666–70.

140. Magro CM, Crowson AN. A clinical and histologic study of 37 cases of immunoglobulin A-associated vasculitis. Am J Dermatopathol 1999;21(3):234–40.

20
Immunodermatology and Viral Skin Infection

Natalia Mendoza, Anita Arora, Cesar A. Arias,
Aron J. Gewirtzman, and Stephen K. Tyring

Key Points

- As a complex immune organ, the skin plays a major part in protecting the body against viruses.
- Innate immunity involves an early response to foreign antigens but is not pathogen specific, whereas an adaptive response is specific for antigen recognition and develops memory but takes longer to activate.
- Viruses have developed methods to evade the skin immune response in order to establish infection or release their progeny.
- Vaccines can protect against viruses by helping to produce a rapid immune response, with high levels of protective antibodies for their target viral antigens.

The skin is the largest organ in the human body and constitutes its first line of defense. It is not only a great physical barrier, but also has an amazing cellular army ready to defend the body from microorganisms such as viruses. This immune capacity was recognized 30 years ago and has since become an important topic of research. There is a wide spectrum of immune responses in the skin, and the mechanisms by which they are triggered are not fully understood. Almost every single microorganism (including bacteria, viruses, fungi, and parasites) is capable of inducing a specific skin response that translates into a particular clinical lesion. This interplay of responses is seen even within organisms of the same family (e.g., human papillomavirus [HPV] type I produces different lesions compared with HPV type 3). Moreover, the viruses are particularly difficult to control due to their ability

to change and adapt to the medium. They have developed the capacity to escape the immune system and in some cases can coexist with the host without being noticed.

Viruses such as the human immunodeficiency virus (HIV), the human herpes simplex virus (HSV), the varicella-zoster virus (VZV), and HPV have high rates of morbidity and mortality, and they have an impact not only on the physical condition of the patient but also generate an enormous psychological trauma. The majority of the populations infected with these viruses are young, sexually active people, and as a result, spread within the population is favored and the socioeconomic impact within the society is significant. Therefore, the development of vaccines against these viruses is one of the priorities of any health care system. The goal of a vaccine is to decrease the rapid and progressive spread of these diseases by producing a rapid immune response with high levels of protective antibodies for the target viral antigen. To achieve this response, the virus's behavior and the immune response it elicits must be properly understood.

The Immune System and the Skin

The skin is a vast immune organ (also known as skin-associated lymphoid tissue [SALT]), and all of its cells are part of an immunologic team (key players include keratinocytes, Langerhans cells [LCs], and skin tropic T cells, among others).[1,2] These cells carry out specific functions and are activated upon infection with certain viruses, and the interplay between them dictates the final immunologic outcome for the infecting virus.

The immune system is divided into two components: innate and adaptive (Table 20.1). Innate immunity is characterized by an early response to foreign antigens and is dependent on the particular environment present during the initial phase of that response.[1] It is the first line of defense against infection and has a broad spectrum of activity (not pathogen specific), including the expression of stimulatory molecules by antigen-presenting cells and the secretion of cytokines and other inflammatory cell products with a limited repertoire of antigen recognition. This initial response does not develop a memory or long-lasting protective immunity. Nonetheless, it is a rapid response and its effectiveness is crucial for the next step (which is more specific and involves antibodies and cytotoxic effector cells).[3,4] The innate immunity detects pathogens and clears the majority of microbial assaults. It is activated by cell injury or cell death, generating inflammation and local vascular responses. The key cellular players recruited in this response are the parenchymal cells and local phagocytic dendritic cells (DCs).[1,3,4] Among the local phagocytes, macrophages are one of the most important cells in this first response. They possess special receptors capable of recognizing the pathogen-associated molecular patterns (PAMPs), known as Toll-like receptors (TLRs).[4] The TLRs activate a variety of signaling pathways involved in antiviral, antibacterial, antitumor, and antiinflammatory activities.[1,5]

TABLE 20.1. Comparison of innate versus adaptive immunity.

Innate	Adaptive
• Early response to foreign antigens	• Occurs within days of infection
• Rapid response is the first line of defense	• Antigen specific
• Broad spectrum (not antigen specific)	• Develops immune memory
• No memory or long-lasting protective immunity	• Aids recovery from viral infection as well as preventing re-infection
• Key players include parenchymal cells and phagocytic dendritic cells	• Key players include T and B lymphocytes

Some of these TLRs involved in the recognition of viruses have been identified. An example is TLR9, which recognizes HSV DNA on DCs and induces antiviral mechanisms that include the secretion of type I interferons (IFNs).[1,6] The interactions between the TLRs and the virus are necessary to guide, in this case, the anti-herpes immunity toward an adaptive (specific) cellular response (T-helper-1 [Th1] type, see below).[7] Other examples of TLR interactions and viruses include the production of IFN-β and different chemokines activated by TLR3 and the induction of phagocytosis and inflammation by TLR4 mediated by the secretion of IFN-β.[6]

The adaptive response is specific for antigen recognition, occurs within days of the infection, and is the result of the interaction of T and B lymphocytes. The immune players are multiple and capable of developing a lasting immune memory. This response not only aids recovery from the primary viral contact but also protects against re-infection. T lymphocytes recognize a processed antigen (short peptides) bound to the major histocompatibility complex (MHC) of the antigen-presenting cells (APCs). There are two major subsets of T cells: CD4 and CD8. CD4 cells recognize antigens bound to MHC class II (exogenous antigens taken from the extracellular milieu and processed in the endosome of the APC), while CD8 cells recognize the antigens bound to MHC class I (usually endogenous antigens).[3] The activation of the CD4 cell results in the secretion of a variety of cytokines. Depending on the pattern of cytokine expression, the immune response is characterized as either a Th1 or Th2 response. Th1 cells secrete IFN-γ, which activates macrophages, natural killer cells, and cytotoxic $CD8^+$ T lymphocytes (cell-mediated immunity). On the other hand, Th2 cells secrete mainly interleukin-4 (IL-4) and IL-10, helping the primed B lymphocytes to differentiate into plasma cells and secrete antibodies (humoral response).[3] Also, an additional type of T cell has been shown to play an important role in the immune response against viruses. These cells, designated the regulatory T (T_{reg}) cells, carry the $CD4^+$ and $CD25^+$ antigens. T_{reg} cells recognize self antigens and prevent autoimmunity responses, regulate the responses to exogenous antigens, and are involved in the chronic and latent phases of viral infections.[8,9]

Viruses have developed a diversity of mechanisms to evade both the innate and adaptive immune response and thus establish an infection (or persist at least until a new progeny of viruses is released). Some of the cutaneous viruses share common evasion mechanisms and others have specialized systems to survive and become latent until they have a new opportunity to flare. Several of these mechanisms are discussed in detail in the sections that follow.

Human Herpes Virus

The human herpes simplex virus (HSV) types 1 and 2 are neurotropic viruses from the α-herpesvirus family. These viruses have a large molecular weight and harbor double-stranded DNA. The genome is in an icosahedral capsid, which is protected by a proteinaceous layer (tegument). The capsid is surrounded by a lipid bilayer with glycoproteins (envelope).[10] Herpes simplex virus is distributed worldwide, affecting developed and developing societies. Animal vectors for human HSV have not been described, and humans appear to be the only reservoir.[11] Usually the first infection is asymptomatic, but this depends on the age and immune status of the host,[12] the amount of the infective dose, and the presence of innate defenses that may abort the infection.[13] About 80% of the adult population in the developed world becomes seropositive to HSV-1 and more than 20% are seropositive to HSV-2. People who experience a primary infection with one or more herpes viruses carry these viruses for the rest of their lives (usually in a latent state). The virus is retained in specific neural reservoirs and may become active with periodic episodes of viral replication and shedding.[7]

Herpes simplex virus infection usually initiates in the mucosa. The virus replicates in epithelial cells and then enters the nervous system through the nerve termini. Control of the acute (and persistent) HSV infection involves the activity of natural killer (NK) cells, virus-specific CD4+ and CD8+ cells, IFNs, and virus-specific antibodies.[14] After entry into the mucosa and skin, HSV establishes a lifelong persistence in the neurons of the sensory ganglia. Herpes simplex virus persi-

stence and latency have been demonstrated in human trigeminal, facial, and vestibular ganglia, and reactivations from these locations can cause herpes labialis, vestibular neuritis, and cranial nerve disorders among others.[15] The mechanisms of viral reactivation are not fully understood but are associated with different events such as ultraviolet (UV) light, stress, fever, infections, and immunosuppression.[16] The role of the immune system during the latent phase is crucial to maintain the virus under control.[17]

Immune Response

Once the virus is in contact with host cellular receptors, the processes leading to viral infection are triggered. Glycoproteins in the lipid bilayer allow the viral envelope to fuse with the epithelial plasma membrane. Viral proteins are released into the cytoplasm and viral DNA enters the nucleus. This process triggers three phases of the innate response: (1) secretion of immune proteins, such as complement and natural antibodies; (2) an early-induced response, in which the main mediators are IFNs produced by the infected epithelial cells and resident DCs; and (3) the activation of inflammatory cells, such as neutrophils, macrophages, and NK cells.[18]

At the site of mucosal contact the virus usually encounters several barriers, including mucus, normal bacterial flora, the glycocalyx, complement proteins, and natural immunoglobulin (IgM) antibodies.[1,18] Although these substances act in concert to decrease the number of infected cells, HSV usually replicates successfully and triggers the early innate immune response. Humans may express different levels of natural antibodies to HSV, which is a reflection of their own past exposure experience.[7,18] The early innate immune response has two goals: (1) limit viral replication and spread of the virus in uninfected cells, and (2) recruit other inflammatory cells.[18] The viral interaction with the epithelial cells may stimulate cell-surface TLR2 (e.g., in the genital mucosa).[1,18] With the activation of this receptor, the epithelial cells activate complement, chemokines, and IFN-α and -β soon (between 8 and 12 hours) after the infection. Interferon-α and -β are produced by most cells types, but the DCs are responsible for the majority of their production. Interferon-α and -β are known to be two of the most important molecules to control HSV infection at this stage. Some studies suggest that resistance or susceptibility to HSV infection is directly correlated with the amount of IFN-α and -β produced.[12]

Complement, chemokines, and IFN-α and -β activate the endothelial cells that express IL-8, tumor necrosis factor-α (TNF–α), IFN-γ, and granulocyte-macrophage colony-stimulating factor (GM-CSF), leading to neutrophil chemotaxis. Figure 20.1 illustrates the chemokine regulation of leukocyte movement.[19] The inflammatory reaction alerts the DCs and resident macrophages to the presence of the virus and induces a "state of aware-ness" or "antiviral status" in the uninfected cells.[7] Infected macrophages that are able to survive acute HSV infection become a significant source of inflammatory chemokines and cytokines including TNF-α, IL-1, IL-6, IL-8, IL-12, IL-18, RANTES (regulated on activation, normal T-cell expressed and secreted; a chemokine that is a chemoattractant

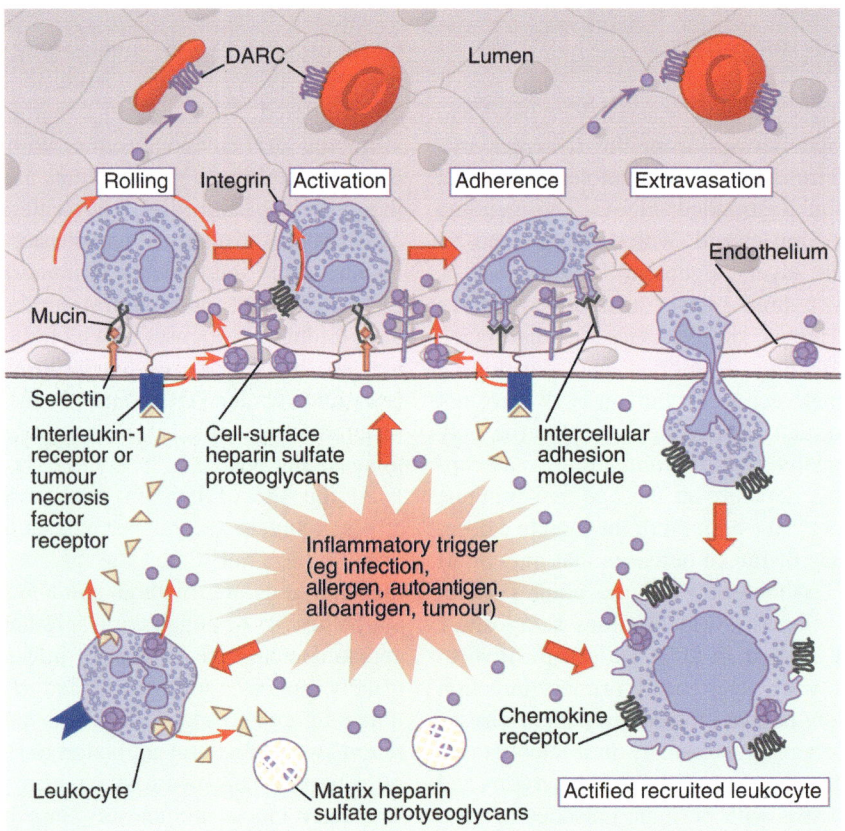

FIG. 20.1. Chemokine regulation of leukocyte movement. Chemokines are secreted at sites of inflammation and infec-tion by resident tissue cells, resident and recruited leukocytes, and cytokine-activated endothelial cells. Chemokines are locally retained on matrix and cell-surface heparin sulfate proteoglycans, establishing a chemokine concentration gradient surrounding the inflammatory stimulus, as well as on the surface of the overlying endothelium. Leukocytes rolling on the endothelium in a selectin-mediated process are brought into contact with chemokines retained on cell-surface heparin sulfate proteoglycans. Chemokine signaling activates leukocyte integrins, leading to firm adher-ence and extravasation. The recruited leukocytes are activated by local proinflammatory cytokines and may become desensitized to further chemokine signaling because of high local concentrations of chemokines. The Duffy antigen receptor for chemokines (DARC), a nonsignaling erythrocyte chemokine receptor, functions as a sink, removing chemokines from the circulation and thus helping to maintain a tissue–bloodstream chemokine gradient. (From Luster.[19] Copyright © 1998 Massachusetts Medical Society. All rights reserved.)

for eosinophils, monocytes, and lymphocytes), and IFN-α and -β. Subsequently, the immature DCs capture viral antigens and transport them to the regional lymph node to alert and stimulate the adaptive immune response.[7]

Once the DC exits the mucosa, the late-induced innate response begins at the infection site. Initially, an influx of neutrophils, monocytes, and NK cells is established. These cells traverse the activated capillary endothelial cells guided by the chemokines present at the infection site. The neutrophils secrete α-defensins that insert into the virion lipid envelope and trigger the degradation of phagocytosed virions.[20] They also secrete TNF-α, which acts synergistically with IFN-α and -β, as well as IFN-γ to produce lysis of the infected cells inhibiting viral replication.[20] Simultaneously, NK cells are activated by the binding of immunoglobulins to the viral antigen (through their Fc receptor [CD16] located on the cell surface) and are recruited by chemokines and cytokines (IFN-α and -β, IL-12, IL-15, IL-18) produced by the activated infected cells within 2 to 3 days after infection. The NKs participate in cytolysis of virus-infected cells by perforin/granzyme-mediated processes that result in phagocytosis and destruction of infected cells and viral particles.[18] The accumulation of viral antigens is followed by complement activation, facilitating the uptake of viral peptides by phagocytes.[21] These phagocytic cells produce antiviral cytokines and defensins such as nitric oxide (NO), which enhance the immune response and promote phagocytosis and destruction of virus particles and infected cells.[18]

One of the key cells for the innate response against HSV is the macrophage. The molecular mechanisms of the immune response within macrophages have been extensively studied. Once HSV infects macrophages, these cells release a series of cell mediators such as TNF-α and IL-12 (which subsequently stimulates the production of IFN-α and -β). Interferon-α and -β induce the NK and T cells to secrete IFN-γ, which eventually controls the HSV replication and initiates the adaptive response.[22,23] At this stage, the site of origin of IL-12 production is controversial. The majority of investigators suggest that DCs are the main producers of IL-12.[7,24] However, other authors indicate that the main source of this molecule is the recruited inflammatory cells.[25]

The adaptive immune response begins when the DCs migrate to the regional lymph nodes. These cells mature and display viral peptides coupled with MHC molecules, secrete cytokines, and regulate the expression of other inflammatory molecules. The cytokines produce differentiation of the Th0 cells to either Th1 or Th2. For HSV, the Th1 response is indispensable for clearance of the infection (particularly for HSV-2).[26] Other cells such as NK cells and macrophages also stimulate the switch from a Th0 to a Th1 response[26] (Table 20.2).

One of the most studied T cells during HSV infection is the CD8$^+$ T cell. These cells are capable of expressing the lymphocyte-associated antigen (cutaneous leukocyte antigen [CLA]).[27,28] During recurrent and symptomatic infection, antigen-specific CD4$^+$ T cells and NK cells infiltrate the dermis by day 2 of the lesion formation, whereas CD8$^+$ dermal infiltration (which implies cytotoxic activity resulting in viral clearance) occurs a few days later.[27,28] Therefore, CD8 cells appear to play an important role in containing HSV infection. Posaved et al.[29] showed that the levels of CD8$^+$ cytotoxic T lymphocytes (CTLs) correlate inversely with the severity of HSV-2 infection and temporally with the local clearance of the virus in lesions. The data from the study of Koelle et al.[27] suggest that the expression of the homing receptor (CLA) by the CD8$^+$ T cells is programmed at the site of the original antigen encounter and promotes migration and immune responses in reactivation. Additional studies indicate that this specific cell has the capacity of T-cell memory and self-renewal that is crucial to control the infection and symptomatic recurrences.[29]

TABLE 20.2. Immune responses to herpes viruses.

- Complement-mediated activation of immune cells
- Antibody mediated activation of immune cells
- Secretion of interferons (IFNs) by the infected epithelial cells
- Activation of neutrophils, macrophages, and natural killer (NK) cells
- Activation of endothelial cells with secretion of tumor necrosis factor-α (TNF-α), interleukin-8 (IL-8), IFN, and granulocyte-macrophage colony-stimulating factor (GM-CSF)
- Secretion of α-defensins by neutrophils
- Activation of NK cells for cytolysis of virus-infected cells
- Secretion of IL-12 and TNF-α by monocytes
- Differentiation into Th1 and Th2 responses

Studies in vivo (mouse model) have demonstrated that CD8$^+$ cells also play a crucial role in controlling the virus during the latent state.[17,30] Latent herpes viral infection in humans in the trigeminal ganglia is accompanied by a chronic inflammatory process that involves elevated levels of cytokine transcripts such as IFN-γ, TNF-α (which affects viral replication), and chemokines, accompanied by persistent lymphocytic cell infiltration (CD8$^+$ T cells, CD68$^+$, and macrophages). It has been suggested that this phenomenon could be due to a low level of expression of viral genes during latency. The CD8$^+$ T cells are capable of controlling the virus through cytokines, and this mechanism is likely to occur in response to the persistence of viruses that are prone to reactivate frequently, providing a survival advantage for both the host and the virus.[17]

Immune Evasion Mechanisms

There appears to be a complex and well-balanced interaction between host cells and HSV. Success for the virus means a delicate balance between infection and latency. Therefore, evasive strategies must be carefully designed to permit viral replication at certain stages that could potentially lead to transmission to other susceptible hosts in order to maintain the viral progeny. Humans and the herpes viruses have evolved together in a symbiotic relationship that has allowed the adaption of the virus to the host and the environment, maintaining a "truce" with the immune system without any serious threats to human life. Some of the identified mechanisms to evade the immune system include the ability of HSV to alter the activity of neutrophils, macrophages, or NK cells.[31] It is known that HSV interferes with monocyte function, suppresses chemotaxis and phagocytosis, and reduces the secretion of IL-1 and TNF-α.[7,18,31] It has also been reported that HSV reduced the activity of NK cells upon contact with infected cells, due in part to the interference with IFN-α and -β production[18,31] (Table 20.3).

Vaccines

A prophylactic HSV vaccine that aims to prevent disease and infection is likely to be more effective at reducing the incidence of genital HSV than interventions such as counseling, condom use, or

TABLE 20.3. Mechanisms of immune evasion in herpes viruses infection.

- Modulation of the activity of neutrophils, macrophages, or natural killer (NK) cells
- Interference with monocyte function
- Suppression of chemotaxis and phagocytosis
- Modulation of the production of IL-1, TNF-α, IFN-α and -β
- Reduced activity of NK cells

even antiviral therapy.[32] Several approaches have been taken in recent decades to developing an effective vaccine with varying results. Two recent studies were carried out by Glaxo Smith Kline, using a recombinant vaccine preparation containing HSV glycoproteins. The first enrolled patients who were seronegative for both HSV-1 and HSV-2. The second study allowed inclusion of HSV-1–seropositive patients.[33] The studies' primary end point was protection against genital HSV-2 clinical disease and the secondary end point was HSV-2 seroconversion. The first study did not show any difference in the primary end point between the group that received vaccine and the group that received a placebo. However, when a gender-stratified analysis was performed, the vaccine proved protective in females only (73%; 95% confidence interval [CI], 19–91%). The sex differences found in these studies might be explained by innate anatomic differences of the genital epithelial layers between men and women. The epithelial layer of male genitals consists mostly of stratum corneum, which is lacking in the genitals of women at the vaginal-cervical mucous membrane. Additionally, the secretions produced by the vagina and the genital mucous membranes contain antibodies and migratory leukocytes. Therefore, women appear to have enhanced immune responses mediated by helper T cells exhibiting a Th1 response, compared to men.[32,34]

The above results indicate that the search for the ideal vaccine should continue. Perhaps the effective vaccine will need to stimulate all the important (or at least the majority of) cellular effectors of the innate and adaptive immune response.

Varicella-Zoster Virus

Varicella-zoster virus (VZV) is also an α-herpesvirus with a genome of ~125,000 base pairs (bp) with at least 70 unique open reading frames (ORFs).[35,36]

It is characterized by a relatively short reproductive cycle, rapid cell-to-cell spread, and significant ability to establish latent infections (primarily in sensory ganglia).[36] Humans are the only known natural reservoir for VZV. This virus causes two different clinical syndromes: varicella (chickenpox) and herpes zoster (shingles). Varicella is usually a self-limited disease of childhood characterized by a very pruritic rash. The disease has a worldwide distribution, and transmission is more pronounced in temperate climates (where it is seen more frequently in children) than in tropical environments.[11] Approximately 20% of those who had varicella later develop herpes zoster, which usually affects adults older than 50 years of age, although it can occur at any age.[11,37]

Immune Response

Initial clinical observations indicate that the primary site of inoculation is the respiratory tract. A rash usually develops after an incubation period of 10 to 12 days.[11,36,37] The entry of the VZV into a host cell requires fusion of the viral envelope with the host cell plasma membrane. This phenomenon is mediated by interactions of viral oligosaccharides with the heparan sulfate proteoglycans (via N-linkage) on the host cell surface. The fusion permits the entry of the viral proteins into the host cell cytosol and then to the nucleus where the nucleocapsid fuses with the outer nuclear membrane, releasing the viral DNA genome into the nucleus.[38] The spread of the virus is controlled by the innate and adaptive responses. The host cell membrane has specific glycoproteins such as gH, gL, gB, and gE that permit the fusion process between cells. These proteins are used by VZV to quickly spread to adjacent epidermal cells by inducing the fusion of the infected cells with noninfected ones.[30] Varicella-zoster virus has a special tropism for three major cell types: the peripheral blood monocytes cells (PBMCs), skin cells, and sensory neurons.[30] This virus not only infects these cells, but also is capable of replicating inside them. This phenomenon of viral replication can be observed in intraepidermal vesicular lesions of the skin, which are loaded with free virus.[11,36,38]

The virus infects the immature DCs of the respiratory mucosa, and these cells transport the virus to the T-cell–draining lymph nodes. From these nodes VZV is subsequently transported to the reticuloendothelial system and then is capable of gaining access to the bloodstream, causing a primary viremia. During this first viremic phase, VZV is able to reach the reticuloendothelial organs where it undergoes a phase of viral amplification. It was previously thought that VZV reached the skin during a second viremic episode that occurred in the late incubation period.[38] However, studies of viral infection in mouse models now suggest that infected T cells from the tonsil area are capable of transferring VZV to the skin immediately after entering the circulation during the primary viremia and that the prolonged interval between exposure and the skin rash reflects the time required for the virus to become recognized by potent innate immune barriers such as IFN-α.[35,38]

Varicella-zoster virus preferentially infects the active memory CD4 T cells that express skin homing markers such as CLA and the chemokine (C-C notif) receptor 4 (CCR4). These T cells are usually programmed for immune surveillance and then may facilitate the transfer of VZV into the skin.[35] It appears that VZV does not trigger any early inflammatory response that might block the appearance of virus-filled vesicles at the skin surface.[35,38] The initial viremia is necessary to ensure that enough cutaneous lesions are formed to transmit the virus efficiently to other individuals as a viral survival mechanism. The T cells trafficking through the skin activate VZV replication at this site, and this process permits infection of more T cells that will return to the circulation.[35]

The innate immune response is induced during the acute VZV infection. This response involves the release of IFN-α and IFN-γ and the secretion of cytokines such as IL-6 (by monocytes) via TLR2.[39] This cell-mediated immune response contains VZV replication and prevents the host from a systemic disease (including severe compromise of organs such as lungs, kidneys, and spleen). The adaptive immune response begins with the presence of CD4+ T cells and the release of IL-2, IL-10, IL-12, and IFN-γ by Th1 and Th2 cells.[40] These cytokines cause the proliferation of VZV specific CD4+ and CD8+ T cells, which express MHC class I and II molecules and recognize the viral glycoproteins gE, gH, and gI, with the subsequent killing of the VZV-infected cells.[41] During the presence of rash, many mononuclear infiltrating cells are present. Most of these cells express CD4 and CD8, including CD45RO+ memory cells, skin homing CLA, and CCR4+ T cells. During this period, the skin shows expression of E-selectin (a cell adhesion molecule and CD antigen that mediates neutrophil, monocyte, and memory T-cell adhesion to cytokine-activated endothelial cells), intercellular adhesion molecule 1 (ICAM-1, a cell-surface ligand involved in leukocyte adhesion and inflammation), and vascular cell adhesion molecule-1 (VCAM-1, a cytokine-induced cell adhesion molecule present on activated endothelial cells, tissue macrophages, and DCs), allowing the migration of the inflammatory cells. The humoral immune response has a reduced role in controlling the virus. Immunoglobulin G (IgG), IgM and IgA appear to respond to some viral proteins. It seems that these antibodies neutralize cell-free virions and contribute in the lysis of infected cells[35] (Table 20.4).

During the resolution of varicella, VZV establishes latency in the trigeminal and dorsal root ganglia where it remains latent through the lifetime of its host. Approximately 20% of infected people develop herpes zoster. Figure 20.2 illustrates the latent virus in a dorsal root ganglion and reactivated virus causing acute vesicular zoster rash.[42] In this period, the VZV multiplies and spreads centrifugally down the sensory nerve, causing neuronal necrosis and intense neuritis. Recent studies have shown that VZV possesses multiple open reading frames (ORFs) that encode proteins present in the cytoplasm of neurons during latency and are localized in the cell nucleus during reactivation.[43] Some of these genes are involved in VZV assembly, replication (such as ORF2),[44] and latency. ORF47 encodes a protein that is part of the VZV virion tegument and is essential for VZV growth in differentiated skin and T cells. Studies of this peptide indicate that the blockage of the kinase function of this protein decreases the VZV virulence in the skin, suggesting interference with the production of complete VZV virions. This peptide has also been implicated as a latency-associated protein along with the products of the ORF4 and ORF63.[45–48] Additionally, the mechanisms of latency appear to be controlled by a group of antisense transcripts called latency-associated transcripts (LATs). However, the exact mechanisms are not well understood.[39]

TABLE 20.4. Immune responses to varicella-zoster virus (VZV).

Acute VZV infection
- Release of IFN-α and IFN-γ
- Secretion of cytokines such as IL-6 (by monocytes) via Toll-like receptor 2 (TLR2)
- Release of IL-2, IL-10, IL-12, and IFN-γ by T-helper-1 (Th1) and Th2 cells
- Proliferation of VZV specific CD4+ and CD8+ T cells

During skin rash
- Expression of E-selectin, intercellular adhesion molecule 1 (ICAM-1) and vascular cell adhesion molecule (VCAM-1)
- Migration of inflammatory cells
- Reduced role of humoral response in controlling the virus

Immune Evasion Mechanisms

Varicella-zoster virus utilizes several mechanisms to overcome the immune response. Major histocompatibility complex class II expression is restricted to APCs and is required to present the viral peptides to CD4 T cells. Usually, the host immune response to the virus produces the release of IFN-γ, which stimulates the expression of MHC II molecules. To evade the immune response and ensure replication, VZV produces a protein that interferes with Stat1 (a signal transducer and activator of transcription that mediates cellular responses to interferons). Stat1 interacts with P53 tumor suppressor protein and regulates expression of genes involved in growth control and apoptosis activation and thereby inhibits antiviral IFN-γ production in foci of infected skin cells.[35] Inhibition of IFN-γ results in decreased MHC II expression, which subsequently affects the efficiency of VZV specific immune responses. Varicella-zoster virus takes advantage of these circumstances, and as a consequence, the initial formation of VZV lesions in skin (varicella or during the VZV reactivation as zoster) is facilitated.[35,49,50] Additionally, VZV has mechanisms to delay clearance of virus-infected cells by interfering with the expression of MHC class I proteins that are necessary for CD4 and CD8 T-cell recognition.[49] This mechanism allows VZV to evade CD8 T-cell lysis during the viremic phase. The precise molecular event is related to the downregulation of MHC I by VZV via interference of its transport from the Golgi compartment to the plasma membrane[35] (Table 20.5)

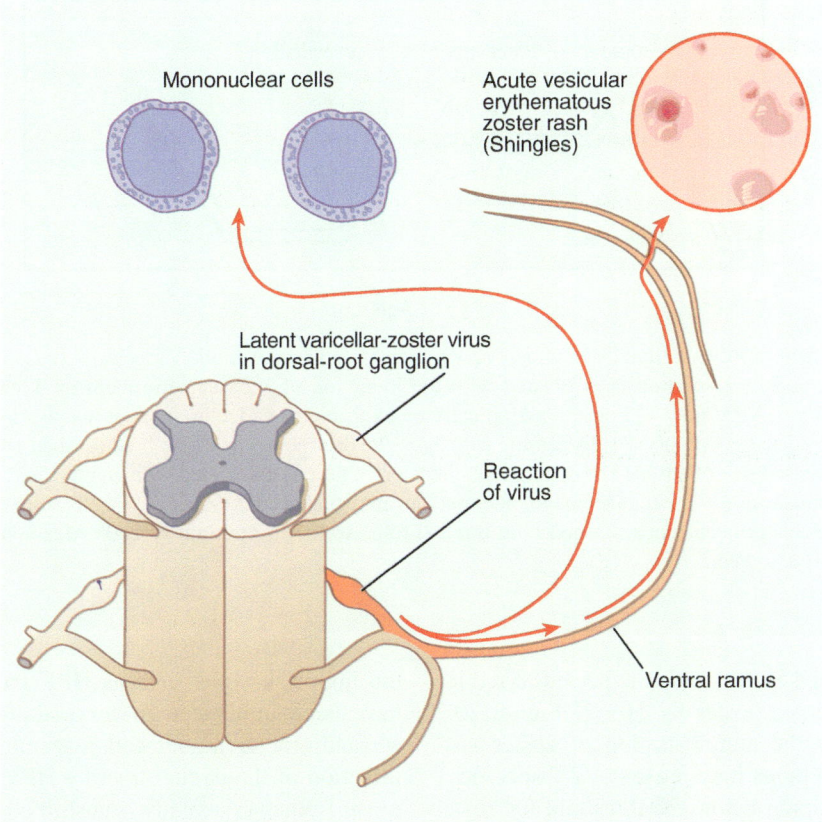

FIG. 20.2. Latent and reactivated varicella–zoster virus. Shown is a latent virus in a dorsal-root ganglion (white fusiform swelling) adjacent to the spinal cord and reactivated virus in a nearby dorsal-root ganglion (orange fusiform swelling) with transaxonal spread to the skin. The reactivated virus causes an acute, vesicular, erythematous zoster rash. (From Gilden et al.[42] Copyright © 2000 Massachusetts Medical Society. All rights reserved.)

TABLE 20.5. Immune evasion mechanisms in varicella-zoster virus infection.

- Interference with signal transduction mechanism through Stat 1
- Decreased major histocompatibility complex class II (MHC II) expression
- Delay of clearance of virus infected cells through interference with MHC expression

Vaccines

Before the introduction in 1995 of VARIVAX, a live attenuated Oka/Merck strain of VZV, millions of children developed primary varicella (chickenpox). VARIVAX is indicated for vaccination against varicella in individuals 12 months of age and older and it is recommended as part of the childhood immunization schedule. Its effectiveness is greater than 95% for varicella prevention. Herpes zoster is the result of the reactivation of latent VZV infection residing in sensory ganglia. In the United States, herpes zoster affects approximately 1,000,000 persons annually, with an incidence of 2.2 cases per 1000 persons of age or older.[51,52] Results from several clinical trials have determined that a live, attenuated VZV vaccine using the Oka/Merck strain (Zostavax) is safe, elevates VZV-specific cell-mediated immunity, and significantly reduces the incidence of herpes zoster and postherpetic neuralgia in immunocompetent people over the age of 60. This vaccine is 14-fold more concentrated than VARIVAX, has been approved for

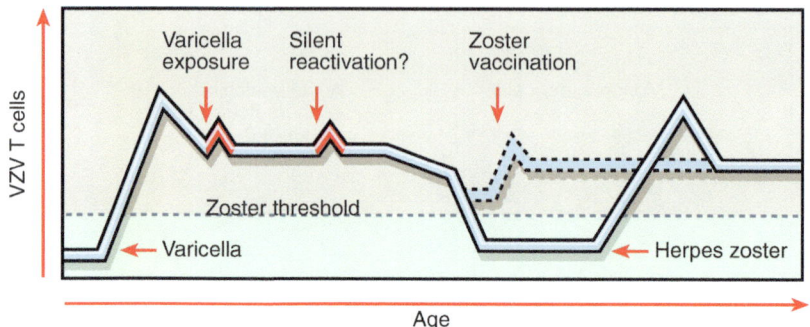

Fig. 20.3. Host factors in varicella-zoster virus (VZV) latency and reactivation. Varicella is the primary infection caused by VZV, and its resolution is associated with the induction of VZV-specific memory T cells (blue line). Memory immunity to VZV may be boosted periodically by exposure to varicella or silent reactivation from latency (red peaks). VZV-specific memory T cells decline with age. The decline below a threshold (dashed green line) correlates with an increased risk of zoster. The occurrence of zoster, in turn, is associated with an increase in VZV-specific T cells. The administration of zoster vaccine to older persons may prevent VZV-specific T cells from dropping below the threshold for zoster occurrence (dashed blue line). (From Arvin.[53] Copyright © 2005 Massachusetts Medical Society. All rights reserved.)

use in the United States, and is expected to reduce the risk for herpes zoster by 50%.[52] Figure 20.3 illustrates how the administration of zoster vaccine to older persons may prevent VZV-specific T cells from dropping below the threshold for zoster occurrence.[53]

Human Papillomavirus

Human papillomaviruses (HPVs) are small DNA tumor viruses that have a circular double-stranded DNA genome of ~8 kb in length. They belong to a large group of recognized oncogenic viruses.[54] Human papillomavirus is a member of the Papillomaviridae family that includes over 120 different genotypes (defined by differences in their nucleotide sequence).[11,55] The HPV genome is composed of three regions: the long control region (LCR), the early region (E), and the late region (L). The early region consists of genes $E1$ to $E8$ (which encode nonstructural proteins for transcription, plasmid replication, and transformation), while the late region codes for the major (L1) and minor (L2) proteins that form the viral capsid. The current vaccines include the protein L1 as the major immunogenic antigen.[56]

The HPVs are commonly categorized as having low or high oncogenic potential. Infections with the high-risk types such as HPV-16 and HPV-18 have been implicated in cervical-anogenital cancer and oral squamous cell carcinomas.[11,57,58] The infection of the genital tract by HPV is one of the most frequent sexually transmitted diseases.[58,59] Approximately 75% of sexually active individuals are infected by HPV during their lifetime. In the United States, it has been calculated that 6.2 million new cases of high-risk HPV infections occur each year, close to 20 million Americans are infected, and 1% of sexually active adults have genital warts.[55,59] It is estimated that >99% of cervical, as well as >70% of anal and vaginal cancers are related to HPV infection (cervical cancer is the second most frequent cause of death due to neoplasia among women worldwide). More specifically, about 30% to 40% of penile, vulvar, and oropharynx cancers are related to the HPV-16 and HPV-18.[58,60–62]

The majority of HPV clinical lesions are located in the genital area (70–90%) in sexually active adolescents and young women. These lesions usually show clearance of the infection within 12 to 30 months.[58] Longer duration of infection is frequently related to the presence of cervical intraepithelial neoplasia (CIN).[63] The prevalence and incidence of the HPV infection varies with age. The cause for this apparent variation is not clear. Many authors postulate that some (but not all) infected individuals develop an adaptive immune response against HPV that prevents future infections.[64]

Immune Response

Human papillomavirus has a special tropism for the epithelial cells (they are epitheliotropic), infecting keratinocytes at a wide range of body sites where they cause aberrant cellular proliferation leading to benign warts or cervical cancer.[3,54,65] Initially, the virus infects primitive basal keratinocytes and starts DNA replication and transcription of the early genes at very low levels.[66] The peak of productive synthesis of virions is reached once the keratinocyte reaches higher strata of the epithelium. Thus, high levels of viral proteins and viral assembly occur only at the upper layers of the squamous epithelia (stratum spinosum and granulosum).[11] At this point the cycle of replication and patterns of gene transcription are dependent on the stage of differentiation of the keratinocyte.[66]

A significant amount of information regarding the immune response has been gathered from observations in animal models. Once the virus has reached the skin, it establishes itself at the basal cells of the epithelia where it starts replication. At this point the replication is minimal but becomes greater once the keratinocyte matures toward desquamation.[67] At the basal layer, there is practically no immune response against the virus (two to several months), but once it is detected by the immune system, replication increases and results in clinically detectable lesions.[68,69] After a few months (which varies depending on the host), the infected keratinocytes express the late viral genes (encoding proteins L1 and L2) that trigger a full immune response.[67–69]

The keratinocytes are able to secrete cytokines, growth factors, and chemokines upon viral stimuli. The host immune response dictates the emergence and characteristics of clinical lesions.[66] Some of the cytokines involved are transforming growth factor-β (TGF-β), TNF-α, and IFNs. TGF-β has been shown to inhibit the growth of nontumorigenic HPV-16 and HPV-18 immortalized cells, and it seems to control the expression of E6 and E7 (although some controversy exists on these facts).[66] In normal cervical cells, TGF-β inhibits viral growth, but HPV can evade this control mechanism.[66] TNF-α, which is another product of the keratinocyte, may have an antiproliferative effect on the HPV-16–infected cells through cell cycle arrest (between the G0 and G1 phases of the cell cycle).[66,70] It has also been suggested that TNF-α acts as a repressor on the expression of E6 and E7 in the immortalized human keratinocytes.[71] The effects attributed to IFNs may be virus-type specific. These molecules also appear to inhibit the production of viral proteins.[66]

The time between HPV infection and the development of a clinical lesion could vary from weeks to more than 9 months. This is an indication that HPV could modulate the immune system as evidenced by the following: (1) HPV infects mainly keratinocytes, which are cells programmed to die and desquamate in a specific and timely manner (apoptosis); and (2) the intracellular location of HPV in these cells allows the virus to hide and avoid immune surveillance. As a consequence, the apoptotic keratinocyte infected with HPV does not trigger a significant inflammatory reaction, eventually resulting in a persistent chronic infection.[68,72]

The adaptive immune response involves two phases: the recognition of antigen and the response to it. This adaptive immune response involves the LCs that capture the virus and its antigen for transport to local lymph nodes and presentation to naive T cells. The T cells return to the infected epithelial tissues via mechanisms that include secretion of chemokines and expression of adhesion molecules to clear the infection. In the recognition phase, the LCs are the major APCs. However, in some HPV infections, a depletion of these cells has been documented, which is associated with enhanced survival of HPV, prolonged courses of infection, and possibly malignancy.[73–75] At this stage, the infected keratinocytes produce IL-1α and TNF, which promote LC migration.

If the immune response is appropriate, the regression of warts usually follows. At this stage, a large infiltrate of T cells (CD4[+] and CD8[+]) and macrophages is present, and the cytokines involved exhibit the Th1 pattern (IL-12, TNF-α, and IFN-γ plus the expression of the adhesion molecules for lymphocyte trafficking) (Table 20.6). A systemic T-cell response to E1 and E6 viral proteins is effective only at the peak of wart regression (although activity is present during the whole infective cycle).[68,69]

In summary, HPV is capable of escaping the immune response for several months by modulating

TABLE 20.6. Immune responses to human papilloma virus.

- Secretion by keratinocytes of cytokines, growth factors, and chemokines (TNF-α, transforming growth factor-β [TGF-β], and IFNs) upon viral stimuli
- Langerhans cells capture of virus and its antigen
- Transport to local lymph nodes and presentation to naive T cells
- Large infiltration of T cells (CD4+ and CD8+) and macrophages
- Th1 pattern of cytokines (IL-12, TNF-α, and IFN-γ)
- Expression of the adhesion molecules for lymphocyte trafficking

---

the inflammatory reaction from the keratinocytes after invasion. Nonetheless, in the majority of cases, the immune system finally catches up and is capable of detecting the virus, (probably when the replication turnover is highest) and thus is able to resolve the infection.

Viral Oncogenesis

It is now accepted that HPV infection is necessary (but not sufficient) to cause cervical cancer, other anogenital neoplasms, and oral squamous cell carcinomas. Several viral types (such as 16 and 18) have been clearly identified as having high oncogenic potential. The majority of infections with these HPV types seem to clear spontaneously. Whether infections clear completely or the virus remains latent in basal cells at undetectable levels is not yet well understood.[55] For high-risk HPV types, the proteins E6 and E7 appear to play a very important role in oncogenesis since they are able to inhibit two well-known oncogenic suppressor genes encoding the pRb (product of retinoblastoma tumor suppressor gene) and p53 proteins.[11] E6 enhances the degradation of p53 via the ubiquitin-mediated proteolysis machinery (E3 ubiquitin ligase, UBE3A) and E7 interacts with the pRb.[76]

Many studies have shown that the absence of mature APCs, CD50, and CD86 and the downregulation of TNF-α represent an inadequate immune response to HPV that leads to persistence of the viral infection in the CIN lesions. The LCs are also decreased in numbers and lack the expression of CD11a/18, CD50, CD54, CD58, and CD86. These changes alter the antigen-presenting capacity and can induce immune tolerance to the viral infec-

tion.[77] The immortalization of epithelial cells in CIN produced by HPV-16 is related to the lack of response to the inhibitory effect of TGF-β and the inhibition in keratinocytes of TNF-α by the HPV-16 E7 protein, resulting in uncontrolled growth of the infected cells and escaping of the virus from the immune system.[66] Figure 20.4 illustrates the changes in cervical squamous epithelium caused by HPV infection.[78]

Immune Evasion Mechanisms

The reasons for the failure of the immune system to recognize HPV are not well understood. It appears that HPV is able to escape detection by the APCs. To survive and have enough time to replicate without detection, HPV has developed many strategies to evade the immune system. The special tropism for keratinocytes (as discussed earlier) is one the first mechanisms of immune evasion.[68]

Keratinocytes are powerful immune cells. They constitute almost 95% of the cervical and skin epithelium and can express MCH II and co-stimulatory signals to T cells (such as ICAM-I) during inflammation.[77] If the immune response is activated, the HPV-infected keratinocytes release TNF-α, which negatively affects the replication of HPV.[60,77] TNF-α upregulates the expression of ICAM-1 levels, which decrease the levels of IFN-γ. In CIN, the keratinocytes express less TNF-α, decreasing the stimulus to the LCs. This alteration also affects the expression of MHC II, and as a consequence the presentation of antigens is altered[58,77] and the expression of the suppressive cytokine IL-10 is increased.[77] These changes in the immunologic microenvironment (with inappropriate T-cell presentation) may contribute to the persistence and progression of the viral infection and development of a CIN lesion.[74,77,79]

Another important mechanism of immune evasion by HPV involves the downregulation of the macrophage inflammatory protein-3α (MIP-3α), which allows the virus to persist in the epithelial cells without being recognized.[80] Macrophage inflammatory protein-3α is one of the most potent attractants of LC precursors and dermal dendritic cells, as well as T cells. It has been shown that infection of keratinocytes by HPV-16 expressing the E6 and E7 proteins decreases the production of MIP-3α.[81] Similarly, it has also been noted that in most cutaneous

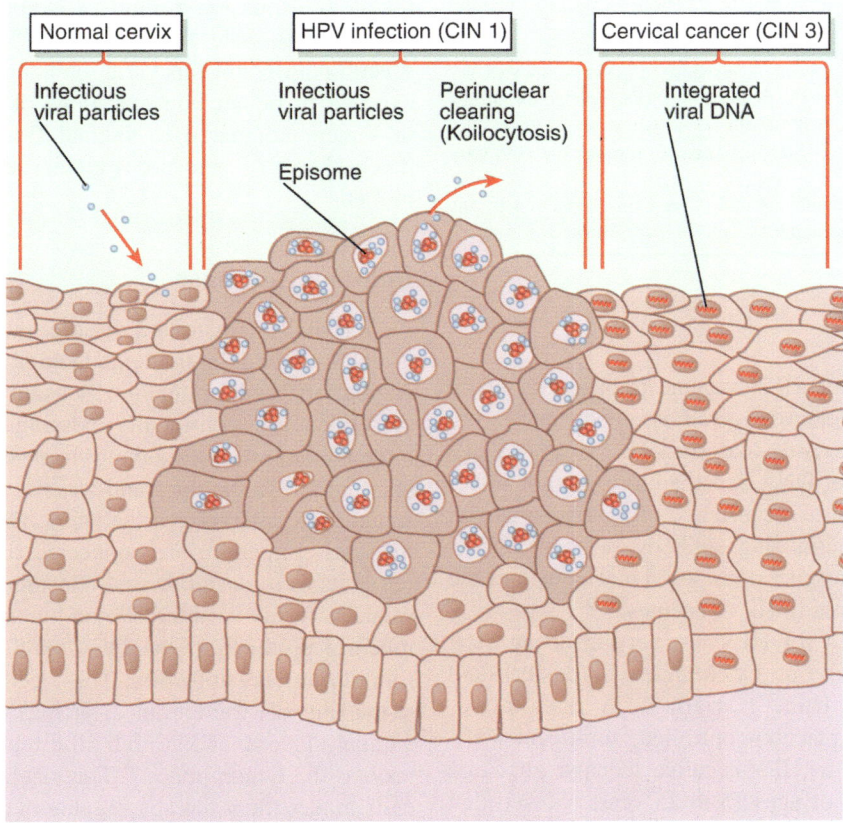

Fig. 20.4. Spectrum of changes in cervical squamous epithelium caused by human papillomavirus (HPV) infection. The left side of the figure shows normal cervical squamous epithelium. When HPV infection occurs (center), the virus exists in the cell nucleus as a circular episome. If the viral genome is intact, new infectious viral particles can be produced; their presence in the cell is indicated by perinuclear clearing, or koilocytosis. In cervical cancer (right), oncogenic portions of HPV DNA become integrated into the host's DNA, with disruption of the *E2* regulatory region and loss of other genes needed to form a complete virus. The cells are undifferentiated and do not show koilocytosis. CIN 1, cervical intraepithelial neoplasia grade 1. (From Goodman and Wilbur.[78] Copyright © 2003 Massachusetts Medical Society. All rights reserved.)

viral infections the number of epidermal LCs is significantly reduced (the decrease in numbers of LCs is more marked in lesions of CIN).[77,81]

Recent studies support the findings that the E5 protein, found in HPV, downregulates the MHC class I molecules, which results in impaired cell lysis by the cytotoxic T lymphocytes. The E5 oncoproteins from multiple types of HPV share similar characteristics; they are small hydrophobic peptides located in the endomembranous compartments of the infected cell that contribute to the activation of growth factor receptors and downregulation of the MHC I.[11,82] The exact mechanisms used by E5

to downregulate MHC I are not completely clear. Two proposed hypotheses include (1) the inhibition of acidification of the Golgi apparatus (where the MHC is assembled),[83] and (2) a direct interaction between E5 and the heavy chain of the MHC.[84]

It has also been shown that the proteins E6 and E7 negatively affect the immune system by inhibiting the production of immune mediators.[74] Both proteins are inversely correlated with the expression of IL-18, which induces the secretion of IFN-γ and IL-8. E6 and E7 also reduce the production of chemokines and monocyte chemoattractant proteins in the genital mucosa of women[66] (Table 20.7).

TABLE 20.7. Mechanisms of immune evasion in human papilloma virus infection.

- Modulation of the immune response in the keratinocytes
- Downregulation of the production of macrophage inflammatory protein-3α (MIP-3α)
- Downregulation of MHC I molecules through the HPV protein E5
- Reduction of chemokine and interleukin production by the HPV proteins E6 and E7

Vaccines

The prophylactic HPV vaccine is based on L1, a major capsid protein that is self-assembled into empty capsids, called virus–like particles (VLPs). VLPs are free of viral DNA and therefore are not infectious, but can provide a source of epitopes that can stimulate a neutralizing antibody response.[3,56,85,86] Figure 20.5 illustrates a proposed mechanism of the immune response to HPV vaccines.[87–90]

The vaccines for HPV are very effective. The studies carried out by Merck (Gardasil®) and Glaxo Smith Kline (Cevarix®) in randomized, double-blind, placebo-controlled, multicenter trials conducted in HPV-negative teenage girls and young women of ages 15 to 25 years showed that the vaccine protected 100% of individuals against infection by HPV strains 16 and 18. The follow-up study performed in the U.S., Canada, and Brazil (776 patients) reported high levels of antibodies for a duration of up to 4.5 years after receiving the vaccine.[56,91] Therefore, the results of these vaccine trials are likely to have an enormous impact in the HPV-associated pathology in the coming years.

Human Immunodeficiency Virus

The human immunodeficiency virus (HIV) pandemic is one of the tragic legacies of the 20th century. HIV is currently one of the leading causes of mortality in sub-Saharan Africa, where more than 5.5 million inhabitants are infected with the virus.[92] The total number of estimated HIV–infected persons worldwide in 2005 was between 33.4 and 46.0 million. Approximately 2.4 to 3.3 million people were estimated to have died as a result of AIDS in 2005.[93]

Women are more susceptible to HIV infection than are men. It seems that the HIV male-to-

female transmission during sex is about twice that of female-to-male transmission.[94,95] Among the several reasons for this variation is that women are exposed to higher concentrations of HIV present in semen (compared to vaginal fluid),[96] and the mucosal area of exposure is greater in women than in men.

Immune Response

As a sexually transmitted disease, the usual portal of entry of the HIV is the anogenital mucosa. The vaginal and anal epithelium is usually moist, and secretions are continually passing through the intercellular spaces, making it more permeable (as opposed to the tight and less easily penetrated squamous epithelium of the skin). The cells in the mucosal epithelium are connected by discontinuous patches of desmosomes (considered one of the weakest forms of intercellular junction).[11] In the mucosal epithelium, the DCs play an important role during HIV infection. These cells are located at the sites of viral entrance, such as the rectal and vaginal mucosa, and at high viral replication sites, such as the lymph nodes.[97] The localization of DC cells makes them the key regulators of HIV transmission and subsequent viral spread.[93,98] The DCs are APCs derived from bone marrow progenitors that home in on peripheral mucosal sites where they become immature DCs. After capturing an antigen and under the effects of the process of infection and inflammation, these cells turn into mature DCs and migrate to the lymph nodes, where the maturation process finalizes, making them capable of presenting the antigen to T cells.[99]

To understand the events and mechanisms of HIV sexual transmission, the most useful animal model has been the rhesus macaque model infected with simian immunodeficiency virus (SIV), which is closely related to HIV. In macaques, the LCs are DCs located within the stratified vaginal squamous epithelia. The LC is the first infected cell after intravaginal exposure to SIV.[100] Extrapolating the animal data to HIV, upon contact with the mucosa, the HIV fuses to the immature DCs through two mechanisms: (1) CD4 cell surface receptors and the chemokine receptors (mostly CCR5), and (2) capture of the virus at the cell surface by DC-specific ICAM-3 grabbing nonintegrin (DC-SIGN) and other C-type lectins.[101] Once inside of the DCs, HIV can replicate and produce

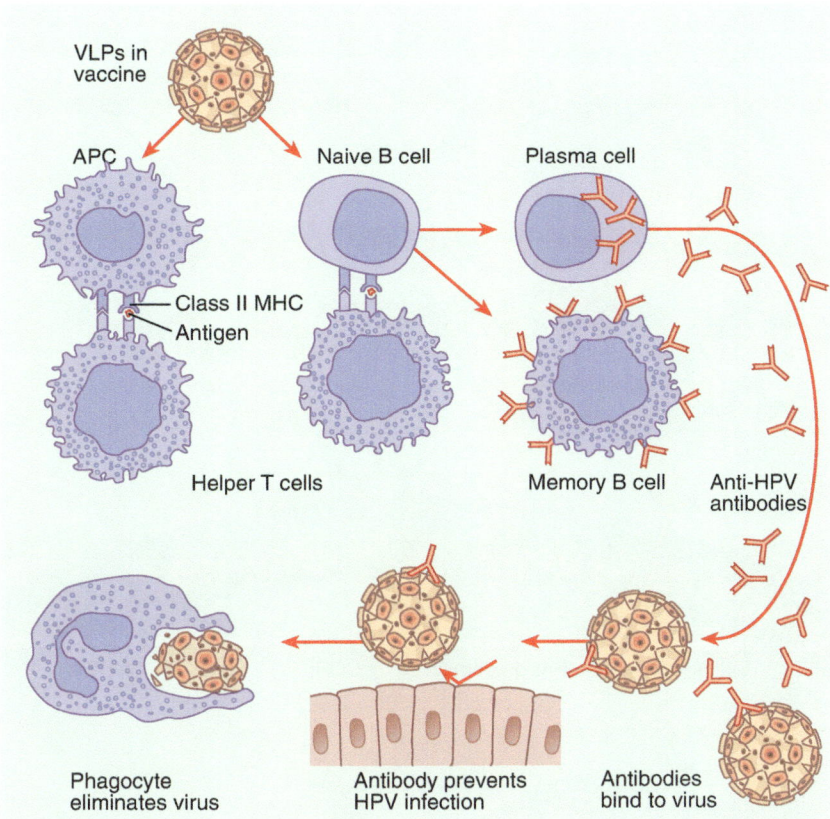

FIG. 20.5. A proposed mechanism for the immune response to HPV vaccines. It has been proposed that HPV L1 virus–like particle (VLP) stimulates an adaptive immune response in humans, resulting in the generation of type-specific neutralizing anti-HPV antibodies. The introduction of VLPs into the systemic circulation via vaccination (upper left) is followed by the ingestion, processing, and display of the VLPs complexed with major histocompatibility class II (MHC II) proteins by antigen-presenting cells (APCs). Naive T-helper cells interact with the aforementioned complex (upper left). The uptake, processing, and display of the VLPs on the B cells are shown (upper middle), which then can interact with T-helper cells that secrete cytokines necessary for B-cell differentiation. Activated B cells differentiate into either memory B cells or plasma cells (upper right). Plasma cells secrete anti-HPV antibodies with high affinity for the target antigen should the antigen enter the body again (upper right). Neutralizing anti-HPV antibodies bind to type-specific neutralizing epitopes on the surface of HPV virus antigens (lower right). The neutralizing anti-HPV antibodies can prevent HPV infection of the host epithelial cell (lower middle). The antibody-coated viruses are eventually eliminated from the body by phagocytes (bottom left).[87–90] (From Merck & Co., Inc. Efficacy and Antibody Response to Human Papilloma Virus [HPV] Vaccines. Powerpoint Presentation. Copyright © 2006 Merck & Co., Inc. All rights reserved.)

intact virions. Figure 20.6 illustrates interactions between HIV and the cell surface).[102] Subsequently, the virus exploits the natural trafficking properties of the DCs to transfer its virion progeny to its primary cellular target, the CD4 cell, located at the draining lymph nodes.[97,103] This strategy explains the rapid and efficient movement of HIV mediated by the LCs from mucosal tissues (the normal sites of LC activation following antigen exposure) to the lymph nodes.[101] This phenomenon also explains the fact that small amounts of infecting viruses (or relatively few infected LCs) could lead to efficient infection of large numbers of CD4+ T cells.[100]

During immune activation, mature LCs and other types of mature DCs have the ability to cluster with the T cells. The microenvironment in these cell clusters

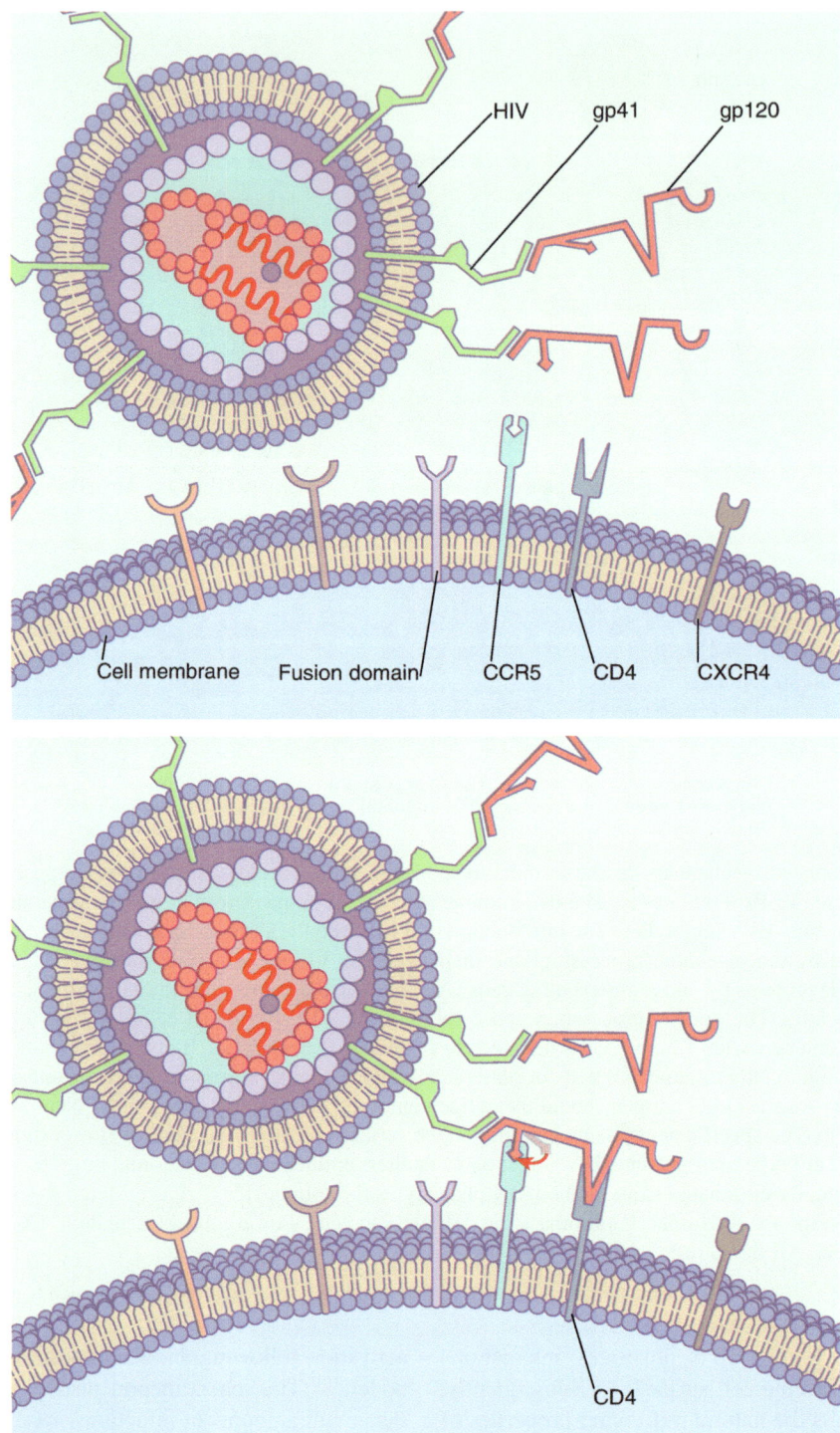

Fig. 20.6. Interactions between HIV and the cell surface. HIV interacts with a cell-surface receptor, primarily CD4, and through conformational changes becomes more closely associated with the cell through interactions with other cell-surface molecules, such as the chemokine receptors CXCR4 and CCR5 (A). Alternatively, some viruses, such as certain strains of HIV-2, could attach to CXCR4 directly.[11] The likely steps in HIV infection are as follows. The CD4–binding site on HIV-1 gp120 interacts with the CD4 molecule on the cell surface (B). Conformational changes in both the viral envelope and the CD4 receptor permit the binding of gp120 to another cell-surface receptor, such as CCR5

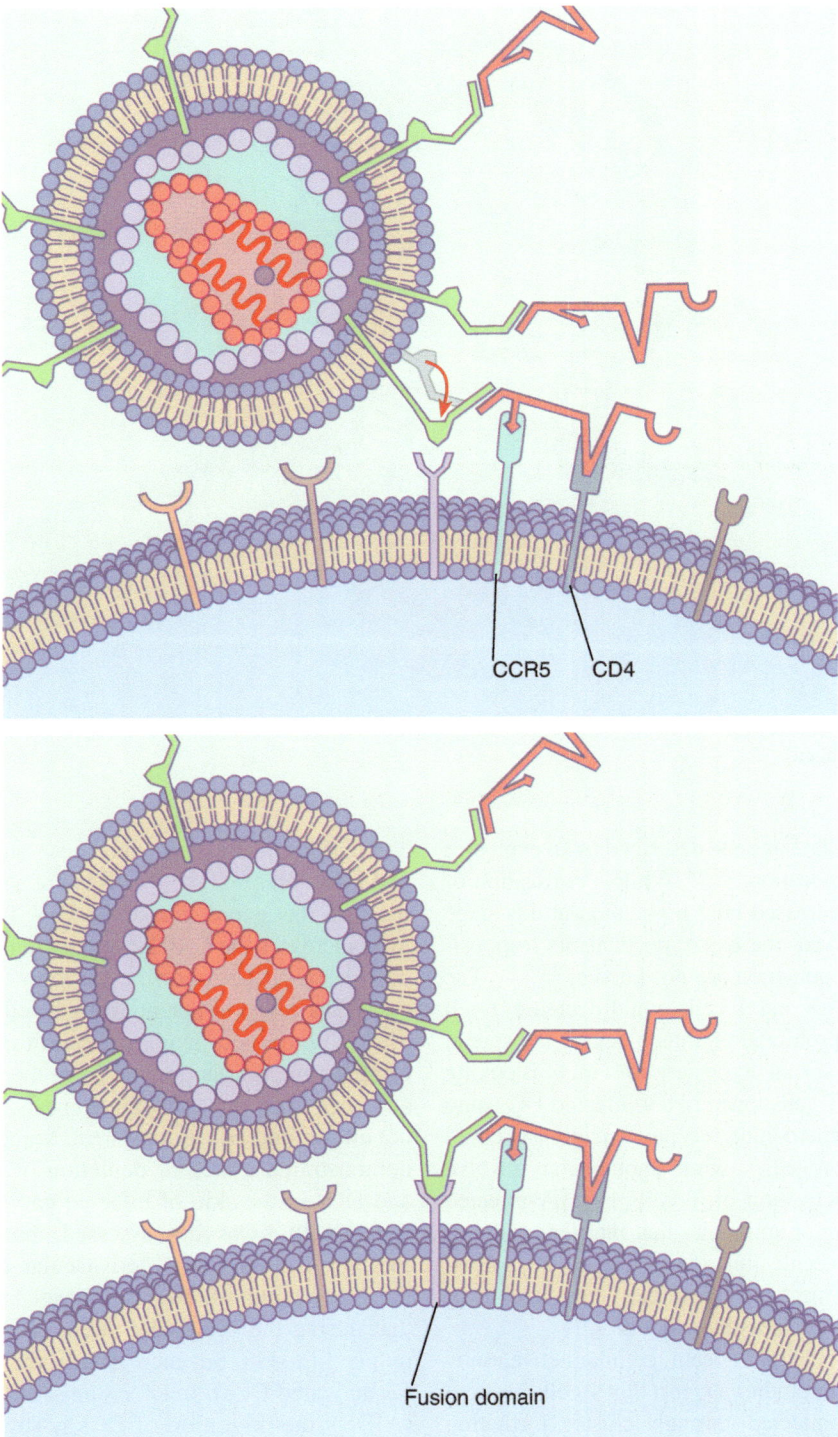

FIG. 20.6. (continued) (C). This second attachment brings the viral envelope closer to the cell surface, allowing interaction between gp41 on the viral envelope and a fusion domain on the cell surface. HIV fuses with the cell (D). Subsequently, the viral nucleoid enters into the cell, most likely by means of other cellular events (E). Once this stage is achieved, the cycle of viral replication begins. (From Levy.[102] Copyright © 1996 Massachusetts Medical Society. All rights reserved.)

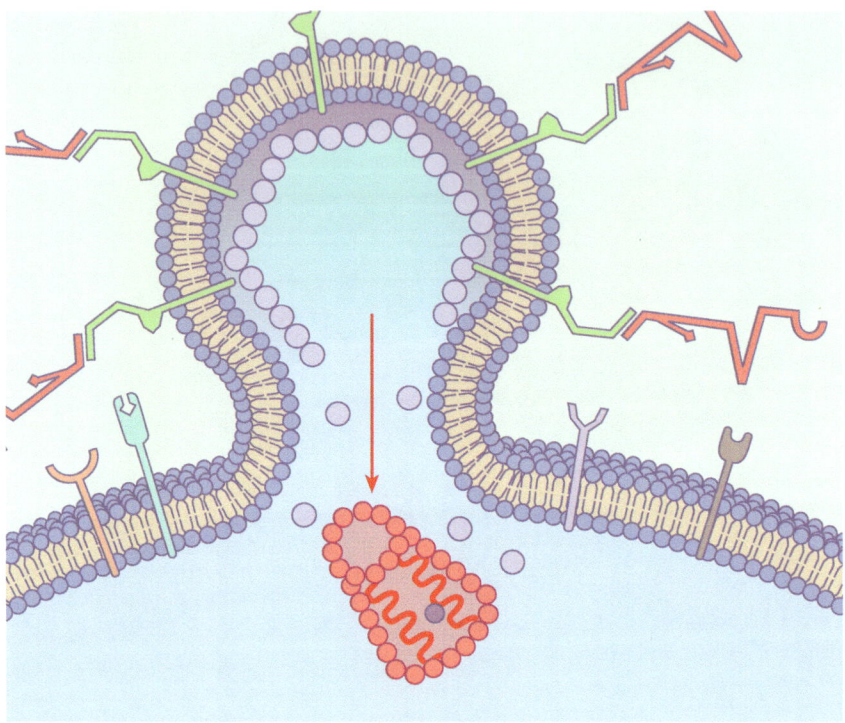

F<small>IG</small>. 20.6. (continued)

(DCs with T cells) has been described as an explosive site for HIV replication.[104–106] While a correlation of the DCs and decreased HIV replication at this stage has been observed, the exact mechanisms responsible for this phenomenon are not known.[98,107,108] The clustering of DCs and T cells could decrease T-cell activation and proliferation, thus blocking the spread of HIV after sexual exposure to virus. Blocking chemotaxis of T cells toward HIV-infected DC using chemokine or chemokine receptor antagonists could be one of the strategies, while another may involve blocking full activation of T cells by HIV-infected DCs by addition of antibodies that interfere with co-stimulatory molecule function.[109] Figure 20.7 illustrates possible mechanisms of the neutralization of HIV at mucosal surfaces by antibodies.[110]

For HIV replication to occur, cellular activation is critical, and some studies suggest that T cells become activated and infected through cluster formation with infected LC and not by direct contact with free viruses produced by infected LCs or T cells.[109] The study of T cells during viral infection suggests that HIV infection of DCs induces expression of chemokines in these cells that differentially attract certain T-cell subsets. Results from these studies indicate that infection of CD4+ T cells is not a random event. It seems that expression of the HIV Tat or Nef proteins increases the CXCR4 expression within monocyte-derived DCs, allowing the virus to gain access to a wider range of potential target cells.[93,111,112]

A hypothesis to explain the skin manifestations of HIV infection is derived from the study of LCs and their role in viral pathogenesis. Nonetheless, not all the studies are consistent. Some studies have demonstrated a lack of depletion of T cells, LCs, and DCs in the skin of infected patients (although functionality was not assessed) but an increase in CD8 T cells in the perivascular dermis.[113] On the other hand, studies in macaques have shown that during the acute SIV infection, LC density is reduced in skin, but increased in the lymph nodes (as activated DCs). In later stages of HIV infection (AIDS), the migration of DCs is suppressed, suggesting that changes in DC function at different stages of viral infection modulate replication, dissemination, and persistence of HIV. The depressed DC function during advanced HIV disease might increase the degree of immunosuppression.[114]

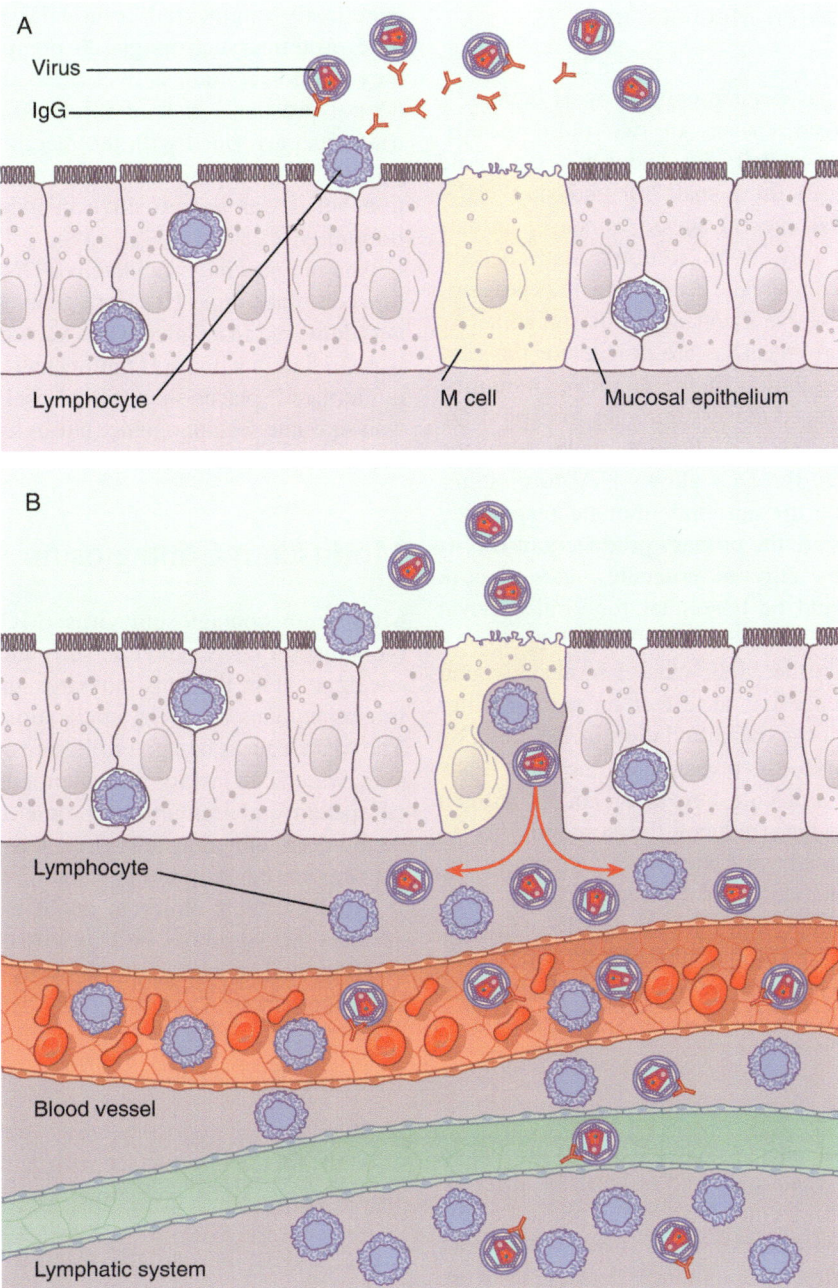

FIG. 20.7. Possible mechanisms of the neutralization of HIV at mucosal surfaces. (A) The transudation of passively infused immunoglobulin G (IgG) from vessels in the submucosa across the epithelium causes it to encounter virus at the mucosal surface. The virus is thus neutralized before it can encounter lymphocytes or M cells associated with the epithelium or underlying lamina propria. (B) IgG circulating in the blood or lymphatic system encounters virus that has been transported across mucosal surfaces by M cells. Antibodies neutralize the virus before it can spread from the site of infection. (From Nabel and Sullivan.[110] Copyright © 2000 Massachusetts Medical Society. All rights reserved.)

Immune Evasion Mechanisms

A simple and useful way to understand viral pathogenesis has been proposed by Hilleman,[115] who categorized viruses in two main groups: (1) those viruses that "hit and run" (e.g., cold viruses), and (2) those that "hit and stay." HIV belongs to the second group, since it infects the host and stays with it until death occurs. Nonetheless, to ensure the persistence of its progeny, it develops effective mechanisms of spread.[115] As specified before, the DCs are crucial for the generation and regulation of the adaptive immunity. HIV has developed clever strategies to exploit the DCs and carry out its replication cycle. Also, the interaction with the DCs allows HIV to disseminate and evade the antiviral immune response.[93] Since the DCs are the primary producers of IFN-α (which is a key antiviral molecule), alterations in these cells could be beneficial for viral survival and evasion.[11] Additionally, HIV is capable of downregulating the MHC class I molecules, and as a consequence has an effect on natural killer cells. HIV reduces the stimulation of NK cells by stabilizing surface expression of the nonclassic MHC class I molecule human leukocyte antigen E (HLA-E), which reduces the susceptibility to NK-cell-mediated cytotoxicity.[116,117] Similarly, the CD8 T lymphocytes (CDL) directed against HIV recognize an important number of HIV epitopes. Mutation of these epitopes alters or abolishes CDL recognition, which results in escape of HIV from the immune system[118] (Table 20.8).

Vaccines

The search for an effective HIV vaccine began more than 15 years ago, and at least 34 different HIV candidate vaccines have begun phase I trials; some have progressed to phase II trials[119] without success. The first recombinant HIV vaccines were genetically engineered from HIV surface envelope proteins, such as gp120 or gp160.[119] Since they do not contain a live virus, these vaccines do not present a risk of infection. One vaccine trial was performed with the recombinant protein gp120. This vaccine stimulated antibody production but it was not effective in inducing cellular immunity.[120,121]

Another vaccine candidate is a DNA preparation that combines three HIV core genes (*gag, pol,* and *nef*) delivered in an adenovirus vector. This vaccine was studied in a phase II multicenter, double-blind, randomized, placebo-controlled trial. The vaccine was safe and immunogenic, but unfortunately was not clinically effective.

Molluscum Contagiosum

Molluscum contagiosum virus (MCV) is a double-stranded DNA poxvirus surrounded by a lipid envelope. It is the only poxvirus that commonly infects humans since the eradication of smallpox. The MCV causes benign proliferative lesions of the skin, which can last for several months in immunocompetent and immunocompromised individuals. Molluscum contagiosum virus has a worldwide distribution but is more prevalent in tropical areas. It usually affects children, but it is also seen in sexually active adults.[122] This virus is the largest of all animal viruses and it is easily visualized on light microscopy.

Immune Response

Molluscum contagiosum virus transmission is through direct skin contact with an infected individual. The MCV infections have a particular location on the epidermis, which makes the virus "safe," almost beyond the reach of the immune system. Lesions in vivo are characterized by a lack of inflammatory cell infiltrates. The typical T or NK cells are usually not found at the base of molluscum lesions. Nonetheless, in the healing stage a mononuclear cell infiltrate is usually observed.[11,123]

Regarding inflammatory mediators, studies have shown that chemokines such as growth regulated oncogene alpha (GRO-α) and IL-8 are inside the molluscum lesions and are released on clearing

TABLE 20.8. Mechanisms of immune evasion in HIV skin and mucosal infection.

- Modulation of the immune activity of dendritic cells
- Downregulation of MHC I molecules and reduced stimulation of NK cells
- Mutations in viral epitopes recognized by CD8 T lymphocytes

of the virus.[124] It is hypothesized that the immune response might be blocked by chemokine antagonists early in MCV infection, and in later stages of the infection the physical barrier (i.e., localization of the epidermis) or the formation of molluscum bodies may prevent detection by the immune system.[122] Some studies indicate that the production of antibodies does not occur in all patients with clinical MCV infection, or the antibody production is not stable during the clinical period.[125]

Immune Evasion Mechanisms

Like many other viruses, MCV uses a variety of methods to escape the immune system. An MCV ORF (designated *mcv148R*) encodes a 104-amino-acid protein with significant homology to β-chemokines such as macrophage inflammatory protein (MIP)-1β. This homology has led investigators to believe that this virally produced chemokine may block the chemotactic activity of the host chemokines.[122] The MCV is also capable of blocking the signal necessary for successful migration of effector cells to the site of infection. Other MCV gene products such as *MC53L* and *MC54L* bind IL-18 with high affinity and prevent IFN-γ production, suggesting that these viral proteins antagonize the development of an inflammatory response to MCV infection in humans.[123–125]

There are no vaccines available to prevent MCV infection, probably because it does not represent an important public health threat and the morbidity is not significant.

Conclusion

The immune response to a viral infection is a complex phenomenon that is specific to each microorganism. Through a highly efficient process of evolution, the viruses have developed several immune evasion mechanisms that allow them to overcome the natural barriers of the skin, cause infection, and establish latency. The delicate balance between the host immune response and viral replication (and dissemination) will eventually dictate the clinical outcome. Factors influencing the host, such as age, immunocompetence, and development of immunity after exposure to the virus, all play a key role in altering this balance.

References

1. Simmons A. Anogenital mucosal immunology and virology. In: Tyring S, ed. Mucosal Immunology and Virology. Singapore: Springer, 2006:7–21.
2. Tigelaar RE, Lewis JM, Bergstresser PR. TCR gamma/delta+ dendritic epidermal T cells as constituents of skin-associated lymphoid tissue. J Invest Dermatol 1990;94(6 suppl):58S-63S.
3. Villa LL. Prophylactic HPV vaccines: reducing the burden of HPV-related diseases. Vaccine 2006;24(suppl 1):S23–8.
4. Medzhitov R, Janeway CA Jr. Decoding the patterns of self and nonself by the innate immune system. Science 2002;296(5566):298–300.
5. Schiller M, et al. Immune response modifiers—mode of action. Exp Dermatol 2006;15(5):331–41.
6. Herbst-Kralovetz M, Pyles R. Toll-like receptors, innate immunity and HSV pathogenesis. Herpes 2006;13(2):37–41.
7. Rouse BT, Gierynska M. Immunity to herpes simplex virus: a hypothesis. Herpes 2001;8(suppl 1): 2A-5A.
8. Serghides L, Vidric M, Watts TH. Approaches to studying costimulation of human antiviral T cell responses: prospects for immunotherapeutic vaccines. Immunol Res 2006;35(1–2):137–50.
9. Rouse BT, Suvas S. Regulatory cells and infectious agents: detentes cordiale and contraire. J Immunol 2004;173(4):2211–5.
10. Cunningham AL, et al. The cycle of human herpes simplex virus infection: virus transport and immune control. J Infect Dis 2006;194(suppl 1):S11–8.
11. Tyring S. Mucocutaneous Manifestations of Viral Diseases, 1st ed. New York: Marcel Dekker, 2002.
12. Ellermann-Eriksen S. Macrophages and cytokines in the early defence against herpes simplex virus. Virol J 2005;2:59.
13. Wald A, et al. Reactivation of genital herpes simplex virus type 2 infection in asymptomatic seropositive persons. N Engl J Med 2000;342(12):844–50.
14. Hukkanen V, et al. Cytokines in experimental herpes simplex virus infection. Int Rev Immunol 2002;21 (4–5):355–71.
15. Theil D, et al. Prevalence of HSV-1 LAT in human trigeminal, geniculate, and vestibular ganglia and its implication for cranial nerve syndromes. Brain Pathol 2001;11(4):408–13.
16. Simmons A, Tscharke D, Speck P. The role of immune mechanisms in control of herpes simplex

virus infection of the peripheral nervous system. Curr Top Microbiol Immunol 1992;179:31–56.

17. Theil D, et al. Latent herpesvirus infection in human trigeminal ganglia causes chronic immune response. Am J Pathol 2003;163(6):2179–84.

18. Duerst RJ, Morrison LA. Innate immunity to herpes simplex virus type 2. Viral Immunol 2003;16(4): 475–90.

19. Luster AD. Chemokines—chemotactic cytokines that mediate inflammation. N Engl J Med 1998;338(7):436–45.

20. Feduchi E, Alonso MA, Carrasco L. Human gamma interferon and tumor necrosis factor exert a synergistic blockade on the replication of herpes simplex virus. J Virol 1989;63(3):1354–9.

21. Guidotti LG, Chisari FV. Noncytolytic control of viral infections by the innate and adaptive immune response. Annu Rev Immunol 2001;19:65–91.

22. Vollstedt S, et al. Interleukin-12– and gamma interferon-dependent innate immunity are essential and sufficient for long-term survival of passively immunized mice infected with herpes simplex virus type 1. J Virol 2001;75(20):9596–600.

23. Leib DA, et al. Interferons regulate the phenotype of wild-type and mutant herpes simplex viruses in vivo. J Exp Med 1999;189(4):663–72.

24. Kanangat S, et al. Herpes simplex virus type 1–mediated up-regulation of IL-12 (p40) mRNA expression. Implications in immunopathogenesis and protection. J Immunol 1996;156(3):1110–6.

25. Kumaraguru U, Rouse BT. The IL-12 response to herpes simplex virus is mainly a paracrine response of reactive inflammatory cells. J Leukoc Biol 2002;72(3):564–70.

26. Bettahi I, et al. Protective immunity to genital herpes simplex virus type 1 and type 2 provided by self-adjuvanting lipopeptides that drive dendritic cell maturation and elicit a polarized Th1 immune response. Viral Immunol 2006;19(2):220–36.

27. Koelle DM, et al. Expression of cutaneous lymphocyte-associated antigen by CD8(+) T cells specific for a skin-tropic virus. J Clin Invest 2002;110(4): 537–48.

28. Arvin AM, et al. Equivalent recognition of a varicella-zoster virus immediate early protein (IE62) and glycoprotein I by cytotoxic T lymphocytes of either CD4+ or CD8+ phenotype. J Immunol 1991;146(1):257–64.

29. Posavad CM, Koelle DM, Corey L. High frequency of CD8+ cytotoxic T-lymphocyte precursors specific for herpes simplex viruses in persons with genital herpes. J Virol 1996;70(11):8165–8.

30. Chen SH, et al. Persistent elevated expression of cytokine transcripts in ganglia latently infected with herpes simplex virus in the absence of ganglionic replication or reactivation. Virology 2000;278(1):207–16.

31. Hayward AR, Read GS, Cosyns M. Herpes simplex virus interferes with monocyte accessory cell function. J Immunol 1993;150(1):190–6.

32. Jones CA, Cunningham AL. Vaccination strategies to prevent genital herpes and neonatal herpes simplex virus (HSV) disease. Herpes 2004;11(1):12–7.

33. Stanberry LR, et al. Glycoprotein-D-adjuvant vaccine to prevent genital herpes. N Engl J Med 2002;347(21):1652–61.

34. Whitacre CC, Reingold SC, O'Looney PA. A gender gap in autoimmunity. Science 1999;283(5406): 1277–8.

35. Ku CC, et al. Varicella-Zoster virus pathogenesis and immunobiology: new concepts emerging from investigations with the SCIDhu mouse model. J Virol 2005;79(5):2651–8.

36. McCrary ML, Severson J, Tyring SK. Varicella zoster virus. J Am Acad Dermatol 1999;41(1):1–14; quiz 15–6.

37. Rockley PF, Tyring SK. Pathophysiology and clinical manifestations of varicella zoster virus infections. Int J Dermatol 1994;33(4):227–32.

38. Quinlivan M, Breuer J. Molecular studies of Varicella zoster virus. Rev Med Virol 2006;16(4):225–50.

39. Wang JP, et al. Varicella-zoster virus activates inflammatory cytokines in human monocytes and macrophages via Toll-like receptor 2. J Virol 2005;79(20):12658–66.

40. Jenkins DE, et al. Interleukin (IL)-10, IL-12, and interferon-gamma production in primary and memory immune responses to varicella-zoster virus. J Infect Dis 1998;178(4):940–8.

41. Arvin AM, et al. Memory cytotoxic T cell responses to viral tegument and regulatory proteins encoded by open reading frames 4, 10, 29, and 62 of varicella-zoster virus. Viral Immunol 2002;15(3):507–16.

42. Gilden DH, Kleinschmidt-DeMasters BK, LaGuardia JJ, et al. Neurologic complications of the reactivation of varicella-zoster virus. N Engl J Med 2000;342(9):635–45.

43. Gary L, Gilden DH, Cohrs RJ. Epigenetic regulation of varicella-zoster virus open reading frames 62 and 63 in latently infected human trigeminal ganglia. J Virol 2006;80(10):4921–6.

44. Hornberger J, Robertus K. Cost-effectiveness of a vaccine to prevent herpes zoster and postherpetic neuralgia in older adults. Ann Intern Med 2006;145(5):317–25.

45. Cohen JI, et al. Varicella-zoster virus ORF4 latency-associated protein is important for establishment of latency. J Virol 2005;79(11):6969–75.

46. Cohen JI, et al. Regions of the varicella-zoster virus open reading frame 63 latency-associated protein important for replication in vitro are also

critical for efficient establishment of latency. J Virol 2005;79(8):5069–77.

47. Sato H, Pesnicak L, Cohen JI. Varicella-zoster virus ORF47 protein kinase, which is required for replication in human T cells, and ORF66 protein kinase, which is expressed during latency, are dispensable for establishment of latency. J Virol 2003;77(20):11180–5.

48. Sato H, Pesnicak L, Cohen JI. Varicella-zoster virus open reading frame 2 encodes a membrane phosphoprotein that is dispensable for viral replication and for establishment of latency. J Virol 2002;76(7):3575–8.

49. Abendroth A, et al. Varicella-zoster virus retains major histocompatibility complex class I proteins in the Golgi compartment of infected cells. J Virol 2001;75(10):4878–88.

50. Abendroth A, et al. Modulation of major histocompatibility class II protein expression by varicella-zoster virus. J Virol 2000;74(4):1900–7.

51. Schmader K. Herpes zoster in older adults. Clin Infect Dis 2001;32(10):1481–6.

52. Mitka M. FDA approves shingles vaccine: herpes zoster vaccine targets older adults. JAMA 2006;296(2):157–8.

53. Arvin A. Aging, immunity, and the varicella-zoster virus. N Engl J Med 2005;352(22):2266–7.

54. Akgul B, Cooke JC, Storey A. HPV-associated skin disease. J Pathol 2006;208(2):165–75.

55. Trottier H, Franco EL. The epidemiology of genital human papillomavirus infection. Vaccine 2006;24(suppl 1):S1–15.

56. Speck LM, Tyring SK. Vaccines for the prevention of human papillomavirus infections. Skin Ther Lett 2006;11(6):1–3.

57. Andersson S, et al. Expression of p16(INK4a) in relation to histopathology and viral load of 'high-risk' HPV types in cervical neoplastic lesions. Eur J Cancer 2006;42(16):2815–20.

58. Ahmed AM, Madkan V, Tyring SK. Human papillomaviruses and genital disease. Dermatol Clin 2006;24(2):157–65, vi.

59. Madkan VK, et al. Sex differences in the transmission, prevention, and disease manifestations of sexually transmitted diseases. Arch Dermatol 2006;142(3):365–70.

60. Palefsky JM, et al. Prevalence and risk factors for human papillomavirus infection of the anal canal in human immunodeficiency virus (HIV)-positive and HIV-negative homosexual men. J Infect Dis 1998;177(2):361–7.

61. Critchlow CW, et al. Effect of HIV infection on the natural history of anal human papillomavirus infection. AIDS 1998;12(10):1177–84.

62. Pinto LA, et al. Cellular immune responses to human papillomavirus (HPV)-16 L1 in healthy volunteers immunized with recombinant HPV-16 L1 virus-like particles. J Infect Dis 2003;188(2):327–38.

63. Ho GY, et al. Natural history of cervicovaginal papillomavirus infection in young women. N Engl J Med 1998;338(7):423–8.

64. Castle PE, et al. A prospective study of age trends in cervical human papillomavirus acquisition and persistence in Guanacaste, Costa Rica. J Infect Dis 2005;191(11):1808–16.

65. Orozco JJ, et al. Humoral immune response recognizes a complex set of epitopes on human papillomavirus type 6 11 capsomers. J Virol 2005;79(15):9503–14.

66. Scott M, Nakagawa M, Moscicki AB. Cell-mediated immune response to human papillomavirus infection. Clin Diagn Lab Immunol 2001;8(2):209–20.

67. Coleman N, et al. Immunological events in regressing genital warts. Am J Clin Pathol 1994;102(6):768–74.

68. Middleton K, et al. Organization of human papillomavirus productive cycle during neoplastic progression provides a basis for selection of diagnostic markers. J Virol 2003;77(19):10186–201.

69. Ghim S, et al. Spontaneously regressing oral papillomas induce systemic antibodies that neutralize canine oral papillomavirus. Exp Mol Pathol 2000;68(3):147–51.

70. Vieira KB, Goldstein DJ, Villa LL. Tumor necrosis factor alpha interferes with the cell cycle of normal and papillomavirus-immortalized human keratinocytes. Cancer Res 1996;56(10):2452–7.

71. Kyo S, et al. Regulation of early gene expression of human papillomavirus type 16 by inflammatory cytokines. Virology 1994;200(1):130–9.

72. Oldak M, et al. Natural cell-mediated cytotoxicity of peripheral blood lymphocytes against target cells transfected with epidermodysplasia verruciformis-specific human papillomavirus type 8 L1 DNA sequences. Int J Mol Med 2004;13(1):187–91.

73. Jimenez-Flores R, et al. High-risk human papilloma virus infection decreases the frequency of dendritic Langerhans' cells in the human female genital tract. Immunology 2006;117(2):220–8.

74. Guess JC, McCance DJ. Decreased migration of Langerhans precursor-like cells in response to human keratinocytes expressing human papillomavirus type 16 E6/E7 is related to reduced macrophage inflammatory protein-3alpha production. J Virol 2005;79(23):14852–62.

75. Fausch SC, et al. Human papillomavirus can escape immune recognition through Langerhans cell phosphoinositide 3–kinase activation. J Immunol 2005;174(11):7172–8.

76. Brimer N, Lyons C, Vande Pol SB. Association of E6AP (UBE3A) with human papillomavirus type 11 E6 protein. Virology 2007;358(2):303–10.

77. Mota F, et al. The antigen-presenting environment in normal and human papillomavirus (HPV)-related premalignant cervical epithelium. Clin Exp Immunol 1999;116(1):33–40.

78. Goodman A, Wilbur DC. Case records of the Massachusetts General Hospital. Weekly clinico-pathological exercises. Case 32–2003. A 37-year-old woman with atypical squamous cells on a Papanicolaou smear. N Engl J Med 2003;349(16):1555–64.

79. Hubert P, et al. E-cadherin-dependent adhesion of dendritic and Langerhans cells to keratinocytes is defective in cervical human papillomavirus-associated (pre)neoplastic lesions. J Pathol 2005;206(3):346–55.

80. Dieu-Nosjean MC, et al. Macrophage inflammatory protein 3alpha is expressed at inflamed epithelial surfaces and is the most potent chemokine known in attracting Langerhans cell precursors. J Exp Med 2000;192(5):705–18.

81. Connor JP, et al. Evaluation of Langerhans' cells in the cervical epithelium of women with cervical intraepithelial neoplasia. Gynecol Oncol 1999;75(1):130–5.

82. Ashrafi GH, et al. Down-regulation of MHC class I is a property common to papillomavirus E5 proteins. Virus Res 2006;120(1–2):208–11.

83. Schapiro F, et al. Golgi alkalinization by the papillomavirus E5 oncoprotein. J Cell Biol 2000;148(2):305–15.

84. Marchetti B, et al. The E5 protein of BPV-4 interacts with the heavy chain of MHC class I and irreversibly retains the MHC complex in the Golgi apparatus. Oncogene 2006;25(15):2254–63.

85. Koutsky LA, et al. A controlled trial of a human papillomavirus type 16 vaccine. N Engl J Med 2002;347(21):1645–51.

86. Roth SD, et al. Characterization of neutralizing epitopes within the major capsid protein of human papillomavirus type 33. Virol J 2006;3:83.

87. Batista FD, Neuberger MS. B cells extract and present immobilized antigen: implications for affinity discrimination. EMBO J 2000;19(4):513–20.

88. Chen XS, et al. Structure of small virus-like particles assembled from the L1 protein of human papillomavirus 16. Mol Cell 2000;5(3):557–67.

89. Stanley M. Immune responses to human papillomavirus. Vaccine 2006;24(suppl 1):S16–22.

90. Tyring SK. Immune-response modifiers: a new paradigm in the treatment of human papillomavirus. Curr Ther Res Clin Exp 2000;61:584–96.

91. Neeper MP, Hofmann KJ, Jansen KU. Expression of the major capsid protein of human papillomavirus type 11 in Saccharomyces cerevisae. Gene 1996;180(1–2):1–6.

92. http://data.unaids.org/pub/globalreport/2006/2006_gr-executivesummary_en.pdf, 2006.

93. Qin S, et al. The chemokine receptors CXCR3 and CCR5 mark subsets of T cells associated with certain inflammatory reactions. J Clin Invest 1998;101(4):746–54.

94. Quinn TC, Overbaugh J. HIV/AIDS in women: an expanding epidemic. Science 2005;308(5728):1582–3.

95. Pope M, Haase AT. Transmission, acute HIV-1 infection and the quest for strategies to prevent infection. Nat Med 2003;9(7):847–52.

96. Ray SC, Quinn TC. Sex and the genetic diversity of HIV-1. Nat Med 2000;6(1):23–5.

97. Steinman RM, et al. The interaction of immunodeficiency viruses with dendritic cells. Curr Top Microbiol Immunol 2003;276:1–30.

98. Cavrois M, et al. Human immunodeficiency virus fusion to dendritic cells declines as cells mature. J Virol 2006;80(4):1992–9.

99. Banchereau J, Steinman RM. Dendritic cells and the control of immunity. Nature 1998;392(6673):245–52.

100. Hu J, Gardner MB, Miller CJ. Simian immunodeficiency virus rapidly penetrates the cervicovaginal mucosa after intravaginal inoculation and infects intraepithelial dendritic cells. J Virol 2000;74(13):6087–95.

101. Kawamura T, et al. R5 HIV productively infects Langerhans cells, and infection levels are regulated by compound CCR5 polymorphisms. Proc Natl Acad Sci USA 2003;100(14):8401–6.

102. Levy JA. Infection by human immunodeficiency virus—CD4 is not enough. N Engl J Med 1996;335(20):1528–30.

103. Berger EA, Murphy PM, Farber JM. Chemokine receptors as HIV-1 coreceptors: roles in viral entry, tropism, and disease. Annu Rev Immunol 1999;17:657–700.

104. Blauvelt A, et al. Productive infection of dendritic cells by HIV-1 and their ability to capture virus are mediated through separate pathways. J Clin Invest 1997;100(8):2043–53.

105. Kawamura T, et al. Decreased stimulation of CD4+ T cell proliferation and IL-2 production by highly enriched populations of HIV-infected dendritic cells. J Immunol 2003;170(8):4260–6.

106. Kawamura T, et al. Candidate microbicides block HIV-1 infection of human immature Langerhans cells within epithelial tissue explants. J Exp Med 2000;192(10):1491–500.

107. Bakri Y, et al. The maturation of dendritic cells results in postintegration inhibition of HIV-1 replication. J Immunol 2001;166(6):3780–8.

108. Granelli-Piperno A, et al. Immature dendritic cells selectively replicate macrophagetropic (M-tropic) human immunodeficiency virus type 1, while

mature cells efficiently transmit both M- and T-tropic virus to T cells. J Virol 1998;72(4):2733–7.

109. Sugaya M, et al. HIV-infected Langerhans cells preferentially transmit virus to proliferating autologous CD4+ memory T cells located within Langerhans cell-T cell clusters. J Immunol 2004;172(4):2219–24.

110. Nabel GJ, Sullivan NJ. Antibodies and resistance to natural HIV infection. N Engl J Med 2000;343(17):1263–5.

111. Bleul CC, et al. The HIV coreceptors CXCR4 and CCR5 are differentially expressed and regulated on human T lymphocytes. Proc Natl Acad Sci USA 1997;94(5):1925–30.

112. Quaranta MG, et al. HIV-1 Nef induces dendritic cell differentiation: a possible mechanism of uninfected CD4(+) T cell activation. Exp Cell Res 2002;275(2):243–54.

113. Galhardo MC, et al. Normal skin of HIV-infected individuals contains increased numbers of dermal CD8 T cells and normal numbers of Langerhans cells. Braz J Med Biol Res 2004;37(5):745–53.

114. Barratt-Boyes SM, Zimmer MI, Harshyne L. Changes in dendritic cell migration and activation during SIV infection suggest a role in initial viral spread and eventual immunosuppression. J Med Primatol 2002;31(4–5):186–93.

115. Hilleman MR. Strategies and mechanisms for host and pathogen survival in acute and persistent viral infections. Proc Natl Acad Sci USA 2004;101(suppl 2):14560–6.

116. Nattermann J, et al. HIV-1 infection leads to increased HLA-E expression resulting in impaired function of natural killer cells. Antivir Ther 2005;10(1):95–107.

117. Wooden SL, et al. Cutting edge: HLA-E binds a peptide derived from the ATP-binding cassette transporter multidrug resistance-associated protein 7 and inhibits NK cell-mediated lysis. J Immunol 2005;175(3):1383–7.

118. Klenerman P, Wu Y, Phillips R. HIV: current opinion in escapology. Curr Opin Microbiol 2002;5(4):408–13.

119. Wu JJ, et al. Vaccines and immunotherapies for the prevention of infectious diseases having cutaneous manifestations. J Am Acad Dermatol 2004;50(4):495–528; quiz 529–32.

120. McCarthy M. HIV vaccine fails in phase 3 trial. Lancet 2003;361(9359):755–6.

121. Evans TG, et al. A canarypox vaccine expressing multiple human immunodeficiency virus type 1 genes given alone or with rgp120 elicits broad and durable CD8+ cytotoxic T lymphocyte responses in seronegative volunteers. J Infect Dis 1999;180(2):290–8.

122. Krathwohl MD, et al. Functional characterization of the C—C chemokine-like molecules encoded by molluscum contagiosum virus types 1 and 2. Proc Natl Acad Sci USA 1997;94(18):9875–80.

123. Viac J, Chardonnet Y. Immunocompetent cells and epithelial cell modifications in molluscum contagiosum. J Cutan Pathol 1990;17(4):202–5.

124. Xiang Y, Moss B. IL-18 binding and inhibition of interferon gamma induction by human poxvirus-encoded proteins. Proc Natl Acad Sci USA 1999;96(20):11537–42.

125. Watanabe T, et al. Antibodies to molluscum contagiosum virus in the general population and susceptible patients. Arch Dermatol 2000;136(12):1518–22.

21
HIV Disease and AIDS

Andrew Blauvelt

Key Points

- The two major glycoprotein subunits on the HIV envelope that interact with target cell surface receptors are gp120 and gp41.
- CD4, as well as co-receptors, on the target cell surface interacts with gp120 to initiate infection.
- The co-receptor used by HIV on T cell targets is primarily CXCR4.
- The co-receptor used by HIV on macrophage targets is primarily CCR5.
- Mucocutaneous manifestations of HIV can be the result of primary infection, but are usually due to opportunistic infections, neoplasia, or various inflammatory conditions.
- Highly active antiretroviral therapy (HAART) includes inhibitors of viral reverse transcriptase, protease, and integrase, as well as blockers of fusion and co-receptors (e.g., CCR5).

Human immunodeficiency virus (HIV) infection continues to be a major pandemic problem, with current estimates of 39.5 million people living with HIV in 2006, 4.3 million newly infected individuals in 2006, and 2.9 million deaths due to AIDS in 2006 worldwide.[1] The widespread use of highly active antiretroviral therapy (HAART), however, over the past 10 years in industrialized nations has provided hope in the fight against HIV disease, in that marked clinical improvement with concomitant drops in death rates have been observed in the majority of individuals receiving this combination drug regimen. The hopes generated by the success of HAART are tempered by the fact that most HIV-infected individuals in the world will never have access to these drugs because of socioeconomic reasons. Thus, the ultimate hope in the war against HIV disease remains a universally accepted vaccine, that is, a vaccine that is safe, inexpensive, easy to administer, and effective. With this goal in mind, understanding basic virologic and immunologic mechanisms in the pathogenesis of HIV disease continues to be of critical importance.

The HIV Life Cycle

Human immunodeficiency virus is a retrovirus. This means that the basic genetic material encoded by HIV is RNA, and that the virus contains an enzyme, reverse transcriptase, which is able to convert viral RNA to viral DNA. Double-stranded viral RNA is contained within the core of the virus, and is immediately surrounded by the viral capsid, which is surrounded by the viral envelope. The viral envelope, which contains two major glycoprotein subunits (gp120 and gp41), interacts with cell-surface receptors on target cells to initiate infection.

The life cycle of HIV begins with viral entry into a new target cell and ends with release of new virions from the infected cell. The first event involves binding of gp120, the major envelope protein of HIV, with the molecule CD4 on the surface of target cells. CD4 extends from the cell membrane, and it is believed that CD4–gp120 interactions induce conformational changes that bring virus close to the cell membrane, and subsequently allows for another region of gp120 to interact with and bind to an HIV co-receptor embedded in the cell membrane.[2] HIV co-receptors are seven-transmembrane-domain molecules, members of the G-protein–coupled receptor family, and normally function as chemokine receptors, helping to mediate chemotaxis during inflammatory processes. The two major HIV co-receptors for HIV are CCR5[3–5] and CXCR4,[6] although several other minor HIV co-receptors with similar structure and function have also been described.[7] Viruses that are predominantly macrophage-tropic use CCR5 for entry (labeled R5 viruses), whereas viruses that are predominantly T-cell-tropic use CXCR4 for entry (labeled X4 viruses). Determination for co-receptor usage is dictated by the amino acid sequence in the co-receptor binding region of gp120. Binding of gp120 to an HIV co-receptor then leads to activation of gp41, the other major envelope glycoprotein, and fusion of the viral envelope with the cell membrane.[2] Following fusion, viral RNA is released into the cytoplasm of the cell. Detailed knowledge of these events has been greatly facilitated by the recent discoveries of HIV co-receptors and by identification of the crystal structures of gp41 and gp120.[8,9] Importantly, these advances in basic research allow for better understanding of HIV disease pathogenesis and have led to design of new therapeutic strategies aimed at blocking viral entry.

Viral RNA is reverse transcribed to DNA in the cytoplasm by the viral enzyme reverse transcriptase. Much of the genetic variability and the development of drug-resistant HIV strains can be attributed to errors introduced into the HIV genome during reverse transcription. Proviral DNA is then transported to the nucleus, where it becomes incorporated into the host genome with the aid of the viral enzyme integrase. Host cellular machinery, in combination with the viral proteins Tat and Rev, drive viral transcription. In cytoplasm, viral messenger RNA (mRNA) is then translated into viral proteins, and viral capsids form around paired strands of viral RNA. Capsids obtain outer envelopes upon budding from cell membranes, which are studded with the viral glycoproteins gp120 and gp41. The viral protease enzyme orchestrates release of virions from infected cell membranes. Currently available antiretroviral drugs were designed to specifically inhibit these various steps in the HIV life cycle.

Virologic, Immunologic, and Clinical Features of HIV Disease

Early-Stage HIV Disease

Langerhans' Cells as Initial Targets for HIV Following Sexual Exposure to Virus

Langerhans' cells are antigen-presenting cells found within skin and in oral, vaginal, cervical, and anal epithelial layers, and normally function as outposts of the immune system within these tissues.[10–13] Here, they capture surface antigens and emigrate from epithelium to draining lymph nodes via afferent lymphatics. Langerhans' cells then present processed antigenic peptides to T cells, thereby leading to antigen-specific T-cell activation. Intraepithelial Langerhans cells' have been shown to be the first cells infected following vaginal exposure to simian immunodeficiency virus (SIV) in a rhesus macaque model of primary HIV infection.[14] Following infection, Langerhans cells' are believed to migrate from mucosal surfaces to draining lymph nodes via afferent lymphatics, where they transmit HIV to paracortical activated CD4+ T cells, thus establishing infection within the lymph node compartment (Fig. 21.1).[15,16]

In situ, immature Langerhans' cells express CD4[17,18] and are CCR5+CXCR4−.[13,18,19] Epithelial cells are CD4− and HIV co-receptor negative, and

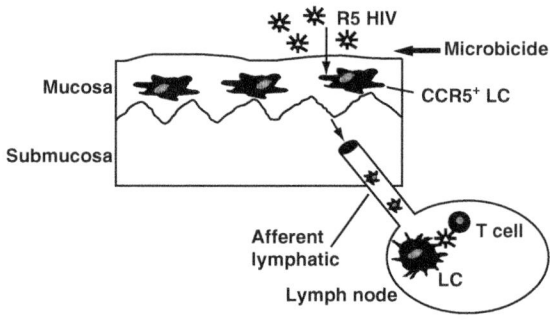

FIG. 21.1. Schematic illustration showing the location of immature Langerhans' cells (LC) within genital mucosal epithelium, their ability to emigrate from tissue to draining lymph nodes following contact with antigen, and the fact that they can interact with and transmit HIV infection to CD4+ T cells. Expression of surface CCR5, the major co-receptor for R5 HIV strains, on Langerhans cells may allow selective sexual transmission of R5 (i.e., macrophage-tropic) viruses

are thus not predicted to be infectable with HIV. This differential surface expression of CCR5 and CXCR4 may explain why macrophage-tropic, or R5 type, viruses are the dominant type of HIV to be sexually transmitted (90% to 95% of cases).[20,21] In vitro, human immature Langerhans' cells are much more easily infected by R5 viruses when compared to X4 viruses, and cells can be completely protected from infection by blocking CCR5.[22–26] The importance of CCR5 in initiating primary HIV infection is underscored by the fact that individuals who have homozygous deletion of their *CCR5* gene are relatively protected from becoming infected by HIV despite numerous exposures.[27–30]

Development of Topical Microbicides to Prevent Sexual Transmission of HIV

In the absence of a prophylactic vaccine against HIV, health measures designed to limit the numbers of new cases of sexually transmitted HIV infection have included abstinence and condom use. Unfortunately, these methods can be impractical in certain countries and social situations where women are not empowered to influence decisions regarding sexual intercourse.[31] Thus, additional means to block sexual transmission of HIV are urgently needed. The use of topical microbicides, drugs or compounds that can be applied to genital tissue prior to sexual intercourse and potentially block sexual transmission of HIV, is being actively investigated.[32]

Most compounds that have been put forth as potential microbicides, including nonoxynol-9, BufferGel, cyanovirin, C31G, and cellulose acetate phthalate, function in a nonspecific virucidal manner when tested in the laboratory. Limitations that hinder the clinical usefulness of these compounds include their potential toxicity to mucosal epithelial cells following sustained use,[33,34] and the requirement that they need to be present within the vaginal vault at the time of HIV exposure. Interestingly, PSC-RANTES (*r*egulated on *a*ctivation, *n*ormal *T*-cell *e*xpressed and *s*ecreted), a CCR5 inhibitor, has the advantages over nonspecific virucidal compounds in that (1) it is not toxic to Langerhans' cells and other cells within epithelial tissue[24,35]; (2) it can lead to rapid down-modulation of CCR5 on cell surfaces for up to 24 hours,[36] potentially allowing it to be used safely many hours before sexual intercourse; and (3) it has been shown to completely protect female

rhesus macaques from SHIV simian-human immunodeficiency virus infection when used topically 15 minutes prior to intravaginal exposure to virus.[35] Of note, initial microbicide acceptability studies in populations of at-risk women have suggested that an effective topical microbicide would likely be used by women,[37,38] potentially making a major impact on improving world health. Further testing of PSC-RANTES as well as other potential topical microbicides to block sexually transmitted HIV infection is urgently needed.

Immunologic Features and Cutaneous Manifestations of Acute Primary HIV Infection

A flu-like illness often develops 2 to 4 weeks following exposure to HIV (Table 21.1).[39–41] The signs and symptoms are often nonspecific. Rash occurs in a relatively high percentage of patients (50% to 75%). Lesions are described as nonpruritic erythematous macules and papules, with a predilection for the upper trunk, head, and neck (Fig. 21.2). The cutaneous eruption is probably caused by infiltration of anti–HIV-specific CD8[+] cytotoxic lymphocytes, as has been shown in the skin of rhesus macaques during acute infection with SIV.[42] Painful oral ulcers are also common in primary HIV infection. Because of the nonspecific nature of these signs and symptoms, clinical diagnosis of acute HIV infection requires a high index of suspicion. Accordingly, it is now suggested that all individuals with known or suspected risk factors for acquiring HIV, who present with rash and fever, should be questioned in detail about possible HIV exposures and have laboratory tests to investigate this possibility.[39]

Characteristically, HIV plasma viremia is high during this acute syndrome, with plasma usually containing >100,000 copies of HIV RNA/mL as measured by standard viral load assays, whereas rou-

TABLE 21.1. Signs and symptoms of primary HIV infection.

Common	Uncommon
Fever (95%)*	Diarrhea (30%)
Lymphadenopathy (75%)	Headache (30%)
Pharyngitis (70%)	Nausea/vomiting (25%)
Rash/oral ulcers (70%)	Hepatosplenomegaly (15%)
Myalgia/arthralgia (55%)	Thrush (10%)
	Neurologic symptoms (10%)

*Approximate incidence.

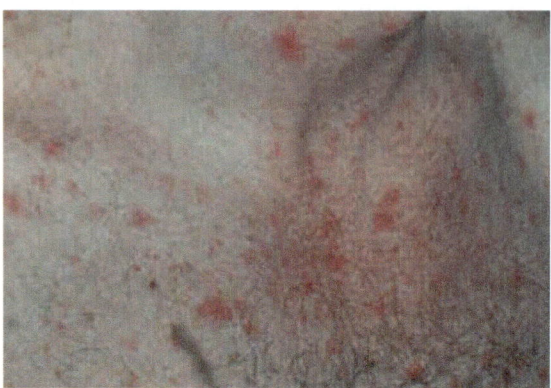

FIG. 21.2. Rash of primary HIV infection. Lesions are characteristically erythematous macules involving the head, neck, and upper trunk. Oral ulcers are also common

tine HIV antibody tests are negative (Fig. 21.3).[39] The combination of a high viral load and no HIV-specific antibodies confirms the diagnosis of primary HIV infection. Signs and symptoms resolve and plasma viremia gradually drops as cellular and humoral immune responses are initiated to control initial infection.[39,41] HIV antibody tests usually become positive within 3 months following infection, although this interval may be prolonged in unusual cases.

Most clinicians and HIV researchers promote the widespread use of antiretroviral therapy at the earliest possible time point following diagnosis of acute HIV infection.[43,44] There are several pieces of data that support this recommendation. First, early use of HAART (often defined as the use of zidovudine, a second reverse-transcriptase inhibitor, and a protease inhibitor) most likely decreases the "viral set point"[45]—the level of plasma viremia following resolution of acute HIV infection. This level of plasma viremia is linked with the ultimate prognosis for a given HIV-infected individual.[39] Second, HAART has been shown to preserve both number and function of anti–HIV-specific CD4+ and CD8+ T cells, believed to be critical in the partial, albeit incomplete, control of HIV replication.[45] Third, early HAART likely blunts loss of antigen-specific memory T cells,[46] which are preferentially lost in early HIV disease. Preservation of cellular immunity to common antigens would be predicted to prevent opportunistic infections. The drawbacks of treatment with HAART in early HIV disease include the possible emergence of drug-resistant strains of HIV, the high cost of medications, and drug-related side effects.[44,47]

Middle-Stage HIV Disease

Virologic and Immunologic Features that Determine Progression to AIDS

Following resolution of acute infection, HIV-infected individuals often go into a prolonged period without

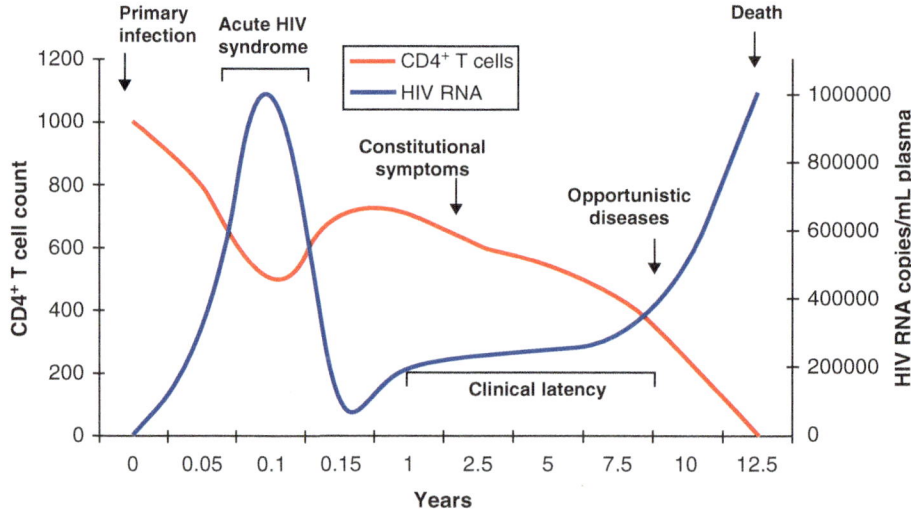

FIG. 21.3. Natural course of HIV disease. Potent highly active antiretroviral therapy (HAART) has a strong influence on this course by prolonging life for HIV-infected individuals

clinical symptoms of HIV disease—the clinical latency period. Although plasma viremia is usually low or undetectable during this asymptomatic stage, viral replication continually occurs unabated within lymph nodes.[48] CD4+ T cell counts during this period range between 200 and 500/μL, with a slow gradual decline often observed (Fig. 21.3). The balance between control of viral replication/preservation of immune function and increased viral replication/loss of immune function is dictated by numerous factors.[49]

The progression to AIDS is often associated with viral mutations that enable HIV to more efficiently infect CD4+ T cells.[50] Specifically, mutations typically develop in the viral envelope protein gp120 that allow HIV to utilize CXCR4 as a co-receptor for cell entry. These viruses, termed X4 viruses, are more cytopathic than macrophage-tropic R5 viruses (i.e., viruses that utilize CCR5 as an HIV co-receptor). The development of X4 viruses is linked to progressive loss of CD4+ T cells and the development of opportunistic disease.[50] Importantly, the future design of synthetic chemokines tailored to block CXCR4 may prevent the progression to AIDS in HIV-infected individuals.

Deletions or polymorphisms in genes encoding HIV co-receptors (i.e., chemokine receptors) and their ligands (i.e., chemokines) have been associated with delayed HIV disease progression. For example, individuals with a particular polymorphism in their *SDF-1* gene, the gene that encodes for the natural chemokine ligand of CXCR4, progress to AIDS less quickly than individuals without this particular polymorphism.[51] Functional studies on the two forms of SDF-1 protein suggest that the variant form is degraded less rapidly than the wild-type form, and would therefore be predicted to have more prolonged binding periods with CXCR4. In addition, heterozygous mutations of the *CCR5* gene or its promoters as well as gene duplications in CCR5 ligands prolong the onset of AIDS, presumably by limiting infection and spread of macrophage-tropic viruses early in HIV disease.[28,52–54]

Cutaneous Manifestations of Middle-Stage HIV Disease

Human immunodeficiency virus–infected individuals with CD4+ T-cell counts in the 200 to 500/μL range are mostly asymptomatic, although this certainly is not always true. Signs and symptoms that belie underlying HIV infection often manifest as cutaneous diseases during this phase.[55] In particular, herpes zoster and treatment-resistant seborrheic dermatitis in young persons should alert clinicians to the possibility of coexisting HIV infection and lead to questioning about known HIV risk factors. Zoster involving multiple dermatomes, zoster involving the head and neck, and prolonged healing of lesions are distinct clues to possible underlying immunosuppression, and thus are more common in HIV-infected individuals. Subtle loss of antigen-specific cell-mediated immunity is believed to be the mechanism by which these diseases occur. Although not limited to patients with particular CD4+ T-cell counts, diagnosis of any sexual transmitted disease (syphilis, condyloma, herpes simplex, etc.) should also prompt questioning about possible concomitant HIV infection.

Acute illnesses, such as herpes simplex reactivation and herpes zoster, lead to tissue inflammation, immune activation, and increases in HIV plasma viremia.[49] The basis for increased plasma viremia is most likely multifactorial. Inflammatory cytokines released during acute inflammation or infection can directly lead to enhanced viral replication within HIV-infected cells. As well, immune activation and cytokine production can stimulate HIV infection of previously uninfected CD4+ T cells. Thus, there is a strong basis for both preventing and aggressively treating all acute infections and illnesses in HIV-infected individuals. Of note, immunizations, which lead to transient activation of the immune system, also trigger transient increases in HIV plasma viremia.[49] The benefits, however, of protecting against future illnesses accorded by immunizations outweigh any potential harm caused by them.

Late-Stage HIV Disease, or AIDS

Virologic and Immunologic Features of AIDS

Viruses of all types (T-cell-tropic, macrophage-tropic, dual-tropic) can be isolated from most AIDS patients.[50] Plasma viremia is also usually high in untreated patients (Fig. 21.3). In addition, destruction of lymph node architecture also contributes to high viral loads in blood. This occurs because many infectious HIV virions previously trapped by follicular dendritic cells are released into blood following breakdown of lymphoid tissue.[48] Viral loads can drop dramatically in AIDS patients who are placed on HAART for the first time,[56,57] although it can be difficult for AIDS patients to get to the point where plasma viremia is undetectable.

Immune defects in advanced-stage HIV disease are profound.[49] CD4+ T-cell counts are less than 200/μL by definition, with preferentially loss of the memory subset of T cells. B cells are activated with consequent hypergammaglobulinemia. Macrophages demonstrate numerous defects. Surprisingly, most studies show that dendritic cell function, including epidermal Langerhans' cell function, remains relatively intact, even in late-stage AIDS patients.[58–61] Peripheral blood mononuclear cells display abnormal cytokine secretion profiles upon stimulation.[49] Predominantly, there is loss of interleukin-2 (IL-2) production, a key cytokine involved in normal T-cell function. Thus, by numerous mechanisms, immune dysregulation in HIV-infected individuals leads to loss of antigen-specific cell-mediated immunity and the development of opportunistic infections. HAART often leads to increases in CD4+ T-cell counts for AIDS patients, although increases do not always occur and are usually only partial.[62,63]

Cutaneous Manifestations of AIDS

Kaposi's Sarcoma

Kaposi's sarcoma (KS) is the most common neoplasm in HIV-infected individuals.[64] Most investigators now believe KS is not a true malignancy, but rather a multicentric proliferative process driven by inflammation and immune dysregulation. In a landmark study from 1994, the husband-and-wife research team of Chang and Moore discovered KS-associated herpesvirus (KSHV), also known as human herpesvirus 8, within lesions of AIDS-associated KS.[65] Subsequently, KSHV was identified in all cases of KS, regardless of HIV status or tissue source.[66] In serologic studies, the presence of KSHV-specific antibodies was shown to correlate with subsequent risk for developing KS. For instance, KSHV seroprevalence is high in gay men, central Africans, and southern Italians,[67,68]—all groups of people in whom the incidence of KS is relatively high regardless of HIV status. Although previous

infection with KSHV is believed to be absolutely required for development of KS, additional factors undoubtedly play roles in KS pathogenesis, including loss of KSHV-specific cell-mediated immune immunity and inflammatory cytokines.[69]

Interestingly, KSHV infects all KS tumor spindle cells.[70] However, only a small number of cells (<2%) within tumors are productively infected with KSHV, demonstrating virions budding from cells upon electron microscopy; the remaining cells are latently infected with virus, that is, they contain viral DNA within nuclei of infected cells but do not produce virions.[71] Most likely, viral genes that are expressed in latently infected cells contribute to the abnormal spindle cell growth observed in KS lesions.[72–74] The precise mechanisms by which KSHV triggers and maintains KS are the current focus of many research teams.

The fact that most KS spindle cells are latently, and not lytically, infected with KSHV means that antiherpesviral therapy is unlikely to be efficacious for established KS. All known drugs in this class, including acyclovir and its derivatives foscarnet, cidofovir, and ganciclovir, act to block active viral replication; they specifically do not have effects on cells latently infected with herpesvirus. Alternatively, antiherpesviral therapy may be extremely useful in the prevention of KS in KSHV-infected individuals.[69] Specifically, all KSHV+HIV+ persons and any KSHV+ individuals undergoing organ transplantation would be candidates for prophylactic antiherpesviral therapy, with the hopes of aborting KSHV infection within dermis and the subsequent development of KS. Incredibly, 30% to 40% of AIDS patients have remissions of KS when placed on HAART.[75,76] This is most likely due to improved KSHV-specific immune function and decreases in HIV-associated inflammatory cytokines that directly stimulate KS spindle cell growth. Other treatments for KS depend on whether disease is localized or widespread, and include local destructive therapy, radiation therapy, interferon-α, and chemotherapy (e.g., paclitaxel).[77]

Other Viral Infections

Loss of cell-mediated immunity predisposes to viral infections. Infection with herpes simplex virus types 1 and 2 or varicella-zoster virus can produce slow-healing painful cutaneous ulcerations, as well as chronic verrucous or crusted lesions in AIDS patients.[55] Treatment and prophylaxis with acyclovir or one of its derivatives is indicated, although clinicians should be wary of the development of acyclovir-resistant strains of these viruses in the setting of AIDS. Lytic replication of Epstein-Barr virus within lingual epithelial cells produces oral hairy leukoplakia.[55] This manifests as white corrugated adherent plaques on the lateral aspects of the tongue. Human papillomavirus and molluscum contagiosum virus infections can be particularly aggressive and treatment-resistant in individuals with AIDS.[55] Of note, anogenital cancer, like cervical cancer, has been linked to human papillomavirus infection and occurs more commonly in HIV-infected persons compared to the general population.[78]

Cutaneous viral infections, like all other cutaneous manifestations of HIV disease, are best treated by first ensuring that patients are on proper HAART, which completely suppresses HIV plasma viremia. Second, specific treatment as dictated by the clinical disease, biopsy findings, and culture results should be instituted. As learned in the era prior to HAART, specific treatment of AIDS-associated dermatoses is unlikely to be optimally effective in face of uncontrolled HIV plasma viremia and continued destruction of the immune system.

Fungal Infections

Loss of cell-mediated immunity also predisposes to fungal infections. Candidiasis is the most common mucocutaneous manifestation of AIDS, often presenting as friable nonadherent white plaques within oral and vaginal mucosa.[55] Esophageal candidiasis is a particularly painful complication and can lead to impaired swallowing. Treatment and prophylaxis with systemic antifungals is often indicated. Dermatophytosis can also be particularly widespread and difficult to treat.[55] Although it is not as common now, dermatologic involvement has been reported in 10% to 15% of AIDS patients with systemic cryptococcosis or histoplasmosis.[79,80] Cutaneous cryptococcosis in this setting usually presents as papules and nodules with central umbilication (i.e., molluscum-like) or necrosis. Histoplasmosis can present with acneiform papules pustules, which often involve the face. As above, fungal infections are best managed by optimizing HAART, making accurate diagnoses, and instituting specific antifungal therapy.

Other Cutaneous Diseases

Eosinophilic folliculitis is an extremely common cutaneous manifestation of AIDS. Patients present with intensely pruritic urticarial papules surmounted by tiny central vesicles (Fig. 21.4A).[81] This morphology may not be preserved at the time of presentation due to scratching of lesions, in which case the lesions appear as excoriated papules or small round scars. Lesions are

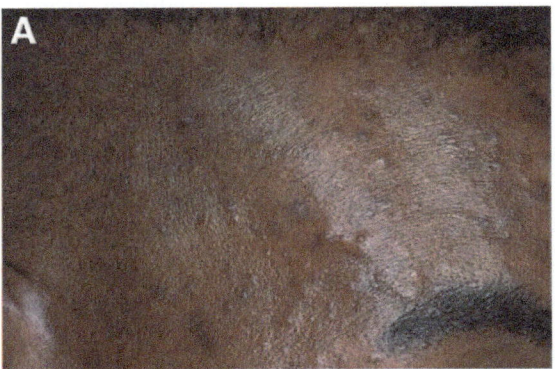
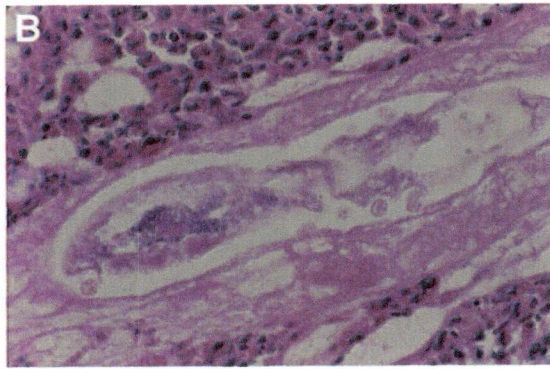

Fig. 21.4. (A) Typical urticarial papules of eosinophilic folliculitis. (B) High-power histologic view of an early lesion of eosinophilic folliculitis. *Demodex* mites are characteristically seen within centers of affected hair follicles surrounded by sheets of eosinophils. Excoriated or older lesions show a mixed infiltrate and will not demonstrate mites

distributed on the face, neck, and upper chest and back. In early nonexcoriated lesions, *Demodex* mites are observed within hair follicles at the center of heavy eosinophilic infiltrates (Fig. 21.4B).[82] In older or excoriated lesions, mites are not present and the inflammation is more mixed. For these reasons, an aberrant immune response directed against *Demodex* mites is believed to trigger eosinophilic folliculitis.[83] Chronic once-daily use of topical permethrin will eventually abort new lesion formation,[82] whereas pruritus and acute eosinophilic inflammation usually respond to ultraviolet light therapy or to potent topical or low-dose systemic corticosteroids.[81,83]

Drug reactions, especially induced by trimetho-prim-sulfamethoxazole, are common in advanced-stage HIV disease; particularly severe reactions, like Stevens-Johnson syndrome and toxic epidermal necrosis, also occur with increased frequency in these patients.[84] Importantly, the antiretro-viral drug nevirapine has been associated with Stevens-Johnson syndrome (Fig. 21.5), occurring in up to 8% of patients treated with this drug.[85] Additionally, patients taking protease inhibitors may develop a syndrome with clinical features resembling Cushing's disease. These individuals have central fat deposition ("buffalo humps," protuberant abdomens, gynecomastia), wasting of facial fat and peripheral fat of the arms and legs, hypertriglyceridemia, glucose intolerance, and increased risk for myocardial infarction (Fig. 21.6).[86–88] Unlike in Cushing's disease, the pituitary axis is unaffected. Facial wasting may be

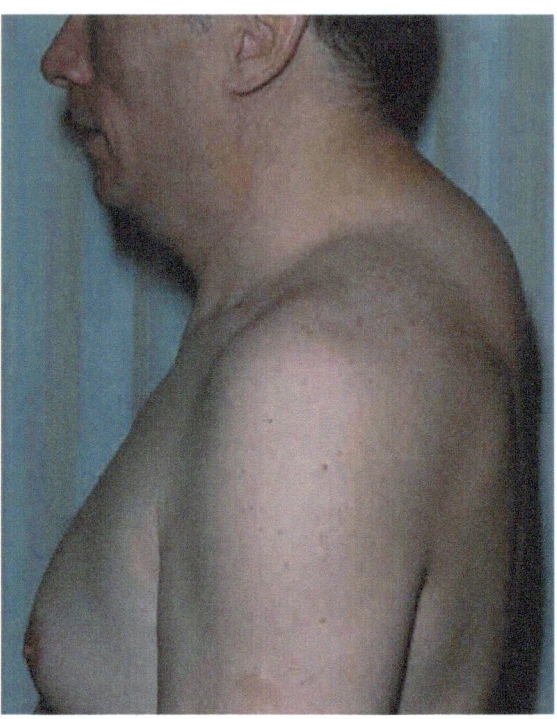

FIG. 21.6. Protease inhibitor-induced lipodystrophy. "Buffalo hump" along with other fat accumulations centrally (i.e., in breast and abdomen) occurs in combination with loss of fat on the face and extremities

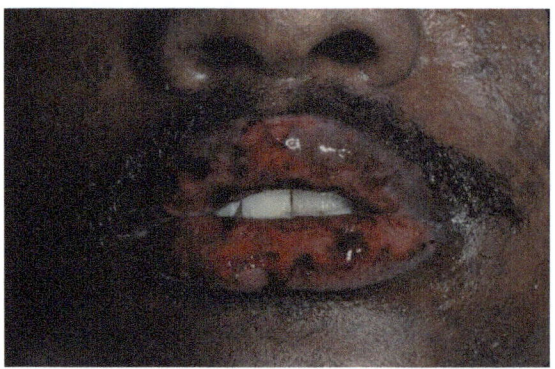

FIG. 21.5. Nevirapine-induced Stevens-Johnson syndrome. This side effect occurs in approximately 8% of individuals treated with this drug

treated by switching drug regimens that have less lipodystrophic effects and by injection of filler substances.[89,90] Other HAART-associated cutaneous drug reactions have also been reported, including abacavir hypersensitivity, zidovudine-associated hyperpigmentation of the nails, and retinoid-like effects due to protease inhibitors (Table 21.2).[91] The pathogenic basis for all of these drug reactions occurring in HIV-infected individuals is unclear.

TABLE 21.2. Major cutaneous manifestations of highly active antiretroviral therapy (HAART).

Hyperpigmentation due to zidovudine
Hypersensitivity due to abacavir
Stevens-Johnson syndrome due to nevirapine
Lipodystrophy due to indinavir, ritonavir, stavudine, or zidovudine
Retinoid-like effects due to indinavir
Injection site reactions to enfuvirtide
Morbilliform eruptions to most drugs

Conclusion

Basic science advances in immunology and virology have led to key advances in the care and management of HIV-infected individuals. For instance, knowledge of the structure and function of the viral proteins and life cycle of HIV has led to the development of novel antiretroviral medications. As well, increased understanding of the initial and later stages of HIV disease through epidemiologic, clinical, immunologic, and genetic studies has provided a solid basis for using these medications in a proper manner. As has been consistently demonstrated in the past, therapeutic advances to combat HIV disease in the future are likely to be based on discoveries in basic virology, biology, and immunology. As evidenced by numerous cutaneous manifestations that can occur throughout the course of HIV disease, the dermatologist remains an important member of the team caring for infected individuals.

References

1. UNAIDS. AIDS epidemic update. World Health Organization, December 2006.
2. Chan DC, Kim PS. HIV entry and its inhibition. Cell 1998;93:681–4.
3. Alkhatib G, Combadiere C, Broder CC, et al. CC CKR5: a RANTES, MIP-1a, MIP-1b receptor as a fusion cofactor for macrophage-tropic HIV-1. Science 1996;272:1955–8.
4. Choe H, Farzan M, Sun Y, et al. The beta-chemokine receptors CCR3 and CCR5 facilitate infection by primary HIV-1 isolates. Cell 1996;85:1135–48.
5. Deng H, Liu R, Ellmeier W, et al. Identification of a major co-receptor for primary isolates of HIV-1. Nature 1996;381:661–6.
6. Feng Y, Broder CC, Kennedy PE, Berger EA. HIV-1 entry cofactor: functional cDNA cloning of a seven-transmembrane, G protein-coupled receptor. Science 1996;272:872–7.
7. Littman DR. Chemokine receptors: keys to AIDS pathogenesis? Cell 1998;93:677–80.
8. Chan DC, Fass D, Berger JM, Kim PS. Core structure of gp41 from the HIV envelope glycoprotein. Cell 1997;89:263–73.
9. Kwong PD, Wyatt R, Robinson J, Sweet RW, Sodroski J, Hendrickson WA. Structure of an HIV gp120 envelope glycoprotein in complex with the CD4 receptor and a neutralizing human antibody. Nature 1998;393:648–59.
10. Bhoopat L, Eiangleng L, Rugpao S, et al. In vivo identification of Langerhans and related dendritic

11. cells infected with HIV-1 subtype E in vaginal mucosa of asymptomatic patients. Mod Pathol 2001;14(12):1263–9.
11. Patton DL, Thwin SS, Meier A, Hooton TM, Stapleton AE, Eschenbach DA. Epithelial cell layer thickness and immune cell populations in the normal human vagina at different stages of the menstrual cycle. Am J Obstet Gynecol 2000;183(4):967–73.
12. Hussain LA, Lehner T. Comparative investigations of Langerhans' cells and potential receptors for HIV in oral, genitourinary and rectal epithelia. Immunology 1995;85:475.
13. Prakash M, Kapembwa MS, Gotch F, Patterson S. Chemokine receptor expression on mucosal dendritic cells from the endocervix of healthy women. J Infect Dis 2004;190(2):246–50.
14. Hu J, Gardner MB, Miller CJ. Simian immuno-deficiency virus rapidly penetrates the cervicovaginal mucosa after intravaginal inoculation and infects intraepithelial dendritic cells. J Virol 2000;74(13):6087–95.
15. Spira AI, Marx PA, Patterson BK, et al. Cellular targets of infection and route of viral dissemination after an intravaginal inoculation of simian immuno-deficiency virus into rhesus macaques. J Exp Med 1996;183:215–25.
16. Piguet V, Blauvelt A. Essential roles for dendritic cells in the pathogenesis and potential treatment of HIV disease. J Invest Dermatol 2002;119(2):365–9.
17. Wood GS, Warner NL, Warnke R. Anti-Leu-3/T4 antibodies react with cells of monocyte/macrophage and Langerhans lineage. J Immunol 1983;131:212–6.
18. Zoeteweij JP, Golding H, Mostowski H, Blauvelt A. Cutting edge: cytokines regulate expression and function of the HIV coreceptor CXCR4 on human mature dendritic cells. J Immunol 1998;161:3219–23.
19. Zaitseva M, Blauvelt A, Lee S, et al. Expression and function of CCR5 and CXCR4 on human Langerhans cells and macrophages: implications for HIV primary infection. Nat Med 1997;3:1369–75.
20. Zhang LQ, MacKenzie P, Cleland A, Brown ECHJ, Simmonds P. Selection for specific sequences in the external envelope protein of human immunodeficiency virus type 1 upon primary infection. J Virol 1993;67:3345–56.
21. Zhu T, Mo H, Wang N, et al. Genotypic and phenotypic characterization of HIV-1 patients with primary infection. Science 1993;261:1179–81.
22. Kawamura T, Cohen SS, Borris DL, et al. Candidate microbicides block HIV-1 infection of human immature Langerhans cells within epithelial tissue explants. J Exp Med 2000;192(10):1491–500.

23. Kawamura T, Gulden FO, Sugaya M, et al. R5 HIV productively infects Langerhans cells, and infection levels are regulated by compound CCR5 polymorphisms. Proc Natl Acad Sci USA 2003;100(14):8401–6.

24. Kawamura T, Bruse SE, Abraha A, et al. PSC-RANTES blocks R5 human immunodeficiency virus infection of Langerhans cells isolated from individuals with a variety of CCR5 diplotypes. J Virol 2004;78(14):7602–9.

25. Sugaya M, Lore K, Koup RA, Douek DC, Blauvelt A. HIV-infected Langerhans cells preferentially transmit virus to proliferating autologous CD4+ memory T cells located within Langerhans cell-T cell clusters. J Immunol 2004;172(4):2219–24.

26. Sugaya M, Hartley O, Root MJ, Blauvelt A. C34, a membrane fusion inhibitor, blocks HIV infection of Langerhans cells and viral transmission to T cells. J Invest Dermatol 2007;127(6):1436–43.

27. Liu R, Paxton WA, Choe S, et al. Homozygous defect in HIV-1 coreceptor accounts for resistance of some multiply-exposed individuals to HIV-1 infection. Cell 1996;86:367–77.

28. Dean M, Carrington M, Winkler C, et al. Genetic restriction of HIV-1 infection and progression to AIDS by a deletion allele of the CKR5 structural gene. Science 1996;273:1856–62.

29. Samson M, Libert F, Doranz BJ, et al. Resistance to HIV-1 infection in Caucasian individuals bearing mutant alleles of the CCR-5 chemokine receptor gene. Nature 1996;382:722–5.

30. Huang Y, Paxton WA, Wolinsky SM, et al. The role of a mutant CCR5 allele in HIV-1 transmission and disease progression. Nat Med 1996;2:1240–3.

31. Grown C, Gupta GR, Pande R. Taking action to improve women's health through gender equality and women's empowerment. Lancet 2005;365(9458):541–3.

32. Lederman MM, Offord RE, Hartley O. Microbicides and other topical strategies to prevent vaginal transmission of HIV. Nat Rev Immunol 2006;6(5):371–82.

33. Dezzutti CS, James VN, Ramos A, et al. In vitro comparison of topical microbicides for prevention of human immunodeficiency virus type 1 transmission. Antimicrob Agents Chemother 2004;48(10):3834–44.

34. Van Damme L, Ramjee G, Alary M, et al. Effectiveness of COL-1492, a nonoxynol-9 vaginal gel, on HIV-1 transmission in female sex workers: a randomised controlled trial. Lancet 2002;360(9338):971–7.

35. Lederman MM, Veazey RS, Offord R, et al. Prevention of vaginal SHIV transmission in rhesus macaques through inhibition of CCR5. Science 2004;306(5695):485–7.

36. Sabbe R, Picchio GR, Pastore C, et al. Donor- and ligand-dependent differences in C-C chemokine receptor 5 reexpression. J Virol 2001;75(2):661–71.

37. Weeks MR, Mosack KE, Abbott M, Sylla LN, Valdes B, Prince M. Microbicide acceptability among high-risk urban U.S. women: experiences and perceptions of sexually transmitted HIV prevention. Sex Transm Dis 2004;31(11):682–90.

38. Bentley ME, Fullem AM, Tolley EE, et al. Acceptability of a microbicide among women and their partners in a 4-country phase I trial. Am J Public Health 2004;94(7):1159–64.

39. Kahn JO, Walker BD. Acute human immunodeficiency virus type 1 infection. N Engl J Med 1998;339:33–9.

40. Kinloch-deLoes S, deSaussure P, Saurat JH, Stalder H, Hirschel B, Perrin LH. Symptomatic primary infection due to human immunodeficiency virus type 1: review of 31 cases. Clin Infect Dis 1993; 17:59–65.

41. Schacker TW, Hughes JP, Shea T, Coombs RW, Corey L. Biological and virologic characteristics of primary HIV infection. Ann Intern Med 1998;128:613–20.

42. Yamamoto H, Ringler DJ, Miller MD, Yasutomi Y, Hasunuma T, Letvin NL. Simian immunodeficiency virus-specific cytotoxic T lymphocytes are present in the AIDS-associated skin rash in rhesus monkeys. J Immunol 1992;149:728–34.

43. Gulick RM, Ribaudo HJ, Shikuma CM, et al. Three- vs four-drug antiretroviral regimens for the initial treatment of HIV-1 infection: a randomized controlled trial. JAMA 2006;296(7):769–81.

44. Cohen OJ, Fauci AS. Current strategies in the treatment of HIV infection. Adv Intern Med 2001;46: 207–46.

45. Rosenberg ES, Billingsley JM, Caliendo AM, et al. Vigorous HIV-1–specific CD4+ T cell responses associated with control of viremia. Science 1997;278:1447–50.

46. Angel JB, Kumar A, Parato K, et al. Improvement in cell-mediated immune function during potent anti-human immunodeficiency virus therapy with ritonavir plus saquinavir. J Infect Dis 1998;177:898–904.

47. Wainberg MA, Friedland G. Public health implications of antiretroviral therapy and HIV drug resistance. JAMA 1998;279:1977–81.

48. Pantaleo G, Graziosi C, Demarest JF. HIV infection is active and progressive in lymphoid tissue during the clinically latent stage of disease. Nature 1993;362:355–8.

49. Cohen OJ, Kinter A, Fauci AS. Host factors in the pathogenesis of HIV disease. Immunol Rev 1997;159:31–48.

50. Connor RI, Sheridan KE, Ceradini D, Choe S, Landau NR. Change in coreceptor use coreceptor use correlates with disease progression in HIV-1–infected individuals. J Exp Med 1997;185:621–8.

51. Winkler C, Modi W, Smith MW, et al. Genetic restriction of AIDS pathogenesis by an SDF-1 chemokine gene variant. Science 1998;279:389–93.

52. McDermott DH, Zimmerman PA, Guignard F, Kleeberger CA, Leitman SF, Murphy PM. CCR5 promoter polymorphism and HIV-1 disease progression. Lancet 1998;352:866–70.

53. Kostrikis LG, Huang Y, Moore JP, et al. A chemokine receptor CCR2 allele delays HIV-1 disease progression and is associated with a CCR5 promoter mutation. Nature Med 1998;4:350–3.

54. Gonzalez E, Kulkarni H, Bolivar H, et al. The influence of CCL3L1 gene-containing segmental duplications on HIV-1/AIDS susceptibility. Science 2005;307(5714):1434–40.

55. Johnson RA. Cutaneous manifestations of human immunodeficiency virus disease. In: Freedberg IM, Eisen AZ, Wolff K, Austen KF, Goldsmith LA, Katz SI, eds. Dermatology in General Medicine, 4th ed. New York: McGraw-Hill, 2003:2138–50.

56. Ho DD, Neumann AU, Perelson AS, Chen W, Leonard JM, Markovitz M. Rapid turnover of plasma virions and CD4 lymphocytes in HIV-1 infection. Nature 1995;373:123–6.

57. Wei X, Ghosh SK, Taylor ME, et al. Viral dynamics in human immunodeficiency virus type 1 infection. Nature 1995;373:117–22.

58. Cameron PU, Forsum U, Teppler H, Granelli-Piperno A, Steinman RM. During HIV-1 infection most blood dendritic cells are not productively infected and can induce allogeneic CD4+ T cells clonal expansion. Clin Exp Immunol 1992;88:226–36.

59. Blauvelt A, Clerici M, Lucey DR, et al. Functional studies of epidermal Langerhans cells and blood monocytes in HIV-infected persons. J Immunol 1995;154:3506–15.

60. Blauvelt A, Chougnet C, Shearer GM, Katz SI. Modulation of T cell responses to recall antigens presented by Langerhans cells in HIV-discordant identical twins by anti-interleukin (IL)-10 antibodies and IL-12. J Clin Invest 1996;97:1550–5.

61. Kawamura T, Gatanaga H, Borris DL, Connors M, Mitsuya H, Blauvelt A. Decreased stimulation of CD4+ T cell proliferation and IL-2 production by highly enriched populations of HIV-infected dendritic cells. J Immunol 2003;170:4260–6.

62. Gulick RM, Mellors JW, Havlir D, et al. Treatment of indinavir, zidovudine, and lamivudine in adults with human immunodeficiency virus infection and prior antiretroviral therapy. N Engl J Med 1997;337:734–9.

63. Hammer SM, Squires KE, Hughes MD, et al. A controlled trial of two nucleoside analogues plus indinavir in persons with human immunodeficiency virus infection and CD4 cell counts of 200 per cubic millimeter or less. N Engl J Med 1997;337:725–33.

64. Antman K, Chang Y. Kaposi's sarcoma. N Engl J Med 2000;342(14):1027–38.

65. Chang Y, Cesarman E, Pessin MS, et al. Identification of herpesvirus-like DNA sequences in AIDS-associated Kaposi's sarcoma. Science 1994;266:1865–9.

66. Moore PS, Chang Y. Detection of herpesvirus-like DNA sequences in Kaposi's sarcoma in patients with and without HIV infection. N Engl J Med 1995;332(18):1181–5.

67. Kedes DH, Operskalski E, Busch M, Kohn R, Flood J, Ganem D. The seroepidemiology of human herpesvirus 8 (Kaposi's sarcoma-associated herpesvirus): distribution of infection in KS risk groups and evidence for sexual transmission. Nature Med 1996;2:918–24.

68. Gao SJ, Kingsley L, Li M, et al. KSHV antibodies among Americans, Italians and Ugandans with and without Kaposi's sarcoma. Nature Med 1996;2:925–8.

69. Blauvelt A. The role of human herpesvirus 8 in the pathogenesis of Kaposi's sarcoma. Adv Dermatol 1999;14:167–207.

70. Boshoff C, Schulz TF, Kennedy MM, et al. Kaposi's sarcoma-associated herpesvirus infects endothelial cells and spindle cells. Nat Med 1995;1:1274–8.

71. Orenstein JM, Alkan S, Blauvelt A, et al. Visualization of human herpesvirus type 8 in Kaposi's sarcoma by light and transmission electron microscopy. AIDS 1997;11:F35–F45.

72. Dittmer D, Lagunoff M, Renne R, Staskus K, Haase A, Ganem D. A cluster of latently expressed genes in Kaposi's sarcoma-associated herpesvirus. J Virol 1998;72(10):8309–15.

73. Watanabe T, Sugaya M, Atkins AM, et al. Kaposi's sarcoma-associated herpesvirus latency-associated nuclear antigen prolongs the life span of primary human umbilical vein endothelial cells. J Virol 2003;77(11):6188–96.

74. Sugaya M, Watanabe T, Yang A, et al. Lymphatic dysfunction in transgenic mice expressing KSHV k-cyclin under the control of the VEGFR-3 promoter. Blood 2005;105(6):2356–63.

75. Murphy M, Armstrong D, Sepkowitz KA, Ahkami RN, Myskowski PL. Regression of AIDS-related Kaposi's sarcoma following treatment with an HIV-1 protease inhibitor. AIDS 1997;11:261–2.

76. Wit FWNM, Sol CJA, Renwick N, et al. Regression of AIDS-related Kaposi's sarcoma associated with clearance of human herpesvirus-8 from peripheral blood mononuclear cells following initiation of antiretroviral therapy. AIDS 1998;12:218–9.

77. Di Lorenzo G, Konstantinopoulos PA, Pantanowitz L, Di Trolio R, De Placido S, Dezube BJ. Management

of AIDS-related Kaposi's sarcoma. Lancet Oncol 2007;8(2):167–76.

78. Frazer IH, Crapper RM, Medley G, Brown TC, Mackay IR. Association between anorectal dysplasia, human papillomavirus, and human immunodeficiency virus infection in homosexual men. Lancet 1986;2:657–60.

79. Paxton WA, Liu R, Kang S, et al. Reduced HIV-1 infectability of CD4+ lymphocytes from exposed-uninfected individuals: association with low expression of CCR5 and high production of beta-chemokines. Virology 1998;244(1):66–73.

80. Bradsher RW. Histoplasmosis and blastomycosis. Clin Infect Dis 1996;22:S102–S11.

81. Rosenthal D, LeBoit PE, Klumpp L, Berger TG. Human immunodeficiency virus-associated eosinophilic folliculitis. Archives of Dermatology 1991;127:206–9.

82. Blauvelt A, Plott RT, Spooner K, Stearn B, Davey RT, Turner ML. Eosinophilic folliculitis associated with the acquired immunodeficiency syndrome responds well to permethrin. Arch Dermatol 1995;131:360–1.

83. Majors MJ, Berger TG, Blauvelt A, Smith KJ, Turner ML, Cruz PD. HIV-related eosinophilic folliculitis: a panel discussion. Semin Cutan Med Surg 1997;16:219–23.

84. Bayard PJ, Berger TG, Jacobsen MA. Drug hypersensitivity reactions and human immunodeficiency virus disease. J AIDS 1992;5:237–57.

85. Warren KJ, Boxwell DE, Kim NY, Drolet BA. Nevirapine-associated Stevens-Johnson syndrome. Lancet 1998;351:567.

86. Lo JC, Mulligan K, Tai VW, Algren H, Schambelan M. "Buffalo hump" in men with HIV-1 infection. Lancet 1998;351:867–70.

87. Miller KD, Jones E, Yanovski JA, Shankar R, Feuerstein I, Falloon J. Visceral abdominal-fat accumulation associated with use of indinavir. Lancet 1998;351:871–5.

88. Carr A, Samaras K, Burton S, et al. A syndrome of peripheral lipodystrophy, hyperlipidaemia and insulin resistance in patients receiving HIV protease inhibitors. AIDS 1998;12:F51–F8.

89. Barragan P, Fisac C, Podzamczer D. Switching strategies to improve lipid profile and morphologic changes. AIDS Rev 2006;8(4):191–203.

90. Mest DR, Humble G. Safety and efficacy of poly-L-lactic acid injections in persons with HIV-associated lipoatrophy: the US experience. Dermatol Surg 2006;32(11):1336–45.

91. Kong HH, Myers SA. Cutaneous effects of highly active antiretroviral therapy in HIV-infected patients. Dermatol Ther 2005;18(1):58–66.

22
Bacterial Infections

Carolyn Senavsky, Noah Craft, and Lloyd S. Miller

Key Points

- Innate immune responses are directed against conserved components of microorganisms called pathogen-associated molecular patterns (PAMPs).
- The host cellular receptors that recognize different PAMPs are called pattern recognition receptors (PRRs).
- Two major families of human antimicrobial peptides are defensins and cathelicidin.
- Toll-like receptors (TLRs) are important PRRs involved in host defense against a variety of pathogenic microorganisms.
- Complement plays a key role in killing of bacteria.
- Neutrophils, monocytes, and macrophages phagocytose opsonized bacteria.

Bacterial skin infections represent a major public health problem, resulting in approximately 11.6 million outpatient/emergency room visits and 464,000 hospital admissions annually in the United States.[1] A recent study found that 76% of all bacterial skin and soft tissue infections presenting to emergency rooms in 11 major U.S. cities were due to *Staphylococcus aureus,* and 78% of these infections were due to community-acquired methicillin-resistant *S. aureus* (CA-MRSA).[2] The importance of the immune response against bacterial skin infections cannot be overemphasized, and many immunocompromised patients are at an increased risk for infection.[3] This chapter focuses on the host defense mechanisms against two of the most common bacterial skin pathogens, *S. aureus* and group A *Streptococcus.*

Staphylococcus aureus

Staphylococcus aureus is a gram-positive extracellular bacterial pathogen that is the most common cause of skin and soft tissue infections such as impetigo, folliculitis, cellulitis, and ecthymas.[4–7] *S. aureus* infections may become more invasive and lead to life-threatening infections such as lymphangitis, septic arthritis, osteomyelitis, pneumonia, abscesses of various organs, meningitis, bacteremia, endocarditis, and sepsis.[4–7] Furthermore, *S. aureus* produces exotoxins that result in staphylococcus scalded skin syndrome and toxic-shock syndrome.[8,9] *S. aureus* colonization of the anterior nares is found in ~30% of the general population and is a major risk factor for infection.[10–13] Patients with atopic dermatitis, diabetes mellitus, renal disease (hemodialysis), HIV infection, a history of intravenous drug abuse, and preexisting tissue injury or inflammation (e.g., ulcer, surgical wound) are particularly predisposed to *S. aureus* infections.[6,7,10–14] Despite advances in antibiotic therapy, the frequencies of both community-acquired and hospital-acquired *S. aureus* infections have steadily increased.[1,2,7] Furthermore, the treatment of these infections is frequently complicated by staphylococcal strains that are resistant to multiple antibiotics, including methicillin (MRSA), gentamicin, and even vancomycin.[15–20]

Clinical Manifestations

Staphylococcus aureus cutaneous infections result in a variably pyogenic immune response characterized by purulent lesions with surrounding erythema, warmth, and induration.[4–7,21] Microscopically, these lesions are composed primarily of collections of neutrophils, a hallmark of *S. aureus* infection.[6,7,21–23] Superficial *S. aureus* infections result in impetigo, an infection confined to the upper layers of the epidermis.[7,21] However, *S. aureus* infections can become more invasive and involve dermal planes and subcutaneous tissues as seen in cellulitis (Fig. 22.1) or deep ulcerative lesions as seen in ecthyma.[4,6,7] *S. aureus* also infects individual hair follicles, leading to folliculitis, furunculosis, and carbuncle formation when multiple follicles become involved (Fig. 22.2).[4,6,7] Lastly, *S. aureus* can cause

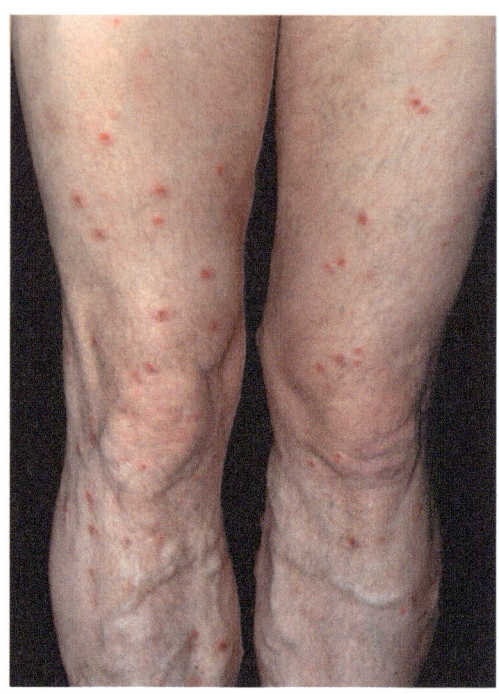

FIG. 22.2. *Staphylococcus aureus* folliculitis/furuncles (boils). Typically, infected hair follicles present as follicularly based erythematous, warm, edematous, and pus-filled nodules. (Courtesy of the Victor D. Newcomer collection at UCLA and Logical Images, Inc.)

superinfection of inflammatory skin diseases such as atopic dermatitis and intertrigo.[7,21,24]

Innate Immune Responses Against *S. aureus*

Innate immune responses are directed against conserved components of microorganisms called pathogen-associated molecular patterns (PAMPs).[25–30] The host cellular receptors that recognize different PAMPs are called pattern recognition receptors (PRRs).[25–30] The PAMPs are predominantly expressed by microorganisms and not by host cells, thus enabling the host's immune system to recognize the pathogen rather than self. This section discusses soluble factors of the innate immune system, such as antimicrobial peptides and complement, and reviews the known PRRs and the role of innate immune system cells in host defense against *S. aureus*.

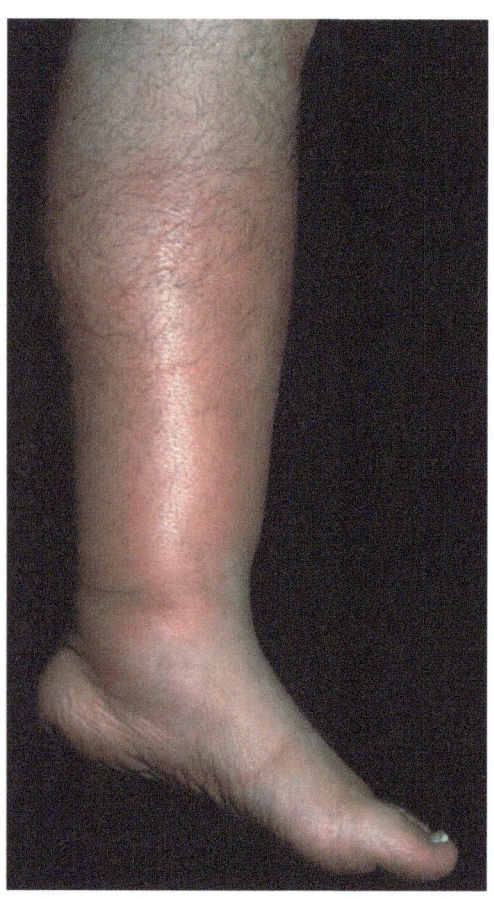

FIG. 22.1. *Staphylococcus aureus* cellulitis on the lower leg. The involved skin characteristically shows signs of inflammation, including erythema, warmth, edema, and pain. (Courtesy of the Victor D. Newcomer collection at UCLA and Logical Images, Inc.)

Soluble Mediators of Innate Immunity Against *S. aureus*

Antimicrobial Peptides

Antimicrobial peptides are polypeptides that have antimicrobial activity at physiologic conditions and are believed to function by disrupting bacterial membranes.[31–36] Two major families of human antimicrobial peptides are defensins (α and β) and cathelicidin. α-defensins (also called human neutrophil peptides, HNPs) are produced by neutrophils, whereas β-defensins are produced predominantly by epithelial cells (including keratinocytes), but are also produced by macrophages and dendritic cells.[31–35] Cathelicidins are produced constitutively by neutrophils and can be induced in epithelial cells, including keratinocytes.[34–36]

There are six known human α-defensins (HNP1–6), which constitute ~50% of the peptides within neutrophil granules.[32,33,37] A recent study demonstrated that only HNPs 2 and 5 (and not HNPs 1, 3, 4, and 6) have antimicrobial activity against *S. aureus* in vitro (Fig. 22.3).[37] Interestingly, *S. aureus* produces proteins such as staphylokinase and MprF that inhibit the activity of α-defensins.[38,39] Thus, the antimicrobial activity of α-defensins may be biologically relevant since *S. aureus* has developed mechanisms to inhibit their activity.

There are four known human β-defensins (HBD1–4), which are expressed by various epithelial cells, including keratinocytes, as well as by activated monocytes/macrophages and dendritic cells. HBDs 1, 2, and 4 have been shown to have only a weak bacteriostatic effect against *S. aureus* in vitro (Fig. 22.3).[40,41] In contrast, HBD3 has strong in vitro bactericidal activity against *S. aureus*.[42] hCAP-18 is the only known member of the human cathelicidin family and is the precursor to the active cleaved C-terminal peptide LL-37.[34–36] Like HBD3, LL-37 has been shown to have potent antimicrobial activity against *S. aureus*.[43–46] Interestingly, *S. aureus* secretes a protein called aureolysin, which is an extracellular metalloproteinase that inhibits LL-37 activity.[47–50]

Keratinocyte production of HBD2, HBD3, and LL-37 can be induced by live or heat-killed *S. aureus* and by *S. aureus* components, including lipopeptides and lipoteichoic acid via activation of TLR2.[42,51–56] Thus, human keratinocytes can upregulate the production of HBD2 and HBD3 in response to *S. aureus* or its components, thereby increasing the innate immune response in the skin. Interestingly, activation of the epidermal growth factor receptor (EGFR) by wounding of human skin in vitro resulted in increased production of HBD3 and antimicrobial activity against *S. aureus*.[57–59] Thus, wounded skin may resist infection by *S. aureus* via production of HBD3. Recently, vitamin D has been shown to increase LL-37 production by keratinocytes, neutrophils, and monocytes/macrophages, suggesting that vitamin D also may play a role in host defense against *S. aureus*.[60–63]

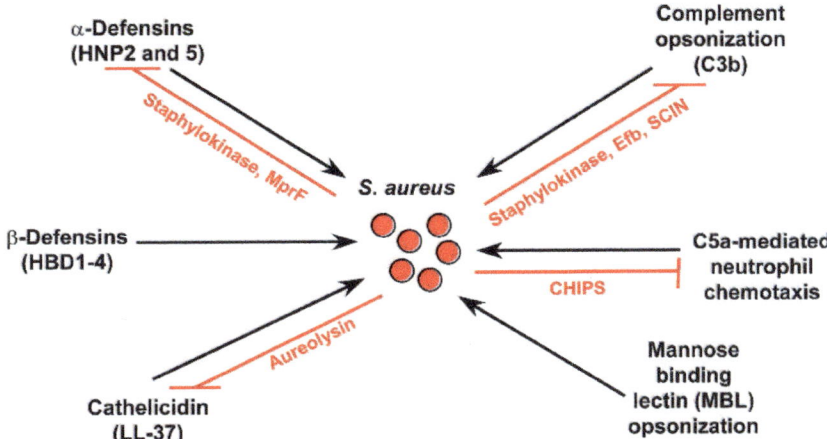

FIG. 22.3. Soluble mediators of the innate immune response against *S. aureus*. The mechanisms that *S. aureus* utilizes to inhibit these soluble mediators are shown in red. CHIPS, chemotaxis inhibitory protein of staphylococci. Efb, extracellular fibrinogen-binding protein; SCIN, staphylococcus complement inhibitor

Antimicrobial peptides may also be involved in the pathogenesis of certain inflammatory skin diseases. HBD2 and HBD3 are expressed at increased levels in the hyperproliferative and inflammatory skin disease, psoriasis, which has been associated with a T-helper-1 (Th1) cytokine profile.[40,42,64,65] In contrast, HBD2, HBD3, and LL-37 are expressed at significantly lower levels in atopic dermatitis, another inflammatory skin disease that is associated with a Th2 cytokine profile.[64,65] These findings may explain why S. aureus superinfection is more frequently seen in lesions of atopic dermatitis and rarely in psoriatic skin lesions.[40,42,64–66]

Lastly, antimicrobial peptides not only have microbicidal activity, but also promote the recruitment of immune system cells to the site of infection. For example, HNPs promote chemotaxis of T cells and immature dendritic cells; HBDs promote chemotaxis of immature dendritic cells and memory CD4 T cells; and LL-37 promotes chemotaxis of neutrophils, monocytes, and T cells.[67–71] The chemotactic activity of HBDs and LL-37 is mediated by the chemokine receptor CCR6 and the formyl peptide receptor-like 1, respectively.[67–71]

Complement Activation and Mannose-Binding Lectin

The complement system includes a family of serum proteins, proteolytic fragments, and cell-surface receptors.[47,72–74] There are three main functions of complement activation: (1) direct killing of bacteria via formation of the membrane attack complex (MAC), which perforates bacterial membranes; (2) promotion of phagocytosis by opsonizing the bacterial surface with complement components such as C3b; and (3) recruitment of immune system cells to the site of infection by generating the complement chemoattractant peptides C3a and C5a.[47,72–74] There are three pathways of complement activation: the classical, alternative, and lectin pathways. Each pathway requires generation of an enzyme complex called the C3 convertase. In the classical pathway, generation of the C3 convertase involves the interaction of complement components with natural IgM antibody or antigen-specific IgG antibody that is bound to antigens of the pathogen. In the alternative pathway, there are low levels of direct activation of the C3 convertase

by components of the pathogen.[47,72–74] In the lectin pathway, the C3 convertase is activated via recognition of carbohydrate groups on the surface of the bacteria via mannose-binding lectin (MBL) or via H-, L-, or M-ficolin and MBL-associated serine proteases (MASP1, 2 and 3).[47,75–77]

There have been several reports demonstrating the key role of complement in host defense against S. aureus (Fig. 22.3).[78–81] First, in a mouse model of S. aureus–induced arthritis and bacteremia, depletion of complement components resulted in higher mortality and significantly decreased neutrophil recruitment and impairment of phagocytosis.[79] In another study, complement-mediated opsonization by C3b as well as activation of complement receptor 1 (CD35) (the primary receptor for C3b) were more critical in controlling S. aureus bacteremia than C5a or generation of the MAC.[80]

Mannose-binding lectin is also important in host defense against S. aureus infections (Fig. 22.3).[82–87] For example, individuals with an MBL gene mutation who have impaired MBL-dependent opsonization suffer from recurrent S. aureus infections.[84] In addition, MBL-deficient mice had only a slightly decreased survival, whereas C3–deficient mice and mice deficient in both MBL and C3 had markedly decreased survival compared with wild-type mice after an intravenous challenge of S. aureus.[82,83] Thus, C3 and complement activation may play a more important role than MBL in host defense against S. aureus. Lastly, MBL can bind to S. aureus in vitro, resulting in increased phagocytosis.[85–87] Taken together, MBL is involved in activation of the lectin complement pathway and in opsonization of S. aureus.

Staphylococcus aureus has developed several mechanisms to counteract complement activity.[47–49] S. aureus produces a protein called staphylococcus complement inhibitor (SCIN), which prevents activation of the complement cascade by inhibiting the C3 convertase.[47–49,88–90] S. aureus also secretes a protein called extracellular fibrinogen-binding protein (Efb), which binds C3 and blocks C3 deposition on the bacterial cell surface.[91,92] Lastly, staphylokinase inhibits opsonization of S. aureus and subsequent phagocytosis by converting plasminogen into plasmin on the bacterial surface, which leads to removal of the antistaphylococcal opsonins IgG and C3b.[93]

Pattern Recognition Receptors that Recognize Components of *S. aureus*

Toll-Like Receptors

Toll-like receptors (TLRs) are important PRRs involved in host defense against a variety of pathogenic microorganisms, including *S. aureus*.[25–30] Activation of TLRs initiates several signaling cascades including nuclear factor κB (NF-κB) activation, ultimately leading to production of cytokines, chemokines, antimicrobial peptides, and upregulation of co-stimulatory and adhesion molecules involved in innate and adaptive immune responses.[25–30]

Of all the known human TLRs (TLR1 to TLR10), TLR2 has been the most implicated in host defense against *S. aureus* (Fig. 22.4). TLR2 is expressed on the surface of numerous cell types in the skin, including keratinocytes, Langerhans cells, monocytes/macrophages, dendritic cells, mast cells, endothelial cells, fibroblasts, and adipocytes.[94–105] TLR2 can be activated by live or heat-killed *S. aureus* as well as the *S. aureus* components, peptidoglycan (PGN), lipoteichoic acid (LTA), and lipopeptides.[102,106–126] However, there have been some conflicting reports regarding the ability of *S. aureus* PGN, LTA, and lipopeptides to activate TLR2.[123,126]

With regard to *S. aureus* skin infections, TLR2–deficient mice develop larger skin lesions than wild-type mice after *S. aureus* skin inoculation.[127,128] Human keratinocytes also express TLR2 and can be activated by live or heat-killed *S. aureus* and *S. aureus* components, resulting

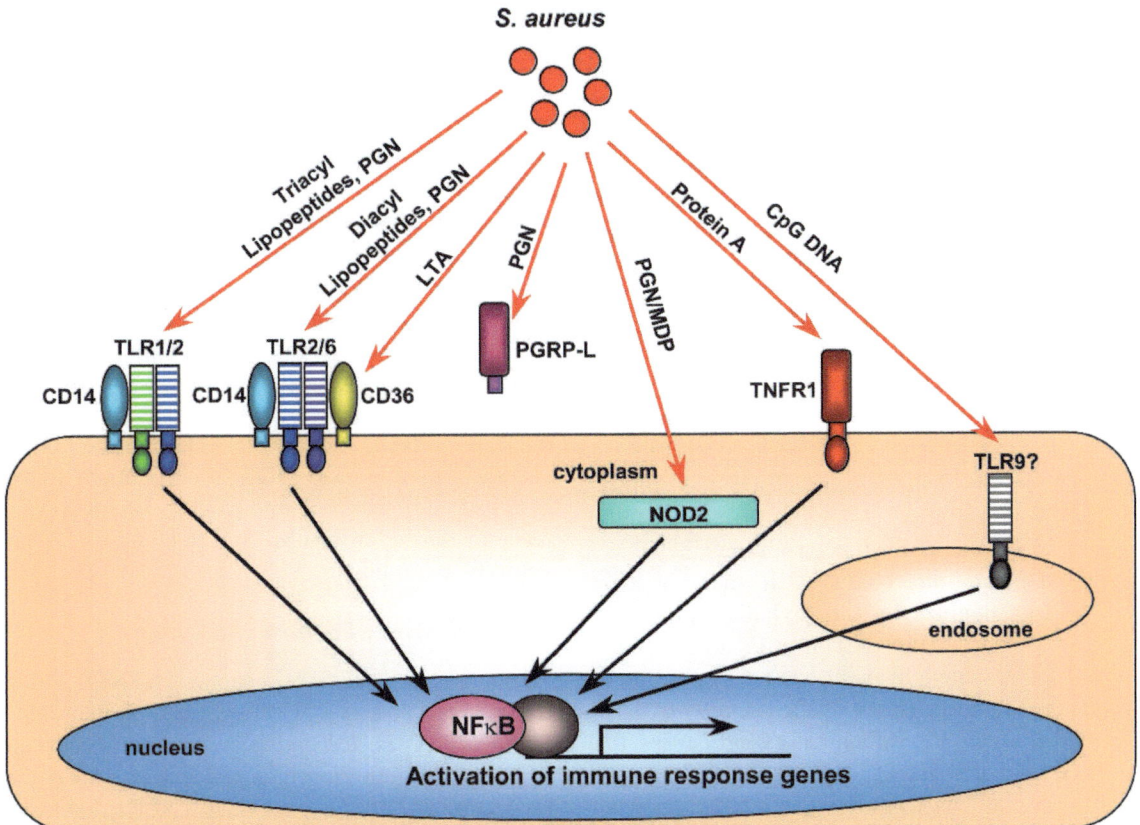

FIG. 22.4. Pattern recognition receptors (PRRs) of host cells involved in recognizing components of *S. aureus* and initiating immune responses. The *S. aureus* components recognized by these PRRs and the cellular localization of these PRRs are shown. LTA, lipoteichoic acid; NF, nuclear factor; PGN, peptidoglycan; TLR, Toll-like receptor; TNFR, tumor necrosis factor receptor

in increased production of cytokines such as interleukin-1β (IL-1β), IL-8, tumor necrosis factor-α (TNF-α), and production of HBD2 and HBD3.[58,95,96,101–103,129,130] Interestingly, a polymorphism in TLR2 has been linked to a severe phenotype of atopic dermatitis, which is frequently associated with superinfection by *S. aureus*.[131–133]

Since *S. aureus* PGN, LTA, and lipopeptides have distinctly different biochemical structures, it was unclear how one receptor could recognize such a broad spectrum of molecules. However, TLR2 interacts with other TLRs and additional co-receptors, which may enable TLR2 to recognize these different ligands (Fig. 22.4). TLR2 heterodimerizes with TLR1 or TLR6 to recognize tri-acyl and di-acyl lipopeptides, respectively.[134–136] Therefore, the ability of the host to recognize certain lipopeptides may depend on the formation of TLR2 heterodimers. Several in vitro studies have indicated that CD14 may act as a TLR co-receptor by interacting with *S. aureus* LTA and PGN and enhancing TLR2 activation.[120,137–147] CD14 is a membrane protein that lacks an intracellular signaling domain and was initially characterized as a TLR4 co-receptor for lipopolysaccharide (LPS) of gram-negative bacteria.[143,148–151] However, CD14 may not play an important host defense role against *S. aureus* in vivo, since CD14–deficient mice and wild-type mice responded similarly in a model of *S. aureus* sepsis.[152] In contrast, using in vitro and in vivo skin and systemic models of infection with *S. aureus*, CD36 was found to be a TLR2 co-receptor involved in the recognition of *S. aureus* LTA (which is diacylated) and in the activation of signaling via the TLR2/6 heterodimer.[128,153]

TLR9 is an intracellular TLR that has been shown to recognize hypomethylated CpG (cytosine-phosphate-guanosine) motifs of bacterial DNA.[154–156] Although TLR9 has not been directly implicated in host defense against *S. aureus*, DNA from *S. aureus* has inflammatory properties that may be mediated via TLR9 (Fig. 22.4). For example, *S. aureus* DNA produces inflammation when injected into the skin.[157] *S. aureus* DNA has also been shown to induce IL-12, TNF-α, interferon-α (IFN-α), and IFN-γ.[158–160] However, it is possible that PRRs other than TLR9 recognize *S. aureus* DNA.[161,162]

Nucleotide-Binding Oligomerization Domain Proteins

In contrast to TLR2, nucleotide-binding oligomerization domain proteins (NOD1 and NOD2) are found free in the cytosol and detect breakdown products of PGN (instead of the whole molecule).[163–166] NOD1 recognizes the breakdown products of gram-negative PGN. In contrast, NOD2 recognizes muramyl dipeptide (MDP), which is a breakdown product of both gram-positive and gram-negative PGN, and has been shown to recognize MDP-derived from *S. aureus* PGN (Fig. 22.4).[163–169] After ligand detection, NODs activate a signaling pathway that results in NF-κB activation and transcription of host genes involved in innate and acquired immune responses.[163–168] Interestingly, activation of NOD2 by MDP resulted in increased expression of HBD2 by keratinocytes, suggesting that NOD2 could play a role in host defense against *S. aureus* skin infection.[170]

The fact that NOD2 is a cytoplasmic receptor calls into question whether an intracellular PRR could be involved in recognition of a *S. aureus* infection, since *S. aureus* has classically been considered an extracellular pathogen. However, several studies have found that *S. aureus* can invade the cytoplasm of various cells, including epithelial cells, enterocytes, endothelial cells, osteoblasts, and neutrophils.[171–177] Once *S. aureus* enters the cytoplasm, host or bacterial enzymes may break down *S. aureus* PGN into MDP that can be recognized by NOD2.[167,168,178–181] Despite the ability of NOD2 to recognize MDP from *S. aureus* PGN, evidence demonstrating that NOD2 is an important receptor during an in vivo *S. aureus* infection has yet to be reported.

Tumor Necrosis Factor-α Receptor 1

Tumor necrosis factor-α receptor 1 (TNFR1) is a receptor for TNF-α that is expressed on many different cell types. Recently, it was discovered that *S. aureus* protein A, which is known to bind the Fc portion of antibody, activates TNFR1 and leads to production of proinflammatory cytokines and chemokines (Fig. 22.4).[182,183] However, TNFR1–deficient mice had no defect in host defense compared with wild-type mice after an in vivo *S. aureus* skin infection, suggesting that activation of TNFR1 may not play an major role in host defense against *S. aureus*.[127]

Peptidoglycan Recognition Proteins

In humans, there are four peptidoglycan recognition proteins (PGRPs) (-S, -L, -Iα, and -Iβ), and all of them are secreted and are not transmembrane proteins.[167,184–186] The precise function of these receptors is unknown, but PGRP-L has amidase activity that may be capable of breaking down *S. aureus* PGN (Fig. 22.4).[187–189] Despite this amidase activity, PGRP-L may not be involved in the immune response against *S. aureus* since there was no difference in cytokine production (IL-6 and TNF-α) or in susceptibility to infection between PGRP-L–deficient mice and wild-type mice after systemic challenge with *S. aureus*.[190]

Cellular Innate Immune Responses Against *S. aureus*

Neutrophils

Pyogenic abscess formation through neutrophil recruitment is a hallmark of *S. aureus* infection.[7,21–23] The importance of neutrophils in host defense against *S. aureus* in humans has been suggested by the recurrent *S. aureus* infections in patients with chronic granulomatous disease (CGD), who have a defect in neutrophil NADPH oxidase.[191,192] The critical role of neutrophils in *S. aureus* infections in humans has been supported by studies of *S. aureus* infections in mice. For example, in a mouse model of *S. aureus* skin infection, neutrophil-depleted mice had a severe defect in bacterial clearance, resulting in nonhealing skin lesions.[22]

Neutrophils are considered first responders of the innate immune system and are recruited to sites of *S. aureus* infection.[193–198] Keratinocytes and other resident skin cells produce neutrophil chemokines such as neutrophil chemotactic factor IL-8 (CXCL8), growth-related oncogene-α, -β, -γ (GRO-α, -β, -γ), neutrophil-activating peptide-2 (NAP-2; CXCL7), and epithelial cell-derived neutrophil-activating peptide-78 (ENA-78, CXCL5) (Fig. 22.5).[199–204] All of these contain glutamic acid-leucine-arginine (ELR) residues preceding the first cysteine and activate the receptors CXCR1 and CXCR2 on neutrophils to promote chemotaxis.[199–204] The antimicrobial peptide LL-37 and

the complement components C3a and C5a are also strong neutrophil chemoattractants. In addition, neutrophils themselves release leukotrienes, which are proinflammatory molecules that are chemoattractant for most leukocytes.[199–201] Activation of the IL-1R, which utilizes the same signaling pathway as TLRs, is critical for recruitment of neutrophils to sites of *S. aureus* infection in the skin (Fig. 22.5).[127]

One of the main neutrophil functions is to engulf microbes into a phagosome, which eventually fuses with a lysosome to form a phagolysosome (Fig. 22.6).[193–198] In the phagosome, reactive oxygen species (ROS) are produced such as superoxide (O_2^-), hydrogen peroxide (H_2O_2), and hyperchlorous acid (HOCl) by the enzymes nicotinamide adenine dinucleotide phosphate (NADPH) oxidase, superoxide dismutase, and myeloperoxidase (MPO), respectively.[205–209] These ROSs are toxic to certain bacterial pathogens, but *S. aureus* is somewhat resistant to ROS-mediated killing alone.[193–198,209] However, ROS also promote killing of bacteria such as *S. aureus* by producing a charge across the phagocytic vacuole membrane, resulting in K^+ influx and release of proteases and antimicrobial peptides from neutrophil granules into the vacuole. Some of the components of neutrophil granules that are important in bacterial killing include proteinases (e.g., cathepsin G, elastase, and proteinase 3), α-defensins, lysozyme, acid hydrolases, lactoferrin (which sequesters iron and copper), transcobalamin II (which binds cyanocobalamin [vitamin B_{12}]), and neutrophil gelatinase-associated lipocalin (NGAL).[193–198,210] NGAL is an antimicrobial protein that binds to bacterial siderophores, and blocks their ability to extract iron needed for bacterial growth.

The critical role of neutrophils in host defense against *S. aureus* is further illustrated by the existence of mechanisms that *S. aureus* has developed to inhibit neutrophil recruitment and function. *S. aureus* secretes a protein called chemotaxis inhibitory protein of staphylococci (CHIPS) that interacts with the C5aR and the formyl peptide receptor to block neutrophil chemotaxis.[211,212] Another *S. aureus*–secreted protein, called extracellular adherence protein (Eap), binds to intercellular adhesion molecule 1 (ICAM-1) on vascular endothelium and prevents neutrophil adhesion and extravasation.[213–215] *S. aureus* also produces factors

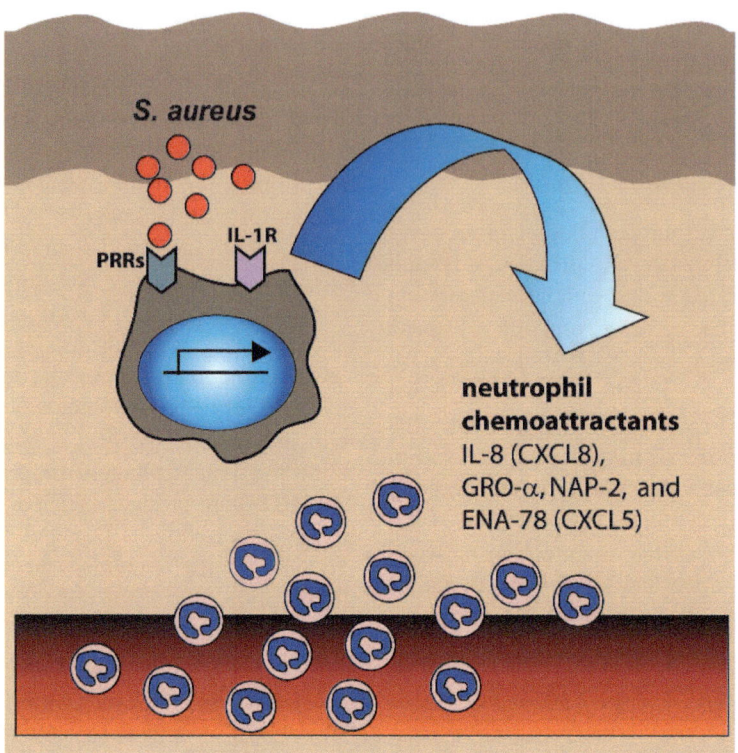

FIG. 22.5. Mechanism of neutrophil recruitment to a site of *S. aureus* infection in the skin. Recognition of *S. aureus* components by pattern recognition receptors (PRRs) and activation of interleukin-1R (IL-1R) signaling leads to resident skin cell production of chemokines that activate chemokine receptors CXCR1 and CXCR2 on neutrophils and promote neutrophil recruitment

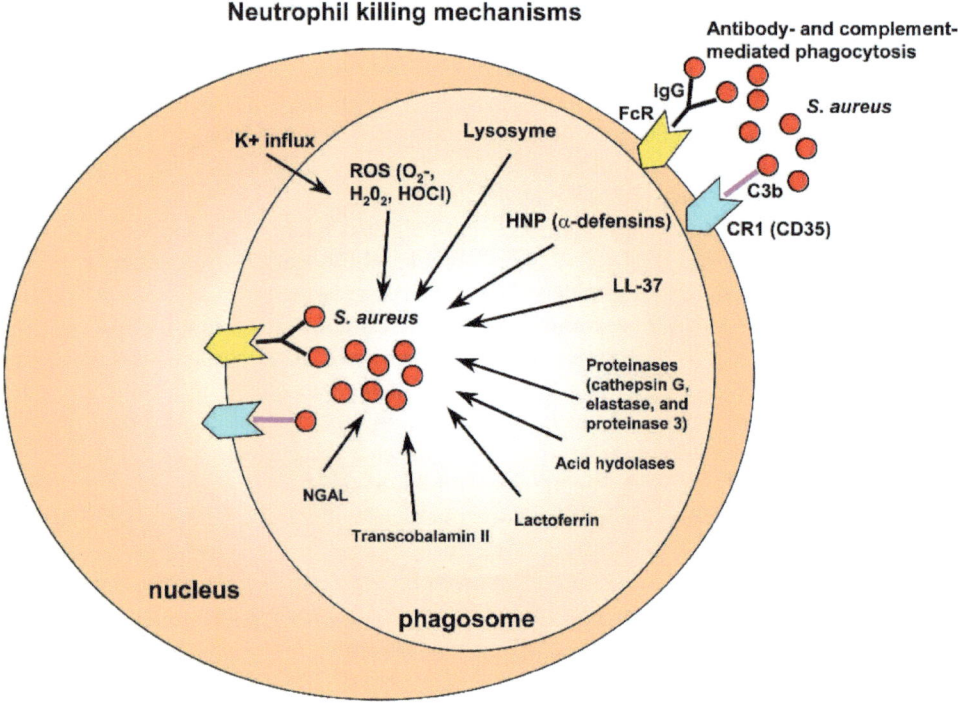

FIG. 22.6. Mechanisms of neutrophil phagocytosis and killing of *S. aureus*. NGAL, neutrophil gelatinase-associated lipocalin; ROS, reactive oxygen species

that inhibit neutrophil function. For example, the yellow carotenoid pigment of *S. aureus* that is responsible for the golden color is an antioxidant that blocks ROS-mediated killing of *S. aureus*.[216] In addition, *S. aureus* produces two superoxide dismutase enzymes that can degrade superoxide and impair ROS-mediated killing.[47-49,217]

Monocytes/Macrophages

Similar to neutrophils, monocytes/macrophages are recruited to the site of an *S. aureus* infection and are important in phagocytosing *S. aureus*.[47-49] Monocytes/macrophages (as well as neutrophils) express Fc and complement receptors that facilitate phagocytosis by recognizing immunoglobulin or complement components opsonized on the bacterial surface. The importance of phagocytosis is exemplified by the existence of several mechanisms that *S. aureus* utilizes to evade this process. For example, *S. aureus* has protein A on its surface that binds the Fc portion of immunoglobulin G (IgG), resulting in the binding of IgG in an incorrect orientation for detection by Fc receptors. In addition, fibrinogen binding proteins and clumping factor A (ClfA) bind fibrinogen and impair macrophage phagocytosis.[47-49,218] *S. aureus* also secretes toxins that are pore-forming proteins that damage membranes of host cells such as macrophages, leading to lysis and the prevention of phagocytosis.[47-49,219-221] There are two main families of these pore-forming toxins: (1) single-component α-hemolysin or α-toxin and (2) biocomponent leukotoxins, including γ-toxin or γ-hemolysin, Panton-Valentine leukocidin (PVL), leukocidin E/D, and leukocidin M/F-PV-like.[47-49,219-221] Panton-Valentine leukocidin has been epidemiologically associated with severe and necrotic skin infections and has been found in certain strains of community-acquired MRSA.[222-226]

Adaptive Immune Responses Against *S. aureus*

The innate immune system provides the first line of defense against microbial pathogens, while the cell-mediated and humoral immune responses of adaptive immunity are recruited later.[74,227-230] The adaptive immune system can be divided into T-cell– and B-cell–mediated immune responses, and the role of these adaptive immune responses against *S. aureus* is discussed in this section.

T-Cell Immune Response

A number of different observations have provided evidence that T cells play an important role in host defense against *S. aureus* skin infections. First, patients with HIV infection are at an increased risk for colonization and skin infection with *S. aureus*.[231-235] In addition, the low serum CD4+ T cell count of HIV patients is a risk factor for *S. aureus* infection.[233,235]

Second, patients with the inflammatory skin disease atopic dermatitis, which is associated with a Th2 cytokine profile (i.e., IL-4, IL-13, and IL-10), have increased colonization and superinfection with *S. aureus*.[132,133] Although the reason for the increased *S. aureus* superinfection in atopic dermatitis is likely multifactorial (including a defective epidermal barrier and impaired innate immune responses such as decreased expression of antimicrobial peptides), Th2 cytokines have also been implicated. For example, IL-4 has been shown to increase the expression of fibronectin and fibrinogen receptors on host cells, which promotes more efficient binding of *S. aureus* to the stratum corneum.[236] In addition, *S. aureus* via the *S. aureus*–derived factors fibronectin-binding protein (fnbp) and clumping factor (Clf, also known as fibrinogen-binding protein) more efficiently bound to skin from atopic dermatitis patients.[237] Also in atopic dermatitis, *S. aureus* produces superantigens such as staphylococcal enterotoxins A and B (SEA and SEB) and toxic shock syndrome toxin-1 (TSST-1), which exacerbate the inflammatory response by nonspecifically activating T cells.[133,238-241] *S. aureus* superantigens also can skew the cutaneous immune response toward the Th2 cytokine profile, thereby increasing *S. aureus* superinfection in atopic dermatitis.[242] Taken together, T cells likely play an important role in colonization and superinfection of atopic dermatitis lesions by increasing levels of Th2 cytokines and via nonspecific activation of T cells by superantigens.

Interestingly, a recent study demonstrated in a mouse model of *S. aureus* skin infection that resident CD4+ T cells in the skin are important in producing neutrophil chemokines that promote neutrophil recruitment to the site of infection.[243]

Thus, T cells may directly promote neutrophil recruitment to a site of *S. aureus* infection in the skin. Additionally, in a preclinical DNA-vaccine study against *S. aureus*, a Th1 immune response and vaccine-specific IFN-γ–producing CD8⁺ T cells were associated with enhanced survival against *S. aureus* challenge.[244] This finding, together with the recent understanding that *S. aureus* may have an important intracellular habitat, suggests that combined Th1 and Th2 immune responses may be required for effective natural or vaccine-induced immunity against *S. aureus* infections.

B-Cell Immune Response

The B-cell–mediated immune response against *S. aureus* involves the production of antibodies directed against specific antigenic components of *S. aureus*. These antibodies play an important role in opsonizing *S. aureus* and facilitating antibody-mediated phagocytosis by neutrophils and macrophages.[47–49] After an acute *S. aureus* infection (including skin infection), antibody levels have been shown to rise, including specific antibodies against protein A, teichoic acid, lipase, ClfA, extracellular fibrinogen binding protein (Efb), and fnbp.[245–249] One study demonstrated that the antibody repertoires differed in patients with superficial versus deep-seated *S. aureus* skin infections.[245] Studies using various animal models of *S. aureus* infection have provided further evidence that antibodies against different *S. aureus* components can provide some level of protection against *S. aureus* infection.[250–258]

The importance of B cell responses and antibodies in host defense against *S. aureus* infections is exemplified by the existence of protein A, an important virulence factor that *S. aureus* uses to counteract antibody-mediated responses.[47–49,259] Protein A of *S. aureus* binds antibody in the incorrect orientation, thus enabling *S. aureus* to evade antibody detection and subsequent antibody-mediated phagocytosis.

There have been attempts to develop vaccines and passive immunization strategies to promote antibody-mediated responses against *S. aureus* in humans. For example, a conjugate vaccine that contains *S. aureus* type 5 and type 8 capsular polysaccharide (StaphVAX), a hyperimmune IgG preparation containing high titers of antibody against ClfA (Veronate), and a humanized monoclonal antibody directed against ClfA (tefibazumab) have all been tested in animals and humans with varying success rates.[259–265] Thus, an effective vaccine that promotes protective antibody-mediated immunity against *S. aureus* infections may be possible in the future.

Group A *Streptococcus*

Group A *Streptococcus* (*Streptococcus pyogenes*) is a gram-positive extracellular bacterial pathogen that causes superficial and invasive skin infections such as impetigo, erysipelas, cellulitis, scarlet fever, and necrotizing fasciitis, and is the most common cause of bacterial pharyngitis (especially in children).[266–269] Group A *Streptococcus* infections can cause other severe infections such as streptococcal toxic shock syndrome, septic arthritis, osteomyelitis, septicemia, pneumonia, and meningitis. Lastly, after a group A *Streptococcus* infection, immunologic-mediated diseases such as guttate psoriasis, acute rheumatic fever, and glomerulonephritis may ensue. The Centers for Disease Control (CDC) estimates that there are approximately 10 million cases of noninvasive pharyngitis and superficial skin infections caused by group A *Streptococcus* per year in the U.S. In addition, there are 10,000 cases of invasive group A *Streptococcus* infections per year in the U.S. (including erysipelas, cellulitis, and necrotizing fasciitis) that result in 1100 to 1300 deaths.[270,271] Thus, group A *Streptococcus* continues to be a major cause of superficial and invasive skin infections in the U.S.

Clinical Manifestations

Group A *Streptococcus* causes superficial skin infections such as impetigo and invasive skin infections such as erysipelas, an infection of the superficial layers of the skin and cutaneous lymphatics (Fig. 22.7), or cellulitis, an infection involving the deep dermis and subcutaneous tissue.[266–271] Group A *Streptococcus* also causes necrotizing fasciitis, which is a severe skin and soft tissue infection that results in total destruction of the deep fat and fascia and often precedes streptococcal sepsis, shock, and multiorgan failure. In addition, scarlet fever, which is usually associated with a streptococcal throat

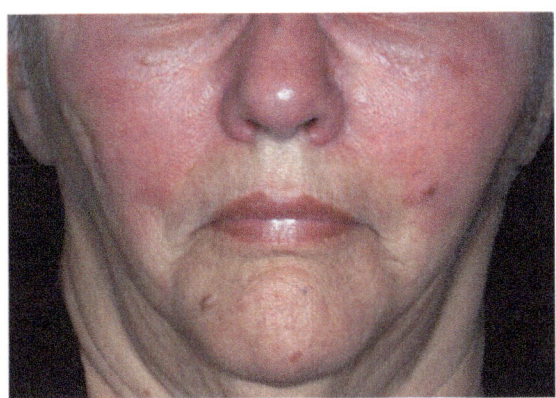

FIG. 22.7. Group A *Streptococcus* erysipelas of the face. The involved skin shows a sharply demarcated, erythematous, and edematous plaque. (Courtesy of the Victor D. Newcomer collection at UCLA and Logical Images, Inc.)

infection, is characterized by a morbilliform rash, strawberry tongue, and desquamation of skin. This constellation of clinical findings in scarlet fever is caused by streptococcal pyrogenic exotoxins A, B, or C, which act as superantigens.

Innate Immune Responses Against Group A *Streptococcus*

The innate immune response against group A *Streptococcus* is similar to that against *S. aureus* and includes soluble factors such as antimicrobial peptides and complement components, PRRs such as TLRs and NOD2, and innate immune system cells such as neutrophils and monocytes/macrophages. However, there are some important differences in the immune response against group A *Streptococcus*, especially with regard to the recognition and activity of M protein expressed by group A *Streptococcus*.

Antimicrobial Peptides

Both α- and β-defensins (HBD1–3) have direct antimicrobial activity against group A *Streptococcus* (Fig. 22.8).[272–275] In addition, stimulation of keratinocytes with group A *Streptococcus* increases production of HBD2.[276]. Cathelicidin also has direct antimicrobial activity against group A *Streptococcus* infections in mouse models of skin infection and in cultures of human keratinocytes or mast cells.[272–275] Cathelicidin production is upregulated in wounded human or mouse skin, which protects the healing wound from infection by group A *Streptococcus*.[277] Thus, both defensins and cathelicidin have antimicrobial activity and play a key role in the innate immune response against group A *Streptococcus*.

The importance of antimicrobial peptides in the innate immune response against group A *Streptococcus* is further illustrated by the existence of several mechanisms that group A *Streptococcus* utilizes to inhibit their function (Fig. 22.8). For example, group A *Streptococcus* produces streptococcal inhibitor of complement (SIC) that inhibits human α-defensin-1, HBDs 1 to 3, LL-37, and lysozyme.[272,273,275] In addition, extracellular proteases released by group A *Streptococcus* can generate dermatan sulfate from host proteoglycans, which subsequently binds to and inactivates α-defensins.[278]

Complement Activation

The importance of complement in the immune response against group A *Streptococcus* is exemplified by the existence of multiple factors produced by group A *Streptococcus* that inhibit complement activity (Fig. 22.8). The M protein of group A *Streptococcus* inhibits complement activity by several different mechanisms. M protein directly binds to and enhances the function of factor H (FH) and FH-like protein, host proteins that inhibit complement activation and prevent C3b-mediated phagocytosis.[279–287] However, this is controversial since one study found FH/FH-like protein-binding activity is mediated by a fibronectin-binding protein (Fba) and not M protein.[288] Group A *Streptococcus* M protein also binds to and enhances the function of C4b-binding protein (C4BP), a host protein that downregulates complement activation by accelerating the decay and preventing formation of C3- and C5-convertases.[289–299] Furthermore, M protein binds fibrinogen, which inhibits complement-mediated phagocytosis by reducing the amount of C3 convertase on the surface of group A *Streptococcus*.[300,301] In addition to M protein, group A *Streptococcus* also secretes C5a peptidase (ScpA), which cleaves C5a and inhibits neutrophil recruitment.[302–310] Lastly, the group A *Streptococcus*–derived protein SIC not only inhibits

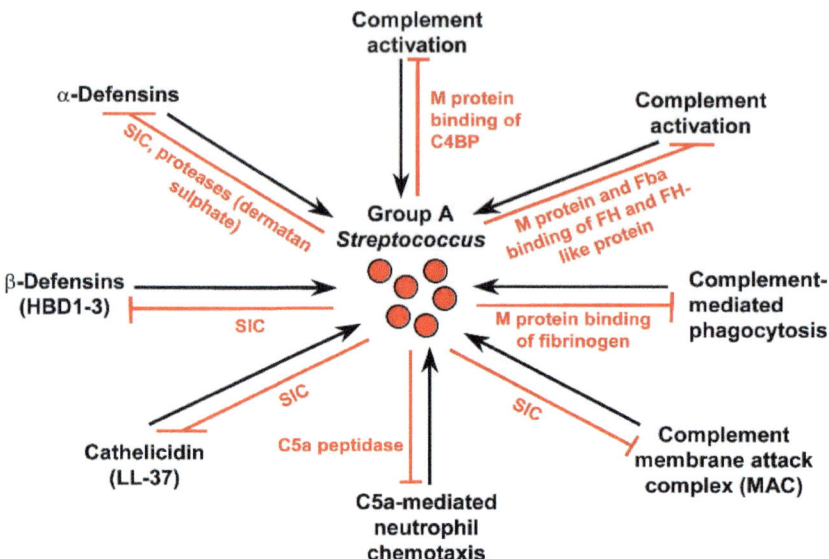

FIG. 22.8. Soluble mediators of the innate immune response against group A *Streptococcus*. The mechanisms that group A *Streptococcus* utilizes to inhibit these soluble mediators and complement activity are shown in red. SIC, streptococcal inhibitor of complement

antimicrobial peptides (see above), but also binds to C5b-C7 complexes and prevents formation of the MAC.[275,311,312]

Pattern Recognition Receptors that Recognize Components of Group A *Streptococcus*

There are only a few reports that have directly tested the ability of specific components of group A *Streptococcus* to be recognized by host PRRs. However, PGN, LTA, and lipopeptides are highly conserved among gram-positive staphylococci and streptococci species and are likely recognized in a similar fashion by PRRs such as TLRs and NODs.[25–30,163–166] In support of this, TLR2 has been shown to play an important role in host defense against group A *Streptococcus* in a mouse model of joint infection.[313] Additionally, TLR2 can be activated by the M protein of group A *Streptococcus*.[314] However, the M protein also binds to CD46 (membrane cofactor protein) on the surface of human keratinocytes, and this interaction facilitates the ability of group A *Streptococcus* to invade these cells.[315–318] Thus, M protein may contribute to protective immunity in some settings and increase pathogenesis in others.

Cellular Innate Immune Responses Against Group A *Streptococcus*

Neutrophils

The importance of neutrophils in host defense against group A *Streptococcus* is demonstrated by the existence of several sophisticated strategies that group A *Streptococcus* utilizes to counteract mechanisms of neutrophil recruitment and function (Fig. 22.9).[193–195,319] With regard to neutrophil recruitment, group A *Streptococcus* not only produces the C5a peptidase (see above), but also produces another peptidase called ScpC that degrades CXC chemokines (including IL-8 in humans and KC and macrophage inflammatory protein-2 [MIP-2] in mice).[320] These chemokines are critical for neutrophil recruitment to sites of infection. Group A *Streptococcus* also directly induces neutrophil lysis or apoptosis, effectively eliminating their antimicrobial activity.[321–323]

Group A *Streptococcus* has developed mechanisms to inhibit both complement- and antibody-mediated phagocytosis (Fig. 22.9). As mentioned above, group A *Streptococcus* prevents complement-mediated phagocytosis via activity of M protein and Fba. In addition, group A *Streptococcus* secretes endoglycosidase (EndoS) and streptococcal

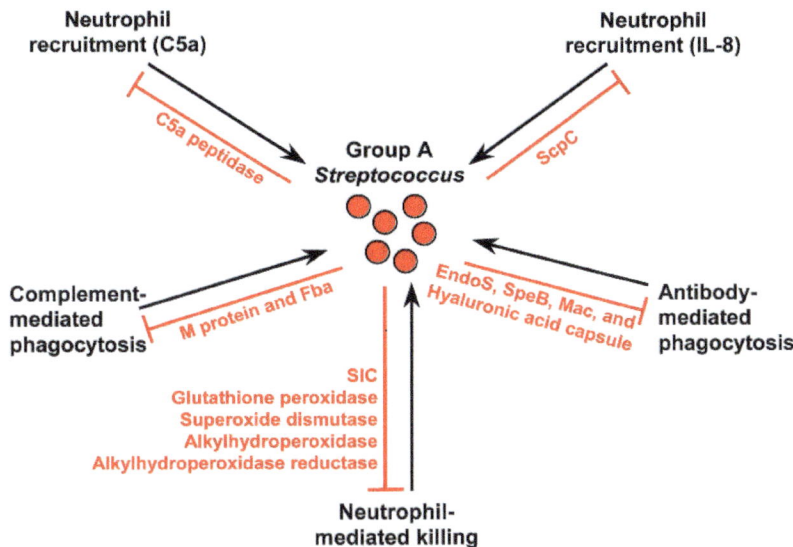

FIG. 22.9. Neutrophil recruitment and function (phagocytosis and killing) in host defense against group A *Streptococcus*. The mechanisms that group A *Streptococcus* utilizes to inhibit these processes are shown in red

pyrogenic exotoxin B (SpeB).[324–326] These bacterial factors inhibit antibody-mediated phagocytosis by hydrolyzing N-linked oligosaccharides on opsonized IgG molecules and by cleaving opsonized IgG molecules into Fab and Fc fragments, respectively. In a mouse skin infection model, group A *Streptococcus* mutant strains expressing protease-inactive SpeB caused significantly less necrosis and demonstrated less efficient systemic dissemination from the initial focus of skin inoculation.[327] The hyaluronic acid capsule of group A *Streptococcus* also acts as a physical barrier that nonspecifically resists phagocytosis.[328,329] In addition, group A *Streptococcus* also resists antibody-mediated phagocytosis by forming large bacterial aggregates via binding fibronectin and recruiting collagen fibers.[330] Lastly, group A *Streptococcus* secretes a protein called Mac (a bacterial homologue of the α-subunit of the β_2–integrin Mac-1) that binds to CD16 (FcγRIIIB) on phagocytes, thus inhibiting Fc-mediated phagocytosis.[331] Taken together, group A *Streptococcus* produces several different factors that can inhibit both complement- and antibody-mediated phagocytosis.

There are several mechanisms that group A *Streptococcus* utilizes to inhibit neutrophil function (Fig. 22.9). In addition to SIC, which inhib-

its antimicrobial peptides (see above), group A *Streptococcus* produces several enzymes that inhibit ROS-mediated microbicidal toxicity such as glutathione peroxidase, superoxide dismutase, alkylhydroperoxidase, and alkylhydroperoxidase reductase.[332–334]

Adaptive Immune Responses Against Group A *Streptococcus*

Both B and T cells play a role in adaptive immune responses against group A *Streptococcus* infections. In particular, antibodies and T cells that recognize antigenic components of M protein have been shown to produce protective immune responses that prevent colonization and infection by group A *Streptococcus*.[335–339] Similar to *S. aureus*, group A *Streptococcus* also produces exotoxins such as streptococcal mitogenic exotoxins SME (A through J, Z-1 and Z-2), and streptococcal superantigen (SSA).[269,340–342] These factors act as superantigens and nonspecifically activate T cells and contribute to the pathogenesis of group A *Streptococcus* infections.[269,340–342]

The important role of adaptive immunity in host defense against group A *Streptococcus* has led to different vaccination strategies to produce protective antibody responses. Since antibodies against

M protein of group A *Streptococcus* have been shown to offer protection against colonization and infection, several vaccines have targeted different antigenic epitopes of the M protein.[335–339] In addition, other vaccine strategies have been directed against the streptococcal immunoglobulin-binding protein Sib35, conserved carbohydrates, C5a peptidase, and lipoproteins.[343–346] These vaccine strategies have had varying successes, and it is hoped that there will be a successful vaccine against group A *Streptococcus* infections in the future.

Conclusion

Recent discoveries involving innate and adaptive immune responses against *S. aureus* and group A *Streptococcus* have greatly improved our understanding of these common skin infections. As antimicrobial resistance increases, strategies to enhance the host immune response to infections are becoming more critical. The mechanisms of bacterial pathogenesis and cutaneous host defense will be important to consider during the development of novel immunotherapies and innovative vaccine strategies against these common bacterial skin pathogens.

References

1. McCaig LF, McDonald LC, Mandal S, Jernigan DB. *Staphylococcus aureus*-associated skin and soft tissue infections in ambulatory care. Emerg Infect Dis 2006;12:1715–1723 http://www.cdc.gov/ncidod/EID/vol12no11/06–0190.htm.
2. Moran GJ, Krishnadasan A, Gorwitz RJ, et al. Methicillin-resistant S. aureus infections among patients in the emergency department. N Engl J Med 2006;355(7):666–674.
3. Lopez FA, Sanders CV. Dermatologic infections in the immunocompromised (non-HIV) host. Infect Dis Clin North Am 2001;15(2):671–702, xi.
4. DiNubile MJ, Lipsky BA. Complicated infections of skin and skin structures: when the infection is more than skin deep. J Antimicrob Chemother 2004;53(suppl 2):ii37–ii50.
5. Stevens DL, Bisno AL, Chambers HF, et al. Practice guidelines for the diagnosis and management of skin and soft-tissue infections. Clin Infect Dis 2005;41(10):1373–1406.
6. Vinh DC, Embil JM. Rapidly progressive soft tissue infections. Lancet Infect Dis 2005;5(8):501–513.
7. Lowy FD. Staphylococcus aureus infections. N Engl J Med 1998;339:520–532.
8. Manders SM. Toxin-mediated streptococcal and staphylococcal disease. J Am Acad Dermatol 1998;39:383–398.
9. Ladhani S. Recent developments in staphylococcal scalded skin syndrome. Clin Microbiol Infect 2001;7:301–307.
10. von EC, Becker K, Machka K, Stammer H, Peters G. Nasal carriage as a source of Staphylococcus aureus bacteremia. Study Group. N Engl J Med 2001;344(1):11–16.
11. Kuehnert MJ, Kruszon-Moran D, Hill HA, et al. Prevalence of Staphylococcus aureus nasal colonization in the United States, 2001–2002. J Infect Dis 2006;193(2):172–179.
12. Kluytmans JA, Wertheim HF. Nasal carriage of Staphylococcus aureus and prevention of nosocomial infections. Infection 2005;33(1):3–8.
13. Wertheim HF, Melles DC, Vos MC, et al. The role of nasal carriage in Staphylococcus aureus infections. Lancet Infect Dis 2005;5(12):751–762.
14. Onorato M, Borucki MJ, Baillargeon G, et al. Risk factors for colonization or infection due to methicillin-resistant Staphylococcus aureus in HIV-positive patients: a retrospective case-control study. Infect Control Hosp Epidemiol 1999;20(1):26–30.
15. Furuya EY, Lowy FD. Antimicrobial-resistant bacteria in the community setting. Nat Rev Microbiol 2006;4(1):36–45.
16. Foster TJ. The Staphylococcus aureus "superbug." J Clin Invest 2004;114(12):1693–1696.
17. Melles DC, Gorkink RF, Boelens HA, et al. Natural population dynamics and expansion of pathogenic clones of Staphylococcus aureus. J Clin Invest 2004;114(12):1732–1740.
18. Lowy FD. Antimicrobial resistance: the example of Staphylococcus aureus. J Clin Invest 2003;111(9):1265–1273.
19. Walsh TR, Howe RA. The prevalence and mechanisms of vancomycin resistance in Staphylococcus aureus. Annu Rev Microbiol 2002;56:657–675.
20. Ferber D. Microbiology. Triple-threat microbe gained powers from another bug. Science 2003;302:1488.
21. Oumeish I, Oumeish OY, Bataineh O. Acute bacterial skin infections in children. Clin Dermatol 2000;18:667–678.
22. Molne L, Verdrengh M, Tarkowski A. Role of neutrophil leukocytes in cutaneous infection caused by Staphylococcus aureus. Infect Immun 2000;68:6162–6167.
23. Verdrengh M, Tarkowski A. Role of neutrophils in experimental septicemia and septic arthritis induced by Staphylococcus aureus. Infect Immun 1997;65(7):2517–2521.

24. Janniger CK, Schwartz RA, Szepietowski JC, Reich A. Intertrigo and common secondary skin infections. Am Fam Physician 2005;72(5):833–838.

25. Akira S, Takeda K. Toll-like receptor signalling. Nat Rev Immunol 2004;4(7):499–511.

26. Modlin RL, Cheng G. From plankton to pathogen recognition. Nat Med 2004;10(11):1173–1174.

27. Sieling PA, Modlin RL. Toll-like receptors: mammalian "taste receptors" for a smorgasbord of microbial invaders. Curr Opin Microbiol 2002;5:70–75.

28. Kang SS, Kauls LS, Gaspari AA. Toll-like receptors: applications to dermatologic disease. J Am Acad Dermatol 2006;54(6):951–983.

29. McInturff JE, Modlin RL, Kim J. The role of toll-like receptors in the pathogenesis and treatment of dermatological disease. J Invest Dermatol 2005;125(1):1–8.

30. Medzhitov R. Toll-like receptors and innate immunity. Nat Rev Immunol 2001;1:135–145.

31. Selsted ME, Ouellette AJ. Mammalian defensins in the antimicrobial immune response. Nat Immunol 2005;6(6):551–557.

32. Oppenheim JJ, Biragyn A, Kwak LW, Yang D. Roles of antimicrobial peptides such as defensins in innate and adaptive immunity. Ann Rheum Dis 2003;62(suppl 2):ii17–ii21.

33. Ganz T. Defensins: antimicrobial peptides of innate immunity. Nat Rev Immunol 2003;3:710–720.

34. Gallo RL, Murakami M, Ohtake T, Zaiou M. Biology and clinical relevance of naturally occurring antimicrobial peptides. J Allergy Clin Immunol 2002;110:823–831.

35. Zasloff M. Antimicrobial peptides of multicellular organisms. Nature 2002;415(6870):389–395.

36. Lehrer RI, Ganz T. Cathelicidins: a family of endogenous antimicrobial peptides. Curr Opin Hematol 2002;9:18–22.

37. Ericksen B, Wu Z, Lu W, Lehrer RI. Antibacterial activity and specificity of the six human {alpha}-defensins. Antimicrob Agents Chemother 2005;49(1): 269–275.

38. Jin T, Bokarewa M, Foster T, Mitchell J, Higgins J, Tarkowski A. Staphylococcus aureus resists human defensins by production of staphylokinase, a novel bacterial evasion mechanism. J Immunol 2004;172(2):1169–1176.

39. Peschel A, Jack RW, Otto M, et al. Staphylococcus aureus resistance to human defensins and evasion of neutrophil killing via the novel virulence factor MprF is based on modification of membrane lipids with l-lysine. J Exp Med 2001;193(9):1067–1076.

40. Harder J, Bartels J, Christophers E, Schroder JM. A peptide antibiotic from human skin. Nature 1997;387:861.

41. Garcia JR, Krause A, Schulz S, et al. Human beta-defensin 4: a novel inducible peptide with a specific salt-sensitive spectrum of antimicrobial activity. FASEB J 2001;15(10):1819–1821.

42. Harder J, Bartels J, Christophers E, Schroder JM. Isolation and characterization of human beta-defensin-3, a novel human inducible peptide antibiotic. J Biol Chem 2001;276:5707–5713.

43. Braff MH, Zaiou M, Fierer J, Nizet V, Gallo RL. Keratinocyte production of cathelicidin provides direct activity against bacterial skin pathogens. Infect Immun 2005;73(10):6771–6781.

44. Turner J, Cho Y, Dinh NN, Waring AJ, Lehrer RI. Activities of LL-37, a cathelin-associated antimicrobial peptide of human neutrophils. Antimicrob Agents Chemother 1998;42(9):2206–2214.

45. Murakami M, Lopez-Garcia B, Braff M, Dorschner RA, Gallo RL. Postsecretory processing generates multiple cathelicidins for enhanced topical antimicrobial defense. J Immunol 2004;172(5):3070–3077.

46. Midorikawa K, Ouhara K, Komatsuzawa H, et al. Staphylococcus aureus susceptibility to innate antimicrobial peptides, beta-defensins and CAP18, expressed by human keratinocytes. Infect Immun 2003;71:3730–3739.

47. Foster TJ. Immune evasion by staphylococci. Nat Rev Microbiol 2005;3(12):948–958.

48. Rooijakkers SH, van Kessel KP, van Strijp JA. Staphylococcal innate immune evasion. Trends Microbiol 2005;13(12):596–601.

49. Celli J, Finlay BB. Bacterial avoidance of phagocytosis. Trends Microbiol 2002;10:232–237.

50. Sieprawska-Lupa M, Mydel P, Krawczyk K, et al. Degradation of human antimicrobial peptide LL-37 by Staphylococcus aureus-derived proteinases. Antimicrob Agents Chemother 2004;48(12):4673–4679.

51. Menzies BE, Kenoyer A. Staphylococcus aureus infection of epidermal keratinocytes promotes expression of innate antimicrobial peptides. Infect Immun 2005;73(8):5241–5244.

52. Liu AY, Destoumieux D, Wong AV, et al. Human beta-defensin-2 production in keratinocytes is regulated by interleukin-1, bacteria, and the state of differentiation. J Invest Dermatol 2002;118(2):275–281.

53. Dinulos JG, Mentele L, Fredericks LP, Dale BA, Darmstadt GL. Keratinocyte expression of human beta defensin 2 following bacterial infection: role in cutaneous host defense. Clin Diagn Lab Immunol 2003;10(1):161–166.

54. Sayama K, Komatsuzawa H, Yamasaki K, et al. New mechanisms of skin innate immunity: ASK1–mediated keratinocyte differentiation regulates the expression of beta-defensins, LL37, and TLR2. Eur J Immunol 2005;35(6):1886–1895.

55. Sumikawa Y, Asada H, Hoshino K, et al. Induction of beta-defensin 3 in keratinocytes stimulated by bacterial lipopeptides through toll-like receptor 2. Microbes Infect 2006;8(6):1513–1521.

56. Menzies BE, Kenoyer A. Signal transduction and nuclear responses in Staphylococcus aureus-induced expression of human beta-defensin 3 in skin keratinocytes. Infect Immun 2006;74(12):6847–6854.

57. Sorensen OE, Thapa DR, Roupe KM, et al. Injury-induced innate immune response in human skin mediated by transactivation of the epidermal growth factor receptor. J Clin Invest 2006;116(7):1878–1885.

58. Sorensen OE, Thapa DR, Rosenthal A, Liu L, Roberts AA, Ganz T. Differential regulation of beta-defensin expression in human skin by microbial stimuli. J Immunol 2005;174(8):4870–4879.

59. Sorensen OE, Cowland JB, Theilgaard-Monch K, Liu L, Ganz T, Borregaard N. Wound healing and expression of antimicrobial peptides/polypeptides in human keratinocytes, a consequence of common growth factors. J Immunol 2003;170:5583–5589.

60. Liu PT, Stenger S, Li H, et al. Toll-like receptor triggering of a vitamin D-mediated human antimicrobial response. Science 2006;311(5768):1770–1773.

61. Wang TT, Nestel FP, Bourdeau V, et al. Cutting edge: 1,25-dihydroxyvitamin D3 is a direct inducer of antimicrobial peptide gene expression. J Immunol 2004;173(5):2909–2912.

62. Gombart AF, Borregaard N, Koeffler HP. Human cathelicidin antimicrobial peptide (CAMP) gene is a direct target of the vitamin D receptor and is strongly up-regulated in myeloid cells by 1,25–dihydroxyvitamin D3. FASEB J 2005;19(9):1067–1077.

63. Weber G, Heilborn JD, Chamorro Jimenez CI, Hammarsjo A, Torma H, Stahle M. Vitamin D induces the antimicrobial protein hCAP18 in human skin. J Invest Dermatol 2005;124(5):1080–1082.

64. Nomura I, Goleva E, Howell MD, et al. Cytokine milieu of atopic dermatitis, as compared to psoriasis, skin prevents induction of innate immune response genes. J Immunol 2003;171:3262–3269.

65. Ong PY, Ohtake T, Brandt C, et al. Endogenous antimicrobial peptides and skin infections in atopic dermatitis. N Engl J Med 2002;347:1151–1160.

66. Henseler T, Christophers E. Disease concomitance in psoriasis. J Am Acad Dermatol 1995;32:982–986.

67. Tjabringa GS, Ninaber DK, Drijfhout JW, Rabe KF, Hiemstra PS. Human cathelicidin LL-37 is a chemoattractant for eosinophils and neutrophils that acts via formyl-peptide receptors. Int Arch Allergy Immunol 2006;140(2):103–112.

68. De Y, Chen Q, Schmidt AP, et al. LL-37, the neutrophil granule- and epithelial cell-derived cathelicidin, utilizes formyl peptide receptor-like 1 (FPRL1) as a receptor to chemoattract human peripheral blood neutrophils, monocytes, and T cells. J Exp Med 2000;192(7):1069–1074.

69. Yang D, Chertov O, Oppenheim JJ. The role of mammalian antimicrobial peptides and proteins in awakening of innate host defenses and adaptive immunity. Cell Mol Life Sci 2001;58(7):978–989.

70. Yang D, Chen Q, Chertov O, Oppenheim JJ. Human neutrophil defensins selectively chemoattract naive T and immature dendritic cells. J Leukoc Biol 2000;68(1):9–14.

71. Yang D, Chertov O, Oppenheim JJ. Participation of mammalian defensins and cathelicidins in antimicrobial immunity: receptors and activities of human defensins and cathelicidin (LL-37). J Leukoc Biol 2001;69:691–697.

72. Walport MJ. Complement. First of two parts. N Engl J Med 2001;344(14):1058–1066.

73. Walport MJ. Complement. Second of two parts. N Engl J Med 2001;344(15):1140–1144.

74. Dempsey PW, Vaidya SA, Cheng G. The art of war: innate and adaptive immune responses. Cell Mol Life Sci 2003;60:2604–2621.

75. Liu Y, Endo Y, Iwaki D, et al. Human M-ficolin is a secretory protein that activates the lectin complement pathway. J Immunol 2005;175(5):3150–3156.

76. Krarup A, Sorensen UB, Matsushita M, Jensenius JC, Thiel S. Effect of capsulation of opportunistic pathogenic bacteria on binding of the pattern recognition molecules mannan-binding lectin, L-ficolin, and H-ficolin. Infect Immun 2005;73(2):1052–1060.

77. Lynch NJ, Roscher S, Hartung T, et al. L-ficolin specifically binds to lipoteichoic acid, a cell wall constituent of gram-positive bacteria, and activates the lectin pathway of complement. J Immunol 2004;172(2):1198–1202.

78. Cunnion KM, Zhang HM, Frank MM. Availability of complement bound to Staphylococcus aureus to interact with membrane complement receptors influences efficiency of phagocytosis. Infect Immun 2003;71(2):656–662.

79. Sakiniene E, Bremell T, Tarkowski A. Complement depletion aggravates Staphylococcus aureus septicaemia and septic arthritis. Clin Exp Immunol 1999;115:95–102.

80. Cunnion KM, Benjamin DK Jr, Hester CG, Frank MM. Role of complement receptors 1 and 2 (CD35 and CD21), C3, C4, and C5 in survival by mice of Staphylococcus aureus bacteremia. J Lab Clin Med 2004;143(6):358–365.

81. Cunnion KM, Frank MM. Complement activation influences Staphylococcus aureus adherence to endothelial cells. Infect Immun 2003;71:1321–1327.

82. Shi L, Takahashi K, Dundee J, et al. Mannose-binding lectin-deficient mice are susceptible to infection with Staphylococcus aureus. J Exp Med 2004;199(10):1379–1390.

83. Takahashi K, Shi L, Gowda LD, Ezekowitz RA. Relative roles of complement factor 3 and mannose-binding lectin in host defense against infection. Infect Immun 2005;73(12):8188–8193.

84. Carlsson M, Sjoholm AG, Eriksson L, et al. Deficiency of the mannan-binding lectin pathway of complement and poor outcome in cystic fibrosis: bacterial colonization may be decisive for a relationship. Clin Exp Immunol 2005;139(2):306–313.

85. Ono K, Nishitani C, Mitsuzawa H, et al. Mannose-binding lectin augments the uptake of lipid A, Staphylococcus aureus, and Escherichia coli by Kupffer cells through increased cell surface expression of scavenger receptor A. J Immunol 2006;177(8):5517–5523.

86. Neth O, Jack DL, Johnson M, Klein NJ, Turner MW. Enhancement of complement activation and opsonophagocytosis by complexes of mannose-binding lectin with mannose-binding lectin-associated serine protease after binding to Staphylococcus aureus. J Immunol 2002;169(8):4430–4436.

87. Neth O, Jack DL, Dodds AW, Holzel H, Klein NJ, Turner MW. Mannose-binding lectin binds to a range of clinically relevant microorganisms and promotes complement deposition. Infect Immun 2000;68(2):688–693.

88. Rooijakkers SH, Ruyken M, van RJ, van Kessel KP, van Strijp JA, van Wamel WJ. Early expression of SCIN and CHIPS drives instant immune evasion by Staphylococcus aureus. Cell Microbiol 2006;8(8):1282–1293.

89. van Wamel WJ, Rooijakkers SH, Ruyken M, van Kessel KP, van Strijp JA. The innate immune modulators staphylococcal complement inhibitor and chemotaxis inhibitory protein of Staphylococcus aureus are located on beta-hemolysin-converting bacteriophages. J Bacteriol 2006;188(4):1310–1315.

90. Rooijakkers SH, Ruyken M, Roos A, et al. Immune evasion by a staphylococcal complement inhibitor that acts on C3 convertases. Nat Immunol 2005;6(9):920–927.

91. Lee LY, Hook M, Haviland D, et al. Inhibition of complement activation by a secreted Staphylococcus aureus protein. J Infect Dis 2004;190(3):571–579.

92. Lee LY, Liang X, Hook M, Brown EL. Identification and characterization of the C3 binding domain of the Staphylococcus aureus extracellular fibrinogen-binding protein (Efb). J Biol Chem 2004;279(49):50710–50716.

93. Rooijakkers SH, van Wamel WJ, Ruyken M, van Kessel KP, van Strijp JA. Anti-opsonic properties of staphylokinase. Microbes Infect 2005;7(3):476–484.

94. Pivarcsi A, Bodai L, Rethi B, et al. Expression and function of Toll-like receptors 2 and 4 in human keratinocytes. Int Immunol 2003;15(6):721–730.

95. Kawai K. Expression of functional toll-like receptors on cultured human epidermal keratinocytes. J Invest Dermatol 2003;121:217–218.

96. Pivarcsi A, Koreck A, Bodai L, et al. Differentiation-regulated expression of Toll-like receptors 2 and 4 in HaCaT keratinocytes. Arch Dermatol Res 2004;296:120–124.

97. Renn CN, Sanchez DJ, Ochoa MT, et al. TLR activation of Langerhans cell-like dendritic cells triggers an antiviral immune response. J Immunol 2006;177(1):298–305.

98. Takeuchi J, Watari E, Shinya E, et al. Down-regulation of Toll-like receptor expression in monocyte-derived Langerhans cell-like cells: implications of low-responsiveness to bacterial components in the epidermal Langerhans cells. Biochem Biophys Res Commun 2003;306(3):674–679.

99. Supajatura V, Ushio H, Nakao A, et al. Differential responses of mast cell Toll-like receptors 2 and 4 in allergy and innate immunity. J Clin Invest 2002;109(10):1351–1359.

100. Lin Y, Lee H, Berg AH, Lisanti MP, Shapiro L, Scherer PE. The lipopolysaccharide-activated toll-like receptor (TLR)-4 induces synthesis of the closely related receptor TLR-2 in adipocytes. J Biol Chem 2000;275(32):24255–24263.

101. Kawai K, Shimura H, Minagawa M, Ito A, Tomiyama K, Ito M. Expression of functional Toll-like receptor 2 on human epidermal keratinocytes. J Dermatol Sci 2002;30(3):185–194.

102. Mempel M, Voelcker V, Kollisch G, et al. Toll-like receptor expression in human keratinocytes: nuclear factor kappaB controlled gene activation by Staphylococcus aureus is toll-like receptor 2 but not toll-like receptor 4 or platelet activating factor receptor dependent. J Invest Dermatol 2003;121(6):1389–1396.

103. Baker BS, Ovigne JM, Powles AV, Corcoran S, Fry L. Normal keratinocytes express Toll-like receptors (TLRs) 1, 2 and 5: modulation of TLR expression in chronic plaque psoriasis. Br J Dermatol 2003;148:670–679.

104. Curry JL, Qin JZ, Bonish B, et al. Innate immune-related receptors in normal and psoriatic skin. Arch Pathol Lab Med 2003;127:178–186.

105. Krutzik SR, Ochoa MT, Sieling PA, et al. Activation and regulation of Toll-like receptors 2 and 1 in human leprosy. Nat Med 2003;9:525–532.

106. Lien E, Sellati TJ, Yoshimura A, et al. Toll-like receptor 2 functions as a pattern recognition receptor for diverse bacterial products. J Biol Chem 1999;274(47):33419–33425.

107. Takeuchi O, Hoshino K, Kawai T, et al. Differential roles of TLR2 and TLR4 in recognition of gram-negative and gram-positive bacterial cell wall components. Immunity 1999;11(4):443–451.

108. Underhill DM, Ozinsky A, Hajjar AM, et al. The Toll-like receptor 2 is recruited to macrophage phagosomes and discriminates between pathogens. Nature 1999;401(6755):811–815.

109. Yoshimura A, Lien E, Ingalls RR, Tuomanen E, Dziarski R, Golenbock D. Cutting edge: recognition of Gram-positive bacterial cell wall components by the innate immune system occurs via Toll-like receptor 2. J Immunol 1999;163(1):1–5.

110. Takeuchi O, Hoshino K, Akira S. Cutting edge: TLR2–deficient and MyD88–deficient mice are highly susceptible to Staphylococcus aureus infection. J Immunol 2000;165(10):5392–5396.

111. Kadowaki N, Ho S, Antonenko S, et al. Subsets of human dendritic cell precursors express different toll-like receptors and respond to different microbial antigens. J Exp Med 2001;194(6):863–869.

112. Mitsuzawa H, Wada I, Sano H, et al. Extracellular Toll-like receptor 2 region containing Ser40–Ile64 but not Cys30–Ser39 is critical for the recognition of Staphylococcus aureus peptidoglycan. J Biol Chem 2001;276(44):41350–41356.

113. Iwaki D, Mitsuzawa H, Murakami S, et al. The extracellular toll-like receptor 2 domain directly binds peptidoglycan derived from Staphylococcus aureus. J Biol Chem 2002;277(27):24315–24320.

114. Morath S, Stadelmaier A, Geyer A, Schmidt RR, Hartung T. Synthetic lipoteichoic acid from Staphylococcus aureus is a potent stimulus of cytokine release. J Exp Med 2002;195(12):1635–1640.

115. Wolfert MA, Murray TF, Boons GJ, Moore JN. The origin of the synergistic effect of muramyl dipeptide with endotoxin and peptidoglycan. J Biol Chem 2002;277(42):39179–39186.

116. Fujita M, Into T, Yasuda M, et al. Involvement of leucine residues at positions 107, 112, and 115 in a leucine-rich repeat motif of human Toll-like receptor 2 in the recognition of diacylated lipoproteins and lipopeptides and Staphylococcus aureus peptidoglycans. J Immunol 2003;171(7):3675–3683.

117. Kristian SA, Lauth X, Nizet V, et al. Alanylation of teichoic acids protects Staphylococcus aureus against Toll-like receptor 2–dependent host defense in a mouse tissue cage infection model. J Infect Dis 2003;188(3):414–423.

118. Lembo A, Kalis C, Kirschning CJ, et al. Differential contribution of Toll-like receptors 4 and 2 to the cytokine response to Salmonella enterica serovar Typhimurium and Staphylococcus aureus in mice. Infect Immun 2003;71(10):6058–6062.

119. McCurdy JD, Olynych TJ, Maher LH, Marshall JS. Cutting edge: distinct Toll-like receptor 2 activators selectively induce different classes of mediator production from human mast cells. J Immunol 2003;170(4):1625–1629.

120. Schroder NW, Morath S, Alexander C, et al. Lipoteichoic acid (LTA) of Streptococcus pneumoniae and Staphylococcus aureus activates immune cells via Toll-like receptor (TLR)-2, lipopolysaccharide-binding protein (LBP), and CD14, whereas TLR-4 and MD-2 are not involved. J Biol Chem 2003;278(18):15587–15594.

121. Lotz S, Aga E, Wilde I, et al. Highly purified lipoteichoic acid activates neutrophil granulocytes and delays their spontaneous apoptosis via CD14 and TLR2. J Leukoc Biol 2004;75(3):467–477.

122. Matsubara M, Harada D, Manabe H, Hasegawa K. Staphylococcus aureus peptidoglycan stimulates granulocyte macrophage colony-stimulating factor production from human epidermal keratinocytes via mitogen-activated protein kinases. FEBS Lett 2004;566(1–3):195–200.

123. Travassos LH, Girardin SE, Philpott DJ, et al. Toll-like receptor 2–dependent bacterial sensing does not occur via peptidoglycan recognition. EMBO Rep 2004;5(10):1000–1006.

124. von AS, Schroder NW, Traub S, et al. Heterozygous toll-like receptor 2 polymorphism does not affect lipoteichoic acid-induced chemokine and inflammatory responses. Infect Immun 2004; 72(3):1828–1831.

125. Dziarski R, Gupta D. Staphylococcus aureus peptidoglycan is a toll-like receptor 2 activator: a reevaluation. Infect Immun 2005;73(8):5212–5216.

126. Hashimoto M, Tawaratsumida K, Kariya H, et al. Not lipoteichoic acid but lipoproteins appear to be the dominant immunobiologically active compounds in Staphylococcus aureus. J Immunol 2006;177(5): 3162–3169.

127. Miller LS, O'Connell RM, Gutierrez MA, et al. MyD88 mediates neutrophil recruitment initiated by IL-1R but not TLR2 activation in immunity against Staphylococcus aureus. Immunity 2006;24(1): 79–91.

128. Hoebe K, Georgel P, Rutschmann S, et al. CD36 is a sensor of diacylglycerides. Nature 2005;433(7025):523–527.

129. Pivarcsi A, Nagy I, Kemeny L. Innate immunity in the skin: how keratinocytes fight against pathogens. Curr Immunol Rev 2005;1:29–42.

130. Kollisch G, Kalali BN, Voelcker V, et al. Various members of the Toll-like receptor family contribute to the innate immune response of human epidermal keratinocytes. Immunology 2005;114(4):531–541.

131. Ahmad-Nejad P, Mrabet-Dahbi S, Breuer K, et al. The toll-like receptor 2 R753Q polymorphism defines a subgroup of patients with atopic dermatitis having severe phenotype. J Allergy Clin Immunol 2004;113(3):565–567.

132. Roll A, Cozzio A, Fischer B, Schmid-Grendelmeier P. Microbial colonization and atopic dermatitis. Curr Opin Allergy Clin Immunol 2004;4(5):373–378.

133. Baker BS. The role of microorganisms in atopic dermatitis. Clin Exp Immunol 2006;144(1):1–9.

134. Takeuchi O, Sato S, Horiuchi T, et al. Cutting edge: role of Toll-like receptor 1 in mediating immune response to microbial lipoproteins. J Immunol 2002;169(1):10–14.

135. Takeda K, Takeuchi O, Akira S. Recognition of lipopeptides by Toll-like receptors. J Endotoxin Res 2002;8(6):459–463.

136. Takeuchi O, Kawai T, Muhlradt PF, et al. Discrimination of bacterial lipoproteins by Toll-like receptor 6. Int Immunol 2001;13(7):933–940.

137. Cleveland MG, Gorham JD, Murphy TL, Tuomanen E, Murphy KM. Lipoteichoic acid preparations of gram-positive bacteria induce interleukin-12 through a CD14–dependent pathway. Infect Immun 1996;64(6):1906–1912.

138. Dziarski R, Tapping RI, Tobias PS. Binding of bacterial peptidoglycan to CD14. J Biol Chem 1998;273(15):8680–8690.

139. Schwandner R, Dziarski R, Wesche H, Rothe M, Kirschning CJ. Peptidoglycan- and lipoteichoic acid-induced cell activation is mediated by toll-like receptor 2. J Biol Chem 1999;274(25):17406–17409.

140. Gupta D, Wang Q, Vinson C, Dziarski R. Bacterial peptidoglycan induces CD14–dependent activation of transcription factors CREB/ATF and AP-1. J Biol Chem 1999;274(20):14012–14020.

141. Rietschel ET, Schletter J, Weidemann B, et al. Lipopolysaccharide and peptidoglycan: CD14–dependent bacterial inducers of inflammation. Microb Drug Resist 1998;4(1):37–44.

142. Gupta D, Kirkland TN, Viriyakosol S, Dziarski R. CD14 is a cell-activating receptor for bacterial peptidoglycan. J Biol Chem 1996;271(38):23310–23316.

143. Pugin J, Heumann ID, Tomasz A, et al. CD14 is a pattern recognition receptor. Immunity 1994;1(6):509–516.

144. Weidemann B, Schletter J, Dziarski R, et al. Specific binding of soluble peptidoglycan and muramyldipeptide to CD14 on human monocytes. Infect Immun 1997;65(3):858–864.

145. Weidemann B, Brade H, Rietschel ET, et al. Soluble peptidoglycan-induced monokine production can be blocked by anti-CD14 monoclonal antibodies and by lipid A partial structures. Infect Immun 1994;62(11):4709–4715.

146. Hermann C, Spreitzer I, Schroder NW, et al. Cytokine induction by purified lipoteichoic acids from various bacterial species–role of LBP, sCD14, CD14 and failure to induce IL-12 and subsequent IFN-gamma release. Eur J Immunol 2002;32(2):541–551.

147. Iwaki D, Nishitani C, Mitsuzawa H, Hyakushima N, Sano H, Kuroki Y. The CD14 region spanning amino acids 57–64 is critical for interaction with the extracellular Toll-like receptor 2 domain. Biochem Biophys Res Commun 2005;328(1):173–176.

148. Haziot A, Ferrero E, Lin XY, Stewart CL, Goyert SM. CD14–deficient mice are exquisitely insensitive to the effects of LPS. Prog Clin Biol Res 1995;392:349–351.

149. Nagai Y, Akashi S, Nagafuku M, et al. Essential role of MD-2 in LPS responsiveness and TLR4 distribution. Nat Immunol 2002;3(7):667–672.

150. Zhang G, Ghosh S. Molecular mechanisms of NF-kappaB activation induced by bacterial lipopolysaccharide through Toll-like receptors. J Endotoxin Res 2000;6(6):453–457.

151. Lien E, Means TK, Heine H, et al. Toll-like receptor 4 imparts ligand-specific recognition of bacterial lipopolysaccharide. J Clin Invest 2000;105(4):497–504.

152. Haziot A, Hijiya N, Schultz K, Zhang F, Gangloff SC, Goyert SM. CD14 plays no major role in shock induced by Staphylococcus aureus but down-regulates TNF-alpha production. J Immunol 1999;162(8):4801–4805.

153. Stuart LM, Deng J, Silver JM, et al. Response to Staphylococcus aureus requires CD36–mediated phagocytosis triggered by the COOH-terminal cytoplasmic domain. J Cell Biol 2005;170(3):477–485.

154. Krieg AM. CpG motifs in bacterial DNA and their immune effects. Annu Rev Immunol 2002;20:709–760.

155. Ashkar AA, Rosenthal KL. Toll-like receptor 9, CpG DNA and innate immunity. Curr Mol Med 2002;2(6):545–556.

156. Krieg AM. CpG motifs: the active ingredient in bacterial extracts? Nat Med 2003;9(7):831–835.

157. Molne L, Collins LV, Tarkowski A. Inflammatogenic properties of bacterial DNA following cutaneous exposure. J Invest Dermatol 2003;121(2):294–299.

158. Neujahr DC, Reich CF, Pisetsky DS. Immunostimulatory properties of genomic DNA from different bacterial species. Immunobiology 1999;200(1):106–119.

159. Sparwasser T, Miethke T, Lipford G, et al. Bacterial DNA causes septic shock. Nature 1997;386(6623):336–337.

160. Yamamoto S, Yamamoto T, Shimada S, et al. DNA from bacteria, but not from vertebrates, induces interferons, activates natural killer cells and inhibits tumor growth. Microbiol Immunol 1992;36(9):983–997.

161. Ishii KJ, Coban C, Kato H, et al. A Toll-like receptor-independent antiviral response induced by double-stranded B-form DNA. Nat Immunol 2006;7(1):40–48.

162. Stetson DB, Medzhitov R. Recognition of cytosolic DNA activates an IRF3–dependent innate immune response. Immunity 2006;24(1):93–103.

163. Strober W, Murray PJ, Kitani A, Watanabe T. Signalling pathways and molecular interactions of NOD1 and NOD2. Nat Rev Immunol 2006;6(1):9–20.

164. Philpott DJ, Girardin SE. The role of Toll-like receptors and Nod proteins in bacterial infection. Mol Immunol 2004;41(11):1099–1108.

165. Boneca IG. The role of peptidoglycan in pathogenesis. Curr Opin Microbiol 2005;8(1):46–53.

166. Fritz JH, Ferrero RL, Philpott DJ, Girardin SE. Nod-like proteins in immunity, inflammation and disease. Nat Immunol 2006;7(12):1250–1257.

167. Fournier B, Philpott DJ. Recognition of Staphylococcus aureus by the innate immune system. Clin Microbiol Rev 2005;18(3):521–540.

168. Girardin SE, Travassos LH, Herve M, et al. Peptidoglycan molecular requirements allowing detection by Nod1 and Nod2. J Biol Chem 2003;278(43):41702–41708.

169. Kapetanovic R, Nahori MA, Balloy V, et al. Contribution of phagocytosis and intracellular sensing for cytokine production by Staphylococcus aureus-activated macrophages. Infect Immun 2006.

170. Voss E, Wehkamp J, Wehkamp K, Stange EF, Schroder JM, Harder J. NOD2/CARD15 mediates induction of the antimicrobial peptide human beta-defensin-2. J Biol Chem 2006;281(4):2005–2011.

171. Bayles KW, Wesson CA, Liou LE, Fox LK, Bohach GA, Trumble WR. Intracellular Staphylococcus aureus escapes the endosome and induces apoptosis in epithelial cells. Infect Immun 1998;66(1):336–342.

172. Gresham HD, Lowrance JH, Caver TE, Wilson BS, Cheung AL, Lindberg FP. Survival of Staphylococcus aureus inside neutrophils contributes to infection. J Immunol 2000;164(7):3713–3722.

173. Hess DJ, Henry-Stanley MJ, Erickson EA, Wells CL. Intracellular survival of Staphylococcus aureus within cultured enterocytes. J Surg Res 2003;114(1):42–49.

174. Hudson MC, Ramp WK, Nicholson NC, Williams AS, Nousiainen MT. Internalization of Staphylococcus aureus by cultured osteoblasts. Microb Pathog 1995;19(6):409–419.

175. Menzies BE, Kourteva I. Internalization of Staphylococcus aureus by endothelial cells induces apoptosis. Infect Immun 1998;66(12):5994–5998.

176. Jarry TM, Cheung AL. Staphylococcus aureus escapes more efficiently from the phagosome of a cystic fibrosis bronchial epithelial cell line than from its normal counterpart. Infect Immun 2006;74(5):2568–2577.

177. Almeida RA, Matthews KR, Cifrian E, Guidry AJ, Oliver SP. Staphylococcus aureus invasion of bovine mammary epithelial cells. J Dairy Sci 1996;79(6):1021–1026.

178. Girardin SE, Boneca IG, Viala J, et al. Nod2 is a general sensor of peptidoglycan through muramyl dipeptide (MDP) detection. J Biol Chem 2003;278(11):8869–8872.

179. Bera A, Herbert S, Jakob A, Vollmer W, Gotz F. Why are pathogenic staphylococci so lysozyme resistant? The peptidoglycan O-acetyltransferase OatA is the major determinant for lysozyme resistance of Staphylococcus aureus. Mol Microbiol 2005;55(3):778–787.

180. Bera A, Biswas R, Herbert S, Gotz F. The presence of peptidoglycan O-acetyltransferase in various staphylococcal species correlates with lysozyme resistance and pathogenicity. Infect Immun 2006;74(8):4598–4604.

181. Bera A, Biswas R, Herbert S, et al. Influence of wall teichoic acid on lysozyme resistance in Staphylococcus aureus. J Bacteriol 2007;189(1): 280–283.

182. Gomez MI, O'Seaghdha M, Magargee M, Foster TJ, Prince AS. Staphylococcus aureus protein A activates TNFR1 signaling through conserved IgG binding domains. J Biol Chem 2006;281(29):20190–20196.

183. Gomez MI, Lee A, Reddy B, et al. Staphylococcus aureus protein A induces airway epithelial inflammatory responses by activating TNFR1. Nat Med 2004;10(8):842–848.

184. Dziarski R, Gupta D. Mammalian PGRPs: novel antibacterial proteins. Cell Microbiol 2006;8(7):1059–1069.

185. Steiner H. Peptidoglycan recognition proteins: on and off switches for innate immunity. Immunol Rev 2004;198:83–96.

186. Liu C, Xu Z, Gupta D, Dziarski R. Peptidoglycan recognition proteins: a novel family of four human innate immunity pattern recognition molecules. J Biol Chem 2001;276(37):34686–34694.

187. Hoijer MA, Melief MJ, Debets R, Hazenberg MP. Inflammatory properties of peptidoglycan are decreased after degradation by human N-acetyl-muramyl-L-alanine amidase. Eur Cytokine Netw 1997;8(4):375–381.

188. Gelius E, Persson C, Karlsson J, Steiner H. A mammalian peptidoglycan recognition protein with N-acetylmuramoyl-L-alanine amidase activity. Biochem Biophys Res Commun 2003;306(4):988–994.

189. Wang ZM, Li X, Cocklin RR, et al. Human peptidoglycan recognition protein-L is an N-acetylmuramoyl-L-alanine amidase. J Biol Chem 2003;278(49):49044–49052.

190. Xu M, Wang Z, Locksley RM. Innate immune responses in peptidoglycan recognition protein L-deficient mice. Mol Cell Biol 2004;24(18):7949–7957.

191. Roos D, van Bruggen R, Meischl C. Oxidative killing of microbes by neutrophils. Microbes Infect 2003;5(14):1307–1315.

192. Heyworth PG, Cross AR, Curnutte JT. Chronic granulomatous disease. Curr Opin Immunol 2003;15(5):578–584.

193. Borregaard N, Theilgaard-Monch K, Cowland JB, Stahle M, Sorensen OE. Neutrophils and keratinocytes in innate immunity—cooperative actions to provide antimicrobial defense at the right time and place. J Leukoc Biol 2005;77(4):439–443.

194. Lehrer RI, Ganz T, Selsted ME, Babior BM, Curnutte JT. Neutrophils and host defense. Ann Intern Med 1988;109(2):127–142.

195. Urban CF, Lourido S, Zychlinsky A. How do microbes evade neutrophil killing? Cell Microbiol 2006;8(11):1687–1696.

196. Thomas EL, Lehrer RI, Rest RF. Human neutrophil antimicrobial activity. Rev Infect Dis 1988;10(suppl 2):S450–S456.

197. Segal AW. How neutrophils kill microbes. Annu Rev Immunol 2005;23:197–223.

198. Mayer-Scholl A, Averhoff P, Zychlinsky A. How do neutrophils and pathogens interact? Curr Opin Microbiol 2004;7(1):62–66.

199. Uchi H, Terao H, Koga T, Furue M. Cytokines and chemokines in the epidermis. J Dermatol Sci 2000;24(suppl 1):S29–S38.

200. Singer AJ, Clark RA. Cutaneous wound healing. N Engl J Med 1999;341(10):738–746.

201. Gillitzer R, Goebeler M. Chemokines in cutaneous wound healing. J Leukoc Biol 2001;69(4):513–521.

202. Walz A, Burgener R, Car B, Baggiolini M, Kunkel SL, Strieter RM. Structure and neutrophil-activating properties of a novel inflammatory peptide (ENA-78) with homology to interleukin 8. J Exp Med 1991;174(6):1355–1362.

203. Walz A, Baggiolini M. Generation of the neutrophil-activating peptide NAP-2 from platelet basic protein or connective tissue-activating peptide III through monocyte proteases. J Exp Med 1990;171(2):449–454.

204. Geiser T, Dewald B, Ehrengruber MU, Clark-Lewis I, Baggiolini M. The interleukin-8–related chemotactic cytokines GRO alpha, GRO beta, and GRO gamma activate human neutrophil and basophil leukocytes. J Biol Chem 1993;268(21):15419–15424.

205. Hampton MB, Kettle AJ, Winterbourn CC. Inside the neutrophil phagosome: oxidants, myeloperoxidase, and bacterial killing. Blood 1998;92(9):3007–3017.

206. Hampton MB, Kettle AJ, Winterbourn CC. Involvement of superoxide and myeloperoxidase in oxygen-dependent killing of Staphylococcus aureus by neutrophils. Infect Immun 1996;64(9):3512–3517.

207. Kobayashi SD, Voyich JM, Deleo FR. Regulation of the neutrophil-mediated inflammatory response to infection. Microbes Infect 2003;5(14):1337–1344.

208. Shao D, Segal AW, Dekker LV. Lipid rafts determine efficiency of NADPH oxidase activation in neutrophils. FEBS Lett 2003;550(1–3):101–106.

209. Reeves EP, Lu H, Jacobs HL, et al. Killing activity of neutrophils is mediated through activation of proteases by K+ flux. Nature 2002;416(6878):291–297.

210. Goetz DH, Holmes MA, Borregaard N, Bluhm ME, Raymond KN, Strong RK. The neutrophil lipocalin NGAL is a bacteriostatic agent that interferes with siderophore-mediated iron acquisition. Mol Cell 2002;10(5):1033–1043.

211. Postma B, Kleibeuker W, Poppelier MJ, et al. Residues 10–18 within the C5a receptor N terminus compose a binding domain for chemotaxis inhibitory protein of Staphylococcus aureus. J Biol Chem 2005;280(3):2020–2027.

212. Postma B, Poppelier MJ, van Galen JC, et al. Chemotaxis inhibitory protein of Staphylococcus aureus binds specifically to the C5a and formylated peptide receptor. J Immunol 2004;172(11):6994–7001.

213. Athanasopoulos AN, Economopoulou M, Orlova VV, et al. The extracellular adherence protein (Eap) of Staphylococcus aureus inhibits wound healing by interfering with host defense and repair mechanisms. Blood 2006;107(7):2720–2727.

214. Chavakis T, Wiechmann K, Preissner KT, Herrmann M. Staphylococcus aureus interactions with the endothelium: the role of bacterial "secretable expanded repertoire adhesive molecules" (SERAM) in disturbing host defense systems. Thromb Haemost 2005;94(2):278–285.

215. Harraghy N, Hussain M, Haggar A, et al. The adhesive and immunomodulating properties of the multifunctional Staphylococcus aureus protein Eap. Microbiology 2003;149(Pt 10):2701–2707.

216. Liu GY, Essex A, Buchanan JT, et al. Staphylococcus aureus golden pigment impairs neutrophil killing and promotes virulence through its antioxidant activity. J Exp Med 2005;202(2):209–215.

217. Karavolos MH, Horsburgh MJ, Ingham E, Foster SJ. Role and regulation of the superoxide dismutases of Staphylococcus aureus. Microbiology 2003;149(Pt 10):2749–2758.

218. Palmqvist N, Patti JM, Tarkowski A, Josefsson E. Expression of staphylococcal clumping factor A impedes macrophage phagocytosis. Microbes Infect 2004;6(2):188–195.

219. Travers JB, Norris DA, Leung DY. The keratinocyte as a target for staphylococcal bacterial toxins. J Invest Dermatol Symp Proc 2001;6(3):225–230.

220. Menestrina G, Serra MD, Prevost G. Mode of action of beta-barrel pore-forming toxins of the staphylococcal alpha-hemolysin family. Toxicon 2001;39(11):1661–1672.

221. Menestrina G, Dalla SM, Comai M, et al. Ion channels and bacterial infection: the case of beta-barrel pore-forming protein toxins of Staphylococcus aureus. FEBS Lett 2003;552(1):54–60.

222. Skiest DJ, Brown K, Cooper TW, Hoffman-Roberts H, Mussa HR, Elliott AC. Prospective comparison of methicillin-susceptible and methicillin-resistant community-associated Staphylococcus aureus infections in hospitalized patients. J Infect 2007;54(5):427–434.

223. Kilic A, Li H, Stratton CW, Tang YW. Antimicrobial susceptibility patterns, Panton-Valentine leukocidin occurrence and staphylococcal cassette chromosome mec types in methicillin resistant Staphylococcus aureus isolates in children versus adults from middle Tennessee. J Clin Microbiol 2006.

224. Frazee BW, Lynn J, Charlebois ED, Lambert L, Lowery D, Perdreau-Remington F. High prevalence of methicillin-resistant Staphylococcus aureus in emergency department skin and soft tissue infections. Ann Emerg Med 2005;45(3):311–320.

225. Yamasaki O, Kaneko J, Morizane S, et al. The association between Staphylococcus aureus strains carrying panton-valentine leukocidin genes and the development of deep-seated follicular infection. Clin Infect Dis 2005;40(3):381–385.

226. Ward PD, Turner WH. Identification of staphylococcal Panton-Valentine leukocidin as a potent dermonecrotic toxin. Infect Immun 1980;28(2):393–397.

227. Medzhitov R, Janeway C Jr. Innate immunity. N Engl J Med 2000;343:338–344.

228. Kupper TS, Fuhlbrigge RC. Immune surveillance in the skin: mechanisms and clinical consequences. Nat Rev Immunol 2004;4(3):211–222.

229. Robert C, Kupper TS. Inflammatory skin diseases, T cells, and immune surveillance. N Engl J Med 1999;341:1817–1828.

230. Clark RA, Chong B, Mirchandani N, et al. The vast majority of CLA+ T cells are resident in normal skin. J Immunol 2006;176(7):4431–4439.

231. Skiest D, Brown K, Hester J, et al. Community-onset methicillin-resistant Staphylococcus aureus in an urban HIV clinic. HIV Med 2006;7(6):361–368.

232. Anderson EJ, Hawkins C, Bolon MK, Palella FJ Jr. A series of skin and soft tissue infections due to methicillin-resistant Staphylococcus aureus in HIV-infected patients. J AIDS 2006;41(1):125–127.

233. Mathews WC, Caperna JC, Barber RE, et al. Incidence of and risk factors for clinically significant methicillin-resistant Staphylococcus aureus infection in a cohort of HIV-infected adults. J AIDS 2005;40(2):155–160.

234. Hidron AI, Kourbatova EV, Halvosa JS, et al. Risk factors for colonization with methicillin-resistant Staphylococcus aureus (MRSA) in patients admitted to an urban hospital: emergence of community-associated MRSA nasal carriage. Clin Infect Dis 2005;41(2):159–166.

235. Manfredi R, Calza L, Chiodo F. Epidemiology and microbiology of cellulitis and bacterial soft tissue infection during HIV disease: a 10-year survey. J Cutan Pathol 2002;29(3):168–172.

236. Cho SH, Strickland I, Tomkinson A, Fehringer AP, Gelfand EW, Leung DY. Preferential binding of Staphylococcus aureus to skin sites of Th2-mediated inflammation in a murine model. J Invest Dermatol 2001;116(5):658–663.

237. Cho SH, Strickland I, Boguniewicz M, Leung DY. Fibronectin and fibrinogen contribute to the enhanced binding of Staphylococcus aureus to atopic skin. J Allergy Clin Immunol 2001;108(2):269–274.

238. Leung DY, Hauk P, Strickland I, Travers JB, Norris DA. The role of superantigens in human diseases: therapeutic implications for the treatment of skin diseases. Br J Dermatol 1998;139(suppl 53):17–29.

239. Taskapan MO, Kumar P. Role of staphylococcal superantigens in atopic dermatitis: from colonization to inflammation. Ann Allergy Asthma Immunol 2000;84(1):3–10.

240. Skov L, Baadsgaard O. Bacterial superantigens and inflammatory skin diseases. Clin Exp Dermatol 2000;25(1):57–61.

241. Herz U, Bunikowski R, Renz H. Role of T cells in atopic dermatitis. New aspects on the dynamics of cytokine production and the contribution of bacterial superantigens. Int Arch Allergy Immunol 1998;115(3):179–190.

242. Laouini D, Kawamoto S, Yalcindag A, et al. Epicutaneous sensitization with superantigen induces allergic skin inflammation. J Allergy Clin Immunol 2003;112(5):981–987.

243. McLoughlin RM, Solinga RM, Rich J, et al. CD4+ T cells and CXC chemokines modulate the pathogenesis of Staphylococcus aureus wound infections. Proc Natl Acad Sci USA 2006;103(27):10408–10413.

244. Gaudreau MC, Lacasse P, Talbot BG. Protective immune responses to a multi-gene DNA vaccine against Staphylococcus aureus. Vaccine 2007;25(5):814–824.

245. Kumar A, Ray P, Kanwar M, Sharma M, Varma S. A comparative analysis of antibody repertoire against Staphylococcus aureus antigens in patients with deep-seated versus superficial staphylococcal infections. Int J Med Sci 2005;2(4):129–136.

246. Dryla A, Prustomersky S, Gelbmann D, et al. Comparison of antibody repertoires against Staphylococcus aureus in healthy individuals and in acutely infected patients. Clin Diagn Lab Immunol 2005;12(3):387–398.

247. Casolini F, Visai L, Joh D, et al. Antibody response to fibronectin-binding adhesin FnbpA in patients with Staphylococcus aureus infections. Infect Immun 1998;66(11):5433–5442.

248. Colque-Navarro P, Palma M, Soderquist B, Flock JI, Mollby R. Antibody responses in patients with staphylococcal septicemia against two Staphylococcus aureus fibrinogen binding proteins: clumping factor and an extracellular fibrinogen binding protein. Clin Diagn Lab Immunol 2000;7(1):14–20.

249. Colque-Navarro P, Soderquist B, Holmberg H, Blomqvist L, Olcen P, Mollby R. Antibody response in Staphylococcus aureus septicaemia—a prospective study. J Med Microbiol 1998;47(3):217–225.

250. Fattom AI, Sarwar J, Ortiz A, Naso R. A Staphylococcus aureus capsular polysaccharide (CP) vaccine and CP-specific antibodies protect mice against bacterial challenge. Infect Immun 1996;64(5):1659–1665.

251. Hall AE, Domanski PJ, Patel PR, et al. Characterization of a protective monoclonal antibody recognizing Staphylococcus aureus MSCRAMM protein clumping factor A. Infect Immun 2003;71(12):6864–6870.

252. Josefsson E, Hartford O, O'Brien L, Patti JM, Foster T. Protection against experimental Staphylococcus aureus arthritis by vaccination with clumping factor A, a novel virulence determinant. J Infect Dis 2001;184(12):1572–1580.

253. LeClaire RD, Hunt RE, Bavari S. Protection against bacterial superantigen staphylococcal enterotoxin B by passive vaccination. Infect Immun 2002;70(5):2278–2281.

254. Lee JC, Park JS, Shepherd SE, Carey V, Fattom A. Protective efficacy of antibodies to the Staphylococcus aureus type 5 capsular polysaccharide in a modified model of endocarditis in rats. Infect Immun 1997;65(10):4146–4151.

255. Mckenney D, Pouliot K, Wang Y, et al. Vaccine potential of poly-1–6 beta-D-N-succinylglucosamine, an immunoprotective surface polysaccharide of Staphylococcus aureus and Staphylococcus epidermidis. J Biotechnol 2000;83(1–2):37–44.

256. Mckenney D, Pouliot KL, Wang Y, et al. Broadly protective vaccine for Staphylococcus aureus based on an in vivo-expressed antigen. Science 1999;284(5419):1523–1527.

257. Nilsson IM, Verdrengh M, Ulrich RG, Bavari S, Tarkowski A. Protection against Staphylococcus aureus sepsis by vaccination with recombinant staphylococcal enterotoxin A devoid of superantigenicity. J Infect Dis 1999;180(4):1370–1373.

258. Senna JP, Roth DM, Oliveira JS, Machado DC, Santos DS. Protective immune response against methicillin resistant Staphylococcus aureus in a murine model using a DNA vaccine approach. Vaccine 2003;21(19–20):2661–2666.

259. Projan SJ, Nesin M, Dunman PM. Staphylococcal vaccines and immunotherapy: to dream the impossible dream? Curr Opin Pharmacol 2006;6(5):473–479.

260. Shinefield HR, Black S. Prospects for active and passive immunization against Staphylococcus aureus. Pediatr Infect Dis J 2006;25(2):167–168.

261. Shinefield H, Black S, Fattom A, et al. Use of a Staphylococcus aureus conjugate vaccine in patients receiving hemodialysis. N Engl J Med 2002;346(7):491–496.

262. Vernachio JH, Bayer AS, Ames B, et al. Human immunoglobulin G recognizing fibrinogen-binding surface proteins is protective against both Staphylococcus aureus and Staphylococcus epidermidis infections in vivo. Antimicrob Agents Chemother 2006;50(2):511–518.

263. Fattom AI, Horwith G, Fuller S, Propst M, Naso R. Development of StaphVAX, a polysaccharide conjugate vaccine against S. aureus infection: from the lab bench to phase III clinical trials. Vaccine 2004;22(7):880–887.

264. Domanski PJ, Patel PR, Bayer AS, et al. Characterization of a humanized monoclonal antibody recognizing clumping factor A expressed by Staphylococcus aureus. Infect Immun 2005;73(8):5229–5232.

265. Patti JM. A humanized monoclonal antibody targeting Staphylococcus aureus. Vaccine 2004;22 (suppl 1):S39–S43.

266. Martin JM, Green M. Group A streptococcus. Semin Pediatr Infect Dis 2006;17(3):140–148.

267. Currie BJ. Group A streptococcal infections of the skin: molecular advances but limited therapeutic progress. Curr Opin Infect Dis 2006;19(2):132–138.

268. Bisno AL, Stevens DL. Streptococcal infections of skin and soft tissues. N Engl J Med 1996;334(4):240–245.

269. Cunningham MW. Pathogenesis of group A streptococcal infections. Clin Microbiol Rev 2000;13(3):470–511.

270. Bisno AL, Brito MO, Collins CM. Molecular basis of group A streptococcal virulence. Lancet Infect Dis 2003;3(4):191–200.

271. O'Brien KL, Beall B, Barrett NL, et al. Epidemiology of invasive group a streptococcus disease in the United States, 1995–1999. Clin Infect Dis 2002;35(3):268–276.

272. Fernie-King BA, Seilly DJ, Lachmann PJ. The interaction of streptococcal inhibitor of complement (SIC) and its proteolytic fragments with the human beta defensins 6. Immunology 2004;111(4):444–452.

273. Frick IM, Akesson P, Rasmussen M, Schmidtchen A, Bjorck L. SIC, a secreted protein of Streptococcus pyogenes that inactivates antibacterial peptides. J Biol Chem 2003;278(19):16561–16566.

274. Fernie-King BA, Seilly DJ, Lachmann PJ. Inhibition of antimicrobial peptides by group A streptococci: SIC and DRS. Biochem Soc Trans 2006;34(Pt 2):273–275.

275. Binks MJ, Fernie-King BA, Seilly DJ, Lachmann PJ, Sriprakash KS. Attribution of the various inhibitory actions of the streptococcal inhibitor of complement (SIC) to regions within the molecule. J Biol Chem 2005;280(20):20120–20125.

276. Chung WO, Dale BA. Innate immune response of oral and foreskin keratinocytes: utilization of different signaling pathways by various bacterial species. Infect Immun 2004;72(1):352–358.

277. Dorschner RA, Pestonjamasp VK, Tamakuwala S, et al. Cutaneous injury induces the release of cathelicidin anti-microbial peptides active against group A Streptococcus. J Invest Dermatol 2001;117(1):91–97.

278. Schmidtchen A, Frick IM, Bjorck L. Dermatan sulphate is released by proteinases of common pathogenic bacteria and inactivates antibacterial alpha-defensin. Mol Microbiol 2001;39(3):708–713.

279. Hong K, Kinoshita T, Takeda J, et al. Inhibition of the alternative C3 convertase and classical C5 convertase of complement by group A streptococcal M protein. Infect Immun 1990;58(8):2535–2541.

280. Hong K, Harada T, Nishimura T, Inoue K. Binding ability of complement receptor CR1 to C3 bound on the surface of M+ group A streptococci. Immunology 1993;80(4):640–644.

281. Perez-Casal J, Okada N, Caparon MG, Scott JR. Role of the conserved C-repeat region of the M protein of Streptococcus pyogenes. Mol Microbiol 1995;15(5):907–916.

282. Kotarsky H, Hellwage J, Johnsson E, et al. Identification of a domain in human factor H and factor H-like protein-1 required for the interaction with streptococcal M proteins. J Immunol 1998;160(7):3349–3354.

283. Backmore TK, Fischetti VA, Sadlon TA, Ward HM, Gordon DL. M protein of the group A Streptococcus binds to the seventh short consensus repeat of human complement factor H. Infect Immun 1998;66(4):1427–1431.

284. Johnsson E, Berggard K, Kotarsky H, et al. Role of the hypervariable region in streptococcal M proteins: binding of a human complement inhibitor. J Immunol 1998;161(9):4894–4901.

285. Giannakis E, Male DA, Ormsby RJ, et al. Multiple ligand binding sites on domain seven of human complement factor H. Int Immunopharmacol 2001;1(3):433–443.

286. Perez-Caballero D, Alberti S, Vivanco F, Sanchez-Corral P, Rodriguez de CS. Assessment of the interaction of human complement regulatory proteins with group A Streptococcus. Identification of a high-affinity group A Streptococcus binding site in FHL-1. Eur J Immunol 2000;30(4):1243–1253.

287. Perez-Caballero D, Garcia-Laorden I, Cortes G, Wessels MR, de Cordoba SR, Alberti S. Interaction between complement regulators and Streptococcus pyogenes: binding of C4b-binding protein and factor H/factor H-like protein 1 to M18 strains involves two different cell surface molecules. J Immunol 2004;173(11):6899–6904.

288. Pandiripally V, Gregory E, Cue D. Acquisition of regulators of complement activation by Streptococcus pyogenes serotype M1. Infect Immun 2002;70(11):6206–6214.

289. Andre I, Persson J, Blom AM, et al. Streptococcal M protein: structural studies of the hypervariable region, free and bound to human C4BP. Biochemistry 2006;45(14):4559–4568.

290. Jenkins HT, Mark L, Ball G, et al. Human C4b-binding protein, structural basis for interaction with streptococcal M protein, a major bacterial virulence factor. J Biol Chem 2006;281(6):3690–3697.

291. Blom AM, Villoutreix BO, Dahlback B. Complement inhibitor C4b-binding protein-friend or foe in the innate immune system? Mol Immunol 2004;40(18):1333–1346.

292. Carlsson F, Berggard K, Stalhammar-Carlemalm M, Lindahl G. Evasion of phagocytosis through cooperation between two ligand-binding regions in Streptococcus pyogenes M protein. J Exp Med 2003;198(7):1057–1068.

293. Blom AM. Structural and functional studies of complement inhibitor C4b-binding protein. Biochem Soc Trans 2002;30(pt 6):978–982.

294. Berggard K, Johnsson E, Morfeldt E, Persson J, Stalhammar-Carlemalm M, Lindahl G. Binding of human C4BP to the hypervariable region of M protein: a molecular mechanism of phagocytosis resistance in Streptococcus pyogenes. Mol Microbiol 2001;42(2):539–551.

295. Morfeldt E, Berggard K, Persson J, et al. Isolated hypervariable regions derived from streptococcal M proteins specifically bind human C4b-binding protein: implications for antigenic variation. J Immunol 2001;167(7):3870–3877.

296. Blom AM. A cluster of positively charged amino acids in the alpha-chain of C4b-binding protein (C4BP) is pivotal for the regulation of the complement system and the interaction with bacteria. Scand J Clin Lab Invest Suppl 2000;233:37–49.

297. Blom AM, Berggard K, Webb JH, Lindahl G, Villoutreix BO, Dahlback B. Human C4b-binding protein has overlapping, but not identical, binding sites for C4b and streptococcal M proteins. J Immunol 2000;164(10):5328–5336.

298. Johnsson E, Thern A, Dahlback B, Heden LO, Wikstrom M, Lindahl G. Human C4BP binds to the hypervariable N-terminal region of many members in the streptococcal M protein family. Adv Exp Med Biol 1997;418:505–510.

299. Accardo P, Sanchez-Corral P, Criado O, Garcia E, Rodriguez de CS. Binding of human complement component C4b-binding protein (C4BP) to Streptococcus pyogenes involves the C4b-binding site. J Immunol 1996;157(11):4935–4939.

300. Horstmann RD, Sievertsen HJ, Leippe M, Fischetti VA. Role of fibrinogen in complement inhibition by streptococcal M protein. Infect Immun 1992;60(12):5036–5041.

301. Carlsson F, Sandin C, Lindahl G. Human fibrinogen bound to Streptococcus pyogenes M protein inhibits complement deposition via the classical pathway. Mol Microbiol 2005;56(1):28–39.

302. Stafslien DK, Cleary PP. Characterization of the streptococcal C5a peptidase using a C5a-green fluorescent protein fusion protein substrate. J Bacteriol 2000;182(11):3254–3258.

303. O'Connor SP, Cleary PP. Localization of the streptococcal C5a peptidase to the surface of group A streptococci. Infect Immun 1986;53(2):432–434.

304. Cleary PP, Prahbu U, Dale JB, Wexler DE, Handley J. Streptococcal C5a peptidase is a highly specific endopeptidase. Infect Immun 1992;60(12):5219–5223.

305. O'Connor SP, Cleary PP. In vivo Streptococcus pyogenes C5a peptidase activity: analysis using transposon- and nitrosoguanidine-induced mutants. J Infect Dis 1987;156(3):495–504.

306. Purushothaman SS, Park HS, Cleary PP. Promotion of fibronectin independent invasion by C5a peptidase into epithelial cells in group A Streptococcus. Indian J Med Res 2004;119 Suppl:44–47.

307. Koroleva IV, Efstratiou A, Suvorov AN. Structural heterogeneity of the streptococcal C5a peptidase gene in Streptococcus pyogenes. J Bacteriol 2002;184(22):6384–6386.

308. Anderson ET, Wetherell MG, Winter LA, Olmsted SB, Cleary PP, Matsuka YV. Processing, stability, and kinetic parameters of C5a peptidase from Streptococcus pyogenes. Eur J Biochem 2002;269(19):4839–4851.

309. Ji Y, McLandsborough L, Kondagunta A, Cleary PP. C5a peptidase alters clearance and trafficking of group A streptococci by infected mice. Infect Immun 1996;64(2):503–510.

310. Chen CC, Cleary PP. Complete nucleotide sequence of the streptococcal C5a peptidase gene of Streptococcus pyogenes. J Biol Chem 1990;265(6):3161–3167.

311. Fernie-King BA, Seilly DJ, Willers C, Wurzner R, Davies A, Lachmann PJ. Streptococcal inhibitor of complement (SIC) inhibits the membrane attack complex by preventing uptake of C567 onto cell membranes. Immunology 2001;103(3):390–398.

312. Akesson P, Sjoholm AG, Bjorck L. Protein SIC, a novel extracellular protein of Streptococcus pyogenes interfering with complement function. J Biol Chem 1996;271(2):1081–1088.

313. Joosten LA, Koenders MI, Smeets RL, et al. Toll-like receptor 2 pathway drives streptococcal cell wall-induced joint inflammation: critical role of myeloid differentiation factor 88. J Immunol 2003;171(11):6145–6153.

314. Pahlman LI, Morgelin M, Eckert J, et al. Streptococcal M protein: a multipotent and powerful inducer of inflammation. J Immunol 2006;177(2):1221–1228.

315. Okada N, Liszewski MK, Atkinson JP, Caparon M. Membrane cofactor protein (CD46) is a keratinocyte receptor for the M protein of the group A streptococcus. Proc Natl Acad Sci USA 1995;92(7):2489–2493.

316. Giannakis E, Jokiranta TS, Ormsby RJ, et al. Identification of the streptococcal M protein binding site on membrane cofactor protein (CD46). J Immunol 2002;168(9):4585–4592.

317. Rezcallah MS, Hodges K, Gill DB, Atkinson JP, Wang B, Cleary PP. Engagement of CD46 and alpha5beta1 integrin by group A streptococci is required for efficient invasion of epithelial cells. Cell Microbiol 2005;7(5):645–653.

318. Darmstadt GL, Mentele L, Podbielski A, Rubens CE. Role of group A streptococcal virulence factors in adherence to keratinocytes. Infect Immun 2000;68(3):1215–1221.

319. Voyich JM, Musser JM, Deleo FR. Streptococcus pyogenes and human neutrophils: a paradigm for evasion of innate host defense by bacterial pathogens. Microbes Infect 2004;6(12):1117–1123.

320. Hidalgo-Grass C, Mishalian I, Dan-Goor M, et al. A streptococcal protease that degrades CXC chemokines and impairs bacterial clearance from infected tissues. EMBO J 2006;25(19):4628–4637.

321. Kobayashi SD, Braughton KR, Whitney AR, et al. Bacterial pathogens modulate an apoptosis differentiation program in human neutrophils. Proc Natl Acad Sci USA 2003;100(19):10948–10953.

322. Miyoshi-Akiyama T, Takamatsu D, Koyanagi M, Zhao J, Imanishi K, Uchiyama T. Cytocidal effect of Streptococcus pyogenes on mouse neutrophils in vivo and the critical role of streptolysin S. J Infect Dis 2005;192(1):107–116.

323. Deleo FR. Modulation of phagocyte apoptosis by bacterial pathogens. Apoptosis 2004;9(4):399–413.

324. Collin M, Svensson MD, Sjoholm AG, Jensenius JC, Sjobring U, Olsen A. EndoS and SpeB from Streptococcus pyogenes inhibit immunoglobulin-mediated opsonophagocytosis. Infect Immun 2002;70(12):6646–6651.

325. Collin M, Olsen A. Effect of SpeB and EndoS from Streptococcus pyogenes on human immunoglobulins. Infect Immun 2001;69(11):7187–7189.

326. Collin M, Olsen A. EndoS, a novel secreted protein from Streptococcus pyogenes with endoglycosidase activity on human IgG. EMBO J 2001;20(12):3046–3055.

327. Lukomski S, Montgomery CA, Rurangirwa J, et al. Extracellular cysteine protease produced by Streptococcus pyogenes participates in the pathogenesis of invasive skin infection and dissemination in mice. Infect Immun 1999;67(4):1779–1788.

328. Moses AE, Wessels MR, Zalcman K, et al. Relative contributions of hyaluronic acid capsule and M protein to virulence in a mucoid strain of the group A Streptococcus. Infect Immun 1997;65(1):64–71.

329. Wessels MR, Moses AE, Goldberg JB, DiCesare TJ. Hyaluronic acid capsule is a virulence factor for mucoid group A streptococci. Proc Natl Acad Sci USA 1991;88(19):8317–8321.

330. Dinkla K, Rohde M, Jansen WT, Carapetis JR, Chhatwal GS, Talay SR. Streptococcus pyogenes recruits collagen via surface-bound fibronectin: a novel colonization and immune evasion mechanism. Mol Microbiol 2003;47(3):861–869.

331. Lei B, Deleo FR, Hoe NP, et al. Evasion of human innate and acquired immunity by a bacterial homolog of CD11b that inhibits opsonophagocytosis. Nat Med 2001;7(12):1298–1305.

332. McMillan DJ, Davies MR, Good MF, Sriprakash KS. Immune response to superoxide dismutase in group A streptococcal infection. FEMS Immunol Med Microbiol 2004;40(3):249–256.

333. Benot A, King KY, Janowiak B, Griffith O, Caparon MG. Contribution of glutathione peroxidase to the virulence of Streptococcus pyogenes. Infect Immun 2004;72(1):408–413.

334. Voyich JM, Sturdevant DE, Braughton KR, et al. Genome-wide protective response used by group A Streptococcus to evade destruction by human polymorphonuclear leukocytes. Proc Natl Acad Sci USA 2003;100(4):1996–2001.

335. Hayman WA, Brandt ER, Relf WA, Cooper J, Saul A, Good MF. Mapping the minimal murine T cell and B cell epitopes within a peptide vaccine candidate from the conserved region of the M protein of group A streptococcus. Int Immunol 1997;9(11):1723–1733.

336. Pruksakorn S, Galbraith A, Houghten RA, Good MF. Conserved T and B cell epitopes on the M protein of group A streptococci. Induction of bactericidal antibodies. J Immunol 1992;149(8):2729–2735.

337. Kotloff KL, Corretti M, Palmer K, et al. Safety and immunogenicity of a recombinant multivalent group a streptococcal vaccine in healthy adults: phase 1 trial. JAMA 2004;292(6):709–715.

338. Batzloff MR, Pandey M, Olive C, Good MF. Advances in potential M-protein peptide-based vaccines for preventing rheumatic fever and rheumatic heart disease. Immunol Res 2006;35(3):233–248.

339. McNeil SA, Halperin SA, Langley JM, et al. Safety and immunogenicity of 26–valent group a streptococcus vaccine in healthy adult volunteers. Clin Infect Dis 2005;41(8):1114–1122.

340. Norrby-Teglund A, Thulin P, Gan BS, et al. Evidence for superantigen involvement in severe group a streptococcal tissue infections. J Infect Dis 2001;184(7):853–860.

341. Fraser J, Arcus V, Kong P, Baker E, Proft T. Superantigens—powerful modifiers of the immune system. Mol Med Today 2000;6(3):125–132.

342. Proft T, Moffatt SL, Berkahn CJ, Fraser JD. Identification and characterization of novel superantigens from Streptococcus pyogenes. J Exp Med 1999;189(1):89–102.

343. Okamoto S, Tamura Y, Terao Y, Hamada S, Kawabata S. Systemic immunization with streptococcal immunoglobulin-binding protein Sib 35 induces protective immunity against group: a

Streptococcus challenge in mice. Vaccine 2005; 23(40):4852–4859.

344. Sabharwal H, Michon F, Nelson D, et al. Group A streptococcus (GAS) carbohydrate as an immunogen for protection against GAS infection. J Infect Dis 2006;193(1):129–135.

345. Cleary PP, Matsuka YV, Huynh T, Lam H, Olmsted SB. Immunization with C5a peptidase from either group A or B streptococci enhances clearance of group A streptococci from intranasally infected mice. Vaccine 2004;22(31–32):4332–4341.

346. Lei B, Liu M, Chesney GL, Musser JM. Identification of new candidate vaccine antigens made by Streptococcus pyogenes: purification and characterization of 16 putative extracellular lipoproteins. J Infect Dis 2004;189(1):79–89.

23
Parasitic Infections

Sidney Klaus

Key Points

- Cell-mediated immunoregulation plays the dominant role in resolving *Leishmania* infections.
- Most promastigotes deposited in the dermis are opsonized by serum complement and killed by complement-mediated lysis.
- The remaining promastigotes are phagocytosed via complement receptors on the macrophage membrane, which binds to gp63 and lipophosphoglycan.
- Macrophages release chemokines that attract more macrophages as well as natural killer (NK) cells and dendritic cells.
- *Wolbachia* bacteria living inside *Onchocerca volvulus* are the essential target of the host's inflammatory response in onchocerciasis.
- The initial reaction in cercarial dermatitis is activation of Langerhans' cells.

Parasitic Infections

Parasitic diseases involving the skin represent an important segment of the globe's emerging disorders that present a threat to the health of millions of people worldwide. Host immune responses to these diseases are complex and display a wide range of variability, involving both the innate and adaptive immune systems. Not all the host's efforts at eliminating the invading parasites are successful, and in some cases the host's immune response causes more damage than the parasite itself.

This chapter examines the immune mechanisms in three widely diverse parasitic diseases that involve the skin: cutaneous leishmaniasis, onchocerciasis, and cercarial dermatitis.

Cutaneous Leishmaniasis

Leishmaniasis, often a debilitating disease of humans, is the result of infection with intracellular protozoan parasites belonging to the genus *Leishmania*. It affects more than 12 million people worldwide, with an additional 350 million at risk of infection. The global yearly incidence of all forms is approaching 2 million cases.[1] Leishmaniasis is found in tropical regions of Africa, Asia, and South and Central America; in the southwestern part of the United States; in the Middle East; and in countries surrounding the Mediterranean Sea.[2] The number of cases increases dramatically in areas of the world undergoing ecologic disruption, associated with rapid major shifts in population. More than 20 species of the genus *Leishmania* have been identified as causative agents of the disease.

The parasites exist in two morphologic forms during their life cycle: as elongated flagellated promastigotes in the gut of the sand fly vector, and as round to oval nonflagellated amastigotes in mammalian hosts.

The skin disorders caused by this parasite have been divided into three clinical syndromes—cutaneous leishmaniasis (CL), diffuse cutaneous leishmaniasis (DCL), and mucocutaneous leishmaniasis (MCL)—each demonstrating a variety of skin manifestations, including localized self-healing skin papules and ulcers, widespread plaques resembling lepromatous leprosy, and disfiguring infections of the mouth, nose, and throat. The outcome of untreated cases depends on the species of *Leishmania* causing the infection as well as on the innate and adaptive immune responses of the host.[3] Although humoral immune responses can be demonstrated during the course of the infection, cell-mediated immunoregulation plays the dominant role in resolving the infection. Many of the details of the immune response have been derived from extensive studies of *Leishmania major* infections in two experimental mouse models: the resistant C57BL/6 strain and the susceptible BALB/c strain.

Early Events in the Immune Response

In humans, the disease is initiated by the bite of an infected female sand fly (of the genus *Phlebotomus* in the Old World and *Lutzomyia* in the New World). During the bite parasites are inoculated into the dermis; in most cases less than 100 parasites are transmitted by a single bite, although the number may reach as high as 1000 or more.[4]

Because the sand fly is a "pool feeder" (it severs capillaries in its hunt for a blood meal) promastigotes are deposited in a small pool of blood within the dermis. The bite of the sand fly initiates a local inflammatory response, with the recruitment of neutrophils, natural killer (NK) cells, eosinophils, and mast cells. The cellular response is rapid; neutrophils are the first cells to arrive at the site of the infection; in mice, they have been found collecting in the skin within 1 hour of a parasite injection.[5]

Most of the promastigotes deposited in the dermis are opsonized by serum complement and killed by complement-mediated lysis. The remaining promastigotes are phagocytosed via complement receptors expressed on the macrophage membrane, which binds to two abundant molecules on the surface of the parasites: gp63, a 63-kd neutral metalloproteinase; and LPG, a lipophosphoglycan.[6]

Macrophages that have engulfed parasites release several chemokines, including CCL2, which attracts NK cells, dendritic cells (DCs), and additional macrophages to the site of the infection.[7]

Components of sand fly saliva also have been shown to affect the immune response by exacerbating lesion development in resistant strains of mice.[8,9] When maxadilan, a vasodilatory peptide isolated from sand fly saliva, was added to human peripheral blood mononuclear cells (PBMCs) the secretion of T-helper-1 (Th1) cytokines (interferon [IFN] and interleukin-12 [IL-12]) was decreased and the secretion of Th2 cytokines enhanced.[10] In addition salivary gland lysates (SGLs) also have been shown to augment the collection of inflammatory cells at the site of the bite and when added to experimental infections caused by *L. major* and *L. braziliensis*.[11]

Once the promastigotes enter the macrophages, they transform into replicative amastigotes over a period of 2 to 5 days and are carried within modified lysosomal compartments known as parisitophorous vacuoles (PVs).[12] A study of the ultrastructure of the vacuoles suggests a significant difference in packaging between Old World and New World leishmania. Amastigotes of *L. major* were found to be segregated into separate vacuoles during replication; in contrast, New World species of *Leishmania* were carried in large vacuoles occupied by many amastigotes.[13]

Once inside the PVs the parasites produce antioxidant enzymes and are able to resist lysosomal hydrolases (the usual mechanism for clearing ingested pathogens). Within the cells the amastigotes replicate rapidly.

Macrophages that accumulate large numbers of replicating amastigotes rupture; the released parasites are taken up by neighboring competent cells. In especially inflamed skin lesions, most parasites are found in extracellular locations. One explanation is that high levels of inflammatory mediators interfere with receptors on the macrophages, blocking re-internalization of the parasites.[14]

Antigen Transport and Presentation

At the same time that macrophages are ingesting parasites, Langerhans cells (LCs), which normally reside in the epidermis and are a potent type of antigen-presenting cell (APC), are stimulated. In a study of *L. major* infections in mice, LCs were found to be the dominant type of APC migrating from the skin to the regional lymph nodes via lymph channels.[15,16]

The ability of LCs (and other APCs) to identify the parasites has been attributed to Toll-like receptor 4 (TLR4), a member of a family of transmembrane receptors implicated in the recognition of a variety of microbial and foreign agents.[17] A study of TLR-deficient mice showed they had larger parasite burdens and were less efficient in the resolution of cutaneous lesions.[18]

The extent to which macrophages also transport parasites and parasite antigen from the skin to the nodes is unresolved, although most studies indicate that LCs are the major carriers and shoulder most responsibility for antigen presentation to CD4+ naive T cells within the lymph nodes.[19]

The initial stages of the uptake of antigen by the LCs is rapid; experiments in mice have demonstrated that LCs can find and engulf parasites within 4 hours of exposure (although the migration to the lymph nodes may take up to 3 weeks).[20] The movement by the LCs to the nodes is influenced by chemokine expression. Studies have indicated that during the migration the level of expression of chemokine receptor CCR7 on the LCs is enhanced, while the level of CCR2 and CCR5 is downregulated.[21]

It is during this stage of the adaptive immune response that naive CD4+ T-helper cells (Th0) are programmed to develop into either Th1 or Th2 cells. Interleukin-12, a cytokine released by DCs, has a critical role at this stage in the immune response[22,23]: IL-12, along with IL-1, serves as a promotor of the differentiation of Th1 cells in the lymph nodes from naive T0 cells. It also enhances chemokine gene expression in mice during the first 3 days of infection with L. major.[24]

It is now clear that the successful clearing of amastigotes from infected macrophages in resistant mouse strains is mediated through the predominance of Th1 cells. The mechanism is through steps that link the production of IFN-γ, a major cytokine of Th1 cells, to the release of nitric oxide (NO), a compound within macrophages harboring amastigotes leading to their destruction. Nitric oxide ordinarily is present within an inactive form in the macrophages (iNO), which needs to be catalyzed by the enzyme NO synthase to become active. Interferon along with IL-12 and tumor necrosis factor (TNF), two other cytokines released by Th1 cells, make up the major upregulators of NO synthase, and the production of NO occurs only when the Th1 cells become predominant.[25]

In contrast to the events within the resistant mice, in susceptible mouse strains (BALB/c) a type 2 response is initiated following infection with L. major, which tends to interfere with the protective activities. Th2 cells that become stimulated produce IL-4, IL-5, and IL-10, which have the capacity through mediators to inhibit the production of IFN-γ, downregulate the expression of iNOS (and consequently NO), and thus inhibit macrophage function.

Although a great deal is known about the process of resistance in mice, much less is known about the human immune response to Leishmania. While mice can mount either a Th1 or Th2 response, Rogers and Titus[26] suggested that in humans the principal response is predominantly if not exclusively a type 1 response. Using an in vitro system they cocultured PBMCs from Leishmania-naive donors with L. major parasites and found that type 1 cytokines were stimulated, (IFN-γ and IL-12), and that when PBMCs were cocultured with macrophages infected with parasites, augmented intracellular killing was observed.[26]

Antibody Response

Anti-Leishmania antibodies, as measured by enzyme-linked immunosorbent assay (ELISA), can be found in low titers in individuals recovering from CL, but their role in recovery from the acute infection and in the prevention of re-infection is debated. Polyclonal activation of human B cells leads to the production of large amounts of parasite specific antibodies, and amastigotes released into the dermis from ruptured macrophages appear to be coated with antiparasite antibodies.[27]

In mice, antibody levels do not correlate in general with resistance to disease, although their effect on the course of the infection may depend on genetic factors. For example, passive transfer of antibody fractions from immune mice to BALB/c mice did not affect their susceptibility to infection,[28] yet ablation of B cells in resistant mice generated a nonhealing response to L. major.[29]

Delayed-Type Hypersensitivity and the Leishmanin Skin Test

Delayed-type hypersensitivity in leishmaniasis can be measured by the leishmanin skin test (LST), in which the extent of a skin reaction is measured 48 to 72 hours after an intradermal injection of 0.2 mL of a killed suspension of cultured leishmania promastigotes in saline. A positive reaction indicates a type 1 CD4[+] cell-specific immune response. Because it is usually positive in individuals who have had CL, it has been used to measure the extent of infection among individuals living in endemic regions who have no history of overt disease. A study of 470 children living in endemic foci of *L. major* infection in Tunisia found that the proportion of asymptomatic infections among this group of children was approximately 10%.[30] The LST also has been used as a predictor of susceptibility to subsequent disease, whether or not the individual had a history of a previous skin lesion.

Persistence of Parasites

In most cases of human cutaneous leishmaniasis it had been assumed that in skin lesions that had "healed" (either spontaneously or following treatment), the parasites had been eliminated by effector mechanisms involving IFN-γ and the generation of NO within the macrophages. It is now recognized that viable *Leishmania* organisms may persist in the skin long after the resolution of the clinical lesions.[31] Persistence has been documented in several ways: in biopsy samples from normal patients who have recovered from CL, in skin lesions of patients who recovered from CL but who later contracted HIV infection, and in skin lesions of patients who recovered from CL but later developed leishmania recidivans.

Schubach et al.[32] examined skin tissue obtained by biopsy at the sites of the scars from two patients from Brazil who had been infected with *Leishmania* 8 and 11 years earlier. The tissues from both patients grew out viable *Leishmania* parasites. A more recent study analyzed skin biopsies from scars of 32 patients with who had CL but who had been treated and clinically cured. *Leishmania* specific DNA was detected by polymerase chain reaction (PCR) in 30 of the patients, and parasites were isolated by culture in three.[33]

The persistence of parasites in postrecovery CL is also evident in patients who later become infected with HIV. Studies of skin biopsies from such immunocompromised patients often show large numbers of amastigotes both within macrophages and free in the dermis. Parasites can also be seen within keratinocytes surrounding sweat ducts, and within the cells of the eccrine glands themselves.[34] Skin lesions in these patients often appear as isolated papules or plaques on exposed areas of the skin and are usually indistinguishable from similar lesions seen in nonimmunosuppressed individuals. Skin lesions in HIV patients may also present as diffuse scaling plaques, which on biopsy show a high concentration of parasites.[35]

Leishmaniasis recidivans (LR) is a rare clinical form of CL in which skin near the site of a previously healed acute CL lesion reappears as a dusky-red granulomatous plaque with active spreading borders. The clinical features resemble lupus vulgaris. Cultures of the skin lesion for *Leishmania* are usually negative, but with perseverance sparse parasites can be detected microscopically or by PCR. Leishmaniasis recidivans patients usually demonstrate high levels of antibodies in the serum and a strongly positive LST.[36]

Vaccine Development

Clinical evidence points to the conclusion that recovery from skin infection with *Leishmania* provides lifelong protection against re-infection despite ongoing exposure to sand flies, suggesting that a vaccine would be of great value in controlling the disease.

For more than 100 years residents of endemic regions in eastern Asia and the Middle East practiced a form of vaccination known as leishmanization, which consisted of the deliberate inoculation of infective material into inconspicuous body areas (especially the buttocks) in the hope of providing protection from a subsequent infection and disfiguring scars on exposed parts of the body. A wide-scale trial of leishmanization was carried out among soldiers in the Iranian army in the 1990s, with more than a million individuals vaccinated, in this case using live *L. major* promastigotes obtained from cultures. Although the degree of protection initially seemed adequate (less than 3% of a cohort of the vaccinated group developed a naturally acquired infection, compared with 14% of unvaccinated volunteers), there was an unacceptable rate of adverse events: 2% to 3% of the subjects developed large nonhealing infections at the site of the vaccinations that required treatment.[37–39]

Today vaccine trials use killed or live-attenuated parasites, genetically modified cells from promastigotes, and DNA encoding recombinant proteins.[40–42]

Other vaccine candidates have included those using specific peptides derived from leishmania proteins such as amino acids derived from gp63, administered with certain adjuvants (such as liposomes or complete Freund's adjuvant).[43] One novel idea was that if components of sand fly saliva were added to a standard mix of antigens, a more effective prophylactic vaccine might result.[44]

Although experimental vaccines to control CL have been studied extensively over the past two decades, inoculation with live *L. major* still remains the only successful vaccine in humans.[45] Currently, vaccine development is hampered by an incomplete understanding of the immune process and by concerns about long-term safety.

Onchocerciasis

Onchocerciasis, also known as river blindness, is an infection caused by the filarial nematode *Onchocerca volvulus,* with significant cutaneous manifestations, including widespread itching, dermatitis, and subcutaneous nodules. It affects more than 18 million people living in endemic zones in Africa, Latin America (including Mexico, Brazil, Venezuela, and Ecuador), Saudi Arabia, and Yemen. It causes significant eye damage, in addition to the skin changes, and is the second most common cause of preventable blindness in sub-Saharan Africa.

The disease is spread by the bite of black flies of the genus *Simulium*; because the flies breed in fast-flowing waters, the disease is located near streams and rivers in tropical countries in both Africa and South America (hence the term *river blindness*).

Humans appear to be the primary host, although the gorilla in the Congo and the spider monkey in Mexico may also be naturally infected.[46]

The disease is initiated when a black fly harboring parasites deposits infective larvae in the dermis of the human host. After two molts over a 9- to 12-month period, the larvae develop into adult worms that become encapsulated deep in the dermis and subcutaneous tissues. They may live for 10 to 15 years and are usually palpable as firm, nontender nodules especially over the bony prominences of the pelvis, or on the scalp.

From these sites, after a prepatent period of 3 to 18 months, fertilized female worms produce thousands of microfilariae daily (millions during a lifetime). The microfilariae (mfs), which can persist for 6 to 36 months, migrate to the subcutaneous and ocular tissues. In the dermis they are accessible to re-ingestion by black flies, restarting the cycle. Most of the skin signs and symptoms of onchocerciasis are related to the body's reaction to dying and degenerating mfs in the dermis.

The clinical features that characterize the disease include itching, commonly occurring over the lower trunk and buttocks, and an eczema-like eruption, which includes lichenification and hyperpigmentation. Individuals who have had the disease for many years may develop lymphedema and postinflammatory depigmentation, often on the anterior tibial surfaces (a sign called "leopard skin"). The prominent change seen on biopsy of affected skin is dermal fibrosis. In time, destruction of elastic tissue occurs, mediated by proteases from the parasites. These changes eventually lead to marked skin atrophy with redundant folds of skin in the inguinal areas, the so-called hanging groin.

Two clinical patterns of reaction are evoked once the process is underway: a generalized form, characterized by widespread itching and dermatitis, and a hyperactive form (Sowda), in which the skin reaction is often intense yet usually localized, often restricted to one limb. A resistant form of the disease is also found among individuals living in hyperendemic areas and who remain unaffected despite being chronically exposed to the bites of infected flies.

Decreased visual acuity is the most serious complication of the disease. The inflammatory reactions within the eye lead to iridocyclitis, choroiditis, and eventually optic atrophy.

The Role of *Wolbachia* Bacteria

Wolbachia bacteria, recently recognized as essential endosymbionts of *O. volvulus* living inside both adult worms and mfs, are now considered to be an essential target of the host's inflammatory response.[47,48] Neutrophil recruitment around the encysted adult worms (onchocercomas) appears to be related to the presence of the bacteria. In patients treated with doxycycline to eliminate the symbionts, the accumulation of neutrophils adjacent to the adult worms was drastically reduced.[49] Antibiotic treatment with doxycycline has also been found to improve skin lesions in hyperergic forms of the disease, and to interrupt embryogenesis of the female adult worms.[50]

Immune Responses

Although early in the course of the disease—in the prepatent phase—inflammatory cells react to protein on the surface of the adult worms, the characteristic cutaneous signs and symptoms of the disease (dermatitis and itching) do not develop until mfs are produced by the gravid female worms.

The mfs represent an ongoing source of antigen; up to 3000 are released daily by the adult female worm, beginning about 6 to 10 months after infection.[51] It is now argued that the predominant portion of the skin reaction in onchocerciasis is a reaction not only to the death and degeneration of the mfs but to their accompanying *Wolbachia* as well.

Early in the course of the infection a polyclonal B-cell activation occurs with the production of parasite-specific immunoglobulins, including IgM, IgG (both IgG1 and IgG4), and IgE. The reaction to the mfs in the dermis and subcutaneous tissue is initiated by antibodies that attach to the surface of the parasites, along with complement. The immune complexes that are formed attract a variety of inflammatory cells, including neutrophils, eosinophils, and later macrophages. Degranulation of eosinophils appears to play the major role in the death of the mfs, but it is likely that proteases secreted by the larvae also add to the tissue damage.

In addition to the effect on B cells, parasite antigens also induce substantial reactions from PBMCs. The initial recognition of these antigens, both the infective larvae themselves and their *Wolbachia* cargo, is mediated by TLRs. TLR4 responds to both the larvae of *O. volvulus* as well as to surface protein of the *Wolbachia*, and initiates a Th2 immune response mediated by IL-4 and IL-5.[52] In addition, TLR2 also responds to surface protein isolated from *Wolbachia*, which mediates the release of TNF-α, IL-12, and IL-8 from PBMCs.[53]

The evolution and final expression of the type of immune reaction that develops (Th1 or Th2) has been attributed to the early presence of specific cytokines; for example, the initial presence of IL-12 directs the immune response toward a Th1 reaction, while a rapid induction of IL-4 promotes the generation of a dominant Th2-type response.[54]

In some individuals an activation of a subset of CD4+ cells known as T regulatory cells (Tr1) occurs, which produce IL-10 and transforming growth factor (TGF), and some IFN.[55]

In the usual generalized, chronic form of the disease, where the microfilarial load in the skin is high (up to 500 microfilaria per milligram of skin), the cutaneous reactions tend to be mild to moderate. In this type of onchocerciasis the cellular reactions are downregulated, with a suppression of Th1 and only a moderate Th2 response.[56] High levels of IL-10 are produced by CD4+ T-regulatory cells (Tr1), which act to inhibit activation of APCs and thus suppress proinflammatory functions. This type of immune response is thought to protect the host from acute skin damage (yet it may also be of benefit to the parasites by protecting them from some of the host's lethal immune responses).[57]

In hyperreactive forms of the disease where the concentration of mfs is low (less than 10 per mg of skin) and the inflammatory reaction of the skin is severe, a strong Th2 response is seen. It is suggested that, in this form of onchocerciasis, inflammatory cells (eosinophils, neutrophils, and macrophages) all combine to kill mfs, under the direction of T cells and APCs.[56]

Up to now HIV infection has been reported to play only a minor role in onchocerciasis, with no significant association with HIV detected in a large case control study.[58] No differences were noted in the density of mfs,[59] although antibody response to the parasite was decreased in HIV-infected individuals, and they tended to lose their reactivity to these antigens over time.[60]

Vaccines

Efforts to conquer onchocerciasis have been directed largely through the control of vectors and the use of drug therapy; only a few vaccine studies have been completed. In one study, three recombinant antigens were identified and used to induce protective immunity in mice.[61] Immunization in mice using DNA encoding of selected parasite genes has also shown promise.[62]

Cercarial Dermatitis

Cercarial dermatitis, also know as swimmer's itch, is a water-borne parasitic infection in which schistosomal cercaria that normally parasitizes birds or small aquatic mammals penetrates the skin of humans. Two of the more common species of trematodes implicated in this disease are *Trichobilharzia* and *Bilharziella*. Due to low species specificity of the penetrating cercaria, humans can be attacked.

The infective form of the parasite is a tiny schistosome larva (cercaria), that hatches from miricidia released by eggs shed into the water by adult worms in the gut of their avian or mammalian host. Within the intermediate snail host the miricidia transform into cercariae, which emerge after a 4- to 6-week period and seek out a warm-blooded host. Swimmer's itch may be contracted in fresh water lakes, brackish inlets, or sea water.

The cercariae attach to the skin by an adhesive mucous material, lose their tails (becoming schistosomulae), and penetrate between the keratinized cells of the stratum corneum.

Although most parasites generally invade no further than the epidermal–dermal basement membrane, a few may migrate beyond the skin.[63] There is evidence, however, that these schistosomes never mature in the human host, and the parasites usually die within 6 to 8 days.

The skin changes usually begin within an hour after invasion, presenting initially as pruritic erythematous macules. Within a few hours the lesions progress to papules, papulovesicles, and pustules. Generally the signs of cutaneous schistosomiasis last for a week to 10 days, though severe cases may last for 2 to 3 weeks.

Based on murine studies, infected percutaneously with the human trematode (*Schistosoma mansoni)* the initial reaction in cercarial dermatitis is likely the activation of epidermal LCs that increase in size and cluster around the schistosomulae.[64] Within hours an influx of leukocytes occurs, including neutrophils, macrophages, mast cells, and CD4+ lymphocytes.[65]

If the infection is a first-time event, the invading parasites produce a mixed Th1/Th2 cytokine response in the skin. During re-infection, however, a Th2 response becomes dominant, and an inflammatory reaction occurs, consisting of an influx of neutrophils, macrophages, CD4+ lymphocytes, and mast cells.[66]

Whether TLRs play a role in cercarial dermatitis has not been examined, although in studies of one of the schistosome species that cause systemic disease in humans (*Schistosoma haematobium*), van der Kleij[67] has found that glycolipids, released by schistosomulae within the epidermis serve as ligands for TLR2.

Conclusion

The immunology of cutaneous parasitic infections can be illustrated by leishmaniasis, onchocerciasis, and cercarial dermatitis. Cell-mediated immunoregulation plays the dominant role in resolving *Leishmania* infections. Most promastigotes deposited in the dermis are opsonized by serum complement and killed by complement-mediated lysis. The remaining promastigotes are phagocytosed via complement receptors on the macrophage membrane, which binds to gp63 and lipophosphoglycan. Macrophages release chemokines, which attract NK cells, dendritic cells, and more macrophages. *Wolbachia* bacteria living inside *Onchocerca volvulus* are the essential target of the host's inflammatory response in onchocerciasis. The initial reaction in cercarial dermatitis is activation of Langerhans cells. Understanding these components of the immune response to parasitic infections will potentially lead to better therapies and possibly to vaccines for prevention.

References

1. Choi C, Lerner E. Leishmaniasis as an emerging infection. J Invest Derm Symp Proc 2001;6:175–182.
2. Klaus S, Frankenburg S, Dhar A. Leishmaniasis and other protozoan infections. In: Freedberg I, Eisen A, Wolff K, et al., eds. Dermatology in General Medicine. New York: McGraw-Hill, 2003:2215–2224.
3. Herwaldt B. Leishmaniasis. Lancet 1999;354:1191–1199.
4. Warburg A, Schlein Y. The effect of post-blood meal nutrition of *Phlebotomus papatasi* on the transmission of *Leishmania major*. Am J Trop Med Hyg 1986;35:926–930.
5. Muller K, et al. Chemokines, natural killer cells and granulocytes in the early course of *Leishmania major* infection in mice. Med Microbiol Immunol 2001;190:73–76.
6. Tait A, Sacks D. The cell biology of parasite invasion and survival. Parasitol Today 1988;4:228–234.
7. Teixeira M, Teixeira C, Bezerril A, et al. Chemokines in host-parasite interactions in leishmaniasis. Trends Parasitol 2006;22:32–40.

8. Theodos C, Ribeiro J, Titus R. Analysis of enhancing effect of sand fly saliva on *Leishmania* infection in mice. Infect Immun 1991;59:1592–1598.

9. Mbow M, Bleyenberg J, Hall L, et al. *Phlebotomus papatasi* sand fly salivary gland lysate down-regulates a Th1, but up-regulates a Th2, response in mice infected with *Leishmania major*. J Immunol 1998;161:5571–5577.

10. Rogers K, Titus R. Immunomodulatory effects of maxadilan and *Phlebotomus papatasi* sand fly salivary gland lysates on human primary in vitro immune responses. Parasite Immunol 2003;25:127–134.

11. Samuelson J, Lerner E, Tesh R, et al. A mouse model of *Leishmania braziliensis braziliensis* infection produced by coinjection with sand fly saliva. J Exp Med 1991;173:49–54.

12. Korner U, Fuss V, Steigerwald J, et al. Biogenesis of *Leishmania major*–harboring vacuoles in murine dendritic cells. Infect Immun 2006;74:1305–1312.

13. Castro R, Scott K, Jordan T, et al. The ultrastructure of parasitophorous vacuole formed by *Leishmania major*. J Parasitol 2006;92:1162–1170.

14. Klaus S. Unpublished data.

15. Baldwin T, Henri S, Curtis J, et al. Dendritic cell populations in *Leishmania major*–infected skin and draining lymph nodes. Infect Immun 2004;72:1991–2001.

16. Meymandi S, Dabiri S, Dabiri D, et al. A quantitative study of epidermal Langerhans cells in cutaneous leishmaniasis caused by *Leishmania tropica*. Int J Dermatol 2004;43:819–823.

17. Moll H. Dendritic cells and host resistance to infection. Cell Microbiol 2003;5:493–500.

18. Kropf P, Freudenberg M, Modolell M, et al. Toll-like receptor 4 contributes to efficient control of infection with the protozoan parasite *Leishmania major*. Infect Immun 2004;72:1920–1928.

19. Udey M, von Stebut E, Mendez S, et al. Skin dendrite cells in murine cutaneous leishmaniasis. Immunobiology 2001;204:590–594.

20. Axelrod O, Klaus S, Frankenburg S. Antigen presentation by epidermal Langerhans cells in experimental cutaneous leishmaniasis. Parasite Immunol 1994;16:593–598.

21. Steigerwald M, Moll H. *Leishmania major* modulates chemokine and chemokine receptor expression by dendritic cells and affects their migratory capacity. Infect Immun 2005;73:2564–2567.

22. Park A, Hondowicz B, Klopf M, et al. The role of IL-12 in maintaining resistance to *Leishmania major*. J Immunol 2002;168:5771–5777.

23. Schopf L, Erickson J, Hayes L, et al. Alterations of intralesional and lymph node gene expression and cellular composition induced by IL-12 administration during leishmaniasis. Parasite Immunol 2001;23:71–84.

24. Zaph C, Scott P. Interleukin-12 regulates chemokine gene expression during the early immune response to *Leishmania major*. Infect Immun 2003;71:1587–1589.

25. Solback W, Laskay T. The host response to *Leishmania* infection. Advances Immunol 2000;74:274–317.

26. Rogers K, Titus R. Characterization of the early cellular immune response to *Leishmania major* using peripheral blood mononuclear cells from *Leishmania*-naïve humans. Am J Trop Med 2004;71:568–576.

27. Peters C, Aebischer T, Stierhof Y, et al. The role of macrophage receptors in adhesion and uptake of *Leishmania mexicana* amastigotes. J Cell Sci 1995;108:3715–3724.

28. Howard J, Nicklin S, Hale C, et al. Prophylactic immunization against experimental leishmaniasis. I. Protection induced in mice genetically vulnerable to fatal *Leishmania tropica* infection. J Immunol 1982;129:2206–2211.

29. Scott P, Natovitz P, Sher A. B-lymphocytes are required for the generation of T-cells that mediate healing of cutaneous leishmaniasis. J Immunol 1986;137:1017–1021.

30. Salah A, Louzir H, Chlif S, et al. The predictive validity of naturally acquired delayed-type hypersensitivity to leishmanin in resistance to *Leishmania major*–associated cutaneous leishmaniasis. J Infect Dis 2005;192:1981–1987.

31. Bogdan C, Rollinghoff M. The immune response to *Leishmania*: mechanisms of parasite control and evasion. Int J Parasitol 1998;28:121–134.

32. Schubach A, Marzochi M, Cuzzi-Maya T, et al. Cutaneous scars in American tegumentary leishmaniasis patients: a site of *Leishmania (Vannia) Braziliensis* persistence and viability eleven years after antimonial therapy and clinical cure. Am J Trop Med Hyg 1998;58:824–827.

33. Mendonca M, de Brito M, Rodrigues E, et al. Persistence of *Leishmania* parasites after clinical cure of American cutaneous leishmaniasis: Is there a sterile cure? J Infect Dis 2004;189:1018–1023.

34. Puig L, Pradinaud R. *Leishmania* and HIV co-infection: dermatological manifestations. Ann Trop Med Parasitol 2002;97:S107–S114.

35. Gillis D, Klaus S, Schnur L, et al. Diffusely disseminated cutaneous *Leishmania major* infection in a child with acquired immunodeficiency syndrome. Pediatr Infect Dis J 1995;14:247–249.

36. Cannavo S, Vaccaro M, Guarneri F. Leishmaniasis recidiva cutis. Int J Dermatol 2000;39:205–206.

37. Khamesipour A, Dowlati Y, Asilian A, et al. Leishmanization: use of an old method for evaluation

of candidate vaccines against leishmaniasis. Vaccine 2005;23:3642–3648.

38. Modabber F. Experiences with vaccines against cutaneous leishmaniasis: of men and mice. Parasitology 1989;98:S49–60.

39. Greenblatt C. Cutaneous Leishmaniasis: the prospects of a killed vaccine. Parasitol Today 1988;4:53–54.

40. Melby P. Vaccination against cutaneous leishmaniasis: current status. Am J Clin Dermatol 2002;3:557–570.

41. Sharifi I, Fekri A, Aflatonian M. Randomized vaccine trial of single dose of killed *Leishmania major* plus BCG against anthroponotic cutaneous leishmaniasis in Bam, Iran. Lancet 1998;351:1540–1543.

42. Handman H. Leishmaniasis: current status of vaccine development. Clin Microbiol Rev 2001;14:229–243.

43. Frankenburg S, Axelrod O, Kutner S, et al. Effective immunization of mice against cutaneous leishmaniasis using an intrinsically adjuvanated synthetic lipopeptide vaccine. Vaccine 1996;14:923–929.

44. Brodskyn C, De Oliveira C, Barral A, et al. Vaccines in leishmaniasis: advances in the last five years. Expert Rev Vaccines 2003;2:705–717.

45. Tabbara K, Peters N, Afrin F, et al. Conditions influencing the efficacy of vaccination with live organisms against *Leishmania major* infection. Infect Immun 2005;73:4714–4722.

46. Cook G. Discovery and clinical importance of the filariases. Infect Dis Clin North Am 2004;18:219–230.

47. Taylor M, Hoerauf A. *Wolbachia* bacterial of filarial nematodes. Parasitol Today 1999;15:437–442.

48. Saint Andre A, Blackwell, Hall L, et al. The role of endosymbiotic *Wolbachia* bacteria in the pathogenesis of river blindness. Science 2002;295:1892–1895.

49. Brattig N, Buttner D, Hoerauf A. Neutrophil accumulation around *Onchocerca* worms and chemotaxis of neutrophils are dependent on *Wolbachia* endobacteria. Microbes Infect 2001;3:439–446.

50. Taylor M, Hoerauf A. A new approach to the treatment of filariasis. Curr Opin Infect Dis 2001;14:727–731.

51. Brattig N. Pathogenesis ands host responses in human onchocerciasis; impact of *Onchocerca* filariae and *Wolbachia* endobacteria. Microbes Infect 2004;6:113–128.

52. Kerepesi L, Leon O, Lustigman S, et al. Protective immunity to the larval stages of *Onchocerca volvulus* is dependent on Toll-like receptor 4. Infect Immun 2005;73:8291–8297.

53. Brattig N, Bazzocchi C, Kirschning C, et al. The major surface protein of *Wolbachia* endosymbionts in filarial nematodes elicits immune responses through TLR2 and TLR4. J Immunol 2004;173:437–445.

54. Constant L, Bottomly K. Induction of Th1 and Th2 CD4+ T cell responses: the alternative approaches. Annu Rev Immunol 1997;15:297–322.

55. Satoguina J, Mempel M, Larbi J, et al. Antigen-specific T regulatory-1 cells are associated with immunosuppression in a chronic helminth infection (onchocerciasis). Microbes Infect 2002;4:1291–1300.

56. Hoerauf A, Brattig N. Resistance and susceptibility in human onchocerciasis—beyond Th1 vs Th2. Trends Parasitol 2002;18:25–31.

57. Hoerauf A, Santoguina J, Saeftel M, et al. Immunomodulation of filarial nematodes. Parasite Immunol 2005;27:417–429.

58. Harms G, Feldmeier H. HIV Infection and tropical parasitic diseases—deleterious interactions in both directions? Trop Med Int Health 2002;7:479–488.

59. Fischer P, Kipp W, Kabwa, et al. Onchocerciasis and HIV in Western Uganda: prevalence and treatment with ivermectin. Am J Trop Med Hyg 1995;53:171–178.

60. Tawill S, Gallin M, Erttmenn K, et al. Impaired antibody responses and loss of reactivity to *Onchocerca volvulus* antigens by HIV-seropositive onchocerciasis patients. Trans R Soc Trop Med Hyg 1996;90:85–89.

61. Abraham D, Leon O, Leon S, et al. Development of recombinant antigen vaccine against infection with the filarial worm *Onchocerca volvulus*. Infect Immun 2001;69:262–270.

62. Harrison R, Bianco A. DNA immunization with Onchocerca volvulus genes, Ov-tmy-1 and OvB20: serological and parasitological outcomes following intramuscular or genegun delivery in a mouse model of onchocerciasis. Parasite Immunol 2000;22:249–257.

63. Horak P, Kolarova L, Adema C. Biology of the schistosome genus *Trichobilharzia*. Adv Parasit 2002;52:155–233.

64. Goodhouse J, Klaus S. Stimulation of Langerhans cells by cercarial penetration of *Schistosoma mansoni* in murine epidermis. J Invest Dermatol 1982;76:330.

65. Mountford A, Trottein F. Schistosomes in the skin: a balance between immune priming and regulation. Trends Parasitol 2004;20: 221–226.

66. Kourilova P, Hogg K, Kolarova L, et al. Cercarial dermatitis caused by bird schistosomes comprises both immediate and late phase cutaneous hypersensitivity reactions. J Immunol 2004;172:3766–3774.

67. van der Kleij D, van den Biggelaar A, Kruize Y, et al. Responses to Toll-like receptor ligands in children living in areas where schistosome infections are endemic. J Infect Dis 2004;189:1044–1051.

24
Fungal Infections

Nahed Ismail and Michael R. McGinnis

Key Points

- The clinical relevance of fungal diseases has increased due to increased populations of immunocompromised patients.
- Fungal infections are classified according to the site of the primary infection: superficial, cutaneous, subcutaneous, and deep or systemic.
- Dimorphic fungi assume both yeast and hyphal states based on environmental conditions and the hosts' immune response.
- Certain fungi can synthesize capsular components, which can affect host immune responses.
- The innate response to fungi serves two purposes: a direct antifungal effector activity, and activation and induction of the specific adaptive immune responses.
- Understanding the immune responses to fungal infections has led to better diagnostic tests and therapeutic interventions for fungal diseases.

Fungi comprise many species that are associated with a wide spectrum of diseases in humans. The clinical relevance of fungal diseases has increased markedly, mainly because of an increasing population of immunocompromised hosts, including individuals infected with HIV, transplant recipients, and patients with cancer. Fungal infections are classified, according to the primary site of infection, as superficial, cutaneous, subcutaneous, and deep or systemic mycosis. Superficial mycosis is limited to the stratum corneum and elicits no or slight inflammation. Cutaneous mycosis involves the integument and its appendages, including hair and nail. Infection of the skin, which is caused by the fungal organisms or its products, may involve stratum corneum or deep layers of the epidermis. Subcutaneous mycosis involves the epidermis and subcutaneous tissues. Subcutaneous mycosis usually follows traumatic inoculation of fungal organisms. The inflammatory response that develops in the subcutaneous tissues usually involves the epidermis. Deep or systemic mycosis usually involves organs such as lung, central nervous system, bones, and abdominal viscera. The portal of entry in deep mycosis is the respiratory tract, gastrointestinal tract, and blood vessels.

Fungi that cause cutaneous, subcutaneous, or disseminated infection with skin involvement exist in a range of morphologic forms that include yeasts and molds. Yeasts (e.g., *Malassezia*) grow as unicellular round- or oval-shaped organisms, whereas molds (e.g., dermatophytes) form long tubular structures termed hyphae that extend into a branch-like network known as a mycelium. Dimorphic fungi (e.g., *Candida albicans, Histoplasma capsulatum, Coccidioides immitis, Blastomyces dermatitis,* and *Sporothrix schenckii*) assume both yeast or spherules and hyphal states of growth based on environmental conditions and interactions with the mammalian immune system. Yeasts and molds are bound by a cell wall composed of polysaccharide polymers (chitin, mannans, and glucans) derived from biosynthetic pathways absent in mammalian cells.[1-2] In addition, certain fungi can synthesize capsular components, melanins, and secondary metabolites that include toxins, for example, gliotoxin and aflatoxin, many of which can affect host immune responses.[3-6]

This chapter discusses the general innate and acquired immune responses against fungi, particularly the cellular and molecular pathways of immune defense mechanisms that have significantly contributed to our present understanding of the host response to fungi and have provided a sound framework for development of effective strategies of immunotherapy against some fungal infections. This chapter also discusses host defenses and specific immune responses against certain fungal pathogens causing cutaneous, subcutaneous, and deep mycosis that either begins with cutaneous or subcutaneous diseases and then disseminates to become a systemic disease that involves also the skin.

Innate Immune Responses to Fungal Infection

The host defense mechanisms against fungi are numerous, and range from nonspecific, germline-encoded immunity that presents early in the evolution of microorganisms, to highly specialized and specific adaptive mechanisms that are induced during infection and disease. The relative importance of specific innate and adaptive defense mechanisms differs, depending on the organism and anatomic site of infection (skin, mucosal sites, or disseminated infection). Additionally, the morphotype of the fungal pathogen (yeast or hyphae) determines the type of host immune response. For example, yeasts and spores are often effectively phagocytosed, while the larger size of hyphae prevents effective ingestion. Pathogenic fungi have also developed mechanisms to subvert host defenses, which allow some intracellular fungi to survive within phagocytes, avoid fungal killing, and then disseminate throughout the host.

The innate response to fungi serves two main purposes: (1) a direct antifungal effector activity by mediating nonspecific elimination of pathogens through either a phagocytic process and intracellular killing of internalized pathogens or through the secretion of microbicidal compounds against undigested fungal molecules; and (2) activation and induction of the specific adaptive immune responses via the production of proinflammatory mediators, including chemokines and cytokines, providing co-stimulatory signals to naive T cells, as well as antigen uptake and presentation to CD4 and CD8 T cells.[7] In addition to the above inducible functions of innate response, the constitutive mechanisms of innate defense that

are present in the skin include the barrier function of body surfaces. Figure 24.1 illustrates the link between innate and acquired (cellular and humoral) immune responses against fungal infections of the skin.

Host innate defenses against fungi are mediated by professional phagocytes, including neutrophils, mononuclear leukocytes (monocytes and macrophages), and dendritic cells (DCs), natural killer (NK) cells, and nonhematopoietic cells, such as keratinocytes and epithelial and endothelial cells. The first step in the innate immunity involves fungal recognition and uptake by germline-encoded pattern recognition receptors (PRRs) expressed on the surfaces of several innate immune cells.[7-10] Figure 24.2 illustrates the different PRRs expressed on phagocytic cells such macrophages and the downstream effector functions of interaction of fungal antigens with these receptors.

The most important classes of PRR are the Toll-like receptors (TLRs),[9,10] dectin-1,[11] the lectin-like receptors,[12,13] Fc receptors,[14] complement receptors,[15] the mannose receptor,[15] and integrins.[16] The microbial ligands of these receptors are called pathogen-associated molecular patterns (PAMPs). Fungal structures such as β-1,3/β-1,6 glucans,[16] glucuronoxylomannan, phospholipomannan, and galactomannan function as ligands for TLR2, TLR4, and TLR6.[17,18] The signaling pathway for mammalian TLR after ligation of PAMPs involves interaction with the adaptor molecule MYD88 (myeloid differentiation primary response gene 88) located in the cytosol.[19,20] The activation of the MYD88 adaptor culminates in the activation and nuclear translocation of nuclear factor κB (NF-κB), which leads to activation of several cytokine and chemokine genes. Recognition of pathogens by TLR in a Myd88-dependent, and sometimes in a Myd88-independent, manner leads to release of proinflammatory cytokines, chemokines, activation of antibacterial mechanisms, and enhancing the T-cell priming ability of professional antigen-presenting cells (APCs) such as dendritic cells. Compared to individual TLRs, Myd88$^{-/-}$ mice had higher levels of fungal growth than control animals.[20,21] The more severe phenotype of Myd88$^{-/-}$ mice compared with mice deficient in individual TLRs probably reflects the broad function of Myd88 as an adaptor for multiple TLR-dependent responses.

Toll-like receptors discriminate between distinct fungal morphotypes. For example, TLR4 and CD14 expressed on human monocytes appear to recognize *Aspergillus* hyphae but not *Candida* hyphae.[22,23]

Similarly, the production of pro-inflammatory and Th1 cytokines such as tumor necrosis factor-α (TNF-α) and interferon-γ (IFN-γ) by macrophages in response to *C. albicans* phospholipomannan

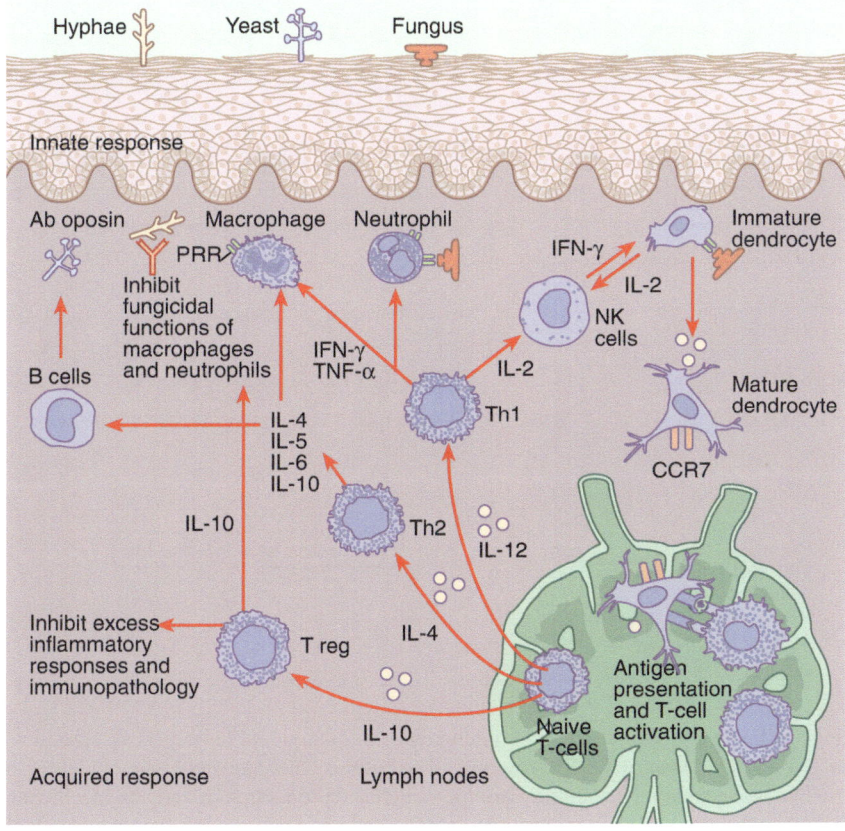

A

FIG. 24.1. Possible pathways for immunologic responses stimulated by fungi. (A) Most fungi are detected and destroyed within hours by innate nonspecific defense mechanisms mediated by phagocytes such as macrophages, neutrophils, immature dendritic cells, and opsonins (antibodies, Ab) through the involvement of distinct pattern-recognition receptors (PRRs). Fungal organisms on the skin surface also release antigens (Ag) that penetrate the skin and are captured by an antigen-presenting cell (APC) such as dendritic cells (DCs). Cross-linking of PRR on the surface of immature DCs by fungal antigen lead to their maturation. In addition, production of inflammatory cytokines such as IFN-γ and TNF-α by other innate cells such as NK cells further enhance activation of microbicidal functions of phagocytic cells as well as maturation of DCs. The DCs sampling fungal antigens from the skin and migrating to secondary lymphoid organs process and present antigens through class I or class II major histocompatibility complex (MHC) molecules to antigen-specific naive T cells endowed with the capacity to recognize the peptide epitopes through specific T-cell receptors (TCRs). This process lead to activation of different antigen-specific T helper (Th) effector cells, regulatory T (T_{reg}) cells and B cells that specifically target the pathogen and induce memory cells. Differentiation of naive CD4+ Th cells in the peripheral lymphoid organs into Th1, Th2, or T_{reg} depend on several factors, among which is the cytokine environment stimulated by different fungal morphotypes. Thus, the production of interleukin-12 (IL-12) by DCs leads to the outgrowth of T-helper-1 (Th1) cells that produce IFN-γ, TNF-α, or both. IFN-γ and TNF-α are required for further activation of fungistatic and fungicidal activities by phagocytes that results in clearance of infection with most, if not all, of these fungal pathogens. The induction of IL-4 (and failure to produce IL-12) by DCs leads to a Th2 response, which blunts the generation of protective immunity.

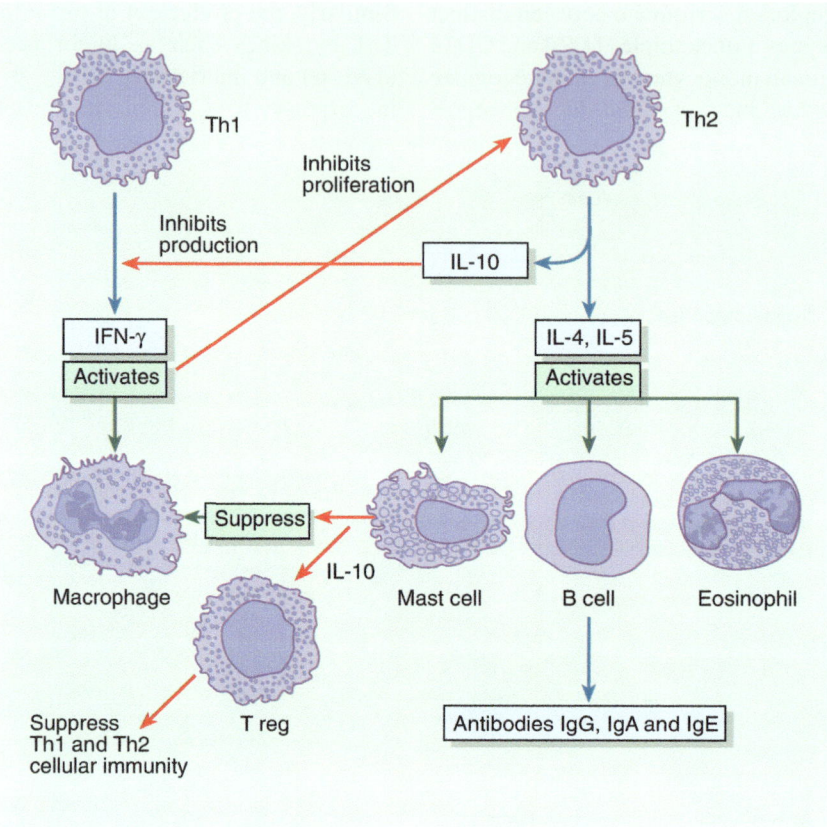

B

Fig. 24.1. (continued) (B) Progressive disease in immunodeficient or susceptible hosts is associated with a shift in the balance between Th1 and Th2, toward the Th2 response. The latter is characterized by upregulation in IL-4, IL-5 and IL-10, an increase in tissue eosinophils, antibody isotype switch and production of antigen-specific antibodies including IgG and IgE. The IgE antibodies bind to mast cells (MCs) and upon subsequent encounter with allergens, trigger degranulation leading to inflammation and clinical features of type I hypersensitivity reactions. IL-10 production by mast cells suppresses cell-mediated immune responses in certain cutaneous fungal diseases. Neutralization of IL-4, IL-5, and IL-10 in vivo can sometimes restore protective immunity. Thus, the activation of the appropriate Th-cell subset is critical in the generation of a successful immune response to fungi. Although IL-4 and IL-10 cytokines block the expression of a protective response against fungi, the elaboration of at least some Th2 cytokines also helps to balance the immune response. Finally, induction of T-regulatory (T_{reg}) cells mediated by IL-10 might serve to dampen the excessive inflammatory reactions through cell contact or secretion of immune suppressive cytokines such as IL-10 (B)

expressed on yeast cells depends on TLR2 and TLR4 signaling, whereas hyphal cells trigger these cytokines in a TLR2-dependent manner only.[18,23–25] In vivo, the role of TLR2 in systemic fungal infection such as systemic candidiasis is less clear: one study reported that TLR2$^{-/-}$ mice are more sensitive to primary infection than control mice,[26] while another study reported no difference between TLR2$^{-/-}$ and TLR2$^{+/+}$ mice, regardless of whether the animals were inoculated with yeast or hyphal forms.[27,28] In addition to their function in fungal recognition, uptake, and production of proinflammatory cytokines, signaling through individual TLR signaling can determine the type of acquired immune responses against fungi. TLR2 ligation by fungal zymosan, and possibly β-glucan, leads

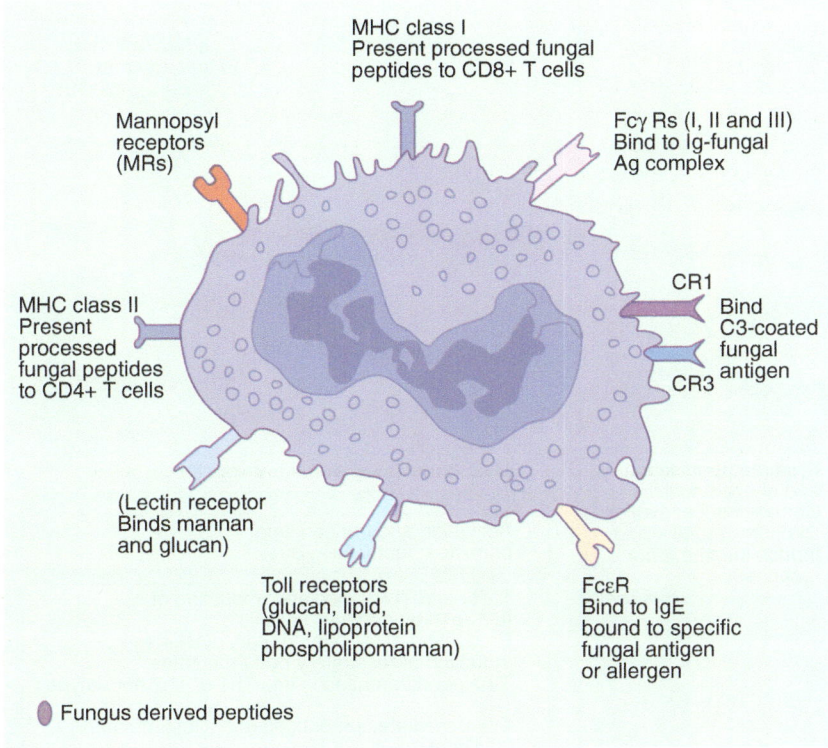

MHC class I
Present processed fungal
peptides to CD8+ T cells

Mannopsyl
receptors
(MRs)

Fcγ Rs (I, II and III)
Bind to Ig-fungal
Ag complex

CR1
Bind
C3-coated
fungal
antigen
CR3

MHC class II
Present
processed
fungal peptides
to CD4+ T cells

(Lectin receptor
Binds mannan
and glucan)

Toll receptors
(glucan, lipid,
DNA, lipoprotein
phospholipomannan)

FcεR
Bind to IgE
bound to specific
fungal antigen
or allergen

● Fungus derived peptides

A

FIG. 24.2. Recognition of fungal ligands by different pattern recognition receptors (PRRs) expressed on the surface of macrophages: the role of Toll-like receptors (TLRs) and other receptors as activators of innate and adaptive immunity to fungi. (A) Innate cells such as macrophages, monocytes, and dendritic cells express several pattern recognition receptors (PRRs) that recognize various fungal ligands, promote fungal internalization, activate intracellular fungicidal effector mechanisms, and play a role in the induction of the acquired immune response against fungi. Concomitant interaction of antibody and complement-coated fungal cells with Fc receptors (FcRs) and complement receptors (CRs) on host phagocytic cell membranes results in prompt ingestion of the fungal cell, which can lead to the death of the ingested fungal cell. Furthermore, phagocytic cells express several TLRs that bind to specific fungal ligands referred to as pathogen-associated molecular patterns (PAMPs). The signaling pathway for mammalian TLRs after ligation of PAMPs involves interaction with the adaptor molecule MyD88 (myeloid differentiation primary response gene 88) located in the cytosol. The activation of MyD88 results in activation and translocation of nuclear transcription factor κB (NF-κB). NF-κB controls the activation of several downstream cytokines and chemokine genes; therefore, its activation is usually linked to production of proinflammatory and antiinflammatory cytokines and chemokines. Although all TLRs signal through MyD88, ligation of certain TLR can result in unique effector functions. For example, TLR2 stimulation leads to production of IL-10, which promotes the expansion and function of immunoregulatory T cells. On the other hand, stimulation of TLR4 or TLR9 leads to the activation of antifungal effector functions in phagocytes, such as respiratory burst and degranulation, and production of interleukin-12p70 (IL-12p70) by dendritic cells. This leads to inflammatory and protective antifungal T-helper-1 (Th1)-cell responses. However, the differential TLR responses could also function by unidentified MyD88–independent pathways (B)

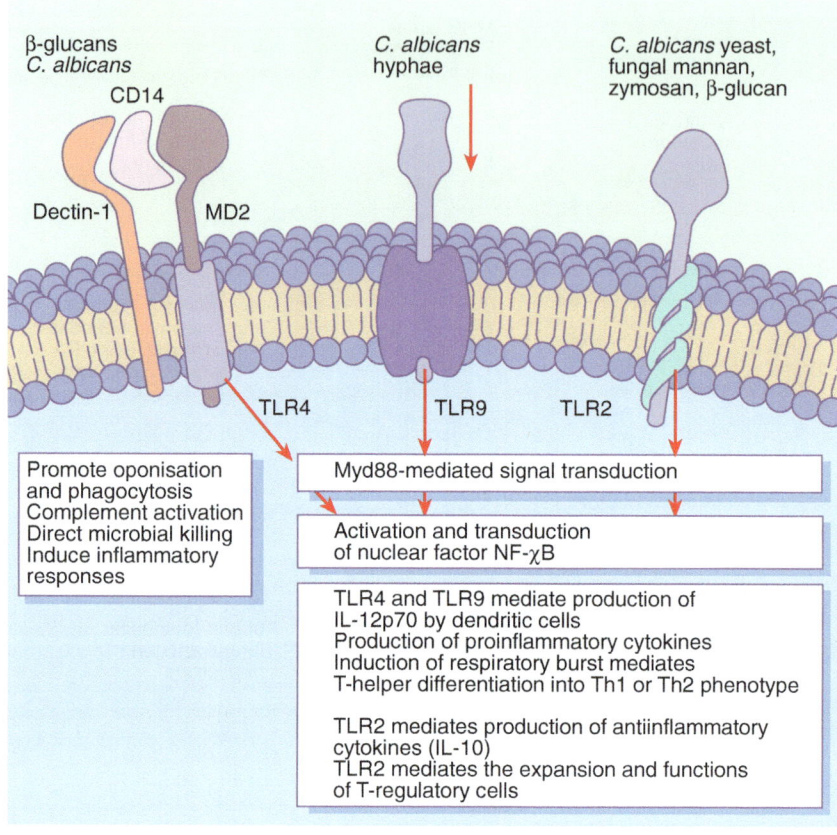

B

FIG. 24.2. (continued)

to the prevalent production of antiinflammatory cytokines such as interleukin-10 (IL-10), which can suppress macrophage microbicidal functions and also derive the induction of Th2 response.[27–30]

Lectin receptors are other PRR receptors on phagocytes that not only play a role in fungal recognition but also mediate distinct downstream intracellular events related to clearance of fungi. Recognition of fungal PAMPs by lectin receptors induces rapid and broad host defense responses such as opsonization, activation of complement, activation of coagulation cascades, phagocytosis, inflammation, and direct microbial killing.[31,32] Among several lectin-like families, galectin-3 binds to β-1,2-linked oligomannan, an uncommon PAMP present on the surface of *C. albicans* but absent on *Saccharomyces cerevisiae*.[33,34] The binding of galectin-3 to yeast cell walls of *C. albicans* is inhibited by *C. albicans* mannans but

not by *S. cerevisiae* mannans. More importantly, binding of galectin-3 results in opsonization of *Candida* expressing different combinations of β-1,2-linked oligomannosides and death of yeast cells.[34] Other fungal receptors such as complement receptors (CRs), mannose receptors (MRs), and dectin-1 receptors mediate fungal internalization following binding of various fungal ligands such as complement-associated products, mannosyle-fucosyl glycoconjugate ligands, and β-glucans, respectively. Internalization through MRs does not lead to effective clearance of fungi in the absence of opsonins. However, MRs expressed by DCs activates specific programs that are relevant to the development of antifungal acquired specific immune responses as will be discussed later. Ligation of CR3 (also known as CD11b/CD18) is one of the most efficient means of engulfing opsonized fungi, but it also has broad recognition capacity for diverse fungal ligands. Interestingly, yeasts such as *Histoplasma capsulatum* establish intracellular fungal parasitism within macrophages when they enter the cells through the CR3. In contrast, a concomitant ligation of both CR3 and FcγIIIR on macrophages triggers an effective phagocytosis and respiratory burst that interferes with fungal infectivity and mediates elimination of fungal pathogens.[35,36]

Neutrophils, macrophages, and monocytes constitute the major cellular effectors of innate immunity against fungal pathogens.[37–40] Following phagocytosis, fungi are killed by intracellular microbicidal effector molecules produced by macrophages and neutrophils, including oxygen-dependent (i.e., nitric oxide, reactive oxygen intermediates, reactive nitrogen intermediates, and peroxynitrite) and oxygen-independent (i.e., release of cationic proteins, lysozyme, and antimicrobial peptides such as defensins, arachidonic acid, myeloperoxidase, and iron sequestration).[40–43] Enzymes such as the reduced nicotinamide adenine dinucleotide phosphate (NADPH) oxidase and inducible nitric oxide synthase initiate the oxygen-dependent pathways known as respiratory burst that produces toxic reactive oxygen intermediates (ROIs).[41–43] In retribution, fungi have evolved strategies to selectively inhibit the respiratory burst through the production of specific scavengers of oxidative killing by phagocytes, such as catalase, mannitol and melanin.

Patients with inherited X-linked chronic granulomatous disease, resulting from a deficiency in oxidant formation due to mutations in any of the four genes that encode the subunits of NADPH oxidase, have increased susceptibility to fungal infection, mainly aspergillosis.[43] These patients could be treated effectively with IFN-γ, which increase the nonoxidative as well as the oxidative intracellular microbicidal mechanisms mediated by phagocytic cells such as macrophages and neutrophils. The involvement of neutrophils or macrophages in host defense against fungi depends on the morphotype of the fungi causing infection. For example, neutrophils play a predominant role in phagocytosis of filamentous fungi,[38–40,43] while macrophages play a predominant role in host dense against fungal yeast.[37,44] In addition to the ability of macrophages to ingest organisms that have been opsonized with antibody, or complement, they are also able to phagocytose unopsonized fungal elements through recognition receptors such as the integrins. Although the main contribution of neutrophils and macrophages resides in their phagocytic and microbicidal functions, they can produce cytokines and chemokines that can modulate the protective immune response. Furthermore, macrophages function also as an APC that activate CD4+ and CD8+ T cells through presentation of fungus-derived peptides in the context of major histocompatibility complex (MHC) class II and I, respectively as well as providing co-stimulatory signals as illustrated in Figure 24.3. Nevertheless, for some intracellular fungal pathogens, such as *H. capsulatum*, their intracellular location protects them from host defenses, and these organisms thrive within macrophages.[35,36]

To overcome the fungal immune evasion mechanism within phagocytic cells, other innate immune cells such as NK,[44–46] NKT, and γδ T cells[44,47,48] play a pivotal role in host defense against fungi. These cells mediate their antifungal response through different mechanisms that include the following: (1) early production of cytokines such as IFN-γ and TNF-α that are important for full activation of macrophages phagocytic and antimicrobial effector functions; (2) direct cytotoxic killing of pathogens or growth inhibition; (3) activation of dendritic cells through either cytokines or cell–cell contact, which in turn mediate activation and differentiation of specific CD4 and CD8+ T cells as described later. Evidence that supports the protective role of NK, NKT, and γδ T cells in immunity against fungi stems from studies conducted in knockout mice that lack a particular cell subset. These mice are susceptible to various fungal infections, mainly *C. albicans*.[46,47]

Langerhans' cells (LCs) and immature dermal DCs are some of the first cells to encounter fungi and play pivotal roles in induction of acquired responses against fungi as well as restriction of fungal growth.[49–51] Immature DCs constantly monitor the epidermal microenvironment by taking up antigen and processing it into fragments that can be recognized by cells of the adaptive immune response. Because of their unique migratory ability, DCs can transport fungal antigen from the epidermis or dermis to regional lymph nodes, where they initiate specific immune responses. Fungal infection provides danger signals, leading

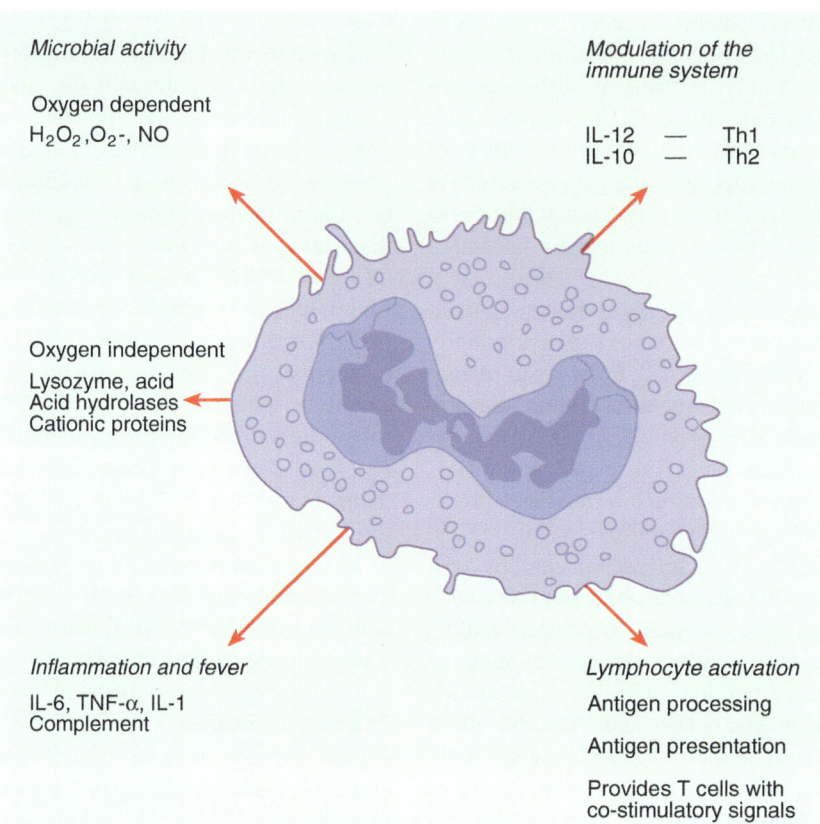

Microbial activity

Oxygen dependent
H_2O_2, O_2-, NO

Oxygen independent
Lysozyme, acid
Acid hydrolases
Cationic proteins

Inflammation and fever

IL-6, TNF-α, IL-1
Complement

Modulation of the
immune system

IL-12   —   Th1
IL-10   —   Th2

Lymphocyte activation

Antigen processing

Antigen presentation

Provides T cells with
co-stimulatory signals

FIG. 24.3. Different functions of macrophages in innate and acquired immune responses against fungal infection. Macrophages play a pivotal role in innate and acquired immune responses against fungal pathogens. Local activation of macrophages at early stages of infection by fungal antigens and later by IFN-γ and TNF-α produced by NK cells or effector CD4[+] Th1 cells results in (1) increased oxygen–dependent and independent fungicidal activities; (2) production of proinflammatory cytokines and chemokines that enhance migration of effector immune cells to the skin as well as play a role in activation of T cells. In addition, macrophages can also function as professional antigen-presenting cells (APC) that process fungal antigens and present fungus-derived peptides in the context of MHC class II and I to CD4[+] and CD8[+] T cells, respectively

to a local production of proinflammatory cytokines that induce local DC maturation.[52,53] Maturation of DCs is associated with a selective change in chemokine receptor profile.[54–62] For example, immature DCs express a number of chemokine receptors for inducible chemokines, such as IL-8 (CXCL8), RANTES (*r*egulated on *a*ctivation, *nor*mal *T*-cell *e*xpressed and *s*ecreted; CCL5), macrophage inflammatory protein 1α (MIP-1α; CCL3), or monocyte chemoattractant protein 3 (MCP-3; CCL7), by which immature DCs are attracted to the site of inflammation (i.e., skin)[58–60]

Following maturation, DCs downregulate these receptors, which may allow them to leave the inflam-

matory site (i.e., the site with the highest chemokine concentration). At the same time, maturing DCs upregulate receptors for constitutively expressed chemokines such as the CXC chemokine receptor 4 and CCR7.[59,60] Interestingly, the CCR7 ligand secondary lymphoid tissue chemokine (SLC; CCL21) is constitutively expressed by stromal cells in T-cell zones of lymph nodes and by lymphatic endothelial cells in the dermis.[58–60] Thus constitutive expression of SLC by lymphatic endothelium seems to provide the first chemotactic gradient for activated CCR7-positive DCs, leading to a selective recruitment of DCs from the epidermis to the afferent lymphatics.[60–62] Once they enter the lymphatics, they are likely to be transported passively with the lymph to the subcapsular region, where they then encounter an additional chemotactic gradient of SLC that directs their migration into the paracortical T-cell zone of the lymph node where they activate T cells specific for the invading fungal pathogen. In the draining lymph nodes, these DC-capturing antigens initiate T-cell immune responses by virtue of their abilities to present fungal antigens to T cells, provide lymphocyte co-stimulatory molecules, and secrete cytokines. The DCs use distinct receptors to recognize each form of a particular fungus, thereby activating different signaling pathways with distinct functional consequences.[52,62–64]

Finally, the noncellular effectors of innate immunity comprise complement and natural antibodies.[65–68] As described before, these molecules mediate opsonization and therefore promote the ingestion of fungi by phagocytes. However, the fate of opsonized fungi can differ from that of unopsonized organisms, because in phagocytes, opsonized fungi may traffic through a different pathway than do the unopsonized organisms.[35,36]

Adaptive Immunity

For many fungal pathogens, the effective immune response to invasion is a cell-mediated immune response. The role of CD4[+] T lymphocytes in protection against fungal infections is underscored by the susceptibility of patients with acquired immunodeficiency syndrome (AIDS) caused by HIV to fungal infections caused by *C. albicans*, *H. capsulatum*, *Cryptococcus neoformans,* and *Aspergillus fumigatus.* For all of the pathogenic fungi, a T-helper-1 (Th1) response characterized by production of IL-2 and IFN-γ is the dominant adaptive protective response. The production of IL-12 by DCs leads to expansion and increased number of Th1 cells that produce IFN-γ or TNF-α.[53,54,69–71] Interestingly, IL-12 secretion seems to be dependent on the morphologic form of the fungi where the yeast form of *C. albicans* stimulates IL-12 production, while the hyphal form inhibits such production.[64,71] Interferon-γ production by Th1 cells is essential for optimal activation of phagocytes (e.g., macrophages, neutrophils, and immature DCs) at sites of infection and enhances their fungicidal effector functions.[63,70] Therefore, deficiency

of this cytokine or Th1 response might predispose patients to overwhelming fungal infections, and also favor fungal persistence. On the other hand, the Th2 response characterized by production of Th2 cytokines (IL-4, IL-13, IL-5, and IL-10) is often associated with a subversion of the host response to fungi. Increases in the Th2 cytokines are commonly observed in progressive disease, and neutralizing their activity restores protective immunity.[71–75]

The role of Th1/Th2 paradigm in outcome of fungal disease is exemplified in skin infection with *Paracoccidioides* (PCM) *brasiliensis*, which stimulates the formation of granulomatous lesions in the skin.[75,76] Presence of well-formed granuloma and local Th1 responses in the skin of PCM patients is associated with mild disease, while the presence of poorly formed granuloma and local Th2 responses is associated with progressive and severe disease. These observations suggest that well-organized granulomas and cutaneous Th1 response reflect a better cellular immune response, while the presence of Th2 cells expressing Th2 cytokine such as IL-4 and IL-5 indicate an ineffective response in PCM skin lesions.

Compared to CD4 T cells, the role of CD8[+] T cells during fungal infection has not been defined as clearly.[77] CD8[+] T cells mediate protection against fungal infection mainly via the production of IFN-γ. However; the role of CD8 T lymphocytes in mediating cytotoxic lysis of fungus-infected target cells is not well delineated.[78] Although CD8[+] T cell activity against filamentous fungi such as *A. fumigatus* has not been demonstrated in mice, the expansion of cytotoxic, class I–restricted, *A. fumigatus*–specific CD8[+] T cell clones from human peripheral blood suggests that CD8[+] T cells might contribute to cell-mediated defense.[78] Interestingly, unlike infection with bacteria and virus, the priming of fungus-specific CD8[+] T cells does not appear to require CD4[+] T-cell help; in fact, CD8 T-cell responses are enhanced in CD4-knockout mice. In the absence of CD4[+] T cells, CD8[+] T cells can protect mice from *H. capsulatum* infections by secretion of IFN-γ.[79–81]

Although Th1-biased responses to fungal infections are protective, Th2-biased responses are deleterious; an excess or unregulated Th1 response may also generate unnecessary tissue damage. The Th1 response can be downregulated by simultaneous elaboration of Th2 cytokines or suppression of Th1 and Th2 responses that usually are associated with either chronic fungal infection or overwhelming infection, respectively. Thus, the induction of regulatory mechanisms in immunity to fungi is pivotal as they ensure that under physiologic conditions, an effective protective antifungal immunity is generated while avoiding immune pathology. One important immunoregulatory cytokine is IL-10, which is a potent immunosuppressive cytokine, produced in non–antigen- specific manner by innate cells such as macrophages and DCs or in an antigen (Ag)-specific manner by regulatory CD4+ T cells.[82,83] Interleukin-10 acts by impairing (1) the antifungal effector functions of phagocytes; (2) the secretion of proinflammatory cytokines such as TNF-α, IL-1, and IL-6; and (3) the production of Th1-promoting cytokines such as IL-12, IFN-γ, and IL-23.[82–85] The IL-10-mediated suppressive functions would result in defective protective antifungal cell-mediated immunity. Production of IL-10 at early stages of infection suppresses immune responses and enhances susceptibility to fungal infection.

Histopathologic and double immunohistochemical examination of skin lesions from patients with severe PCM infection revealed an increased number of mast cells expressing IL-10.[86,87] Early production of IL-10 by mast cells, as part of the innate system, could contribute to an ineffective response against fungal antigens. It is of interest that IL-10 expressing mast cells were detected only in skin lesions characterized by loose granuloma and local Th2 response, but not in lesions that are characterized by compact granuloma and Th1 response. Other studies have shown that patients treated with anti–TNF-α antibodies, which resulted in increases in IL-10 production are susceptible to fungal pneumonia. On the other hand, production of IL-10 at later stages of infection by CD4 T regulatory cells is beneficial by contributing to resolution of excessive inflammatory responses, thus avoiding immune-mediated tissue damage.[88–91]

Role of Antibodies in Protective Immunity Against Fungi

Nearly all fungi elicit an antibody response; however, the role of these antibodies in pathogenesis or protective immunity is not completely clear. The absence of an association between deficiencies in antibodies and susceptibility to infections with fungal pathogens and the presence of specific antibodies in patients with progressive fungal infections have provided evidence against a protective role of antibodies in fungal infections. However, studies involving opportunistic fungal diseases, mainly candidiasis and aspergilosis, provided evidence that supports a role for antibodies in protective immunity against fungal diseases.[92–95] Possible targets for these protective antibodies included fungal cell-wall polysaccharides of *Candida* and *Aspergillus* species, heat shock protein 90, histone like proteins, and mannoprotein in *C. albicans*.[92–96]

Recently, another fungal cell-wall polysaccharide, β-glucan, has been identified as a possible target for the induction of protective antibodies.[97] The conserved structure suggested that β-1,3-glucan could be part of a universal antifungal vaccine. In the light of known inverse relationship between Th1 and Th2 cytokines and immunregulation of the Th1 and Th2 responses, a role for antibodies in defense against fungal disease might seem to be in conflict with the underlying Th1-directed response that is the most widely accepted explanation for host-acquired specific immunity against fungi. However, some studies show that Th2-derived antibodies have a protective effect by augmenting cell-mediated immunity.

Antibodies can function as opsonins, promoting fungal ingestion and even killing by phagocytes, and several antibodies are directly fungicidal.[98–100] These kinds of activities are complementary, rather than exclusive, to cell-mediated mechanisms. The central importance of granulocytes and macrophages in innate defense against opportunistic fungal pathogens, and of activated neutrophils and macrophages against fungi in general, is consistent with an expectation that opsonic antibodies facilitate host defence. Antifungal antibodies also contribute to the activation of the classic complement system and antibody-mediated cytotoxicity by NK cells.[101,102]

The question that remains to be answered is whether these antibodies that react to specific fungal ligands and provide protective immunity upon immunization with whole fungal cells or specific fungal antigens such as glucan in mice are truly playing a protective role in humans. As discussed before, the finding that patients typically have antibodies before and after the disease suggested that antibodies play a minor role in protection against fungi. However, it is necessary to consider certain factors that are known to influence the protective functions of antibodies such as the amount, specificity, isotype, and idiotype of antibodies generated in vivo before drawing such a conclusion. Thus, the differences in antibody isotype may explain the discrepant results between different studies on the role of antibodies in host defense. Th1-derived antibodies are usually of immunoglobulin G2 (IgG2) isotype, which are excellent opsonins that promote fungal ingestion and even killing by phagocytes. In contrast, the association of antibodies with nonprotective response or progressive fungal diseases could be due to the possibility that these antibodies are of Th2 isotype (usually IgG1), which is produced by antigen-specific B cells interacting with antigen specific CD4[+] Th2 cells producing Th2 cytokines such as IL-4 or IL-10. In that case, Th2-derived antibodies are associated with a Th2 response that causes suppression of protective Th1 and cell-mediated immunity.[103,104]

Cutaneous Fungal Diseases

Cutaneous Candidiasis

Clinical Manifestations and Pathogenesis of the Fungal Disease

Cutaneous candidiasis is an infection of the skin that is caused by the yeast *C. albicans* and can be either acute or chronic in nature. Cases of cutaneous candidiasis caused by other *Candida* species such as *C. parapsilosis* or *C. tropicalis* are sometimes seen, but these are rare. *Candida albicans* is part of the normal flora of the gastrointestinal tract rather than of the skin, although it can be found on the skin.[105–107] This organism can grow as either yeast cells or filamentous forms, with mixtures of the two phases generally seen in tissue infections. Acute cutaneous candidiasis may present as lesions with intense erythema, edema, creamy exudate, and satellite pustules within folds of the skin. Other infections may be more chronic, as in the feet, where there can be a thick, white layer of infected stratum corneum overlaying the epidermis of the interdigital spaces. *Candida* paronychia is marked by infections of the periungual skin and the nail itself, resulting in the typical swelling and redness of this type of candida infection. The virulence of *C. albicans* has been attributed variously to its ability to grow at particular temperatures, its ability to produce filamentous forms, its adherence capabilities, and the activity of different enzymes. In some cases superficial *C. albicans* infections may be particularly severe and refractory to treatment, producing the uncommon disorder known as chronic mucocutaneous candidiasis (CMC),[108–110] which consists of persistent and recurrent infections of the mucous membranes, skin, and nails. Oral thrush and *Candida* vaginitis are fairly common in patients with CMC. There is often infection of the esophagus, although further extension into the viscera is unusual. The typical skin lesions are generally red, raised, and hyperkeratotic but usually are not painful. Epidermal neutrophilic microabscesses, which are common in acute cutaneous candidiasis, are rare in the lesions of CMC. Nail involvement can be severe in this condition, producing marked thickening, distortion, and fragmentation of the nails, with chronic swelling of the distal phalanx.

Immune Responses and Host Defenses Against Candida

The initial events in stimulation of both innate and acquired immune responses against cutaneous *Candida* infection include recognition of fungal ligands and phagocytosis. The immunoreactive components of *C. albicans* are thought to be the carbohydrate derivatives found on the yeast surface, including glucans, mannans, and chitin. The activation of TLRs by these fungal products presumably contributes to the inflammatory tissue injury seen in mucocutaneous candidiasis by signaling the release of proinflammatory cytokines and by directing the recruitment and activation of other inflammatory cells.[111–116]

Recognition of mannan by the mannose receptor on macrophages results in the internalization of *Candida*. Mannan drives TNF-α production by murine alveolar macrophages in vitro and increases the serum TNF-α level upon intravenous administration in vivo. Earlier studies of the immune response against yeasts have relied heavily on the use of zymosan, an insoluble fungal cell wall preparation, which contains large amounts of β-glucan and mannan.[21–29] It was shown that TLR6 and TLR2 formed heterodimers to coordinate the macrophage activation by zymosan.[29,119] These findings also suggested that immunity against *C. albicans* requires the collaboration between receptors responsible for phagocytosis (e.g., mannose or complement receptors) and TLRs designed to induce proinflammatory cytokines. Recent studies highlighted the role of Myd88,[11–18,117,118] a signaling molecule for TLR in the phagocytosis of *C. albicans*.[19–21] Macrophages harvested from Myd88–deficient mice and challenged with live *C. albicans* showed a diminished capacity to engulf and kill the yeast, and produce TNF-α when compared to wild-type cells.[21]

In contrast to immune mechanisms involved in protection against widespread, systemic candidiasis, where cells of the innate immune system, particularly neutrophils, are crucial,[16,36] it has long been recognized, based on both clinical and experimental data, that in the mucocutaneous form of candidiasis, cell-mediated immunity is essential for protection. Chronic mucocutaneous candidiasis represents a group of syndromes with a variety of predisposing or secondary abnormalities in host defense function. The most common deficiency appears to be one of cell-mediated immune responses against candida antigens, although abnormalities in chemotaxis or phagocytic cell function have also been reported.[108–114] Other host defense mechanisms, such as humoral immunity and the complement system, have generally been found to be normal in these patients.[115] Although treatment of this condition with amphotericin B could be successful in prompt clearance of the cutaneous lesions, relapses usually occurred, presumably because of the underlying immunodeficiency state. HIV infection or severe combined immune deficiencies affecting cell-mediated immunity predispose to mucocutaneous candidiasis. Evidence of impaired cell-mediated immunity to *Candida* spp. in these patients is represented by negative delayed-type hypersensitivity skin tests, absent or low T-cell proliferation in vitro, and impaired production of leukocyte/macrophage inhibitory factor.[120]

Several human and murine studies suggest that impaired clearance of *Candida* spp. in patients with CMC is due to imbalance between Th1 and Th2 responses with bias toward the Th2 phenotype. Appropriate and timely induction of Th1 responses characterized by production of Th1 cytokines such as IL-2, IFN-γ, TNF-α,[121,122] and IL-12,[63,70,123] which activate and recruit effector cells such as macrophages or CD8+ cytotoxic T cells, are of major importance for protection and clearance of the yeast.[120,121] In contrast, induction of Th2 responses marked by production of Th2 cytokines such as IL-4 and IL-10, which are necessary for mounting an antibody response but also downregulate type 1 cytokine production, had opposite detrimental effects.[122] Peripheral blood mononuclear cells from patients with CMC produce high levels of IL-10, but normal levels of IL-4 and IL-5, upon in vitro stimulation with carbohydrate and mannan fractions of *C. albicans*. Although Th1 cytokines such as IL-12 and IFN are also decreased in CMC patients, receptors for IL-12 and IFN are shown to be intact.[122]

Two possibilities can account for the bias toward Th2 response in CMC patients. The first possibility is that altered cytokine environment caused by interaction of the yeast or hyphal forms of *Candida* with innate immune cells could inversely influence the induction of CD4 Th1 cells producing IFN-γ and IL-2. The second possible mechanism could lie more upstream, involving the co-stimulatory functions of APCs such as DCs or macrophages.[30,123] In support of the first possibility, recent evidence in mice indicates that innate immune cells such as neutrophils and macrophages discriminate between the hyphal and yeast forms of the fungus through binding to different PRRs such as TLR and lectin, being able to produce IL-12 in response to *C. albicans* yeasts, and IL-10 in response to *C. albicans* hyphae.[30,63] The production of IL-12 and IL-10 can thus bias the CD4 Th response to Th1 or Th2 phenotype, respectively.

Interestingly, in vitro culture of DCs with the two forms showed that hyphae escaped the phagosome and were lying free in the cytoplasm of the cells, while the yeast form remained within the phagosome. The differences in fungal localization within DCs, therefore, may influence the access of fungal antigens to MHC class I (cytoplasmic) or II (phagosomal) pathways of antigen presentation to CD8 and CD4 T cells, respectively, which influences the ability of each fungal form to stimulate CD4 or CD8 T cells. Therefore, DCs, by discriminating between yeast and hyphal forms of the fungus, through different TLRs and the downstream effect of differential TLR ligation on cytokine environment, as well as differential fungal localization within DC, can influence the type of specific immune response.

Nevertheless, it remains to be identified whether the differential immune responses to different phenotypes of *Candida* is due to altered responses of immune cells or to expression of different virulent genes that allow evasion of host immune response and persistence. In support of the latter possibility, several studies suggested that phenotypic switching represents a pathogenic strategy for the combinatorial expression of batteries of genes leading to a variety of pathologic states. This conclusion was based on the findings that the process of phenotype switching between yeast and hyphal forms, which is characterized by different colony morphology, regulates the expression of a number of phase-specific genes, including *PEP1* (*SAP1*), *SAP3*, *OP4*, *CDR3*, *CDR4*, *NIK1*, *WH11*, and *EFG1*.[124–126] High-frequency phenotypic switching has also been demonstrated to regulate a number of phenotypic characteristics that have been implicated in pathogenesis, including antigenicity, sensitivity to neutrophils and oxidants, adhesion, and susceptibility to common antifungal agents.[126,127] Whether similar host-microbial interaction involving putative inherent defects of dendritic cells in terms of different dendritic cell subsets or receptors on the cells or differential gene expression upon phenotype switch exists in CMC patients is not yet known.

Dermatophytosis

Clinical Manifestations and Pathogenesis of the Fungal Disease

The dermatophytes include a group of fungi (ringworm) that under most conditions have the ability to infect and survive only on dead keratin, that is, the top layer of the skin (stratum corneum or keratin layer), the hair, and the nails. Dermatophytes cannot survive on mucosal surfaces such as the mouth or vagina where the keratin layer does not form. Very rarely, dermatophytes undergo deep local invasion and multivisceral dissemination in the immunosuppressed host. Dermatophytes are responsible for the vast majority of skin, nail, and hair fungal infections. These types of infections, termed "dermatophytoses," are widespread and increasing in prevalence on a global scale.[128,129] Reasons for this increase are not clear, although it may be due, in part, to an aging

process. This observation is consistent with the view that changes in the immune response that occur with advancing age lead to disease susceptibility. In keeping with this, fungal nail infections are more frequent in immunocompromised patients such as those who are HIV positive and those who have diabetes.[130,131] Alternatively, age-related changes in peripheral vasculature may be important in predisposing to infection. In addition to the effects of aging, genetic susceptibility has been proposed to contribute to infection. Although *Trichophyton rubrum* infection has been reported to show a familial pattern of autosomal dominant inheritance, more recent epidemiologic findings challenge this view.[131] Other factors that have been implicated include those associated with a modern lifestyle, including the use of footwear made from synthetic materials and exposure to dermatophytes in communal areas with damp environments that favor fungal growth, such as swimming pools and school gymnasiums.[131–133] Despite the identification of multiple predisposing factors, there is no consensus of opinion regarding a single mechanism to explain the increased incidence of foot disease that has occurred in recent years.

Dermatophytes are classified in several ways. The ringworm fungi belong to three genera: *Microsporum, Trichophyton,* and *Epidermophyton.* There are several species of *Microsporum* and *Trichophyton,* and one species of *Epidermophyton.* The inflammatory response to dermatophytes varies.[129–134] In general, zoophilic and geophilic dermatophytes elicit a brisk inflammatory response on skin and in hair follicles. The inflammatory response to anthropophilic fungi is usually mild. One very characteristic pattern of inflammation is the active border of infection. The highest numbers of hyphae are located in the active border, and this is the best area to obtain a sample for a potassium hydroxide examination. Typically the active border is scaly, red, and slightly elevated. Vesicles appear at the active border when inflammation is intense. This pattern is present in all locations except the palms and soles. Infections of the feet are particularly troublesome and affect both the skin (athlete's foot) and nails (tinea unguium). Despite the availability of new systemic antifungal therapies, nail infections are difficult to eradicate, with recurrence reported in up to 25% to 40% of cases. Since lesions vary in presentation and closely resemble other diseases, laboratory confirmation is often required.

Innate Immune Responses to Dermatophytes

Interaction of dermatophytes with many dermal and epidermal immune cell types including keratinocytes results in a cascade of chemokines and proinflammatory and antiinflammatory cytokine responses.[135–138] Activation of the alternative complement pathway by dermatophytes such as the case with *Trichophyton mentagrophytes* also results in production of chemotactic factors. These chemotactic events and inflammatory responses are thus responsible for the observed macroscopic changes associated with dermatophyte infections including scaling, vesicles, pustules, annular dermatitis, and severe inflammatory reactions (kerions). Microscopically, the lesions are characterized by an accumulation of neutrophils in the infected skin of acute infections or a mononuclear cell infiltrate in the dermis of the more chronic ones.[135–138] The acute inflammatory responses may be manifested as epidermal microabscesses, while chronic dermatophyte infection is usually manifested as epidermal hyperkeratosis and parakeratosis.[131–135]

Similar to other cutaneous mycosis, neutrophils mediate elimination of dermatophyte infections by a variety of microbicidal processes, including (1) microbicidal oxidants such as superoxide, hydrogen peroxide, hypochlorous acid, and monochloramine; and (2) nonoxidative microbicidal granules such as cathepsins, defensins, lactoferrin, lysozyme, elastase, azurocidin, and a number of other proteins.[136] Furthermore, neutrophils inhibit the growth of dermatophytes through release of large amounts of calcium and zinc-binding protein, called calprotectin that has potent microbiologic static activity against these fungi. This protein is released into inflammatory exudates as neutrophils degranulate at sites of infection.[136,137]

Acquired Immune Responses Against Dermatophytes: Immediate and Delayed-Type Hypersensitivity Reactions

Several of dermatophyte antigens are cross-reactive with airborne molds. These antigens stimulate IgE production, which mediates immediate hypersensitivity (IH) reaction in infected patients, mainly those with chronic dermatophytosis. The IH reaction in these patients is mediated by IgE antibody, and is characterized by a local wheal and flare occurring 5 to 20 minutes after injection of antigen into the skin. In this process, binding of antigen to IgE antibody (Ab) on the surface of mast cells results in cross-linking of IgE Ab, which, in turn, triggers the degranulation of mast cells and release of histamine and other proinflammatory mediators.[137,138]

The IH skin tests to *Trichophyton* are associated with the presence of serum IgE and IgG Ab to *Trichophyton* antigens. IgG4 Ab is a major component of the IgG Ab response.[132] Thus, IH reactions to dermatophytes bear the hallmarks of a Th2 response. In this type of response, IL-4 produced by CD4+ Th2 cells induces antibody isotype switching to IgG4 and IgE.[138,139] A role for fungal antigens (Ags) in allergic disease is strongly supported by the association between chronic dermatophytosis and allergic respiratory symptoms, and the improvement of late-onset asthma after antifungal therapy in patients with IH to *Trichophyton*.

By contrast, *Trichophyton* antigens are also able to induce delayed-type hypersensitivity (DTH) response in some patients.[129,139] Delayed-type hypersensitivity is a form of cell-mediated immunity in which the ultimate effector cell is the activated macrophage. In the classic DTH reaction, activation of macrophages is mediated by IFN-γ–producing Th1 CD4+ T lymphocytes.[138–140] These T cells recognize and respond to foreign antigen presented in the form of peptide complexed with MHC class II molecules expressed on the surface of APCs. This cell-mediated response is characterized by induration at the injection site, which is maximal at 48 hours. There is considerable evidence that DTH is pivotal in the eradication of dermatophyte infection. This conclusion is based on data showing (1) the development of DTH in association with inflammatory responses in primary infections, (2) the association between acute highly inflamed lesions and DTH, and (3) the failure to develop infection after experimental inoculation when DTH is present. Interestingly, DTH to *Trichophyton* extract is associated with lower titers of IgG Ab to *Trichophyton* antigens and no IgE or IgG4.[138,140,141] These observations suggest that humoral response to *Trichophyton* is less protective. A subset of patients also mounts "dual" skin test responses in which a DTH response follows the

IH reaction. Whether this represents a transitional stage in DTH-to-IH conversion (or vice versa) is not known.

Several hypotheses have been proposed to explain the mechanism of induction or suppression of protective DTH responses in different individuals. One study suggested that development of IH suppresses DTH responses in patients with chronic dermatophytosis since most IH responses occur in the absence of DTH.[141,142] Treatment of chronic dermatophytosis associated with IH responses with the systemic antifungal terbinafine can restore DTH responsiveness to intradermal trichophytin antigen. Another study proposed that prolonged antigen exposure can induce immunologic unresponsiveness, or anergy, by activating suppressor T cells, which then downregulate cell-mediated responses. However, several studies have failed to demonstrate diminished T-cell proliferative responses to dermatophyte antigens in patients with IH.[139,141,143,144]

An alternative hypothesis was that the properties of the fungus itself may prevent the development of cell-mediated responses. For example, mannans derived from *T. rubrum* have been proposed to inhibit DTH by interfering with antigen-processing pathways required for T-cell activation. However, despite all these data, it is not yet clear whether chronic infection results from a lack of DTH or from the presence of an IH response. Thus, a major question is whether IH is a prerequisite for the development of chronic infection and, if so, whether it reflects a more broad-based immune dysregulation. The answer to this question is complicated by the fact that host factors, such as integrity of the skin barrier as well as immune status of the host, play a central role in determining the outcome of dermatophyte infection. Indeed, it is well recognized that patients with HIV infection or those receiving immunosuppressive therapy are predisposed to develop chronic dermatophytosis and sometimes an invasive disease. This observation is consistent with impairment of cell-mediated immunity associated with these conditions.

Changes in the balance between Th1 and Th2 responses with bias toward Th2 response have been implicated in the progression of several diseases such as HIV infection associated with chronic dermatophytosis.[141] Indeed, this would be consistent with the dogma that Th2 polarization contributes

to disease progression in HIV-infected subjects. Similarly, chronic *T. rubrum* infection associated with IH and a markedly elevated total IgE level in the serum was proposed to contribute to the development of severe measles infection by favoring the development of Th2 responses.[139–142] However, this does not explain the paradoxical association between chronic dermatophytosis and Th1-mediated diseases such as diabetes. Nevertheless, the association between diabetes and dermatophytosis is also complex, as diabetic complications such as peripheral vascular disease could contribute to persistent dermatophyte infection.

Although immune mechanisms involved in the natural resolution of infection have yet to be resolved, recent findings suggest that T cells with a defined specificity for *Trichophyton* antigens or epitopes are critical for development of DTH or IH responses in different individuals. This conclusion was based on comparison of the T-cell repertoire in subjects with distinct immune responses to a single Ag such as the 29-kd Tri-r-2 derived from *T. rubrum*. Interestingly, the differences in the T-cell repertoire between patients with IH and those with DTH were independent of human leukocyte antigen (HLA) haplotype.[139,140,145,147,148] The clinical relevance of different T-cell repertoires remains to be determined. However, it is possible that certain antigenic peptides derived from *Trichophyton* antigens contain an epitope that specifically promotes the development of a DTH response, making progression to chronic dermatophytosis unlikely.[145–147]

Malassezia Infection

Clinical Manifestation and Pathogenesis of Fungal Diseases

Yeasts of the genus *Malassezia* undergo asexual reproduction by monopolar budding. The yeast cell is actually a phialide that has a small collarette at its apex, which gives it an overall bottle-shaped appearance. Some of the species are able to undergo a phase transition from yeasts to hyphae, although the factors that control this transition are not clearly understood. The genus *Malassezia* is known to include at least seven species of yeast (*M. furfur, M. pachydermatis, M. sympodialis, M. globosa, M. obtusa, M. restricta,* and *M. slooffiae*). Except for *M. pachydermatis*, the species require an exogenous source of lipid owing to their inability to synthesise C14–C16 saturated fatty acids because of a block in the de novo synthesis of myristic acid.[148] Although *Malassezia* can be found on normal human skin, it has implicated in a range of both cutaneous and systemic diseases such as seborrheic dermatitis, dandruff, folliculitis, atopic dermatitis (recently renamed atopic eczema/dermatitis syndrome [AEDS]), psoriasis, confluent reticulate papillomatosis, and seborrheic blepharitis.[149–156] *Malassezia* is most frequently associated with pityriasis (tinea) versicolor (PV), which is one of the most common disorders of pigmentation seen in dermatologic clinics worldwide.[149,150] PV is a chronic superficial fungal infection of the skin. The *Malassezia* species that have been isolated from patients with PV include *M. furfur, M. globosa, M. restricta, M. slooffiae,* and *M. sympodialis,* with more than one species of *Malassezia* being present. PV most often occurs on the trunk, neck, and proximal extremities. It is characterized by scaly hypopigmented or hyperpigmented macules and patches with minimal pruritic reaction.[148–150]

Malassezia folliculitis is characterized by follicular papules and pustules localized to the trunk, upper arms, neck, and, less often, the face.[154–156] These lesions are generally pruritic. Diagnosis is based on clinical signs, cytology, and culture in combination with histopathology. Although it has been suggested that follicular occlusion was the primary cause of *Malassezia* folliculitis with a secondary overgrowth of *Malassezia* organisms, colonization of normal pilosebaceous units by these yeasts can also be extensive. The exact role of *Malassezia* in *Malassezia* folliculitis, therefore, awaits further elucidation. Therapy for *Malassezia* folliculitis is similar to that described for PV. As with PV, recurrence tends to be a common problem.

Seborrheic dermatitis and dandruff are other diseases caused by *Malassezia*. Seborrheic dermatitis is characterized by inflammation and desquamation in areas that are rich in sebaceous glands such as the scalp, face, and upper trunk, whereas dandruff is a noninflammatory scaling condition of the scalp. Dandruff is now generally considered the mildest form or a variant of seborrheic dermatitis.[155,156] The decreased severity of these diseases upon fungal therapy, the increase in the number of *Malassezia* organisms, and relapse upon discontinuation of therapy support a role of *Malassezia*

as the etiologic agents in these two conditions. The species that have been isolated from patients with seborrheic dermatitis are similar to those causing PV, with *M. furfur* and *M. globosa* being most common. Atopic dermatitis is another chronic, multifactorial, inflammatory allergic skin disease associated with abnormal immunologic regulation and is associated with *Malassezia* infection.[156–158] Similar to dermatophyte antigens, allergens from *Malassezia* organisms have been implicated in its pathogenesis.[157–159] For atopic patients with a hypersensitivity response to *Malassezia* spp., antifungal therapy should be included in the treatment regime. In addition to the diseases described above, *Malassezia* spp. have also been shown to cause more deep-seated infections, including mastitis, sinusitis, septic arthritis, malignant otitis externa, fungemia, pulmonary vasculitis, peritonitis, and meningitis.[154–157]

Immunology of Malassezia-Associated Diseases

There have been large numbers of studies examining the innate and acquired (cellular and humoral) immune responses to *Malassezia* in patients with many *Malassezia*-associated diseases.[160] For many of the diseases, the responses reported have varied widely. The innate response against *Malassezia* involves several components such as complement, phagocytosis, and NK-mediated lysis. Several groups have reported the ability of *Malassezia* to activate the complement system, via either the alternative pathway or the classic pathway.[161–163] The extent of activation of the alternative pathway was cell concentration and time dependent, reaching a plateau after 30 minutes. Although the molecule responsible for triggering the alternative pathway is not well defined, ß-glucan in the cell wall may be involved.[163] The ability to activate complement has been suggested as a mechanism responsible for the inflammation associated with seborrheic dermatitis. Phagocytosis and intracellular killing of the yeast, mainly by neutrophils, is another important innate mechanism by which nonspecific effector cells play a role in host defense against *Malassezia*.[164,165]

The importance of phagocytosis in protection against fungal infections is highlighted by the increased susceptibility of neutropenic patients to many mycoses. In vitro, neutrophils take up

Malassezia in a complement-dependent process. On the other hand, the receptors involved in phagocyte–yeast cell binding have been characterized in a human monocytic cell line as the mannose receptor, ß-glucan receptor, and complement receptor type 3.[166] Recent studies have shown that when a monocytic cell line, THP1, was stimulated with either live or heat-killed *Malassezia*, the production of IL-8 was increased, while stimulation of a granulocytic cells line, HL-60, resulted in increased levels of both IL-8 and IL-1β.[167] The effects of IL-1β in host defense against cutaneous fungal organisms include the activation of lymphocytes, chemotaxis, and neutrophils and the induction of inflammation.[167–169] Interleukin-8 also induces chemotaxis and activation of neutrophils and T cells. Therefore, the interaction of *Malassezia* with phagocytic cells may serve to amplify the inflammatory response and encourage further recruitment of phagocytic cells.

Opsonized live *Malassezia* yeast cells are more stimulatory than were nonopsonized or heat-killed *Malassezia* yeast cells. However, the ability of neutrophils to kill *Malassezia* seems limited compared to efficient killing of *C. albicans* yeast cells and other fungal genera. The mechanism by which *Malassezia* may resist or prevent phagocytic killing is not completely clear. In addition to escaping phagolysosomal killing, in vitro studies suggested an immunosuppressive effect of *Malassezia* on activation of different innate effector cells.[169,170] *M. furfur* was able to invade human keratinocytes and resist phagolysosomal fusion, which allows their survival inside host cells. In addition, culture of yeast cells of *M. furfur* with normal human keratinocytes did not also stimulate cytokines or chemokines production.

Low levels of monocyte chemotactic protein 1 (MCP-1), TNF-α, and IL-1β (IL-1β) were found, which were associated with overproduction of immunosuppressive cytokines IL-10 and tumor growth factor-β (TGF-β).[170] It was further postulated that the suppression of proinflammatory cytokines might allow *Malassezia* to survive within host cells without causing an inflammatory response. Suppression of IL-1β, IL-6, and TNF-α also has been reported when *Malassezia* was cocultured with peripheral blood mononuclear cells (PBMCs), and that the suppression was IL-10 dependent.[170] This correlates with the situation seen in normal healthy skin and also with the limited inflammation seen in PV, despite the large fungal burden seen in the lesions.[171,172] It is known that the immunosuppressive effects of *Malassezia* on PBMCs can be reversed by removal of the lipid-rich capsular-like layer around the organism, and it will be interesting to determine if this is also the case with keratinocytes.[173]

The role of DC and NK cells in innate and acquired immune responses against *Malassezia* in atopic and nonatopic individuals has been extensively studied. Uptake of whole *M. furfur* yeast cells and various allergenic components from the yeast, including *M. furfur* extracts, recombinant *M. furfur* allergen 5 (Mal-f-5), and *M. furfur* mannan by immature monocyte-derived dendritic cells (MDDCs) has been demonstrated in vitro.[174,175] The internalization of *Malassezia* was shown to occur via binding to the mannose receptor (other receptors may also be involved) or pinocytosis and is not influenced by IgE. The presence of *M. furfur* was also shown to induce maturation of immature MDDCs by upregulation of CD83 expression, and increase in expression of the co-stimulatory molecules CD80 and CD86.[174–176]

The uptake of the yeast by the DCs also induced a significant production of TNF-α, IL-1β, and IL-18, but not IL-10 or IL-12, after 46 hours of coculture. Although immature DCs are highly phagocytic, mature DCs are excellent at presenting antigen-derived peptides on MHC molecules to T cells.[177] Thus, the DCs that had been exposed to *Malassezia* induced proliferation of autologous T lymphocytes in a dose-dependent way.[177–179] The interaction of *Malassezia*-infected mature DCs with NK cells in atopic patients also has been examined by comparing the numbers of NK cells in the normal skin of healthy controls with those in the atopic skin of atopic dermatitis or AEDS patients.[174,180] These studies showed that there were only scanty NK cells in normal skin, but that they were numerous in the atopic skin, and they were in close apposition with DCs. Dendritic cells that had been preincubated with *Malassezia* for 46 hours were less susceptible to NK-mediated lysis, and this resistance to NK lysis was mediated by soluble factors.[180–184]

This protection of DCs against NK-mediated lysis, if it were to occur in vivo, would allow the mature dendritic cells to remain in the epidermis, presenting *Malassezia* antigens to T cells and hence contributing to the maintenance of the inflammatory response in AEDS lesions.[183,184] The effect of different forms of *Malassezia* on the responses of DCs has been examined. Similar to that described in immunity against *C. albicans*, the yeast phase elicits production of IL-12 and priming of Th1 cells, while the hyphal phase inhibits IL-12 and Th1 priming, and induces production of IL-4, a Th2-type cytokine.[185–187] Similar to other fungi, Th1 T-cell–mediated immunity is important in the prevention and recovery from infections. A deficiency in cell-mediated Th1 responses could therefore predispose the host to overgrowth of *Malassezia*. Atopic patients with specific IgE antibodies against *M. furfur* were shown to have increased synthesis of the Th2-related cytokines IL-4, IL-5, and IL-10 by *Malassezia*-stimulated PBMCs.[185–187]

In regard to humoral immune responses against *Malassezia,* it is clear that IgG responses to *Malassezia* yeasts are common in both healthy individuals and patients with *Malassezia*-associated diseases. This probably reflects exposure of the immune system to antigens produced by commensal organisms.[188] However, enhanced IgG responses can be seen in humans with atopic dermatitis. The role of this IgG response in the pathogenesis of skin disease is currently unclear. IgG antibodies are known to be able to act as opsonins coating microorganisms and to activate phagocytes, which in turn ingest and destroy extracellular pathogens. This could in theory provide protection for the host. However, as overgrowth with *Malassezia* does not appear to be a self-resolving condition, it seems likely that these antibodies are not protective.[189,190] Alternatively, IgG antibodies could activate the complement system, as has been demonstrated with *Pityrosporum ovale* and *P. orbiculare,* and exacerbate the inflammatory response.[191] A final possibility is that IgG responses to the yeast are merely an association and neither contributes to nor inhibits the ongoing disease process.[190] Further studies are therefore required to determine the precise role played by these antibodies in *Malassezia*-induced skin disease. Using in vitro serologic tests such as enzyme-linked immunosorbent assay (ELISA), the radioallergosorbent test (RAST), and Western immunoblotting, *Malassezia*-specific IgE has been detected in human atopic patients for over a decade.[189,190] Stimulation with *Malassezia* extracts and IL-4

led to a dose-dependent increase in IgE synthesis from PBMCs only in RAST(+) atopic patients, indicating a Th2-type skewed response towards *Malassezia* in these patients.[192,193] The *Malassezia*-specific IgE antibodies in human atopic patients could play a key role in enhancement of immune responses.[191–193] The allergen-specific IgE antibodies could bind to Langerhans' cells in the skin, thus enhancing their allergen capturing and presentation capacity upon a second encounter with the allergen. In addition, IgE could mediate mast cell-mediated hypersensitivity responses to *Malassezia* allergens, and that may be involved in the pathogenesis, and contribute to the clinical signs, in some cases of human atopic dermatitis.

Subcutaneous Mycosis

Chromoblastomycosis

Clinical Manifestations and Pathogenesis of the Disease

Chromoblastomycosis is a term that designates a group of chronic cutaneous and subcutaneous mycoses caused by several species of dematiaceous (darkly pigmented) fungi. As a member of the heterogeneous group of subcutaneous mycoses, chromoblastomycosis commonly presents the following typical features: lesions beginning at the site of a transcutaneous trauma, chronic evolution associated with survival of the fungal agent, and fibrotic reaction.[194–196] In tissues, all agents form thick-walled, dark multiseptate structures—the muriform (sclerotic) cells. It is common worldwide but occurs mostly in tropical and subtropical areas of Africa, Asia, and South America. Chromoblastomycosis is considered an occupational disease in many tropical and temperate countries (Madagascar, northern Venezuela, and the Amazon region of Brazil).[197–199]

The disease is caused by a large number of fungi that exist in the soil, plants, flowers, and wood. The most common agents are *Fonsecaea pedrosoi* and *Cladophialophora carrionii*. The latter is considered to be the most important etiologic agent in deserts in South Africa and Australia.[197–199] Less frequently, the disease is caused by *Phialophora verrucosa*, *Rhinocladiella aquaspersa*, or *Wangiella Exophiala dermatitidis*. Other etiologic agents that were discovered recently are *Exophiala jeanselmei* and *Exophiala spinifera*. *Fonsecaea compacta* has also been observed in lesions of chromoblastomycosis. The etiologic agents enter the host through cutaneous puncture wounds, usually on a thorn or a splinter. Other kinds of trauma such as animal-associated trauma (insect bite or sting) are identified as the portal of entry of the fungus.

A primary lesion is represented by a papule that slowly enlarges over time and can ulcerate. The primary lesion can progress to polymorphic skin lesions, including nodular and verrucous lesions. Sometimes the lesions can heal as sclerotic plaques, scars, or keloid formations.[194–199] The most frequent clinical presentation is a cauliflower-like lesion that develops at the site of inoculation, and satellite lesions gradually arise from scratching autoinoculation and spread via the lymphatic system. Secondary lymph edema and pruritus are common findings, but the disease remains confined to the subcutaneous tissue and does not invade underlying muscles and bone, except in immunosuppressed patients such as those on high-dose corticosteroids. The lower limb is the most common site followed by the upper limb, ear pinna, and nose.[194–199] The diagnosis can be made by detection of multiform cells, referred to as sclerotic bodies, from tissue biopsies or from fungal culture. Hydrogen peroxide and hematoxylin and eosin (H&E) are recommended stains for elucidation of the sclerotic bodies in tissues.[199,200] The hyphae and budding cells are usually seen in the surface of the lesion, while the muriform cells are often seen in the deep part of the lesion. The treatment of chromoblastomycosis is difficult due to its limited response to oral antifungal therapy.[201,202] Medical treatment usually includes combined use of antifungal drugs such as itraconazole with terbinafine. Other treatment strategies include a combination of cryotherapy, fluorocytosine, and amphotericin B. Surgical treatment is the ultimate effective therapy, which involves surgical removal of lesions, electrodesiccation, and cryosurgery.

Immunology of Chromoblastomycosis

The host defense mechanism in chromoblastomycosis has not been extensively investigated. Some studies have focused on fungus–host interactions, showing a predominantly cell-mediated immune response, with activated macrophages involved in fungus phagocytosis.[203–205] The highly organized inflammatory reaction and chronic nature of chromoblastomycosis is characterized by the presence of a granulomatous reaction in association with neutrophil-rich purulent abscesses. This granulomatous reaction shows extensive phagocytosis of brown thick-wall fungal cells, which is considered the main factor explaining the chronic and inflammatory nature of the disease.[199,206]

Macrophages (referred to as epithelioid or giant cells) are highly activated as marked by higher expression of TNF-α and their enhanced in vitro antifungal activities marked by H_2O_2 and NO production.[207,208] Inhibition of NO synthesis by macrophages by fungus-produced melanin has been proposed as an immune evasion mechanism that prevents the host from clearing *F. pedrosoi*, leading to a chronic disease.[209] CD4 Th1 cells and type 1 response is important for host defense against causative agents of chromoblastomycosis.[210] Patients with a mild form of the disease have predominant production of IFN-γ, low levels of IL-10, and efficient T-cell proliferation, consistent with a type 1 response, while patients with the severe form of the disease have predominant production of IL-10, low levels of IFN-γ, and inefficient T-cell proliferation, consistent with an immunosuppression rather than Th2 response.[210,211]

Histopathologic and immunohistochemical staining of skin tissues from patients with the verrucous form of the disease has identified CD4 T lymphocytes at the periphery of the granulomas, with immunostaining for IL-10. These findings suggest that either a Th2 phenotype or immunosuppression is linked to severe or verrucous forms. Furthermore, patients with chromoblastomycosis produce specific IgM, IgG, and IgA antibodies.[203] Several cell wall and secreted immunoreactive antigens of *F. pedrosoi* have been identified. Antifungal antibodies specific to secreted melanin inhibit fungal development, support fungal internalization, and enhance macrophage functions as marked by greater degrees of oxidative burst.[212] Sera from infected human patients also reacted with secreted melanins, suggesting that *F. pedrosoi* synthesizes melanin in vivo.[212] Antibodies against melanin purified from patients' sera also reacted with sclerotic cells from patients' lesions as well as with sclerotic bodies cultivated in vitro—conidia, mycelium, and digested residues.[213] Taken together, these results indicate that melanin from *F. pedrosoi* is an immunologically active fungal structure that activates humoral and cellular responses that could help the control of chromoblastomycosis. Glucosylceramide (GlcCer) is another immunoreactive conserved lipid component in the cell wall of many fungi including dark fungi. Antifungal antibodies specific to GalCer directly inhibit fungal development, which supported the use of monoclonal antibodies to GlcCer as potential tools in antifungal immunotherapy.[214,215] However, unlike the clear correlation between mild disease and cell mediated type 1 response, evidence that supports a protective role of the humoral immune response in host defense in chromoblastomycosis is inconclusive.

Mycetoma

Clinical Manifestation and Pathogenesis of Fungal Disease

Mycetoma is a chronic granulomatous infection caused by fungi (eumycetoma) or actinomycetes (actinomycetoma). The first description of a case of mycetoma is usually attributed to Dr. John Gill, who reported "Madura foot" in a report of the Madras Medical Service of the British Army in India in 1842.[216–219] The mycetoma lesion is characterized by a subcutaneous mass and multiple sinuses draining pus, blood, and fungal grains. The morphologic characteristics and color of the grains provides clues about the species of the agents. The mycetoma infection has a prolonged and indolent course. The mycetoma lesion might ultimately extend to deeper tissues and bones, leading to deformity of the affected site and subsequent disability for the patient. This disease has been reported in many countries including Sudan, Somalia, Senegal, Mauritania, Kenya, Niger, Nigeria, Ethiopia, Chad, Cameroon, Djibouti, India, Yemen, Mexico, Venezuela, Columbia, and Argentina.[216–220]

Mycetoma infection is not self-curing and, if untreated, leads to massive lesions, which in the end necessitate surgical amputation. Mycetoma initially presents as a slowly progressive and painless subcutaneous swelling, sometimes in combination with a history of preceding trauma.[220–222] However, the incubation time before classic signs develop is not well defined because in many cases the patients usually present at later stages of disease when most of early clinical symptoms have disappeared.

The duration of the disease, the type of causative organism, the site of the infection, and the immune response of the host can all affect the clinical presentation of mycetoma. However, patients with a short disease history might present with massive lesions and severe destruction of deep tissues and even of bones. The subcutaneous swelling is usually firm and rounded but it can also be soft and lobular. It is rarely cystic and is often movable. The subcutaneous nodule increases in size, and secondary nodules might evolve as well. The nodules might suppurate and drain through multiple sinus tracts, which can close transiently after discharge during the active phase of the disease. The disease process involves opening of fresh adjacent sinuses while the old ones heal completely. The nodules are connected to the skin surface and to each other through deep sterile abscesses.

Mycetoma can affect any part of the body. Most cases are usually seen in the feet, followed by the hands, legs, and knee joints. Rarely, the chest and abdominal walls, facial bones, paranasal sinuses, eyelid, orbit, scrotum, and old surgical incisions might also be affected.[219–223] Mycetoma spreads locally or through the lymphatic system, and, rarely, through the bloodstream. Compared to actinomycetoma where secondary nodules, which represent lymphatic metastasis, are common, eumycetoma is rarely associated with secondary nodules.[224] Mycetoma is usually painless, and the mycetoma lesion has been suggested to produce substances that have an anesthetic effect. At a late stage of the disease, the absence of pain might be due to nerve damage by the tense fibrous tissue reaction or endarteritis obliterans, or alternatively, poor vascularization of the nerves. In the final stages of the disease, pain might be due to invasion of the bone or to secondary bacterial infection. As the mycetoma granuloma increases in size, the skin may become smooth and shiny, and areas of hypopigmentation or hyperpigmentation can develop.[221–225]

Diagnosis of mycetoma is based on the presence of subcutaneous mass, sinuses, and granular discharge in patients from an endemic area. *Madurella* species, the causative agents for eumycetoma, in general are slow-growing fungi that produce dark colonies composed of a dense, melanized, and mostly sterile mycelium. *Madurella* species are well-known agents of black-grain mycetoma. Two species are recognized, *M. mycetomatis* and *M. grisea*.

In different culture media, *M. mycetomatis* strains show various colonies and moderate growth rate. The colonies, which are white and woolly at first, becoming olivaceous, yellow, or brown, and produce a brownish, diffusing pigment. Colonies are mostly sterile, composed of dense melanized mycelium. No efficient sporulation has ever been seen.[226,227] However, phialides with minute conidia in balls and collarettes may be seen. Species-differentiation of *M. mycetomatis* and *M. grisea* can be made by differences in sugar assimilation and optimal growth temperature. *M. mycetomatis* assimilates lactose but not sucrose, whereas *M. grisea* assimilates sucrose but not lactose. *M. mycetomatis* grows well at 37°C, while *M. grisea* does not grow at 37°C (growth is seen at 30°C). This finding might also explain the observed difference in virulence.

Molecular tests have recently been developed and have significantly improved the diagnosis. The polymerase chain reaction (PCR) test is useful for detection and identification of *M. mycetomatis* in patients.[228] The test showed that a wide range of agents can actually cause eumycetoma. When different isolates of *M. mycetomatis* deriving from patients originating from endemic areas were genetically compared, they did not show major differences, despite differences in phenotypes seen when cultured.[226–228] The diverse clinical presentations thus seem to be due to differences in host susceptibility rather than gross genetic differences among the fungal strains involved. In addition to culture, biochemical, and molecular identification of the fungal etiologic agents of mycetoma, other diagnostic tests are important in developing an appropriate plan of treatment.[229–231] Magnetic resonance imaging has been shown to be valuable in the detection and even identification of fungal grains and for the assessment of therapeutic success.[231] Furthermore, radiology helps in clinical diagnostics, especially in the follow-up of disease progression, development of a surgical strategy, and assessing the clinical cure. At the level of the fungus, direct examination of grains might be useful in determining the type of mycetoma.[229,230] The large numbers of causative organisms and the poor in-vitro differentiation of fungi that cause mycetoma complicate the identification process. Histopathologic examination is generally not useful for differentiation of fungi, although some of the pigmented fungi may be categorized to a certain extent.[232] Fine-needle aspiration cytologic methods for mycetoma have also been described and are considered to be useful. Finally, serodiagnosis also can be helpful in identification of the etiologic agent.[233–237] The common serologic tests are immunodiffusion and ELISA; however, due to possible cross-reactivity between some species, the specificity of these assays is compromised.[224,233–237]

In tissues, *M. mycetomatis* forms numerous black sclerotia (grains). Grains are vegetative aggregates of the fungal mycelium embedded in a hard brown matrix, which consists of extracellular cement that seems to be 1,8-dihydroxynaphthalene melanin in combination with host tissue debris. This rigid matrix might act as a barrier protecting the fungus from the natural immunity of the host and antifungal agents. Melanins are thought to be protective in cases of host-induced oxidative stress. Two types of grains have been identified: filamentous and, less commonly, vesicular. Triple-layered tissue reaction zones have been described around the grains. An inner neutrophil zone immediately around the grain, an intermediate zone containing mainly macrophages, and an outer zone consisting of lymphocytes and plasma cells mainly can be seen under the microscope.[229,230,232] The medical treatment of eumycetoma is difficult, as the in-vivo activity of azoles is often poor especially in late, advanced cases, but lesions of patients under ketoconazole treatment remain localized and well encapsulated. Thus, long-term treatment with itraconazole seems to be the best therapeutic regimen at present. Treatment of advanced cases usually implies amputation of the infected limb.

Immune Responses in Mycetoma

In 1964, Mahgoub[233] was able to demonstrate that eumycetoma patients developed Abs against *M. mycetomatis*. Counterimmunoelectrophoresis, immunodiffusion, and ELISA were developed to detect Abs raised against different mycetoma causative agents, using crude culture extracts as Ag.[234–236] This did not identify the type of Abs produced or the nature of the Ags involved. It was not until the second half of the 1980s that it was experimentally demonstrated that the cytoplasm, organelles, and, predominantly, the cell wall of *M. mycetomatis* were antigenic. About the same time it was also determined that IgM and IgG were the dominant immunoglobulins resulting from mycetoma. In 1991, the first attempts were made to characterize the nature of the epitopes present in the crude extracts used for the initial experiments. Cytoplasmic proteins were extracted from several eumycetoma agents, and, although the different *M. mycetomatis* isolates had very heterogeneous protein profiles by sodium dodecyl sulfate–polyacrylamide gel (SDS-PAGE), the antigenic makeup was quite similar within the species.[237] However, information about the individual immunoreactive Ags was not examined at this study.[234–237]

A recent study identified the first immunogenic Ag, a protein homologous to the translational controlled tumor protein (TCTP), a well-conserved histamine release factor in a range of eukaryotes.[238] The gene for this Ag was demonstrated to be present in two variants in *M. mycetomatis*, with 13% amino acid difference between the two proteins encoded. In vitro, TCTP was secreted into the culture medium. In vivo, this protein was found to be expressed on hyphae present in developing stages of the eumycetoma-characteristic black grain. Significant IgG and IgM immune responses, against the whole protein and selected *M. mycetomatis*–specific peptides, were detected. The Ab levels correlated with lesion size and disease duration. Overall, the patients with the largest lesions had the highest Ab level, which lowered with decreasing size of the lesion. Similarly, prolonged duration of the disease was associated with the highest Ab levels. Whether these TCTP-specific antibodies are markers of progressive and chronic disease or they play a protective role in host defenses against *M. mycetomatis* infection is not yet known. Nevertheless, this TCTP is considered to be the first well-characterized immunogenic Ag that can be used as a monomolecular vaccine candidate against *M. mycetomatis*.

Dimorphic Fungi with Cutaneous Involvement

Sporotrichosis

Clinical Manifestations and Pathogenesis of the Disease

Sporotrichosis is caused by a thermo-dependent dimorphic fungus, *Sporothrix schenckii*. The hyphal form that is present in the normal environment consists of both conidia and hyphae, while the yeast form develops at 37°C.[239] The conidia or hyphae enter the body through either traumatic implantation or inhalation. However, *S. schenckii* is observed only as the yeast form in biopsies or excised specimens. Such conversion from hyphal to yeast form seems to occur in both the implantation and inhalation sites. Clinical manifestations of sporotrichosis are variable.[239–243] The major clinical manifestations occur in the skin and present primarily as either fixed cutaneous or lymphocutaneous forms. However, cases of disseminated cutaneous or visceral forms in immunosuppressed patients have been reportedly increased.

Immune Responses in Cutaneous and Visceral Sporotrichosis

Both virulence factors of the individual *S. schenckii* strains and the immunologic status of the host determine the clinical manifestations of sporotrichosis.[244,245] From the host perspective, cell-mediated immunity to *S. schenckii* antigen is a key immunologic defense mechanism that controls infection with *S. schenckii*.[244,245] Both CD4+ Th1 cells producing IFN-γ and macrophages are required for the development of granuloma formation, which is a critical and essential component of normal host defense against the pathogens. Interferon-γ messenger RNA (mRNA) is detected in the granulomatous skin lesions of sporotrichosis,[246] and immunohistochemical analysis demonstrated the existence of IFN-γ–producing CD4+ T cells in the periphery of such lesions.[247] The Th1 response activates macrophages to kill intracellular *S. schenckii*. Other studies demonstrated a CD83+ DC subpopulation in the granulation tissue of sporotrichosis, which indicates that activated DCs that express co-stimulatory molecules such as CD83 may play important roles in the Th1 immune response against *S. schenckii*.[248]

From the fungal pathogen perspective, infection with different strains of *S. schenckii* possessing special virulence factors is a critical factor that contributes to different clinical manifestations of individual *S. schenckii* strains (cutaneous versus visceral strains).[249,250] *S. schenckii* of cutaneous origin and yeast forms are more potent at activating DCs to induce subsequently stronger Th1-prone immune responses than those of visceral origin as evidenced by (1) higher expressions of HLA-DR and co-stimulatory molecules such as OX40L on DC and (2) higher induction of Th1 cytokines (IFN-γ and TNF-α). In contrast, *S. schenckii* of visceral origin positively induced a Th2 cytokine environment as evidenced by significantly higher IL-4 production and the inability to induce strong Th1 immune responses. Thus, similar to immune responses generated against other fungi described in this chapter, the Th1/Th2 balance may explain the differential clinical manifestations observed in cutaneous versus systemic or visceral sporotrichosis.[249–252]

Although the exact mechanism that accounts for differential Th1/Th2 responses following cutaneous and visceral sporotrichosis is not known, two possibilities are postulated: (1) different efficacies for the internalization of individual *S. schenckii* strains may affect the immunostimulatory response of DCs; and (2) differential expressions of surface molecules on *S. schenckii* could contribute to differential abilities of these strains to stimulate DCs via TLR or other PRRs such as lectin.[253–255] Examination of fungal internalization reveals no difference between the cutaneous and visceral strains. Therefore, the second possibility involving differential interaction of different strains with different PRRs on various APCs is the most likely mechanism that accounts for different clinical manifestations between the two strains of *Sporothrix*.[256–259] The PRRs that recognize *S. schenckii* have not yet been identified; however, TLR2 and TLR4 appear to be plausible because many fungi such as *C. albicans*, *Aspergillus* spp., and *S. cerevisiae* are recognized through TLR2 and TLR4. Recognition of fungi via TLR2 and TLR4 activates several signaling molecules including JNK, ERK, p38 MAPK, and NF-κB pathways. While TLR induces release of proinflammatory cytokines such as IL-6 and TNF-α, TLR2 signals mediate antiinflammatory effect by release of IL-10 that shifts the immune responses toward the Th2 phenotype. Since IL-10 was not detected in studies involving interaction of *S. schenckii* with DCs, these studies suggested that TLR4, but not TLR2, might be the receptor to recognize *S. schenckii* of cutaneous, but not visceral, origin, which induces a strong Th1 immune response. In conclusion, *S. schenckii* of cutaneous, but not visceral, origin may be localized to the skin due to stimulation of

protective Th1- responses.[256–260] Nevertheless, the immune status of the host might be another contributing factor that accounts for the limited versus disseminated disease in cutaneous and visceral sporotrichosis, respectively.

Coccidioidomycosis

Clinical Manifestations and Pathogenesis of Cutaneous and Systemic Disease

Coccidioidomycosis (San Joaquin Valley fever) is a mycotic disease caused by *Coccidioides immitis* and the newly proposed phylogenetic species *C. posadasii*. The fungus propagates in soil in the regions of the southwestern United States, Mexico, and Central and South America, in a region corresponding to the Lower Sonoran Life Zone.[261] The saprobic phase is characterized by mycelia that give rise to infectious arthroconidia, which become aerosolized when the soil is disturbed. Humans acquire the infection by inhalation of the arthroconidia, which differentiate into large, endosporulating spherules once they are in the host. The disease presents a diverse clinical spectrum that includes inapparent infection, primary respiratory disease (usually with uncomplicated resolution), stabilized or progressive chronic pulmonary disease, and extrapulmonary dissemination involving skin, which can be acute, chronic, or progressive. The degree of severity varies considerably within each category and depends, in part, on the dose of inhaled arthroconidia, the genetic predisposition of the host, and the host's immunologic status.[261–265] Cutaneous infection with *Coccidioides* can also be acquired via a percutaneous route. Most infections occur in laboratory workers as a result of a hypodermic injection of *Coccidioides*. Primary cutaneous coccidioidomycosis is characterized by a painful suppurative lesion at the site of inoculation, often with regional lymphadenopathy. Most of the cutaneous coccidioidomycosis acquired via this route is self-limited, and most cases have remained localized.[261–265]

Immune Response Against Cutaneous and Systemic Coccidioides

Polymorphonuclear leukocytes (PMNLs) comprise the earliest cellular influx to arthroconidia. Ingestion of the arthroconidia is followed by a respiratory burst. However, fewer than 20% of the arthroconidia are killed by this mechanism, and some studies suggest that PMNL may promote the maturation of arthroconidia into endosporulating spherules. Transformation of arthroconidia into spherules renders the latter impervious to phagocytosis and killing by PMNLs.[266,267] Rupture of the spherules and release of the endospores triggers an influx of PMNLs. Ingestion of the endospores triggers an oxidative burst, and the level of intracellular killing is less effective compared to that observed in the killing of arthroconidia by PMNLs.[266] Both arthroconidia and endospores are phagocytosed by monocytes/macrophages, but less than 1% of the phagocytosed cells are killed. One mechanism that *Coccidioides* might use to survive intracellularly is the inhibition of phagosome-lysosome fusion, a strategy used by many intracellular pathogens to evade the antimicrobial effects of phagocytes. Co-incubation of monocytes/macrophages with immune T lymphocytes or IFN-γ significantly enhanced their anticoccidioidal activity.[266–268]

Natural killer (NK) cells are a major component of innate immunity against *Coccidioides*. On activation, NK cells secrete cytokines, notably IFN-γ, and chemokines that induce inflammatory responses and control the activation of monocytes and granulocytes. Before adaptive immunity has fully developed, NK cells are thought to the main source of IFN-γ, in response to macrophage-derived IL-12 and IL-18.[269] In addition, some studies suggest a direct cytotoxicity of NK cells to *Coccidioides*. Dendritic cells also play a pivotal role in innate immunity and adaptive immunity against *Coccidioides*. As described before, DCs are sentinel cells that trigger T-cell responses against several fungi. A study has shown the potential immunotherapeutic use of DCs when the anergy demonstrated by peripheral blood lymphocytes from patients with disseminated coccidioidomycosis could be reversed by the addition of DCs pulsed with coccidioidal antigen.[270] Although the study was conducted in vitro, additional studies of the restoration of immunity by DC immunotherapy in animal models could reveal a new avenue for adjunctive therapy in severe coccidioidomycosis.[275,276]

Proinflammatory and Th1 cytokines play a dominant protective role in antifungal host defense. It has been reported that heat-killed spherules and arthroconidia of *Coccidioides* induced the production of TNF-α by adherent mononuclear cells from healthy human donors. TNF-α has several biologic functions, including its ability to activate neutrophils, enhance the cytolytic activity of macrophages, augment NK-cell activity, and promote T- and B-cell proliferation. TNF-α has also been implicated as a major component in host-mediated destruction of host tissue. Similarly, IFN-γ production is associated with protection against *Coccidioides* infection and significantly lowers levels of IFN-γ, which is detected more frequently in patients with disseminated disease than in healthy, skin test–positive persons. Incubation of the monocytes with recombinant human IFN-γ or recombinant TNF-α augmented the fungicidal capabilities of the monocytes via increases in phagosome-lysosome fusion.[268–272] The mechanism by which IFN-γ or TNF-α activates human monocytes to kill *Coccidioides* is not known, but in studies with other intracellular pathogens such as those examining responses of human alveolar macrophages from tuberculosis patients, IFN-γ and TNF-α activate the macrophages to generate nitric oxide and related reactive nitrogen intermediates via nitric oxide synthase, using L-arginine as the substrate.

Different profiles of adaptive immune responses in persons with various clinical forms of coccidioidomycosis have been characterized. Persons with primary, asymptomatic, or benign disease characteristically have strong skin test reactivity to coccidioidin (the classic antigen preparation that was used in the early skin test and serologic studies), and low or nondemonstrable levels of anti-*Coccidioides* complement fixation (CF) antibody.[271–273] The converse pattern develops in patients who develop severe, chronic, or progressive pulmonary or disseminated disease. Typically, these persons, in particular those with disease involving two or more organ systems, are hyporesponsive or show anergy to coccidioidal skin testing but have high levels of anti-*Coccidioides* IgG to the CF antigen. Recovery from active disease, either spontaneous or in response to antifungal therapy, is in many patients associated with a reacquisition of T-cell reactivity to *Coccidioides* antigens and decreased CF antibody titers.[271–273]

Chronic or progressive coccidioidomycosis is associated with a polyclonal B-lymphocyte activation, as evidenced by elevated levels of IgG, IgA, and IgE in serum. Antibodies reactive with coccidioidal antigens have been demonstrable within each of these Ig classes.[274–276] Serum IgG levels directly correlate with disease involvement, being highest in patients with multifocal involvement. The serum IgA level is elevated in approximately 20% of patients, being manifested most often in patients with chronic pulmonary disease. Hyperproduction of IgE would be consistent with a Th2 response and has been demonstrated in approximately 23% of patients with active disease, with the highest incidence occurring in patients with disseminated disease and, within this group, in patients who have disease involving two or more organ systems.[272–274]

Longitudinal studies of coccidioidomycosis patients with excessive IgE levels revealed that, in most patients, IgE production diminished to normal or near-normal levels after clinical remission, suggesting that IgE hyperproduction is a consequence of the disease.[273] This interpretation is countered, however, by the report that atopic persons are at greater risk of developing symptomatic coccidioidomycosis than are persons who are nonatopic.[277] Circulating immune complexes complement products binding have been detected in sera from coccidioidomycosis patients and shown to correlate with disease severity. Whereas 33% of sera from patients with disease involving a single organ system had elevated immune complex levels, 67% of sera from patients with disseminated multifocal disease showed circulating immune complexes. The role, if any, of immune complexes in the immunopathogenesis of coccidioidomycosis is not known.

Investigators reported suppression of lymphocyte proliferation responses when lymphocytes from healthy coccidioidin skin test–positive persons were assayed in the presence of patient sera and, conversely, augmentation of the responses of patient lymphocytes when assayed in sera from healthy subjects (versus autologous serum). However, addition of immune complexes formed in vitro (by the addition of coccidioidin to a serum sample with high levels of anti-*Coccidioides* IgG) to cultured mononuclear cells from healthy, coccidioidin skin test–positive persons did not suppress their proliferation response to coccidioidin. These results, taken together, argue against suppression by immune complexes and raise the question of whether the suppression observed with

patient sera was merely attributable to the neutralization of coccidioidin in such a manner that it was not available to stimulate lymphocytes.[275–277]

Cutaneous Histoplasmosis

Clinical Manifestations and Pathogenesis of Cutaneous and Systemic Histoplasmosis

Histoplasmosis, caused by the dimorphic fungus *Histoplasma capsulatum*, is a deep mycosis endemic to regions in the Western Hemisphere, including southern Mexico and some areas of the southeastern United States. The infection is acquired by the inhalation of spores from soil contaminated by bird and bat excreta. *Histoplasma capsulatum* is an opportunistic pathogen residing in the macrophage phagolysosome. *Histoplasma* infection commonly results in mild or inapparent clinical symptoms in immune-competent individuals.[278–280] However, in immune-compromised individuals deficient in CD4+ T-cell function, failure of adequate granuloma function formation allows the fungus to disseminate systemically and can lead to a life-threatening disease. Thus, in endemic areas, histoplasmosis affects a susceptible population of patients with secondary immune defects due to HIV infection, immune suppression after transplantation, or anti–TNF-α immunotherapy

Three forms of histoplasmosis in susceptible individuals, including acute pulmonary, chronic cavitary, and disseminated histoplasmosis, have been described. In the pre-AIDS era, disseminated histoplasmosis was rare and the cutaneous manifestations were reported infrequently, mainly in patients at the extremes of age and in those with decreased cell immunity secondary to inborn errors of immunity, malignancies, and cytotoxic or steroid therapy. Whether HIV-associated disseminated histoplasmosis is a manifestation of progressive primary infection or whether it represents reactivation of old infection, is currently unknown. The cutaneous manifestations of histoplasmosis are reported to occur in 10% to 25% of AIDS patients with disseminated histoplasmosis.[281,284] Clinical manifestation of cutaneous histoplasmosis varies depending on the stage of the disease and immune status of the host. The cutaneous lesions usually have not only different morphologic appearances in different patients but also varying morphology in the same patient. The cutaneous histopatho-logic spectrum comprises necrotizing tuberculoid and nonnecrotizing granulomatous inflammation with focal organisms, diffuse dermal histiocytosis (DDH), and diffuse dermal karyorrhexis (DDK) characterized by the presence of sheets of heavily parasitized histiocytes.[281–284] Clumps of *H. capsu-latum* var. *capsulatum,* released from disintegrat-ing macrophages, are identified predominantly extracellularly in an interstitial location in DDK, while a dense infiltrate of heavily parasitized histiocytes is identified in biopsies demonstrating DDH. Exfoliative dermatitis and cutaneous vascu-litis have not been documented in AIDS patients with disseminated histoplasmosis. The lesions are usually painless unless they ulcerate. The skin lesions are widely disseminated, but they are common on the trunk, face, and upper limbs. In the majority of patients, cutaneous histoplasmosis is accompanied by disseminated histoplasmosis involving lung, bone marrow, esophagus, duode-num, and liver.[281–284]

Since the clinical lesions of histoplasmosis are nondiagnostic and the morphologic spectrum is shared by a range of infective and noninfective dis-eases that are common in AIDS patients, the gold standard of differentiating disseminated cutaneous histoplasmosis (DCH) from other processes is the identification and isolation of the infective agent in tissue sections and in fungal cultures, respec-tively.[285–289] Cutaneous histoplasmosis entails dis-ease caused by two morphologically different forms of the fungus, *H. capsulatum* var. *capsulatum and H. capsulatum* var. *duboisii. H. capsulatum* var. *duboisii* infection causes a relatively indolent form of histoplasmosis with skin, bone, and lymph node involvement, and rarely fatal disseminated disease, while *H. capsulatum* var. *capsulatum* causes wide-spread visceral (including pulmonary) involvement that is commonly fatal. However, the cutaneous clinical spectrum of *H. capsulatum* var. *capsu-latum* is similar to that caused by *H. capsulatum* var. *duboisii* infection in some features including isolated or disseminated papules, nodules, plaques, or large subcutaneous nodules. The most impor-tant distinguishing feature is the larger size of *H. capsulatum* var. *duboisii* yeasts (i.e., 8–15 μm) and their predominant location within foreign body giant cells. *H. capsulatum* var. *capsulatum,* 2–4 μm in diameter, is located predominantly

within histiocytes and less commonly in giant cells. Under special circumstances, *H. capsulatum* var. *capsulatum* is known to transform to a larger size that mimics *H. capsulatum* var. *duboisii.* Both organisms may be identified extracellularly. Round and oval configuration of the yeasts is common to both variants.[285–289]

The yeast forms of *B. dermatitidis* may resem-ble *H. capsulatum* var. *capsulatum;* however, the former forms are multinucleate and demonstrate broad-based budding, while *H. capsulatum* var. *capsulatum* is uninucleate with narrow-necked budding. Other fungal pathogens with similar mor-phology are encapsulated and nonencapsulated *C. neoformans* that stains black or dark brown with the Fontana–Masson stain, while *H. capsulatum* var. *capsulatum* is characteristically negative. Intracellular small yeast forms have also been doc-umented in sporotrichosis. *S. schenckii,* however, grows easily in cultures as dark brown colonies at 25°C within 5 days.[285–289] Furthermore, identifica-tion of *Sporothrix schenckii* within microabscesses is facilitated when a Splendore–Hoeppli phenom-enon is present. The presence of pseudohyphae, and intercellular location of the yeast cells in tissues allow the differentiation of *Candida* species that have a comparable size range to *H. capsulatum* var. *capsulatum.* Finally, *H. capsulatum* var. *capsulatum* must be distinguished from *Leishmania* species, which may be difficult on low-power examination, as both organisms share a 2- to 4-μm size range, round and oval morphology, and intracellular location. High-power examination, however, demonstrates the kinetoplast of *Leishmania* amastigotes, which on Giemsa-stained sections appears red and is not seen in *H. capsulatum* var. *capsulatum.*[289]

Immune Response Against *Histoplasma Capsulatum*

Histopathologic examination of skin biopsies from HIV patients with disseminated cutaneous histo-plasmosis demonstrated granulomatous inflamma-tion with a histiocytic palisade bordering central necrosis. Although intracellular organisms were identified focally within histiocytes and giant cells, they were not numerous as in the biopsies that lacked a granulomatous component.[290,291] The granuloma is a form of delayed-type hypersensitiv-ity. Localized inflammatory lesions composed of infected macrophages and fused giant cells can subsequently form granulomata with the help of CD4[+] T lymphocytes. CD4[+] T cells are very important for initiating and regulating granuloma function, but macrophages are the dominant cell type. The benefit of granuloma formation for the host is that it isolates the inflammation, protects the surrounding healthy tissue, controls the growth of pathogens, and prevents systemic dissemination. At the same time, the microorganism may also benefit from localization to the granuloma.

As an isolated microenvironment, granuloma presents a special environment for the pathogen in the host.[290–292] The chronic granulomatous lesion may be the reservoir from which surviving pathogens emerge to reactivate the infection after a long-term latency is broken by a compromised immune system. Thus, granulomata formed in response to macrophages infected by *Histoplasma* are most likely a dominant component of the highly effective antifungal immune response. Conversely, the progressive, disseminated histoplasmosis observed in immune-compromised persons arises in large part from failures of established granulomas and failure to form new inflammatory lesions in response to recently infected macrophages. While there is growing knowledge about the nature of systemic immunity during the course of histoplasmosis, there is little known about local immune responses within granulomas despite these lesions representing the main interaction between the fungi and the host. A recent study in mice isolated *H. capsulatum*–induced granulomas in order to determine the cellular composition and cytokine milieu of granuloma-infiltrating cells during the course of disseminated infection that involves multiple organs.[284] The average granuloma size reaches a maximum at day 10 of the infection and subsequently declines. Furthermore, this study shows that IL-10 and TGF-β were elevated in the *Histoplasma* granuloma, mainly at early stages of granuloma formation. The main source of TGF-β were macrophages. In addition to production of IL-10, the decreased granuloma size in this animal model of histoplasmosis was postulated to be due to fungal clearance leading to decreased antigenic stimuli, inflammatory agents, chemoattractants, and attenuated cellular recruitment. Although the new granuloma formation was detected after clearance of the yeast, it is not completely clear whether granulomatous

protection is completely sterilizing. However, it is possible that very low numbers of yeast survive within granuloma similar to *Mycobacterium tuberculosis* and serve as a source for reactivation during immune deficiency.

Identification of the type of cells infiltrating the granuloma indicates that macrophages are the dominant cell type in the lesion reaching up to 70% of the granuloma. The local expressions of IFN-γ and TNF-α in the lesion indicate that most of infiltrating macrophages are activated. The main cellular source of IFN-γ in the granulomas is CD4[+] and CD8[+] T cells. Interferon-γ plays a central role in the immunity against *H. capsulatum* as marked by findings that IFN-γ–deficient animals are killed by *H. capsulatum* infection.[293] Local IFN-γ activates macrophage to produce reactive radicals crucial to control of the yeast. The primary cellular source of TNF-α is the macrophage, and T cells contribute little if any to local TNF-α levels. Therapeutic anti-TNF-α treatments induced reactivation of latent *H. capsulatum* infection in some patients, emphasizing the role of this mediator in control of the yeast and preventing dissemination.[294] The H&E-stained sections suggest that most lesions have few, if any, neutrophils, and flow cytometry analysis indicates that only a low percentage of granuloma-infiltrating cells express a dendritic cell phenotype (CD11c[+]DEC205[+]).[284] The latter could be due to the fact that DCs are professional APCs that sample antigens from peripheral sites of infection, and migrate to lymph nodes where they stimulate T cells.

The presence of DCs may provide a local reactivation for the recruited effector T cells and raises the possibility that they sample granuloma Ags and may carry them to draining lymph nodes. The idea that Ags in granulomas contained might prime systemic T cells needs further investigation. Both effector CD25[low] CD4[+] and CD8[+] T cells are recruited to the lesions. At early stages, there was more CD4[+] T cells present, but later the ratio was close to 1:1. This temporal change in the CD4/CD8 T-cell ratio likely reflects the somewhat earlier systemic activation of CD4[+] T cells relative to activation of CD8[+] T cells. Interestingly, in HIV patients with disseminated cutaneous histoplasmosis, a predominant infiltration of CD8[+] T cells was detected in biopsy samples from skin lesions.[284] Both T cells contribute to the cytokine milieu of the granulomas.

In contrast to high infiltration with CD4+CD25^{low} T cells, CD25^{high}CD4$^+$ T cells, thought to be regulatory T cells, are present at much lower levels in the granuloma relative to both infected spleen and naive spleen, suggesting an exclusion of those cells from the local inflammatory site. Thus, the role of regulatory T cells in *Histoplasma*-induced granuloma formation warrants more investigation since these cells are reported to regulate *Leishmania*- and *Schistosoma*-induced lesions.

However, due to the limitation of regulatory T-cell classification based on CD25 expression alone, additional phenotypic and functional characterization will be needed in further studies of regulatory T cells in *Histoplasma* infection. The level of γδ T cells was also lower in granulomas compared with systemic sites; γδ T cells have been reported in granulomas affecting granuloma size during the chronic stage of infection. A low level of B cells was also present having a conventional B cell phenotype (CD5$^-$, Mac-1$^-$) characteristic of peripheral blood.[284] The local Ab production in the granuloma could be potentially important since there are reports that Abs can protect against intracellular yeasts. Taken altogether, local granuloma responses in histoplasmosis at infection site(s) are similar to systemic responses represented by the spleen where responses against *Histoplasma* infection are dominated by CD4$^+$ Th1 cell responses and require IFN-γ and TNF-α for activation of macrophages.

Conclusion

Due to the increased populations of immunocompromised patients, the clinical relevance of fungal infections has risen in the last three decades. Fungal diseases are classed according to the site of the primary infection: superficial, cutaneous, subcutaneous, and deep or systemic. Dimorphic fungi assume both yeast and hyphal states based on environmental conditions and the hosts' immune response. Certain fungi can synthesize capsular components, which can affect host immune responses. The innate response to fungi serves both a direct antifungal effector activity and an activation and induction of the specific adaptive immune responses. Understanding the immune response to fungal infections has led to better diagnostic tests and therapeutic interventions for fungal diseases. In the future, it is hoped that this knowledge will lead to vaccines for their prevention.

References

1. Wang Z, et al. WdChs4p, a homolog of chitin synthase 3 in Saccharomyces cerevisiae, alone cannot support growth of Wangiella (Exophiala) dermatitidis at the temperature of infection. Infect Immun 1999;67:6619–30.

1a. Kozel TR, et al. Biological activities of naturally occurring antibodies reactive with *Candida albicans* mannan. Infect Immun 2004;72:209–18.

2. Gardiner DM, Howlett BJ. Bioinformatic and expression analysis of the putative gliotoxin biosynthetic gene cluster of *Aspergillus fumigatus*. FEMS Microbiol Lett 2005;248:241–248.

3. Hagens WI, et al. Gliotoxin non-selectively induces apoptosis in fibrotic and normal livers. Liver Int 2006;26:232–239.

4. Johannessen LN, Nilsen AM, Lovik M. The mycotoxins citrinin and gliotoxin differentially affect production of the pro-inflammatory cytokines tumour necrosis factor-alpha and interleukin-6, and the anti-inflammatory cytokine interleukin-10. Clin Exp Allergy 2005;35:782–789.

5. Niide O, et al. Fungal metabolite gliotoxin blocks mast cell activation by a calcium- and superoxide-dependent mechanism: implications for immunosuppressive activities. Clin Immunol 2006;118:108–116.

6. Janeway CA Jr, Medzhitov R. Innate immune recognition. Annu Rev Immunol 2002;20: 197–206.

7. Romani L. In: Calderone RA, Cihlar LR, eds. Innate Immunity Against Fungal Pathogens: Principles and Clinical Applications. New York: Marcel Dekker, 2002:401–432.

8. Akira S. Mammalian Toll-like receptors. Curr Opin Immunol 2003;15:5–11.

9. O'Neill LA, Fitzgerald KA, Bowie AG. The Toll-IL-1 receptor adaptor family grows to five members. Trends Immunol 2003;24:286–290.

10. Gantner BN, et al. Collaborative induction of inflammatory responses by Dectin-1 and Toll-like receptor 2. J Exp Med 2000;197:1107–1117.

11. Brown GD, et al. Dectin-1 mediates the biological effects of β-glucans. J Exp Med 2003;197:1119–1124.

12. Netea MG, et al. Immune sensing of *Candida albicans* requires cooperative recognition of mannans and glucans by lectin and Toll-like receptors. J Clin Invest 2006;116:1642–50.

13. Sato K, et al. Dectin-2 is a pattern recognition receptor for fungi that couples with the Fc receptor gamma

chain to induce innate immune responses. J Biol Chem 2006;281:38854–66.

14. Jimenez MP, et al. Importance of complement 3 and mannose receptors in phagocytosis of *Paracoccidioides brasiliensis* conidia by Nramp1 congenic macrophages lines. FEMS Immunol Med Microbiol 2006;47:56–66.

15. Lavigne LM, Albina JE, Reichner JS. Beta-glucan is a fungal determinant for adhesion-dependent human neutrophil functions. J Immunol 2006;177:8667–75.

16. Tada H, et al. *Saccharomyces cerevisiae*- and *Candida albicans*-derived mannan induced production of tumor necrosis factor by human monocytes in a CD14– and Toll-like receptor 4–dependent manner. Microbiol Immunol 2002;46:503–512.

17. Jouault T, et al. *Candida albicans* phospholipomannan is sensed through toll-like receptors. J Infect Dis 2003;188:165–172.

18. Marr KA, et al. Differential role of MyD88 in macrophage-mediated responses to opportunistic fungal pathogens. Infect Immun 2003;71:5280–5286.

19. Tauszig-Delamasure S, et al. L. *Drosophila* MyD88 is required for the response to fungal and Gram-positive bacterial infections. Nature Immunol 2002;3:91–97.

20. Marr KA, et al. Differential role of MyD88 in macrophage-mediated responses to opportunistic fungal pathogens. Infect Immun 2003;71:5280–5286.

21. Wang JE, et al. Involvement of CD14 and Toll-like receptors in activation of human monocytes by *Aspergillus fumigatus* hyphae. Infect Immun 2001;69: 2402–2406.

22. Tada H, et al. *Saccharomyces cerevisiae*- and *Candida albicans*-derived mannan induced production of tumor necrosis factor-α by human monocytes in a CD14– and Toll-like receptor 4–dependent manner. Microbiol Immunol 2002;46:503–512.

23. Netea MG, et al. The role of toll-like receptor (TLR) 2 and TLR4 in the host defense against disseminated candidiasis. J Infect Dis 2002;185:1483–1489.

24. Van der Graaf CA, et al. Differential cytokine production and Toll-like receptor signaling pathways by *Candida albicans* blastoconidia and hyphae. Infect Immun 2005;73:7458–64.

25. Villamon E, et al. Toll-like receptor-2 is essential in murine defenses against *Candida albicans* infections. Microbes Infect 2004;6:1–7.

26. Gil ML, Gozalbo D. The role of TLR2 and TLR4 in cytokine secretion by murine macrophages in response to *Candida albicans*. FEMS Immunol Med Microbiol 2006;46:1–2.

27. Sutmuller RP, et al. Toll-like receptor 2 controls expansion and function of regulatory T cells. J Clin Invest 2006;116:485–94.

28. Goodridge HS, Simmons RM, Underhill DM. Dectin-1 stimulation by *Candida albicans* yeast or zymosan triggers NFAT activation in macrophages and dendritic cells. J Immunol 2007;178:3107–15.

29. Netea MG, Sutmuller R, Hermann C, et al. Toll-like receptor 2 suppresses immunity against Candida albicans through induction of IL-10 and regulatory T cells. J Immunol 2004;172:3712–8.

30. Willment JA, Gordon S, Brown GD. Characterization of the human β-glucan receptor and its alternatively spliced isoforms. J Biol Chem 2001;276:43818–43823.

31. Brown GD, Gordon S. Immune recognition: a new receptor for β-glucans. Nature 2001;413:36–37.

32. Cooper DN, et al. Fungal galectins, sequence and specificity of two isolectins from Coprinus cinereus. J Biol Chem 1997;272:1514–1521.

33. Kohatsu L, Hsu DK, Jegalian AG, Liu FT, Baum LG. Galectin-3 induces death of *Candida* species expressing specific beta-1, 2-linked mannans. J Immunol 2006;177:4718–26.

34. Long KH, Gomez FJ, Morris RE, Newman SL. Identification of heat shock protein 60 as the ligand on *Histoplasma capsulatum* that mediates binding to CD18 receptors on human macrophages. J Immunol 2003;170:487–494.

35. Glidea LA, et al. *Histoplasma capsulatum* yeasts are phagocytosed via very late antigen-5, killed, and processed for antigen presentation by human dendritic cells. J Immunol 2001;166:1049–1056.

36. Huffnagle GB, Deepe GS. Innate and adaptive determinants of host susceptibility to medically important fungi. Curr Opin Microbiol 2003;6:344–350.

37. Romani L, et al. Neutrophil production of IL-12 and IL-10 in candidiasis and efficacy of IL-12 therapy in neutropenic mice. J Immunol 1997;158:5349–5356.

38. Rolston KV. Management of infections in the neutropenic patient. Annu Rev Med 2004;55:519–526.

39. Mencacci A, et al. CD80+ Gr-1+ myeloid cells inhibit development of antifungal T_H1 immunity in mice with candidiasis. J Immunol 2002;169:3180–3190.

40. Mansour MK, Levitz SM. Interactions of fungi with phagocytes. Curr Opin Microbiol 2002;5:359–365.

41. Hamilton AJ, Holdon MD. Antioxidant systems in the pathogenic fungi of man and their role in virulence. Med Mycol 1999;37:375–389.

42. Heyworth PG, Cross AR, Curnutten JT. Chronic granulomatous disease. Curr Opin Immunol 2003;15:578–584.

43. Herring AC, Huffnagle GB. In: Kaufmann SHE, Sher A, Ahmed R, eds. Innate immunity to fungi. Immunology of Infectious Diseases. Washington, DC: ASM Press, 2001:127–137.

44. Arancia G, et al. Interaction between human interleukin-2–activated natural killer cells and heat-killed germ tube forms of *Candida albicans*. Cell Immunol 1998;186:28–38.

45. Tran P, Ahmad R, Xu J, Ahmad A, Menezes J. Host's immune response to fungal and bacterial agents in vitro: up-regulation of interleukin-15 gene expression resulting in enhanced natural killer cell activity. Immunology 2003;109:263–270.

46. Algarra I, Ortega E, Serrano MJ, Alvarez de Cienfuegos G, Gaforio JJ. Suppression of splenic macrophage *Candida albicans* phagocytosis following in vivo depletion of natural killer cells in immunocompetent BALB/c mice and T-cell-deficient nude mice. FEMS Immunol Med Microbiol 2002;33: 159–63.

47. Uezu K, et al. Accumulation of gammadelta T cells in the lungs and their regulatory roles in Th1 response and host defense against pulmonary infection with *Cryptococcus neoformans*. J Immunol 2004;172:7629–34.

48. Claudia M, et al. The interaction of fungi with dendritic cells: implications for TH immunity and vaccination. Curr Mol Med 2002;2:507–524.

49. Huang Q, et al. The plasticity of dendritic cell responses to pathogens and their components. Science 2001;294:870–875.

50. Sotto MN, et al. Antigen distribution and antigen-presenting cells in skin biopsies of human chromoblastomycosis. J Cutan Pathol 2004;31:14–8.

51. Sotto MN, De Brito T, Ana Maria G, Martins LG. Antigen distribution and antigen-presenting cells in skin biopsies of human chromoblastomycosis. J Cutan Pathol 2002;31:14–18.

52. Romani L, Bistoni F, Puccetti P. Fungi, dendritic cells and receptors: a host perspective of fungal virulence. Trends Microbiol 2002;10:508–514.

53. Romani L, Puccetti P, Bistoni F. Interleukin-12 in infectious diseases. Clin Microbiol Rev 1997;10: 611–636.

54. Cumberbatch M, Kimber I. Dermal tumour necrosis factor-α induces dendritic cell migration to draining lymph nodes, and possibly provides one stimulus for Langerhans cell migration. Immunology 1992;75:257–63.

55. Jakob T, Udey MC. Regulation of E-cadherin-mediated adhesion in Langerhans cell-like dendritic cells by inflammatory mediators that mobilize Langerhans cells in vivo. J Immunol 1998;160: 4067–73.

56. Sallusto F, Schaerli P, Loetscher P, Schanie C, Lenig D, Mackay CR. Rapid and coordinated switch in chemokine receptor expression during dendritic cell maturation. Eur J Immunol 1998;28:2760–9.

57. Lin CL, Suri RM, Rahdon RA, Austyn JM, Roake J. A. Dendritic cell chemotaxis and transendothelial migration are induced by distinct chemokines and are regulated on maturation. Eur J Immunol 1998;28:4114–22.

58. Yanagihara S, Komura E, Nagafune J, Watarai H, Yamaguchi Y. EBI1/ CCR7 is a new member of dendritic cell chemokine receptor that is upregulated upon maturation. J Immunol 1998;161:3096–102.

59. Saeki H, Moore AM, Brown MJ, Hwang ST. Secondary lymphoid-tissue chemokine (SLC) and CC chemokine receptor 7 (CCR7) participate in the emigration pathway of mature dendritic cells from the skin to regional lymph nodes. J Immunol 1999;162:2472–5.

60. Gunn MD, et al. Chemokine expressed in lymphoid high endothelial venules promotes the adhesion and chemotaxis of naive T lymphocytes. Proc Natl Acad Sci USA 1998;95:258–63.

61. Gunn MD, et al. Mice lacking expression of secondary lymphoid organ chemokine have defects in lymphocyte homing and dendritic cell localization. J Exp Med 1999;189:451–60.

62. Bellocchio S, et al. The contribution of the Toll-like receptor superfamily to innate and adaptive immunity to fungal pathogens in vivo. J Immunol 2006;76:2345–8.

63. d'Ostiani CF, et al. Dendritic cells discriminate between yeasts and hyphae of the fungus *Candida albicans*. Implications for initiation of T helper cell immunity in vitro and in vivo. J Exp Med 2000;191:1661–1674.

64. Romani L. Immunity to fungal infections. Nat Rev Immunol 2004;4:1–23.

65. Kozel TR. Activation of the complement system by pathogenic fungi. Clin Microbiol Rev 1996;9: 34–46.

66. Taborda CP, Casadevall A. CR3 (CD11/CD18) and CR4 (CD11c/CD18) are involved in complement-independent antibody-mediated phagocytosis of *Cryptococcus neoformans*. Immunity 2002;16:791–802.

67. Casadevall A, Feldmesser M, Pirofski LA. Induced humoral immunity and vaccination against major human fungal pathogens. Curr Opin Microbiol 2002;5:386–391.

68. Magee DM, Cox RA. In: Calderone RA, Cihlar LR, eds. Fungal Pathogenesis: Principles and Clinical Applications. New York: Marcel Dekker, 2002: 279–292

69. Netea MG, Stuyt RJ, Kim SH, Van der Meer JW, Kullberg BJ, Dinarello CA. The role of endogenous interleukin (IL)-18, IL-12, IL-1 β, and tumor necrosis factor- in the production of interferon-v induced by *Candida albicans* in human whole-blood cultures. J Infect Dis 2002;185:963–970.

70. Romani L, Mencacci A, Cenci E, et al. Neutrophil production of IL-12 and IL-10 in candidiasis and efficacy of IL-12 therapy in neutropenic mice. J Immunol 1997;158:5349–5356.

71. Gildea LA, Morris RE, Newman SL. *Histoplasma capsulatum* yeasts are phagocytosed via very late antigen-5, killed, and processed for antigen presentation by human dendritic cells. J Immunol 2001;166:1049–1056.

72. Lijin L, Dial SM, Rennels MA, Ampel NM. Cellular immune suppressor activity resides in lymphocyte cell clusters adjacent to granulomata in human coccidiodomycosis. Infect Immun 2005;73:3923–3928.

73. Pilar-Jimenez M, Walls L, Fierer J. High levels of interleukin-10 impair resistance to pulmonary coccidioidomycosis in mice in part through control of nitric oxide synthase 2 expression. Infect Immun 2006;74:3387–3395.

74. Romano CC, et al. The role of interleukin-10 in the differential expression of interleukin-12p70 and its beta2 receptor on patients with active or treated paracoccidioidomycosis and healthy infected subjects. Clin Immunol 2005;114:86–94.

75. Pagliari C, Sotto MN. Dendritic cells and pattern of cytokines in paracoccidioidomycosis skin lesions. Am J Dermatopathol 2003;25:107–12.

76. Fierer J, Waters C, Walls L. Both CD4+ and CD8+ T cells can mediate vaccine-induced protection against *Coccidioides immitis* infection in mice. J Infect Dis 2006;193:1323–31.

77. Stanzani M, et al. *Aspergillus fumigatus* suppresses the human cellular immune response via gliotoxin-mediated apoptosis of monocytes. Blood 2005;105:2258–65.

78. Lin JS, et al. Dendritic cells cross-present exogenous fungal antigens to stimulate a protective CD8 T cell response in infection by *Histoplasma capsulatum*. J Immunol 2005;174:6282–91.

79. Wuthrich M, et al. Vaccine immunity to pathogenic fungi overcomes the requirement for CD4 help in exogenous antigen presentation to CD8+ T cells: implications for vaccine development in immunedeficient hosts. J Exp Med 2003;197:1405–16.

80. Schnizlein-Bick C, et al. Effects of CD4 and CD8 T lymphocyte depletion on the course of histoplasmosis following pulmonary challenge. Med Mycol 2003;41:189–97.

81. Netea MG, Van der Meer JW, Kullberg BJ. Role of the dual interaction of fungal pathogens with pattern recognition receptors in the activation and modulation of host defence. Clin Microbiol Infect 2006;5:404–9.

82. Brouard J, et al. Influence of interleukin-10 on *Aspergillus fumigatus* infection in patients with cystic fibrosis. J Infect Dis 2005;191:1988–91.

83. Willment JA, et al. Dectin-1 expression and function are enhanced on alternatively activated and GM-CSF-treated macrophages and are negatively regulated by IL-10, dexamethasone, and lipopolysaccharide. J Immunol 2003;171:4569–73.

84. Roilides E, et al. Suppressive effects of interleukin-10 on human mononuclear phagocyte function against *Candida albicans* and *Staphylococcus aureus*. J Infect Dis 1998;178:1734–42.

85. Pagliari C, Fernandes ER, Guedes F, Alves C, Sotto M N. Role of mast cells as IL10 producing cells in paracoccidioidomycosis skin lesions. Mycopathologia 2006;162:331–5.

86. Romano CC, Mendes-Giannini MJ, Duarte AJ, Benard G. IL-12 and neutralization of endogenous IL-10 revert the in vitro antigen-specific cellular immunosuppression of paracoccidioidomycosis patients. Cytokine 2002;18:149–57.

87. McGuirk P, Mills KH. Pathogen-specific regulatory T cells provoke a shift in the Th1/Th2 paradigm in immunity to infectious diseases. Trends Immunol 2002;23:450–5

88. Montagnoli C, et al. B7/CD28–dependent CD4+CD25+ regulatory T cells are essential components of the memory-protective immunity to *Candida albicans*. J Immunol 2002;169:6298–308.

89. Blaser K, Akdis CA. Interleukin-10, T regulatory cells and specific allergy treatment. Clin Exp Allergy 2004;34:328–31.

90. Weiss E, et al. The role of interleukin 10 in the pathogenesis and potential treatment of skin diseases. J Am Acad Dermatol 2004;50:657–75.

91. Pearsall NN, Adams BL, Bunni R. Immunologic responses to *Candida albicans*. III. Effects of passive transfer of lymphoid cells or serum on murine candidiasis. J Immunol 1978;120:1176–1180.

92. Casadevall A. Antibody immunity and invasive fungal infections. Infect Immun 1995;63:4211–4218.

93. Cutler JE. Defining criteria for anti-mannan antibodies to protect against candidiasis. Curr Mol Med 2005;5:383–392.

94. Taborda CP, Rivera J, Zaragoza O, Casadevall A. More is not necessarily better: prozone-like effects in passive immunization with IgG. J Immunol 2003;170:3621–3631.

95. Nosanchuk JD, et al. Antibodies to a cell surface histone-like protein protect against *Histoplasma capsulatum*. J Clin Invest 2003;112:1164–1175.

96. Torosantucci A, et al. A novel glyco-conjugate vaccine against fungal pathogens. J Exp Med 2005;202:597–606.

97. Grappel SF, Calderone RA. Effect of antibodies on the respiration and morphology of *Candida albicans*. S Afr Med J 1976;14:51–60.

98. Casanova M, Martinez JP, Chaffin WL. Fab fragments from a monoclonal antibody against a germ tube mannoprotein block the yeast-to-mycelium

transition in *Candida albicans*. Infect Immun 1990;58:3810–3812.

99. Moragues MD, et al. A monoclonal antibody directed against a *Candida albicans* cell wall mannoprotein exerts three anti- *C. albicans* activities. Infect Immun 2003;71:5273–5279.

100. Pirofski LA, Casadevall A. Use of licensed vaccines for active immunization of the immunocompromised host. Clin Microbiol Rev 1998;11:1–26.

101. Han Y, et al. Complement is essential for protection by an IgM and an IgG3 monoclonal antibody against experimental hematogenously disseminated candidiasis. J Immunol 2001;167:1550–1557.

102. Magliani W, et al. Therapeutic potentials of antiidiotypic single chain antibodies with yeast killer toxin activity. Nature Biotech 1997;15:155–158.

103. Moragues MD, et al. A monoclonal antibody directed against a *Candida albicans* cell wall mannoprotein exerts three anti-C. albicans activities. Infect Immun 2003;71:5273–5279.

104. Eggimann P, Garbino J, Pittet D. Epidemiology of *Candida* species infections in critically ill non-immunosuppressed patients. Lancet Infect Dis 2003;3:685702.

105. Hajjeh RA, et al. Incidence of bloodstream infections due to *Candida* species and in vitro susceptibilities of isolates collected from 1998 to 2000 in a population-based active surveillance program. J Clin Microbiol 2004;42:151927.

106. Pfaller MA, Diekema DJ. Twelve years of fluconazole in clinical practice: global trends in species distribution and fluconazole susceptibility of bloodstream isolates of *Candida*. Clin Microbiol Infect 2004;10:1123.

107. Kirkpatrick CH. Chronic mucocutaneous candidiasis. Pediatr Infect Dis J 2001;20:197–206.

108. Rowen JL. Mucocutaneous candidiasis. Semin Perinatol 2003;5:406–13.

109. Lilic D. New perspectives on the immunology of chronic mucocutaneous candidiasis. Curr Opin Infect Dis 2002;2:143–7.

110. Lilic D. New perspectives on the immunology of CMC. Curr Opin Infect Dis 2002;15:143–147.

111. Bodey GP. Candidiasis. Pathogenesis, Diagnosis and Treatment, 2nd ed. New York: Raven Press, 1993.

112. Krutzik SR, Sieling PA, Modlin RL. The role of Toll-like receptors in host defense against microbial infection. Curr Opin Immunol 2001;13:104–108.

113. Lilic D, Cant AJ, Abinun M, Calvert JE, Spickett GP. Chronic mucocutaneous candidiasis. I. Altered-antigen stimulated IL-2, IL-4, IL-6 and IFN-γ production. Clin Exp Immunol 1996;105:205–212.

114. Lilic D, Calvert JE, Cant AJ, Abinun M, Spickett GP. Chronic mucocutaneous candidiasis. II. Class

and subclass of specific antibody responses in vivo and in vitro. Clin Exp Immunol 1996;105:213–219.

115. Medzhitov R, Janeway C. Innate immunity. N Engl J Med 2000;343:338–344.

116. Underhill DM, et al. The Toll-like receptor 2 is recruited to the macrophage phagosomes and discriminates between pathogens. Nature 1999;401:811–815.

117. Roeder A, et al. Toll-like receptors as key mediators in innate antifungal immunity. Med Mycol 2004;42:485–98.

118. Gantner BN, Simmons RM, Underhill DM. Dectin-1 mediates macrophage recognition of *Candida albicans* yeast but not filaments. EMBO J 2005;24:1277–86.

119. Lewandowski D, et al. Altered CD4+ T cell phenotype and function determine the susceptibility to mucosal candidiasis in transgenic mice expressing HIV-1. J Immunol 2006;177:479–91.

120. Cenci E, et al. IFN-gamma is required for IL-12 responsiveness in mice with *Candida albicans* infection. J Immunol 1998;161:3543–50.

121. Lilic D, et al. Deregulated production of protective cytokines in response to *Candida albicans* infection in patients with chronic mucocutaneous candidiasis. Infect Immun 2003;71:5690–9.

122. Bacci A, et al. Dendritic cells pulsed with fungal RNA induce protective immunity to *Candida albicans* in hematopoietic transplantation. J Immunol 2002;168:2904–13.

123. Schaller M, et al. The secreted aspartyl proteinases Sap1 and Sap2 cause tissue damage in an in vitro model of vaginal candidiasis based on reconstituted human vaginal epithelium. Infect Immun 2003;71:3227–34.

124. Van der Graaf CA, et al. Differential cytokine production and Toll-like receptor signaling pathways by *Candida albicans* blastoconidia and hyphae. Infect Immun 2005;73:7458–64.

125. Kvaal CA, Srikantha T, Soll DR. Misexpression of the white-phase-specific gene WH11 in the opaque phase of *Candida albicans* affects switching and virulence. Infect Immun 1997;65:4468–75.

126. Geiger J, Wessels D, Lockhart SR, Soll DR. Release of a potent polymorphonuclear leukocyte chemoattractant is regulated by white-opaque switching in *Candida albicans*. Infect Immun 2004;72:667–77.

127. Seebacher R. The change of dermatophyte spectrum in dermatomycoses. Mycoses 2003;46:42–46.

128. Woodfolk JA. Allergy and dermatophytes. Clin Microbiol Rev 2005;18:30–43.

129. Shimada A, Charlton B, Rohane P, Taylor-Edwards C, Fathman CG. Immune regulation in type 1 diabetes. J Autoimmun 1996;9:263–269.

130. Wagner DK, Sohnle PG. Cutaneous defenses against dermatophytes and yeasts. Clin Microbiol Rev 1995;8:317–35.

131. Weitzman I, Summerbell RC. The dermatophytes. Clin Microbiol Rev 1995;8:240–59.

132. Summerbell RC. Epidemiology and ecology of onychomycosis. Dermatology 1997;194:32–36

133. Meymandi S, Silver SG, Crawford RI. Intraepidermal neutrophils—a clue to dermatophytosis? J Cutan Pathol 2003;30:253–5.

134. Calderon RA, Hay RJ. Fungicidal activity of human neutrophils and monocytes on dermatophyte fungi, *Trichophyton quinckeanum* and *Trichophyton rubrum*. Immunology 1987;61:289–95.

135. Tan BH, et al. Macrophages acquire neutrophil granules for antimicrobial activity against intracellular pathogens. J Immunol 2006;177:1864–71.

136. Duek L, Kaufman G, Ulman Y, Berdicevsky I. The pathogenesis of dermatophyte infections in human skin sections. J Infect 2004;48:175–180.

137. Woodfolk JA, et al. Definition of a *Trichophyton* protein associated with delayed hypersensitivity in humans: evidence for immediate (IgE and IgG4) and delayed type hypersensitivity to a single protein. J Immunol 1996;156:1695–1701.

138. Woodfolk JA, Sung SJ, Benjamin DC, Lee JK, Platts-Mills TAE. Distinct human T cell repertoires mediate immediate and delayed-type hypersensitivity to the *Trichophyton* antigen, Tri r 2. J Immunol 2000;165:4379–4387

139. Woodfolk JA, Platts-Mills TAE. Diversity of the human allergen-specific T cell repertoire associated with distinct skin test reactions: delayed-type hypersensitivity-associated major epitopes induce Th1– and Th2–dominated responses. J Immunol 2001;167:5412–5419.

140. Leibovici V, et al. Imbalance of immune responses in patients with chronic and widespread fungal skin infection. Clin Exp Dermatol. 1995;20:390–4.

141. Faergemann J. Atopic dermatitis and fungi. Clin Microbiol Rev 2002;15:545–63.

142. Dahl MV, Grando SA. Chronic dermatophytosis: what is special about *Trichophyton rubrum*? Adv Dermatol 1994;9:97–109.

143. Hay RJ, Shennan G. Chronic dermatophyte infections. II. Antibody and cell-mediated immune responses. Br J Dermatol 1982;106:191–198.

144. Gao J, Takashima A. Cloning and characterization of *Trichophyton rubrum* genes encoding actin, Tri r2, and Tri r4. J Clin Microbiol 2004;42:3298–9.

145. Deuell B, Arruda LK, Hayden ML, Chapman MD, Platts-Mills TAE. *Trichophyton tonsurans* allergen I: characterization of a protein that causes immediate but not delayed hypersensitivity. J Immunol 1991;147:96–99

146. Woodfolk JA, et al. *Trichophyton* antigens associated with IgE antibodies and delayed type hypersensitivity: sequence homology to two families of serine proteinases. J Biol Chem 1998;273: 2948–2952.

147. De Luca C, et al. Lipoperoxidase activity of Pityrosporum:characterisation of by-products and possible role in pityriasis versicolor. Exp Dermatol 1996;5:49–56.

148. Schwartz RA. Superficial fungal infections. Lancet 2004;364:1173–82.

149. Crespo-Erchiga V, Florencio VD. *Malassezia* yeasts and pityriasis versicolor. Curr Opin Infect Dis 2006;19:139–47.

150. Faergemann J. Treatment of seborrhoeic dermatitis with oral terbinafine? Lancet 2001;358:170–174.

151. Mickelsen PA, Viano-Paulson MC, Stevens DA, Diaz PS. Clinical and microbiological features of infection with *Malassezia pachydermatis* in high-risk infants. J Infect Dis 1988;157:1163–8.

152. Pierard GE, et al. A pilot study on seborrheic dermatitis using pramiconazole as a potent oral anti-Malassezia agent. Dermatology 2007;214:162–9.

153. Aytimur D, Sengoz V. *Malassezia* folliculitis on the scalp of a 12–year-old healthy child. J Dermatol 2004;31:936–8.

154. Ljubojevic S, Skerlev M, Lipozencic J, Basta-Juzbasic A. The role of *Malassezia furfur* in dermatology. Clin Dermatol 2002;20:179–82.

155. Gupta AK, Batra R, Bluhm R, Boekhout T, Dawson TL Jr. Skin diseases associated with *Malassezia* species. J Am Acad Dermatol 2004;51:785–98.

156. Schmid-Grendelmeier P, Scheynius A, Crameri R. The role of sensitization to *Malassezia sympodialis* in atopic eczema. Chem Immunol Allergy 2006;91:98–109.

157. Bayrou O, Pecquet C, Flahault A, Artigou C, Abuaf N, Leynadier F. Head and neck atopic dermatitis and *Malassezia furfur*-specific IgE antibodies. Dermatology 2005;211:107–13.

158. Johansson C, Tengvall Linder M, Aalberse RC, Scheynius A. Elevated levels of IgG and IgG4 to *Malassezia* allergens in atopic eczema patients with IgE reactivity to Malassezia. Int Arch Allergy Immunol 2004;135:93–100.

159. Ashbee HR, Evans EGV. Immunology of diseases associated with *Malassezia* species. Clin Microbiol Rev 2002;15:21–57.

160. Belew PW, Rosenberg EW, Jennings BR. Activation of the alternative pathway of complement by *Malassezia ovalis (Pityrosporum ovale)*. Mycopathologia 1980;70:187–191.

161. Sohnle PG, Collins-Lech C. Activation of complement by *Pityrosporum orbiculare*. J Invest Dermatol 1983;80:93–97.

162. Suzuki T, Ohno N, Ohshima Y. Activation of complement system, alternative and classical pathways, by *Malassezia furfur*. Pharm Pharmacol Lett 1998;45:388–393.

163. Richardson MD, Shankland GS. Enhanced phagocytosis and intracellular killing of *Pityrosporum ovale* by human neutrophils after exposure to ketoconazole is correlated to changes of the yeast cell surface. Mycoses 1991;34:29–33.

164. Murphy JW. Mechanisms of natural resistance to pathogenic fungi. Annu Rev Microbiol 1991;45:509–538.

165. Suzuki T, Ohno N, Ohshima Y, Yadomae T. Soluble mannan and beta-glucan inhibit the uptake of *Malassezia furfur* by human monocytic cell line, THP-1. FEMS Immunol Med Microbiol 1998;21:223–230.

166. Suzuki T, et al. Enhancement of IL-8 production from human monocytic and granulocytic cell lines, THP-1 and HL-60, stimulated with *Malassezia furfur*. FEMS Immunol Med Microbiol 2000;28:157–162.

167. Austyn JM, Wood KJ, ed. Principles of Cellular and Molecular Immunology. Oxford, UK: Oxford University Press, 1993.

168. Walters CE, et al. In vitro modulation of keratinocyte-derived interleukin 1α (IL-1α) and peripheral blood mononuclear cell-derived IL-1β release in response to cutaneous commensal micro-organisms. Infect Immun 1995;63:1223–1228.

169. Kesavan S, Walters CE, Holland KT, Ingham E. The effects of *Malassezia* on pro-inflammatory cytokine production by human peripheral blood mononuclear cells in vitro. Med Mycol 1998;36:97–106

170. Pierard-Franchimont C, Pierard GE, Arrese JE, De Doncker P. Effect of ketoconazole 1% and 2% shampoos on severe dandruff and seborrhoeic dermatitis: clinical, squamometric and mycological assessments. Dermatology 2001;202:171–6.

171. Brasch J, Martens H, Sterry W. Langerhans cell accumulation in chronic tinea pedis and pityriasis versicolor. Clin Exp Dermatol 1993;18:329–332.

172. Kesavan S, Holland KT, Ingham E. The effect of lipid extraction on the immunomodulatory activity of Malassezia species in vitro. Med Mycol 2000;38:239–247.

173. Buentke E, D'Amato M, Scheynius A. *Malassezia* enhances natural killer cell-induced dendritic cell maturation. Scand J Immunol 2004;59:511–6.

174. Buentke E, Scheynius A. Dendritic cells and fungi. APMIS 2003;111:789–96.

175. Lechmann M, et al. CD83 on dendritic cells:more than just a marker for maturation. Trends Immunol 2002;23:273–5.

176. Banchereau J, et al. Immunobiology of dendritic cells. Annu Rev Immunol 2000;18:767–811.

177. De Jong EC, et al. Microbial compounds selectively induce Th1 cell-promoting or Th2 cell-promoting dendritic cells in vitro with diverse the cell-polarizing signals. J Immunol 2002;168:1704–9.

178. Weiner HL. Induction and mechanism of action of transforming growth factor-beta-secreting Th3 regulatory cells. Immunol Rev 2001;182:207–14.

179. Buentke E, et al. Natural killer and dendritic cell contact in lesional atopic dermatitis skin – *Malassezia*-influenced cell interaction. J Invest Dermatol 2002;119:850–7.

180. Gerosa F, Baldani-Guerra B, Nisii C, Marchesini V, Carra G, Trinchieri G. Reciprocal activating interaction between natural killer cells and dendritic cells. J Exp Med 2002;195:327–33.

181. Ferlazzo G, Tsang ML, Moretta L, Melioli G, Steinman RM, Munz C. Human dendritic cells activate resting natural killer (NK) cells and are recognized via the NKp30. J Exp Med 2002;195:343–51.

182. Scheynius A, Johansson C, Buentke E, Zargari A, Tengvall-Linder M. Atopic eczema/dermatitis syndrome and *Malassezia*. Int Arch Allergy Immunol 2002;127:161–9.

183. Gabrielsson S, Buentke E, Lieden A, et al. *Malassezia sympodialis* stimulation differently affects gene expression in dendritic cells from atopic dermatitis patients and healthy individuals. Acta Dermatol Venereol 2004;45:367–370.

184. Kanda N, Tani K, Enomoto U, Nakai K, Watanabe S. The skin fungus-induced Th1– and Th2–related cytokine, chemokine and prostaglandin E2 production in peripheral blood mononuclear cells from patients with atopic dermatitis and psoriasis vulgaris. Clin Exp Allergy 2002;32:1243–50.

185. Johansson C, Eshaghi H, Linder MT, Jakobson E, Scheynius A. Positive atopy patch test reaction to *Malassezia furfur* in atopic dermatitis correlates with a T helper 2–like peripheral blood mononuclear cells response. J Invest Dermatol 2002;118:1044–51.

186. Allam JP, Bieber T. A review of recent journal highlights focusing on atopic dermatitis. Clin Exp Dermatol 2003;28:577–8.

187. Sohnle PG, Collins-Lech C, Huhta KE. Class specific antibodies in young and aged humans against organisms producing superficial fungal infections. Br J Dermatol 1983;108:69–76.

188. Johansson S, Faergemann J. Enzyme linked immunosorbent assay for detection of antibodies against *Pityrosporum orbiculare*. J Med Vet Mycol 1990;28:257–260

189. Faggi E, Pini G, Campisi E, Gargani G. Anti-*Malassezia furfur* antibodies in the population. Mycoses 1998;41:273–275.

190. Lindgren L, et al. Occurrence and clinical features of sensitization to *Pityrosporum orbiculare* and other allergens in children with atopic dermatitis. Acta Dermato-Venereol 1995;75:300–304.

191. Lintu P, Savolainen J, Kalimo K. IgE antibodies to protein and mannan antigens of *Pityrosporum ovale* in atopic dermatitis. Clin Exp Allergy 1997;27:87–95.

192. Lintu P, et al. Cross reacting IgE and IgG antibodies to *Pityrosporum ovale* mannan and other yeasts in atopic dermatitis. Allergy 1999;54:1067–1073.

193. McGinnis MR. Chromoblastomycosis and phaeohyphomycosis: new concepts, diagnosis, and mycology. J Am Acad Dermatol 1983;8:1–16.

194. De Hoog GS, et al. Black fungi: clinical and pathogenic approaches. Med Mycol 2000;38:243–250.

195. Brandt ME, Warnock DW. Epidemiology, clinical manifestations and therapy of infections caused by dematiaceous fungi. J Chemother 2003;152:36–47.

196. Fader RC, McGinnis MR. Infections caused by dematiaceous fungi: chromoblastomycosis and phaeohyphomycosis. Infect Dis Clin North Am 1988;2:925–938

197. McGinnis MR, Hilger AE. Infections caused by black fungi. Arch Dermatol 1987;123:1300–2.

198. Burks JB, Wakabongo M, McGinnis MR. Chromoblastomycosis. A fungal infection primarily observed in the lower extremity. J Am Podiatr Med Assoc 1995;85:260–4.

199. Da Silva P, et al. Comparison of *Fonsecaea pedrosoi* sclerotic cells obtained in vivo and in vitro: ultrastructure and antigenicity. FEMS Immunol Med Microbiol 2002;33:63–69.

200. Andrade TS, Castro LGM, Nunes RS, Gimenes VMF, Cury AE. Susceptibility of sequential *Fonsecaea pedrosoi* isolates from chromoblastomycosis patients to antifungal agents. Mycoses 2004;47:216–221.

201. Esterre P, Queiroz-Telles F. Management of chromoblastomycosis: novel perspectives. Curr Opin Infect Dis 2006;19:148–152.

202. Esterre P, Jahevitra M, Andriantsimahavandy A. Humoral immune response in chromoblastomycosis during and after therapy. Clin Diag Lab Immunol 2000;7:497–500.

203. Kurita N. Cell mediated immune responses in mice infected with *Fonsecaea pedrosoi*. Mycopathologia 1979;68:9–12.

204. D'Avila SC, Pagliari C, Duarte MI. The cell-mediated immune reaction in the cutaneous lesion of chromoblastomycosis and their correlation with different clinical forms of the disease. Mycopathologia 2003;156:51–60.

205. Kwon-Chung KJ, Bennett JE, eds. Chromoblastomycosis. In: Medical Mycology. Philadelphia: Lea and Febiger, 1992:337–55.

206. Hayakawa M, et al. Phagocytosis, production of nitric oxide and pro-inflammatory cytokines by macrophages in the presence of dematiaceous fungi that cause chromoblastomycosis. Scand J Immunol 2006;64:382–7.

207. Rozental S, Alviano CS, de Souza W. The in vitro susceptibility of *Fonsecaea pedrosoi* to activated macrophages. Mycopathologia 1994;126:85–91.

208. Bocca AL, et al. Inhibition of nitric oxide production by macrophages in chromoblastomycosis: a role for *Fonsecaea pedrosoi* melanin. Mycopathologia 2006;161:195–203.

209. Teixeira de Sousa Mda G, Ghosn EE, Almeida SR. Absence of CD4+ T cells impairs host defence of mice infected with *Fonsecaea pedrosoi*. Scand J Immunol 2006;64:595–600.

210. Gimenes VMF, et al. Cytokine and lymphocyte proliferation in patients with different clinical forms of chromoblastomycosis. Microbes Infect 2005;7:708–13.

211. Alviano DS, Franzen AJ, Travassos LR, et al. Melanin from *Fonsecaea pedrosoi* induces production of human antifungal antibodies and enhances the antimicrobial efficacy of phagocytes. Infect Immun 2004;72:229–37.

212. Sotto MN, De Brito T, Silva AM, Vidal M, Castro LG. Antigen distribution and antigen-presenting cells in skin biopsies of human chromoblastomycosis. J Cutan Pathol 2004;31:14–8.

213. Nimrichter L, Cerqueira MD, Leitao EA, et al. Structure, cellular distribution, antigenicity, and biological functions of *Fonsecaea pedrosoi* ceramide monohexosides. Infect Immun 2005;73: 7860–8.

214. Nimrichter L, et al. Monoclonal antibody to glucosylceramide inhibits the growth of *Fonsecaea pedrosoi* and enhances the antifungal action of mouse macrophages. Microbes Infect 2004;6:657–65.

215. McGinnis MR. Mycetoma. Dematol Clin 1996;14:97–104.

216. Agaña M. Mycetoma. Dermatol Clin 1989;7: 203–217.

217. Boiron P, et al. *Nocardia*, nocardiosis and mycetoma. Med Mycol 1998;36:26–37.

218. Dieng MT, et al. Mycetoma: 130 cases. Ann Dermatol Venereol 2003;130:16–22.

219. Ahmed A, Adelmann D, Fahal A, Verbrugh H, van Belkum A, de Hoog S, Environmental occurrence of *Madurella mycetomatis*, the major agent of human eumycetoma in Sudan. J Clin Microbiol 2002;40:1031–1036.

220. Queiroz-Telles F, McGinnis MR, Salkin I, Graybill J. R. Subcutaneous mycoses. Infect Dis Clin North Am 2003;17:59–85

221. McGinnis MR, Padhye AA. Fungi causing eumycotic mycetoma. In: Manual of Clinical Microbiology, 7th ed. Washington, DC: ASM Press, 2003:1848–1856.

222. Mariat F, Destombes P, Segretain G. The mycetomas: clinical features, pathology, etiology and epidemiology. Contrib Microbiol Immunol 1977;5:1–38.

223. Gugnani HC, et al. "Nocardia asteroides" mycetoma of the foot. J Eur Acad Dermatol Venereol 2002;16 :640–642

224. Chaveiro MA, Vieira R, Cardoso J, Afonso A. Cutaneous infection due to Scedosporium apiospermum in an immunosuppressed patient. J Eur Acad Dermatol Venereol 2003;17:47–49.

225. Ahmed AO, et al. Mycetoma caused by Madurella mycetomatis: a neglected infectious burden. Lancet Infect Dis 2004;4:566–574.

226. Fahal AH. Mycetoma: a thorn in the flesh. Trans R Soc Trop Med Hyg 2004;98:3–11.

227. Ahmed AO, et al. Development of a species-specific PCR-restriction fragment length polymorphism analysis procedure for identification of Madurella mycetomatis. J Clin Microbiol 1999;37:3175–3178.

228. Maslin J, Morand JJ, Civatte M. The eumycetomas (fungal mycetomas with black or white grains). Med Trop 2001;61:111–114.

229. Fahal AH, El Sheik H, El Hassan AM. Pathological fracture in mycetoma. Trans R Soc Trop Med Hyg 1996;90:675–676.

230. Sarris I, Berendt AR, Athanasous N, Ostlere SJ. MRI of mycetoma of the foot: two cases demonstrating the dot-in-circle sign. Skeletal Radiol 2003;32:179–183.

231. El Hassan AM, Faha AH, El Hag IA, Khalil EAG. The pathology of mycetoma: light microscopic and ultrastructural features. Sud Med J 1994;32:23–45.

232. Kaplan W, Gonzalez-Ochoa A. Application of the fluorescent antibody technique to the rapid diagnosis of sporotrichosis. Lab Clin Med 1963;62:835–884.

233. Mahgoub ES. The value of gel diffusions in the diagnosis of mycetoma. Trans R Soc Trop Med Hyg 1964;58:560–563.

234. Gumaa SA, Mahgoub ES. Counterimmunoelectrophoresis in the diagnosis of mycetoma and its sensitivity as compared to immunodiffusion. Sabouraudia 1975;13:309–315.

235. McLaren ML, Mahgoub ES, Georgakopoulos E. Preliminary investigation of the use of the enzyme linked immunosorbent assay (ELISA) in the serodiagnosis of mycetoma. Sabouraudia 1978;16:225–228.

236. Murray IG, Mahgoub ES. Further studies on the diagnosis of mycetoma by double diffusion in agar. Sabouraudia 1968;6:106–110.

237. van de Sande WW, et al. Translationally controlled tumor protein from Madurella mycetomatis, a marker for tumorous mycetoma progression. J Immunol 2006;177:1997–2005.

238. Travassos LR. Sporothrix schenckii. In: Szaniszlo PJ, ed. Fungal Dimorphism with Emphasis on Fungi Pathogenic for Humans. New York: Plenum Press, 1985:121.

239. Carvalho MTT, de Castro AP, Baby C, Werner B, Neto JF, Queiroz-Telles F. Disseminated cutaneous sporotrichosis in a patient with AIDS: report of a case. Rev Soc Bras Med. Trop 2002;35:655–659.

240. Ware AJ, et al. Disseminated sporotrichosis with extensive cutaneous involvement in a patient with AIDS. J Am Acad Dermatol 1999;40:350–355.

241. Hay RJ, Moore M. Sporotrichosis. In: Champion RH, Burton JL, Burns DA, Breathnach SM, eds. Rook/Wilkinson/Ebling Textbook of Dermatology, 6th ed. London: Blackwell Science UK, 1998:1351.

242. Weedon D. Sporotrichosis. In: Weedon D, ed. Skin Pathology. New York: Churchill Livingstone, 1997:569.

243. Carlos IZ, et al. Detection of cellular immunity with the soluble antigen of the fungus Sporothrix schenckii in the systemic form of the disease. Mycopathologia 1992;117:139–145.

244. Tachibana T, Matsuyama T, Mitsuyama M. Involvement of CD4+ T cells and macrophages in acquired protection against infection with Sporothrix schenckii in mice. Med Mycol 1999;37:397–401.

245. Fujimura T, Asai T, Muguruma K, Masuzawa M, Katsuoka K. Local expression of migration inhibitory factor and Th1 type cytokine mRNA in sporotrichosis lesions. Acta Dermato-Venereol 1996;76:321–325.

246. Koga T, Duan H, Furue M. Immunohistochemical detection of interferon-γ-producing cells in granuloma formation of sporotrichosis. Med Mycol 2002;40:111–114.

247. Koga T, Duan H, Urabe K, Furue M. Immunohistochemical localization of activated and mature CD83+ dendritic cells in granulomas of sporotrichosis. Eur J Dermatol 2001;11:527–529.

248. Maia DC, Sassa MF, Placeres MC, Carlos IZ. Influence of Th1/Th2 cytokines and nitric oxide in murine systemic infection induced by Sporothrix schenckii. Mycopathologia 2006;161:11–9.

249. Uenotsuchi T, et al. Differential induction of Th1-prone immunity by human dendritic cells activated with Sporothrix schenckii of cutaneous and visceral origins to determine their different virulence. Int Immunol 2006;18:1637–46.

250. Kajiwara H, Saito M, Ohga S, Uenotsuchi T, Yoshida S. Impaired host defense against Sporothrix schenckii in mice with chronic granulomatous disease. Infect Immun 2004;72:5073–9.

251. Romani L, Francesco B, Puccetti P. Fungi, dendritic cells and receptors: a host perspective of fungal virulence. Trends Microbiol 2002;10:508–513.

252. Buentke E, Scheynius A. Dendritic cells and fungi. Acta Pathol. Microbiol Immunol Scand 2003;111:789–792.

253. Netea MG, et al. Recognition of fungal pathogens by Toll-like receptors. Eur J Clin Microbiol Infect Dis 2004;23:672–675.

254. Brown GD. Dectin-1: a signaling non-TLR pattern-recognition receptor. Nat Rev Immunol 2006;6: 33–39.

255. Shoham S, Lavitz SM. The immune response to fungal infections. Br J Haematol 2004;129: 569–574.

256. Takeda K, Akira S. TLR signaling pathways. Semin Immunol 2004;16:3–7.

257. Roeder A, Kirschning CJ, Rupoc RA, Schaller M, Weindl G, Korting HC. Toll-like receptors as key mediators in innate antifungal immunity. Med Mycol 2004;42:485–489.

258. Kisho T, Akira S. Toll-like receptor function and signaling. J Allergy Clin Immunol 2006;117: 979–985.

259. Netea MG, Van der Meer JWM, Kullberg BJ. Role of the dual interaction of fungal pathogens with pattern recognition receptors in the activation and modulation of host defence. Clin Microbiol Infect 2006;12:404–408.

260. De Hoog GS, et al. Molecular phylogeny and taxonomy of medically important fungi. Med Mycol 1998;36:52–56.

261. Standaert SM, et al. Coccidioidomycosis among visitors to a *Coccidioides immitis*-endemic area: an outbreak in a military reserve unit. J Infect Dis 1995;171:1672–1675.

262. Cole GT, et al. A vaccine against coccidioidomycosis is justified and attainable. Med Mycol 2004;42:189–216.

263. Johnson RH, Einstein HE. Coccidioidal meningitis. Clin Infect Dis 2006;42:103–107

264. Dismukes WE. Antifungal therapy: lessons learned over the past 27 years. Clin Infect Dis 2006;42:1289–1296.

265. Ampel NM, Kramer LA. In vitro modulation of cytokine production by lymphocytes in human coccidioidomycosis. Cell Immunol 2003;221(2): 115–21.

266. Ampel NM, Christian L. In vitro modulation of proliferation and cytokine production by human peripheral blood mononuclear cells from subjects with various forms of coccidioidomycosis. Infect Immun 1997;65:4483–4488.

267. Corry DB, Ampel NM, Christian L, Locksley RM, Galgiani JN. Cytokine production by peripheral blood mononuclear cells in human coccidioidomycosis. J Infect Dis 1996;174:440–443.

268. Ampel NM, Bejarano GC, Galgiani JN. Killing of *Coccidioides immitis* by human peripheral blood mononuclear cells. Infect Immun 1992;60:4200–4.

269. Dionne SO, et al. Spherules derived from *Coccidioides posadasii* promote human dendritic cell maturation and activation. Infect Immun 2006;74:2415–22.

270. Cox RA, Brummer E, Lecara G. In vitro lymphocyte responses of coccidioidin skin test-positive and -negative persons to coccidioidin, spherulin, and a coccidioides cell wall antigen. Infect Immun 1977;15:751–753.

271. Hung CY, et al. Major cell surface antigen of *Coccidioides immitis* which elicits both humoral and cellular immune responses. Infect Immun 2000;68:584–593.

272. Ward ER, et al. Delayed-type hypersensitivity responses to a cell wall fraction of the mycelial phase of *Coccidioides immitis*. Infect Immun 1975;12:1093–1097.

273. Delgado N, Xue J, Yu JJ, Hung CY, Cole GT. A recombinant β-1,3–glucanosyltransferase homolog of *Coccidioides posadasii* protects mice against coccidioidomycosis. Infect Immun 2003;71: 3010–3019.

274. Awasthi S, Awasthi V, Magee DM, Coalson JJ. Efficacy of antigen 2/proline-rich antigen cDNA-transfected dendritic cells in immunization of mice against *Coccidioides posadasii*. J Immunol 2005;175:3900–6.

275. Shubitz LF, Yu JJ, Hung CY, et al. Improved protection of mice against lethal respiratory infection with *Coccidioides posadasii* using two recombinant antigens expressed as a single protein. Vaccine 2006;26;24:5904–11.

276. Ampel NM, Hector RF, Lindan CP, Rutherford GW. An archived lot of coccidioidin induces specific coccidioidal delayed-type hypersensitivity and correlates with in vitro assays of coccidioidal cellular immune response. Mycopathologia 2006;161:67–72.

277. Couppie P, et al. Acquired immunodeficiency syndrome-related oral and/or cutaneous histoplasmosis: a descriptive and comparative study of 21 cases in French Guiana. Int J Dermatol 2002;41:571–576.

278. Ramdial P, et al. Disseminated cutaneous histoplasmosis in patients infected with human immunodeficiency virus. J Cutan Pathol 2002;29:215–25.

279. Rappleye CA, Eissenberg LG, Goldman WE. *Histoplasma capsulatum* alpha-(1,3)-glucan blocks innate immune recognition by the beta-glucan receptor. Proc Natl Acad Sci USA 2007;104: 1366–70.

280. Wheat LJ, et al. disseminated histoplasmosis in the acquired immune deficiency syndrome: clinical findings, diagnosis and treatment, and review of the literature. Medicine (Baltimore) 1990;69:361–370.

281. Wu-Hsieh BA, Howard DH. Histoplasmosis. In: Murphy J Jr, Friedman H Jr, Bendinelli M Jr, eds. Fungal Infections and Immune Responses. New York: Plenum Press, 1993:213–250.

282. Body BA. Cutaneous manifestations of systemic mycoses. Dermatol Clin 1996;14:125–35.

283. Heninger E, et al. Characterization of the *Histoplasma capsulatum*-induced granuloma. J Immunol 2006;177:3303–13.

284. Akpek G, et al. Bone marrow aspiration, biopsy, and culture in the evaluation of HIV-infected patients for invasive mycobacteria and *histoplasma* infections. Am J Hematol 2001;67:100–106.

285. Sahapatayavongs B, et al. Clinical and laboratory features of disseminated histoplasmosis during two large urban outbreaks. Medicine (Baltimore) 1983;62:263–270.

286. Unis G, da Silva VB, Severo LC. Disseminated histoplasmosis and AIDS: the role of culture medium for the bronchoscopic clinical specimens. Rev Soc Bras Med Trop 2004;37:234–237.

287. Santiago AR, Hernandez B, Rodriguez M, Romero H. A comparative study of blood culture conventional method vs a modified lysis/centrifuga-

tion technique for the diagnosis of fungemias. Rev Iberoam Micol 2004;21:198–201.

288. Castro R, et al. The ultrastructure of the parasitophorous vacuole formed by Leishmania major. J Parasitol 2006;92:1162–70.

289. Wu-Hsieh BA, Howard DH. Inhibition of the intracellular growth of *Histoplasma capsulatum* by recombinant murine interferon. Infect Immun 1987;55:1014–1016.

290. Kugler S, Schurtz Sebghati T, Groppe Eissenberg L, Goldman WE. Phenotypic variation and intracellular parasitism by *Histoplasma capsulatum*. Proc Natl Acad Sci USA 2000;97:8794–8798.

291. Gildea LA, Morris RE, Newman SL. Histoplasma capsulatum yeasts are phagocytosed via very late antigen-5, killed, and processed for antigen presentation by human dendritic cells. J Immunol 2001;166:1049–1056.

292. Clemons KV, et al. Experimental histoplasmosis in mice treated with anti-murine interferon–gamma antibody and in interferon gamma gene knockout mice. Microbes Infect 2000;2:997–1001.

293. Allendoerfer R, Deepe GS Jr. Blockade of endogenous TNF-alpha exacerbates primary and secondary pulmonary histoplasmosis by differential mechanisms. J Immunol 1998;160:6072–6082.

294. Belkaid Y, et al. CD4+CD25+ regulatory T cells control *Leishmania* major persistence and immunity. Nature 2002;420:502–507.

25
Cutaneous T-Cell Lymphoma

Ellen J. Kim, Camille E. Introcaso, Stephen K. Richardson, and Alain H. Rook

Key Points

- Cutaneous T-cell lymphomas are a group of extranodal non-Hodgkin's lymphomas that present initially in the skin.
- The incidence of this condition is approximately 0.52–0.64/100,000 person-years.
- Cutaneous T-cell lymphomas usually present as indolent patches and plaques, but may also present with more aggressive tumors or erythroderm. The survival is highly dependent on the stage of the disease.
- The diagnosis is made with clinical findings and histology. Staging of this disease is critical, and this may include history and physical examination, blood tests, peripheral blood flow cytometry, and Sézary cell preparations, and scans for internal involvement.
- Cell trafficking of malignant T cells into the skin and the epidermis is critical in the pathophysiology of this disease, and involves chemokines and chemokine receptors.
- The immunology of this condition suggests that T-helper-2 (Th2) lymphocyte cytokine patterns are associated with the malignant cells, and there is a progressive loss of cellular immunity with advancing disease.
- There are two major categories of treatments for this condition: skin-directed therapies or systemic therapies. Combination therapies are effective and have immunomodulatory effects.
- Bone marrow transplantation is an emerging therapy for patients with advanced disease that is refractory to skin and systemic therapy.

Cutaneous T-cell lymphomas (CTCLs) are a group of extranodal non-Hodgkin's lymphomas (NHLs) that present primarily in the skin. The most common type of CTCLs, mycosis fungoides (MF) and Sézary syndrome (SS), were first described over two centuries ago, and since that time, the clinical characteristics, pathophysiology, and immunobiology have been characterized in detail. Derived from skin-homing, mature, effector T cells that usually express CLA/CD4/CCR4/CCR10 and lack T-cell markers CD7 and CD26, the malignant MF/SS cells typically have a T-helper-2 (Th2) phenotype. With more advanced disease, Th2 cytokines predominate and result in decreased host cell-mediated immunity that likely contributes to increased susceptibility to infection and disease progression. Early aggressive systemic chemotherapy has not been shown to improve overall survival in MF/SS, and over the past 30 years the therapeutic approach has undergone a paradigm shift, such that skin-directed therapies (SDTs) and systemic immune-modifying biologics play a central role in MF/SS management.[1] This chapter reviews MF/SS clinical presentation, staging workup, pathophysiology, and immunobiology, and discusses how these factors have shaped current treatment strategies. In particular, this chapter highlights MF/SS chemokine biology, immune defects, and immune-modifying therapies, including the new frontier of hematopoietic stem cell transplantation.

Clinical Presentation

Cutaneous T-cell lymphomas are a heterogeneous group of extranodal lymphomas, and they were recently the subject of a new joint classification system by the World Health Organization (WHO) and the European Organization for Research and

TABLE 25.1. World Health Organization (WHO) and the
European Organization for Research and Treatment
of Cancer (EORTC) classification of cutaneous T- and
natural killer (NK)/T-cell lymphomas, 2005.

Mycosis fungoides and variants/subtypes
Sézary syndrome
Primary cutaneous CD30[+] lymphoproliferative disorders
Subcutaneous panniculitis-like T-cell lymphoma
Extranodal NK/T-cell lymphoma, nasal type
Adult T-cell leukemia/lymphoma
Primary cutaneous peripheral T-cell lymphoma, unspecified
• Aggressive epidermotropic CD8[+] T-cell lymphoma
• Cutaneous γδ T-cell lymphoma
• PC CD4[+] small/medium-sized pleomorphic T-cell lymphoma
• Peripheral T-cell lymphoma, other

Source: Willemze,[2] with permission of the American Society
of Hematology.

Treatment of Cancer (EORTC) (Table 25.1).
Mycosis fungoides/Sézary syndrome is relatively
uncommon, and comprises approximately 1% of all
NHLs. A recent study of lymphoma incidence patterns in the United States (1992–2001, Surveillance,
Epidemiology, and End Results [SEER] data),
demonstrated that the incidence of MF/SS has
remained unchanged at 0.52 per 100,000 person-
year.[3] More recently Criscione and Weinstock
demonstrated a similar disease incidence of 0.64
per 100,00 person-year but this was increased over
the time period studied (1973–2002).[3a] The cause
of the vast majority of MF/SS cases is unknown,
despite numerous environmental and infectious
etiologies having been investigated as potential
sources of chronic antigenic stimulation. These
include human T-cell lymphotrophic virus (HTLV),
cytomegalovirus (CMV), Borrelia burgdorferi,
human herpes virus-8 (HHV-8), Staphylococcus
aureus, Chlamydia species, and chemical exposures
such as aromatic/halogenated hydrocarbons.[4,5]

Mycosis fungoides classically presents as scaly
oval or annular patches/plaques on sun-protected
areas ("bathing trunk" distribution) such as the
trunk, buttocks, axillae, groin, proximal extremities, with or without pruritus (Fig. 25.1A–C).
Typically, it has indolent behavior and in early
disease when host immunity is intact, lesions may
wax and wane spontaneously. Because of this,
early disease may take years before definitive
diagnosis is made, and multiple skin biopsies may
demonstrate nonspecific dermatitis. Lesions may

also less commonly affect sun-exposed areas such
as the face and can also result in localized hair loss.
They may also progress to thicker, more infiltrated plaques (Fig. 25.1C), ulcerated tumors (Fig.
25.1D), or coalesce into a confluent erythema on
>80% of the body surface area ("erythroderma")
(Fig. 25.1E). In these cases, the disease can cause
more symptoms and behave more aggressively.

In addition to the classic presentation, MF has
myriad other clinical morphologies and histologic
variants (classic Alibert-Bazin subtype, erythro-
dermic/Sézary syndrome, unilesional, hypopigmented, pagetoid reticulosis, follicular/follicular
mucinosis, syringotropic, granulomatous/slack
skin, bullous/vesicular, palmoplantar, pigmented
purpuric dermatosis–like, interstitial, ichthyosiform, hyperkeratotic/verrucous, vegetating/papil-
lomatous),[6] and has been referred to as one of the
great clinical imitators, similar to cutaneous syphilis
and sarcoidosis. Subtypes may be characterized by
more indolent behavior (hypopigmented MF) vs.
more aggressive behavior (follicular, granulomatous) depending on their clinical course. Follicular
MF, even with limited lesions, can be recalcitrant to
therapy given the depth of the malignant infiltrate.

Sézary syndrome typically has a more aggressive
course than MF from its onset, and typically presents
as de novo erythroderma with leukemic peripheral
blood involvement by the atypical, hyperconvoluted,
cerebriform, malignant T cells known as Sézary
cells (also previously referred to as Lutzner cells or
cells monstreuse). This is in contrast to patients who
have MF that evolves into erythroderma over time
(erythrodermic MF). Originally, SS was described
with the clinical triad of erythroderma, lymphadenopathy, and palmoplantar keratoderma (Fig. 25.1F).
Sézary syndrome patients may also have severe
pruritus, active scaling/desquamation, prominent
conjunctival eversion of the eyelids (referred to as
ectropion), diffuse alopecia, chills, low-grade fevers,
night sweats, or fatigue.

Mycosis fungoides/Sézary syndrome patients,
particularly erythrodermic patients, are heavily
colonized by skin bacteria and are susceptible to
recurrent infections with Staphylococcus aureus,
which often are methicillin-resistant (MRSA).
Patients with ulcerated tumors are also at high risk
for bacterial sepsis, and in general, infections have
previously been the leading cause of mortality in
MF/SS patients.[7]

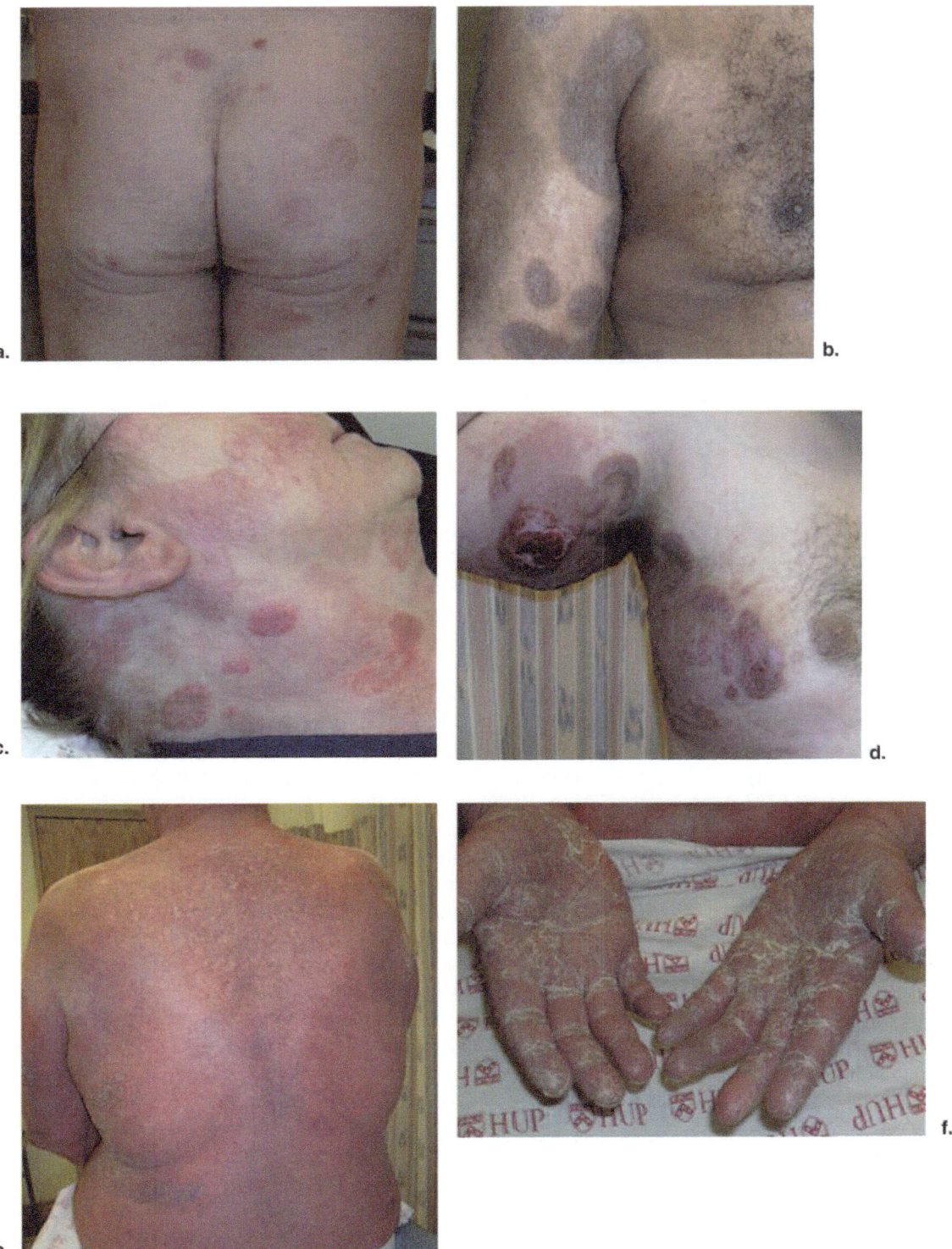

FIG. 25.1. Skin lesions in mycosis fungoides (MF)/Sézary syndrome (SS). Oval patches of MF in typical sun-protected areas of the buttocks (A) and proximal arms/axillae (B). (C) Raised, annular plaques of MF. (D) MF plaques and an ulcerated tumor. SS patient with erythroderma (E) and palmar keratoderma (F)

Mycosis fungoides/Sézary syndrome patients may also present with other concomitant skin conditions, such as the chronic, recurrent primary cutaneous CD30[+] lymphoproliferative disorders (LPDs) such as lymphomatoid papulosis (LyP) or CD30[+] primary cutaneous anaplastic large cell lymphoma (ALCL).[8] Patients with MF/SS may also be at higher risk for having secondary malignancies, such as other skin cancers (nonmelanoma and melanoma) as well as secondary lymphomas.[9]

Diagnosis

Early diagnosis of MF can be elusive, as the clinical and histopathology of early MF lesions can mimic benign dermatoses, such as eczematous dermatitis, allergic contact dermatitis, psoriasis, and parapsoriasis. Traditionally, the diagnosis is made when a patient presents clinically with typical lesions, and skin biopsy reveals atypical lymphocytes (with large, hyperchromatic and hyperconvoluted nuclei) within the epidermis, in the absence of epidermal spongiosis, and often associated with epidermal dendritic cells (DCs) to form the pathognomonic "Pautrier's microabscesses." Currently there are sophisticated laboratory tools to aid in diagnosis, which include tissue immunohistochemistry and flow cytometry (which can demonstrate CD3 expression, CD4 > CD8 expression of greater than 4:1, as well as characteristic T-cell lineage antigen loss of CD5, CD7, CD26, and less often CD3). Molecular detection of clonal T-cell receptor (TCR) gene rearrangements (β or γ chains) in more than one skin lesion or in skin lesions and another tissue (blood, lymph node) can also further strengthen the diagnosis.[10] These days, the standard evaluation of early MF often involves assessment of multiple criteria (clinical, histopathologic, molecular).[11] However, it must be noted that T-cell clonality can also be detected in benign and autoimmune inflammatory dermatoses and should not be automatically equated with neoplasia.[12,13]

In SS, leukemic blood involvement was traditionally measured by the Sézary preparation, visual examination of a peripheral blood buffy coat smear for the atypical Sézary cells (Sézary count >5% total lymphocytes was considered significant). However, this method was laborious and was subject to considerable interobserver variability. More sensitive and specific tools to measure peripheral blood involvement include anti-TCR Vβ-specific monoclonal antibodies, or T-cell surface marker antibodies (CD3, CD4, CD7, CD8, CD26) using fluorescence-activated cell-sorting (FACS) analysis and flow cytometry. Other markers recently reported useful in flow cytometric analysis include CD158k and vimentin.[14] In SS, molecular testing for TCR gene rearrangements can often detect the identical clonal T-cell population in the blood and the skin. In general, T-cell monoclonality detectable in several different skin lesions or tissues (skin, nodes, blood) in a patient over time is suggestive of CTCL.[15]

Disease Staging

Since 1979, a tumor, node, and metastasis blood (TNMB) classification and staging system has been used for MF/SS, and TNMB stage has proven to be an important prognostic measure (Tables 25.2 and 25.3).[16] Recent modifications have been proposed by the International Society for Cutaneous Lymphomas (ISCL) regarding further stratifying blood involvement parameters, to reflect the newer, more sensitive assays.[17,18] The current B classification proposed by the ISCL includes B0, no clinically significant blood involvement; B1, clinically significant "minimal" blood involvement with Sézary cells <1.0 K/μL; and B2, leukemic blood involvement detectable either as (1) Sézary cells > 1.0 K/μL, (2) CD4/CD8 ratio >10 and CD4[+]CD7[−] population > 40% or CD4[+]CD30[−] population >30%, (3) lymphocytosis with molecular genetic evidence of a clonal T-cell population, or (4) chromosomally abnormal T-cell clones. These newer blood involvement parameters may affect staging and prognosis of patients. Currently the ISCL proposes that in patients with erythroderma (T4 skin classification), the B2 classification be considered the equivalent to nodal involvement (hence T4N0-1M0B2 would be upgraded from stage III to stage IVA). A recent retrospective study by Vonderheid et al.[18] demonstrated that using modified B criteria improved prognostication in erythrodermic patients; prospective studies are needed for further validation.

TABLE 25.2. Tumor, node, and metastasis blood (TNMB) classification for mycosis fungoides and Sézary syndrome, National Cancer Institute (NCI) workshop, 1978.

T (Skin)
T1 Limited patch/plaque (<10% body surface area)
T2 Generalized patch/plaque (≥10% body surface area)
T3 Tumors
T4 Generalized erythroderma
N (Lymph Node)
N0 Clinically uninvolved
N1 Clinically abnormal, histologically uninvolved
N2 Clinically uninvolved, histologically involved
N3 Clinically abnormal, histologically involved
M (Viscera)
M0 No visceral involvement
M2 Visceral involvement
*B (Blood)**
B0 No circulating atypical (Sézary) cells
B1 Circulating atypical (Sézary) cells

*See International Society for Cutaneous Lymphomas (ISCL) 2002 consensus report on the B Classification changing this to B0, B1, B2 as discussed in text section Disease Staging
Source: Lamberg and Bunn,[16] with permission of the American Medical Association.

Once patients have an established diagnosis of MF/SS, a typical staging workup includes complete skin and physical examination, complete blood count with differential, comprehensive metabolic panel, lactate dehydrogenase (LDH), and either peripheral blood flow cytometry or Sézary cell prep. Computed tomography (CT) or positron emission tomography (PET) scanning is appropriate for patients with systemic symptoms, clinically palpable lymphadenopathy (>1.5 cm), or more advanced T classification (T3/tumors or T4/erythrodermic disease). These tests are useful to assess nodal or visceral involvement by MF/SS. The role

TABLE 25.3. Clinical staging system for mycosis fungoides and Sézary syndrome, NCI Workshop 1978.

Clinical stages			
IA	T1	N0	M0
IB	T2	N0	M0
IIA	T1–2	N1	M0
IIB	T3	N0–1	M0
IIIA	T4	N0	M0
IIIB	T4	N1	M0
IVA	T1–4	N2–3	M0
IVB	T1–4	N0–3	M1

Source: Lamberg and Bunn,[16] with permission of the American Medical Association.

of staging bone marrow biopsy remains controversial.[19] In the United States, bone marrow biopsy is typically reserved only for patients with advanced disease with some evidence of other hematologic abnormalities (e.g., other cytopenias).

Overall survival in MF/SS is highly dependent on the initial disease stage. Several studies have demonstrated that early-stage disease (i.e., skin disease only, limited to <10% of the body surface area) if treated has overall median survival comparable to healthy control populations. However, with more advanced disease, overall survival also decreases, with stage IV disease having a 27% 5-year survival and Sézary syndrome patients having a 30% 5-year survival.[20] In retrospective studies, the risk of disease progression ranged from 10% (stage IA) to 25% (stages IB or higher) over a 30-year period.[21,22] Recently a series of MF patients from England were demonstrated to have significantly improved overall survival over the past 20 years.[23] However, the reasons for this improvement are unclear from their data (increased diagnosis of early-stage disease patients vs. advent of new therapies in MF/SS).

Various clinical prognostic factors have been demonstrated including patient age, initial stage, T classification, visceral disease, elevated LDH, eosinophilia, and the presence of Sézary cells. Important histologic factors that indicate poor prognosis include "large cell transformation" (presence of >30% large atypical CD30+ T cells in the infiltrate seen in the skin or lymph node or blood), folliculotropic or granulomatous infiltrate; in contrast, the presence CD8+ tumor infiltrating cytotoxic lymphocytes (TILs) in the infiltrate has been demonstrated to be a favorable prognostic marker. T-cell clonality has been shown to be useful in MF/SS diagnosis; however, its role as an independent prognostic marker remains to be fully determined.

Unlike the field of nodal NHLs, validated prognostic indices have not been used in the field of MF/SS for risk stratification. Recently, however, the CTCL severity index (CTCL-SI) had been proposed as a point-based system to assess disease severity (based on lesion body surface area, number of tumors, nodal/visceral/blood involvement), and also to predict 5-year survival.[24] If validated, the CTCL-SI could supplement the current National Cancer Institute (NCI) staging system and be useful as a prognostic index for individual patients and for making comparisons between different groups of patients in clinical trials.

Perhaps the most potentially powerful prognostic tool currently being developed in MF/SS is complementary DNA (cDNA) microarray analysis. Previously, MF/SS patients were shown to have a distinct gene expression profile that was distinguishable from other benign inflammatory dermatoses.[25] In addition, such profiles could also identify high-risk patients with <6 months' survival. The panel of genes identified included upregulated *GATA3* (involved in Th2 differentiation), downregulated *STAT4* (involved in Th1 differentiation), and *CD26* (dipeptidylpeptidase IV, which regulates T-cell entry into the epidermis; see Chemokines and Their Receptors, below). Recently, quantitative real-time polymerase chain reaction (PCR) using a similar panel of genes has also been shown to be capable of molecularly diagnosing MF/SS patients.[26]

Pathophysiology

Chemokines and Their Receptors

As mentioned previously, CTCL is a malignancy in which tumor cells exhibit an affinity for the skin. This affinity is dependent on their expression of cell surface trafficking molecules, which mediate their migration to the cutaneous microenvironment. Chemokines and their receptors are included in this family of molecules and play a critical role in mediating tissue-specific trafficking of leukocytes to the skin.

Chemokines are chemotactic cytokines that are produced by a wide array of tissues and range from 8 to 17 kd in size. They are divided into families in accordance with the positioning of cysteine residues in their chemical structure. Aside from their role in cell migration, they have also been shown to play a role in the mediation of inflammatory responses, angiogenesis, and cellular proliferation.[27]

Chemokine receptors are seven-transmembrane-spanning G-protein–coupled proteins that are capable of recognizing more than one chemokine. Several chemokines and their receptors have been identified to play a critical role in the trafficking of immune cells to the skin, more specifically, thymus and activation-regulated chemokine (TARC), macrophage-derived chemokine (MDC), stromal-derived factor-1 (SDF-1), and cutaneous T-cell–attracting chemokine (CTACK). These chemokines have been shown to be produced by multiple cell types (including keratinocytes, fibroblasts, and endothelial cells), and are upregulated at sites of cutaneous inflammation. Skin-trafficking T cells have been shown to express receptors for these chemokines.

Lymphocyte trafficking to the skin requires that the cell undergo a sequential series of events that begins with an initial tethering interaction with the endothelial surface, followed by rolling, activation, firm adhesion, and diapedesis into the dermal microenvironment. The tethering and rolling events are mediated by interactions between cutaneous lymphocyte-associated antigen (CLA) and E-selectin;[28] CLA is expressed on the surface of skin-trafficking T cells and E-selectin is expressed by endothelial cells at sites of cutaneous inflammation.

Activation of the arrest stage of lymphocyte trafficking is mediated by interactions between chemokines and their receptors. Upon engagement of the chemokine receptor, signals are transduced that activate downstream events, including a change in cellular morphology, such that integrins on the surface of the leukocyte are sufficiently exposed to contact their ligands on the dermal microvasculature (e.g., lymphocyte function–associated antigen 1 [LFA-1] binding to intercellular adhesion molecule 1 [ICAM-1]). This leads to the arrest of the rolling cell, which may then migrate into the dermis along a chemotactic gradient generated by chemokines produced in the skin.

The malignant cells in CTCL have been shown to express skin-trafficking molecules, which include CLA and an array of chemokine receptors. Although frequently elevated, we and others have observed that CLA expression may be more variable among circulating malignant cells,[29] whereas chemokine receptors involved in skin trafficking are more consistently expressed at high levels among this population.

It appears somewhat counterintuitive that cells expressing skin-trafficking molecules may remain confined to the circulation, as is noted among patients with advanced disease such as in SS.

This confinement of malignant cells to the blood compartment may in part be accounted for by significantly elevated chemokine levels (such as TARC) in the skin and circulation of patients. It is plausible that TARC levels in the blood may exceed a threshold concentration required for effective chemotaxis, and thus abolish a skin-derived chemotactic gradient. This idea is supported by the work of Poznansky et al.,[30] who reported the potential for T cells to exhibit movement away from a chemotactic gradient established at concentrations above which normal directional migration is detected. This finding, in combination with the variable expression levels of other skin-trafficking molecules (such as CLA) among the malignant population in CTCL may provide an explanation for the high percentage of neoplastic cells detected in the circulation of patients with advanced disease.

Several studies have evaluated the expression of chemokine receptors by malignant cells in the skin and circulation of CTCL patients. Flow cytometric analysis and immunohistochemical studies revealed preferential expression of the chemokine receptors CCR4, CXCR3, and CXCR4 among MF cells and the surrounding reactive T cells in patients with early patch and plaque stage disease. Interestingly, patients with tumor stage disease exhibit a loss of CXCR3 (and rarely, CCR4), while expressing high levels of the chemokine receptor, CCR7.[31] CXCR4 and CCR4 have both been shown to play a role in lymphocyte migration to the skin, while CCR7 mediates the migration of T cells to lymphatic tissue and may account for the nodal disease observed among patients with advanced disease. CCR7 recognizes secondary lymphoid tissue chemokine (SLC/CCL21) produced within the nodal microenvironment. Preferential expression of CCR10 has also been reported among tumor cells of MF patients. CCR10 is the receptor for the cutaneous T-cell attracting chemokine (CTACK/CCL27) which is constitutively produced by epidermal keratinocytes.[32]

Similar to the MF cells in tumor-stage disease, the malignant cells in patients with peripheral blood disease have been shown to express elevated levels of CCR4, CCR7, CXCR4, and CCR10.[33] In addition, the circulating malignant cells are also characterized by their loss of the cluster of differentiation markers CD7 and CD26.[34] The absence of

CD26 is believed to contribute to the accumulation of malignant cells in the skin of Sézary syndrome patients.[35]

CD26 is a dipeptidyl transferase expressed as both a soluble factor in the circulation and as a cell-surface protein expressed by lymphocytes. CD26 mediates the cleavage of the chemokine stromal-derived factor-1 (SDF-1), produced by inflamed skin (Fig. 25.2A). SDF-1 is the natural ligand for the chemokine receptor CXCR4, which is expressed by the malignant population in Sézary syndrome. The absence of CD26 leads to elevated levels of SDF-1, which in turn contribute to the trafficking of malignant cells to skin (Fig. 25.2B).

A CD26-negative population of greater than 30% among erythrodermic patients is believed to be sufficient to support a diagnosis of Sézary syndrome, and thus differentiate such patients from individuals suffering from benign inflammatory dermatoses.[36] We have recently reported a correlation between the percentage of circulating CD4+CD26− T cells and changes in clinical status among Sézary syndrome patients. More specifically, a reduction in this population typically heralds improved clinical status, whereas an increase frequently precedes disease progression characterized by a greater than 20% increase in affected body surface area, or a greater than 10% increase in body surface area accompanied by progressive lymphadenopathy or hepatosplenomegaly.[37]

While chemokine receptors are necessary for tissue-specific lymphocyte trafficking to the skin, expression of their chemokine ligands plays an essential role in this process. In the absence of chemokines, engagement and activation of the chemokine receptor do not occur. The epidermotropism exhibited by neoplastic cells in CTCL has been attributed, in part, to the production of chemokines by epidermal cells. Whether their production arises secondary to the accumulation of malignant cells in the skin or precedes the infiltration has not been established.

Elevated levels of the chemokine cutaneous T-cell–attracting chemokine (CTACK/CCL27) has recently been reported in the serum of patients with CTCL. The highest levels were detected among patients with more advanced disease (tumor stage and erythroderma), and improved in response to successful treatment.[38] CTACK has been shown to be produced by epidermal keratinocytes and

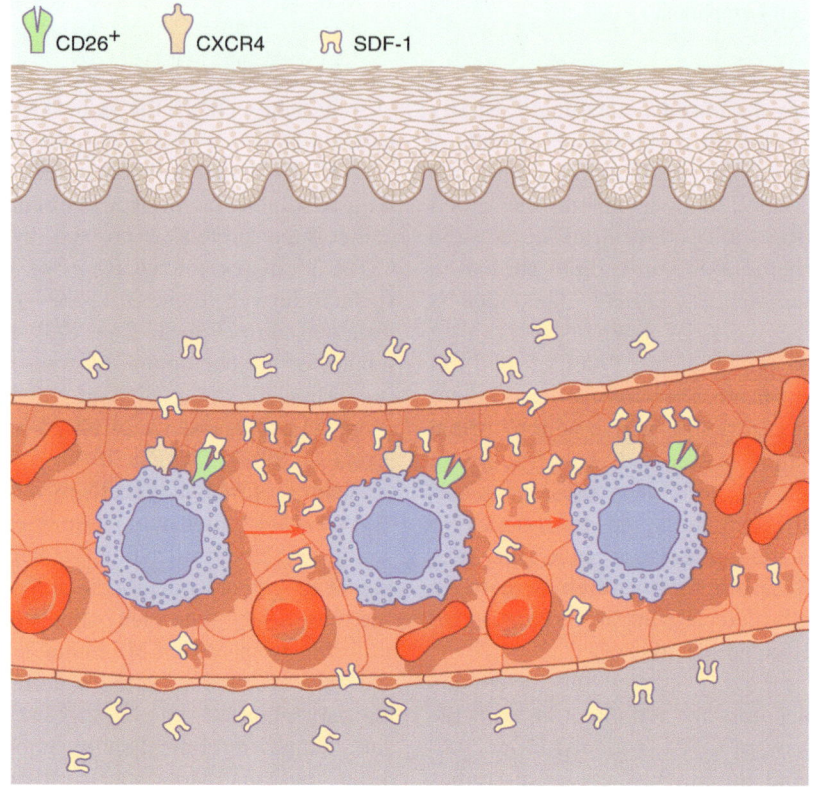

A

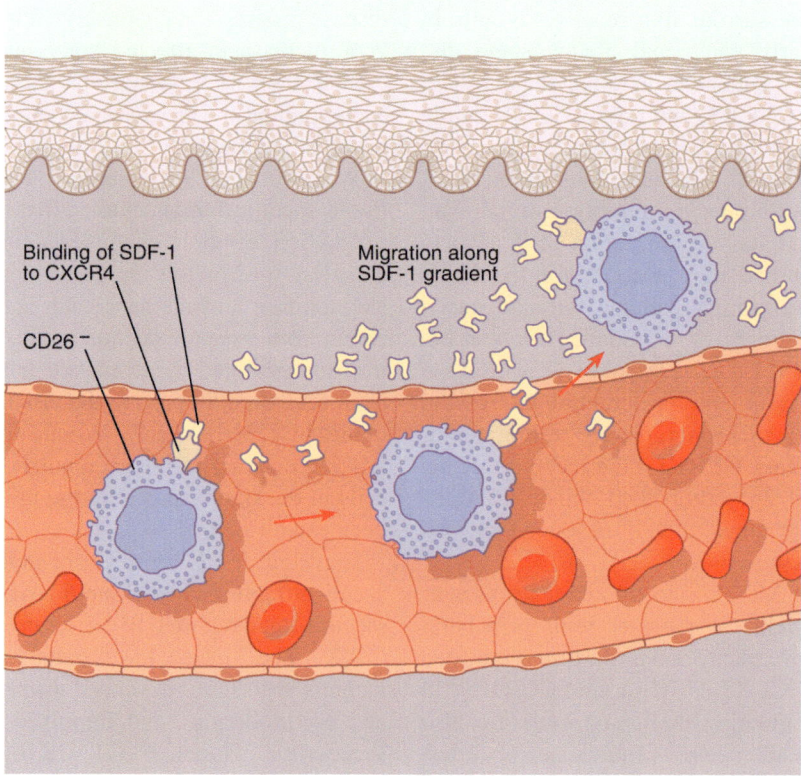

B

is presented on the surface of dermal endothelial cells.[32,39] It is recognized by the chemokine receptor CCR10, which, as mentioned previously, is expressed by the malignant population.[40]

Thymus and activation-regulated chemokine (TARC/CCL17), the ligand for CCR4, was shown to be elevated in CTCL patients compared to normal individuals and patients with psoriasis vulgaris.[41] More specifically, an increase in serum TARC levels was shown to correlate with more advanced disease, being greatest among tumor-stage patients as compared to patch- and plaque-stage patients. Immunohistochemistry revealed TARC expression by lesional keratinocytes at all stages of disease. These findings support a functional role for CCR4 in the accumulation of malignant cells in the skin of CTCL patients.

Preferential expression of messenger RNA (mRNA) for the chemokine interferon-γ inducible protein 10 (IP-10) has been reported in the epidermis of patients with early-stage epidermotropic CTCL.[42] IP-10 is the ligand for CXCR3, which is expressed by MF cells in early patch/plaque-stage disease.[31] CXCR3 and its ligand, IP-10, are considered to be Th1-associated molecules given their ability to recruit Th1 cells to sites of inflammation. Thus, levels of IP-10 and CXCR3 positive cells may reflect the host antitumor response. Patients with more advanced disease exhibit a depression in CXCR3 levels, whereas expression of the Th2-associated chemokine-receptor CCR4 and its ligand (TARC) remains elevated and skews the cutaneous cytokine milieu in favor of Th2 cytokine production, which likely contributes to the pathogenesis of disease in CTCL.

Once the malignant T cells have been recruited to the skin, their growth appears to be supported by the in situ production of cutaneous cytokines. Yamanaka and colleagues[43] have demonstrated that lesional skin of CTCL patients overproduces interleukin-7 (IL-7). IL-7 itself clearly exhibits pro-proliferative effects on malignant T cells derived from CTCL patients.

Chromosomal and Genetic Abnormalities

Mycosis fungoides/Sézary syndrome is not considered a primary genetic disorder attributable to discrete mutation(s); however, with disease progression, several genetic abnormalities have been detected. Cytogenetic studies have demonstrated chromosomal deletions (1p, 17p, 10q, 19) and gains (4q, 18, 17q).[44] Even early MF lesions have been shown to have *STAT3* constitutively activated or defects in their apoptosis pathways (decreased Fas expression).[45–47] In more advanced disease, such as tumor-stage MF or SS, other genetic perturbations include *p15/16* and *p53* defects, microsatellite instability, hypermethylation of tumor suppressor genes *(p14, p15, p16, BCL7a, PTPRG, p73)*,[48,49] and constitutive activation of nuclear factor κB (NF-κB).[50] In addition to these, epigenetic factors (which affect gene expression through modification of histones and other chromatin-associated proteins) appear to play a role in CTCL development/progression, given the clinical activity of histone deacetylase inhibitors (HDIs) in CTCL.[51]

Mycosis fungoides/Sézary syndrome malignant T cells also can variably express the IL-2 receptor (IL-2R), which binds the cytokine IL-2. IL-2R is composed of three subunits: IL-2Rα (CD25/p55), IL-2Rβ (CD122/p75), and IL-2Rγ (CD132/p64). IL-2Rα has been viewed as a marker of cell activation and is significantly expressed in approximately 20% of MF/SS patients, particularly in later-stage disease,[52] and soluble IL-2R can be detected in the peripheral blood.[53] The T cells can also express other activation markers such as CD45RO or proliferating-cell nuclear antigen (PCNA).

Fig. 25.2. (A) CD26 is a bipeptidyl transferase expressed by normal T lymphocytes that induces the cleavage and inactivation of the chemokine stromal-derived factor-1 (SDF-1). This cleavage prevents the binding of SDF-1 to its receptor, CXCR4, thus interfering with SDF-1/CXCR4-mediated chemotaxis into the skin. CD26+ T cells are resistant to the chemotactic effects of SDF-1 via CD26-mediated inactivation (top). (B) The absence of CD26 is reported among circulating malignant cells in Sézary syndrome. In the absence of CD26, SDF-1 may efficiently establish a chemotactic gradient that promotes the migration of malignant cells into the skin via engagement of CXCR4. Engagement of CXCR4 by SDF-1 in the cutaneous microvasculature and subsequent chemotaxis of the cell into the dermal microenvironment are demonstrated (top).

Immunobiology

Immune Dysregulation in CTCL: Clues to Understanding Disease Progression

It has long been known that patients with advanced MF/SS typically exhibit abnormalities in a variety of parameters of cell-mediated immunity. Moreover, the malignant T cells have been implicated as the cause of the endogenous immune deficiency. Earlier observations by Vowels and colleagues[54] demonstrated that the malignant CD4+ T cells observed in most cases of MF/SS appear to exhibit a Th2 phenotype (Fig. 25.3). In vitro stimulation of peripheral blood cells derived from SS patients routinely results in increased levels of measurable IL-4 expression.[54] Furthermore, Vowels et al. demonstrated levels of IL-4 and IL-5 mRNA in clinically involved skin, even among patients with early patches or plaques, while uninvolved skin and the skin of normal volunteers did not have detectable levels of Th2 cytokine mRNA.[55] Increasing levels of IL-10 mRNA in parallel with an increasing density of the malignant T-cell infiltrate as lesions progressed from patch to plaque to tumor has also been demonstrated.[56] cDNA microarray analysis of the malignant T cells isolated from patients with SS have shown that the Th2 cell–specific transcription factors such as GATA-3 and Jun B are highly overexpressed.[25] Thus, despite evidence of a vigorous host response

in skin lesions in early disease, characterized by the presence of interferon-α (IFN-α)–secreting CD8+/TiA-1+ T cells,[57] the chronic production of Th2 cytokines such IL-4, IL-5, and IL-10 by the malignant T-cell population likely represents one mechanism by which the tumor cells circumvent the antitumor immune response.

The host antitumor response, although effete, may play a small role in containment of disease progression, even among those with advanced disease. This is supported by the observation of rapid progression of SS associated with the use of immunosuppressive agents such as cyclosporine.[58] In addition to enhanced Th2 cytokine production during disease progression, patients with circulating malignant T cells also manifest defects in Th1 cytokine production. Wysocka et al.[59] observed a progressive decline in the production of IL-12 and IFN-α by peripheral blood cells that correlated with an increase in the peripheral blood burden of malignant T cells.[59] Furthermore, the decline in production of these cytokines appeared to be linked to a decline in the numbers of peripheral blood myeloid and plasmacytoid DCs, respectively. Accompanying the decrease in DCs and a defect in IL-12 production is a deficit in production of other products of myeloid DCs, including IL-15, which is an important IFN-α–stimulating agent and powerful booster of Th1 responses. In contrast, however, Yamanaka et al.[60] observed increased serum IL-18 and IL-18 mRNA within CTCL skin

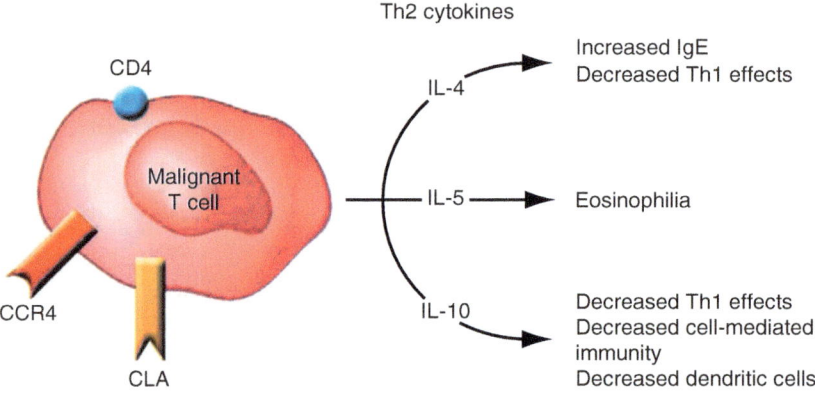

FIG. 25.3. The malignant T cell in MF/SS expresses CD4/CLA/CCR4/CCR10 and produces the cytokines IL-4/IL-5/IL-10, which results in Th2 predominance and subsequent multiple abnormalities in cellular immunity. (From Kim et al.,[5] with permission of the American Society for Clinical Investigation. Copyright 2005.)

samples, suggesting alternative potential sources for this IFN-inducing cytokine. Nevertheless, peripheral blood cells of SS patients clearly manifest marked decreases in IFN-α production.[54]

Intense interest has recently focused on the possible contributory role of T-regulatory (T_{reg}) cells in the endogenous immunosuppression in advanced CTCL. Berger and colleagues[61] have demonstrated that under certain conditions the malignant T cells may assume properties of T_{reg}s, including the expression of Foxp3 and production of transforming growth factor-β (TGF-β) and IL-10.[61] Similarly, Walsh et al.[62] were able to demonstrate increased Foxp3 expression among the peripheral blood cells of some patients with SS and among the circulating cells of all patients with HTLV-1–associated CTCL. The cells of such patients were found to produce increased concentrations of TGF-β. Wong et al.[63] observed increased expression of CTLA-4 upon activation of the circulating cells of patients with CTCL, indicating that this molecule, which is typically associated with T_{reg}s, was upregulated and a sign of increased numbers of T_{reg} cells. These findings remain controversial, as Tiemessen et al.[64] observed that the Foxp3-positive T_{reg}s of some CTCL patients are dysfunctional and exhibit a reduced ability to inhibit the proliferation of CD4+/CD25− T cells, while Yamano and colleagues[65] have made similar observations in regard to HTLV-1 infected CD4+ cells. Despite these disparate findings, many investigators involved in studies of the immunobiology of CTCL feel that T_{reg}s likely play some role in the pathogenesis of the immune suppression. Thus, as discussed below, elimination of T_{reg}s is just one of several new therapeutic strategies under investigation.

Other mechanisms that could account for abnormalities in DC maturation, and thus for diminished IL-12 production, have been highlighted by recent studies by French et al.,[66] which demonstrated a defect in expression of CD40 ligand upon activation of malignant T cells derived from patients with SS. CD40 ligand is not expressed on resting T cells but is normally upregulated on the cell surface upon engagement of the TCR. By contrast, malignant CD4+/CD7− T cells fail to express CD40 ligand upon engagement of the TCR by anti-CD3. Clearly, the absence of CD40 ligand interaction with CD40 on antigen-presenting cells (APCs) during an immune response can lead to a profound reduction in DC activation and cytokine production. Through the in vitro addition of recombinant hexameric CD40 ligand, French and colleagues demonstrated reconstitution of IL-12 and tumor necrosis factor (TNF) production by the cells of patients with SS. These findings provide obvious insights regarding potential strategies for correcting defects in immune dysregulation related to diminished numbers and function of DCs associated with advancing MF/SS.

Derangements in T-cell diversity may also play a role in the immune suppression of CTCL. Yawalkar et al., using β-variable complementarity-determining region 3 spectratyping, determined that patients with both early as well as late disease exhibit loss of the normal T-cell repertoire.[67,68] These findings are reminiscent of a chronic retroviral infection, as similar observations have been made in HIV infection. Loss of T-cell repertoire may partially account for the failure of advanced-stage CTCL patients to respond normally to a variety of antigens.

The result of the diverse abnormalities of DC and T-cell function during progressive MF/SS is multiple abnormalities in cellular immunity (Fig. 25.4). Marked defects in cellular cytotoxicity occur that correlate with the burden of circulating malignant T cells.[69] Progression from early to more advanced MF/SS is typically associated with a marked decline in natural killer (NK) cell numbers and activity that could partially be due to a decline in myeloid DC production of IL-15, which is critical for the normal growth of these cells. Similarly, a decline in the number of peripheral blood CD8+ T cells accompanies an increasing burden of circulating malignant T cells. Furthermore, the percentage of these cytotoxic cells that express activation markers, such as CD69, is also significantly reduced compared to NK and CD8+ T cells from MF patients without overt peripheral blood involvement.[70] A reduction in the number of functioning NK and CD8+ T cells is almost certainly associated with a deterioration of both host antitumor immunity and immune surveillance against microbial organisms. Examples of these phenomena include infections such as disseminated herpes simplex/zoster or progressive multifocal leukoencephalopathy among SS patients who have never been iatrogenically immunosuppressed by chemotherapy or other immunosuppressive medications.[7,71,72] As mentioned earlier, other malignant neoplasms, includ-

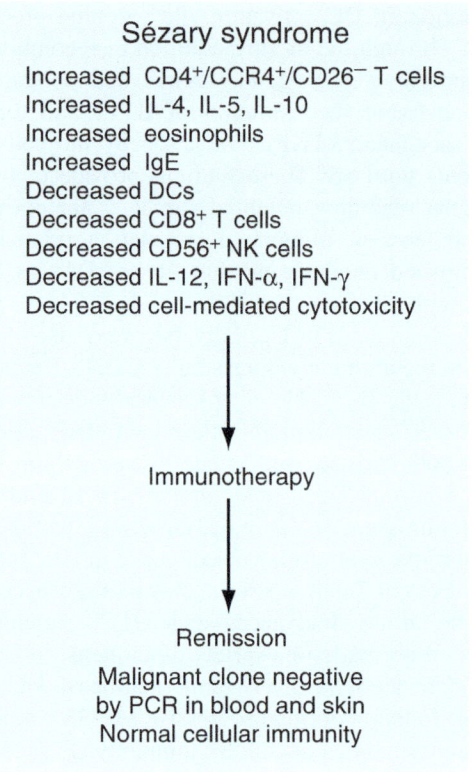

Sézary syndrome

Increased CD4+/CCR4+/CD26⁻ T cells
Increased IL-4, IL-5, IL-10
Increased eosinophils
Increased IgE
Decreased DCs
Decreased CD8+ T cells
Decreased CD56+ NK cells
Decreased IL-12, IFN-α, IFN-γ
Decreased cell-mediated cytotoxicity

Immunotherapy

Remission
Malignant clone negative
by PCR in blood and skin
Normal cellular immunity

Fig. 25.4. Elimination of the malignant T-cell clone during immunotherapy leads to a restoration of a normal immune response. Studies of numerous patients with SS have demonstrated that induction of complete remission with clearing of the malignant T-cell clone during multimodality immunotherapy leads to a restoration of normal host immune function. (From Kim et al.,[5] with permission of the American Society for Clinical Investigation. Copyright 2005.)

ing melanoma and nonmelanoma skin cancers as well as Hodgkin's lymphoma also appear to be more common in MF/SS patients independent of the history of previous predisposing therapy (such as phototherapy or radiation therapy).[9,73,74] These findings reflect an overall impairment in immune surveillance against cancer.

Other characteristic immunologic findings associated with the progression of MF/SS include development of peripheral eosinophilia and elevated levels of serum IgE.[54,75] Peripheral eosinophilia has been determined to be an independent marker for poor prognosis and disease progression.[76] In one study, peripheral blood cells from patients with SS and eosinophilia produced markedly higher levels of

IL-5 upon stimulation than did the cells of patients or normal volunteers without eosinophilia.[77] A finding of importance in this study indicated that culture of the patients' cells with either recombinant IFN-α or IL-12 significantly inhibited the excess production of IL-5. These observations suggest that these cytokines could be useful therapeutic tools to prevent continued proliferation of eosinophils under the influence of IL-5, thus possibly preventing at least some of the adverse effects associated with high eosinophil counts.

It is particularly noteworthy that after successful treatment of SS with immunotherapeutic agents, with resolution of evidence for skin disease and disappearance of the malignant clone from the blood, virtually all abnormal immune parameters are restored to normalcy (Fig. 25.4).[69] One implication of these observations is that the malignant clone is likely responsible for much of the immune dysregulation that occurs in SS. Moreover, these findings indicate that SS patients who experience remission will have their immune system at least partially reconstituted. Thus, such patients should be less likely to experience severe consequences of microbial infection in comparison to those with advanced SS.

Treatment

Treatment of MF/SS can be divided into two major categories: skin-directed therapies (SDTs) and systemic therapies. As listed in Table 25.4, there are numerous options. Therapeutic approaches can vary widely from center to center, and the availability of many newer therapies varies among countries. It is useful to divide the discussion of therapies into those for early-stage disease and those for late-stage disease (Table 25.5).

Early Stage

It has become quite clear during the past several decades that traditional systemic chemotherapy has not resulted in durable remissions in MF/SS.[1] As a consequence, emerging therapeutic efforts have focused on targeted biologic agents and immune modifications using a multimodality approach. Numerous arms of the immune system must cooperate to generate a sufficient host antitumor response

TABLE 25.4. Treatment options in MF/SS.

Therapy	Mechanism of action
Skin-directed therapy	
Topical corticosteroids	Tumor cell apoptosis, decrease skin LCs
Topical chemotherapy (nitrogen mustard, BCNU)	Tumor cell apoptosis
Topical retinoids (bexarotene, tazarotene)	Tumor cell apoptosis
Topical imiquimod	TLR7 agonist, triggers innate and adaptive antitumor immunity
Phototherapy (UVB, PUVA, excimer laser)	Tumor cell apoptosis
	Decrease skin LCs
Electron-beam therapy (EBT)	Tumor cell apoptosis
Biologic therapy	
RXR retinoid (bexarotene)	Tumor cell apoptosis
	Inhibit tumor cell IL-4 production
RAR retinoid (isotretinoin, all-*trans* retinoic acid)	Tumor cell apoptosis
	Induce interferon-γ
Interferons (alpha, gamma)	Enhanced cell-mediated cytotoxicity
	Inhibit tumor cell Th2 cytokine production
GM-CSF	Enhanced circulating dendritic cell numbers and function
Extracorporeal photopheresis	Circulating tumor cell apoptosis
	Induction of DC differentiation
Fusion protein/toxin (denileukin diftitox)	Targets and kills CD25 (IL-2 receptor) expressing tumor cells.
Histone deacetylase inhibitors (vorinostat, romidepsin)	Affects tumor cell gene transcription, non-histone effects.
Other systemic therapy	
Cytotoxic chemotherapy (MTX, pegylated doxorubicin, gemcitabine, etoposide, pentostatin)	Cytotoxic agents
Hematopoietic stem cell transplantation (allogeneic)	Cytotoxic agents (induction)
	Graft-vs-tumor effect
Experimental therapy	
Transimmunization ECP	Enhances DCs antigen processing of apoptotic tumor cells
Targeted monoclonal antibodies (CD4, CD52, CD40, CCR4)	Targets tumor cells (CD4, CD52, CCR4)
	Activates dendritic cells (CD40)
Cytokines (IL12, IL2, IL15)	Augments cell mediated antitumor immunity
Toll-like receptor agonists (CpG-ODN, imidazoquinolones)	TLR agonists, augment innate and adaptive antitumor immunity
Tumor vaccines	Clonotypic TCR as antigen
	Dendritic cell–based vaccines

Source: Kim et al.,[5] with permission of the American Society for Clinical Investigation. Copyright 2005.

such that the proliferation of the malignant T-cell population in MF/SS patients can be controlled and, ideally, eradicated (Fig. 25.5).

Patients with patches or plaques limited to less than 10% of the skin surface area (stage IA or T1 disease) tend to exhibit normal cellular immune responses. Therefore, use of skin-directed therapies, including topical chemotherapy,[78,79] superpotent topical corticosteroids, topical retinoid application,[80]

psoralen plus ultraviolet A phototherapy (PUVA),[81,82] or electron-beam radiation therapy,[83] which target the tumor burden in the skin by directly inducing apoptosis of malignant T cells, is often sufficient to induce complete clearing of disease. At this stage, the systemic immune response is intact, and it may contribute to controlling disease burden from going beyond the skin. In the event that clearing is not complete, the addition of a single-agent systemic

TABLE 25.5. Treatment of MF/SS by clinical stage.

Stage	Initial therapy	Subsequent therapy	Therapy for refractory disease
IA (early stage)	Skin-directed therapies		
IB/IIA	Topical chemotherapy Phototherapy Electron-beam therapy (+/− low dose biologic agents)	Interferons Retinoids Multimodality rx • Topical chemo + biologic agent • Phototherapy + biologic agent • Two biologic agents Denileukin diftitox Histone deacetylase inhibitors	Experimental therapies
IIB (advanced stage)	Few tumors • Localized EBT • Intralesional IFN • Topical chemotherapy + biologic agent Generalized tumors • Total skin EBT • Denileukin diftitox • Multimodality therapies	Multimodality therapy Denileukin diftitox Histone deacetylase inhibitors Single-agent chemotherapy	Experimental therapies
IIIA, B	PUVA Retinoids Interferons Methotrexate ECP Histone deacetylase inhibitors Multimodality therapies	Multimodality therapies Denileukin diftitox Histone deacetylase inhibitors Single-agent chemotherapy	Experimental therapies
IVA, B	Single agent systemic therapy Multimodality therapy (+ skin-directed therapy)	Adjuvant palliative local radiation for extracutaneous disease Bone marrow/stem cell transplant Chemotherapy	Experimental therapies

Source: Kim et al.,[5] with permission of the American Society for Clinical Investigation. Copyright 2005.

immunomodulator, such as recombinant IFN-α or the retinoid bexarotene (Targretin), typically leads to a better clinical response.

For patients who do not yet manifest overt peripheral blood disease but who exhibit more extensively infiltrated cutaneous plaques or a greater extent of skin surface area involvement, multimodality therapeutic approaches appear to result in more rapid responses.[84–87] Interferon-α, produced by plasmacytoid DCs, is a product of the innate immune response, and appears to be one of the most highly active biologic agents used in the therapy of MF/SS.[88] It is now well accepted that PUVA plus IFN-α administration can produce higher clinical response rates than the use of PUVA alone.[87,89,90] Several small studies have also suggested that a combination of IFN-α with oral retinoids, including bexarotene or 13-cis retinoic acid, may induce rapid responses among patients with extensive skin lesions.[84,91]

Mechanistically, IFN-α induces a variety of beneficial effects on the host immune response that may lead to disease clearing. It directly enhances cell-mediated cytotoxicity; both CD8[+] T cells and CD56[+] NK cells exhibit rapid activation as assessed by upregulation of CD69, and the cytotoxic effects

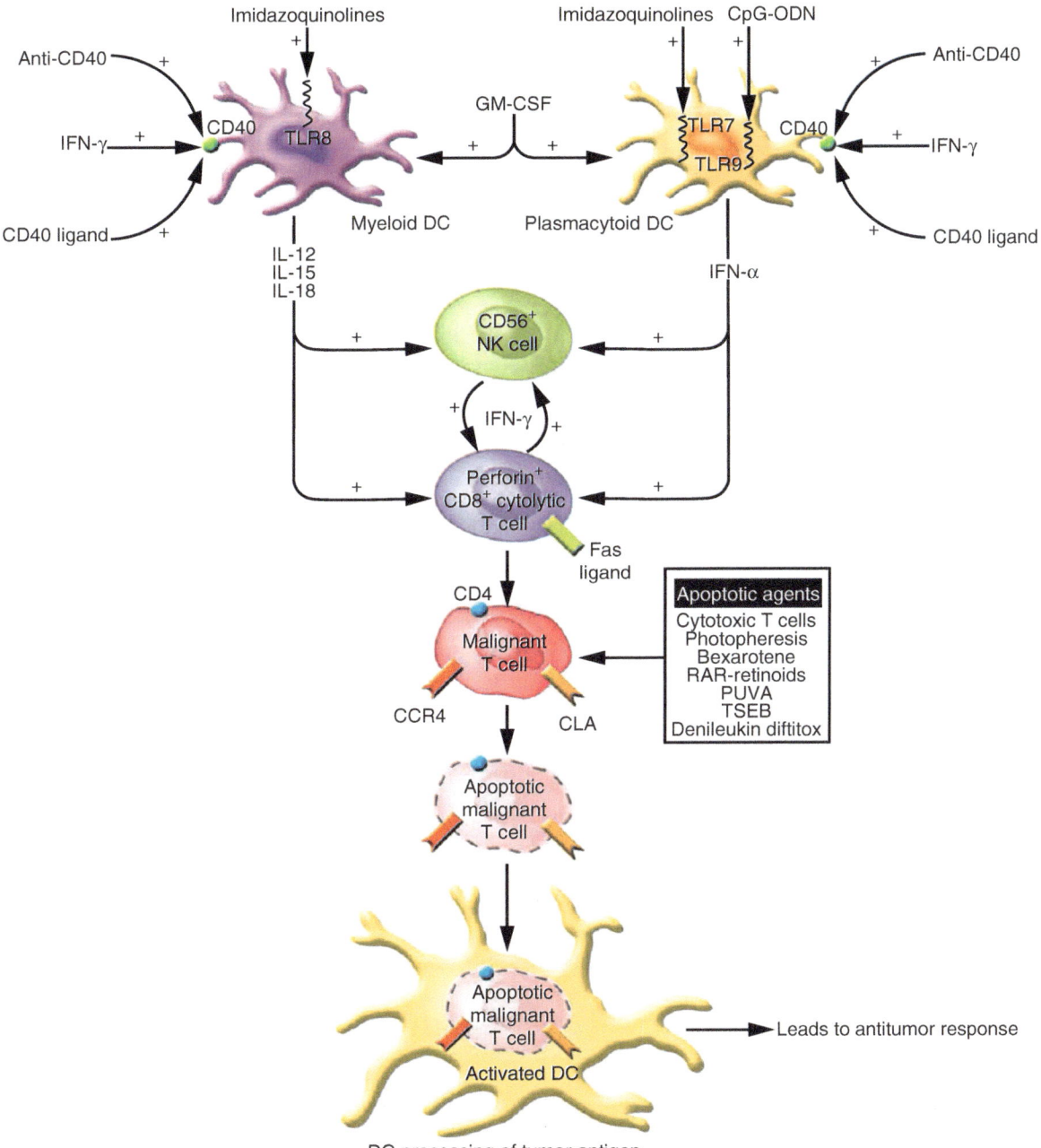

FIG. 25.5. Multimodality strategy for enhancing the antitumor response using immunotherapeutics. A multimodality approach encompasses the activation of multiple arms of the immune response through the use of agents to activate DCs, CTLs (CD8+), and NK cells (CD56+). Granulocyte-macrophage colony-stimulating factor (GM-CSF) may enhance the numbers of DCs while agents that enhance CD40 expression (IFN-γ) and activation (CD40 ligand; activating anti-CD40 antibody) and TLR ligands (CpG-ODNs; imidazoquinolines) lead to DC cytokine production and to enhanced DC processing of apoptotic malignant T cells. Cytokines produced by DCs as well as exogenously administered cytokines augment CD8+ T-cell cytokine production. Proapoptotic agents, including bexarotene, RAR-specific retinoids, PUVA, photopheresis, topical chemotherapy, total skin electron beam irradiation (TSEB), and denileukin diftitox can assist in the development of an antitumor immune response by reducing the overall tumor burden and by providing a source of apoptotic malignant cells and tumor antigens for uptake by DCs. (From Kim et al.,[5] with permission of the American Society for Clinical Investigation. Copyright 2005.)

of NK cells are significantly boosted.[70] Interferon-α also suppresses Th2 cytokine production by malignant T cells, which may lead to abrogation of the suppressive effects of IL-4 and IL-10 on antitumor immunity

Bexarotene, which recently received Food and Drug Administration (FDA) approval, is a retinoid X receptor–specific compound that has also been determined to have valuable immunomodulatory effects that are of benefit in the treatment of MF/SS, particularly when used in combination therapy. Bexarotene has the ability to induce apoptosis within the malignant population of T cells.[92,93] This effect may account for the nearly 50% response rate of MF/SS patients when high-dose, single-agent oral bexarotene is administered.[94] Nevertheless, Budgin et al.[93] have demonstrated that although the malignant cells of most patients with SS are susceptible to the apoptotic effects of bexarotene in vitro, purified Sézary cells from approximately one third of patients demonstrate significant resistance to apoptosis.[93] This finding may account for the failure of a subset of patients to respond clinically to this compound. Furthermore, recent observations suggest that chronic bexarotene use may be associated with emergence of malignant clones of T cells that lack the specific RXR-responsive receptor and that exhibit resistance to the apoptotic effects of this retinoid.[94a] In regard to cytokine production, bexarotene has the capacity to inhibit IL-4 production, and possibly other Th2 cytokines, in vitro by stimulated peripheral blood cells of SS patients. The net effect would be to negate the suppressive effects of these cytokines on cellular immunity.

In contrast to bexarotene, retinoic acid receptor (RAR)-specific retinoids may have modest direct immune potentiating properties. Using a number of different RAR-specific retinoids, including all-*trans*-retinoic acid and 13-*cis*-retinoic acid, Fox et al.[95] demonstrated that these compounds exhibited the capacity to induce IL-12–dependent IFN-α production.[95] Moreover, synergistic production of IFN-α occurred when low concentrations of IL-2 were added to the RAR-specific retinoids. In contrast, bexarotene does not induce IFN-α production.[93] These findings support the use of an RAR-specific retinoid as another component of the combined therapeutic approach.

Late Stage

Current Therapies

In contrast to patients with early-stage MF, patients with late-stage MF/SS exhibit a broad array of abnormalities affecting every arm of the immune response that participates in antitumor immunity (CD8+ T cells, NK cells, and DCs). Thus, more aggressive therapy is required to adequately restore the host immune response. Accordingly, evidence is now emerging that multimodality immunotherapy can frequently induce complete clinical responses in advanced disease that are both durable and sufficient to eradicate the malignant clone.[69,96,97]

Central to the strategy for elimination of the malignant T-cell population is the use of agents that can induce apoptosis of these cells while simultaneously enhancing the host's ability to process the apoptotic cells so that a robust cytotoxic T-cell response can be generated. For patients with circulating malignant T cells, extracorporeal photopheresis (ECP) can result in massive apoptosis of cells within this compartment.[98,99] Extracorporeal photopheresis is an FDA-approved leukapheresis procedure for the treatment of SS in which approximately 10^{10} peripheral blood mononuclear cells are collected from the patient, treated with 8-methoxypsoralen, exposed to 1 to 2 joules of ultraviolet A light in the photopheresis machine, and re-infused back to the patient. In addition to inducing malignant T-cell apoptosis, ECP also induces monocyte differentiation into DCs capable of phagocytosing and processing the apoptotic tumor cell antigens.[100] Repeated cycles of ECP for two consecutive days every 3 to 4 weeks with readministration of the treated cells is occasionally sufficient to induce a complete clinical response in SS. One potential modification to ECP, called transimmunization, is currently being studied and has completed phase I clinical trial testing; during ECP, the apoptotic malignant T cells and the newly formed DCs are co-incubated prior to re-infusion to optimize the above antigen processing and more efficient induction of tumor-targeted immunity.[100]

Nevertheless, administration of large numbers of apoptotic cells as generated by ECP can compromise dendritic cell functions, including cytokine production, and therefore, has the potential to exacerbate the preexisting immune-depressed state.[101] Such observations support the rationale for the adjunctive use of multiple agents that can enhance both the afferent immune response (events related to processing of apoptotic malignant cells) as well as the efferent response (direct cytolytic attack on the tumor cells).

In support of this approach, Richardson and colleagues[96] have recently demonstrated high response rates of SS patients when ECP was combined with the administration of multiple immune adjuvants. As part of this regimen, IFN-α and bexarotene were routinely used in combination with ECP. In some cases, granulocyte-macrophage colony-stimulating factor (GM-CSF) was administered following each ECP treatment to enhance APC function. The monthly administration of 125 μg of GM-CSF on two consecutive days resulted in significant increases in circulating DC numbers compared to DC numbers in ECP-treated SS patients who did not received GM-CSF.[59] In one patient, administration of GM-CSF three times per week for 6 months resulted in the persistent normalization of DC numbers, indicating that APC functions might be markedly augmented in this patient population with the long-term use of GM-CSF.

In addition to IFN-α, additional approaches to enhance the effector phase of antitumor immunity are presently being utilized. Although limited results have been reported following the administration of recombinant IFN-γ, recent evidence suggests that it has significant potential for the treatment of MF/SS and it is clearly well tolerated, particularly by the elderly who experience frequent cognitive dysfunction and fatigue with IFN-α treatment.[102–104] In addition to enhancing the cytolytic lymphocyte function of patients with MF/SS, IFN-γ suppresses the excess cytokine production, enhances CD40 expression, and primes their abnormal DCs for IL-12 and IL-15 production, particularly in response to CD40 ligation[59] and Toll-like receptor agonistic stimulation.[105] In our Cutaneou s Lymphoma Program at the University of Pennsylvania, when possible we are presently routinely using IFN-γ for SS patients who appear to be refractory to IFN-α. In several cases, addition of IFN-γ to a multimodality regimen that included photopheresis and bexarotene appeared to be associated with the induction of a sustained complete clinical response.[103,104]

Alternative routes exist for the administration of IFN-γ. In a small pilot study, Dummer and colleagues[106] have demonstrated clinical efficacy of IFN-γ cDNA administered subcutaneously in an adenoviral vector. The local intralesional injection resulted in significant responses rates of individual lesions in both MF and SS patients. Moreover, elevated serum levels of IFN-γ were observed and appeared to be associated with regression of lesions distant from the injection sites. This study further suggests that elevation of IFN-γ levels can beneficially alter disease progression.

Removal of the Immunologic Brake: Elimination of T_{reg} Activity

As indicated above, increasing evidence exists for the role of enhanced CD4⁺CD25⁺ T_{reg} function in CTCL as a contributory mechanism for depressed cellular immunity.[61,62] Although strategies for the elimination of suppressor activity in MF/SS remain untested, several potential approaches are possible. Currently, denileukin diftitox (Ontak), a diphtheria toxin–IL-2 protein conjugate, is available for targeting IL-2 receptor–bearing T cells.[107] After binding to the IL-2 receptor, it undergoes endocytosis followed by release of the diphtheria toxin, which results in arrest of protein synthesis and, ultimately, apoptosis of T cells. Intravenous administration of denileukin diftitox to patients with MF results in the regression of plaques and tumors.[108] Its major mechanism of action is thought to be mediated by direct killing of malignant T cells. However, it is entirely possible that at least a portion of its activity is mediated through the elimination of CD25-bearing T_{reg}s as suggested during recent studies of ovarian cancer treatment.[109]

Because T_{reg}s express CTLA-4, another potential approach to their inhibition is through the use of anti–CTLA-4 antibody.[110] This therapeutic approach, although promising for metastatic melanoma,[111] remains untested so far for CTCL. T_{reg}s may also suppress immunoreactivity by production of IL-10 or TGF-β. Antibodies with neutralizing activity for these factors could be utilized to reverse their inhibitory effects on the immune response.

Experimental Therapy

Numerous alternative strategies exist for the enhancement of antigen-presenting cell function. These include the administration of a variety of

Toll-like receptor (TLR) agonists, which are presently in clinical development.[112,113] Imiquimod, a member of the imidazoquinoline family, which is presently FDA approved to treat basal cell carcinoma, actinic keratoses, and condyloma, has recently been demonstrated to have substantial clinical activity when applied topically to skin lesions of MF patients.[114,115] Imiquimod potently triggers TLR7, expressed on plasmacytoid DCs, which results in IFN-α and TNF-α production.[116,117] Imiquimod may also directly induce cells of some tumor types to undergo apoptosis.[118]

Several newer members of the imidazoquinoline family have the capacity to trigger TLR8 in addition to TLR7.[119] This would be expected to result in a broader activation of both myeloid as well as plasmacytoid DCs with the release of a more extensive array of immune activating cytokines, including IL-12, IL-15, IL-18, and IFN-α. Because T_{reg}s also express TLR8, triggering of this receptor by the appropriate ligand can lead to inhibition of these suppressive cells, the net effect being immune augmentation. Thus, such compounds would likely broadly activate multiple compartments of the immune response and make them highly desirable compounds to use as systemic therapeutic agents either alone or as part of a multimodality approach.

Recent clinical trials have tested the effects of an alternative class of DC-activating agents, synthetic oligodeoxynucleotides that contain CpG motifs (CpG-ODNs). CpG-ODNs have been recognized as immune stimulatory agents through their activation of DCs following binding to TLR9 expressed on plasmacytoid DCs.[120] The immunostimulatory potential of CpG-ODNs has been tested in murine tumor models and has been observed to lead to the generation of strong antitumor T-cell responses, resulting in complete remission of certain established solid tumors.[121] Thus, there is substantial rationale to study the activity of CpG-ODNs in human tumor systems. In this regard, in vitro data indicate that CpG-ODNs can potently activate CTCL patients' DCs, leading to IFN-α production, increased expression of critical immune accessory molecules, and enhanced cell-mediated cytotoxicity.[70] Moreover, Kim and colleagues[122] have shown in a phase II clinical trial for refractory advanced CTCL that CpG-ODNs administered subcutaneously as a single agent demonstrate therapeutic

efficacy, in some cases inducing complete clinical responses in advanced stage patients. Therefore, application of CpG-ODNs in a multimodality therapeutic approach that uses photopheresis or transimmunization might also yield significant therapeutic benefit. It is noteworthy that antiviral vaccination strategies that incorporate the use of CpG-ODNs along with viral antigen appear to be markedly superior to those that use antigen alone.[123] Since ECP represents an immunization procedure utilizing apoptotic tumor cells, such findings support the use of CpG-ODNs at the time of re-infusion of the treated tumor cells in an effort to directly target the tumor antigens to DCs for processing.

Other mechanisms for activating the DCs of patients with MF/SS that are under preclinical investigation include strategies for the engagement of CD40. As stressed above, there is substantial evidence that a defect in CD40 ligand expression by malignant T cells plays some role in the depressed production of DC-dependent cytokines.[66] Furthermore, coculture of peripheral blood cells of SS patients with hexameric recombinant CD40 ligand resulted in substantial production of IL-12. Clinical trials using this approach have yet to be undertaken. Another strategy that appears promising for the treatment of solid tumors but that awaits clinical testing for CTCL, involves the use of an activating anti-CD40 antibody. Animal models using this approach indicate that enhanced generation of tumor-specific T cells can occur.[124,125]

Interleukin-12 is a cytokine known to induce IFN-α release and to enhance cytolytic T cell and NK cell activities, and thus has the potential to enhance the antitumor immune response of MF/SS patients. In a small phase I study followed by a limited phase II study, the subcutaneous administration of recombinant IL-12 to a total of 32 patients with MF resulted in approximately a 50% response rate.[126,127] Since malignant T cells lack the IL-12 β_2 receptor[128] and are thus incapable of signaling in response to IL-12, it is presumed that the clinical response was not due to the direct effects of the cytokine on the malignant cells. Indeed, serial biopsies of cutaneous plaques during treatment revealed dense infiltrates of CD8+ T cells that appeared near the time of initial signs of lesional regression.[126] Thus, it is believed that CD8+ T cells with augmented cytolytic activity are the predominant "workhorses" activated in response to IL-12. Whether IL-12 administration has advantages over IFN-α use is presently unknown, but it is hoped that in the future, IL-12 will also find its place in a multimodality therapeutic approach.

Future Strategies for Enhancing the Host Immune Response

Tumor Vaccines

Most vaccination strategies for MF/SS utilize the clonotypic TCR as a source of tumor-specific antigen. Immunogenic epitopes are found within both the variable (V-region) and the constant (C-region) regions of the clonotypic TCR-α and TCR-β receptor.[129,130] In some experiments, immunogenic peptides have been directly isolated from the major histocompatibility complex (MHC) class I molecules on the surface of the malignant clone. This confirms that the antigen-processing pathway for endogenous proteins remains intact in the malignant clone, and that the clonotypic TCR is subjected to antigen processing and presentation by MHC class I. Consequently, the TCR peptide-MHC complex on the surface of a malignant cell can serve as a target for recognition by CD8+ CTLs (cytolytic T-cell lymphocyte). This has been demonstrated in both normal donors and patients with MF/SS, where immunogenic peptides derived from the clonotypic TCR induced tumor-specific CD8+ T cells that were capable of secreting TNF-α,[129] as well as lysing autologous tumor cells in vitro.[130]

Dendritic-cell–based vaccines have also been developed for CTCL.[131] Sources of antigen used to pulse DCs prior to vaccination may include tumor-cell lysates, peptides, "mimotopes," tumor-derived DNA or RNA, apoptotic tumor cells and even tumor cell–DC fusions. Maier et al.[132] reported on 10 CTCL patients treated with weekly intranodal injections of autologous DCs pulsed with tumor lysate. In this study, 50% of patients had a clinical response to the vaccine, accompanied by an infiltration of CD8+ and TIA-1+ cytotoxic cells at the site of regressing lesions as well as molecular remission in some cases. Of note, clinical responses in this study were associated with a low tumor burden, which underscores the importance of instituting immunotherapy early in the course of the disease and prior to the development of significant immune dysregulation.

The addition of an immune adjuvant(s) may be used in an attempt to enhance the efficacy of the vaccine. Cytokines such as IL-12,[126,133] IL-15,[70,134] IL-18,[135] and IL-21[136] can augment the development, the effectiveness, and the maintenance of antitumor CTL responses. Moreover, these same cytokines have also been shown to enhance NK-cell activity, which may play an important role in controlling tumor growth in vivo. Granulocyte-macrophage colony-stimulating factor is another cytokine that has been used as a cancer vaccine adjuvant to enhance both the number and function of dendritic cells.[137,138] As discussed earlier, other immune activating agents including TLR agonists (i.e., imidazoquinolines, CPG-ODNs), anti-CD40, and anti-CTLA-4 could be used in conjunction with a tumor vaccine for patients with CTCL.

Monoclonal Antibodies

Monoclonal antibodies and fusion toxins directed against a variety of cell-surface markers have been tested in patients with SS/MF. In addition to denileukin diftitox as described earlier, examples of such antibodies include anti-CD4 (zanolimumab, currently in pivotal phase II clinical trials)[139] and anti-CD52 (alemtuzumab).[140,141] These two agents have direct potent antitumor activity; anti-CD52 mAb treatment has been associated with prolonged immunosuppression and 20% risk of opportunistic infections as it also removes DCs, monocytes, NK, and B cells.

Chemokine receptors and their ligands may serve as potential targets for antitumor therapy in MF/SS. Antibody-based therapeutics targeting chemokine receptors and compounds with the potential to downregulate chemokine receptor expression hold great promise as potential therapies. A novel humanized-CCR4 monoclonal antibody has recently been developed and is currently being investigated as a potential therapeutic for the treatment of patients with CCR4+ T-cell leukemia/lymphoma.[142] The CCR4+ cells in these conditions have been shown to exhibit features of regulatory T cells with the ability to suppress antitumor immune responses. In addition to lysing CCR4+ T cells in vitro, this antibody reduced the expression of Foxp3 mRNA suggesting a possible role in depleting T_{reg}s.[143] It is plausible that this antibody may potentially serve as a therapeutic modality for the treatment of CTCL patients with advanced disease among which the majority of malignant cells express CCR4.

As mentioned earlier, IFN-α can be combined with other biologic response modifiers to achieve high clinical response rates among SS patients.[96] In addition to its ability to enhance cell-mediated cytolytic activity and suppress Th2 cytokine production, IFN-α may also significantly increase production of the Th1 associated chemokine, monokine induced by interferon-γ (Mig), a CXC chemokine recognized by CXCR3.[144] Aside from its expression by MF cells in early-stage disease (as discussed earlier), it is also expressed by cytotoxic T cells, and thus contributes to the accumulation of tumoricidal cytolytic T cells in lesional skin.

In recent work, we have observed the ability of the rexinoid bexarotene to preferentially decrease CCR4 levels among malignant cells in vitro.[145] This reduction was associated with a decrease in malignant cell chemotaxis in response to TARC. Our findings, may in part, explain the marked clearing of cutaneous erythroderma we have noted among patients treated with this therapeutic agent,[146] and suggest a potential role for such compounds in the management of inflammatory and neoplastic diseases of the skin in the near future.

Histone Deacetylase Inhibitors

Histone deacetylase (HDAC) inhibitors represent a novel class of compounds that modulate gene expression by shifting the balance toward acetylation of nucleosomal histones.[147] Compounds such as suberoylanilide hydroxyamic acid[147,148] and depsipeptide (FK228/romidepsin)[149–151] have been shown to induce differentiation or apoptosis of malignant lymphocytes. HDAC inhibitors also likely affect nonhistone targets that may contribute to their antitumor effects. Suberoylanilide hydroxamic acid (vorinostat/Zolinza) was FDA approved in late 2006 for the treatment of refractory CTCL,[152] and romidepsin is currently in phase II clinical trials. In addition, recent data indicate that HDAC inhibitors may upregulate the expression of the IL-2 receptor on malignant T cells, resulting in enhanced susceptibility to killing by denileukin diftitox.[150,153] Some evidence exists

suggesting that HDAC inhibitors may stimulate the induction of T_{reg}s, thus leading to heightened immune suppression. One manifestation of this effect may be the increased frequency of reactivation of herpes viruses during therapy. However, the overall immunologic effects of the HDAC inhibitors remains to be elucidated.

Stem Cell Transplant Therapy

Advanced-stage CTCL patients, with multiple tumors, erythroderma, or reticuloendothelial system involvement who are refractory to the above therapies, are increasingly being considered for hematopoietic stem cell transplantation (HSCT). Originally, HSCT was conceived as a replacement for a patient's own diseased hematopoietic system, which theoretically had been destroyed by a pretransplant regimen of chemoradiation. This concept of eliminating the abnormal cells and supporting hematopoiesis with transplanted stem cells continues to be the basis for autologous stem cell transplants, in which patients' own reserved stem cells are returned after chemoradiation. In fact, some authors support *high-dose chemotherapy with hematopoietic progenitor cell support* as a more appropriate term for autologous stem cell transplant.[154]

However, allogeneic HSCT has evolved conceptually into an immunologic therapy with the observation that donor transplanted T cells can elicit a graft-versus-tumor effect against the host's tumor cells.[155] The immunologic basis of the disorder graft-versus-host disease (GVHD), which causes a significant amount of transplant-related morbidity and mortality, also supports the concept that the engrafted immune system, even when human leukocyte antigen (HLA) matched, is active against host tissue.[154] Based on this model, investigators have employed strategies of pre- and posttransplant immunosuppression that are less toxic to the host's other organ systems and have had success with nonmyeloablative conditioning regimens for allogeneic stem cell transplants.[156] A truly nonmyeloablative conditioning regimen results in mixed chimerism of both donor and host hematopoiesis posttransplant, and it allows for transplantation in elderly patients and those with comorbidities that may not survive the pancytopenia and organ toxicities that accompany a myeloablative transplant.

Stem cell transplants have achieved long-term complete responses in many types of hematologic malignancies, and there are reports of autologous and allogeneic, as well as myeloablative and non-myeloablative, stem cell transplants for advanced CTCL. In the two largest series of advanced MF/SS patients undergoing autologous stem cell transplant, almost all patients did achieve a complete response. However, out of 13 reported patients with a complete response, 12 relapsed, with the longest time to relapse being 14 months, and the median time to relapse in the larger study being 7 months.[157,158] Several other case reports of autologous stem cell transplant for advanced CTCL have been published, and although patients do achieve a safe and complete response overall, more than half of reported cases have relapsed within 6 months.[154] Active disease was present in all reported patients at the time of conditioning and transplant. Further studies are needed to elucidate if there might be a role for autologous stem cell transplant in advanced CTCL, but these early reports indicate relapse may be a significant problem limiting their use for this disease.

There have been 17 reported cases of allogeneic bone marrow transplant in advanced CTCL, and the small amount of data gathered so far indicates that if the patient and the graft are able to survive the transplant period, complete responses can be achieved and sustained.[159–164] All of these cases represented patients with MF or SS, with one exceptional case of an advanced cutaneous CD30⁻ large T-cell lymphoma.[164] All of the patients had active disease at the time of conditioning and transplantation and had been heavily pretreated, in many instances with multiple courses of cytotoxic chemotherapy. Of these reported cases, three patients died due to infections, similar to the reported mortality rate of 15% to 40% for other types of patients undergoing allogeneic stem cell transplant.[154] However, of 14 patients who have survived, complete responses have been maintained for as many as 9 years, and the single patient who was reported to have relapsed had her disease brought under good control after donor lymphocyte infusion.[162,163] These responses are evidence of a graft versus tumor effect, which in most cases is accompanied by some degree of GVHD. In all allogeneic stem cell transplant patients, a bal-ance between disease relapse and GVHD must be achieved using some degree of posttransplant immunosuppression. In the reported cases discussed here, 16 patients developed at least grade II acute GVHD. Information was available regarding chronic GVHD, which occurred in 11 cases, while two had no chronic GVHD and six had limited GVHD.[160,161,163,164] In some cases, patients have been able to discontinue immunosuppression entirely, without evidence of recurrent CTCL or GVHD.[163] More extensive studies are needed to assess the safety and efficacy of these promising therapies.

Conclusion

Cutaneous T-cell lymphoma is a skin-homing extranodal non-Hodgkin's lymphoma. It is a slowly progressive disease, in which cellular immunity gradually declines. The pathogenesis of the disease includes skin-homing malignant lymphocytes that become progressively more resistant to programmed cell death. Current therapies involve skin-directed treatments, systemic treatments, and immune adjuvants. Experimental treatments include dendritic cell–based immunization strategies against the TCR derived from malignant clones, as well as cytokine therapies such as IL-12.

References

1. Kaye FJ, et al. A randomized trial comparing combination electron-beam radiation and chemotherapy with topical therapy in the initial treatment of mycosis fungoides. N Engl J Med 1989;321(26):1784–90.
2. Willemze R, et al. WHO-EORTC classification for cutaneous lymphomas. Blood 2005;105(10):3768–85.
3. Morton LM, et al. Lymphoma incidence patterns by WHO subtype in the United States 1992–2001. Blood 2006;107(1):265–76.
3a. Criscione VD, Weinstock MA. Incidence of cutaneous T-cell lymphoma in the United States, 1973–2002. Arch Dermatol. 2007;143(7):854–9.
4. Girardi M, Heald PW, Wilson LD. The pathogenesis of mycosis fungoides. N Engl J Med 2004350(19):1978–88.
5. Kim EJ, et al. Immunopathogenesis and therapy of cutaneous T cell lymphoma. J Clin Invest 2005;115(4):798–812.

6. Kazakov DV, Burg G, Kempf W. Clinicopathological spectrum of mycosis fungoides. J Eur Acad Dermatol Venereol 2004;18(4):397–415.

7. Axelrod PI, Lorber B, Vonderheid EC. Infections complicating mycosis fungoides and Sezary syndrome. JAMA 1992;267(10):1354–8.

8. Liu HL, et al. CD30+ cutaneous lymphoproliferative disorders: the Stanford experience in lymphomatoid papulosis and primary cutaneous anaplastic large cell lymphoma. J Am Acad Dermatol 2003;49(6):1049–58.

9. Huang KP, et al. Second lymphomas and other malignant neoplasms in patients with mycosis fungoides and Sezary syndrome: evidence from population-based and clinical cohorts. Arch Dermatol 2007;143(1):45–50.

10. Wood GS, et al. Detection of clonal T-cell receptor gamma gene rearrangements in early mycosis fungoides/Sezary syndrome by polymerase chain reaction and denaturing gradient gel electrophoresis (PCR/DGGE). J Invest Dermatol 1994;103(1):34–41.

11. Pimpinelli N, et al. Defining early mycosis fungoides. J Am Acad Dermatol 2005;53(6):1053–63.

12. Ponti R, et al. T-cell receptor gamma gene rearrangement by multiplex polymerase chain reaction/heteroduplex analysis in patients with cutaneous T-cell lymphoma (mycosis fungoides/Sezary syndrome) and benign inflammatory disease: correlation with clinical, histological and immunophenotypical findings. Br J Dermatol 2005;153(3):565–73.

13. Alessi E, et al. The usefulness of clonality for the detection of cases clinically and/or histopathologically not recognized as cutaneous T-cell lymphoma. Br J Dermatol 2005;153(2):368–71.

14. Ortonne N, et al. Significance of circulating T-cell clones in Sezary syndrome. Blood 2006;107(10):4030–8.

15. Guitart J. Beyond clonal detection: defining the T-cell clone. Arch Dermatol 2005;141(9):1159–60.

16. Lamberg SI, Bunn PA Jr. Cutaneous T-cell lymphomas. Summary of the Mycosis Fungoides Cooperative Group-National Cancer Institute Workshop. Arch Dermatol 1979;115(9):1103–5.

17. Vonderheid EC, Bernengo MG. The Sezary syndrome: hematologic criteria. Hematol Oncol Clin North Am 2003;17(6):1367–89, viii.

18. Vonderheid EC, Pena L, Nowell P. Sezary cell counts in erythrodermic cutaneous T-cell lymphoma: implications for prognosis and staging. Leuk Lymphoma 2006;47(9):1841–56.

19. Beylot-Barry M, et al. Is bone marrow biopsy necessary in patients with mycosis fungoides and Sezary syndrome? A histological and molecular study at diagnosis and during follow-up. Br J Dermatol 2005;152(6):1378–9.

20. Kim YH, et al. Long-term outcome of 525 patients with mycosis fungoides and Sezary syndrome: clinical prognostic factors and risk for disease progression. Arch Dermatol 2003;139(7):857–66.

21. Kim YH, et al. Clinical stage IA (limited patch and plaque) mycosis fungoides. A long-term outcome analysis. Arch Dermatol 1996;132(11):1309–13.

22. Kim YH, et al. Clinical characteristics and long-term outcome of patients with generalized patch and/or plaque (T2) mycosis fungoides. Arch Dermatol 1999;135(1):26–32.

23. Morales MM, et al. Survival of mycosis fungoides in patients in the Southeast of England. Dermatology 2005;211(4):325–9.

24. Klemke CD, et al. Prognostic factors and prediction of prognosis by the CTCL Severity Index in mycosis fungoides and Sezary syndrome. Br J Dermatol 2005;153(1):118–24.

25. Kari L, et al. Classification and prediction of survival in patients with the leukemic phase of cutaneous T cell lymphoma. J Exp Med 2003;197(11):1477–88.

26. Nebozhyn M, et al. Quantitative PCR on 5 genes reliably identifies CTCL patients with 5–99% circulating tumor cells with 90% accuracy. Blood 2006;107(8):3189–96.

27. Murdoch C, Finn A. Chemokine receptors and their role in inflammation and infectious diseases. Blood 2000;95(10):3032–43.

28. Robert C, Kupper TS. Inflammatory skin diseases, T cells, and immune surveillance. N Engl J Med 1999;341(24):1817–28.

29. Ferenczi K, et al. Increased CCR4 expression in cutaneous T cell lymphoma. J Invest Dermatol 2002;119(6):1405–10.

30. Poznansky MC, et al. Active movement of T cells away from a chemokine. Nat Med 2000;6(5):543–8.

31. Kallinich T, et al. Chemokine receptor expression on neoplastic and reactive T cells in the skin at different stages of mycosis fungoides. J Invest Dermatol 2003;121(5):1045–52.

32. Morales J, et al. CTACK, a skin-associated chemokine that preferentially attracts skin-homing memory T cells. Proc Natl Acad Sci U S A 1999;96(25):14470–5.

33. Sokolowska-Wojdylo M, et al. Circulating clonal CLA(+) and CD4(+) T cells in Sezary syndrome express the skin-homing chemokine receptors CCR4 and CCR10 as well as the lymph node-homing chemokine receptor CCR7. Br J Dermatol 2005;152(2):258–64.

34. Sokolowska-Wojdylo M, et al. Absence of CD26 expression on skin-homing CLA+ CD4+ T lymphocytes in peripheral blood is a highly sensitive marker for early diagnosis and therapeutic moni-

toring of patients with Sezary syndrome. Clin Exp Dermatol 2005;30(6):702–6.

35. Narducci MG, et al. Skin homing of Sezary cells involves SDF-1–CXCR4 signaling and down-regulation of CD26/dipeptidylpeptidase IV. Blood 2006;107(3):1108–15.

36. Bernengo MG, et al. The relevance of the CD4+ CD26– subset in the identification of circulating Sezary cells. Br J Dermatol 2001;144(1):125–35.

37. Introcaso CE, et al. Association of change in clinical status and change in the percentage of the CD4+CD26– lymphocyte population in patients with Sezary syndrome. J Am Acad Dermatol 2005;53(3):428–34.

38. Kagami S, et al. Elevated Serum CTACK/CCL27 Levels in CTCL. J Invest Dermatol 2006;126(5): 1189–91.

39. Homey B, et al. CCL27–CCR10 interactions regulate T cell-mediated skin inflammation. Nat Med 2002;8(2):157–65.

40. Notohamiprodjo M, et al. CCR10 is expressed in cutaneous T-cell lymphoma. Int J Cancer 2005;115(4):641–7.

41. Kakinuma T, et al. Thymus and activation-regulated chemokine (TARC/CCL17) in mycosis fungoides: serum TARC levels reflect the disease activity of mycosis fungoides. J Am Acad Dermatol 2003;48(1):23–30.

42. Tensen CP, et al. Epidermal interferon-gamma inducible protein-10 (IP-10) and monokine induced by gamma-interferon (Mig) but not IL-8 mRNA expression is associated with epidermotropism in cutaneous T cell lymphomas. J Invest Dermatol 1998;111(2):222–6.

43. Yamanaka K, et al. Skin-derived interleukin-7 contributes to the proliferation of lymphocytes in cutaneous T-cell lymphoma. Blood 2006;107(6):2440–5.

44. Smoller BR, et al. Histopathology and genetics of cutaneous T-cell lymphoma. Hematol Oncol Clin North Am 2003;17(6):1277–311.

45. Sommer VH, et al. In vivo activation of STAT3 in cutaneous T-cell lymphoma. Evidence for an antiapoptotic function of STAT3. Leukemia 2004;18(7):1288–95.

46. Dereure O, et al. Infrequent Fas mutations but no Bax or p53 mutations in early mycosis fungoides: a possible mechanism for the accumulation of malignant T lymphocytes in the skin. J Invest Dermatol 2002;118(6):949–56.

47. Ni X, et al. Resistance to activation-induced cell death and bystander cytotoxicity via the Fas/Fas ligand pathway are implicated in the pathogenesis of cutaneous T cell lymphomas. J Invest Dermatol 2005;124(4):741–50.

48. van Doorn R, et al. Epigenetic profiling of cutaneous T-cell lymphoma: promoter hypermethylation of multiple tumor suppressor genes including BCL7a, PTPRG, and p73. J Clin Oncol 2005;23(17): 3886–96.

49. Nagasawa T, et al. Multi-gene epigenetic silencing of tumor suppressor genes in T-cell lymphoma cells; delayed expression of the p16 protein upon reversal of the silencing. Leuk Res 2006;30(3): 303–12.

50. Sors A, et al. Down-regulating constitutive activation of the NF-kappaB canonical pathway overcomes the resistance of cutaneous T-cell lymphoma to apoptosis. Blood 2006;107(6):2354–63.

51. Rosato RR, Grant S. Histone deacetylase inhibitors: insights into mechanisms of lethality. Expert Opin Ther Targets 2005;9(4):809–24.

52. Talpur R, et al. CD25 expression is correlated with histological grade and response to denileukin diftitox in cutaneous T-cell lymphoma. J Invest Dermatol 2006;126(3):575–83.

53. Wasik MA, et al. Increased serum concentration of the soluble interleukin-2 receptor in cutaneous T-cell lymphoma. Clinical and prognostic implications. Arch Dermatol 1996;132(1):42–7.

54. Vowels BR, et al. Aberrant cytokine production by Sezary syndrome patients: cytokine secretion pattern resembles murine Th2 cells. J Invest Dermatol 1992;99(1):90–4.

55. Vowels BR, et al. Th2 cytokine mRNA expression in skin in cutaneous T-cell lymphoma. J Invest Dermatol 1994;103(5):669–73.

56. Asadullah K, et al. Progression of mycosis fungoides is associated with increasing cutaneous expression of interleukin-10 mRNA. J Invest Dermatol 1996;107(6):833–7.

57. Hoppe RT, et al. CD8–positive tumor-infiltrating lymphocytes influence the long-term survival of patients with mycosis fungoides. J Am Acad Dermatol 1995;32(3):448–53.

58. Zackheim HS, et al. Psoriasiform mycosis fungoides with fatal outcome after treatment with cyclosporine. J Am Acad Dermatol 2002;47(1):155–7.

59. Wysocka M, et al. Sezary syndrome patients demonstrate a defect in dendritic cell populations: effects of CD40 ligand and treatment with GM-CSF on dendritic cell numbers and the production of cytokines. Blood 2002;100(9):3287–94.

60. Yamanaka K, et al. Expression of interleukin-18 and caspase-1 in cutaneous T-cell lymphoma. Clin Cancer Res 2006;12(2):376–82.

61. Berger CL, et al. Cutaneous T cell lymphoma, malignant proliferation of T-regulatory cells. Blood 2005;105(4):1640–7.

62. Walsh PT, et al. A role for regulatory T cells in cutaneous T-Cell lymphoma; induction of a CD4 + CD25 + Foxp3+ T-cell phenotype associated with HTLV-1 infection. J Invest Dermatol 2006;126(3):690–2.

63. Wong HK, et al. Increased expression of CTLA-4 in malignant T-cells from patients with mycosis fungoides–cutaneous T cell lymphoma. J Invest Dermatol 2006;126(1):212–9.

64. Tiemessen MM, et al. Lack of suppressive CD4+CD25+FOXP3+ T cells in advanced stages of primary cutaneous T-cell lymphoma. J Invest Dermatol 2006;126(10):2217–23.

65. Yamano Y, et al. Virus-induced dysfunction of CD4+CD25+ T cells in patients with HTLV-I-associated neuroimmunological disease. J Clin Invest 2005;115(5):1361–8.

66. French LE, et al. Impaired CD40L signaling is a cause of defective IL-12 and TNF-{alpha} production in Sezary syndrome: circumvention by hexameric soluble CD40L. Blood 2005;105(1):219–225.

67. Yawalkar N, et al. Profound loss of T-cell receptor repertoire complexity in cutaneous T-cell lymphoma. Blood 2003;102(12):4059–66.

68. Yamanaka K, et al. Decreased T-cell receptor excision circles in cutaneous T-cell lymphoma. Clin Cancer Res 2005;11(16):5748–55.

69. Yoo EK, et al. Complete molecular remission during biologic response modifier therapy for Sezary syndrome is associated with enhanced helper T type 1 cytokine production and natural killer cell activity. J Am Acad Dermatol 2001;45(2):208–16.

70. Wysocka M, et al. Enhancement of the host immune responses in cutaneous T-cell lymphoma by CpG oligodeoxynucleotides and IL-15. Blood 2004;104(13):4142–9.

71. Goldgeier MH, et al. An unusual and fatal case of disseminated cutaneous herpes simplex. Infection in a patient with cutaneous T cell lymphoma (mycosis fungoides). J Am Acad Dermatol 1981;4(2):176–80.

72. Lee J, et al. Progressive Multifocal Leukoencephalopathy (JC Virus) in a patient with advanced Mycosis Fungoides. J Am Acad Dermatol (submitted) 2007;57(5):893–5.

73. Evans AV, et al. Cutaneous malignant melanoma in association with mycosis fungoides. J Am Acad Dermatol 2004;50(5):701–5.

74. Pielop JA, Brownell I, Duvic M. Mycosis fungoides associated with malignant melanoma and dysplastic nevus syndrome. Int J Dermatol 2003;42(2):116–22.

75. Molin L, Thomsen K, Volden G. Serum IgE in mycosis fungoides. Br Med J 1978;1(6117):920–1.

76. Tancrede-Bohin E, et al. Prognostic value of blood eosinophilia in primary cutaneous T-cell lymphomas. Arch Dermatol 2004;140(9):1057–61.

77. Suchin KR, et al. Increased interleukin 5 production in eosinophilic Sezary syndrome: regulation by interferon alfa and interleukin 12. J Am Acad Dermatol 2001;44(1):28–32.

78. Kim YH, et al. Topical nitrogen mustard in the management of mycosis fungoides: update of the Stanford experience. Arch Dermatol 2003;139(2):165–73.

79. Zackheim HS. Topical carmustine (BCNU) for patch/plaque mycosis fungoides. Semin Dermatol 1994;13(3):202–6.

80. Zhang C, Duvic M. Retinoids: therapeutic applications and mechanisms of action in cutaneous T-cell lymphoma. Dermatol Ther 2003;16(4):322–30.

81. Herrmann JJ, et al. Treatment of mycosis fungoides with photochemotherapy (PUVA): long-term follow-up. J Am Acad Dermatol 1995;33(2 pt 1):234–42.

82. Querfeld C, et al. Long-term follow-up of patients with early-stage cutaneous T-cell lymphoma who achieved complete remission with psoralen plus UV-A monotherapy. Arch Dermatol 2005;141(3):305–11.

83. Jones G, Wilson LD, Fox-Goguen L. Total skin electron beam radiotherapy for patients who have mycosis fungoides. Hematol Oncol Clin North Am 2003;17(6):1421–34.

84. McGinnis KS, et al. Psoralen plus long-wave UV-A (PUVA) and bexarotene therapy: An effective and synergistic combined adjunct to therapy for patients with advanced cutaneous T-cell lymphoma. Arch Dermatol 2003;139(6):771–5.

85. McGinnis KS, et al. Low-dose oral bexarotene in combination with low-dose interferon alfa in the treatment of cutaneous T-cell lymphoma: clinical synergism and possible immunologic mechanisms. J Am Acad Dermatol 2004;50(3):375–9.

86. Singh F, Lebwohl MG. Cutaneous T-cell lymphoma treatment using bexarotene and PUVA: a case series. J Am Acad Dermatol 2004;51(4):570–3.

87. Rupoli S, et al. Long-term experience with low-dose interferon-alpha and PUVA in the management of early mycosis fungoides. Eur J Haematol 2005;75(2):136–45.

88. Rook AH, Kuzel TM, Olsen EA. Cytokine therapy of cutaneous T-cell lymphoma: interferons, interleukin-12, and interleukin-2. Hematol Oncol Clin North Am 2003;17(6):1435–48, ix.

89. Kuzel TM, et al. Effectiveness of interferon alfa-2a combined with phototherapy for mycosis fungoides and the Sezary syndrome. J Clin Oncol 1995;13(1):257–63.

90. Chiarion-Sileni V, et al. Phase II trial of interferon-alpha-2a plus psolaren with ultraviolet light A in patients with cutaneous T-cell lymphoma. Cancer 2002;95(3):569–75.

91. Knobler RM, et al. Treatment of cutaneous T cell lymphoma with a combination of low-dose interferon alfa-2b and retinoids. J Am Acad Dermatol 1991;24(2 pt 1):247–52.

92. Zhang C, et al. Induction of apoptosis by bexarotene in cutaneous T-cell lymphoma cells: relevance to mechanism of therapeutic action. Clin Cancer Res 2002;8(5):1234–40.

93. Budgin JB, et al. Biological effects of bexarotene in cutaneous T-cell lymphoma. Arch Dermatol 2005;141(3):315–21.

94. Duvic M, et al. Bexarotene is effective and safe for treatment of refractory advanced-stage cutaneous T-cell lymphoma: multinational phase II–III trial results. J Clin Oncol 2001;19(9):2456–71.

94a. Lin J, et al. Clinical and in-vitro resistance to bexarotene in Adult T-cell leukemia: loss of RXR-alpha receptor. Blood 2008 (in press).

95. Fox FE, et al. Retinoids synergize with interleukin-2 to augment IFN-gamma and interleukin-12 production by human peripheral blood mononuclear cells. J Interferon Cytokine Res 1999;19(4):407–15.

96. Richardson SK, et al. High clinical response rate with multimodality immunomodulatory therapy for Sezary syndrome. Clin Lymphoma Myeloma 2006;7(3):226–32.

97. Suchin KR, et al. Treatment of cutaneous T-cell lymphoma with combined immunomodulatory therapy: a 14-year experience at a single institution. Arch Dermatol 2002;138(8):1054–60.

98. Yoo EK, et al. Apoptosis induction of ultraviolet light A and photochemotherapy in cutaneous T-cell Lymphoma: relevance to mechanism of therapeutic action. J Invest Dermatol 1996;107(2):235–42.

99. Heald PW, Edelson RL. Photopheresis for T cell mediated diseases. Adv Dermatol 1988;3:25–40.

100. Girardi M, et al. Transimmunization for cutaneous T cell lymphoma: a Phase I study. Leuk Lymphoma 2006;47(8):1495–503.

101. Kim S, Elkon KB, Ma X. Transcriptional suppression of interleukin-12 gene expression following phagcytosis of apoptotic cells. Immunity 2004;21(5):643–53.

102. Kaplan EH, et al. Phase II study of recombinant human interferon gamma for treatment of cutaneous T-cell lymphoma. J Natl Cancer Inst 1990;82(3):208–12.

103. McGinnis KS, et al. The addition of interferon gamma to oral bexarotene therapy with photopheresis for Sezary syndrome. Arch Dermatol 2005;141(9):1176–8.

104. Shapiro M, et al. Novel multimodality biologic response modifier therapy, including bexarotene and long-wave ultraviolet A for a patient with refractory stage IVa cutaneous T-cell lymphoma. J Am Acad Dermatol 2002;47(6):956–61.

105. Wysocka M, et al. Synthetic imidazoquinolines potently and broadly activate the cellular immune response of patients with cutaneous T-cell lymphoma: synergy with interferon-gamma enhances production of interleukin-12. Clin Lymphoma Myeloma 2007;7(8):524–34.

106. Dummer R, et al. Adenovirus-mediated intralesional interferon-gamma gene transfer induces tumor regressions in cutaneous lymphomas. Blood 2004;104(6):1631–8.

107. vanderSpek JC, et al. Structure/function analysis of the transmembrane domain of DAB389–interleukin-2, an interleukin-2 receptor-targeted fusion toxin. The amphipathic helical region of the transmembrane domain is essential for the efficient delivery of the catalytic domain to the cytosol of target cells. J Biol Chem 1993;268(16):12077–82.

108. Olsen E, et al. Pivotal phase III trial of two dose levels of denileukin diftitox for the treatment of cutaneous T-cell lymphoma. J Clin Oncol 2001;19(2):376–88.

109. Dannull J, et al. Enhancement of vaccine-mediated antitumor immunity in cancer patients after depletion of regulatory T cells. J Clin Invest 2005;115(12):3623–33.

110. Camacho LH, Ribas A, Glaspy JA, et al. Phase 1 clinical trial of anti-CTLA4 human monoclonal antibody CP-675,206 in patients with advanced solid malignancies. J Clin Oncol 2004;22(14 S):2505.

111. Phan GQ, et al. Cancer regression and autoimmunity induced by cytotoxic T lymphocyte-associated antigen 4 blockade in patients with metastatic melanoma. Proc Natl Acad Sci USA 2003;100(14):8372–7.

112. Wu JJ, Huang DB, Tyring SK. Resiquimod: a new immune response modifier with potential as a vaccine adjuvant for Th1 immune responses. Antiviral Res 2004;64(2):79–83.

113. Dockrell DH, Kinghorn GR. Imiquimod and resiquimod as novel immunomodulators. J Antimicrob Chemother 2001;48(6):751–5.

114. Suchin KR, Junkins-Hopkins JM, Rook AH. Treatment of stage IA cutaneous T-Cell lymphoma with topical application of the immune response modifier imiquimod. Arch Dermatol 2002;138(9):1137–9.

115. Dummer R, et al. Imiquimod induces complete clearance of a PUVA-resistant plaque in mycosis fungoides. Dermatology 2003;207(1):116–8.

116. Hurwitz DJ, Pincus L, Kupper TS. Imiquimod: a topically applied link between innate and

acquired immunity. Arch Dermatol 2003;139(10): 1347–50.

117. Kawai T, et al. Interferon-alpha induction through Toll-like receptors involves a direct interaction of IRF7 with MyD88 and TRAF6. Nat Immunol 2004;5(10):1061–8.

118. Schon MP, Schon M. Immune modulation and apoptosis induction: two sides of the antitumoral activity of imiquimod. Apoptosis 2004;9(3): 291–8.

119. Jones T. Resiquimod 3M. Curr Opin Invest Drugs 2003;4(2):214–8.

120. Krieg AM. CpG motifs: the active ingredient in bacterial extracts? Nat Med 2003;9(7):831–5.

121. Lonsdorf AS, et al. Intratumor CpG-oligodeoxy-nucleotide injection induces protective antitumor T cell immunity. J Immunol 2003;171(8):3941–6.

122. Kim YH, et al. TLR9 agonist immunomodulator treatment of cutaneous T-cell lymphoma (CTCL) with CPG7909 [abstract]. American Society of Hematology Meeting, 2004.

123. Tritel M, et al. Prime-boost vaccination with HIV-1 Gag protein and cytosine phosphate guanosine oligodeoxynucleotide, followed by adenovirus, induces sustained and robust humoral and cellular immune responses. J Immunol 2003;171(5): 2538–47.

124. Bergstrom RT, et al. CD40 monoclonal antibody activation of antigen-presenting cells improves therapeutic efficacy of tumor-specific T cells. Otolaryngol Head Neck Surg 2004;130(1): 94–103.

125. Watanabe S, et al. The duration of signaling through CD40 directs biological ability of dendritic cells to induce antitumor immunity. J Immunol 2003;171(11):5828–36.

126. Rook AH, et al. Interleukin-12 therapy of cutaneous T-cell lymphoma induces lesion regression and cytotoxic T-cell responses. Blood 1999;94(3):902–8.

127. Duvic M, et al. A phase II open-label study of recombinant human interleukin-12 in patients with stage IA, IB, or IIA mycosis fungoides. J Am Acad Dermatol 2006;55(5):807–13.

128. Zaki MH, et al. Dysregulation of lymphocyte interleukin-12 receptor expression in Sezary syndrome. J Invest Dermatol 2001;117(1):119–27.

129. Berger CL, et al. Tumor-specific peptides in cutaneous T-cell lymphoma: association with class I major histocompatibility complex and possible derivation from the clonotypic T-cell receptor. Int J Cancer 1998;76(3):304–11.

130. Winter D, et al. Definition of TCR epitopes for CTL-mediated attack of cutaneous T cell lymphoma. J Immunol 2003;171(5):2714–24.

131. Muche JM, Sterry W. Vaccination therapy for cutaneous T-cell lymphoma. Clin Exp Dermatol 2002;27(7):602–7.

132. Maier T, et al. Vaccination of patients with cutaneous T-cell lymphoma using intranodal injection of autologous tumor-lysate-pulsed dendritic cells. Blood 2003;102(7):2338–44.

133. Rook AH, et al. The potential therapeutic role of interleukin-12 in cutaneous T-cell lymphoma. Ann N Y Acad Sci 1996;795:310–8.

134. Berard M, et al. IL-15 promotes the survival of naive and memory phenotype CD8+ T cells. J Immunol 2003;170(10):5018–26.

135. Son YI, et al. Interleukin-18 (IL-18) synergizes with IL-2 to enhance cytotoxicity, interferon-gamma production, and expansion of natural killer cells. Cancer Res 2001;61(3):884–8.

136. Strengell M, et al. IL-21 in synergy with IL-15 or IL-18 enhances IFN-gamma production in human NK and T cells. J Immunol 2003;170(11):5464–9.

137. Miller G, et al. Endogenous granulocyte-macrophage colony-stimulating factor overexpression in vivo results in the long-term recruitment of a distinct dendritic cell population with enhanced immunostimulatory function. J Immunol 2002;169(6):2875–85.

138. Chang DZ, et al. Granulocyte-macrophage colony stimulating factor: an adjuvant for cancer vaccines. Hematology 2004;9(3):207–15.

139. Kim YH, et al. Clinical efficacy of zanolimumab (HuMax-CD4): two Phase II studies in refractory cutaneous T-cell lymphoma. Blood 2007;109(11):4655–62.

140. Lundin J, et al. CAMPATH-1H monoclonal antibody in therapy for previously treated low-grade non-Hodgkin's lymphomas: a phase II multicenter study. European Study Group of CAMPATH-1H Treatment in Low-Grade Non-Hodgkin's Lymphoma. J Clin Oncol 1998;16(10):3257–63.

141. Lundin J, et al. Phase 2 study of alemtuzumab (anti-CD52 monoclonal antibody) in patients with advanced mycosis fungoides/Sezary syndrome. Blood 2003;101(11):4267–72.

142. Ishida T, Ueda R. CCR4 as a novel molecular target for immunotherapy of cancer. Cancer Sci 2006;97(11):1139–46.

143. Ishida T, et al. The CC chemokine receptor 4 as a novel specific molecular target for immunotherapy in adult T-Cell leukemia/lymphoma. Clin Cancer Res 2004;10(22):7529–39.

144. Hino R, Shimauchi T, Tokura Y. Treatment with IFN-gamma increases serum levels of Th1 chemokines and decreases those of Th2 chemokines in patients with mycosis fungoides. J Dermatol Sci 2005;38(3):189–95.

145. Richardson SK, et al. Bexarotene blunts malignant T-cell chemotaxis in Sezary syndrome: reduction of chemokine receptor 4 (CCR4)-positive lymphocytes and decreased chemotaxis to thymus and activation regulated chemokine (TARC). Am J Hematol 2007;82(9):792–7.

146. Richardson S, et al. Low-dose bexarotene and low-dose interferon alfa-2b for adult T-cell leukemia/lymphoma associated with human T-lymphotropic virus 1. Arch Dermatol 2005;141(3):301–4.

147. Mitsiades N, et al. Molecular sequelae of histone deacetylase inhibition in human malignant B cells. Blood 2003;101(10):4055–62.

148. Kelly WK, et al. Phase I clinical trial of histone deacetylase inhibitor: suberoylanilide hydroxamic acid administered intravenously. Clin Cancer Res 2003;9(10 Pt 1):3578–88.

149. Piekarz RL, et al. Inhibitor of histone deacetylation, depsipeptide (FR901228), in the treatment of peripheral and cutaneous T-cell lymphoma: a case report. Blood 2001;98(9):2865–8.

150. Piekarz RL, et al. T-cell lymphoma as a model for the use of histone deacetylase inhibitors in cancer therapy: impact of depsipeptide on molecular markers, therapeutic targets, and mechanisms of resistance. Blood 2004;103(12):4636–43.

151. Piekarz R, Bates S. A review of depsipeptide and other histone deacetylase inhibitors in clinical trials. Curr Pharm Des 2004;10(19):2289–98.

152. Duvic M, et al. Phase 2 trial of oral vorinostat (suberoylanilide hydroxamic acid, SAHA) for refractory cutaneous T-cell lymphoma (CTCL). Blood 2007;109(1):31–9.

153. Shao RH, et al. Arginine butyrate increases the cytotoxicity of DAB(389)IL-2 in leukemia and lymphoma cells by upregulation of IL-2Rbeta gene. Leuk Res 2002;26(12):1077–83.

154. Oyama Y, et al. High-dose therapy and bone marrow transplantation in cutaneous T-cell lymphoma. Hematol Oncol Clin North Am 2003;17(6):1475–83, xi.

155. Storb R, et al. Allogeneic hematopoietic stem cell transplantation: from the nuclear age into the twenty-first century. Transplant Proc 2000;32(7):2548–9.

156. Baron F, Sandmaier BM. Current status of hematopoietic stem cell transplantation after nonmyeloablative conditioning. Curr Opin Hematol 2005;12(6):435–43.

157. Bigler RD, et al. Autologous bone marrow transplantation for advanced stage mycosis fungoides. Bone Marrow Transplant 1991;7(2):133–7.

158. Olavarria E, et al. T-cell depletion and autologous stem cell transplantation in the management of tumour stage mycosis fungoides with peripheral blood involvement. Br J Haematol 2001;114(3):624–31.

159. Burt RK, et al. Allogeneic hematopoietic stem cell transplantation for advanced mycosis fungoides: evidence of a graft-versus-tumor effect. Bone Marrow Transplant 2000;25(1):111–3.

160. Masood N, et al. Induction of complete remission of advanced stage mycosis fungoides by allogeneic hematopoietic stem cell transplantation. J Am Acad Dermatol 2002;47(1):140–5.

161. Soligo D, et al. Treatment of advanced mycosis fungoides by allogeneic stem-cell transplantation with a nonmyeloablative regimen. Bone Marrow Transplant 2003;31(8):663–6.

162. Guitart J, et al. Long-term remission after allogeneic hematopoietic stem cell transplantation for refractory cutaneous T-cell lymphoma. Arch Dermatol 2002;138(10):1359–65.

163. Molina A, et al. Durable clinical, cytogenetic, and molecular remissions after allogeneic hematopoietic cell transplantation for refractory Sezary syndrome and mycosis fungoides. J Clin Oncol 2005;23(25):6163–71.

164. Fijnheer R, et al. Complete remission of a radio-chemotherapy-resistant cutaneous T-cell lymphoma with allogeneic non-myeloablative stem cell transplantation. Bone Marrow Transplant 2003;32(3):345–7.

26
Graft-Versus-Host Disease

Edward W. Cowen

Key Points

- Over 15,000 patients per year are treated with allogeneic stem cell transplantation as an intervention for cancer, primary immunodeficiency, and other serious heritable and acquired disease states.
- Graft-versus-host disease (GVHD) is a potentially life-threatening complication of allogeneic transplantation, with risk factors stem cell related to human leukocyte antigen (HLA) compatibility, the age and sex of the donor and recipient, the conditioning regimen used to prepare the graft and the donor, as well as the T-cell composition of the graft.
- The frequency of acute GVHD, even in haploidentical transplants can be as high as 30%; chronic GVHD may occur in 30% to 80% of transplant recipients.
- Acute graft-versus-host disease is a syndrome of skin, liver, and gastrointestinal dysfunction, which is a result of donor T lymphocyte activation by host antigen-presenting cells, resulting in an immune-mediated inflammatory response.
- There are a variety of morphologic changes that can occur in the skin in the setting of chronic GVHD, ranging from erythema, to lichenoid lesions, to fibrotic conditions and fasciitis.
- Systemic treatments such as glucocorticosteroids, calcineurin inhibitors extracorporeal photopheresis, and biologic therapies have been applied with varying success to ameliorate the signs and symptoms of cutaneous and systemic disease.

Hematopoietic Stem Cell Transplantation

Allogeneic hematopoietic stem cell transplantation (HSCT) is a potentially curative intervention for more than 15,000 patients each year suffering from cancer, primary immunodeficiency, and other serious heritable and acquired disorders (Table 26.1). However, allogeneic HSCT may lead to graft-versus-host disease (GVHD), a complex multiorgan disease that is a major cause of posttransplant non-relapse morbidity and mortality. Although it occurs most frequently in association with allogeneic HSCT, GVHD may also result from autologous HSCT, allogeneic liver transplantation, or blood transfusion. Practically every organ system may be affected by GVHD, but the skin is the most common site of involvement, and chronic cutaneous GVHD is perhaps most remarkable for its variable cutaneous manifestations.

The first step in allogeneic HSCT is the identification of a suitable stem cell donor. The donor is selected based on the similarity of his/her histocompatibility antigen (human leukocyte antigen [HLA]) profile to that of the recipient. There are three major class I HLA antigens, HLA-A, -B, and –C, and three major class II HLA antigens, HLA-DP, -DQ, and –DR. Because the alleles in each HLA class tend to be inherited together, there is approximately a 25% chance that a sibling donor will be a 6/6 HLA-identical match. If no related donor is available, a bone marrow registry is utilized to search for an unrelated donor. International registries now contain over 9 million

TABLE 26.1. Conditions treated with allogeneic hematopoietic stem cell transplantation (HSCT).

Autoimmune disorders
Autoimmune lymphoproliferative syndrome (ALPS)
Immune dysregulation, polyendocrinopathy, X-linked
  syndrome (IPEX)

Hematologic malignancy
Acute myeloid leukemia
Acute lymphoblastic leukemia
Chronic lymphocytic leukemia
Chronic myeloid leukemia
Hodgkin's lymphoma
Multiple myeloma
Non-Hodgkin's lymphoma

Bone marrow failure
Aplastic anemia
Diamond-Blackfan syndrome
Fanconi anemia
Dyskeratosis congenita/Hoyeraal-Hreidarsson syndrome
Myelodysplastic syndrome
Shwachman-Diamond syndrome

Immunodeficiency
Ataxia-telangiectasia
Chediak-Higashi syndrome
Chronic granulomatous disease
Complete interferon-γ receptor 1 deficiency
DiGeorge syndrome
Familial hemophagocytic lymphohistiocytosis
Griscelli's syndrome
Hyper-IgM syndrome
Kostmann syndrome
Leukocyte adhesion deficiency
Severe combined immunodeficiency
Wiskott-Aldrich syndrome
X-linked proliferation syndrome

Metabolic disorders
Fucosidosis
Gaucher's disease
Mucopolysaccharidoses
Osteopetrosis

Other disorders
Congenital erythropoietic porphyria (Günther's disease)
Essential thrombocytopenia
Histiocytoses
Idiopathic hypereosinophilic syndrome
Myelofibrosis
Polycythemia vera
Paroxysmal nocturnal hemoglobinuria
Sickle cell disease
Thalassemia
Waldenström's macroglobulinemia

potential donors and identify an unrelated donor for approximately 50% of patients.[1] The risk of GVHD is directly proportional to the degree of mismatch in major HLA alleles between donor and recipient. In addition, mismatch of minor HLA antigens is more likely to occur in the setting of unrelated-donor HSCT, which also contributes to the development of GVHD. Once a suitable donor is identified, the stem cells are collected from the donor's bone marrow, or colony-stimulating factor (CSF) is administered to the donor in order to mobilize stem cells from the marrow prior to pheresis from the peripheral blood. Umbilical cord blood is also used for stem cell transplantation but currently accounts for a small percentage of transplants performed worldwide. The source of the stem cell graft is an important factor in the development of GVHD, as peripheral blood grafts may be associated with a higher risk of GVHD than bone marrow–derived grafts.[2] After harvesting, donor stem cells are selected by physical and immunologic sorting methods. Specific T-cell depletion of the graft may be performed in order to decrease the risk of GVHD [prior to transfusion].

Pretreatment of the recipient's marrow before transplantation is necessary in order to allow engraftment of the donor stem cells. Traditional myeloablative regimens utilize a combination of total-body irradiation and chemotherapeutic agents such as cyclophosphamide to permit engraftment. These regimens create an immunosuppressed state, preventing the host from rejecting the foreign stem cells. Myeloablative preparative regimens may reduce tumor burden through a direct effect on the cancer; however, they are associated with a high rate of toxicity.[3] Over the last several years, reduced-intensity (nonmyeloablative) preparative regimens have resulted in less acute toxicity and have expanded the use of allogeneic transplantation to higher risk groups including older patients or those with significant organ dysfunction. Reduced-intensity regimens rely primarily on the transplanted graft for antileukemic activity rather than the direct cytotoxicity of the preparative regimen.[1]

Autologous stem cell transplantation, which utilize the patient's own stem cells following ablation of the hematopoietic system, is an important treatment for certain malignancies such as non-Hodgkin's lymphoma and multiple myeloma. More than 30,000 autologous procedures are performed worldwide each year. Although the risk of GVHD and overall nonrelapse mortality are greatly reduced following autologous transplantation when compared with allogeneic transplantation, autologous procedures are associated with an increased rate of malignancy relapse.[4]

Acute Versus Chronic Graft-Versus-Host Disease

Traditionally, acute and chronic GVHD are designations based on the timing of the onset of GVHD symptoms; the onset of acute GVHD occurs on or before the 100th day following transplantation, and the onset of chronic GVHD occurs after the 100th day. However, this temporal distinction is somewhat arbitrary, as patients may manifest classic signs of acute GVHD even after day 100, and chronic manifestations may occur before 100 days posttransplantation. Whereas acute cutaneous GVHD typically presents as an exanthematous skin eruption with gastrointestinal and hepatic involvement, chronic cutaneous GVHD is remarkable for its protean skin presentation, and it is associated with variable but potentially widespread organ dysfunction and immunodsyregulation. Changes in transplant protocols have also impacted the onset of acute and chronic symptoms. Nonmyeloablative conditioning regimens commonly delay the onset of manifestations of acute GVHD until after 100 days following transplantation.[5] Similarly, the use of donor lymphocyte infusions (DLI), wherein additional stem cells are administered weeks or months following transplantation to augment the graft-versus-tumor response, may induce symptoms of acute GVHD after the 100-day period.

Clinical Manifestations of Graft-Versus-Host Disease

Acute Graft-Versus-Host Disease

Acute GVHD is a potentially life-threatening complication of allogeneic transplantation. The risk of developing acute GVHD depends on a number of factors, including HLA compatibility, the age and sex of the donor and recipient, the prophylactic regimen used, and the T-cell composition of the graft. Without prophylactic immunosuppression, acute GVHD develops in nearly every allogeneic HSCT recipient. Therefore, a calcineurin inhibitor

(cyclosporine or tacrolimus) is commonly used in combination with methotrexate in the first several weeks to months following transplantation, during which time the risk of acute GVHD is greatest.

Despite prophylactic immunosuppressive therapy, nearly 30% of HLA-identical related transplant procedures result in significant acute GVHD.[6] This risk is significantly higher in HLA-matched unrelated and mismatched transplants. Because the skin is often the earliest clinical sign of acute GVHD and long-term survival from acute GVHD is directly related to the severity of skin, liver, and gut involvement, a quick and accurate diagnosis of GVHD is helpful to guide important management decisions. The 1994 Consensus Conference grading for acute GVHD is listed in Table 26.2.[7]

Acute GVHD primarily involves the skin, liver, and gastrointestinal tract, although other organ systems may be affected less frequently. Skin involvement most often occurs within 2 to 4 weeks after transplantation and is usually the first manifestation of acute GVHD. Cutaneous involvement may range in severity from an asymptomatic maculopapular erythematous eruption to widespread necrolysis, but most commonly presents with an exanthem-like eruption that preferentially involves the head, ears, palms, and soles (Fig. 26.1). In early GVHD, there may be involvement of the hair follicle, creating a folliculocentric appearance.[8]

TABLE 26.2. Staging and grading of acute graft-versus-host disease (GVHD).

Stage	Skin	Liver	Gut
1	Rash <25% BSA	Bilirubin 2 mg/dL to <3 mg/dL	Diarrhea 500–1000 mL/day or persistent nausea
2	Rash 25–50% BSA	Bilirubin 3–6 mg/dL	Diarrhea >1000–1500 mL/day
3	Rash >50% BSA	Bilirubin 6–15 mg/dL	Diarrhea >1500 mL/day
4	Erythroderma w/ bullae formation	Bilirubin >15 mg/dL	Severe abdominal pain with or without ileus
Grade			
I	Stage 1–2	None	None
II	Stage 3 or	Stage 1 or	Stage 1
III		Stege 2–3 or	Stage 2–4
IV	Stage 4 or	Stage 4	

BSA, body surface area.
Adapted from Przepiorka et al.[7]

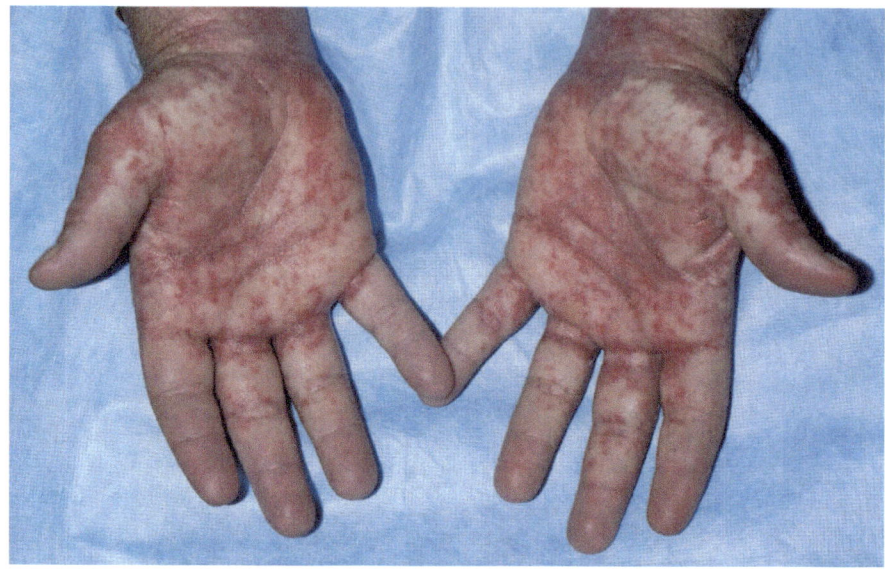

Fɪɢ. 26.1. Acute graft-versus-host disease (GVHD) of the palms

When severe, diffuse erythroderma or bullae with epidermal necrolysis may occur (Fig. 26.2).

Histologically, acute GVHD is characterized by widespread keratinocyte necrosis with a dermal lymphocytic infiltrate and basal cell hydropic degeneration (Fig. 26.3). Histologic changes mimicking GVHD may be found following high-dose chemo/radiotherapy, in the setting of drug hypersensitivity, and with the eruption of lymphocyte recovery.[9] In cases in which the clinical and histologic diagnosis of acute skin GVHD is nondiagnostic, the presence of hyperbilirubinemia or symptoms of nausea, vomiting, diarrhea, or abdominal pain are important indicators of hepatic and gastrointestinal involvement. Even in the setting of equivocal cutaneous and histologic findings, the mortality associated with severe acute GVHD necessitates a low threshold for initiating empiric corticosteroid therapy.

Chronic Graft-Versus-Host Disease

Chronic GVHD occurs in 30% to 80% of allogeneic HSCT recipients and is the leading cause of nonre-

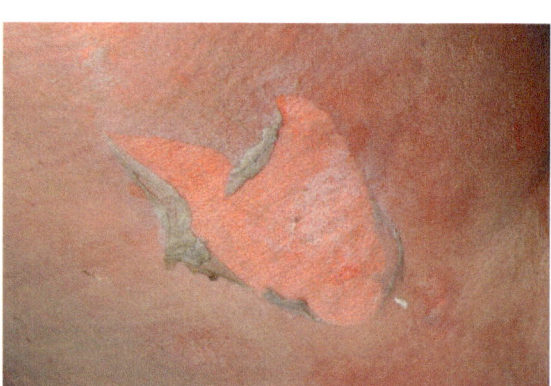

Fɪɢ. 26.2. Acute GVHD with necrolysis

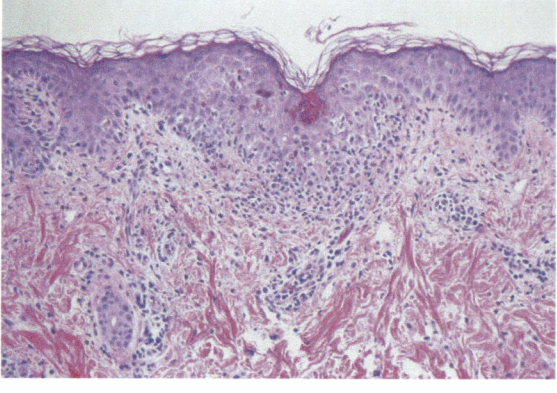

Fɪɢ. 26.3. Scattered necrotic epidermal keratinocytes with vacuolization of the basal cell layer and lymphocytic infiltration in the papillary dermis in a patient with acute GVHD (hematoxylin and eosin, 20×)

lapse mortality in survivors more than 2 years after transplantation.[10] Skin involvement may progress directly from acute disease, may occur following a period of disease quiescence, or occur de novo without a history of previous acute involvement. The greatest predictor of chronic GVHD is a history of prior acute GVHD.[11] Other risk factors include older patient age, a female donor for a male patient, a mismatched or unrelated donor, a peripheral blood graft, a T-cell replete graft, and use of donor lymphocyte infusions. A flare of chronic cutaneous GVHD may be triggered by a number of factors, most commonly tapering of immunosuppression, but may also occur following a drug eruption or sunburn, or in the setting of a systemic viral or bacterial infection.

One of the greatest hurdles to improving survival in patients who develop chronic GVHD stems from the clinical and immunologic complexity of the disorder. In an effort to facilitate clinical research in the field of chronic GVHD, the National Institutes of Health Chronic GVHD Consensus Project published a series of articles providing a standardized approach for diagnosis and staging,[12] histopathology,[13] disease biomarkers,[14] response criteria,[15] supportive care,[16] and clinical trial design.[17] Traditionally, chronic cutaneous GVHD has been described as either "lichenoid" or "sclerodermoid" involvement. However, these terms do not accurately portray the variability in the currently recognized cutaneous manifestations of chronic GVHD.[18] The Consensus Project diagnosis and staging guidelines provide a classification system of the clinical manifestations of chronic cutaneous GVHD (Table 26.3). Poikiloderma, lichen-planus–like lesions, and sclerotic skin changes including fasciitis are considered diagnostic features of chronic cutaneous GVHD when they occur in the setting of allogeneic

TABLE 26.3. Clinical manifestations of chronic GVHD.

Dermatologic and mucosal features			
Skin	Alopecia		Ulcer
	Angiomatous papules		Xerostomia
	Bullae	Genital mucosa	Lichen-planus–like*
	Erythema		Vulvar erosions/fissures
	Hypo- or hyperpigmentation		Vaginal scarring/stenosis*
	Ichthyosis-like	*Other organ system involvement in chronic*	
	Keratosis-pilaris-like	*GVHD*	
	Lichen-planus-like*	Cardiovascular	Pericardial effusion
	Lichen-sclerosus-like*	Ophthalmologic	Cicatricial conjunctivitis
	Maculopapular		Sicca symptoms
	Morphea-like*		Confluent punctuate keratopathy
	Poikiloderma*		Photophobia
	Scleroderma-like*		Blepharitis
	Sweat impairment	Gastrointestinal	Esophageal web
	Ulceration		Esophageal stricture/stenosis
Nails	Brittleness	Hematopoietic	Thrombocytopenia
	Longitudinal ridging or splitting		Eosinophilia
	Onycholysis		Lymphopenia
	Pterygium unguis		Hypo- or hypergammaglobulinemia
Subcutaneous tissue	Fasciitis*		Autoantibodies
	Panniculitis	Hepatic	Elevated total bilirubin
Oral mucosa	Erythema		Elevated alkaline phosphatase
	Gingivitis		Elevated transaminases
	Hyperkeratotic plaques*	Musculoskeletal	Myositis or polymyositis
	Lichen-planus–like*		Edema
	Mucocele		Myalgia
	Mucosal atrophy		Arthralgia, arthritis
	Mucositis	Neurologic	Peripheral neuropathy
	Pseudomembrane		Myasthenia gravis
	Restriction of oral opening from	Pulmonary	Bronchiolitis obliterans +/− organizing
	sclerosis*		pneumonia
			Pleural effusion

*Diagnostic feature; other signs and symptoms listed are not considered sufficient to establish a diagnosis of chronic GVHD without further testing or other organ involvement.

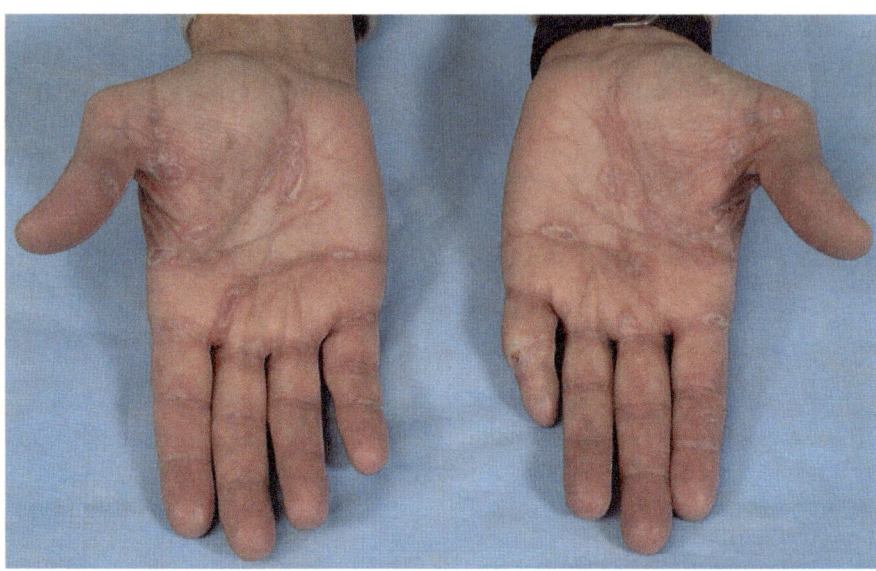

FIG. 26.4. Chronic GVHD; scaling violaceous papules and plaques on the hands

HSCT. Other cutaneous features, such as ichthyosis, dyspigmentation, and alopecia are also well-recognized manifestations but are not considered diagnostic of skin involvement.[12]

Given the variety of epidermal changes associated with GVHD, the term *lichenoid* is better reserved for use as a histologic descriptor of GVHD rather than as a clinical disease classification. Discrete lichen-planus–like violaceous papules are relatively uncommon in chronic GVHD, but may be seen most commonly on the palms and soles (Fig. 26.4). In the past, the term *lichenoid* has been used most commonly to describe cutaneous GVHD which manifests as poorly defined interconnecting erythematous papules and plaques with overlying scale. This eruption may localize to sites of previous ultraviolet (UV) exposure, such as the posterior and lateral neck, and may spare UV-protected areas such as the buttocks. Underlying sclerotic changes resembling lichen sclerosus or morphea may also be present. Resolution of this manifestation of chronic GVHD results in a distinct reticulate pattern of hyperpigmentation, reflecting the pigment incontinence induced by the epidermal-dermal interface reaction.

Sclerotic changes associated with chronic GVHD may develop at any layer of the dermal and subcutaneous tissue. Chosidow et al.[19] estimated the incidence of sclerodermatous GVHD to be 3.6% based on a review of 196 HSCT patients. However, the true frequency of sclerotic changes associated with GVHD may be higher if all forms of sclerosis are included. Sclerosis may be present on multiple levels in a single patient, and the changes may or may not occur in the presence of overlying epidermal involvement. The most superficial level of sclerotic changes resembles lichen sclerosus and consists of atrophic gray patches with epidermal atrophy, often distributed symmetrically on the upper back. Morpheaform GVHD represents the next deeper level of sclerosis and mimics morphea with patchy areas of prominent dermal sclerosis, often with overlying pigmentation. Dermal sclerosis results in a decreased ability to pinch the skin. Morpheaform GVHD often occurs preferentially at sites of skin friction or pressure such as the waistband area (Fig. 26.5). Scleroderma-like GVHD represents full-thickness sclerosis with the complete inability to pinch skin and a hidebound appearance. Involvement over joints may significantly limit range of motion of the affected joint. In contrast to scleroderma, scleroderma-like GVHD does not begin with symmetric distal hand involvement and proceed proximally, and Raynaud's phenomenon is uncommon. Chronic sclerosis may be complicated by bullae formation as well as spontaneous erosions and ulceration (Fig. 26.6). Benign angiomatous papules and nodules may develop in patients with chronic disease (Fig. 26.7).[20]

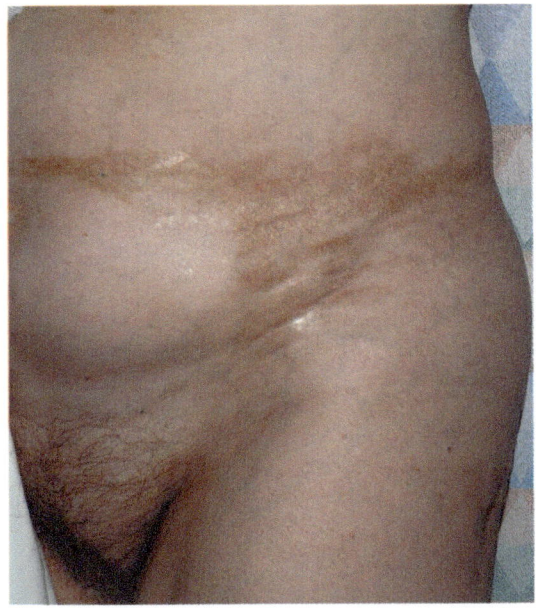

FIG. 26.5. Tan sclerotic plaques with koebnerization at site of waistband in patient morpheaform chronic GVHD

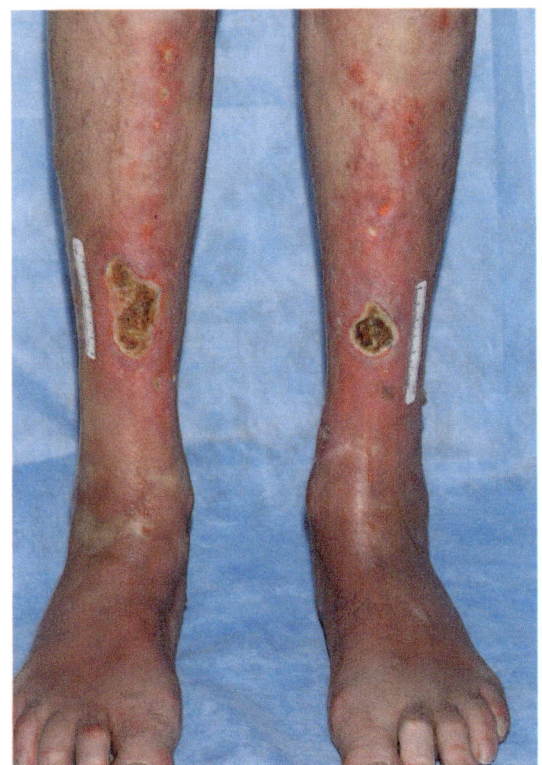

FIG. 26.6. Hidebound sclerosis with skin ulceration in a patient with scleroderma-like chronic GVHD

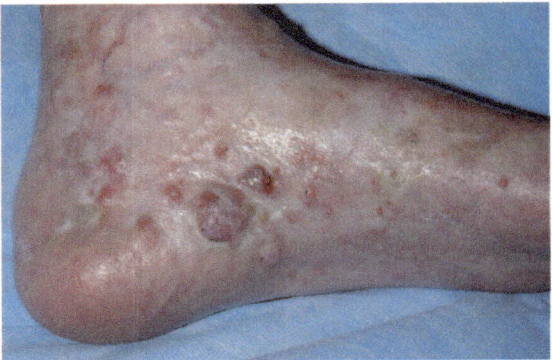

FIG. 26.7 Numerous angiomatous papules and nodules in a patient with chronic sclerotic GVHD of the legs

The histologic of "lichenoid" chronic GVHD resembles that of lichen planus with a bandlike lymphoplasmacytic infiltrate. Sclerotic GVHD resembles scleroderma with homogenization of collagen and loss of adnexal structures. The level and degree of fibrosis observed histologically reflects the clinical type of sclerosis. In patients with primary rippling to the skin consistent with subcutaneous disease, sclerosis and inflammation will be seen primarily at the interface between the reticular dermis and the subcutaneous fat.

Chronic Graft-Versus-Host Disease–Related Fasciitis

Graft-versus-host disease–related panniculitis and fasciitis represent sclerosis of the deep subcutaneous tissue and fascia. Although GVHD-related fasciitis is thought to be an uncommon presentation, it may present in an insidious manner and may result in marked functional limitations. Patients with GVHD-related fasciitis often manifest overlapping features of both panniculitis and fasciitis, and the histologic diagnosis may depend on the depth and extent of the tissue biopsy. Patients may complain of muscle pain or weakness,[21] or may demonstrate limited range of motion at affected joints at the time of presentation. Graft-versus-host disease–associated fasciitis shares many similarities with eosinophilic fasciitis, an uncommon disorder of unknown etiology first described by Shulman[22] in 1974. Graft-versus-host disease–associated fasciitis presents with prominent induration and rippling of

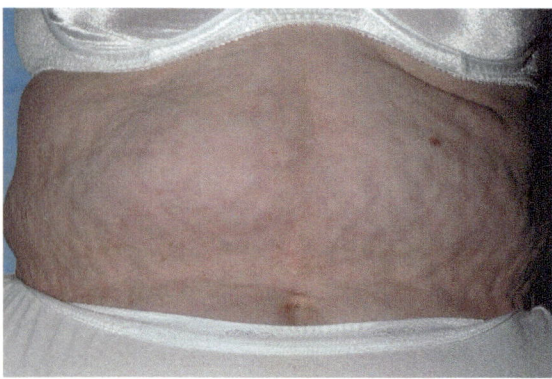

FIG. 26.8. Subcutaneous sclerosis from chronic GVHD; there is prominent rippling and nodularity of the subcutaneous tissue appreciable by deep palpation. The overlying skin is normal in texture and color

tissue, visible grooves demarcating fascial bundles or underlying superficial veins, and decreased range of motion (Fig. 26.8). The first indications of subcutaneous involvement may be edema of the affected limb. Magnetic resonance imaging may facilitate the diagnosis of subcutaneous involvement.[23]

Genital Graft-Versus-Host Disease

Assessment of genital involvement is important in the management of GVHD patients. Genital involvement is most commonly associated with sclerotic cutaneous disease, but may occur with other forms of cutaneous involvement, or in the absence of other cutaneous involvement. Genital tract involvement may be present in as many as 49% of female patients 2 years posttransplantation and may seriously impact the quality of life of affected individuals.[24] Manifestations include burning and irritation, discharge, erosions and fissures, or vaginal stricture (Fig. 26.9). Involvement of the male genitalia may result in phimosis.[25]

Oral Graft-Versus-Host Disease

The second most common organ system involved with chronic GVHD after the skin is the mouth. Chronic oral GVHD may affect the oral mucosa and salivary glands. Lichen-planus–like oral involvement is common, and manifests as erythema, hyperkeratotic plaques, and erosions. Sclerosis of

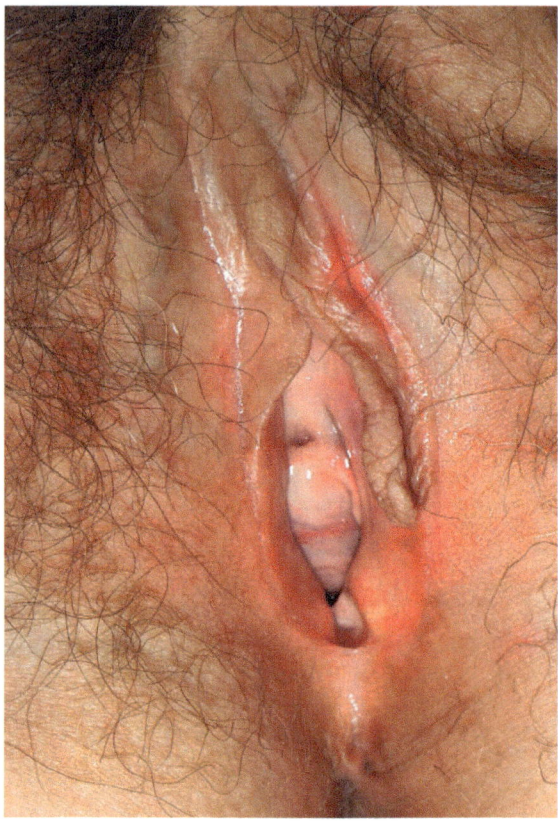

FIG. 26.9. Chronic vulvar GVHD; resorption of labia minora; pallor and sclerosis of vulvar vestibule; fissuring of the interlabial sulcus

the skin surrounding the mouth or the frenulum can cause difficulty opening the mouth or protruding the tongue, respectively. Persistent erosions and fissures cause burning pain, particularly upon contact with acidic foods. Salivary gland involvement from chronic GVHD results in decreased saliva production and sicca symptoms. Loss of taste is also commonly reported by patients.

Immunology of Graft-Versus-Host Disease

Acute Graft-Versus-Host Disease

Acute GVHD is a reaction of immunocompetent donor cells against the cells and organs of the host. Billingham[26] described three features necessary for the development of GVHD: (1) the transplanted graft must be immunologically competent, (2) the recipient must not be capable of rejecting the graft, and (3) the recipient must express antigens that are recognized as foreign by the graft. Grafted cells recognize the host as foreign through differences between the donor and host in major and minor HLA expression.

Proinflammatory Environment

Ferrara and Reddy[27] proposed a three-step model for the immunopathophysiology of acute GVHD. The first phase occurs prior to transplantation of the graft, during which time chemoradio-therapy, the underlying disease state, and other factors activate host antigen-presenting cells (APCs). Total body irradiation in particular plays an important role in priming the immune response by inducing epithelial cell damage in the gastrointestinal tract, which leads to host secretion of inflammatory cytokines (tumor necrosis factor-α [TNF-α], interleukin-1 [IL-1]) and exposure to microbial products such as lipopolysaccharide.

In the second phase of acute GVHD, host APCs expressing major histocompatibility complex (MHC) class I and II molecules are recognized as foreign by donor T cells. In murine studies, host dendritic cells are sufficient to activate donor T cells.[28] Differences in minor histocompatibility antigens (mHags), such as those encoded on the Y chromosome, may also play an important role in propagating acute GVHD, particularly in the setting of HLA-identical transplantation. Activation of natural killer (NK) cells, which eliminate APCs, abrogates the development of GVHD, suggesting a crucial role for host APCs in the propagation of acute GVHD.[29] The three major organ systems involved in acute GVHD—the skin, liver, and gut—contain large numbers of APCs, which may in part be responsible for the localization of tissue damage to these organ systems.[30]

In the final effector phase, inflammatory mediators and cell-mediated killing work together to induce the clinical manifestations typical of acute GVHD. CD8+ cytotoxic T lymphocytes (CTLs) utilize perforin/granzyme–mediated cytolysis, whereas CD4+ T cells utilize Fas/FasL signaling, which may be particularly important for inducing

hepatic damage.[27] Tumor necrosis factor-α and IL-1 signaling play a prominent role in cellular damage in acute gastrointestinal GVHD. Cytokine gene polymorphisms may influence the expression of GVHD. A polymorphism in the TNF-α gene has been associated with an increased risk of severe acute GHVD,[31] whereas polymorphisms in IL-10, a potent suppressor of TNF-α, IL-1, and other inflammatory cytokines, has been associated with a decreased incidence of acute GVHD.[32]

Regulatory T Cells

Acute GVHD is mediated by donor T cells that expand following transplantation in response to the recipient environment. Regulatory T (T_{reg}) cells constitute a subset of the T-cell population that exerts control over the allogeneic T-cell response against the host. T_{reg}s express FOXP3, a key transcription factor for T_{reg} function, as well as CD25, the IL-2 receptor α-chain that is also expressed by activated T cells. Donor grafts with a low percentage of CD4+Foxp3+ T_{reg}s are associated with an increased risk of acute GVHD. In addition, the ratio of CD4+FOXP3+ cells to CD4+FOXP3−CD25+ in patients after transplant is significantly reduced in patients with acute GVHD, suggesting an important role for T_{reg}s in control of effector function.[33] Manipulation of specific T-cell subsets in donor grafts may allow for modulation of the GVHD and graft-versus-leukemia response.

Chronic Graft-Versus-Host Disease

In contrast to acute disease, our understanding of the pathogenesis of chronic GVHD is somewhat incomplete. Chronic GVHD demonstrates a complex interplay of immunologic processes with features of alloimmunity, autoimmunity, and immunodeficiency. The heterogeneity of clinical manifestations and disease course in chronic GVHD makes human studies more challenging than studies of acute disease. In addition, correlations between murine models of GVHD and human chronic GVHD are difficult because marked differences in immune reactions are observed by the intensity of the conditioning regimen, disparity between strains, donor graft composition, and endogenous microbes of the animals.[34] The best characterized murine model of GVHD is the parent-into-F_1 mouse. In this model, parental lymphocytes are injected into the F_1 recipient offspring. Because the parental lymphocytes are genetically related to the recipient, they are not recognized as foreign. However, the donor lymphocytes recognize the F_1 mouse as foreign, inducing a GVHD reaction. The parent-into-F_1 model has several limitations as a model for GVHD, including the absence of a conditioning regimen, which is known to significantly impact the pathogenesis of GVHD.

In chronic GVHD, autoreactive T cells are thought to arise from impairment of the negative selection process in the thymus due to thymic damage incurred from chemotherapy, acute GVHD, or age-related atrophy.[35] The clinical similarity of chronic GVHD to autoimmune diseases such as Sjögren's syndrome and scleroderma and the reported benefit of treatment of chronic GVHD with anti-CD20 monoclonal antibody[36] also suggest an important role for B cells in chronic GVHD. Circulating autoantibodies were described in one of the first series describing the clinical features of chronic GVHD in 1980[37]; however, the relevance of antibody formation to disease activity remains unclear. In a prospective study of autoantibody formation following transplantation, the cumulative incidence of antinuclear antibodies (ANAs) in patients with extensive chronic GVHD was 94% after a median follow-up of 26 months.[38] The presence of ANA with a nucleolar pattern and the detection of other antibodies in association with ANA are associated with an increased risk of extensive chronic GVHD, but the presence and titer of specific autoantibodies does not predict the type of organ involvement.[38] Antibodies targeting minor HLA antibodies on the Y chromosome in male recipients of stem cell grafts from female donors correlate with the presence of chronic GVHD, suggesting a potentially important interplay between T and B cells in the pathogenesis of chronic GVHD.[39]

Cytokine Dysregulation

Chronic GVHD is associated with elevated levels of IL-1(β), IL-6, transforming growth factor-β (TGF-β), TNF-α, and interferon-γ (IFN-γ), and decreased levels of IL-10.[40,41] Transforming growth factor-β is the cytokine that has been most strongly implicated in GVHD-related fibrosis. Tissue fibrosis is a common manifestation in sev-

eral organ systems involved with chronic GVHD, including the liver and pulmonary system (bronchiolitis obliterans) as well as the skin. Transforming growth factor-β is a pleiotropic cytokine that in the acute posttransplant period regulates donor engraftment and graft-versus-leukemia effect.[42] In the chronic period, TGF-β appears to the major driving force for collagen synthesis and the development of fibrosis. In the murine sclerodermatous GVH model, treatment with anti–TGF-β antibody prevents lung and skin fibrosis.[43]

Platelet-Derived Growth Factor

In scleroderma, platelet-derived growth factor (PDGF) appears to play a key role in the increased proliferative capacity of fibroblasts, an effect that is enhanced by the presence of TGF-β.[44] Increased gene expression of PGDF has been also detected in the skin in the murine sclerodermatous GVHD model.[45] Recently, Baroni et al.[46] reported stimulatory autoantibodies to the platelet-derived growth factor receptor (PDGFR) in a group of 46 patients with systemic sclerosis. Ten additional patients with scleroderma-like GVHD were also reported to have agonistic antibodies (this group was not further described in the paper). In this study, production of reactive oxygen species (ROS) and tyrosine phosphorylation was reversed with the use of PDGFR tyrosine kinase inhibitors, suggesting that agents such as imatinib with activity against the PDGFR may have potential utility for targeting this signaling pathway in the setting of scleroderma and sclerotic GVHD. In addition, bronchiolitis obliterans, a fibrosing pulmonary complication that may occur in patients with chronic GVHD, has also been associated with PDGF expression[47] and has been reported to respond to treatment with imatinib.[48] Activation of angiogenic cytokine signaling through PDGF or vascular endothelial growth factor (VEGF) has been proposed as the mechanism for the development of angiomatous skin lesions that have been described in patients with chronic GVHD (Fig. 26.7).[20]

Donor Lymphocyte Infusion and Graft-Versus-Tumor Effect

An important barrier to the effective control of acute and chronic GVHD is the risk of inhibiting the activity of the stem cell graft against the donor's primary malignancy (graft vs. leukemia effect). Numerous studies have demonstrated that the risk of tumor relapse is lower in patients with GVHD than in those who do not develop GVHD.[49] Similarly, T-cell depletion of the donor graft and aggressive multiagent GVHD prophylaxis reduces the risk of developing GVHD, but does so at the expense of the antileukemic effect, resulting in an increased relapse rate.[50] Donor lymphocyte infusions (DLIs) have been utilized to augment the antitumor response of the graft, but are also associated with an increased rate of GVHD.[51] Ideally, our understanding of chronic GVHD will progress to the point where separation of the graft versus host and graft versus leukemia (tumor) effect would be possible. In reality, it is a constant struggle to balance these competing forces in the management of these patients.

Treatment of Cutaneous Graft-Versus-Host Disease

Acute Graft-Versus-Host Disease

Acute GVHD is treated with systemic steroids, resulting in a 40% to 50% response rate. There is no consensus as to the appropriate second-line agent in those patients who do not respond adequately to corticosteroid therapy. A variety of salvage therapies have been utilized in patients with steroid refractory GVHD, but no single agent has proven to be a superior option (Table 26.4).[52] The major limitation of most acute GVHD therapies arises from the use of systemic immunosuppression and attendant risk of infection. Newer biologic agents, such as those targeting TNF-α, have shown some benefit in acute GVHD; however, these agents have also been linked to invasive fungal infections.[53]

Topical agents play a limited role in the management of acute cutaneous GVHD. However, high-potency topical corticosteroids may be of benefit in patients with limited skin involvement. Proper skin hygiene and surveillance for the development of cutaneous infections is needed.

For patients manifesting primarily cutaneous involvement, phototherapy is a potential treatment option in lieu of additional systemic immunosuppression. Psoralen in combination with UVA

(PUVA) resulted in a disease response in 15 of 20 patients treated for acute skin GVHD.[54] Wetzig et al.[55] reported improvement with UVA1 in five of seven patients with acute skin GVHD. Narrowband UVB administered five times weekly resulted in complete response in seven of 10 patients and a partial response in the remaining three patients after 3 to 5 weeks.[56]

Extracorporeal Photopheresis

Extracorporeal photopheresis (ECP) is a leukopheresis procedure that is approved by the U.S. Food and Drug Administration for the treatment of cutaneous T-cell lymphoma. Following leukopheresis, the mononuclear cell sample is mixed with 8-methoxypsoralen and exposed to a UVA light source before re-infusion into the patient. This procedure spares the patient the risk of serious infection associated with systemic immunosuppression and is particularly effective for skin GVHD.[57] Greinix et al.[57] reported a 65% complete response rate for acute skin GVHD after 3 months of treatment. Similarly, Messina et al.[58] reported a 76% response rate for acute skin involvement in 33 pediatric patients. The optimal frequency and duration of ECP for GVHD is unclear. Apoptosis of alloreactive T cells is the presumed mechanism for the efficacy of ECP in GVHD, despite the fact that only a small percentage of circulating lymphocytes are treated at each ECP session.[59] Extracorporeal photopheresis requires a large, double-lumen pheresis catheter and is not available at all medical centers. In addition, very small children are not able to undergo this procedure because of the fluid volume extracted for the procedure. However, modifications in the pheresis process may soon allow this therapy utilizing smaller fluid volumes.

Chronic Graft-Versus-Host Disease

Skin-Directed Versus Systemic Therapy

Infection is the leading cause of death in patients with chronic GVHD. Patients are immunosuppressed from their disease state as well as from the immunosuppressive regimens required to treat their disorder. Treatment recommendations for chronic cutaneous GVHD must include a consideration of the type and extent of skin involvement, the potential for long-term morbidity (e.g., sclerotic

TABLE 26.4. Treatment for acute and chronic mucocutaneous GVHD.

Treatment	Type of GVHD	
	Acute	Chronic (L/Sc/Oral)
Antithymocyte globulin	Remberger et al.[84]	–
Azathioprine	–	Penas et al.[85](Sc)
		Epstein et al.[82](Oral)
Basiliximab	Funke et al.[86]	–
Clofazimine	–	Lee et al.[87](L/Sc)
Corticosteroids (systemic)	Doney et al.[88]	Goerner et al.[90]*
	Ruutu et al.[89]	
Cyclosporine	Aschan[91]	Goerner et al.[90]*
		Epstein and Reece[81](Oral)
Daclizumab	Bordigoni et al.[92]	Teachey et al.[93]*
Denileukin diftitox	Shaughnessey et al.[94]	
Etanercept	Uberti et al.[95]	Chiang et al.[96]*
Etretinate	–	Marcellus et al.[78](Sc)
Extracorporeal photopheresis	Greinix et al.[57]	Couriel et al.[67](L/Sc)[97]
	Messina et al.[58]	Seaton[97] (L/Sc)
Hydroxychloroquine	–	Gilman et al.[98](L)+
Infliximab	Patricarca et al.[99]	–
	Couriel et al.[100]	
Mycophenolate mofetil	Basara et al.[101]	Basara[101]*
	Baudard et al.[102]	Baudard et al.[102](L/Sc)
Pentostatin	Bolanos-Meade et al.[103]	Goldberg et al.[104](L/Sc)
Pimecrolimus (topical)	–	Schmoook[62](L)
PUVA	Wiesmann et al.[54]	Leiter et al.[74](L/Sc)#
		Vogelsang et al.[105](L/Sc)
Rapamycin (sirolimus)	Benito et al.[106]	Johnston et al.[107](L/Sc)
Rituximab	Kamble et al.[108]	Cutler et al.[36](L/Sc)
Tacrolimus [systemic]	Furlong et al.[109]	Carnevale-Schianca[110](L/Sc)
Tacrolimus [topical]	–	Choi and Ngheim[60](L)
		Elad et al.[61](L/Sc)
		Eckardt et al. (Oral)[63]
Thalidomide	–	Kulkarni et al.[111]*
		Browne et al.[112]*
UVA1:	Wetzig et al.[55]	Calzavara Pinton et al.[77](L/Sc)
		Stander et al.[113](Sc)
UVB:	Grundmann-Kollmann et al.[56]†	Enk et al.[114](L/Sc)

L, lichenoid or erythematous skin involvement; Sc, sclerotic skin involvement.
*Type of chronic cutaneous GVHD not specified.
+In this study, both lichenoid and sclerotic-type cutaneous GVHD were treated; however, none of the sclerotic patients responded to therapy.
#Bath PUVA.
†Narrowband UVB.

disease), and the presence of other organ system involvement. Other important factors include the presence of high-risk features such as thrombocytopenia and progressive onset of disease, risk of infection, and the status of the underlying disease state/malignancy.

Limited cutaneous involvement in the absence of high-risk features or other systemic involve-ment may be addressed with topical measures. Nonsclerotic disease may respond well to mid- to ultra-high potency topical steroids (triamcinolone 0.1%–clobetasol 0.05% cream/ointment), but care should be taken to avoid skin atrophy with prolonged use.[16] Topical emollients and antipru-ritic agents may provide additional symptomatic relief. Choi and Nghiem[60] reported improvement in pruritus and erythema in 18 patients treated with tacrolimus 0.1% ointment. However, all patients eventually required systemic therapy or phototherapy to control their skin disease. Subsequent reports have also described a modest benefit from tacrolimus ointment 0.1%/0.03% as well as pimecrolimus 1% cream.[61,62] These agents have some limited utility for the treatment of superficial involvement, particularly in areas at high risk of skin atrophy with topical steroids. A response to topical tacrolimus 0.01% has also been reported for oral GVHD.[63] However, treatment of oral GVHD with tacrolimus 0.1% ointment markedly elevated the serum drug level in a patient taking systemic tacrolimus.[64] Systemic toxicity after three applications of topical tacrolimus has also been reported in a pediatric patient with acute GVHD who was not on systemic tacrolimus therapy.[65] The risk of cutaneous malignancy following long-term treatment with topical calcineurin inhibitors in the setting of chronic GVHD is unknown.

Preventative strategies, including sun avoidance and the use of sunblock and protective clothing, decrease the risk of a UV-radiation associated flare in symptoms. Surveillance should be done at regular intervals, looking for signs of cutaneous malignancy, and skin biopsy should be performed as appropriate. Diffuse or patchy postinflammatory pigmentation is a frequent sequela of chronic GVHD, particularly in darkly pigmented individuals. Following resolution of GVHD activity, this pigmentation fades gradually. Topical hydroquinone with or without retinoids or corticosteroid-containing compounds offer very limited benefit.[16]

Treatment of eroded tissue and skin ulcerations in the setting of skin sclerosis is challenging. Aggressive wound management utilizing protective films, dressings, and wound healing products such as becaplermin may be beneficial.[16] Regular supervision in a dedicated wound care clinic may maximize the likelihood of achieving wound healing. As patients may be relatively immunosuppressed by the presence of GVHD or by therapies aimed at controlling GVHD, it is important to rule out an infectious source. Bacterial, viral, mycobacterial, and fungal cultures should be performed as indicated. Similarly, consideration should be given to other noninfectious source of skin breakdown other than GVHD, including vasculitis, bullous drug reaction, neuropathy, primary cutaneous malignancy, and metastatic disease.

Systemic treatment of chronic GVHD utilizes many of the same systemic modalities as for acute GVHD (Table 26.4). Unfortunately, interpretation of therapeutic responses in clinical trials is hampered by the lack of standardized evaluative indices for skin involvement. In addition, responses to epidermal (lichenoid) and sclerotic skin disease are frequently reported together without the use of response criteria specific for the different skin manifestations.[66]

Extracorporeal Photopheresis

In a retrospective review of 71 patients with chronic GVHD treated with ECP, 59% of patients with cutaneous involvement responded to therapy, including 67% of those patients categorized as having "scleroderma."[67] The precise mechanism by which ECP treatment affects chronic GHVD is still unclear, but ECP causes an increase in the plasmacytoid DC2 dendritic cell population and a corresponding decrease in the monocytoid DC1 population, which may result in a shift from a primarily T-helper-1 (Th1) to a Th2 cytokine profile.[68] Increased production of IL-10, in particular, may play an important role in the mitigation of the GVHD response, through inhibition of antigen presentation and promotion of regulatory T-cell differentiation.[69,70] Although GVHD-related fasciitis resembles eosinophilic fasciitis, in contrast to eosinophilic fasciitis, it does not respond well to steroid therapy and may result in significant long-term functional disability. Extracorporeal photopheresis has been used successfully for the treatment of eosinophilic fasciitis,[71] and appears to be an attractive treatment option for GVHD-related fasciitis.[72]

Phototherapy

As with acute GVHD, chronic GVHD may respond to PUVA therapy. "Lichenoid" chronic GVHD has been reported to respond to PUVA therapy in several small series.[73] Improvement in both lichenoid and sclerotic chronic GVHD has also been reported in a small series following treatment with PUVA bath therapy.[74] It must be kept in mind, however, that chronic GVHD results in immunodeficiency that is often further compounded by iatrogenic immunosuppression and may result in an increased risk of skin neoplasia. Multiple squamous cell carcinomas have been reported following PUVA treatment for chronic GVHD.[75] The risk of melanoma in patients following HSCT is also significantly elevated.[76] UVA1 therapy has been used in small numbers of patients with lichenoid and sclerotic disease; however, relapse after therapy was seen in both types of cutaneous involvement.[77]

Systemic Retinoids

Marcellus et al.[78] describe the Johns Hopkins GVHD group's experience with etretinate for treatment-refractory sclerotic GVHD. Twenty of 27 evaluable patients had a subjective response. Six patients could not tolerate the medication due to scaling or skin breakdown. Further prospective studies are needed to determine the utility of systemic retinoids for superficial disease.

Treatment of Genital Graft-Versus-Host Disease

As mentioned earlier, genital involvement should be assessed by history and physical examination in the dermatologic evaluation of all female patients. Standard recommendations in all female patients regardless of the presence of GVHD include the use of a vaginal topical estrogen to decrease atrophy of mucosal tissue, discussion of the risks/benefits of systemic hormonal therapies, education regarding self-examination, and regular gynecologic symptom review, pelvic examination, and cervical cytology. External genital involvement may be treated with high-potency topical glucocorticoids (betamethasone dipropionate cream 0.05% gel or ointment) applied once or twice daily for up to 12 weeks.[16] Topical calcineurin inhibitors (cyclosporine, tacrolimus) are also beneficial in mild-moderate disease.[16,79] The presence of vulvar disease or symptoms of vaginal involvement should prompt consultation with a gynecologist experienced in the evaluation and management of genital GVHD for a comprehensive internal examination. Hydrocortisone acetate 10% rectal foam for 4 to 6 weeks may be used for intravaginal application.[24] Severe vaginal stenosis may result in hematocolpos and

requires the use of aggressive topical steroids and vaginal dilator insertion. Surgical lysis of extensive vaginal synechiae may be necessary in severe cases.[16] Transplant patients may also be at higher risk for cervical dysplasia and require close surveillance for the presence of vulvar human papillomavirus (HPV) infection along with regular cervical cytology.[80]

Treatment of Oral Graft-Versus-Host Disease

Localized oral disease should be treated with alcohol-based high-potency corticosteroid gels. Tacrolimus ointment is preferable for lip involvement due to the risk of atrophy with topical steroid use. Widespread oral disease may be treated with dexamethasone rinse formulation (0.5 mg/mL) four to six times a day. Cyclosporine[81] and azathioprine[82] rinses have been used in steroid-resistant cases. Oral phototherapy (PUVA, UVB, narrowband UVB) may be effective, but the specialized equipment required for oral phototherapy is not readily available.[16] Patients with oral sicca symptoms are treated with salivary stimulants (e.g., sugar-free gum), saliva substitutes, and frequent sipping of water.[16] Patients with oral dryness are at increased risk of tooth decay, and meticulous oral hygiene is advised as well as surveillance for candidal infection. An increased incidence of squamous cell carcinoma of the oral cavity has been reported in patients with chronic GVHD following HSCT,[83] and therefore a high degree of suspicion is required for oral lesions that do not respond appropriately to therapy.

Conclusion

Graft-versus-host disease is a serious complication stem cell of allogeneic transplantation cells. The skin is a frequently involved target organ in a systemic inflammatory response that is triggered by donor T cells recognition of host alloantigens on host antigen-presenting cells. A wide variety of dermatologic manifestations may occur in the acute and chronic phases of this disease. Further study is needed to determine the optimum treatment strategy for the various cutaneous features of chronic GVHD.

References

1. Copelan EA. Hematopoietic stem-cell transplantation. N Engl J Med 2006;354(17):1813–26.
2. Cutler C, Giri S, Jeyapalan S, et al. Acute and chronic graft-versus-host disease after allogeneic peripheral-blood stem-cell and bone marrow transplantation: a meta-analysis. J Clin Oncol 2001;19(16):3685–91.
3. Tabbara IA, Ingram RM. Nonmyeloablative therapy and allogeneic hematopoietic stem cell transplantation. Exp Hematol 2003;31(7):559–66.
4. Kersey JH. Historial background to hematopoietic stem cell transplantation. In: Atkinson K Champlin R, Ritz J, Fibbe WE, Ljungman P, Brenner MK, eds. Clinical Bone Marrow and Blood Stem Cell Transplantation, 3rd ed. Cambridge: Cambridge University Press, 2004:1–10.
5. Couriel DR, Saliba RM, Giralt S, et al. Acute and chronic graft-versus-host disease after ablative and nonmyeloablative conditioning for allogeneic hematopoietic transplantation. Biol Blood Marrow Transplant 2004;10(3):178–85.
6. Couriel D, Caldera H, Champlin R, et al. Acute graft-versus-host disease: pathophysiology, clinical manifestations, and management. Cancer 2004;101(9):1936–46.
7. Przepiorka D, Weisdorf D, Martin P, et al. 1994 Consensus Conference on Acute GVHD Grading. Bone Marrow Transplant 1995;15(6):825–8.
8. Friedman KJ, LeBoit PE, Farmer ER. Acute follicular graft-vs-host reaction. A distinct clinicopathologic presentation. Arch Dermatol 1988;124(5):688–91.
9. Zhou Y, Barnett MJ, Rivers JK. Clinical significance of skin biopsies in the diagnosis and management of graft-vs-host disease in early postallogeneic bone marrow transplantation. Arch Dermatol 2000;136(6):717–21.
10. Sullivan KM, Agura E, Anasetti C, et al. Chronic graft-versus-host disease and other late complications of bone marrow transplantation. Semin Hematol 1991;28(3):250–9.
11. Lee SJ, Vogelsang G, Flowers ME. Chronic graft-versus-host disease. Biol Blood Marrow Transplant 2003;9(4):215–33.
12. Filipovich AH, Weisdorf D, Pavletic S, et al. National Institutes of Health consensus development project on criteria for clinical trials in chronic graft-versus-host disease: I. Diagnosis and staging working group report. Biol Blood Marrow Transplant 2005;11(12):945–56.
13. Shulman HM, Kleiner D, Lee SJ, et al. Histopathologic diagnosis of chronic graft-versus-host disease: National Institutes of Health Consensus Development Project on Criteria for Clinical Trials in Chronic Graft-versus-Host Disease: II. Pathology Working Group Report. Biol Blood Marrow Transplant 2006;12(1):31–47.
14. Schultz KR, Miklos DB, Fowler D, et al. Toward biomarkers for chronic graft-versus-host disease: National Institutes of Health consensus development project on criteria for clinical trials in chronic graft-versus-host disease: III. Biomarker Working Group Report. Biol Blood Marrow Transplant 2006;12(2):126–37.
15. Pavletic SZ, Martin P, Lee SJ, et al. Measuring therapeutic response in chronic graft-versus-host disease: National Institutes of Health Consensus Development Project on Criteria for Clinical Trials in Chronic Graft-versus-Host Disease: IV. Response Criteria Working Group report. Biol Blood Marrow Transplant 2006;12(3):252–66.
16. Couriel D, Carpenter PA, Cutler C, et al. Ancillary therapy and supportive care of chronic graft-versus-host disease: national institutes of health consensus development project on criteria for clinical trials in chronic graft-versus-host disease: V. Ancillary Therapy and Supportive Care Working Group Report. Biol Blood Marrow Transplant 2006;12(4):375–96.
17. Martin PJ, Weisdorf D, Przepiorka D, et al. National Institutes of Health Consensus Development Project on Criteria for Clinical Trials in Chronic Graft-versus-Host Disease: VI. Design of Clinical Trials Working Group report. Biol Blood Marrow Transplant 2006;12(5):491–505.
18. Hymes SR, Turner ML, Champlin RE, Couriel DR. Cutaneous manifestations of chronic graft-versus-host disease. Biol Blood Marrow Transplant 2006;12(11):1101–13.
19. Chosidow O, Bagot M, Vernant JP, et al. Sclerodermatous chronic graft-versus-host disease. Analysis of seven cases. J Am Acad Dermatol 1992;26(1):49–55.
20. Adamski H, Le Gall F, Cartron L, et al. Eruptive angiomatous lesions associated with graft-versus-host disease. Br J Dermatol 2003;149(3):667–8.
21. Carroll CB, Hilton DA, Hamon M, et al. Muscle cramps and weakness secondary to graft versus host disease fasciitis. Eur J Neurol 2005;12(4):320–2.
22. Shulman L. Diffuse fasciitis with hypergamma-globulinemia and eosinophilia: A new syndrome. J Rheumatol 1974;1(suppl 1):46.
23. Dumford K, Anderson JC. CT and MRI findings in sclerodermatous chronic graft vs. host disease. Clin Imaging 2001;25(2):138–40.
24. Zantomio D, Grigg AP, MacGregor L, et al. Female genital tract graft-versus-host disease: incidence, risk factors and recommendations for management. Bone Marrow Transplant 2006;38(8):567–72.
25. Kami M, Kanda Y, Sasaki M, et al. Phimosis as a manifestation of chronic graft-versus-host disease

after allogeneic bone marrow transplantation. Bone Marrow Transplant 1998;21(7):721–3.

26. Billingham RE. The biology of graft-versus-host reactions. Harvey Lect 1966;62:21–78.

27. Ferrara JL, Reddy P. Pathophysiology of graft-versus-host disease. Semin Hematol 2006;43(1):3–10.

28. Duffner UA, Maeda Y, Cooke KR, et al. Host dendritic cells alone are sufficient to initiate acute graft-versus-host disease. J Immunol 2004;172(12):7393–8.

29. Ruggeri L, Capanni M, Urbani E, et al. Effectiveness of donor natural killer cell alloreactivity in mismatched hematopoietic transplants. Science 2002;295(5562):2097–100.

30. Zhang Y, Shlomchik WD, Joe G, et al. APCs in the liver and spleen recruit activated allogeneic CD8+ T cells to elicit hepatic graft-versus-host disease. J Immunol 2002;169(12):7111–8.

31. Mullighan C, Heatley S, Doherty K, et al. Non-HLA immunogenetic polymorphisms and the risk of complications after allogeneic hemopoietic stem-cell transplantation. Transplantation 2004;77(4):587–96.

32. Lin MT, Storer B, Martin PJ, et al. Relation of an interleukin-10 promoter polymorphism to graft-versus-host disease and survival after hematopoietic-cell transplantation. N Engl J Med 2003;349(23):2201–10.

33. Rezvani K, Mielke S, Ahmadzadeh M, et al. High donor FOXP3–positive regulatory T-cell (Treg) content is associated with a low risk of GVHD following HLA-matched allogeneic SCT. Blood 2006;108(4):1291–7.

34. Blazar BR, Murphy WJ. Bone marrow transplantation and approaches to avoid graft-versus-host disease (GVHD). Philos Trans R Soc Lond 2005;360(1461):1747–67.

35. Sakoda Y, Hashimoto D, Asakura S, et al. Donor-derived thymic-dependent T cells cause chronic graft-versus-host disease. Blood 2007;109(4):1756–64.

36. Cutler C, Miklos D, Kim HT, et al. Rituximab for steroid-refractory chronic graft-versus-host disease. Blood 2006;108(2):756–62.

37. Shulman HM, Sullivan KM, Weiden PL, et al. Chronic graft-versus-host syndrome in man. A long-term clinicopathologic study of 20 Seattle patients. Am J Med 1980;69(2):204–17.

38. Patriarca F, Skert C, Sperotto A, et al. The development of autoantibodies after allogeneic stem cell transplantation is related with chronic graft-vs-host disease and immune recovery. Exp Hematol 2006;34(3):389–96.

39. Miklos DB, Kim HT, Miller KH, et al. Antibody responses to H-Y minor histocompatibility antigens correlate with chronic graft-versus-host disease and disease remission. Blood 2005;105(7):2973–8.

40. Barak V, Levi-Schaffer F, Nisman B, et al. Cytokine dysregulation in chronic graft versus host disease. Leuk Lymphoma 1995;17(1–2):169–73.

41. Korholz D, Kunst D, Hempel L, et al. Decreased interleukin 10 and increased interferon-gamma production in patients with chronic graft-versus-host disease after allogeneic bone marrow transplantation. Bone Marrow Transplant 1997;19(7):691–5.

42. Banovic T, MacDonald KP, Morris ES, et al. TGF-beta in allogeneic stem cell transplantation: friend or foe? Blood 2005;106(6):2206–14.

43. McCormick LL, Zhang Y, Tootell E, et al. Anti-TGF-beta treatment prevents skin and lung fibrosis in murine sclerodermatous graft-versus-host disease: a model for human scleroderma. J Immunol 1999;163(10):5693–9.

44. Bonner JC. Regulation of PDGF and its receptors in fibrotic diseases. Cytokine Growth Factor Rev 2004;15(4):255–73.

45. Zhou L, Askew D, Wu C, et al. Cutaneous gene expression by DNA microarray in murine sclerodermatous graft-versus-host disease, a model for human scleroderma. J Invest Dermatol 2007;127(2):281–92.

46. Baroni SS, Santillo M, Bevilacqua F, et al. Stimulatory autoantibodies to the PDGF receptor in systemic sclerosis. N Engl J Med 2006;354(25):2667–76.

47. Hertz MI, Henke CA, Nakhleh RE, et al. Obliterative bronchiolitis after lung transplantation: a fibroproliferative disorder associated with platelet-derived growth factor. Proc Natl Acad Sci USA 1992;89(21):10385–9.

48. Majhail NS, Schiffer CA, Weisdorf DJ. Improvement of pulmonary function with imatinib mesylate in bronchiolitis obliterans following allogeneic hematopoietic cell transplantation. Biol Blood Marrow Transplant 2006;12(7):789–91.

49. Weiden PL, Sullivan KM, Flournoy N, et al. Antileukemic effect of chronic graft-versus-host disease: contribution to improved survival after allogeneic marrow transplantation. N Engl J Med 1981;304(25):1529–33.

50. Marmont AM, Horowitz MM, Gale RP, et al. T-cell depletion of HLA-identical transplants in leukemia. Blood 1991;78(8):2120–30.

51. Sullivan KM, Storb R, Buckner CD, et al. Graft-versus-host disease as adoptive immunotherapy in patients with advanced hematologic neoplasms. N Engl J Med 1989;320(13):828–34.

52. Bolanos-Meade J, Vogelsang GB. Novel strategies for steroid-refractory acute graft-versus-host disease. Curr Opin Hematol 2005;12(1):40–4.

53. Marty FM, Lee SJ, Fahey MM, et al. Infliximab use in patients with severe graft-versus-host disease and

other emerging risk factors of non-Candida invasive fungal infections in allogeneic hematopoietic stem cell transplant recipients: a cohort study. Blood 2003;102(8):2768–76.

54. Wiesmann A, Weller A, Lischka G, et al. Treatment of acute graft-versus-host disease with PUVA (psoralen and ultraviolet irradiation): results of a pilot study. Bone Marrow Transplant 1999;23(2):151–5.

55. Wetzig T, Sticherling M, Simon JC, et al. Medium dose long-wavelength ultraviolet A (UVA1) phototherapy for the treatment of acute and chronic graft-versus-host disease of the skin. Bone Marrow Transplant 2005;35(5):515–9.

56. Grundmann-Kollmann M, Martin H, Ludwig R, et al. Narrowband UV-B phototherapy in the treatment of cutaneous graft versus host disease. Transplantation 2002;74(11):1631–4.

57. Greinix HT, Volc-Platzer B, Kalhs P, et al. Extracorporeal photochemotherapy in the treatment of severe steroid-refractory acute graft-versus-host disease: a pilot study. Blood 2000;96(7):2426–31.

58. Messina C, Locatelli F, Lanino E, et al. Extracorporeal photochemotherapy for paediatric patients with graft-versus-host disease after haematopoietic stem cell transplantation. Br J Haematol 2003;122(1):118–27.

59. Bladon J, Taylor PC. Extracorporeal photopheresis induces apoptosis in the lymphocytes of cutaneous T-cell lymphoma and graft-versus-host disease patients. Br J Haematol 1999;107(4):707–11.

60. Choi CJ, Nghiem P. Tacrolimus ointment in the treatment of chronic cutaneous graft-vs-host disease: a case series of 18 patients. Arch Dermatol 2001;137(9):1202–6.

61. Elad S, Or R, Resnick I, et al. Topical tacrolimus–a novel treatment alternative for cutaneous chronic graft-versus-host disease. Transpl Int 2003;16(9):665–70.

62. Schmook T, Kraft J, Benninghoff B, et al. Treatment of cutaneous chronic graft-versus-host disease with topical pimecrolimus. Bone Marrow Transplant 2005;36(1):87–8.

63. Eckardt A, Starke O, Stadler M, et al. Severe oral chronic graft-versus-host disease following allogeneic bone marrow transplantation: highly effective treatment with topical tacrolimus. Oral Oncol 2004;40(8):811–4.

64. Conrotto D, Carrozzo M, Ubertalli AV, et al. Dramatic increase of tacrolimus plasma concentration during topical treatment for oral graft-versus-host disease. Transplantation 2006;82(8):1113–5.

65. Neuman DL, Farrar JE, Moresi JM, et al. Toxic absorption of tacrolimus [corrected] in a patient with severe acute graft-versus-host disease. Bone Marrow Transplant 2005;36(10):919–20.

66. Greinix HT, Volc-Platzer B, Knobler R. Criteria for assessing chronic GVHD. Bone Marrow Transplant 2000;25(5):575.

67. Couriel DR, Hosing C, Saliba R, et al. Extracorporeal photochemotherapy for the treatment of steroid-resistant chronic GVHD. Blood 2006;107(8):3074–80.

68. Gorgun G, Miller KB, Foss FM. Immunologic mechanisms of extracorporeal photochemotherapy in chronic graft-versus-host disease. Blood 2002;100(3):941–7.

69. Craciun LI, Stordeur P, Schandene L, et al. Increased production of interleukin-10 and interleukin-1 receptor antagonist after extracorporeal photochemotherapy in chronic graft-versus-host disease. Transplantation 2002;74(7):995–1000.

70. Fimiani M, Di Renzo M, Rubegni P. Mechanism of action of extracorporeal photochemotherapy in chronic graft-versus-host disease. Br J Dermatol 2004;150(6):1055–60.

71. Romano C, Rubegni P, De Aloe G, et al. Extracorporeal photochemotherapy in the treatment of eosinophilic fasciitis. J Eur Acad Dermatol Venereol 2003;17(1):10–3.

72. Sbano P, Rubegni P, De Aloe GB, et al. Extracorporeal photochemotherapy for treatment of fasciitis in chronic graft-versus-host disease. Bone Marrow Transplant 2004;33(8):869–70.

73. Jampel RM, Farmer ER, Vogelsang GB, et al. PUVA therapy for chronic cutaneous graft-vs-host disease. Arch Dermatol 1991;127(11):1673–8.

74. Leiter U, Kaskel P, Krahn G, et al. Psoralen plus ultraviolet-A-bath photochemotherapy as an adjunct treatment modality in cutaneous chronic graft versus host disease. Photodermatol Photoimmunol Photomed 2002;18(4):183–90.

75. Altman JS, Adler SS. Development of multiple cutaneous squamous cell carcinomas during PUVA treatment for chronic graft-versus-host disease. J Am Acad Dermatol 1994;31(3 pt 1):505–7.

76. Curtis RE, Rowlings PA, Deeg HJ, et al. Solid cancers after bone marrow transplantation. N Engl J Med 1997;336(13):897–904.

77. Calzavara Pinton P, Porta F, Izzi T, et al. Prospects for ultraviolet A1 phototherapy as a treatment for chronic cutaneous graft-versus-host disease. Haematologica 2003;88(10):1169–75.

78. Marcellus DC, Altomonte VL, Farmer ER, et al. Etretinate therapy for refractory sclerodermatous chronic graft-versus-host disease. Blood 1999;93(1):66–70.

79. Spiryda LB, Laufer MR, Soiffer RJ, et al. Graft-versus-host disease of the vulva and/or vagina: diagnosis and treatment. Biol Blood Marrow Transplant 2003;9(12):760–5.

80. Sasadeusz J, Kelly H, Szer J, et al. Abnormal cervical cytology in bone marrow transplant recipients. Bone Marrow Transplant 2001;28(4):393–7.

81. Epstein JB, Reece DE. Topical cyclosporin A for treatment of oral chronic graft-versus-host disease. Bone Marrow Transplant 1994;13(1):81–6.

82. Epstein JB, Nantel S, Sheoltch SM. Topical azathioprine in the combined treatment of chronic oral graft-versus-host disease. Bone Marrow Transplant 2000;25(6):683–7.

83. Bhatia S, Louie AD, Bhatia R, et al. Solid cancers after bone marrow transplantation. J Clin Oncol 2001;19(2):464–71.

84. Remberger M, Aschan J, Barkholt L, Tollemar J, Ringden O. Treatment of severe acute graft-versus-host disease with anti-thymocyte globulin. Clin Transplant 2001;15(3):147–53.

85. Penas PF, Jones-Caballero M, Aragues M, et al. Sclerodermatous graft-vs-host disease: clinical and pathological study of 17 patients. Arch Dermatol 2002;138(7):924–34.

86. Funke VA, de Medeiros CR, Setubal DC, et al. Therapy for severe refractory acute graft-versus-host disease with basiliximab, a selective interleukin-2 receptor antagonist. Bone Marrow Transplant 2006;37(10):961–5.

87. Lee SJ, Wegner SA, McGarigle CJ, et al. Treatment of chronic graft-versus-host disease with clofazimine. Blood 1997;89(7):2298–302.

88. Doney KC, Weiden PL, Storb R, et al. Treatment of graft-versus-host disease in human allogeneic marrow graft recipients: a randomized trial comparing antithymocyte globulin and corticosteroids. Am J Hematol 1981;11(1):1–8.

89. Ruutu T, Niederwieser D, Gratwohl A, et al. A survey of the prophylaxis and treatment of acute GVHD in Europe: a report of the European Group for Blood and Marrow, Transplantation (EBMT). Chronic Leukaemia Working Party of the EBMT. Bone Marrow Transplant 1997;19(8):759–64.

90. Goerner M, Gooley T, Flowers ME, et al. Morbidity and mortality of chronic GVHD after hematopoietic stem cell transplantation from HLA-identical siblings for patients with aplastic or refractory anemias. Biol Blood Marrow Transplant 2002;8(1):47–56.

91. Aschan J. Treatment of moderate to severe acute graft-versus-host disease: a retrospective analysis. Bone Marrow Transplant 1994;14(4):601–7.

92. Bordigoni P, Dimicoli S, Clement L, et al. Daclizumab, an efficient treatment for steroid-refractory acute graft-versus-host disease. Br J Haematol 2006;135(3):382–5.

93. Teachey DT, Bickert B, Bunin N. Daclizumab for children with corticosteroid refractory graft-versus-host disease. Bone Marrow Transplant 2006;37(1):95–9.

94. Shaughnessy PJ, Bachier C, Grimley M, et al. Denileukin diftitox for the treatment of steroid-resistant acute graft-versus-host disease. Biol Blood Marrow Transplant 2005;11(3):188–93.

95. Uberti JP, Ayash L, Ratanatharathorn V, et al. Pilot trial on the use of etanercept and methylprednisolone as primary treatment for acute graft-versus-host disease. Biol Blood Marrow Transplant 2005;11(9):680–7.

96. Chiang KY, Abhyankar S, Bridges K, et al. Recombinant human tumor necrosis factor receptor fusion protein as complementary treatment for chronic graft-versus-host disease. Transplantation 2002;73(4):665–7.

97. Seaton ED, Szydlo RM, Kanfer E, et al. Influence of extracorporeal photopheresis on clinical and laboratory parameters in chronic graft-versus-host disease and analysis of predictors of response. Blood 2003;102(4):1217–23.

98. Gilman AL, Chan KW, Mogul A, et al. Hydroxychloroquine for the treatment of chronic graft-versus-host disease. Biol Blood Marrow Transplant 2000;6(3A):327–34.

99. Patriarca F, Sperotto A, Damiani D, et al. Infliximab treatment for steroid-refractory acute graft-versus-host disease. Haematologica 2004;89(11):1352–9.

100. Couriel D, Saliba R, Hicks K, et al. Tumor necrosis factor-alpha blockade for the treatment of acute GVHD. Blood 2004;104(3):649–54.

101. Basara N, Kiehl MG, Blau W, et al. Mycophenolate Mofetil in the treatment of acute and chronic GVHD in hematopoietic stem cell transplant patients: four years of experience. Transplant Proc 2001;33(3):2121–3.

102. Baudard M, Vincent A, Moreau P, et al. Mycophenolate mofetil for the treatment of acute and chronic GVHD is effective and well tolerated but induces a high risk of infectious complications: a series of 21 BM or PBSC transplant patients. Bone Marrow Transplant 2002;30(5):287–95.

103. Bolanos-Meade J, Jacobsohn DA, Margolis J, et al. Pentostatin in steroid-refractory acute graft-versus-host disease. J Clin Oncol 2005;23(12):2661–8.

104. Goldberg JD, Jacobsohn DA, Margolis J, et al. Pentostatin for the treatment of chronic graft-versus-host disease in children. J Pediatr Hematol Oncol 2003;25(7):584–8.

105. Vogelsang GB, Wolff D, Altomonte V, et al. Treatment of chronic graft-versus-host disease with ultraviolet irradiation and psoralen (PUVA). Bone Marrow Transplantation 1996;17(6):1061–7.

106. Benito AI, Furlong T, Martin PJ, et al. Sirolimus (rapamycin) for the treatment of steroid-refractory acute graft-versus-host disease. Transplantation 2001;72(12):1924–9.

107. Johnston LJ, Brown J, Shizuru JA, et al. Rapamycin (sirolimus) for treatment of chronic graft-versus-host disease. Biol Blood Marrow Transplant 2005;11(1):47–55.

108. Kamble R, Oholendt M, Carrum G. Rituximab responsive refractory acute graft-versus-host disease. Biol Blood Marrow Transplant 2006; |12(11):1201–2.

109. Furlong T, Storb R, Anasetti C, et al. Clinical outcome after conversion to FK 506 (tacrolimus) therapy for acute graft-versus-host disease resistant to cyclosporine or for cyclosporine-associated toxicities. Bone Marrow Transplant 2000;26(9): 985–91.

110. Carnevale-Schianca F, Martin P, Sullivan K, et al. Changing from cyclosporine to tacrolimus as salvage therapy for chronic graft-versus-host disease. Biol Blood Marrow Transplant 2000;6(6): 613–20.

111. Kulkarni S, Powles R, Sirohi B, et al. Thalidomide after allogeneic haematopoietic stem cell transplantation: activity in chronic but not in acute graft-versus-host disease. Bone Marrow Transplant 2003;32(2):165–70.

112. Browne PV, Weisdorf DJ, DeFor T, et al. Response to thalidomide therapy in refractory chronic graft-versus-host disease. Bone Marrow Transplant 2000;26(8):865–9.

113. Stander H, Schiller M, Schwarz T. UVA1 therapy for sclerodermic graft-versus-host disease of the skin. J Am Acad Dermatol 2002;46(5):799–800.

114. Enk CD, Elad S, Vexler A, et al. Chronic graft-versus-host disease treated with UVB phototherapy. Bone Marrow Transplant 1998;22(12):1179–83.

27
Allergic Urticaria

Laura M. Gober and Sarbjit S. Saini

Key Points

- Urticaria can be acute or chronic, and may be allergic (mediated by immunoglobulin E) or nonallergic (mediated by pharmacologic effects of drugs such as aspirin or an acute-phase response).
- There are variants of urticaria that are caused by physical factors such as exposure of the skin to pressure, vibration, cold, or even water (aquagenic urticaria).
- Urticarial lesions are produced in the skin by the degranulation of mast cells. Urticaria can be a presenting sign of urticarial vasculitis.
- Chronic urticaria is the common presentation of this condition, and in most instances it is not possible to identify an etiology (idiopathic urticaria).
- There are a multitude of causes of urticaria, including food or medication allergies, infections, as well as in association with autoimmune diseases such as thyroid disease. Histamine-releasing autoantibodies are thought to be one of the possible causes of urticaria.
- Treatment is based on identifying a trigger factor. If this is not possible, short courses of glucocorticosteroids are warranted. Antihistamines are a cornerstone of treatment. For more severe cases, immune modulating drugs such as cyclosporine may be necessary to control signs and symptoms of this process. Biologic agents such as rituximab and omalizumab are promising.

Acute and Chronic Urticaria

Urticaria, commonly known as hives, is characterized by the episodic appearance of pruritic, erythematous papules or plaques with superficial swelling of the dermis (Fig. 27.1). Acute urticaria entails a symptom duration of less than 6 weeks, and chronic urticaria entails a symptom duration of 6 weeks or longer. Acute urticaria occurs in an estimated 15% to 23% of the population, although cases are likely to be underreported due to the short-lived nature of the disease.[1] The prevalence of acute urticaria increases to 50% in individuals with allergic rhinitis, asthma, or atopic dermatitis.[2] Chronic urticaria can be further defined as physical or chronic idiopathic urticaria (CIU). Physical urticarias comprise many subtypes in which a specific trigger can quickly induce hives, while CIU lacks a known trigger.[3] The prevalence of physical urticarias is not well established, but it is thought to account for 20% to 35% of all chronic urticarias.[4,5] Chronic idiopathic urticaria occurs in approximately 0.1% to 3% of the population and has a female predominance, as do many forms of chronic urticaria.[1,6,7]

Clinical and Cellular Features of Urticaria

Clinically, urticarial lesions are intensely pruritic and can appear anywhere on the body, typically appearing quickly and typically lasting 1 to 24 hours.[8] Unlike other pruritic skin diseases such as atopic dermatitis, patients with urticaria find relief from rubbing the skin versus scratching, making excoriated skin an unusual finding in CIU.[6] Lesions

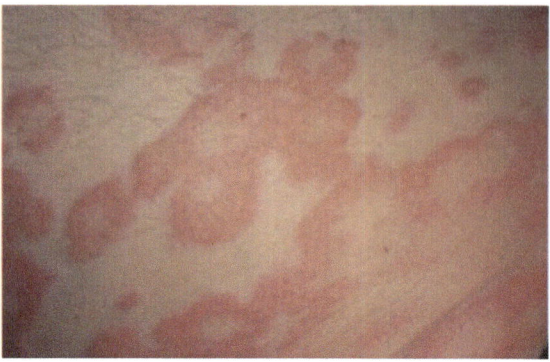

FIG. 27.1. Urticarial lesions. (Courtesy of Carrie McCann, RN, Dermatlas; http://www.dermatlas.org.)

can vary in size and can be confluent (Fig. 27.1). The swelling observed with urticaria results from the movement of plasma from small blood vessels into adjacent connective tissue.[5] Angioedema, or deeper, swelling of the dermis, subcutaneous, and submucosal tissues, often coexists with urticaria but has a slower resolution time, typically longer than 24 hours, although large areas of swelling may take even longer to resolve (Fig. 27.2).[6] Angioedema is described as painful or burning in quality, and not pruritic; this is likely due to the presence of fewer mast cells and sensory nerve endings in the lower dermis and subcutis.[9] It frequently involves mucous membranes, with common locations being the face, lips, tongue, pharynx, and extremities (Fig. 27.2).[6] In contrast, urticaria, both acute and chronic, rarely involves mucosal surfaces with the

exception of cold urticaria, which may involve the tongue or palate.[6]

The classic wheal observed in both acute and chronic urticaria represents dermal edema with dilatation of postcapillary venules and lymphatic vessels (Fig. 27.3A,B).[10] In biopsies, the leukocyte infiltrate is characteristically perivascular and classically consists of neutrophils, macrophages, lymphocytes, and occasionally eosinophils (Fig. 27.3A,B).[11,12] By immunohistochemistry, tumor necrosis factor-α (TNF-α) and interleukin-3 (IL-3) protein expression are increased in acute and chronic urticarial lesions.[13] Tumor necrosis factor-α is a cytokine made by epithelial cells, leukocytes, and mast cells.[14,15] It can induce mast cell mediator release and increase endothelial adhesion molecule expression, and thus an increase of this cytokine in urticaria may contribute to the leukocyte infiltrate observed.[15–17] Interleukin-3 is a cytokine produced by mast cells, T cells, monocytes, and granulocytes, and can increase expression of the endothelial adhesion molecule P-selectin.[18–21] P-selectin expression is elevated in both the skin and serum of chronic urticaria patients.[22] Two endothelial adhesion molecules, integrins endothelial leukocyte adhesion molecule 1 (ELAM-1) and intercellular adhesion molecule 1 (ICAM-1), were upregulated in acute and chronic urticarial lesions.[11] The persistent expression of ELAM-1 and ICAM-1 in lesions older than 6 hours may help to explain the long duration of urticarial wheals.[11]

History and Physical Exam

In diagnosing either acute or chronic urticaria, a good history is the most important element (Fig. 27.4). It is important to assess the time of onset of hives, as some patients may experience diurnal variation, as well as the days affected in association with certain environmental exposures or stressors. Patients should provide a description of lesions including elements such as shape, size, distribution, color, pigmentation, and the quality of pain or itch. Urticarial lesions are typically pruritic and usually demonstrate complete resolution without skin pigment changes. A clinician also must determine the presence of angioedema in association with urticaria. In patients with isolated angioedema without urticaria, family history is critical to determine the presence of hereditary angioedema, an

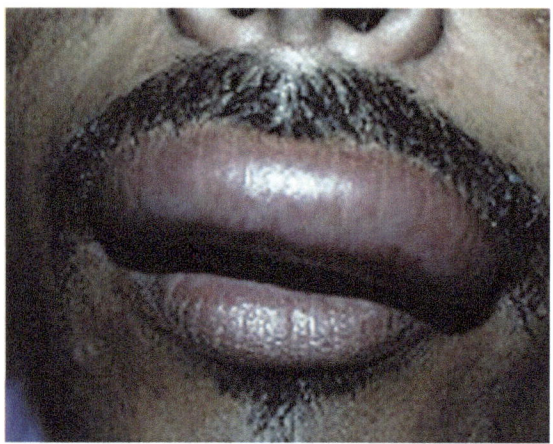

FIG. 27.2. Angioedema. (Courtesy of Kosman S. Zikry, MD, Dermatlas; http://www.dermatlas.org.)

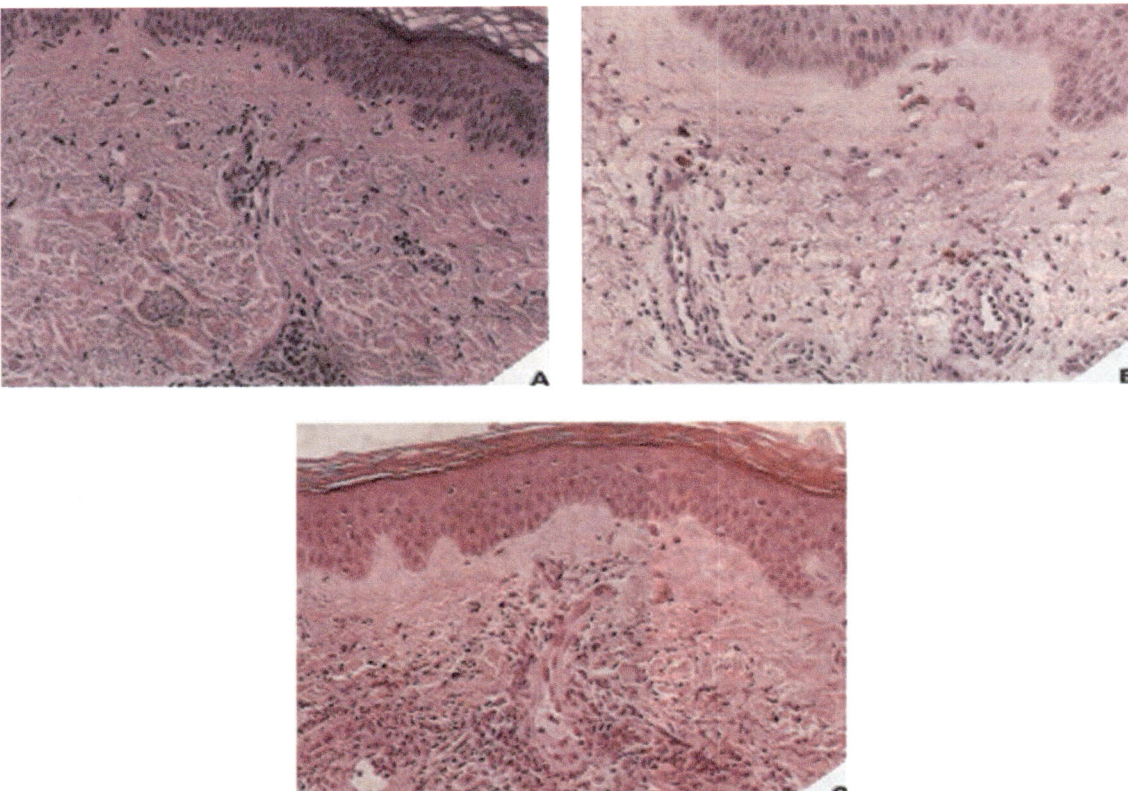

FIG. 27.3. Biopsy of urticarial lesion. (A) Representative of acute urticaria with dermal edema and a perivascular mononuclear infiltrate. (B) Chronic urticaria may also have infiltration of neutrophils or eosinophils without evidence of vasculitis. (C) Urticarial vasculitis is shown with a large perivascular infiltration of neutrophils, and even some neutrophilic damage. (From Fireman, Savin. Atlas of Allergies, 2nd ed. 1996, Elsevier Publisher.)

autosomal dominant trait involving a defect in C1 esterase inhibitor function. Atopic history is useful, especially for acute urticaria, since (1) atopic individuals have a higher prevalence of acute urticaria, and (2) this may uncover a possible trigger. The most important role of history-taking is to identify the inducing agent of the patient's urticaria or angioedema. This involves questions regarding recent use of medications, including antibiotics, nonsteroidal antiinflammatory agents, and aspirin. A history of food ingested shortly prior to symptom occurrence, possible insect stings, or changes in environment should also be sought. Additional questions should include recent infections, thyroid disease symptoms, surgical history of implantable devices, and, for females, the relationship of hives to their menstrual cycle or pregnancy. Further evaluation of life stressors, including patient's work and a history of tobacco smoking, may assist

in understanding the timing or exacerbation of lesions. It is also important to evaluate how the patient is coping and what therapeutics, including nonprescription medications and dietary regimens, are being used and if they are providing any relief.

Along with the detailed history, the physical exam in a patient with urticaria can be helpful in excluding other disorders. It is important to do a complete exam as well as determine the presence of dermatographism (Fig. 27.5). Physical urticarias may require additional maneuvers in the physical exam, such as an ice-cube test to evaluate cold urticaria, and should be tailored to the suspected type of urticaria (Fig. 27.6 and Table 27.1).[1] The size, distribution, and color of lesions should be noted. Wheals are characteristically pink or red due to histamine-induced dilatation of vessels in the skin, while vasculitic lesions have a darker red or purple appearance resulting from vascular damage and

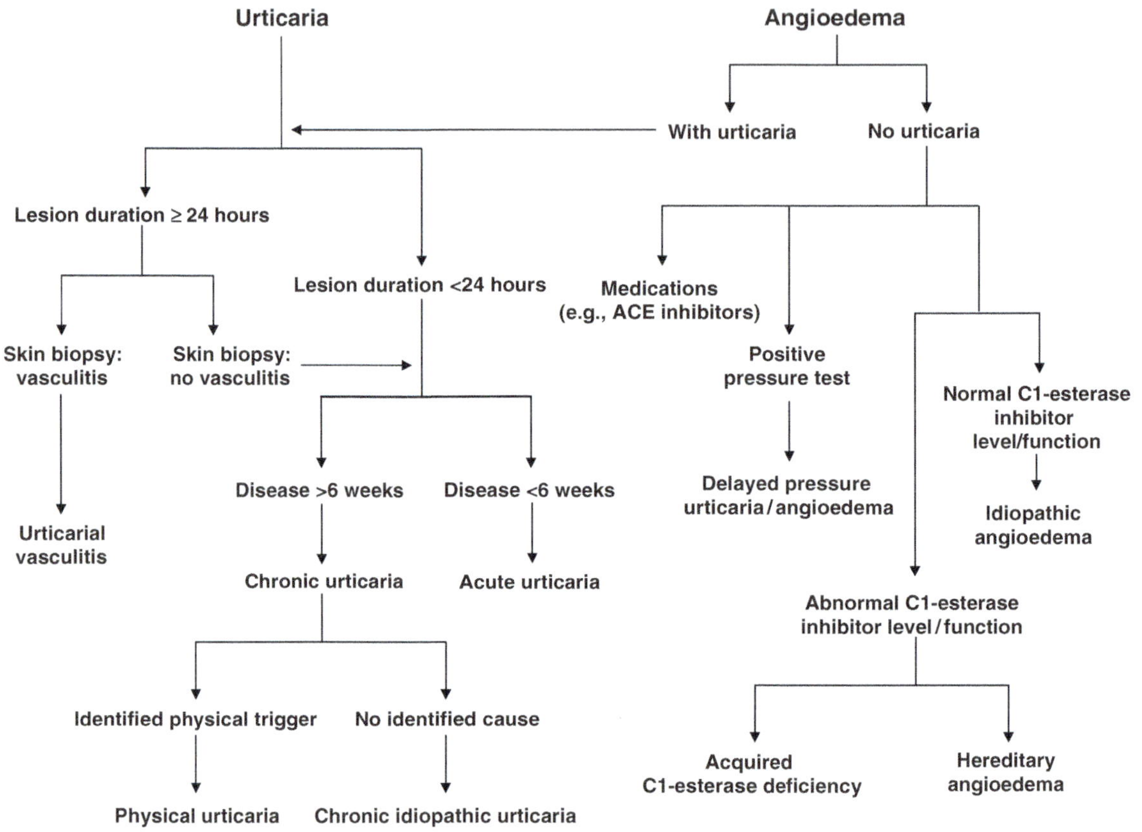

```
                    Urticaria                                    Angioedema

                                                        ┌──────────────┬──────────────┐
                                   ◄────────────── With urticaria    No urticaria
              ┌─────────────┴──────────┐
                                       │                ┌──────────┬──────────────┬──────────┐
    Lesion duration ≥ 24 hours         │                │
                                       │           Medications
       ┌──────────┴─────────┐   Lesion duration <24 hours  (e.g., ACE inhibitors)
                                 ┌──────────┘
  Skin biopsy:    Skin biopsy:  │              Positive                    Normal C1-esterase
  vasculitis      no vasculitis │           pressure test                    inhibitor
                              ┌──┴──────────┐                                level/function
     │                  Disease >6 weeks  Disease <6 weeks
                                                │          Delayed pressure      Idiopathic
  Urticarial                                    │        urticaria/angioedema   angioedema
  vasculitis          Chronic urticaria    Acute urticaria

                ┌─────────────┴─────────┐                Abnormal C1-esterase
                                                          inhibitor level/function
      Identified physical trigger   No identified cause
                                                    ┌──────────────┴──────────────┐
                                                  Acquired                    Hereditary
       Physical urticaria    Chronic idiopathic urticaria  C1-esterase deficiency   angioedema
```

FIG. 27.4. Diagnosis algorithm for urticaria. ACE, angiotensin-converting enzyme.

leakage (see Fig. 27.1).[23] Urticarial lesions can be easily blanched. The physician should also inspect mucous membranes for the presence of angioedema (see Fig. 27.2).[4] Patients should also be evaluated for thyroid gland abnormalities on physical exam. No specific laboratory testing is needed for all patients with urticaria; the testing to be done depends on the

subtype (e.g., acute, chronic idiopathic, or physical) of urticaria as indicated below.

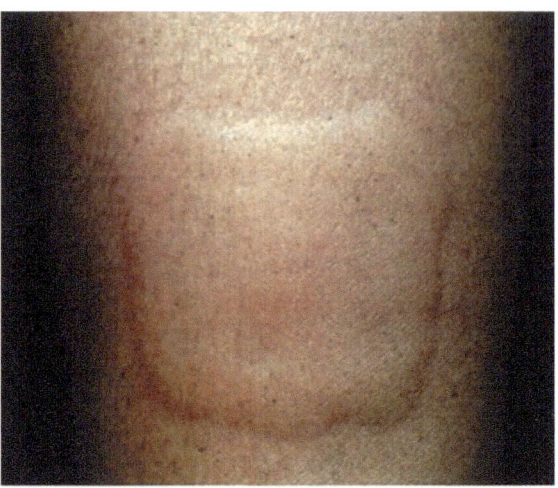

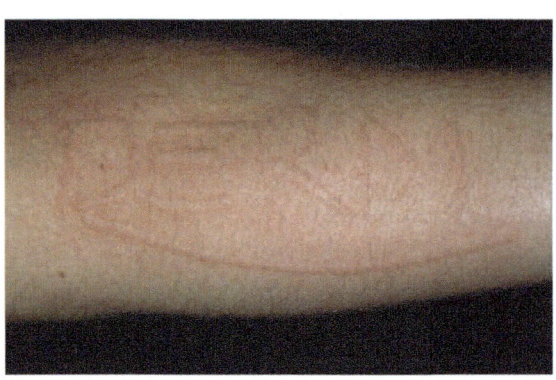

FIG. 27.5. Dermatographism. (Courtesy of Bernard Cohen, MD, Dermatlas; http://www.dermatlas.org.)

FIG. 27.6. Ice-cube test for cold urticaria. (From Greaves,[3] with permission of Allergy.)

Acute Urticaria

Acute urticaria is classified as hives of less than 6 weeks' duration and accounts for up to two thirds of cases of urticaria.[24] Lesions are short-lived, lasting less than 24 hours, but they can return.[25] Clinically, acute urticaria cannot be distinguished from chronic urticaria by physical exam alone. No routine laboratory testing should be done except to identify the trigger, such as in suspected food or drug reactions.

Acute urticaria can be classified as an allergic or immunoglobulin E (IgE)-mediated allergic response, such as observed in food, insect, and drug allergies; a non–IgE-mediated response to a "pseudoallergen" such as aspirin; or an immunologic response as seen with blood transfusions and febrile illnesses.[26] Urticaria related to food allergy should occur within 30 minutes to 2 hours following exposure. Testing for food allergies is appropriate in acute urticaria if the patient history reveals urticaria associated with other symptoms such as nausea or vomiting, but food allergies are not a common cause in adults. One prospective study of adults with acute urticaria demonstrated that 63% suspected a food as the causative agent, but only one of 109 had confirmation of a food allergy.[2] In children, food allergy plays a larger role in acute urticaria, such as with milk, egg, soy, peanuts, and wheat.[27,28] Some beverages and foods containing vasoactive amines (e.g., wine, beer, and cheese) and pseudoallergens (e.g., food additives) have been implicated in acute urticaria, although IgE-mediated food hypersensitivity is more common.[29] Drugs can also be responsible for acute urticaria, acting as either allergens or pseudoallergens. Penicillin is an example of an allergen, IgE-mediated, that can elicit urticaria, while acetyl salicylic acid (aspirin) is a frequent non–IgE-mediated stimulus for histamine release.[8] Angiotensin-converting enzyme (ACE) inhibitors have also been implicated as triggers for angioedema through effects on the bradykinin pathway.[30] Viral infections are the most common reason for acute urticaria, with hive onset occurring a few days after the start of viral symptoms, with coexistence of acute urticaria and upper respiratory infections reported in 28% to 62% of cases.[2,27,28,31,32] Surprisingly, no identifiable trigger is found in more than 50% of cases of acute urticaria.[26]

Chronic Urticaria

Chronic urticaria by definition is wheals occurring at least 2 days per week of at least 6 weeks' duration.[3] In chronic urticaria, IgE-mediated allergic reactions are unlikely causes of symptoms.[29,33] Studies assessing the role of non–IgE-mediated reactions, such as seen with salicylates in foods, demonstrated inconclusive results.[8] One study showed a decrease in symptoms in 30% of patients after 2 weeks on an elimination diet, but the patients had not received a prior workup and only 15% had complete resolution of symptoms.[29]

Chronic urticaria can be divided into two subtypes: chronic idiopathic urticaria (65% to 35%) and physical urticaria (20% to 35%).[4,5] Chronic idiopathic urticaria (CIU) usually lacks an identifiable and consistent trigger and is a disease that waxes and wanes. In contrast, physical urticaria is categorized into subtypes by specific triggers that can elicit hives within minutes with a life span limited to a few hours.[6] In contrast, CIU lesions typically are present for at least 6 to 8 hours without clear trigger factors.[3,5] Some crossover exists between CIU and physical urticarias, with 40% of CIU patients displaying dermatographism.[34]

Physical Urticaria

Physical urticaria is defined by the ability of a physical stimulus to reproducibly elicit urticarial lesions. Physical urticaria can be further divided into many subtypes depending on the physical stimulus (Table 27.1), and more than one subtype can exist simultaneously in one individual.[3] Unlike CIU, in which lesions may last up to 1 day, hives in physical urticaria are short-lived.[35] Features of physical urticarias can be common in the general population, with dermatographism reported in approximately 45% of patients with no history of chronic urticaria.[36]

Evaluation of physical urticaria is strongly guided by the patient's history and provocative testing. Mechanical shearing forces, such as rubbing or scratching the skin, are the catalyst for *dermatographic urticaria*, the most frequent type of physical urticaria, in which lesions arise a few minutes following application of the trigger.[8,26] *Delayed pressure urticaria* and *angioedema* result

TABLE 27.1. Classification of physical urticaria.

Type	% of All Urticaria	Pathogenesis	Features	Reaction Times	Provocation Test	Differences on Biopsy	Treatment
Dermatographic	7–10%	Unknown, but elevated plasma histamine levels and positive passive transfer experiments, indicate an IgE-mediated process.	Mechanical shearing forces lead to lesions. Koebner's phenomenon, a wheal and flare reaction at pressure sites (e.g. waistband), is present. Higher frequency in young adults.	1) Immediate–Within 2–5 min.; lasting 30 min. 2) Intermediate–Within 30 min.–2 hrs.;lasting 3–9 hrs. 3) Late onset (rare)–Within 4–6 hrs;lasting 24–48 hrs.	Stroke forearm or back with tongue blade	Scant leukocytic infiltrate in upper dermis.	Nonsedating H$_1$ blocker.
Delayed pressure	3–5%	Unknown	Constant application of pressure to skin results in erythema and superficial and deep swelling. Pressure areas commonly affected. Male predominance.	Within 3–12 hrs; lasting up to 48 hrs.	Application of weight to one area for minimum 10 minutes	Infiltrate typically located in mid- to lower dermis. Neutrophils may be seen in lower dermis.	Nonsedating H$_1$ blocker.Short course of corticosteroids, leukotriene antagonists may also be used.
Vibratory	rare	Unknown, but elevated histamine levels and mast cell degranulation reported following application of stimuli. Familial cases have autosomal dominant inheritance.	Occurs after vibratory stimuli (e.g. lawn mowing or motorcycling).	Within minutes; lasting up to 24 hrs.	Challenge with vibratory stimuli (e.g. vortex mixer) for 5 min.		Avoidance of trigger.
Familial cold		Gene alteration at CIAS1 on chromosome 1q.44. Autosomal dominant inheritance.	Immediate type characterized by burning papules or macules and systemic symptoms such as arthralgias and fever. Delayed type follows cold exposure.	Delayed occurs within 9–18 hrs. of cold exposure, lasting 2–3 days.		1) Immediate– Polymorphonuclear infiltrates. 2) Delayed– Mononuclear infiltrates.	
Cold contact	3–5%	IgE-mediated histamine release with IgM and IgG antibodies reported.	Occurs with skin cold exposure. May have angioedema. Rare cases of anaphylaxis after total body exposure to cold.	Within 2–5 min. as skin re-warms.	Ice cube placement to area for 10–20 minutes	Loose lymphocytic and leukocytic infiltrates. Platelet infiltrates and vascular changes may also be present.	Nonsedating H$_1$ blocker. Leukotriene antagonist may be added.

Type	Prevalence	Mechanism	Clinical features	Time course	Test	Histology	Treatment
Heat contact		Unknown, but complement system is affected.	Occurs at sites of heat application. Divided into immediate nonfamilial and delayed familial.	1) Immediate–Within 5 min.; up to 1 hr. 2) Delayed–Within 6–18 hrs.; lasting 12–24 hrs	Local contact with hot water or object		Avoidance of trigger.
Solar	rare	Unknown, but thought to be IgE-mediated with increased serum histamine levels, mast cell and eosinophil degranulation, and photoallergen production. Secondary solar urticaria is characterized by a porphyrin metabolism abnormality leading to complement activation.	Induced by sunlight or indoor lighting exposure (wavelengths 280–760 nm). Most common in 3rd and 4th decades of life, commonly affecting young adults.	Within 2–3 min.; lasting 3–4 hrs.	Expose to UV light		Avoidance of sun exposure and skin protection. Nonsedating H_1 blocker.
Cholinergic	2–7%	Unknown, but acetylcholine, released by exercise, can release histamine. Elevated histamine and eosinophil and neutrophil chemotactic factors reported.	Due to a rise in core body temperature. Usually start on face and neck, then spreading. The pruritic wheals are small (1–5 mm) with "fried egg" appearance. More common in young adults.	Within minutes; lasting less than 1 hr.	Physical activity (e.g. running in place for 5 min.)	Loose lymphocytic and leukocytic infiltrates in upper dermis.	Nonsedating H_1 blocker. Increase dose if necessary. In addition, danazol can be used.
Aquagenic	rare	Unknown, but a proposed mechanism is that water induces formation of histamine-releasing substances.	Contact with water induces small hives similar to those seen in cholinergic urticaria. More common in young adults.	Within 2 min.; lasting up to 1 hr.	Apply water compress for 30 min.	Mast cell degranulation noted in challenged skin.	Avoidance of trigger.
Contact		May be IgE-mediated.	Inciting triggers are plants, foods, drugs, and chemicals.	Within minutes; lasting less than a few hours.			Avoidance of trigger.
Adrenergic		Unknown	Pin-sized wheals elicited by stress.	Within minutes; lasting less than 1 hr.			Propanolol

Source: Data from Zuberbier[8]; Kaplan[9]; Haas, Toppe, and Henz.[10] From Kontou-Fili K, Borici-Mazi R, Kapp A, et al. Physical urticaria: classification and diagnostic guidelines. An EAACI position paper. Allergy 1997;52:504–13.

after vertical pressure is applied to the skin, with lesions, often painful, appearing several hours after application and persisting for up to 48 hours; this subtype of urticaria predominantly affects the palms, soles, buttocks, and back and has a male predominance.[8,26] *Vibratory urticaria* is instigated by vibratory forces, is quite rare, and can be described as familial with autosomal dominant inheritance or sporadic.[9] *Familial cold urticaria* is an autosomal dominant disease mainly affecting young adults and is due to gene alteration *CIAS1* at chromosome 1q.44, which is also the gene locus involved in Muckle-Wells syndrome and autosomal dominant periodic fever syndrome, both diseases that demonstrate cold-sensitivity.[9,37,38]

Cold contact urticaria, which occurs after direct contact of skin to a cold object or air, also occurs predominantly in young adults, women, and cold climates and can be idiopathic, or incited by bacterial or viral infections (see Fig. 27.6).[8] *Heat contact urticaria* results after the skin directly comes in contact with a warm object or air and is rare.[9] Ultraviolet (UV) light is the trigger for *solar urticaria*, an IgE-dependent subtype that occurs at wavelengths of 280 to 760 nm and more commonly affects females and young adults.[8] *Cholinergic urticaria* is aggravated by a rise in body temperature and thus is triggered by exercise, bathing, and emotions, and less by alcohol or spicy food consumption.[9] Cholinergic urticaria typically involves adolescents and young adults, with a prevalence of 11% reported in those ages 15 to 35 years and is characterized by small, pin-sized wheals (1- to 5-mm diameter), sometimes with a white halo, or "fried egg" appearance, that last for less than an hour and can be mild so that an estimated 80% of people with this urticarial subtype do not seek medical advice.[8,26,39] *Adrenergic urticaria* is also described as pin-sized wheals, but, unlike cholinergic urticaria, it is elicited by stress and can by treated with propranolol.[8] *Aquagenic urticaria*, which is elicited by any exposure to water regardless of its temperature, mimics cholinergic urticaria in the appearance of its lesions but has a female predominance and affects young adults.[8] *Contact urticaria* can be IgE-mediated, with the inciting triggers being plants such as grass, foods (e.g., peanuts), drugs, cosmetics, chemicals, and textiles, and it is of short duration as with the cholinergic and adrenergic urticarial subtypes, occurring within minutes of exposure with resolution within a few hours.[5,8] Systemic symptoms can be present with contact urticaria, especially if IgE-mediated.[8]

Chronic Idiopathic Urticaria

Chronic idiopathic urticaria accounts for approximately 80% of all chronic urticaria.[4] It is episodic and persistent in nature, with a typical disease duration of 3 to 5 years.[40] One prospective study of CIU demonstrated that 94% of patients were still active at 6 months, 75% at 12 months, 52% at 24 months, 43% at 36 months, and 14% at 5 years.[4] Disease duration was directly correlated to the presence of severe disease, angioedema, and autoimmune features, such as a positive autologous serum skin test (see below) and the presence of antithyroid antibodies.[4] Angioedema coexists with urticaria in approximately 40% to 50% of people affected with CIU.[40,41] The most common and disturbing symptom for patients with CIU is pruritus, which usually adversely affects their sleep, and while fatigue and gastrointestinal symptoms have been previously described with exacerbations, respiratory and arthralgic complaints are rare.[6,42] Chronic idiopathic urticaria can be a socially and financially disabling disease, with an impact on quality of life comparable to that of coronary heart disease.[43] One study of 170 chronic urticaria patients reported a moderate quality of life impairment in those suffering from CIU alone using the Dermatology Life Quality Index (DLQI), while those with CIU and a history of angioedema and delayed pressure features had a significantly greater quality of life impairment leading to disability in the realms of work and study, emotional well-being, and social or leisure activities.[44] Compared to other debilitating dermatologic diseases, the quality of life impairment in chronic urticaria is similar to that in patients with severe atopic dermatitis and greater than that in patients with psoriasis, acne, and vitiligo.[44] Part of the frustration in treating urticaria is the lack of an identifiable trigger for urticarial exacerbations, leading to an unpredictable disease. Chronic idiopathic urticaria also entails an economic burden for patients, with multiple medications, medical evaluations, work absence, and use of the emergency department.[45]

Aspirin and nonsteroidal antiinflammatory drugs (NSAIDs) can aggravate urticaria and angioedema via inhibition of prostaglandin synthesis. Selective cyclooxygenase-2 (COX-2) inhibitors lead to fewer symptoms when compared to aspirin and traditional NSAIDs and provide a choice for analgesics in these patients.[46] One study of chronic urticaria patients undergoing aspirin challenge demonstrated that approximately 20% of CIU patients had a positive challenge while those with physical urticaria were left unaffected.[47] A patient history of suspected aspirin sensitivity correlates very well, with 92% of cases confirmed by positive aspirin challenge in one study.[48] Patients need to be advised of this potential exacerbating factor and be knowledgeable that salicylates may be an occult ingredient in medications, supplements, or foods, including fruits, vegetables, herbs, and spices.[49]

Thyroid disease coexists with CIU at a higher incidence than in the general population, with a higher presence of thyroid antibodies, specifically antimicrosomal and antithyroglobulin antibodies. Hashimoto's thyroiditis and, less commonly, Graves' disease are the only reported systemic diseases with a correlation to CIU.[50–53] A reported 27% of CIU patients have thyroid autoantibodies, nearly twice the rate observed in the normal population, and typically, the majority are euthyroid, although some can be hypothyroid and rarely hyperthyroid.[52,54,55] Currently, these autoantibodies are not thought to be pathogenic in urticaria but may support an autoimmune cause to CIU.[56] Studies of thyroid hormone replacement in patients with coexistent CIU and thyroid autoantibodies have yielded mixed results.[51,57,58] The current recommendation is to screen patients for underlying thyroid disease and to treat any underlying thyroid disease, but at this time no clear evidence exists for the use of thyroid hormone in euthyroid patients with thyroid autoantibodies present.

Histology

Histologically, CIU shares lesional features with acute urticaria consisting of a lymphocytic-predominant perivascular infiltrate. The lymphocytes present mainly express human leukocyte antigen (HLA) DR or DQ.[59] Occasionally, neutrophils are seen within capillary or postcapillary venules' walls, but unlike the neutrophilic infiltrate seen in urticarial vasculitis, there is no evidence of vascular damage, nuclear debris, or red cell extravasation (see Fig. 27.3B,C).[1] The presence of intradermal CD3+, CD4+, CD8+ and CD25+ T-cells, as well as eosinophils, neutrophils, basophils, and macrophages, is significantly higher in CIU skin as compared to normal skin.[60] Although this cellular infiltrate of CIU resembles that seen in allergen-induced late-phase skin biopsies, the cytokine profile in CIU is T-helper-1 (Th1) and Th2 with higher expression of interferon-γ (IFN-γ) as well as IL-4 and IL-5.[60]

Pathophysiology of Urticaria

Whereas the pathophysiology of allergic urticaria supports allergen interacting with IgE bound on skin mast cells, the pathophysiology of physical urticaria is unknown. Although mast cell degranulation is a clear component in some subtypes of physical urticaria, such as dermatographic, cholinergic, cold, and solar urticaria, a serum immunoglobulin may also play a role as demonstrated by passive transfer experiments.[5,8,55] An acute rise in serum histamine levels has been observed in cold urticaria following cold exposure.[61] In CIU, there is also evidence for mast cell degranulation observed on skin biopsies. Mast cell number appears to be similar in nonlesional and lesional CIU skin and normal skin, using tryptase and chymase staining.[62] Although mast cell number is not altered, increased mast cell releasability has been demonstrated in patients with CIU with active disease, which resolves when in disease remission, suggesting that the mast cell alteration is reversible.[63] Unlike acute urticaria, chronic urticarias do not appear to involve IgE binding to allergen.[5]

More recently, there has been evidence that basophils play a role in CIU. Basophils have been reported in both lesional and nonlesional CIU skin using Basogranulin antibody (BB1) staining.[60,64] Also, basopenia is a feature of active CIU disease, and the reduction in basophil number correlates inversely with disease severity.[65,66] Also, as is seen with allergen late-phase reactions, basophils that have migrated to the skin may play a role in the duration as well as the magnitude of urticarial lesions.[67]

Select basophil surface markers correlate with basophil activation and have been measured in CIU, in particular CD63, CD69, and CD203c.[68–71] CD63 is a member of the transmembrane-4 superfamily and is rapidly mobilized onto the basophil surface by IL-3, allergen, anti-IgE, and other stimuli of degranulation, while CD69 is slowly induced following IL-3 stimulation.[68,72] CD203c, also known as ectonucleotide pyrophosphatase, is unique to basophils, mast cells, and their progenitors, and is mobilized by allergen and anti-IgE.[73–77] One study showed that CIU patients demonstrated enhanced basophil surface expression of CD63 and CD69 when compared to nonallergic controls, while no difference was noted in CD203c expression between groups.[71]

Furthermore, CIU basophils demonstrated a decreased functional response to IgE receptor stimulation but not to other stimuli.[78–80] One study showed that histamine release mediated via the basophil high-affinity IgE receptor FcεRI was diminished in patients with CIU versus controls.[78] This finding is paradoxical since antihistamines are used to treat CIU, and pruritus, the predominant symptom in CIU, is histamine-dependent. A recent study has shown that basophils in CIU have altered FcεRI-mediated histamine release and have found two patterns of histamine release in patients with active CIU disease.[79] Approximately 50% of patients with CIU tested were found to be "responders," releasing greater than 10% of complete histamine when triggered with a polyclonal anti-IgE stimulus, and 50% were "nonresponders," releasing less than 10% of total histamine.[79] Also, these basophil phenotypes appear to be stable over time as patients maintain active disease, but this altered basophil function changes with disease remission.[78,79,81]

Autoimmune Urticaria

In a subset of CIU referred to as autoimmune urticaria, histamine-releasing autoantibodies have been reported and hypothesized to be pathogenic, although this remains controversial.[56,82–86] The autoantibodies are thought to activate mast cells and basophils via complement and act by C5a to potentiate histamine release. These autoantibodies are detected in 30% to 40% of patients with CIU, and the majority of these autoantibodies are directed against the α-subunit of the high-affinity receptor, FcεRI, while the remainder target IgE.[42,84] In favor of autoimmune mechanisms is an increased incidence in CIU of thyroid autoantibodies, specifically antimicrosomal and antithyroglobulin, as well as the report that certain HLA class II alleles (DR4, DQ8) occurred at higher frequencies in CIU patients with autoantibodies.[50–52,54,59]

Also in support of the autoantibody theory is that autologous serum injected into a CIU patient's skin may result in a wheal-and-flare response.[87,88] This autologous serum skin test (ASST) is reduced by pretreatment with antihistamines or 48/80, a mast cell degranulating compound.[89] However, a recent study demonstrated the presence of an ASST in healthy controls and patients with allergic rhinitis as well as in those with CIU, causing doubt about the usefulness of the ASST in the diagnosis of urticaria.[90] Also, the presence of an ASST response alone does not prove that autoantibodies are present, thus further studies were done and demonstrated that sera from ASST-positive CIU patients also had histamine-releasing activity (HRA) from healthy donor basophils.[84,91] A large study found that 40% of CIU patients' sera exhibit HRA when performed in vitro on donor basophils.[83] Although HRA is reported to indicate the presence of autoantibodies, the presence of HRA is inconsistent with the presence of autoantibodies by Western blotting in CIU patients.[79,92,93] The presence of serum HRA had no effect on the character of the leukocyte infiltrates of new (<4 hours) or established (>12 hours) skin lesions, even though autoantibody presence has been previously linked to increased disease severity.[60,93,94] In addition, serum HRA has been demonstrated in normal sera, and there is no correlation between HRA and CIU basophil FcεRI function.[79] Another problem with the autoantibody hypothesis is that anti-FcεRIα autoantibodies are also found at a similar frequency in other autoimmune diseases such as systemic lupus and dermatomyositis as well as in normal subjects.[95] Also, anaphylaxis is rarely seen in CIU, which is a skin-limited disease, but would be expected to occur more often if autoantibodies directed against basophils and mast cells are present.

Evaluation

In most cases of urticaria, a history and physical are sufficient for diagnosis.[1,96] A thorough history may identify potential triggers such as medications. Patients with chronic urticaria and disease resistant to conventional therapies or uncharacteristic lesions may need further evaluation to exclude secondary causes of hives. The laboratory testing should evaluate general health with a complete blood count with differential, complete metabolic panel, and urinalysis and screen for autoimmune or inflammatory disorders, such as a vasculitis, with an erythrocyte sedimentation rate (ESR) and antinuclear antibody (ANA) test.[97] Patients with significant angioedema without urticaria should have complement levels checked along with C1 inhibitor testing to screen for hereditary and acquired angioedema due to C1 esterase inhibitor deficiency, which would result in low complement C4 levels. Patients who have symptoms or a family history of thyroid disease also warrant thyroid screening by measuring thyroid-stimulating hormone and possibly thyroid autoantibodies. Atypical lesions also should have complement screening.

Infections have been implicated in urticaria. As previously mentioned, viral infections, especially viral upper respiratory infections, are a common cause of acute urticaria. A study in a Japan, which has a high prevalence of hepatitis C, demonstrated that this infection may manifest with chronic urticarial lesions, but further work in areas with lower prevalence has not supported this finding.[98,99] It is recommended that individuals with risk factors for infectious hepatitis should have the appropriate testing. Bacterial cultures are rarely necessary, as bacterial infections are not a common cause of urticaria.[100] In recent years, *Helicobacter pylori*, linked closely to gastritis and gastroesophageal reflux disease (GERD), has been implicated in CIU and may trigger autoantibody production and hives via molecular mimicry, but controlled studies have not been able to establish this link.[101–104] Patients with symptoms of GERD or gastritis may benefit from *H. pylori* serology or may be tested via endoscopy if this procedure is otherwise medically relevant.[29,105,106] The complete blood count also serves to check for peripheral eosinophilia, which may result from a parasitic infection. These infections are a rare cause of urticaria that should be investigated by stool examination for ova and parasites. Fungal testing should not be routinely performed, as this is not a common cause of urticaria.

Radioallergosorbent tests (RASTs) or skin testing may be beneficial in if a type I hypersensitivity reaction or allergic urticaria is suspected. Skin testing is difficult to perform in chronic urticaria patients due to the high prevalence of dermatographism and delayed pressure features in this group as well as their dependence on antihistamines. Another skin test used in the past to define autoimmune urticaria is ASST. Since the presence or absence of autoantibodies does not alter treatment options in patients, the ASST should not be used as a diagnostic tool for chronic urticaria.[26] Also, recent study demonstrated an ASST sensitivity of 53% to 55% and specificity of 28% to 31% in CIU when compared to healthy controls or patients with allergic rhinitis.[90] Newer basophil-based assays that check for serum histamine-releasing activity also lack specificity and validation for clinical use.[107,108]

For physical urticarias, patients are unlikely to benefit from further laboratory testing.[34,109,110] The physical exam can assist substantially in defining the type of physical urticaria that is present based on provocative tests (see Table 27.1). There are other diseases associated with urticarial lesions, and patients presenting with appropriate symptoms should be evaluated for these disorders. Urticarial vasculitis must be excluded in patients with chronic urticaria unresponsive to conventional therapy. The duration of urticarial vasculitis lesions is characteristically greater than 24 hours and they may be painful and purpuric, leaving residual skin changes.[1] These patients may also complain of systemic symptoms and have laboratory findings consistent with an inflammatory process, such as an elevated ESR or C-reactive protein or low complement levels.[1] To rule out urticarial vasculitis, the definitive test is a skin biopsy. The features of urticarial vasculitis on biopsy are leukocytoclasia, extravasation of red blood cells, fibrin deposition, leukocyte invasion of the vascular endothelium, and endothelial edema, of which the latter three features may also be observed in chronic urticaria.[1] Also, urticarial pigmentosa, a subtype of mastocytosis, may mimic urticarial lesions, except that these are pigmented and typically longer-lasting lesions than those in urticaria. Schnitzler's syndrome is associated with recurrent urticarial lesions, arthralgia, fever, and a high ESR and IgM monoclonal gammopathy, and should be considered in the differential and evaluated by serum protein electrophoresis as indicated.[111]

Treatment

For acute urticaria the most important step is to eliminate the trigger, if one is identified. Also, avoidance of certain potential triggers such as aspirin,

NSAIDs, ACE inhibitors, and codeine-containing products that can directly stimulate skin mast cells is recommended.[5,26] Patients can use antihistamines to help with symptom alleviation until resolution of the episode. Typically, nonsedating H1-blockers are utilized, although H2-blockers and classic sedating H1-blockers, such as diphenhydramine or hydroxyzine, may be used. Approximately 44% to 91% of all urticaria patients treated with H1-blockers found a benefit.[112,113] Similarly, the treatment of physical urticaria involves nonsedating H1-blockers and avoidance of triggers. Nonsedating H1-blockers can be used to cover daytime symptoms, while sedating H1-blockers, such as hydroxyzine, may be beneficial to assist with sleep at night. The major risk associated with administration of H1-blockers is somnolence. Some past studies in CIU patients demonstrated an improvement in dermatographism and pruritus with the simultaneous use of an H1-blocker and H2-blocker versus and H1-blocker alone, although this may be a result of the H2-blocker's increasing the serum concentration of the H1-blocker.[114–119]

For severe cases of acute urticaria, a short course of systemic corticosteroids may provide quicker control.[8] One study reported that acute urticaria exacerbations lasted only 3 days in approximately 94% of studied patients compared to only 66% of patients not receiving steroids.[2] Topical steroids play no role in the treatment of urticaria since application would involve a large area of skin with minimal benefit, with the exception of reported benefit in localized delayed pressure urticaria.[26,120]

The treatment of CIU is a greater challenge than that of acute and physical urticarias. The physician should explain to the patient the natural history of CIU and the lack of a cause, as this may lessen patient frustration. Patients should avoid triggers, but these are rarely identified in CIU. H1-blockers as well as H2-blockers are used to control the intense pruritus associated with the disease. One study reported that 94% of patients with urticaria had some itch relief with use of H1-blockers, with the majority of the sedating type.[121] Different H1-blockers can be tried since one may work better in one patient than another, and many patients are on multiple H1-blockers simultaneously. H1-blocker dosing is variable with supratherapeutic dosing of these medications currently under investigation.[56,122] Doxepin, a tricyclic antidepressant with some H1- and H2-receptor antagonist properties,

may be useful for nighttime itch, as well as helping with disease-associated depression, and has been shown to be more effective than diphenhydramine in the treatment of CIU.[123] Drugs such as cimetidine, macrolides, and some antifungals may be less effective when used with doxepin, and the drug should not be used with monoamine oxidase (MAO) inhibitors due to a risk for prolonged QT syndrome.[26]

Evidence of leukotriene receptor antagonist use in CIU, although conflicting, has been reported for CIU and physical urticaria of the cold-induced and delayed pressure types, as well as aspirin-sensitive or food-induced acute urticaria.[124–126] Various randomized, placebo-controlled studies reported that montelukast provided symptom alleviation in CIU patients when used as a monotherapy or in conjunction with cetirizine or desloratadine, but another placebo-controlled study demonstrated that montelukast plus desloratidine was equal to desloratidine alone, while montelukast monotherapy offered no benefit over placebo.[124,127–129] Another leukotriene receptor antagonist, zafiruklast, failed to show benefit over placebo in CIU.[130] Some studies have only shown a benefit with leukotriene receptor antagonists in a subset of CIU patients with a positive ASST.[131,132] Overall, leukotriene receptor antagonists may be added to antihistamines in urticaria patients as a limited trial and have a side effect profile similar to placebo.

As in acute urticaria, systemic corticosteroids also have a role in severe, antihistamine-resistant CIU when rapid control is warranted or with episodes of significant angioedema. The mechanism for disease alleviation with corticosteroids is not known, but they can lower tissue mast cell number, possibly changing mast cell migration to tissues, although this is controversial in skin.[133] Also, corticosteroids are known to (1) significantly decrease peripheral basophil counts due to apoptosis as well as demargination, and (2) diminish the basophil response to an IgE-dependent stimulus with no effect on a non–IgE-dependent pathway.[133,134] Chronic idiopathic urticaria patients treated with steroids have a transient rise in peripheral basophil counts, perhaps suggesting decreased recruitment of basophils to the skin.[66] The use of systemic corticosteroids should be sparse due to the side-effect profile with prolonged use, including a greater risk of osteoporosis, peptic ulcer disease, diabetes, and hypertension, to name a few.

More recently, immunomodulators have been used for the treatment of antihistamine-unresponsive and steroid-dependent CIU. Cyclosporine has shown some success in CIU patients.[135–137] Cyclosporine reduces the Th1 lymphocyte response, inhibits antibody formation, and inhibits basophil and mast cell anti-IgE–induced histamine release.[135,138] One of the studies reported that cyclosporine treatment did not change the presence of the ASST in patients who entered drug remission.[137] In various case reports, sulfasalazine has also shown some benefits in CIU as well as in delayed pressure urticaria.[139–141] One recent study of patients with antihistamine unresponsive CIU reported that 74% of patients treated with sulfasalazine had significant improvement in disease, with an additional 21% showing minimal improvement, and all patients treated either discontinued or decreased their steroid use.[142] Although the mechanism of action is unknown, it is hypothesized that sulfasalazine may alter IgE-mediated mast cell histamine release, with one study demonstrating reduced release in mast cells and two prior studies demonstrating enhanced release in mast cells as well as basophils.[143–145]

Dapsone, which exhibits antiinflammatory properties and inhibits neutrophil function, showed promising results in one open-label study and may be beneficial for patients with neutrophil-predominant infiltrates on skin biopsy.[146,147] Small case reports of cyclophosphamide and methotrexate have also shown a potential role for immunomodulating drugs in CIU.[148,149] Colchicine and hydroxychloroquine have also been suggested as therapeutics.[150,151] Plasmapheresis has been used with the intended purpose of removing autoantibodies with temporary effects on disease activity.[6] One study in HRA-positive CIU patients demonstrated a reduction in ASST in treated patients but a positive ASST response with use of preinfusion autologous serum.[152] Intravenous immunoglobulin infusions was studied in patients with reported functional anti-FcεRI or anti-IgE autoantibodies and had a reported benefit, but a subsequent study demonstrated that the improvement with intravenous immunoglobulin (IVIG) was temporary and that IVIG is likely not an effective therapy for CIU.[153–155]

Other therapies, although less studied, have also been used in CIU. A 3-week pseudoallergen-free diet has been studied with limited success.[8] Psoralen UVA (PUVA) or UVB phototherapy has no proven beneficial use in CIU, although PUVA is known to reduce skin mast cell number.[96,156–159] Zileuton, a 5-lipoxygenase inhibitor, inhibits leukotriene B_4 and C_4 production and has shown success in a small case study of chronic urticaria patients.[160,161] Warfarin therapy was studied due its ability to alter proteases of the complement, kinin, clotting, or fibrinolytic systems, which may be activated in vivo and lead to vasoactive mediator release in CIU, but further work needs to be done to assess the benefit as well as the mechanism of action.[162] Some other therapeutics that have been mentioned are interferon, mycophenolate mofetil, and danazol.[163–166]

Unfortunately, with all of the therapeutics so far mentioned, some patients still have active disease; thus, novel therapies are needed. Rituximab, a monoclonal anti-CD20, has had success in the treatment of SLE, and due to CD20's role in B-cell development, it may decrease autoantibodies, thus making it a potential therapeutic for CIU.[166,167] The TNF-α antagonists, which have known antiinflammatory properties, are currently used for autoimmune diseases such as rheumatoid arthritis, as well as inflammatory skin diseases such as psoriasis, and they may be a potential therapeutic for CIU.[168,169] Another potential therapeutic that is Food and Drug Administration (FDA) approved for allergic asthma is omalizumab, a monoclonal anti-IgE. A few case reports in chronic urticaria have demonstrated significant improvement in disease activity.[170–172] Omalizumab is known to alter mast cell and basophil anti-IgE induced histamine release and is known to decrease free IgE and FcεRI expression on mast cells and basophils, which decreases the potential targets of anti-FcεRI and anti-IgE autoantibodies.[173]

Urticaria, especially chronic urticaria, takes a large toll on patient quality of life, and presents a medical and financial burden, with the high cost of multiple medical visits, specialists, lab testing, and medications. The current available therapies for urticaria fall short, especially for patients with chronic urticaria, which only increases patient frustration. A greater understanding of the disease mechanism is necessary for both acute and chronic urticaria, which may lead to new therapeutics.

Conclusion

Urticaria is produced by the degranulation of mast cells in the skin, and has immunologic (IgE-mediated) and nonimmunologic mechanisms. Chronic urticaria is a troublesome condition that can adversely affect the quality of life of an afflicted individual. Evaluations to identify and remove trigger factors are critical to the management of this condition. If this is not possible, glucocorticosteroids, antihistamines, immunosuppressive drugs, and biologics can be used to treat severe cases.

References

1. Greaves MW. Chronic urticaria. N Engl J Med 1995;332:1767–72.
2. Zuberbier T, Ifflander J, Semmler C, et al. Acute urticaria: clinical aspects and therapeutic responsiveness. Acta Derm Venereol 1996;76:295–7.
3. Greaves MW. Chronic urticaria in childhood. Allergy 2000;55:309–20.
4. Toubi E, Kessel A, Avshovich N, et al. Clinical and laboratory parameters in predicting chronic urticaria duration: a prospective study of 139 patients. Allergy 2004;59:869–73.
5. Grattan CE, Sabroe RA, Greaves MW. Chronic urticaria. J Am Acad Dermatol 2002;46:645–57.
6. Greaves M. Chronic urticaria. J Allergy Clin Immunol 2000;105:664–72.
7. Sibbald RG, Cheema AS, Lozinski A, et al. Chronic urticaria. Evaluation of the role of physical, immunologic, and other contributory factors. Int J Dermatol 1991;30:381–6.
8. Zuberbier T. Urticaria. Allergy 2003;58:1224–34.
9. Kaplan AP. Urticaria and angioedema. In: Adkinson, NF, Yunginger JW, Busse WW, et al, eds. Middleton's Allergy: Principles and Practice, 6th ed. Philadelphia: Mosby, 2003:1537–58.
10. Haas N, Toppe E, Henz BM. Microscopic morphology of different types of urticaria. Arch Dermatol 1998;134:41–6.
11. Haas N, Schadendorf D, Henz BM. Differential endothelial adhesion molecule expression in early and late whealing reactions. Int Arch Allergy Immunol 1998;115:210–4.
12. Haas N, Motel K, Czarnetzki BM. Comparative immunoreactivity of the eosinophil constituents MBP and ECP in different types of urticaria. Arch Dermatol Res 1995;287:180–5.
13. Hermes B, Prochazka AK, Haas N, et al. Upregulation of TNF-alpha and IL-3 expression in lesional and uninvolved skin in different types of urticaria. J Allergy Clin Immunol 1999;103:307–14.
14. Luger TA, Beissert S, Schwarz T. The epidermal cytokine network. In: Bos JD, ed. Skin Immune System, 2nd ed. Boca Raton, FL: CRC Press, 1997:271–310.
15. Galli SJ, Nakae S, Tsai M. Mast cells in the development of adaptive immune responses. Nat Immunol 2005;6:135–42.
16. Van Overveld FJ, Jorens PG, Rampart M, et al. Tumour necrosis factor stimulates human skin mast cells to release histamine and tryptase. Clin Exp Allergy 1991;21:711–4.
17. Walsh LJ, Trinchieri G, Waldorf HA, et al. Human dermal mast cells contain and release tumor necrosis factor alpha, which induces endothelial leukocyte adhesion molecule 1. Proc Natl Acad Sci USA 1991;88:4220–4.
18. Moller A, Henz BM, Grutzkau A, et al. Comparative cytokine gene expression: regulation and release by human mast cells. Immunology 1998;93:289–95.
19. Schrader JW. The panspecific hemopoietin of activated T lymphocytes (interleukin-3). Annu Rev Immunol 1986;4:205–30.
20. Kita H, Ohnishi T, Okubo Y, et al. Granulocyte/macrophage colony-stimulating factor and interleukin 3 release from human peripheral blood eosinophils and neutrophils. J Exp Med 1991;174:745–8.
21. Khew-Goodall Y, Butcher CM, Litwin MS, et al. Chronic expression of P-selectin on endothelial cells stimulated by the T-cell cytokine, interleukin-3. Blood 1996;87:1432–8.
22. Zuberbier T, Schadendorf D, Haas N, et al. Enhanced P-selectin expression in chronic and dermographic urticaria. Int Arch Allergy Immunol 1997;114:86–9.
23. Zuberbier T, Bindslev-Jensen C, Canonica W, et al. EAACI/GA2LEN/EDF guideline: definition, classification and diagnosis of urticaria. Allergy 2006;61: 316–20.
24. Bingham CO. Diagnostic evaluation of urticaria. UpToDate in Medicine (CD-ROM). Wellesley: UpToDate Inc., 2004.
25. Greaves MW, Sabroe RA. Histamine: the quintessential mediator. J Dermatol 1996;23:735–40.
26. Kozel MM, Sabroe RA. Chronic urticaria: aetiology, management and current and future treatment options. Drugs 2004;64:2515–36.
27. Legrain V, Taieb A, Sage T, et al. Urticaria in infants: a study of forty patients. Pediatr Dermatol 1990;7:101–7.
28. Kauppinen K, Juntunen K, Lanki H. Urticaria in children. Retrospective evaluation and follow-up. Allergy 1984;39:469–72.
29. Zuberbier T, Chantraine-Hess S, Hartmann K, et al. Pseudoallergen-free diet in the treatment of chronic urticaria. A prospective study. Acta Derm Venereol 1995;75:484–7.

30. Sabroe RA, Black AK. Angiotensin-converting enzyme (ACE) inhibitors and angio-oedema. Br J Dermatol 1997;136:153–8.

31. Simons FE. Prevention of acute urticaria in young children with atopic dermatitis. J Allergy Clin Immunol 2001;107:703–6.

32. Aoki T, Kojima M, Horiko T. Acute urticaria: history and natural course of 50 cases. J Dermatol 1994;21:73–7.

33. Juhlin L. Recurrent urticaria: clinical investigation of 330 patients. Br J Dermatol 1981;104:369–81.

34. Barlow RJ, Warburton F, Watson K, et al. Diagnosis and incidence of delayed pressure urticaria in patients with chronic urticaria. J Am Acad Dermatol 1993;29:954–8.

35. Kaplan AP. Chronic urticaria: pathogenesis and treatment. J Allergy Clin Immunol 2004;114:465–74.

36. Henz BM, Jeep S, Ziegert FS, et al. Dermal and bronchial hyperreactivity in urticarial dermographism and urticaria factitia. Allergy 1996;51:171–5.

37. Hoffman HM, Wanderer AA, Broide DH. Familial cold autoinflammatory syndrome: phenotype and genotype of an autosomal dominant periodic fever. J Allergy Clin Immunol 2001;108:615–20.

38. Hoffman HM, Mueller JL, Broide DH, et al. Mutation of a new gene encoding a putative pyrin-like protein causes familial cold autoinflammatory syndrome and Muckle-Wells syndrome. Nat Genet 2001;29:301–5.

39. Zuberbier T, Althaus C, Chantraine-Hess S, et al. Prevalence of cholinergic urticaria in young adults. J Am Acad Dermatol 1994;31:978–81.

40. Champion RH, Roberts SO, Carpenter RG, et al. Urticaria and angio-oedema. A review of 554 patients. Br J Dermatol 1969;81:588–97.

41. Charlesworth EN. Urticaria and angioedema. Allergy Asthma Proc 2002;23:341–5.

42. Sabroe RA, Seed PT, Francis DM, et al. Chronic idiopathic urticaria: comparison of the clinical features of patients with and without anti-FcεRI or anti-IgE autoantibodies. J Am Acad Dermatol 1999;40:443–50.

43. O'Donnell BF, Lawlor F, Simpson J, et al. The impact of chronic urticaria on the quality of life. Br J Dermatol 1997;136:197–201.

44. Poon E, Seed PT, Greaves MW, et al. The extent and nature of disability in different urticarial conditions. Br J Dermatol 1999;140:667–71.

45. DeLong LK, Saini S, Beck LA, Chen SC. Annual direct and indirect healthcare costs in patients with chronic idiopathic urticaria: a cost analysis. J Am Acad Dermatol 2007;56:AB103.

46. Grattan CE. Aspirin sensitivity and urticaria. Clin Exp Dermatol 2003;28:123–7.

47. Moore-Robinson M, Warin RP. Effect of salicylates in urticaria. Br Med J 1967;4:262–4.

48. Grzelewska-Rzymowska I, Szmidt M, Rozniecki J. Aspirin-induced urticaria—a clinical study. J Invest Allergol Clin Immunol 1992;2:39–42.

49. Swain AR, Dutton SP, Truswell AS. Salicylates in foods. J Am Diet Assoc 1985;85:950–60.

50. Leznoff A, Josse RG, Denburg J, et al. Association of chronic urticaria and angioedema with thyroid autoimmunity. Arch Dermatol 1983;119:636–40.

51. Leznoff A, Sussman GL. Syndrome of idiopathic chronic urticaria and angioedema with thyroid autoimmunity: a study of 90 patients. J Allergy Clin Immunol 1989;84:66–71.

52. Kaplan AP, Finn A. Autoimmunity and the etiology of chronic urticaria. Can J Allergy Clin Immunol 1999;4:286–92.

53. Verneuil L, Leconte C, Ballet JJ, et al. Association between chronic urticaria and thyroid autoimmunity: a prospective study involving 99 patients. Dermatology 2004;208:98–103.

54. Kikuchi Y, Fann T, Kaplan AP. Antithyroid antibodies in chronic urticaria and angioedema. J Allergy Clin Immunol 2003;112:218.

55. Gruber BL, Baeza ML, Marchese MJ, et al. Prevalence and functional role of anti-IgE autoantibodies in urticarial syndromes. J Invest Dermatol 1988;90:213–7.

56. Kaplan AP. Clinical practice. Chronic urticaria and angioedema. N Engl J Med 2002;346:175–9.

57. Gaig P, Garcia-Ortega P, Enrique E, et al. Successful treatment of chronic idiopathic urticaria associated with thyroid autoimmunity. J Invest Allergol Clin Immunol 2000;10:342–5.

58. Rumbyrt JS, Katz JL, Schocket AL. Resolution of chronic urticaria in patients with thyroid autoimmunity. J Allergy Clin Immunol 1995;96:901–5.

59. O'Donnell BF, O'Neill CM, Francis DM, et al. Human leucocyte antigen class II associations in chronic idiopathic urticaria. Br J Dermatol 1999;140:853–8.

60. Ying S, Kikuchi Y, Meng Q, et al. TH1/TH2 cytokines and inflammatory cells in skin biopsy specimens from patients with chronic idiopathic urticaria: comparison with the allergen-induced late-phase cutaneous reaction. J Allergy Clin Immunol 2002;109:694–700.

61. Ormerod AD, Kobza Black A, Dawes J, et al. Prostaglandin D2 and histamine release in cold urticaria unaccompanied by evidence of platelet activation. J Allergy Clin Immunol 1988;82:586–9.

62. Smith CH, Kepley C, Schwartz LB, et al. Mast cell number and phenotype in chronic idiopathic urticaria. J Allergy Clin Immunol 1995;96:360–4.

63. Jacques P, Lavoie A, Bedard PM, et al. Chronic idiopathic urticaria: profiles of skin mast cell histamine release during active disease and remission. J Allergy Clin Immunol 1992;89:1139–43.

64. Caproni M, Giomi B, Volpi W, et al. Chronic idiopathic urticaria: infiltrating cells and related cytokines in autologous serum-induced wheals. Clin Immunol 2005;114:284–92.

65. Grattan CE. Basophils in chronic urticaria. J Invest Dermatol Symp Proc 2001;6:139–40.

66. Grattan CE, Dawn G, Gibbs S, et al. Blood basophil numbers in chronic ordinary urticaria and healthy controls: diurnal variation, influence of loratadine and prednisolone and relationship to disease activity. Clin Exp Allergy 2003;33:337–41.

67. Charlesworth EN, Hood AF, Soter NA, et al. Cutaneous late-phase response to allergen. Mediator release and inflammatory cell infiltration. J Clin Invest 1989;83:1519–26.

68. Knol EF, Mul FP, Jansen H, et al. Monitoring human basophil activation via CD63 monoclonal antibody 435. J Allergy Clin Immunol 1991;88:328–38.

69. Bochner BS. Systemic activation of basophils and eosinophils: markers and consequences. J Allergy Clin Immunol 2000;106:S292–302.

70. Ebo DG, Hagendorens MM, Bridts CH, et al. In vitro allergy diagnosis: should we follow the flow? Clin Exp Allergy 2004;34:332–9.

71. Vasagar K, Vonakis BM, Gober LM, et al. Evidence of in vivo basophil activation in chronic idiopathic urticaria. Clin Exp Allergy 2006;36:770–6.

72. Yoshimura C, Yamaguchi M, Iikura M, et al. Activation markers of human basophils: CD69 expression is strongly and preferentially induced by IL-3. J Allergy Clin Immunol 2002;109:817–23.

73. Buehring HJ, Seiffert M, Giesert C, et al. The basophil activation marker defined by antibody 97A6 is identical to the ectonucleotide pyrophosphatase/phosphodiesterase 3. Blood 2001;97:3303–5.

74. Boumiza R, Monneret G, Forissier MF, et al. Marked improvement of the basophil activation test by detecting CD203c instead of CD63. Clin Exp Allergy 2003;33:259–65.

75. Hauswirth AW, Natter S, Ghannadan M, et al. Recombinant allergens promote expression of CD203c on basophils in sensitized individuals. J Allergy Clin Immunol 2002;110:102–9.

76. Binder M, Fierlbeck G, King T, et al. Individual hymenoptera venom compounds induce upregulation of the basophil activation marker ectonucleotide pyrophosphatase/phosphodiesterase 3 (CD203c) in sensitized patients. Int Arch Allergy Immunol 2002;129:160–8.

77. Buehring H-J, Simmons PJ, Pudney M, et al. The monoclonal antibody 97A6 defines a novel surface antigen expressed on human basophils and their multipotent and unipotent progenitors. Blood 1999;94:2343–2356.

78. Kern F, Lichtenstein LM. Defective histamine release in chronic urticaria. J Clin Invest 1976;57:1369–77.

79. Vonakis BM, Vasagar K, Gibbons SP Jr, et al. Basophil FcεRI histamine release parallels expression of Src-homology 2–containing inositol phosphatases in chronic idiopathic urticaria. J Allergy Clin Immunol 2007;119:441–8.

80. Sabroe RA, Francis DM, Barr RM, et al. Anti-Fcε)RI auto antibodies and basophil histamine releasability in chronic idiopathic urticaria. J Allergy Clin Immunol 1998;102:651–8.

81. Gober LM, Sterba PM, Baker R, et al. Longitudinal examination of basophil functional phenotypes and disease activity in chronic idiopathic urticaria (CIU). J Allergy Clin Immunol 2007;119:S312.

82. Fiebiger E, Maurer D, Holub H, et al. Serum IgG autoantibodies directed against the alpha chain of Fc epsilon RI: a selective marker and pathogenetic factor for a distinct subset of chronic urticaria patients? J Clin Invest 1995;96:2606–12.

83. Ferrer M, Kinet JP, Kaplan AP. Comparative studies of functional and binding assays for IgG anti-FcεRIα (α-subunit) in chronic urticaria. J Allergy Clin Immunol 1998;101:672–6.

84. Hide M, Francis DM, Grattan CE, et al. Autoantibodies against the high-affinity IgE receptor as a cause of histamine release in chronic urticaria. N Engl J Med 1993;328:1599–604.

85. Niimi N, Francis DM, Kermani F, et al. Dermal mast cell activation by autoantibodies against the high affinity IgE receptor in chronic urticaria. J Invest Dermatol 1996;106:1001–6.

86. Sheikh J. Autoantibodies to the high-affinity IgE receptor in chronic urticaria: how important are they? Curr Opin Allergy Clin Immunol 2005;5:403–7.

87. Sabroe RA, Grattan CE, Francis DM, et al. The autologous serum skin test: a screening test for autoantibodies in chronic idiopathic urticaria. Br J Dermatol 1999;140:446–52.

88. Grattan CE, Wallington TB, Warin RP, et al. A serological mediator in chronic idiopathic urticaria—a clinical, immunological and histological evaluation. Br J Dermatol 1986;114:583–90.

89. Grattan CEH, Francis DM. Autoimmune urticaria. Adv Dermatol 1999;15:311–40.

90. Guttman-Yassky E, Bergman R, Maor C, et al. The autologous serum skin test in a cohort of chronic idiopathic urticaria patients compared to respiratory allergy patients and healthy individuals. J Eur Acad Dermatol Venereol 2007;21:35–9.

91. Grattan CE, Francis DM, Hide M, et al. Detection of circulating histamine releasing autoantibodies with functional properties of anti-IgE in chronic urticaria. Clin Exp Allergy 1991;21:695–704.

92. Kikuchi Y, Kaplan AP. Mechanisms of autoimmune activation of basophils in chronic urticaria. J Allergy Clin Immunol 2001;107:1056–62.

93. Sabroe RA, Fiebiger E, Francis DM, et al. Classification of anti-FcεRI and anti-IgE autoantibodies in chronic idiopathic urticaria and correlation with disease severity. J Allergy Clin Immunol 2002;110:492–9.

94. Sabroe RA, Poon E, Orchard GE, et al. Cutaneous inflammatory cell infiltrate in chronic idiopathic urticaria: comparison of patients with and without anti-FcεRI or anti-IgE autoantibodies. J Allergy Clin Immunol 1999;103:484–93.

95. Fiebiger E, Hammerschmid F, Stingl G, et al. Anti-FcεRIα autoantibodies in autoimmune-mediated disorders. Identification of a structure-function relationship. J Clin Invest 1998;101:243–51.

96. Grattan C, Powell S, Humphreys F. Management and diagnostic guidelines for urticaria and angiooedema. Br J Dermatol 2001;144:708–14.

97. Buss YA, Garrelfs UC, Sticherling M. Chronic urticaria—which clinical parameters are pathogenetically relevant? A retrospective investigation of 339 patients. J Dtsch Dermatol Ges 2007; 5:22–7.

98. Kanazawa K, Yaoita H, Tsuda F, et al. Hepatitis C virus infection in patients with urticaria. J Am Acad Dermatol 1996;35:195–8.

99. Cribier B. Urticaria and hepatitis. Clin Rev Allergy Immunol 2006;30:25–9.

100. Champion RH. Urticaria: then and now. Br J Dermatol 1988;119:427–36.

101. Greaves MW. Chronic idiopathic urticaria (CIU) and *Helicobacter pylori*—not directly causative, but could there be a link? Allergy Clin Immunol Int 2001;13:23–6.

102. Schnyder B, Helbling A, Pichler WJ. Chronic idiopathic urticaria: natural course and association with Helicobacter pylori infection. Int Arch Allergy Immunol 1999;119:60–3.

103. Hook-Nikanne J, Varjonen E, Harvima RJ, et al. Is Helicobacter pylori infection associated with chronic urticaria? Acta Derm Venereol 2000; 80:425–6.

104. Valsecchi R, Pigatto P. Chronic urticaria and Helicobacter pylori. Acta Derm Venereol 1998;78:440–2.

105. Wedi B, Kapp A. Helicobacter pylori infection in skin diseases: a critical appraisal. Am J Clin Dermatol 2002;3:273–82.

106. Gaig P, Garcia-Ortega P, Enrique E, et al. Efficacy of the eradication of Helicobacter pylori infection in patients with chronic urticaria. A placebo-controlled double blind study. Allergol Immunopathol 2002;30:255–8.

107. Yasnowsky KM, Dreskin SC, Efaw B, et al. Chronic urticaria sera increase basophil CD203c expression. J Allergy Clin Immunol 2006;117:1430–4.

108. Altrich ML, Halsey JF, Altman LC. Evaluation of a functional assay for the diagnosis of autoimmune chronic urticaria. J Allergy Clin Immunol 2007;119:S199.

109. Breathnach SM, Allen R, Ward AM, et al. Symptomatic dermographism: natural history, clinical features laboratory investigations and response to therapy. Clin Exp Dermatol 1983;8:463–76.

110. Commens CA, Greaves MW. Tests to establish the diagnosis in cholinergic urticaria. Br J Dermatol 1978;98:47–51.

111. Venzor J, Lee WL, Huston DP. Urticarial vasculitis. Clin Rev Allergy Immunol 2002;23:201–16.

112. Humphreys F, Hunter JA. The characteristics of urticaria in 390 patients. Br J Dermatol 1998;138: 635–8.

113. Nettis E, Pannofino A, D'Aprile C, et al. Clinical and aetiological aspects in urticaria and angiooedema. Br J Dermatol 2003;148:501–6.

114. Bleehen SS, Thomas SE, Greaves MW, et al. Cimetidine and chlorpheniramine in the treatment of chronic idiopathic urticaria: a multi-centre randomized double-blind study. Br J Dermatol 1987;117:81–8.

115. Harvey RP, Wegs J, Schocket AL. A controlled trial of therapy in chronic urticaria. J Allergy Clin Immunol 1981;68:262–6.

116. Mansfield LE, Smith JA, Nelson HS. Greater inhibition of dermographia with a combination of H1 and H2 antagonists. Ann Allergy 1983;50:264–5.

117. Kaur S, Greaves M, Eftekhari N. Factitious urticaria (dermographism): treatment by cimetidine and chlorpheniramine in a randomized double-blind study. Br J Dermatol 1981;104:185–90.

118. Paul E, Bodeker RH. Treatment of chronic urticaria with terfenadine and ranitidine. A randomized double-blind study in 45 patients. Eur J Clin Pharmacol 1986;31:277–80.

119. Simons FE, Sussman GL, Simons KJ. Effect of the H2-antagonist cimetidine on the pharmacokinetics and pharmacodynamics of the H1-antagonists hydroxyzine and cetirizine in patients with chronic urticaria. J Allergy Clin Immunol 1995;95:685–93.

120. Vena GA, Cassano N, D'Argento V, et al. Clobetasol propionate 0.05% in a novel foam formulation is safe and effective in the short-term treatment of patients with delayed pressure urticaria: a randomized, double-blind, placebo-controlled trial. Br J Dermatol 2006;154:353–6.

121. Yosipovitch G, Ansari N, Goon A, et al. Clinical characteristics of pruritus in chronic idiopathic urticaria. Br J Dermatol 2002;147:32–6.

122. Asero R. Chronic unremitting urticaria: is the use of antihistamines above the licensed dose effective? A preliminary study of cetirizine at licensed and above-licensed doses. Clin Exp Dermatol 2007;32:34–8.

123. Greene SL, Reed CE, Schroeter AL. Double-blind crossover study comparing doxepin with diphenhydramine for the treatment of chronic urticaria. J Am Acad Dermatol 1985;12:669–75.

124. Pacor ML, Di Lorenzo G, Corrocher R. Efficacy of leukotriene receptor antagonist in chronic urticaria. A double-blind, placebo-controlled comparison of treatment with montelukast and cetirizine in patients with chronic urticaria with intolerance to food additive and/or acetylsalicylic acid. Clin Exp Allergy 2001;31:1607–14.

125. Bonadonna P, Lombardi C, Senna G, et al. Treatment of acquired cold urticaria with cetirizine and zafirlukast in combination. J Am Acad Dermatol 2003;49:714–6.

126. Berkun Y, Shalit M. Successful treatment of delayed pressure urticaria with montelukast. Allergy 2000;55:203–4.

127. Nettis E, Colanardi MC, Paradiso MT, et al. Desloratadine in combination with montelukast in the treatment of chronic urticaria: a randomized, double-blind, placebo-controlled study. Clin Exp Allergy 2004;34:1401–7.

128. Erbagci Z. The leukotriene receptor antagonist montelukast in the treatment of chronic idiopathic urticaria: a single-blind, placebo-controlled, crossover clinical study. J Allergy Clin Immunol 2002;110:484–8.

129. Di Lorenzo G, Pacor ML, Mansueto P, et al. Randomized placebo-controlled trial comparing desloratadine and montelukast in monotherapy and desloratadine plus montelukast in combined therapy for chronic idiopathic urticaria. J Allergy Clin Immunol 2004;114:619–25.

130. Reimers A, Pichler C, Helbling A, et al. Zafirlukast has no beneficial effects in the treatment of chronic urticaria. Clin Exp Allergy 2002;32:1763–8.

131. Bagenstose SE, Levin L, Bernstein JA. The addition of zafirlukast to cetirizine improves the treatment of chronic urticaria in patients with positive autologous serum skin test results. J Allergy Clin Immunol 2004;113:134–40.

132. Nettis E, Dambra P, D'Oronzio L, et al. Comparison of montelukast and fexofenadine for chronic idiopathic urticaria. Arch Dermatol 2001;137:99–100.

133. Schleimer RP, Spahn JD, Covar R, et al. Glucocorticoids. In: Adkinson, NF, Yunginger JW, Busse WW, et al, eds. Middleton's Allergy: Principles and Practice, 6th ed. Philadelphia: Mosby, 2003:870–904.

134. Schleimer RP, MacGlashan DW Jr, Gillespie E, et al. Inhibition of basophil histamine release by anti-inflammatory steroids. II. Studies on the mechanism of action. J Immunol 1982;129:1632–6.

135. Grattan CE, O'Donnell BF, Francis DM, et al. Randomized double-blind study of cyclosporin in chronic "idiopathic" urticaria. Br J Dermatol 2000;143:365–72.

136. Fradin MS, Ellis CN, Goldfarb MT, et al. Oral cyclosporine for severe chronic idiopathic urticaria and angioedema. J Am Acad Dermatol 1991;251065–7.

137. Toubi E, Blant A, Kessel A, et al. Low-dose cyclosporin A in the treatment of severe chronic idiopathic urticaria. Allergy 1997;52:312–6.

138. Stellato C, de Paulis A, Ciccarelli A, et al. Anti-inflammatory effect of cyclosporin A on human skin mast cells. J Invest Dermatol 1992;98: 800–4.

139. Jaffer AM. Sulfasalazine in the treatment of corticosteroid-dependent chronic idiopathic urticaria. J Allergy Clin Immunol 1991;88:964–5.

140. Engler RJ, Squire E, Benson P. Chronic sulfasalazine therapy in the treatment of delayed pressure urticaria and angioedema. Ann Allergy Asthma Immunol 1995;74:155–9.

141. Hartmann K, Hani N, Hinrichs R, et al. Successful sulfasalazine treatment of severe chronic idiopathic urticaria associated with pressure urticaria. Acta Derm Venereol 2001;81:71.

142. McGirt LY, Vasagar K, Gober LM, et al. Successful treatment of recalcitrant chronic idiopathic urticaria with sulfasalazine. Arch Dermatol 2006;142: 1337–42.

143. Lee EH, Kim HM. Inhibition of anaphylaxis by sulfasalazine in rats. Pharmacology 1998;56:223–9.

144. Fox CC, Moore WC, Lichtenstein LM. Modulation of mediator release from human intestinal mast cells by sulfasalazine and 5-aminosalicylic acid. Dig Dis Sci 1991;36:179–84.

145. Barrett KE, Tashof TL, Metcalfe DD. Inhibition of IgE-mediated mast cell degranulation by sulphasalazine. Eur J Pharmacol 1985;107:279–81.

146. Cassano N, D'Argento V, Filotico R, et al. Low-dose dapsone in chronic idiopathic urticaria: preliminary results of an open study. Acta Derm Venereol 2005;85:254–5.

147. Boehm I, Bauer R, Bieber T. Urticaria treated with dapsone. Allergy 1999;54:765–6.

148. Gach JE, Sabroe RA, Greaves MW, et al. Methotrexate-responsive chronic idiopathic urticaria: a report of two cases. Br J Dermatol 2001;145:340–3.

149. Bernstein JA, Garramone SM, Lower EG. Successful treatment of autoimmune chronic idiopathic urti-

caria with intravenous cyclophosphamide. Ann Allergy Asthma Immunol 2002;89:212–4.

150. Reeves GE, Boyle MJ, Bonfield J, et al. Impact of hydroxychloroquine therapy on chronic urticaria: chronic autoimmune urticaria study and evaluation. Intern Med J 2004;34:182–6.

151. Lawlor F, Black AK, Ward AM, et al. Delayed pressure urticaria, objective evaluation of a variable disease using a dermographometer and assessment of treatment using colchicine. Br J Dermatol 1989;120:403–8.

152. Grattan CE, Francis DM, Slater NG, et al. Plasmapheresis for severe, unremitting, chronic urticaria. Lancet 1992;339:1078–80.

153. O'Donnell BF, Barr RM, Black AK, et al. Intravenous immunoglobulin in autoimmune chronic urticaria. Br J Dermatol 1998;138:101–6.

154. Asero R. Are IVIG for chronic unremitting urticaria effective? Allergy 2000;55:1099–101.

155. Asero R, Tedeschi A. Emerging drugs for chronic urticaria. Expert Opin Emerg Drugs 2006;11: 265–74.

156. Sharma JK, Miller R, Murray S. Chronic urticaria: a Canadian perspective on patterns and practical management strategies. J Cutan Med Surg 2000;4:89–93.

157. Berroeta L, Clark C, Ibbotson SH, et al. Narrowband (TL-01) ultraviolet B phototherapy for chronic urticaria. Clin Exp Dermatol 2004;29:97–8.

158. Hannuksela M, Kokkonen EL. Ultraviolet light therapy in chronic urticaria. Acta Derm Venereol 1985;65:449–50.

159. Olafsson JH, Larko O, Roupe G, et al. Treatment of chronic urticaria with PUVA or UVA plus placebo: a double-blind study. Arch Dermatol Res 1986;278:228–31.

160. Ellis MH. Successful treatment of chronic urticaria with leukotriene antagonists. J Allergy Clin Immunol 1998;102:876–7.

161. Spector S, Tan RA. Antileukotrienes in chronic urticaria. J Allergy Clin Immunol 1998;101:572.

162. Parslew R, Pryce D, Ashworth J, et al. Warfarin treatment of chronic idiopathic urticaria and angio-oedema. Clin Exp Allergy 2000;30:1161–5.

163. Czarnetzki BM, Algermissen B, Jeep S, et al. Interferon treatment of patients with chronic urticaria and mastocytosis. J Am Acad Dermatol 1994;30:500–1.

164. Parsad D, Pandhi R, Juneja A. Stanozolol in chronic urticaria: a double blind, placebo controlled trial. J Dermatol 2001;28:299–302.

165. Shahar E, Bergman R, Guttman-Yassky E, et al. Treatment of severe chronic idiopathic urticaria with oral mycophenolate mofetil in patients not responding to antihistamines and/or corticosteroids. Int J Dermatol 2006;45:1224–7.

166. Frieling U, Luger TA. Mycophenolate mofetil and leflunomide: promising compounds for the treatment of skin diseases. Clin Exp Derm 2002;27:562–70.

167. Isenberg DA. B cell targeted therapies in autoimmune diseases. J Rheumatol Suppl 2006;77:24–8.

168. Williams JD, Griffiths CE. Cytokine blocking agents in dermatology. Clin Exp Dermatol 2002;27:585–90.

169. Magerl M, Philipp S, Manasterski M, et al. Successful treatment of delayed pressure urticaria with anti-TNF-alpha. J Allergy Clin Immunol 2007;119:752–4.

170. Boyce JA. Successful treatment of cold-induced urticaria/anaphylaxis with anti-IgE. J Allergy Clin Immunol 2006;117:1415–8.

171. Shapiro CA, Kapetanos NS, Sarmiento E. Successful treatment of chronic idiopathic urticaria and angioedema, with Xolair. J Allergy Clin Immunol 2007;119:S274.

172. Rafi A, Do L, Mangat R, et al. Efficacy of omalizumab for the treatment of allergic urticaria and angioedema. J Allergy Clin Immunol 2007;119:312.

173. Beck LA, Marcotte GV, MacGlashan D, et al. Omalizumab-induced reductions in mast cell Fce psilon RI expression and function. J Allergy Clin Immunol 2004;114:527–30.

Section III
Immunopharmacology

28
Biologic Therapies for Inflammatory Disease

Emily M. Berger and Alice B. Gottlieb

Key Points

- Biologics are approved for the therapy of psoriasis and psoriatic arthritis as well as a number of nondermatologic indications.
- Biologics include cell adhesion molecule antagonists (alefacept and efalizumab) and cytokine antagonists (etanercept, infliximab, and adalimumab).
- Biologics appear relatively safe, but clinical and laboratory monitoring of safety is recommended.
- Cytokine (i.e., tumor necrosis factor) antagonists have other potential uses in dermatology, including pyoderma gangrenosum, hidrandenitis suppurativa, and sarcoidosis.
- Future biologics will include interleukin-12/interleukin-23–targeted therapies.

Biologic therapies, or biologics, are substances created by scientists from living cells for the treatment or prevention of human diseases.[1] To treat disease, biologics can add back missing proteins such as enzymes or hormones, or they can neutralize or combat pathogenic organisms, cells, or immune mediators.[1] In inflammatory diseases such as psoriasis and psoriatic arthritis (PsA), biologics are recombinant proteins that alter a patient's immune system to interfere with a specific step along the pathogenesis of either disease at the level of cells or cytokines in the skin, joints, or blood.[2] Biologics currently used to treat psoriasis and PsA include monoclonal antibodies and fusion proteins.

An antibody, or immunoglobulin (Ig), is a soluble protein made by and released from plasma B-cell lymphocytes as part of an organism's acquired immunity.[3] An antibody is composed of two light chains as well as two heavy chains, and it can be divided both into an Fc fragment joined at a hinge to two Fab fragments as well as into a constant region merged with a variable region (Fig. 28.1). The Fc fragment (crystallizable fragment) facilitates the biologic functions of an antibody such as the lysis, opsonization, and degranulation of cells by binding to either complement or different cell receptors. The two Fab fragments (fragment antigen binding) facilitate the binding of antigen, as the antigen binding sites are at their tips. The variable region of an antibody is made from parts of the light and heavy chains, and it binds specifically to an antigen. The constant region is also made up of light and heavy chains, where the latter chains are common to one class of antibody (e.g., IgG, IgA, IgM, IgE, or IgD). In the laboratory, scientists can produce several kinds of antibodies, including chimeric, humanized, or human sequence antibodies that differ from each other by how much of their structure is made from mouse vs. human proteins.[2] Chimeric antibodies combine mouse and human proteins such that mouse protein makes up the variable region and human protein makes up the constant region.[1] Humanized antibodies have mouse and human proteins interspersed in the variable region, which is attached to a human protein constant region.[1] Human sequence antibodies, or fully human antibodies, are entirely human proteins made inside genetically engineered mice.[2]

As its name implies, a fusion protein is made by combining two genes together to create a single new protein coded for by information from each of the two genes. Fusion proteins usually combine a receptor domain (to attach to a specific target, as

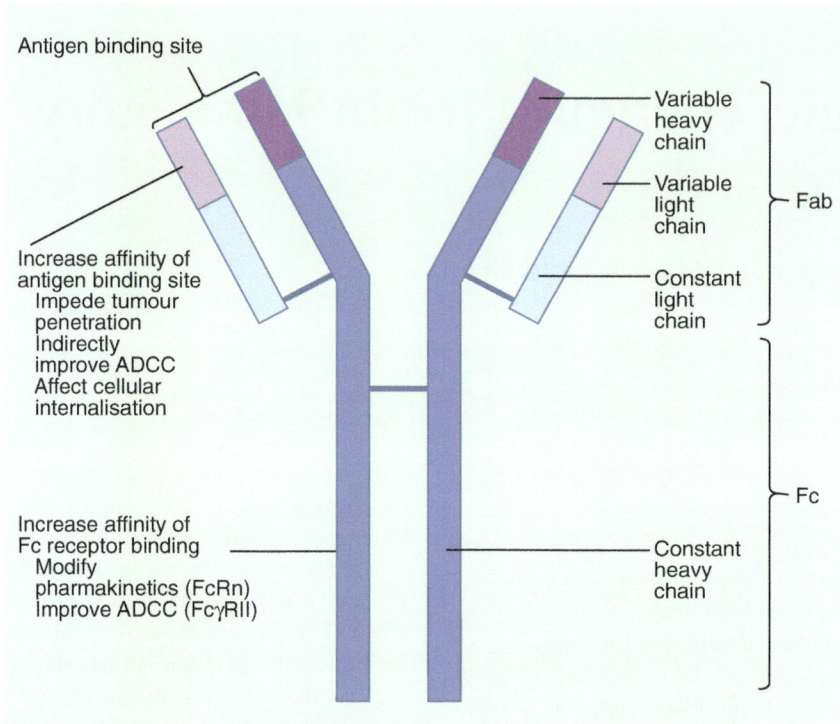

FIG. 28.1. Antibody structure. An antibody is composed of two light chains and two heavy chains. It is divided both into an Fc fragment joined at a hinge to two Fab fragments as well as into a constant region merged with a variable region.

would a receptor to a ligand or co-receptor), and the constant region sequences of human IgG (for the fusion protein to be soluble in plasma, as is human IgG).[2]

The World Health Organization (WHO) maintains an organized schematic for naming biologic therapies and biotechnologic substances including antibodies and fusion proteins.[1] The names of monoclonal antibodies have a common stem of "-mab" with different sub-stems added before the common stem, depending on both the disease/target of therapy as well as the animal(s) of origin of the protein. For example, antibodies that are immunomodulators such as those that treat psoriasis and PsA have the sub-stem "-li(m)-," followed by an additional sub-stem to indicate if the source of the antibody is mouse, human, or both. Fusion proteins all end in "-cept," where a specific "infix" may specify its target. For example, in this schematic, a fusion protein targeted against lymphocyte function–associated antigen 3 (LFA-3) has the infix "-lefa-" followed by the pre-stem "-cept," whereas

a fusion protein targeted against tumor necrosis factor (TNF) has the common stem "-nercept" (Table 28.1).

Traditional Therapies for Psoriasis and Psoriatic Arthritis and the Need for Biologic Therapies

As demonstrated both by animal models[4–12] and by human clinical research,[13–23] psoriasis vulgaris is a type 1 immune disease of the skin that is mediated by subsets of T cells, dendritic cells (DCs), and cytokines (including TNF-α, interferon-γ [IFN-γ], and interleukin-12 [IL-12]/IL-23). Clinical research showed that T cells, DCs, and cytokines are similarly important in the immunopathogenesis of PsA,[24–27] a potentially debilitating seronegative inflammatory arthritis that affects patients with all degrees of severity of psoriasis.[28] According to recent estimates, PsA occurs in approximately 11%

TABLE 28.1. Naming a biologic therapy for psoriasis or psoriatic arthritis.

Type of biologic therapy	Sub-stem (if applies, to indicate that the agent is of the immunomodulator disease or target class)	Sub-stem (if applies, to indicate the source of product, i.e., the animals of origin)	Infix (if applies, to indicate the agent's target)	Common stem (or pre-stem)	Available agents (with complete stem)
Chimeric antibody	-li(m)-	-xi-	n/a	-mab	Infliximab (Remicade®)
Humanized antibody	-li(m)-	-zu-	n/a	-mab	Efalizumab (Raptiva®)
Human sequence antibody	-li(m)-	-u-	n/a	-mab	Adalimumab (Humira®)
Fusion protein (receptor molecule targeted against lymphocyte function–associated antigen 3 [LFA-3])	n/a	n/a	-lefa-	(-cept)	Alefacept (Amevive®)
Fusion protein (receptor molecule targeted against tumor necrosis factor [TNF] antagonist)	n/a	n/a	n/a	-nercept	Etanercept (Enbrel®)

Data from International Nonproprietary Names (INN) for Biological and Biotechnological Substances (A Review). World Health Organization (WHO) Web site: http://www.who.int/medicines/services/inn/BioRevforweb.pdf.

to one third[29] of psoriasis patients, but it can be as common as 55% in psoriasis patients who present to the clinic with joint pain.[30] Psoriasis patients report persistent joint pain or stiffness even before the diagnosis of PsA,[31] which develops approximately 10 years after the development of skin disease in most patients.[32,33] Thus, the timeline for the development of PsA allows dermatologists the unique opportunity to interfere with the progression to PsA and the development of disability.[32,34]

Typically, phototherapy and systemic agents are used to treat moderate-severe psoriasis, which afflicts one third of psoriasis patients.[32] These therapies include ultraviolet B (UVB) phototherapy, psoralen plus UVA irradiation (PUVA), acitretin, methotrexate (MTX), and cyclosporine, all of which must be used as repeated courses of short-term therapy, for they are inconvenient and globally toxic to a patient's system. When psoriasis patients were asked about their level of satisfaction with common conventional systemic therapies, they indicated that these agents do not completely meet their needs or provide great treatment satisfaction.[35] Thus, the risk-to-benefit ratio of traditional treatments is high. Therapies traditionally used to treat PsA are nonsteroidal antiinflammatory drugs (NSAIDs) and disease-modifying antirheumatic drugs (DMARDs), which include the off-label use of cyclosporine, MTX, and leflunomide.[36] Although DMARDs may be dual-purpose agents that can treat symptoms associated with both psoriasis and PsA, they do not slow the development/progression of joint disease. A most important potential function of biologic therapies is thus to provide a more convenient and less toxic maintenance therapy for sustained skin clearance in psoriasis; relief from pain and prevention of disability in PsA; and improved quality of life for patients with skin or joint disease.[32]

Clinical trials of the biologic agents most often include patients with moderate and more severe disease based on quality of life and physical parameters.[37] More severe psoriasis typically involves a Psoriasis Area and Severity Index (PASI), percent of affected body surface area (BSA), and a Dermatology Life Quality Index (DLQI) score greater than 10[38] (see Appendix). Accordingly, physicians frequently employ biologics to treat patients with moderate-severe psoriasis or PsA who are candidates for systemic therapy.[34] Such

patients have often failed or have a contraindication to traditional systemic therapies.[38] In addition, biologics are an emerging treatment modality for patients with less common forms of psoriasis, as demonstrated by their off-label use to treat patients with palmoplantar psoriasis,[39–44] erythrodermic psoriasis,[39,45] and generalized pustular psoriasis.[46–50]

Discovering Therapeutic Targets: Targeting the T-Cell

By studying skin biopsies of psoriasis patients, scientists discovered that there are many activated T cells in the dermal infiltrate of psoriasis lesions.[51] Scientists knew that drugs that interfere with T-cell activation such as cyclosporine improve psoriasis but also affect other cells such as keratinocytes (epidermal skin cells).[32] Thus, for years there had been an association between psoriasis and T cells, but there was no definitive proof that the T cell was mainly responsible for skin lesions. The T-cell–targeted drug denileukin diftitox/DAB389IL-2 is a fusion protein specific to activated T cells that is made from portions of diphtheria toxin and the T-cell–activating cytokine IL-2.[15] It attaches to the IL-2 receptor expressed on activated T cells and ultimately leads to the toxin-mediated destruction of these cells, the histologic improvement of psoriasis lesions, and the clinical clearance of psoriasis plaques.[15] Its use determined that T cells were central to the pathogenesis of psoriasis, and thus was born a new era for treating psoriasis and PsA with such targeted biologic therapies.[2,32] Such therapies aim to halt T-cell and DC activation and neutralize inflammatory cytokines.[32] They fall into one of two main therapeutic classes: (1) cell adhesion molecule antagonists or (2) cytokine antagonists.

Cell Adhesion Molecule Antagonists

Normal T-cell activation requires two main steps.[32] First, the T-cell receptor (TCR) interacts with a peptide antigen attached to a human leukocyte antigen (HLA) protein that is either a class I or class II major histocompatibility complex (MHC

I or MHC II) on an antigen-presenting cell (APC) such as a Langerhans' cell or a dermal DC. Second, co-stimulation occurs where pairs of molecules on the surface of the T cell and the APC interact. The interaction between LFA-1 on the T cell and intercellular adhesion molecule 1 (ICAM-1) on the APC anchor the two cells together for cellular activation to occur. The interactions between molecule pairs, including CD2 on the T cell with LFA-3 on the APC, and CD28 on the T cell with B7.1 (CD80) and B7.2 (CD86) on the APC lead to cellular activation. When activation is complete, there are signals for cellular downregulation including

the interaction of cytotoxic T-lymphocyte antigen 4 (CTLA4) on the T cell with B7 on the APC[32] (Fig. 28.2).

In psoriasis plaques, there is increased expression of HLA molecules capable of presenting antigen to T cells and contributing to their activation, and there are increased numbers of Langerhans' cell APCs.[51] Similarly, DCs bearing the maturation markers CD11c and CD83 are upregulated in psoriatic skin and contribute substantially, in addition to T cells, to the inflammation characteristic of psoriasis lesions.[19,22] Scientists believe that APCs react to an unknown self antigen in the skin

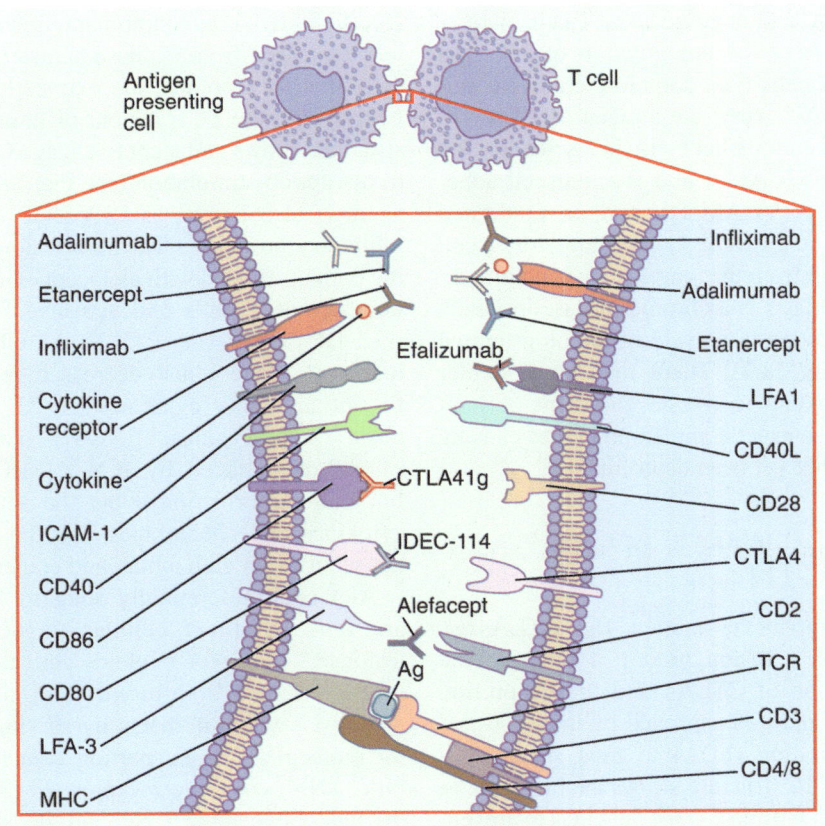

Fig. 28.2. Known sites of action of psoriasis therapies. Interactions between antigen-presenting cells (such as dendritic cells) and T cells have a key role in the pathogenesis of psoriasis. Several biologic therapies target molecules expressed on the surface of these cells, as shown here. Alefacept is a fusion protein that binds to CD2; efalizumab is a monoclonal antibody that binds to lymphocyte function–associated antigen 1 (LFA-1); cytotoxic T-lymphocyte antigen immunoglobulin (CTLAIg) is a fusion protein that binds to CD86 and CD80; and IDEC-114 is a monoclonal antibody that binds to CD80. These four therapies target T-cell co-stimulation or antigen-presenting cell–T-cell interactions. Infliximab and adalimumab are monoclonal antibodies that target the inflammatory cytokine tumor necrosis factor-α (TNF-α), which is also the target of etanercept, a fusion protein. Ag, antigen; ICAM-1, intercellular adhesion molecule 1; MHC, major histocompatibility complex; TCR, T-cell antigen receptor.

of hereditarily predisposed patients and then move to lymph nodes to activate T cells to differentiate and proliferate.[2,32] T cells then return to the skin for reactivation and production of inflammatory lesions. As a result of activation, mature T cells produce cytokines such as IL-2 that proliferate, and mature DCs make chemokines and cytokines such as IL-12 and IL-23. IL-12 influences T-cell differentiation into type 1 (T1) cells, which will in turn manufacture and secrete cytokines including TNF-α, IFN-γ, and granulocyte-monocyte colony-stimulating factor (GM-CSF).[2] In the T1 cytokine milieu, keratinocytes become activated, and they release chemokines to attract inflammatory cells, cytokines, and growth factors to encourage skin cell proliferation and angiogenesis. T-cell maturation also influences the upregulation of adhesion molecules on T cells (i.e., common leukocyte antigen [CLA], LFA-1, very late antigen 4 [VLA-4]), on blood vessel endothelial cells (i.e., selectins and integrins such as ICAM-1 and vascular cell adhesion molecule 1 [VCAM-1]), and on epidermal keratinocytes (i.e., ICAM-1) to allow for T-cell return to the skin from the lymph nodes and blood.[2] Ultimately, psoriasis is a chronic disease in which T cells and DCs are in a cycle of ongoing mutual activation[32] (Fig. 28.3). There may be a similar set of steps leading to the development of joint involvement. The exact complex processes causing psoriasis have not yet been determined.

Cytotoxic T-Lymphocyte Antigen 4Ig and IDEC-114

Cytotoxic T-lymphocyte antigen 4Ig (CTLA4Ig), or abatacept, is a fusion protein combining the peripheral portion of CTLA4 and the Fc portion of human IgG, and it is approved by the Food and Drug Administration (FDA) to treat rheumatoid arthritis (RA).[52] Its structure allows the molecule to bind B7 (both CD80 and CD86) on APCs to prevent the CD28-B7 interaction that is required for T-cell activation[32] (see Fig. 28.2). In a phase I investigation for the treatment of psoriasis, intravenous (IV) infusions of CTLA4Ig resulted in dose-related clinical improvement in psoriasis patients and histologic changes in psoriatic lesions including decreases in skin thickness, T-cell number,[16,17] DC activation and number, and vascular adhesion molecules.[17] This use of CTLA4Ig pointed to the role of CD28-B7 co-stimulation in the immunopathogenesis and maintenance of psoriasis lesions.

Similarly, IDEC-114, or galiximab, an anti-B7.1 monoclonal antibody, enacted clinical improvement and histologic changes in psoriatic lesions in a phase I/II study, further solidifying the importance of the CD28-B7 co-stimulatory interaction.[18,53] The understanding of co-stimulation paved the way for the development of alefacept, the first biologic therapy approved by the FDA for the treatment of moderate-severe plaque-type psoriasis.

Alefacept

Alefacept, or Amevive® (Astellas Pharma US, Inc., Deerfield, IL), is a recombinant dimeric fusion protein expressed from Chinese hamster ovary (CHO) cells that incorporates the extracellular region of LFA-3 with the Fc fragment of human IgG$_1$.[54] Its structure allows alefacept to engage CD2 on T cells to disrupt co-stimulation (see Fig. 28.2). Thus, the agent is also known as LFA-3TIP (LFA-3 T-cell inhibitory protein).[55] The skin lesions of responding patients treated with alefacept exhibit decreased numbers of T cells and activated "mature" DCs (i.e., DCs expressing CD83[+] and CD11c[+] surface markers). There is also decreased gene expression for inflammatory cytokines (IL-23 and inducible nitric oxide synthase [iNOS]) and chemokines (monokine induced by IFN-γ [MIG] and IL-8). For more information about the actions of these cytokines and chemokines, see the discussion in the sections on efalizumab and etanercept, below.

Alefacept preferentially binds to T cells, which are thus its direct cellular target in psoriatic lesions.[55] Alefacept depletes activated CD45RO[+] memory T cells both in vitro and in vivo through apoptosis, which it enacts by serving as an effector molecule.[56] Its Fc portion connects to natural killer (NK) cells' Fc receptor (FcγR) to serve as the link between the T cell and the NK cell, which subsequently kills the T cell by lysing it with toxic molecules such as granzyme and perforin.[56,57] Although alefacept exerts a number of effects to counteract psoriatic pathology, exactly how these effects improve psoriasis is not known.[32,55] Although clinical improvement correlates with the depletion of T cells in skin lesions,[58,59] clinical improvement may[60–63] or may not[58] correlate as well with the depletion of CD4[+] and CD8[+] memory

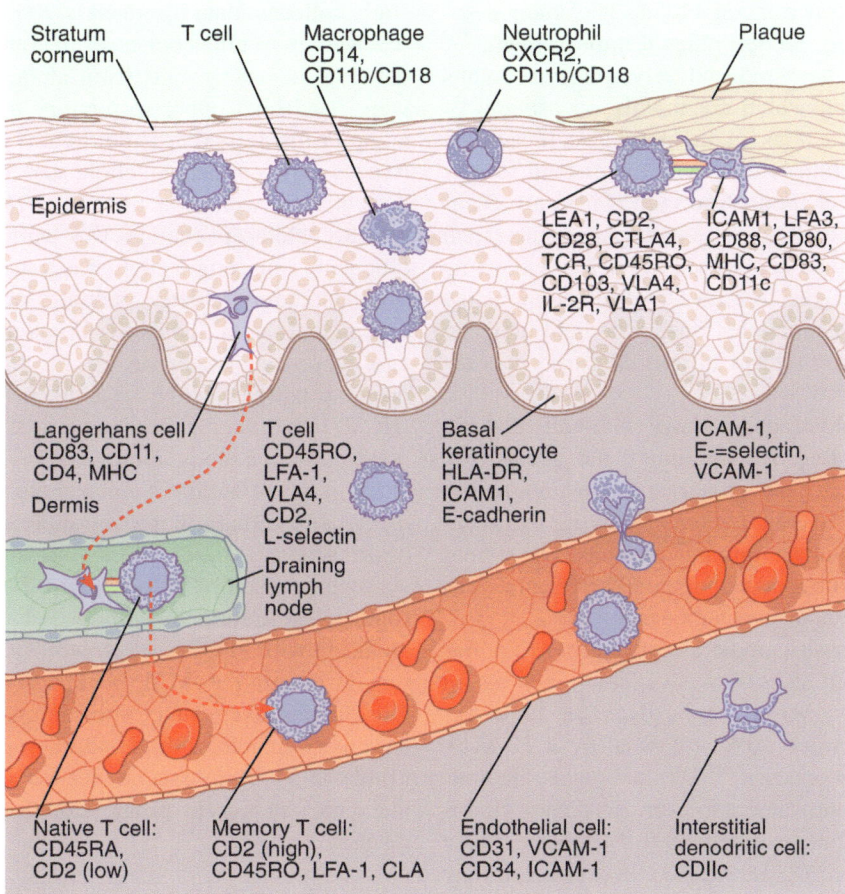

Fɪɢ. 28.3. Immunopathogenesis of psoriasis: a selected view. Some key cell types thought to be involved in the pathogenesis of psoriasis are shown, together with important molecules expressed on the surface of these cells. After a stimulus, dendritic cells and T cells become activated through the formation of an immunologic synapse. T-cell and dendritic-cell activation result in nuclear factor-κB (NF-κB) activation, and the release of cytokines, such as tumor necrosis factor-α, chemokines, proteases, and other inflammatory mediators, which induce a wound-healing–like phenotype in the epidermis that is characterized by keratinocyte proliferation. A key event is the migration of T cells into the epidermis, which involves interactions between T cells and endothelial cells (for example, mediated by lymphocyte function–associated antigen 1 [LFA-1] on T cells and intercellular adhesion molecule 1 [ICAM-1] on endothelial cells) and between T cells and basement membrane constituents (for example, very late antigen 1 [VLA-1] on T cells interacting with collagen type 4 in basement membranes). In a chronic psoriatic plaque, as shown in the top right, it is thought that there is a cycle of continuous T-cell and dendritic-cell activation. CTLA4, cytotoxic T-lymphocyte antigen 4; CXCR2, CXC chemokine receptor 2; HLA-DR, human leukocyte antigen DR; IL, interleukin; MHC, major histocompatibility complex; TCR, T-cell antigen receptor; VCAM, vascular cell adhesion molecule.

T cells in the peripheral blood. The latter association does not foretell clinical improvement.[32,63] Patients may have reduced T-lymphocyte counts from treatment, which are mainly on account of reversible reductions in memory T cell subsets, but overall serum lymphocyte values tend to stay above the lower limit of normal.[61,62] As a precaution, a baseline CD4+ cell count is measured, and a CD4+ cell count is obtained every 2 weeks while on therapy[54] (Table 28.2). A CD4+ cell count below 250 cells/μL requires that dosing be held until the CD4+ cell count returns to normal during weekly blood counts.

Although alefacept interferes with cells that are involved in protective immunity, the agent does not appear to cause global immunosuppression. In a randomized trial, patients receiving treatment demonstrated intact immune responses to initial vaccination with a new antigenic bacteriophage as well as to a tetanus booster vaccine.[64]

When originally studied, alefacept was administered IV, but it is now available only as an intramuscular (IM) injection, given for 12 weeks at 15 mg per week (QW) followed by a 12-week period of observation.[54] Clinical trials demonstrated that improvement in psoriasis occurs gradually and continues even after a full 12-week course is administered[63,65] (Table 28.3). In practice, it may take a couple of months until patients experience significant clinical effects. This delay in clinical response may be accounted for by a late onset of T-cell apoptosis some 16 to 22 weeks after the administration of alefacept.[66]

Alefacept is a remittive therapy, which means that it induces significant remission in patients that allows them to experience a period of continuous disease clearance without having to take continuous therapy.[65,67] In a study that aimed to assess the remission period following one IV course of the agent, investigators noted a median of 10 months before patients needed further treatment for their psoriasis.[67] In clinical trials, patients did not experience tachyphylaxis; thus upon relapse, successive courses of alefacept could be administered successfully after the 12-week observation period.[65,68,69] And, for patients who did not respond to a first course of therapy, an additional course provided them with relief from psoriasis symptoms.[70]

An analysis of 13 clinical trials assessed the long-term safety of therapy for up to 5 years.[71] This study collected data from nearly 2000 patients who received up to nine courses of treatment. The most common adverse events from alefacept treatment were headache, upper respiratory tract infection, and pruritus. Less that 1% of treated patients experienced any serious infection, and infections did not correlate with reductions in CD4+ cell counts. Notably, alefacept therapy was well tolerated and efficacious in certain high-risk treatment populations including elderly patients, obese patients, and patients with diabetes.[72] In addition, there are case reports supporting its use for the treatment of psoriasis patients who have active hepatitis C virus (HCV) infection, patients who are especially sensitive to immune modulation.[73]

Initial investigation of alefacept for the treatment of PsA found that it improved signs and symptoms of arthritis and decreased inflammation in the PsA synovium, resulting in decreased T-cell and macrophage infiltration.[74] A phase II study combining alefacept with MTX for the treatment of PsA found that the addition of IM alefacept enacted significant clinical improvement in arthritis and in skin disease as compared with the addition of a placebo[75] (Table 28.3). More data are needed to determine if alefacept can halt the progression of psoriatic joint disease.

Efalizumab

Efalizumab, or Raptiva® (Genentech, Inc., San Francisco, CA) is a recombinant humanized monoclonal antibody expressed from CHO cells that is directed against the CD11a subunit of the LFA-1 adhesion molecule (see Fig. 28.2).[76] By binding to CD11a on leukocytes, it interferes with the interaction between LFA-1 and ICAM-1 and thus has the ability to act at the level of the leukocyte, the blood, and the skin.[2,76,77] Antigen-presenting cells display ICAM, thus efalizumab would disrupt the process of T-cell activation.[76,77] Endothelial cells express ICAM, thus efalizumab would interfere with T-cell movement through vasculature, and epithelial cells have ICAM, thus efalizumab would interfere with T-cell exocytosis and travel into the skin. Indeed, scientists have shown that the agent prevents T cells,[23] specifically memory CD8+ T cells from entering the skin.[78] This action causes a peripheral lymphocytosis with an increase mostly in CD3+ cells, where CD8+ memory T cells are the most

TABLE 28.2. Biologic therapies for psoriasis and psoriatic arthritis.

Agent (common name)	Agent (commercial name)	Date of FDA approval (or current phase of clinical trials) for treatment of psoriasis	Date of FDA approval (or current phase of clinical trials) for treatment of PsA	Structure and target	Dosing for psoriasis treatment	Dosing for PsA treatment	Common or concerning adverse events associated with treatment	Suggested clinical monitoring (if monitoring is suggested by the manufacturer, citation follows; otherwise, monitoring is an example of clinical practice performed by author Gottlieb)	Contraindications to therapy
Alefacept	Amevive[54]	January 2003	Phase II completed[202]	Recombinant fusion protein of LFA-3 and Fc portion of human IgG1[1]	15 mg IM weekly × 12 weeks[1]	N/A	- Headache, URI, pruritus[1] - Reversible reduction in CD4+ T-cell count[1]	- PGA, BSA, physical exam, & assess for PsA q 3 months - Labs: CD4+ T-cell count @ baseline then q 2 weeks[1] LFTs at baseline then q 3 months	- Severe hypersensitivity reaction[1] - CD4 T-cell count <250 cells/μL[1] - Active infection, including HIV[1] - Active hepatitis or liver injury[1] - Active cancer[1] - Pregnancy (category B) is a relative contraindication[1] - Live vaccines are contraindicated during therapy[1]
Efalizumab	Raptiva[76]	October 2003	N/A	Humanized monoclonal antibody against the CD11a subunit of the LFA1 adhesion molecule[4]	Conditioning dose of 0.7 mg/kg SC injection→ 1 mg/kg/wk self-administered SC injection (max 200 mg/dose)[4]	N/A	- Flu-like symptoms (within 24–48 hours, decrease over time)[4]	- PGA, BSA, physical exam, & assess for PsA q 3 months - Labs: CBC (platelet Count)	- Severe hypersensitivity reaction[4] - Active infection[4] - Thrombocytopenia[4] - Active cancer[4]

(continued)

TABLE 28.2. (continued)

Agent (common name)	Agent (commercial name)	Date of FDA approval (or current phase of clinical trials) for treatment of psoriasis	Date of FDA approval (or current phase of clinical trials) for treatment of PsA	Structure and target	Dosing for psoriasis treatment	Dosing for PsA treatment	Common or concerning adverse events associated with treatment	Suggested clinical monitoring (if monitoring is suggested by the manufacturer, citation follows; otherwise, monitoring is an example of clinical practice performed by author Gottlieb)	Contraindications to therapy
							- Reversible thrombocytopenia[4] - Psoriasis events[1]	@ baseline, q month × 3 months, then q 3 months[4] LFTs @ baseline then q 3 months	- Relative contraindications:PsA, pregnancy (category C)[4] - Live vaccines are contraindicated during therapy[4]
Etanercept	Enbrel[115]	April 2004	January 2002	Recombinant fusion protein of p75 TNF receptor and Fc portion of human IgG1, forming a soluble human TNF receptor[6]	50 mg SC injection self-administered BIW for 3 months → SC injection self-administered as 25 mg BIW or 50 mg QW[6]	SC injection self-administered as 50 mg QW or 25 mg BIW[6]	- Injection site reaction[6] - Headache, injection site bruising, URIs[1]	- PGA, BSA, physical exam, & assess for PsA q 3 months - Screen for latent TB with PPD (a positive test requires beginning TB treatment prior to starting therapy) - Screen for HBV status[6] - Labs: CBC, LFTs q 3 months ANA titers at baseline and periodically	- Severe hypersensitivity reaction[6] - Active infection including TB, HBV[6] - Moderate-severe CHF (NYHA Class III/IV)[8] - CNS demyelinating disorders (such as MS)[1] - Lupus[6] - Relative contraindications: pregnancy (category B), active cancer[1] - Live vaccines are contraindicated during therapy[6]

				Dosing	Side effects	Monitoring	Contraindications/warnings
Adalimumab	Humira[202]	Phase III trials[202]	October 2005	Fully human, recombinant monoclonal antibody against TNF-α[10]	40 mg SC injection self-administered QoW (+/– MTX)[10]	- Injection site reaction/ pain[10] - URI, headache, nausea[10] - Anti-adalimumab antibody formation[10]	- PGA, BSA, physical exam, & assess for PsA q 3 months - Test for latent TB with PPD (a positive screening test requires initiation of TB treatment prior to starting therapy)[10] - Screen for HBV status[10] - Labs: CBC, LFTs Q 3 months ANA titers at baseline and periodically	- Hypersensitivity reaction[10] - Active infection including TB, HBV[10] - Moderate-severe CHF (NYHA class III/IV)[8] - CNS demyelinating disorders[8] - lupus[10] - relative contraindications: active cancer, pregnancy (category B)[9] - Live vaccines are contraindicated during therapy[10]
Infliximab	Remicade[202]	September 2006	May 2005	Chimeric monoclonal antibody against TNF-α[12]	5 mg/kg IV infusion @ wks 0, 2, 6 → 5 mg/kg IV infusion q 8 wks[12]	5 mg/kg IV infusion @ wks 0, 2, 6 → 5 mg/kg IV infusion q 8 wks (+/– MTX)[12]	- Infusion reaction[12] - Serum sickness/delayed reaction[12] - Anti-infliximab antibody formation[12] - Elevation of aminotransferase levels[12] - Possibly increased risk for cancer[12]	- PGA, BSA, physical exam, & assess for PsA q 3 months - Test for latent TB with PPD and CXR (a positive PPD or CXR requires TB treatment prior to starting therapy)[12] - Screen for HBV status[12] - Labs: CBC, LFTs Q 3 months - ANA titers at baseline and periodically

(Infliximab contraindications column)
- Hypersensitivity reaction[12]
- Active infection including TB, HBV[12]
- Jaundice/LFT elevation >5× the upper limit of normal[12]
- Moderate-severe CHF (NYHA Class III/IV)[8]
- CNS demyelinating disorders[8]
- Lupus[12]
- Relative contraindications: active cancer, pregnancy (category B)[9]
- Exercise caution in COPD patients and young patients on immunosuppressive therapy[12]
- Live vaccines are contraindicated during therapy[12]

TABLE 28.3. Efficacy and safety of biologic therapies for the treatment of psoriasis and psoriatic arthritis: data from selected phase II and III clinical trials

Agent	Trial design, phase, & number (n) of subjects	Disease investigated	Investigators	Treatment regimen	Primary endpoint(s) of efficacy Note: 1 + asterisk (*) indicate the significant p value vs. placebo	Other endpoints of efficacy Note: 1 + asterisk (*) indicate the significant p value vs. placebo	Adverse events (AEs)	Additional points and notes regarding presented data
Alefacept	Phase 3 RCT 553	Chronic plaque-type psoriasis	Krueger GG, Papp KA, Stough DB, et al.[65]	Cohort 1:alefacept 7.5 mg IV injection QW × 12 wks→ 12 week follow-up → alefacept 7.5 mg IV injection QW × 12 wks	(Wk 14) Alefacept: PASI-75 = 14%* Placebo: PASI-75 = 4%	(Wk 14) alefacept: PGA (clear or almost clear)= 11%* Placebo: PGA (clear or almost clear) = 4%	- 1st 12 wks: chills in alefacept patients (10%) > placebo patients (1%), soon after treatment and decreasing in frequency with time - Last 12 wks: accidental injury in alefacept patients (20%) > placebo patients (15%)	After 1 course of alefacept, the median duration to relapse was >7 months After 2 courses of alefacept, less than ½ of patients relapsed after 1 year of follow-up
				Cohort 2: alefacept 7.5 mg IV injection QW × 12 wks→ 12 week follow-up → placebo QW × 12 wks	(p <.001)*	(p <.001)*	- CD4+ counts <250 cells/μL: 10% of alefacept patients after 1st 12 weeks of treatment; no relation to infections - Infections: mostly "common cold," no opportunistic infection	Patients receiving alefacept continued to improve during treatment and during the 12-week follow-up period No disease rebound after therapy
				Cohort 3: placebo QW × 12 wks→ 12 week follow-up → alefacept 7.5 mg IV injection QW × 12 wks		Note: After 2 courses of alefacept, PASI-75 = 40% in cohort 2	- Alanine aminotransferase (ALT) elevation (<3× upper limit of normal): 17% of alefacept patients vs. 8% of placebo patients during second course - ≤1% developed anti-alefacept antibodies - No allergy	

| Alefacept | Phase 3 RCT 507 | Chronic plaque-type psoriasis | Lebwohl M, Christophers E, Langley R, et al.[63] | Alefacept 15 mg IM injection or 10 mg IM injection QW × 12 wks vs. placebo → 12-week follow-up | (Wk 18) 15 mg alefacept: Mean Δ PASI = 46%[*]

10 mg alefacept: Mean Δ PASI = 41%[*]

Placebo: Mean Δ PASI = 25%
(p <.001)[*]

(Throughout the study period): 15 mg alefacept: PASI-75 = 33%[*]
10 mg alefacept: PASI-75 = 28%[*]
Placebo: PASI-75 = 13%
PGA (clear or almost clear) = 24%[*]
PGA (clear or almost clear) = 22%[*]
PGA (clear or almost clear) = 8%[*] | - AEs in alefacept groups > placebo group (by at least 5%): headache, pruritus, infection, rhinitis, injection site pain, mild injection site inflammation
- CD4+ counts <250 cells/μL: 5% of 15 mg alefacept patients, 3% of 10 mg alefacept patients; no relation to infections
- Infections: mostly "common cold," no opportunistic infection
- Cancer: 2 BCC (alefacept), 1 prostate cancer (placebo)
- Aspartate aminotransferase (AST) elevation (<3× upper limit of normal): 13% of 15 mg alefacept patients, 8% of 10 mg alefacept patients, 9% of placebo patients.
- 4% developed anti-alefacept antibodies
- No allergy | Patients receiving alefacept continued to improve after the 12-week dosing period
Nearly ¾ of patients in the 15 mg alefacept group did not relapse during the 12-week follow-up period
No disease rebound after therapy
Antibodies were not neutralizing |
| Alefacept | Phase 2 RCT 185 | Active PsA, despite MTX treatment for 3+ mos | Mease PJ, Gladman DD, Keystone EC[75] | MTX (10–25 mg/wk) + alefacept 15 mg IM injection vs. MTX + placebo QW × 12 wks → 12-week follow-up | Effects on psoriasis (n = 87): (wk 14) MTX + alefacept: PASI-50 = 53%[*]
MTX + placebo: PASI-50 = 17%
(p <.001)[*]

(Wk 24) MTX + alefacept: ACR-20 = 54%[*]
MTX + placebo: ACR-20 = 23%
(p <.001)[*] | - AEs in % alefacept similar to % placebo patients
- AEs in >5% of patients: ALT elevation, back pain, nasopharyngitis, URI, nausea
- CD4+ cell count reductions not related to infections | |

(continued)

TABLE 28.3. (continued)

Agent	Trial design, phase, & number (*n*) of subjects	Disease investigated	Investigators	Treatment regimen	Primary endpoint(s) of efficacy Note: 1 + asterisk (*) indicate the significant *p* value vs. placebo	Other endpoints of efficacy Note: 1 + asterisk (*) indicate the significant *p* value vs. placebo	Adverse events (AEs)	Additional points and notes regarding presented data
Efalizumab	Phase 3 RCT 556	Moderate-severe plaque-type psoriasis	Gordon KB, Papp KA, Hamilton TK, et al.[92]	Efalizumab 1 mg/kg SC injection QW × 12 wks vs. placebo	(Wk 12) efalizumab: PASI-75 = 27%* Placebo: PASI-75 = 4% (*p* <.001)*	(Wk 12) efalizumab: PGA (excellent or cleared) = 33%* DLQI = 47% improvement* Placebo: PGA (excellent or cleared) = 5% DLQI = 14% improvement (*p* <.001)*	- AEs in efalizumab > placebo patients (by at least 5%, *p* <.05): mild-moderate flu-like symptoms (headache, chills, myalgia, fever, pain) with 1st 1 to 2 injections - Infections: efalizumab > placebo patients (by >1%): viral URI, strep throat, bacterial skin infection, yeast infection; no opportunistic infections - Cancer: 1 BCC, 1 SCC - 2% developed anti-efalizumab antibodies - No allergy	Improvement in efalizumab vs. placebo patients by week 4 (*p* <.001)
Efalizumab	Phase 3 RCT 597	Moderate-severe plaque-type psoriasis	Lebwohl M, Tyring SK, Hamilton TK, et al.[88]	First treatment (wk 0– wk 12): efalizumab 2 mg/kg or 1 mg/kg SC injection QW vs. placebo Extended treatment (wks 13–24): subjects w/ at least a PASI-50 response: efalizumab 2 mg/kg QW or 2 mg/kg QoW vs. placebo	(Wk 12) 1 mg/kg efalizumab: PASI-75 = 22%* 2 mg/kg efalizumab: PASI-75 = 28%* Placebo: PASI-75 = 5%	(Follow-up): 2/3 of patients relapsed Time to relapse = 84 days with a "gradual loss of benefit"	- AEs in efalizumab > placebo patients (by at lease 1%, *p* <.05): flu-like symptoms (mild-moderate headache, chills, pain, fever, back pain), with 1st 1 to 2 injections - Transient elevation in WBC, absolute lymphocytes, eosinophils - 5% developed anti-efalizumab antibodies	

Drug	Study	Disease	Methods	Results		Adverse events	Comments
			Subjects with less than a PASI-50 response: efalizumab 4 mg/kg QW vs. placebo Follow-up (wks 25–36): observation × 12 wks	$(p <.001)^*$ (Wk 24): 2 mg/kg QW efalizumab: maintenance of wk 12 PASI-75 = 77%* 2 mg/kg QoW efalizumab: maintenance of wk 12 PASI-75 = 78%* Placebo: maintenance of wk 12 PASI-75 = 20% $(p <.001)^*$		- Steady low rate of infections, no increase in AEs, slowed rate of acute AEs	
Efalizumab	Phase 3 RCT (556)→ Open-label study (516)	Moderate-severe plaque-type psoriasis	RCT (wks 0–12) efalizumab 0.7 mg/kg SC conditioning dose × 1 then 1 mg/kg SC injection QW × 11 wks vs. placebo → Open-label study (wks 13–24) efalizumab 1 mg/kg SC injection QW × 12 wks	(Wk 12) efalizumab: PASI-75 = 26.6%* Placebo: PASI-75 = 4.3% $(p <.001)^*$ (Wk 24) all efalizumab patients: PASI-75 = 43.8%	(Wk 24) continuous efalizumab patients: sPGA (minimal or clear) = 35.9% DLQI = 49.2% improved from baseline Pruritus = 42.2% improved from baseline	- Wks 0–12: AEs in efalizumab > placebo patients (by at least 5%): flu-like symptoms (headache, chills, fever, myalgia, pain), with 1st 1 to 2 injections, within 48 hours - Wks 13–24: AEs in >5% of patients: arthritis (5.6%), headache (6.1%), nonspecific infection (11.1%) - No increase in infection, SAEs, or AEs leading to withdrawal	Improvement in mean PASI response in efalizumab vs. placebo patients by week 2 $(p <.001)$ Menter A, Gordon K, Carey W, et al.[89]
Efalizumab	Phase 3 RCT → +/– extended therapy 498	Moderate-severe plaque-type psoriasis	Efalizumab 0.7 mg/kg SC conditioning dose × 1 then 1 mg/kg or 2 mg/kg SC injection QW × 11 wks vs. placebo→	(Wk 12) 1 mg/kg efalizumab: PASI-75 = 39%* 2 mg/kg efalizumab: PASI-75 = 27%* Placebo: PASI-75 = 2%	(Wk 12) 1 mg/kg efalizumab: PGA (excellent or clear) = 38.9%* 2 mg/kg efalizumab: PGA (excellent or clear) = 30.1 %* Placebo: PGA (excellent or clear) = 4.1%	- AEs in efalizumab > placebo patients (by at least 1%): mild-moderate flu-like symptoms (headache, chills, myalgia, fever, nausea), with 1st 1 to 2 injections - Reversible thrombocytopenia (1 efalizumab patient) - Transient increase in WBC, RBC, lymphocyte counts	Antibodies were not neutralizing Leonardi CL, Papp KA, Gordon KB, et al.[90]

(continued)

TABLE 28.3. (continued)

Agent	Trial design, phase, & number (n) of subjects	Disease investigated	Investigators	Treatment regimen	Primary endpoint(s) of efficacy Note: 1 + asterisk (*) indicate the significant p value vs. placebo	Other endpoints of efficacy Note: 1 + asterisk (*) indicate the significant p value vs. placebo	Adverse events (AEs)	Additional points and notes regarding presented data
				Extended treatment If <PASI-75 response at wk 12, re-randomized to efalizumab 1 mg/kg or efalizumab 2 mg/kg vs. placebo SC injection QW × 12 wks & placebo patients from the 1st 12 wks transitioned to efalizumab QW × 12 wks	(p <.001)*	(p <.001)* (Wk 24) re-randomized efalizumab patients: PASI-75 = 20.3%** PGA (excellent or clear) = 29.3%*** Placebo patients PASI-75 = 6.7% PGA (excellent or clear) = 10% (p = .018)** (p = .005)***	- 4% of patients developed anti-efalizumab antibodies - No increase in adverse events over 24 weeks	
Efalizumab	Phase 3 RCT 793 Clear	Moderate-severe plaque-type psoriasis	Dubertret L, Sterry W, Bos JD, et al.[83]	Efalizumab 0.7 mg/kg SC conditioning dose ×1 then 1 mg/kg SC injection QW × 11 wks vs. placebo	(Wk 12) efalizumab: PASI-75 = 31.4%* Placebo: PASI-75 = 4.2% (p <.0001)*	Efalizumab patients demonstrated significant changes in sPGA* (minimal or clear) & reduction in affected BSA (p <.001)*	- Acute AEs in efalizumab (40.1%) > placebo (22.3%) patients: flu-like symptoms (mild-moderate headache, chills, fever, nausea/vomiting, myalgia, diarrhea), within 1 to 2 days of injection	Data include 526 "high-need" patients, who could not use 2 or more systemic psoriasis therapies because of a contraindication, intolerance, or resistance "High-need" patients @ wk 12: 1. Effects on psoriasis: -Efalizumab: PASI-75 = 29.5%*

Drug	Design	Condition	Intervention	Efficacy	Results/Notes
					- Placebo: PASI-75 = 2.7% ($p < .001$)* 2. Quality of life assessment: -Efalizumab patients significantly improved vs. placebo as measured by DLQI, SF-36, itching VAS[202]	- Psoriasis events (including erythroderma) in efalizumab (5.7%) > placebo (3.6%) patients - Transient increase in WBC & total lymphocyte counts - SAEs of "musculoskeletal events" (psoriatic arthropathy, arthralgia, arthritis, back pain, joint swelling, stiffness, or neck pain) lead to study termination in 12 efalizumab patients (vs. 0 placebo patients) - No opportunistic infection, no TB
Etanercept	Phase 3 RCT 652	Moderate-severe plaque-type psoriasis	Wks 0–12 High-dose etanercept (50 mg BIW) or medium-dose etanercept (25 mg BIW) or low-dose etanercept (25 mg QW) SC injection vs. placebo × 12 wks→ Wks 13–24 continued etanercept dose × 12 wks & placebo group transitioned to medium dose etanercept	(Wk 12) High dose: PASI-75 = 49%* Medium dose: PASI-75= 34%* Low dose: PASI-75 = 14%* Placebo: PASI-75 = 4% ($p < .001$)* (Wk 24)- See Note 1 high dose: PASI-75 = 59% Medium dose: PASI-75 = 44% Low dose: PASI-75 = 25% (Wk 12) PGA (clear or almost clear) -High dose = 49%*	Note 1: Sustained/improved efficacy with continued therapy Statistically significant improvement in mean PASI response in etanercept vs. placebo by 2 weeks Data from a subsequent extension study demonstrated: -No rebound - 3 months median time to relapse - Response to original dose of etanercept therapy was maintained upon readministration after relapse (83% of patients with a PASI-50	- AEs in >5% of patients (% etanercept similar to % placebo): URI, headache, injection site bruising, accidental injury - Mild-moderate ISRs in % etanercept > % placebo patients - No opportunistic infections, no TB - No neutralizing antibodies

(continued)

TABLE 28.3. (continued)

Agent	Trial design, phase, & number (n) of subjects	Disease investigated	Investigators	Treatment regimen	Primary endpoint(s) of efficacy Note: 1 + asterisk (*) indicate the significant p value vs. placebo	Other endpoints of efficacy Note: 1 + asterisk (*) indicate the significant p value vs. placebo	Adverse events (AEs)	Additional points and notes regarding presented data
						- Medium dose = 34%* - Low dose = 23%* - Placebo = 5% DLQI in all etanercept groups improved by wk 2* Patient Global Assessment in all etanercept groups improved by wk 2* (p <.001)*		response at wk 12 of treatment achieved a PASI-50 response at wk 12 of re-treatment[202]
Etanercept	Phase 3 RCT → extended therapy 583	Moderate-severe plaque-type psoriasis	Papp KA, Tyring S, Lahfa M, et al.[104]	RCT etanercept 25 mg SC injection or 50mg SC injection BIW × 12 wks vs. placebo→ Extended therapy etanercept 25 mg SC injection BIW × 12 wks	(Wk 12) Etanercept 50mg BIW: PASI-75 = 49%* Etanercept 25 mg BIW: PASI-75= 34%* Placebo: PASI-75= 3% (p <.0001)*	(Wk 24) Original 50mg BIW cohort: PASI-75 = 54% Original 25 mg BIW cohort: PASI-75 = 45% Original placebo cohort PASI-75 = 28% (Wk 12) Etanercept 50 mg BIW: sPGA (clear or almost clear) = 57%* Etanercept 25 mg BIW: sPGA (clear or almost clear) = 39%* Placebo: sPGA (clear or almost clear) = 4% (p <.0001)*	- AEs in at least 5% of any treatment group (% etanercept similar to % placebo): URI, headache, injection site bruise, accidental injury, flu-like symptoms - Mild-moderate ISRs in etanercept 50 BIW (18%) > etanercept 25 BIW (13%) > placebo (6%) - No neutralizing antibodies	Significant improvement in mean PASI response in both etanercept cohorts vs. placebo by 2 weeks (p <.0001) 97% of patients who reached PASI-75 maintained at least PASI-50 response at 24 wks No loss of efficacy by wk 24 with dose reduction @ wk 12

| Etanercept | Phase 3 RCT 618 | Moderate-severe plaque-type psoriasis | Tyring S, Gottlieb A, Papp K, et al.[107] | Etanercept 50 mg SC injection BIW × 12 wks vs. placebo | (Wk 12) Etanercept: PASI-75 = 47%* Placebo: PASI-7 5 = 5% ($p <.0001$)* | (Wk 12) Patients on etanercept demonstrated improvement in depression (at least 50% improvement in Ham-D or BDI) * (see Note 1) & improvement in fatigue (FACIT-F score)* (see Notes 1 and 2)* ($p <.0001$)* | - AEs in >3% of either group (% etanercept similar to% placebo): headache, injection site bruising, fatigue, arthralgia, URI | Note 1: These data reinforce the role TNF-α has in producing depression and fatigue in psoriasis patients and the importance of TNF blockade for improving quality of life Note 2: Improvements in fatigue correlated with improvements in joint pain |
| Etanercept | Phase 3 RCT (N=205) → open-label extension study 186 | Active PsA | Mease PJ, Kivitz AJ, Burch FX, et al.[124] | RCT etanercept 25 mg SC injection BIW × 24 wks vs. placebo Open-label extension study etanercept 25 mg SC injection BIW × 48 wks | (Wk 12) Etanercept: ACR-20 = 59%* Placebo: ACR-20 = 15% ($p <.0001$)* | (12 months) Radiographic progression (rate of change in Sharp score): -Etanercept patients = -0.03 unit* - Placebo patients = +1.00 unit ($p = .0001$)* | - AEs in >5% of either group (% etanercept similar to % placebo): URI, injection site bruising, accidental injury, headache, sinusitis, rash, UTI - ISRs in etanercept (36%) > placebo (9%) patients (p <.001) - No neutralizing antibodies | Allowed concomitant medications: stable doses of MTX (25 mg/wk or less), prednisone (10 mg/day or less), and/or NSAIDs Data from a subsequent extension study that followed 141 patients receiving up to 2 years of etanercept therapy (25 mg SC BIW) revealed[202]: radiographic progression (rate of change in Sharp score) remained inhibited at 2 years |

(continued)

TABLE 28.3. (continued)

Agent	Disease investigated	Investigators	Treatment regimen	Primary endpoint(s) of efficacy Note: 1 + asterisk (*) indicate the significant p value vs. placebo	Other endpoints of efficacy Note: 1 + asterisk (*) indicate the significant p value vs. placebo	Adverse events (AEs)	Additional points and notes regarding presented data
					(Wk 24) Disability: etanercept patients demonstrated improvement from baseline in HAQ scores[**] - Effects on psoriasis (n = 128 for PASI-75 assessment): -Etanercept: PASI-75 = 23%[***] sPGA (clear or almost clear) = 47%[**] - Placebo: PASI-75 = 3% sPGA (clear or almost clear) = 11% (p <.001)[**] (p = .001)[***]	- No increase in AEs in extension study - 1 case of MS (etanercept)	
Etanercept	Active PsA (and psoriasis)	Mease PJ, Goffe BS, Metz J, et al.[108]	Etanercept 25 mg SC injection BIW × 12 wks vs. placebo	(Wk 12) Effects on joint disease: - Etanercept: PsARC = 87%[*] - Placebo: PsARC = 23% (p <.0001)[*] Effects on psoriasis: (n = 38) - Etanercept: PASI-75 = 26%[**] - Placebo: PASI-75 = 0 (p = .015)[**]	(Wk 12) Etanercept: ACR-20 = 73%[*] Placebo: ACR-20 = 13% (p <.0001)[*]	- Most common AEs (% etanercept similar to % placebo): ISR, URI, injection site bruise, headache - Flu-like symptoms in % etanercept > % placebo patients (p = .0237)	Allowed concomitant medications: stable doses of MTX (25 mg /wk), prednisone (10 mg/day), and/ or NSAIDs

Drug	Study	Condition	Authors	Intervention	Results (PASI-75)	Results (PGA)	Adverse Events	Conclusions
Infliximab	Phase 2 RCT → +/– re-treatment 249 "SPIRIT"	Severe plaque-type psoriasis; patients were previously treated with PUVA or other systemic therapy	Gottlieb AB, Evans R, Li S, et al.[111]	Induction infliximab 3 mg/kg or 5 mg/kg IV infusion @ wks 0, 2, 6 vs. placebo → follow-up for 20 wks Re-treatment infliximab IV infusion × 1 @ wk 26 if PGA = moderate or severe	(Wk 10) 3 mg/kg infliximab: PASI-75 = 72%* 5 mg/kg infliximab: PASI-75 = 88%* Placebo: PASI-7 5 = 6% (p <.001)*	(Wk 10) 3 mg/kg infliximab: PGA (minimal or cleared) = 71.7%* 5 mg/kg infliximab: PGA (minimal or cleared) = 89.9%* Placebo: PGA (minimal or cleared) = 9.8% (p <.001)*	- AEs in infliximab 5 mg/kg (79%) > 3 mg/kg (78%) > placebo (63%) - IRs: 3 mg/kg = 18% 5 mg/kg = 22% (2 were severe) Placebo = 2% - Antibody formation: 3 mg/kg = 27% 5 mg/kg = 20% - Aminotransferase elevations (of more than 25% from baseline): ALT:infliximab = 34%, placebo = 16% AST: infliximab = 24%, placebo = 14% - Anti-dsDNA antibody formation: infliximab = 3.8%, placebo = 2.1% (no lupus-like or drug-induced lupus syndromes)	Significant improvement in PASI scores by 2 week Response to treatment decreased after wk 10 assessment in infliximab 3 mg/kg group and after wk 14 assessment in infliximab 5 mg/kg group
Infliximab	Phase 3 RCT → extended therapy 378 "EXPRESS"	Moderate-severe plaque-type psoriasis	Reich K, Nestle FO, Papp K, et al.[112]	Induction infliximab 5 mg/kg IV infusion @ wks 0, 2, & 6 vs. placebo → Maintenance -wks 12–24: infliximab 5 mg/kg IV infusion q 8 wks vs. placebo - wks 24– 46: infliximab 5 mg/kg IV infusion q 8 wks with placebo crossover to induction and maintenance infusions	(Wk 10→ wk 24→ wk 50) See Note 1 infliximab: PASI-75 = 80%* → 82%* → 61% Placebo: PASI-75 = 3% → 4% (p <.0001)*	(Wk 10→ wk 24→ wk 50) See Note 1 infliximab: PGA (minimal or cleared) = 83%* → 74%* → 53% Placebo: PGA (minimal or cleared) = 4% → 3%	- AEs (including SAEs) in infliximab (82%) > placebo (71%) patients - Overall, infection and IRs in % infliximab similar to % placebo - No TB, opportunistic infection, demyelinating disease, new-onset CHF, or hematologic events	Significant PASI-75 response by 3rd infusion Note 1: Decreased efficacy of infliximab treatment over trial duration was associated with decreased drug levels and increased prevalence of human antichimeric antibodies

(continued)

TABLE 28.3. (continued)

Agent	Trial design, phase, & number (n) of subjects	Disease investigated	Investigators	Treatment regimen	Primary endpoint(s) of efficacy Note: 1 + asterisk (*) indicate the significant p value vs. placebo	Other endpoints of efficacy Note: 1 + asterisk (*) indicate the significant p value vs. placebo	Adverse events (AEs)	Additional points and notes regarding presented data
						(p <.0001)* Effects on nail psoriasis: improvement in NAPSI score in infliximab group at wk 10* & wk 24, with continued improvement through wk 50 (p <.0001)*	Infliximab group: -Serious IRs (4) - Delayed hypersensitivity reactions (3) - + Anti-dsDNA with lupus-like reaction and arthralgia (2) - 27% of patients developed human antichimeric antibodies - 6% elevated AST & 2% elevated ALT in infliximab vs. 0 placebo patients	
Infliximab	Phase 3 RCT → extended therapy 835 "EXPRESS II"	Moderate-severe plaque-type psoriasis	Menter A, Feldman SR, Weinstein GD, et al.[113]	Induction infliximab 3 mg/kg or 5 mg/kg IV infusion @ wks 0, 2, 6 vs. placebo→ Maintenance -wk 14: infliximab q 8 wk or PRN IV infusion therapy -wk 16–50: placebo cross-over to infliximab induction and maintenance infusions	(Wk 10) 3 mg/kg infliximab: PASI-75 = 70.3%* 5 mg/kg infliximab: PASI-75 = 75.5%* Placebo: PASI-75 = 2% (p <.001)*	(Wk 10) 3 mg/kg infliximab: PGA (clear or excellent) = 69.8%* 5 mg/kg infliximab: PGA (clear or excellent) = 76%* Placebo: PGA (clear or excellent) = 1%	- AEs in infliximab 5 mg/kg > 3 mg/kg - IRs: 1. 3 mg/kg > 5 mg/kg > placebo 2. Intermittent > continuous therapy 3. Increased over time 4. Highest in Ab-positive patients - Anti-infliximab antibody formation (see Note 3): 5 mg/kg maintenance = 35.8%	Note 1: Decreased efficacy of infliximab treatment over trial duration Note 2: q 8 wk dosing vs. PRN dosing achieved a higher % of PASI-75 responses Note 3: Antibody formation may be lowest in the patients with the most consistent exposure to infliximab Antibody formation imparted an increased risk of failure to maintain PASI-75 response and of experienc-

Drug	Study/Design	Population	Reference	Intervention	Results	Notes/Adverse Events
					5 mg/kg PRN = 41.5% 3 mg/kg maintenance = 51.5% 3 mg/kg PRN = 46.2% (p <.001)* (Wk 50) See Notes 1 and 2 3 mg/kg infliximab (continuous): PASI-75 = 43.8% 3 mg/kg infliximab (intermittent PRN): PASI-75 = 25.4% 5 mg/kg infliximab (continuous): PASI-75 = 54.5% 5 mg/kg infliximab (intermittent PRN): PASI-75 = 38.1%	Infliximab groups: -TB (2) - Cancer (12– mainly NMSC) - Reversible marked elevations in AST (3.1%) or ALT (4.9%) - Lupus-like syndromes (2)- 1 with pulmonary disease & 1 with CNS vasculitis - Serious IRs (5) - Serious delayed hypersensitivity reactions (4)
Infliximab	Phase 3 RCT → extended therapy 104 "IMPACT I"	Active PsA, unresponsive to 1 or more DMARD(s)	Antoni CE, Kavanaugh A, Kirkham B, et al.[26]	RCT infliximab 5 mg/kg IV infusion @ wks 0, 2, 6, 14 vs. placebo Wk 16–50 infliximab 5 mg/kg IV infusion q 8 wks with placebo cross-over to infliximab induction and maintenance infusions	(Wk 16) Infliximab: ACR-20 = 65%* Placebo: ACR-20 = 10% (p <.001)* Effects on psoriasis (n = 39): infliximab group: PASI-75 = 68%* (Wk 16) Infliximab patients demonstrated clinically significant improvements in enthesitis & dactylitis Disability: - Infliximab: DAS28 improvement (mean) = 45.5%* - Placebo: DAS28 improvement (mean) = 2.8%	- AEs in % infliximab similar to % placebo - No opportunistic infections, TB, autoimmune disease, demyelinating disease, or hematologic abnormalities Allowed concomitant medications: stable doses of NSAID, prednisone (<10mg/day), and/or DMARD [MTX (>15mg/kg), leflunomide, sulfasalazine, hydroxychloroquine, IM gold, penicillamine, or azathioprine] Topical agents allowed for psoriasis Significant improvement in ACR response in infliximab vs. placebo patients by 2 weeks

(continued)

TABLE 28.3. (continued)

Agent	Trial design, phase, & number (n) of subjects	Disease investigated	Investigators	Treatment regimen	Primary endpoint(s) of efficacy Note: 1 + asterisk (*) indicate the significant p value vs. placebo	Other endpoints of efficacy Note: 1 + asterisk (*) indicate the significant p value vs. placebo	Adverse events (AEs)	Additional points and notes regarding presented data
					Placebo group: PASI-75 = 0% (p <.001)*	(p <.001)* [Wk 50] In continuous infliximab cohort, ACR-20 = 69.4%		A 1-year follow-up showed that infliximab inhibited radiographic progression of joint disease on hand and foot films[202]
Infliximab	Phase 3 RCT 200 "IMPACT II"	Active PsA. unresponsive to DMARD(s) or NSAID(s)	Antoni C. Krueger GG, de Vlam K, et al.[27]	Infliximab 5 mg/kg IV infusion @ wks 0, 2, 6, 14 and 22 vs. placebo	(Wk 14 → wk 24) infliximab: ACR-20 = 58%* → 54%* Placebo: ACR-20 = 11% → 16% (p <.001)*	Effects on psoriasis (wk 14 → wk 24): (n = 70) infliximab: PASI-75 = 64%* → 60%* Placebo: PASI-75 = 2% → 1% (p <.001)* (Wk 14 & wk 24) Infliximab patients demonstrate significant improvements in dactylitis, enthesopathy & quality of life (SF-36 physical and mental components & HAQ score)	- AEs in % infliximab similar to % placebo - No opportunistic infections, TB, new-onset CHF, new autoimmune disease, demyelinating disease, hematologic abnormalities, anaphylaxis, serious IRs, or delayed hypersensitivity reactions Infliximab group: -Reversible marked elevations in aminotransferase levels in 5 patients (vs. 0 of placebo). -4.5% of patients developed human anti-chimeric Abs -9.9% of patients became ANA + (vs. 2.6% of placebo) -3 patients became anti-dsDNA Ab + (vs. 0 placebo)	Allowed concomitant medications: stable doses of NSAID, prednisone (10mg/day), and/or MTX (25 mg/kg weekly) Significant improvement in skin and joint assessments by 2 weeks

Drug	Study	Patients	Intervention	Results	Adverse Events	Notes
Adali-mumab	Phase 3 RCT 315 "ADEPT"	Active PsA, patients with inadequate response to NSAID(s)	Adalimumab 40 mg SC injection QoW × 24 wks vs. placebo	(Wk 12) adalimumab: ACR-20 = 58%* Placebo: ACR-20 = 14% (Wk 24) adalimumab: Δ Sharp score = −0.2* Placebo: Δ Sharp score = 1.0 (p <.001)*	- Most common AEs (% adalimumab similar to % placebo): URIs, ISRs, headache, HTN, arthropathy - (Transient) ALT elevations in adalimumab > placebo	Allowed concomitant medications: stable doses of MTX (<30 mg), and/or prednisone (10 mg/ day max) Significant ACR-20 responses in adalimumab vs. placebo by 2 weeks, maintained through wk 24 Significant PASI-75 responses in adalimumab vs. placebo by 4 weeks, peaking at wk 16 A subsequent open-label extension study ("ADEPT II") followed patients for up to 48 weeks on adalimumab treatment and demonstrated maintenance of joint and skin responses[202]
	Mease PJ, Gladman DD, Ritchlin CT, et al.[140]			(Wk 24) Effects on psoriasis (n = 138–140) adalimumab: PASI-75 = 59%* PGA (clear or almost clear) = 67%* Placebo: PASI-75 = 1% PGA (clear or almost clear) = 10% Quality of life: adalimumab patients experienced improvement @ wk 12 (HAQ DI & SF-36 PCS) & wk 24 (HAQ DI, SF-36, DLQI & FACIT-F)* (p <.001)*		
Adalimumab	Phase 2	Moderate-severe plaque-type psoriasis	RCT (wks 0–12) low-dose adalimumab (80 mg × 1 wk → 40 mg QoW SC × 11 wks) or high-dose adalimumab (80 mg × 2 wks→ 40 mg QW SC × 10 wks) vs. placebo	(Wk 12* → wk 24 → wk 36 → wk 60) (Wk 12→ wk 60)	- Most common AEs (% adalimumab similar to % placebo): nasopharyngitis, URI	Significant PASI-75 responses in adalimumab vs. placebo by wk 4
	Gordon KB, Langley RG, Leonardi C, et al.[141]					

(continued)

TABLE 28.3. (continued)

Agent	Disease investigated	Investigators	Trial design, phase, & number (n) of subjects	Treatment regimen	Primary endpoint(s) of efficacy Note: 1 + asterisk (*) indicate the significant p value vs. placebo	Other endpoints of efficacy Note: 1 + asterisk (*) indicate the significant p value vs. placebo	Adverse events (AEs)	Additional points and notes regarding presented data
			RCT → placebo cross-over → extension study 147	Placebo cross-over (wks 13–24) adalimumab dose continued with placebo cross-over to low dose adalimumab Extension study (wks 25–60) adalimumab dose continued with "dose escalation" available if patients achieved <PASI-50 response at QoW dosing	See Note 1 Low-dose adalimumab: PASI-75 = 53%* → 64% → 62% → 56% High-dose adalimumab: PASI-75 = 80%* → 72% → 68% → 64% Placebo/40mg QoW: PASI-75 = 4% → 55% → 57% → 45% (p <.001)*	See Note 1 Low-dose adalimumab: PGA (clear or almost clear) = 49% → 44% High-dose adalimumab: PGA (clear or almost clear) = 76% → 52%	- AEs in adalimumab > placebo: dyspepsia, nausea, mildly elevated triglycerides - Mild-moderate, transient pain with injection: high dose > low dose > placebo - No lupus or demyelinating diseases - Cancer: MM (1), SCC (1) - Infection: TB (1), coccidioidomycosis (1) - Transient elevations of LFTs to 3–3.5 × normal, returning to normal upon discontinuation of adalimumab (2)	Note 1: Decreased efficacy of adalimumab treatment sometime between wk 12 & wk 60

affected.[78] Thus, as opposed to other agents that target co-stimulation including alefacept, efalizumab does not deplete T cells in the blood.[32,77]

When scientists first explored the agent's effects on psoriatic pathology, they discovered that one dose of IV efalizumab could completely block CD11a in the blood and skin, and it effected changes in psoriasis plaques including decreases in skin thickness, reduced T-cell numbers, and down-regulation of ICAM-1 on keratinocytes and blood vessels.[23] Similar improvements were achieved from multiple doses of IV efalizumab.[79] The agent displayed a dose-response effect in which increasing doses had greater ability to block and downregulate CD11a. These pharmacodynamic effects correlated with both clinical and histologic responses. In addition, investigators observed a notable decrease in the expression of K16, a protein expressed by keratinocytes in response to damage/inflammation that indicates disordered skin cell differentiation and hyperplasia. In a separate study, a 12-week course of subcutaneous (SC) efalizumab decreased the expression of CD11a in addition to other co-stimulatory molecules on circulating T cells including LFA-1 (both CD11a and CD18 subunits) and B7.[78] Scientists have since discovered that improvements in skin disease following efalizumab therapy also correlated with decreased numbers of activated inflammatory DCs (i.e., DCs expressing CD83+ and CD11c+ surface markers),[22,80] in addition to decreased expression of messenger RNA (mRNA) for iNOS in the skin.[80] Inducible NOS is an enzyme that is expressed from DCs and produces the molecule nitric oxide (NO) to mediate cell damage and small blood vessel dilation.[19] Thus, in psoriasis, iNOS results in abnormal differentiation of skin cells, lesion erythema, and inflammation.[19,35]

Among the biologics, efalizumab is frequently used for treating patients in whom TNF blockade is contraindicated[38] (see Table 28.2). Efalizumab is administered by weight as an SC injection.[76] Administration starts with a conditioning dose of 0.7 mg/kg to allay the flu-like symptoms that patients could experience in the first 1 to 2 days after receiving the initial few treatments.[81] Treatment continues as weekly SC self-injections of 1 mg/kg,[76] which is the maintenance dose that most effectively blocked and downregulated CD11a molecules in clinical studies. During conditioning and mainte-nance, the maximum amount of efalizumab that should be administered in one dose is 200 mg.[76] In phase III clinical trials, 12 weeks of efalizumab therapy at 1 mg/kg/wk resulted in a PASI-75 (75% improvement in PASI score) response in 22% to 39% of patients (see Table 28.3). A retrospective analysis of phase III trials noted that the efficacy and safety of efalizumab were similar in patients who weighed more than 100 kg as compared with leaner patients.[82] Efalizumab can also benefit high-need patients who cannot be on an alternate systemic therapy.[83,84] In a phase III trial of efalizumab for the treatment of psoriasis, 526 of 793 patients were high-need patients who had either failed or had a contraindication or intolerance to two or more systemic therapies. After 12 weeks of efalizumab therapy, these patients experienced significant improvements in skin disease[83] and in quality of life measures.[84]

Efalizumab is a continuous therapy.[85] An open-label trial investigated the use of efalizumab in patients on continuous therapy for up to 36 months.[86] The agent maintained efficacy after 3 years, and some patients continued to improve over time.[87] Whereas at 3 months of treatment a PASI-75 response was achieved in 41% of all patients (n = 339), at 27 months of treatment a PASI-75 response was achieved in 56% of patients who continued to receive maintenance therapy (n = 290).[86] In this study and in other phase III trials, continuation of therapy was well tolerated without new adverse events or an increase in the number of adverse events.[88–90] In the event that patients are discontinued from therapy, they can be re-treated because the agent is not associated with tachyphylaxis.[91] Patients who completed various clinical trials and were without the agent for 1 month or longer were retreated with efalizumab and still experienced a good clinical response.

In phase III trials, the most common adverse event associated with the use of efalizumab was a flu-like syndrome (see Table 28.3). Other adverse events of concern were worsening of psoriasis and reversible changes in CBC values including transient thrombocytopenia and reversible increases in white blood count (WBC), red blood count (RBC), and lymphocyte counts (see Table 28.3). Flu-like symptoms included headache, chills, fever, nausea and vomiting, and myalgia.[83,88–90,92] Because platelet counts decreased with treatment in some patients treated with efalizumab,[76,93] a baseline blood count is performed, and platelet counts are monitored monthly at first and then about every 3 months during maintenance therapy[76] (see Table 28.2). The thrombocytopenia associated with treatment likely has an immune-mediated pathogenesis.[93] There can be psoriasis-adverse events, or a worsening of skin disease during therapy.[85] There can also be worsening of skin disease after discontinuing treatment.

An analysis of several clinical trials found that 3.2% of patients experienced an "event" during therapy (vs. 1.4% of placebo-treated patients), where an event was either a localized mild breakthrough of psoriasis papules in areas not covered by psoriasis plaques or a generalized inflammatory flare (GIF) of skin disease.[85] The same analysis found that after discontinuing treatment, up to 86% of patients experienced relapse (i.e., lost ≥50% of the improvement in PASI score achieved during treatment) in a median time period of just over 2 months. Additionally, 14% of patients experienced disease rebound (i.e., developed erythrodermic psoriasis, inflammatory psoriasis, generalized pustular psoriasis, or disease worsening such that the PASI score was ≥125% of the baseline PASI score within 3 months of discontinuing therapy). The majority of patients experiencing GIF or rebound were nonresponders, that is, they did not achieve a meaningful improvement in their psoriasis during efalizumab therapy. Thus, providers may choose to switch patients to a different therapy to treat psoriasis if no response is noted after about 3 months of efalizumab treatment. The exact mechanism for disease worsening is unknown, but a flare does not appear to be caused by an allergic hypersensitivity reaction or neutralizing antibodies.[94]

The use of efalizumab to treat psoriasis in patients with PsA is controversial. In a phase II clinical trial investigating the use of efalizumab for the treatment of PsA in which all subjects were on a concomitant systemic therapy, efalizumab failed to enact a significant 20% improvement in the American College of Rheumatology score of inflammatory arthritis response (ACR-20) when compared with placebo.[95] However, the study may not have been sufficiently powered to detect a meaningful difference between these groups.[95] Of note, when compared with placebo patients, patients treated with efalizumab did not experience more flares of PsA or psoriasis either during therapy or after withdrawal of treatment.

A pooled analysis of safety data from phase II, III, and IV studies of efalizumab found no significant increase in arthropathy (i.e., arthritis and joint pain) associated with efalizumab therapy versus placebo administration during initial dosing or extended treatment for up to 3 years.[96] A different analysis of phase III trials and their extension studies included data from more than 3000 patients and also reached the conclusion that arthropathy adverse events were not more common in patients treated with efalizumab versus placebo.[97] Arthropathy was most common in patients who had a history of joint disease and in patients whose skin disease did not improve on efalizumab therapy. However, there are cases in which new-onset PsA occurred during treatment with efalizumab.[97a] In general, caution should be exercised when administering efalizumab for the treatment of psoriasis in patients with joint disease.[76] Periodic questioning regarding joint symptoms and a careful joint exam are necessary during therapy, and the agent is a relative contraindication especially in patients who have more severe PsA.

Cytokine Antagonists

In a normal immune response, at the immunologic synapse in lymphoid tissue,[32] DCs present T cells with antigen that the APCs detected during their innate immune function of immune surveillance.[98] Antigen presentation then activates adaptive immunity. Thus, DCs bridge a gap between the innate and the adaptive immune systems. Accordingly, in psoriasis and PsA, DCs in the lymphoid tissue and the target organs (i.e., skin and joints) may link adaptive immunity as targeted by the cell adhesion molecule antagonists alefacept and efalizumab and innate immunity as targeted by cytokine antagonists.[32] Cytokine antagonists aim to neutralize or reduce production of inflammatory cytokines in part by targeting the mature DC. Cytokine antagonists approved by the FDA for the treatment of psoriasis or PsA target TNF-α, and those in advanced stages of drug development target the p40 subunit of the cytokines IL-12 and IL-23.

Tumor Necrosis Factor Blockade

Tumor necrosis factor-α is the proinflammatory cytokine that contributes to multiple disease states such as septic shock[99] and inflammatory disorders such as psoriasis, PsA, RA, ankylosing spondylitis (AS), and inflammatory bowel disease (IBD), including Crohn's disease (CD) and ulcerative colitis (UC).[100] Tumor necrosis factor-α is released by immune cells including activated T cells[100] as well as stimulated keratinocytes.[101] It binds to either its p55 or p75 receptor.[32] It then acts through nuclear transcription factor κB (NF-κB)[100] to promote the expression of inflammatory mediators including IL-1, IL-8, IL-6,[32,100] and iNOS[32] as well as to upregulate adhesion molecules on inflammatory cells.[32] TNF-α,[20] NF-κB,[102] and the inflammatory mediators named above are all upregulated in lesions of psoriasis.[32,100] Similarly, TNF-α and NF-κB have been detected in the joints of patients with PsA.[103] The ability of TNF-blocking agents to enact significant and sustainable clinical improvement in patients with psoriasis and PsA reinforces the fact that TNF-α is a main orchestrater of the immunopathogeneses of these disease states.[25–27,104–114] Two TNF-blocking agents are approved by the FDA and the European Medicines Agency (EMEA) for the treatment of psoriasis and PsA, including the fusion protein etanercept (Enbrel®, Amgen and Wyeth Pharmaceuticals, Immunex Corp., Thousand Oaks, CA),[115] and the chimeric monoclonal antibody infliximab (Remicade®, Centocor, Inc., Malvern, PA).[116] In addition, the human monoclonal antibody adalimumab (Humira®, Abbott Laboratories, North Chicago, IL) is approved to treat PsA.[117] A novel anti-TNF agent, certolizumab pegol (Cimzia™, UCB, Brussels, Belgium) is in development.[118] Certolizumab is the PEGylated Fab' fragment of a humanized monoclonal antibody directed against TNF-α. In a phase II clinical trial, investigators administered certolizumab SC as a loading dose of 400mg followed by either 200- or 400-mg maintenance doses every other week (QoW) for 12 weeks. At 12 weeks, a PASI-75 response was achieved by 74.6% of patients in the 200mg QoW treatment group and 82.8% of patients in the 400mg QoW treatment group as compared with 6.8% of placebo-treated patients ($p < .001$).

Etanercept

Etanercept is a dimeric fusion protein expressed by CHO cells that combines the extracellular domain of the p75 TNF receptor with the Fc fragment of human IgG$_1$ to form a soluble receptor that can attach to and neutralize two molecules of TNF-α or TNF-β/lymphotoxin[115] (see Fig. 28.2). Etanercept is FDA approved to treat moderate-severe plaque-type psoriasis in candidates for systemic therapy and to reduce signs and symptoms, improve physical function, and inhibit disease progression of PsA with or without the use of MTX. It is also approved to treat DMARD-resistant, polyarticular juvenile rheumatoid arthritis (JRA); to decrease signs and symptoms, inhibit radiographic progression, and improve functioning in RA; and to improve signs and symptoms of AS.

In a study that advanced the understanding of how TNF-blocking agents help improve skin disease, ten psoriasis patients were followed with repeated biopsy of lesional skin during 6 months on etanercept therapy.[19] Researchers recorded changes in histology, inflammatory gene expression, and cellular infiltration in plaques and found a rapid and complete reduction of IL-1 and IL-8 (immediate/early genes), followed by progressive reductions in many other inflammation-related genes, and finally somewhat slower reductions in infiltrating myeloid cells (CD11c$^+$ cells) and T cells. The observed decreases in the expression of mRNA for chemokines such as IL-8, IFN-γ–inducible protein-10 (CXCL10), and macrophage inflammatory protein 3α (MIP-3α; CCL20) may account for decreased infiltration of neutrophils, T cells, and DCs, respectively. Dendritic cells may be less activated with therapy, as suggested by decreased IL-23 mRNA and decreased iNOS mRNA and protein. Thus, a reduction in DC-mediated T-cell activation may account for decreases in T-cell numbers and decreases in T-cell expression of inflammatory genes such as IFN-γ, STAT1, and granzyme B. In this way, etanercept-induced TNF-α/lymphotoxin blockade may break the potentially self-sustaining cycle of DC activation and maturation, subsequent T-cell activation, and cytokine, growth factor, and chemokine production by multiple cell types including lymphocytes, neutrophils, DCs, and keratinocytes. Tumor necrosis factor inhibition then results in reversal of the epidermal hyperplasia and cutaneous inflammation that is characteristic of psoriatic plaques. In a separate analysis of skin samples from these 10 patients, etanercept caused downregulation of NF-κB activity in keratinocytes that correlated with clinical and histologic improvements, such as decreased epidermal thickness and decreased K16 expression.[102] Most recently, researchers found that by 1 month of therapy, even before maximal histologic changes and clinical responses were experienced by these patients, etanercept caused apoptosis of dermal DCs without affecting apoptosis of T cells in the blood or skin in patients subsequently achieving a PASI-75 response.[119] Taken together, these results reinforce the finding that TNF and DCs are essential to the immunopathogenesis of psoriasis and that they are important disease targets for drug development.

Among the biologic agents, etanercept is frequently used in psoriasis patients with stable disease who have elected to begin TNF blockade as well as in patients who have significant, uncontrolled psoriatic arthritis.[38] It is an SC injection that can be self-administered.[115] The indicated dosing for psoriasis is 50 mg twice a week (BIW) for 3 months followed by 25 mg BIW (or 50 mg QW), and the indicated dosing for PsA is 50 mg weekly as 25 mg BIW (or 50 mg QW).

Etanercept effects a major clinical improvement in psoriasis signs and symptoms (see Table 28.3). In phase III clinical trials, significant improvements in PASI scores were noted as early as 2 weeks into 6 months of etanercept therapy, and 49% of patients receiving 50 mg BIW etanercept therapy achieved a PASI-75 response during their initial 3 months of treatment.[104,105] Although many patients achieved a clinical response after a short time on etanercept therapy, approximately half of the patients who lacked a clinical response after 6 months on etanercept (i.e., failed to achieve at least 50% improvement in PASI score) were able to experience significant clinical improvement with an extended course of open-label etanercept therapy after a phase III trial.[120] An additional phase III trial demonstrated that etanercept improved skin disease as well as physical and emotional symptoms.[107] The agent relieved symptoms of fatigue associated with psoriasis from early in the course of treatment and reduced symptoms of documented depression in psoriasis patients. The fact that inflammatory cytokines such as TNF-α are activated in patients with major depressive disorder and that TNF blockade helps improve symptoms of fatigue and depression implies that depressive symptoms in psoriasis patients are mediated by TNF-α and reaffirms the importance of TNF blockade for improving quality of life in psoriasis patients.[32,107]

Etanercept therapy is not associated with disease rebound, the typical time to relapse after discontinuation of therapy is 3 months, and patients can be re-treated after relapse without experiencing tachyphylaxis.[121] Although etanercept could thus be used as an intermittent therapy,[32] the current package labeling in the United States,[115] as well as clinical data,[122] support continuous administration of the agent. In a 24-week study of 2546 psoriasis patients, treatment with etanercept 50 mg SC BIW for 12 weeks was followed by either etanercept as continuous therapy at 50 mg SC QW for an additional 12 weeks or etanercept as intermittent therapy, readministered at 50 mg SC QW upon relapse of skin lesions through week 24. Although both the continuous and intermittent therapy groups responded with improvements in their psoriasis, the patients who were treated continuously had a significantly greater rate of response than the patients who were treated intermittently. An open-label extension study following phase III clinical trials speaks to the safety of continuous administration.[123] This study followed 591 patients with psoriasis on continuous 50 mg BIW etanercept therapy, a high dose that is more than the recommended stepdown to 25 mg BIW (or 50 mg QW) after 3 months of therapy. Etanercept maintained efficacy without an increase in the rate of exposure-adjusted adverse events and infections over a total of 96 weeks.

Clinical trials indicate that etanercept is an effective treatment for PsA (see Table 28.3). In a phase III trial in which patients were able to continue their regular doses of MTX, low-dose prednisone, or NSAIDs, an ACR-20 response was achieved at 3 months by 59% of patients given 25 mg BIW etanercept therapy.[25] As measured by the change in Sharp score (a measurement of radiographic progression of joint disease), radiographic progression was slowed significantly in patients who received etanercept therapy for 1 year as compared with patients who initially received placebo. Continued follow-up found that after 2 years of etanercept therapy, radiographic progression remained inhibited.[124] In an observational study, etanercept enacted clinical improvement in signs and symptoms of PsA in patients who failed to respond to at least one DMARD (MTX, sulfasalazine, or cyclosporine).[125]

Experience with treating psoriasis and PsA with etanercept in the community nearly mirrors the success of etanercept in clinical trials.[33] A phase IV, open-label study collected clinical data from 1122 patients with PsA being treated with etanercept (50 mg SC QW) for 24 weeks. Patients were followed in dermatology clinics, the majority of which were in the community versus academic institutions. The Physician Global Assessment (PGA) of psoriasis was improved to where the skin was clear or almost clear in 41% of patients at 12 weeks and in 57% of patients at 24 weeks. These improvements are comparable to the PGA responses seen in phase III clinical trials[25,104,105] (see Table 28.3). Regarding the benefit from etanercept for PsA, patients reported improvement in symptoms such as joint pain and morning stiffness, and investigators observed improvement in clinical signs such as tender and swollen joint counts.[33] During the study, there was a decrease in the use of concomitant MTX and systemic corticosteroids. Etanercept was well tolerated, there were no deaths, and serious adverse events (SAEs) including serious infections were rare.

Regarding the short-term safety of etanercept, a multistudy database pooled the results from the first 3 months of three phase II or III clinical trials in which 1347 patients were treated with etanercept.[126] Adverse events were not dose-dependent, and the most common side effect seen more often in etanercept-treated patients (14%) as compared with patients receiving placebo (6%) was a mild to moderate injection-site reaction (ISR) characterized by erythema, pruritus, or edema that decreased in frequency over time. Evaluation of skin biopsies from patients receiving etanercept treatment who had ISRs found that the ISR is likely a T-cell–mediated, delayed-type hypersensitivity reaction.[127] In the pivotal phase III trials, other than ISR, the most frequently experienced adverse events (seen in at least 5% of either etanercept- or placebo-treated patients) were headache, injection-site bruising, upper respiratory infection (URI), flu-like symptoms, and accidental injury[104,105] (see Table 28.3). There were no opportunistic infections, tuberculosis, or apparent increases in the frequency of cancers in etanercept-treated patients as compared with patients who received placebo. Although a small number of patients developed antibodies against etanercept, antibodies were not

neutralizing (i.e., they did not bind to the drug to render it ineffective).

Given that etanercept deactivates immune cells and decreases the production of immune mediators, there is the concern that it could prevent a patient from mounting a proper immune response against harmful antigens.[128] A report in the literature describes a man with psoriasis who was on etanercept therapy (25 mg SC BIW) for 5 months and developed acute contact dermatitis to poison ivy, suggesting that this aspect of type IV immunity may be intact during etanercept therapy. In a randomized trial, investigators studied the antibody response to the 23-valent pneumococcal vaccine in patients with PsA on etanercept therapy.[129] The PsA patients treated with etanercept 25 mg SC BIW were as likely as placebo-treated patients to mount an expected humoral immune response to the pneumococcal vaccine.

More study is needed to examine the safety and efficacy of etanercept for the treatment of psoriasis and PsA in high-risk patients such as children, the elderly, the obese, and hepatitis C patients, but current data are promising. Etanercept is approved for the treatment of DMARD-resistant polyarticular JRA in children over 4 years, but it is otherwise not approved to treat inflammatory diseases in the pediatric population.[115] Currently, a phase III trial is underway to examine the safety and efficacy of etanercept for the treatment of psoriasis in pediatric patients.[130] An analysis of two phase III clinical trials showed that elderly patients (age >65) were as likely as younger patients to experience clinical benefit as demonstrated by PASI responses and quality of life improvements, with no increase in ISRs and an increase only in SAEs that were not related to treatment.[131] There are case reports in the literature that suggest that etanercept could help improve psoriasis and PsA without having deleterious effects on transaminase levels in patients with HCV infection.[132–134] Psoriasis is not uncommon in this population, as the treatments for HCV infection can worsen or invoke psoriasis or PsA, and more safe options for therapy of skin/joint disease in this population are needed because traditional systemic therapies for psoriasis/PsA can be toxic to the liver or immune system. In theory, overweight or obese patients are at a disadvantage as far as the degree of clinical improvement they can experience on etanercept therapy because the agent is not dosed by weight and TNF-α can be made by fat cells. Clinical trial data suggest that patients with a high body mass index (BMI) respond to etanercept treatment.[135] However, patients with a higher BMI demonstrated a smaller clinical response compared with leaner patients over 48 weeks of therapy with 50 mg BIW etanercept.

Infliximab

Infliximab is a recombinant chimeric monoclonal IgG$_1$ antibody directed against TNF-α that binds specifically to TNF-α (both soluble and transmembrane types) to prevent receptor-binding[116] (see Fig. 28.2). Infliximab is able to induce the lysis of cells that display TNF-α on their surface, including activated T cells, via complement-mediated or via antibody-dependent/cell-mediated toxicity.[32,116] As of September 2006, in addition to EMEA approval, infliximab gained FDA approval for the treatment of adults with chronic and severe plaque-type psoriasis in whom other systemic treatments are not appropriate and who are closely monitored with routine follow-up by their physicians.[116] Among the biologics, it is an excellent agent for the immediate relief of skin disease "in clinical circumstances requiring rapid disease control," that is, in very severe, unstable, erythrodermic, or pustular psoriasis.[38] In addition to its psoriasis indication, infliximab is FDA approved to reduce signs and symptoms, inhibit radiographic progression, and improve physical functioning in adults with PsA (with or without MTX) and adults with RA (in combination with MTX); to reduce signs and symptoms of AS; and as an induction and maintenance therapy for resistant IBD including CD in adults and children, fistulizing CD in adults, and UC in adults.[116]

For psoriasis and PsA, treatment is administered as IV infusions that last approximately 2 to 3 hours each.[116] Induction therapy of 5 mg/kg IV infusions is given at weeks 0, 2, and 6, and maintenance therapy of 5 mg/kg IV infusions is given every 8 weeks thereafter. In the phase II and III randomized clinical trials that led to the approval of infliximab for the treatment of psoriasis, 75% to 88% of patients achieved a PASI-75 response after induction therapy at 5 mg/kg.[111–113] Maintenance therapy is best administered on a continuous basis.[113] In a phase III trial that compared continuous

versus intermittent (PRN) maintenance therapy for 1 year following the typical induction regimen, patients treated with continuous maintenance therapy every 8 weeks at 5 mg/kg best maintained PASI-75 responses[113] (see Table 28.3). In clinical trials investigating infliximab for the treatment of PsA (Infliximab Multinational Psoriatic Arthritis Controlled Trials [IMPACT] I and II), infliximab enacted significant ACR-20 responses, inhibition in radiographic progression, and improvement in dactylitis, enthesopathy, and physical functioning in patients resistant to therapy with one or more DMARD(s)[26, 27,136] (see Table 28.3).

Researchers are discovering more and more about how infliximab clears psoriasis, thus providing new insight into how TNF-α produces the psoriatic phenotype. In a pharmacodynamic and pharmacokinetic study of infliximab, the first infusion induced swift decreases in CD3$^+$ T cells and in the thickness of the epidermis in psoriasis plaques even before the occurrence of skin clearance.[109] Subsequent PASI-75 responses and improvements in PGA scores correlated with changes in the skin such as decreased T-cell number in the epidermis, decreased epidermal thickness, normalization of K16, and downregulation of ICAM-1 on keratinocytes. In a separate study, improvements in PASI scores correlated with the apoptosis-like programmed cell death of keratinocytes in psoriasis plaques of patients receiving infliximab.[137] Similarly, researchers administered infliximab induction therapy and linked subsequent improvements in joint disease and reductions in PASI scores to parallel decreases in the protein survivin, an inhibitor of apoptosis-like protein present in psoriasis lesions around blood vessels in the dermis and basal cells in the epidermis.[138] One of the functions of survivin is to inhibit apoptosis of keratinocytes and endothelial cells to support the keratinocyte hyperplasia and new blood vessel formation that is characteristic of psoriasis. Infliximab induction therapy disturbed angiogenesis in a study that linked clinical and histologic improvements to changes in skin biopsies including decreased vascularity, decreased endothelial cell activation, and decreased mRNA or protein expression of growth factors for angiogenesis (i.e., vascular endothelial growth factor [VEGF], angiopoietin 1 and 2, and the angiopoietin receptor Tie 2).[139] The above findings indicate that infliximab works directly (i.e., on

T cells) or indirectly (i.e., on DCs, keratinocytes, and endothelial cells) to quickly improve psoriatic skin and joint disease,[109,137–139] typically by the third infusion or earlier in clinical trials.[26,27,112] These results reinforce the idea that psoriasis results from the functions of multiple cell types working in concert.

Regarding adverse effects, treatment is sometimes associated with loss of efficacy over time[112,113] (see Table 28.3). In addition, patients may experience one or more infusion reaction (IR), defined as any event that occurs within 1 hour of an infusion.[116] An immediate IR can be a hypersensitivity reaction or a non–immune-mediated reaction. A delayed reaction can also occur in the form of a delayed hypersensitivity/serum sickness-like reaction within 2 weeks of an infusion. Loss of efficacy and IRs are in part the result of human antichimeric antibodies that patients may raise against infliximab, which is nearly one fifth mouse protein.[112,113,116] Across indications, about 10% of infliximab-treated patients in clinical trials developed antibodies to the drug during typical induction and maintenance therapy for 1 to 2 years.[116] In psoriasis trials, the incidence of anti-infliximab antibodies was somewhat higher than this average, ranging from approximately 27% to 36% in patients treated with 5 mg/kg induction and maintenance therapy every 8 weeks.[112,113] These higher percentages were probably because of a lack of concomitant MTX treatment. As compared with patients who were antibody-negative, a smaller percentage of patients who were antibody-positive experienced a PASI-75 response or sustained a PASI-75 response throughout the course of these studies. Consistent with trials studying infliximab therapy for other inflammatory diseases,[116] there was an increased incidence of IRs in patients on infliximab treatment who were antibody-positive.[111,113] Patients should be monitored closely during infusions and may benefit from a slow infusion rate in addition to premedication with antihistamines, acetaminophen, or corticosteroids,[116] although corticosteroids are the least attractive option because of the potential for psoriasis to flare upon their cessation. As noted by the manufacturer in Remicade's package insert, the frequency of antibodies to infliximab can be attenuated if a patient takes a concomitant immunosuppressive therapy (i.e., MTX or AZA). In addition, antibody formation was lowest in patients with the most consistent exposure to infliximab.[113] Because not all patients who raise antibodies against the drug experience adverse effects on efficacy or IRs, more research is needed to elucidate the mechanisms of these events.

Additional adverse events of concern include elevations in aminotransferase levels and a possibly increased risk for cancer. In two phase III clinical trials investigating the use of infliximab for the treatment of psoriasis, 8% of patients experienced aminotransferase elevations to over three times the upper limit of normal (versus <1% of placebo patients), and 3% of patients experienced elevations to over five times the upper limit of normal (versus 0% of placebo patients).[116] The development of jaundice or alanine aminotransferase (ALT) elevations to over five times the upper limit of normal in any patient requires discontinuation of the agent and warrants further investigation (see Table 28.2). Regarding the risk of cancer associated with infliximab therapy, in clinical trials for the agent's multiple indications more patients treated with infliximab developed cancer as compared with patients given placebo treatment. Cancers of the lung, head, and neck are of greatest concern, and adult patients with chronic obstructive pulmonary disease (COPD) may be at greatest risk, as shown in an exploratory trial that evaluated infliximab for the treatment of moderate-severe COPD. In addition, the treatment of adolescents with CD on concomitant immunosuppressive therapy with azathioprine (AZA) or 6-MP (6-mercaptopurine) resulted in six cases of the uncommon but highly life-threatening cancer hepatosplenic T-cell lymphoma.

Adalimumab

Adalimumab is a fully human recombinant monoclonal IgG_1 antibody directed exclusively against TNF-α[117] (see Fig. 28.2). It thus prevents TNF-α from binding to its receptors, and it binds TNF bound to cells to cause complement-mediated cell lysis. In addition, it causes the downregulation of selected adhesion molecules. In addition to having EMEA approval, it is FDA approved for use as monotherapy or as combination therapy with DMARDs such as MTX for the treatment of PsA or RA to inhibit progression and reduce signs, symptoms, and physical limitations. It is also approved to reduce signs and symptoms of AS. For the treatment of PsA, adalimumab is administered as a 40 mg SC injection QoW that patients can self-inject. Adalimumab was studied for the treatment of PsA in the Adalimumab Effectiveness in Psoriatic Arthritis Trial (ADEPT).[114] Adalimumab was administered by SC injection QoW for 24 weeks, and patients were allowed to continue MTX (<30 mg per week) or prednisone (<10 mg per day) during treatment. Significant ACR-20 responses were reached by patients treated with adalimumab versus placebo by 2 weeks of therapy, and after 12 weeks of treatment 58% of patients treated with adalimumab achieved an ACR-20 response. At 24 weeks, there was significant inhibition of joint destruction (as measured by change in Sharp score) in the patients treated with adalimumab (see Table 28.3). An open-label extension study followed patients from ADEPT for up to 48 weeks on adalimumab treatment and found that patients maintained improvements in PsA signs, symptoms, and radiographic progression.[140] Over 48 weeks of therapy, adverse events were similar to placebo.[114,140]

Adalimumab is currently in phase III study to investigate its efficacy and safety for the treatment of moderate-severe psoriasis (go to ClinicalTrials. gov, ID NCT00237887, ID NCT00235820, ID NCT00195676). Fifty-nine percent of the 69 patients assessed for improvement of psoriasis in the ADEPT trial demonstrated a significant PASI-75 response at the week 24 assessment and maintained this response through 48 weeks[114] (see Table 28.3). A phase II trial investigated adalimumab for the treatment of psoriasis over 60 weeks.[141] The first 12 weeks of treatment was a randomized controlled trial comparing high-dose adalimumab (40 mg SC QW) versus low-dose adalimumab (40 mg SC QoW) versus placebo. During weeks 13 to 24 high-dose versus low-dose adalimumab was studied, and placebo patients were crossed over to receive low-dose adalimumab. Weeks 25 to 60 were an open label extension study in which patients continued to receive their respective dose of adalimumab, and patients on low-dose therapy with less than a PASI-50 response became eligible for dose escalation to QW therapy. At the week 12 assessment, 53% of low-dose patients and 80% of high-dose patients achieved a PASI-75 response, whereas only 4% of placebo patients achieved a PASI-75 response (p <.001). Impressive clinical responses ensued

for the remainder of the trial; however, at the 24 week assessment of the high-dose group and the 36 week assessment of the low-dose group, a lower percentage of patients achieved a PASI-75 response as compared with the percentage of patients with a PASI-75 response only 12 weeks earlier for each treatment group (see Table 28.3). This apparent loss of efficacy with adalimumab therapy may be in part a result of antibodies raised against the drug, so-called human antihuman antibodies (HAHAs) that developed in about 5% of patients with RA treated with adalimumab in clinical trials (1% of patients on concomitant MTX versus 12% of patients on adalimumab monotherapy).[117] Even though the product is entirely human and therefore it is not expected to be immunogenic (i.e., elicit an antibody response), the presence of HAHAs is believed to account at least in part for the loss of efficacy or lack of response to adalimumab that was experienced by some RA patients being treated with this agent.[142]

How adalimumab helps to control plaque-type psoriasis is not fully understood. Whereas untreated skin has a characteristically low number of epidermal Langerhans' cells, the skin of patients treated with adalimumab demonstrates a rapid increase in the number of Langerhans' cells present in the psoriatic epidermis within 7 days of therapy.[143] This finding demonstrates that TNF-α could cause the initial decreased number of Langerhans' cells, the absence of which may contribute to psoriasis pathogenesis because the Langerhans' cell might be antiinflammatory or help regulate keratinocyte differentiation.

Regarding the agent's safety when administered to psoriasis patients, in the phase II trial cited above,[141] the most common adverse events seen more frequently in adalimumab-treated patients as compared with placebo-treated patients were dyspepsia, nausea, and mildly elevated triglycerides. In addition, mild to moderate transient pain with injection was experienced by twice as many patients in the high-dose group (12%) as in the low-dose group (6.7%) or placebo group (5.8%). Although there was no evidence of lupus or demyelinating diseases in this trial, there were two instances of cancer, including one malignant melanoma (MM) and one squamous cell carcinoma (SCC) that were likely preexistent, two instances of serious infection including one case of TB and one case of coccidioidomycosis, and two instances of reversible liver function test (LFT) elevation to 3 to 3.5 times the upper limit of normal. The most common side effect observed in clinical trials for any of adalimumab's indications was a mild ISR consisting of redness, pruritus, bleeding, pain, or swelling at the injection site.[117] Patients may also experience URI, headache, or nausea (see Table 28.2).

Contraindications to and Long-Term Safety of Tumor Necrosis Factor Blockade

In general, TNF-blocking therapy is contraindicated in patients with serious active infections including TB, moderate to severe congestive heart failure (CHF) (New York Heart Association class III or IV), multiple sclerosis (MS) or similar demyelinating disease, and lupus.[38,115–117] There are no prospective clinical trials investigating therapy in patients with active cancer or in patients during pregnancy.[32] Although animal models (the agents are pregnancy category B),[115–117] safety database information,[144] and case reports[145–147] of women treated for IBD or RA during pregnancy speak to the overall lack of teratogenicity of TNF-blocking agents, there are no data that specifically address the immune system integrity in children born to women using TNF blockade during pregnancy.

Given the distinctive benefits of therapy, long-term safety is of concern to patients and to the medical community. Safety concerns with the TNF-blocking agents include autoimmunity, cancer (especially lymphoma and skin cancer), and serious infections.

There are numerous reports in the literature of patients on TNF blockade for various indications who developed drug-induced systemic lupus erythematosus (SLE) or lupus-like syndromes,[148–159] discoid lupus,[160,161] or cutaneous lupus.[162,163] In clinical trials of infliximab (for CD, RA, psoriasis, and PsA), drug-induced lupus-like syndromes and full-blown lupus (with central nervous system [CNS] and renal manifestations) were quite rare, even though about 50% of patients on active therapy (versus 20% of placebo-treated patients) converted from antinuclear antibody (ANA)-negative at baseline to ANA-positive in the course of therapy, and about 20% of patients (versus 0% of placebo patients) converted from antinuclear double-stranded DNA (anti-dsDNA)-negative at

baseline to anti-dsDNA-positive in the course of therapy.[116] Of the available TNF inhibitors, infliximab carries the highest risk for development of autoantibodies. In clinical trials of adalimumab therapy, one of 2334 patients had drug-induced lupus and no patients had renal manifestations suggestive of SLE despite 12% of adalimumab-treated patients (versus 7% of placebo-treated patients) converting from ANA-negative at baseline to ANA-positive in the course of therapy.[164] Among patients with RA who were treated with etanercept, there were few reports of lupus-like syndromes, whereas ANA seroconversion occurred in 11% of etanercept-treated patients (versus 5% of placebo-treated patients).[115] It is prudent to check the ANA titer prior to beginning treatment, to monitor titers periodically during therapy, and to monitor for signs and symptoms of lupus while a patient is on TNF-blocking therapy.

Etanercept, infliximab, and adalimumab carry FDA-mandated warnings of infection and malignancy on their labelings.[115–117] A meta-analysis of nine clinical trials involving nearly 3500 patients with RA treated for at least 12 weeks with an anti-TNF antibody provides some data regarding the risk of serious infections and cancer associated with adalimumab and infliximab.[165] Data demonstrated that therapy with anti-TNF antibodies put patients at an increased risk for acquiring a serious infection (126 of 3493 patients on active treatment versus 26 of 1512 patients taking placebo, odds ratio versus placebo = 2.0) and at an increased risk for developing cancer (24 of 3493 patients on active treatment versus 2 of 1512 of patients on placebo, odds ratio versus placebo= 3.3). The latter relationship was related to the dose of the agent administered. These results represent the pooling of data from a few of the trials performed in RA patients, and data do not reflect adjustment for duration of drug exposure to account for time spent in open-label extensions without placebo control. Patients included in this meta-analysis were clinically heterogeneous, meaning that their disease ranged in chronicity and severity, and patients may have received immunosuppressive therapies that could affect their risk for infection or malignancy. Patients with chronic inflammatory diseases such as RA and psoriasis are at high risk for developing certain cancers at baseline. Rheumatoid arthritis patients have at least twice the risk of acquiring lymphoma when compared with people in the general population, with higher degrees of risk based on increasing disease severity.[166] Similarly, psoriasis patients are at an increased risk of developing lymphoma as compared with the general population.[167] This baseline risk cannot be discounted when considering the safety of TNF blockade.

Regarding the safety of etanercept therapy, Amgen and Wyeth Pharmaceuticals reported that etanercept-treated and placebo-treated patients were at a similar risk (1%) for developing serious infections in clinical trials.[115] There have been nine cases of lymphoma and 67 other cancers out of nearly 4500 patients with RA treated with etanercept in clinical trials. Patients were observed for an average of 27 months and up to 5 years without an increase in the rate of cancers during this time. Lymphomas occurred at a rate three times that in the general population but similar to that in RA patients, and other cancers were common cancers (e.g., colon, breast, lung, prostate) and occurred at a rate likely to be seen in the general population. An FDA-requested meta-analysis of clinical trials investigating etanercept therapy demonstrated a relative risk for malignancy of 0.86 (95% confidence interval [CI], 0.56–1.31) for patients treated with etanercept versus patients who received control treatment.[168] In clinical experience with RA patients on etanercept therapy for up to 8.2 years, infections and cancer rates did not increase with time on therapy.[169] Similarly, in psoriasis patients, there does not appear to be an increased risk of SAEs such as serious infections or malignancy with prolonged use of etanercept at BIW or QW dosing, as demonstrated in an open-label extension study of etanercept administration for up to 2.5 years, in which 591 of 912 patients were on etanercept 50 mg SC BIW.[170]

Researchers have separately investigated the relationship between TNF-α inhibitors and the development of nonmelanoma skin cancer (NMSC) in RA patients.[171] The RA patients have a greater risk of developing NMSC as compared to patients with osteoarthritis. This risk is further elevated by therapy with TNF blockade and even further elevated by therapy with MTX in addition to a TNF-α inhibitor (but not by MTX as monotherapy).

As a precaution, physicians should monitor for infection and cancer while a patient is on a TNF-blocking agent. Patients require screening for TB (as indicated in the package inserts for adalimumab and infliximab and as standard of care for etanercept even though there is no explicit recommendation in the package insert). Patients require initiation of treatment for a positive TB screening test indicating latent TB before they can be treated with a TNF-blocking agent. In addition, patients should be screened for hepatitis B virus (HBV) status prior to starting treatment.[115–117] As indicated by the manufacturers, caution should be exercised when administering these agents to patients who are HBV carriers, and TNF blockade should not be administered in patients with active HBV infection. In general, patients should not receive live vaccines during treatment. To monitor for infection and malignancy, physicians can check complete blood count (CBC) values, LFT values, and perform periodic skin checks as part of a complete physical exam (see Table 28.2).

Emerging Dermatologic Uses for Tumor Necrosis Factor Blockade

Tumor necrosis factor blockers are increasingly being used off-label to treat dermatologic conditions including but not limited to pyoderma gangrenosum, hidradenitis suppurativa, and sarcoidosis, especially in patients with disease that is severe or resistant to traditional therapies.

Patients with pyoderma gangrenosum (PG) have experienced benefit from treatment with adalimumab,[172] as well as with etanercept.[173,174] There are numerous case reports in the literature in which patients with PG who had active IBD, inactive IBD, or no history of IBD experienced improvement in skin disease from infliximab therapy.[175–178] These reports prefaced a multicenter, randomized, double-blind, placebo-controlled trial that investigated the treatment of PG with infliximab infusion in 30 patients including patients with and without IBD.[179] Infliximab demonstrated significant improvement in 46% (six of 13) of patients after one 5 mg/kg infusion versus 6% (one of 17) of placebo patients at the week 2 assessment of disease activity (p = .025), and a second infusion provided relief in the majority of patients who did not demonstrate an adequate response at the week 2 assessment. In total, 69% (20 of 29) of patients who received at least one infliximab infusion experienced a benefit from therapy.

For the treatment of hidradenitis suppurativa (HS), etanercept was associated with improvements in self-reported disease activity and DLQI scores in patients with severe, recalcitrant HS who took part in a small open-label study of 25 mg BIW therapy for 12 to 24 weeks.[180] Infliximab benefited patients with HS who were evaluated as part of a retrospective chart review.[181] Similarly, several case reports of patients with HS describe beneficial effects of infliximab therapy.[182–186] Case reports support a similar benefit from treatment with adalimumab.[187,188]

Patients with various manifestations of cutaneous sarcoidosis who were previously resistant to treatment have experienced improvement in disease with infliximab therapy,[189–191] adalimumab therapy,[192,193] and etanercept therapy.[194,195] The successful treatment of these skin (and systemic) diseases points out the role that TNF and the immune system have in their pathogeneses and opens the door for an emerging area of research.

Interleukin-12/Interleukin-23 p40-Targeted Therapies

The p40 subunit of the type 1 cytokines IL-12 and IL-23 is emerging as a pathogenic target for inflammatory disease therapy. Improvement of psoriasis lesions in patients on traditional therapies has been accompanied by downregulation of type 1 inflammatory cytokine expression in psoriatic skin. For example, expression of IFN-γ–inducing cytokines such as IL-12, IL-23, and IL-18 was found to be decreased along with decreases in PASI scores in the skin of psoriasis patients after UVB light box therapy,[196] and IL-12 expression was found to be reduced after systemic therapy with cyclosporin A.[197] Interleukin-23 is made up of two subunits, its own p19 subunit and a p40 subunit that is has in common with IL-12.[198] Investigators have found that the IL-12 p40 subunit is significantly overexpressed in psoriasis lesions as opposed to unaffected skin of psoriasis patients and normal skin.[199] It was determined that IL-23 as opposed to just IL-12 contributes greatly to inflammation in psoriasis when investigators found that both the p40 and p19 subunits were upregulated in the skin of psoriasis patients, whereas the p35 subunit that is unique to IL-12 was not.[198] Investigators subsequently found that IL-23 was produced at an accelerated pace in psoriatic skin by keratinocytes and APCs including epidermal Langerhans' cells, dermal DCs, and macrophages.[200] Here, it augments memory T-cell synthesis/secretion of IFN-γ and thus

plays an important role in maintaining the robust inflammatory response of psoriasis. Overexpression of type 1 cytokines including the p40 subunit may have a genetic basis.[201]

A phase I clinical study has evaluated the use of CNTO-1275 (Centocor, Inc., Malvern, PA), a fully human IgG$_1$ monoclonal antibody directed against IL-12/IL-23 p40.[21] This agent thus engages the p40 subunit to prohibit the cytokines from binding to their shared receptor IL-12Rβ1, and it thus decreases the activation of T cells and NK cells. One IV infusion produced significant improvements in patients with moderate-severe plaque-type psoriasis. Patients were dosed at 0.1 mg/kg, 0.3 mg/kg, 1.0 mg/kg, or 5.0 mg/kg, and 67% of patients (12 of 18) experienced a PASI-75 response and maintained this response over the 16-week evaluation period. Adverse events were mostly mild and included decreased T-cell counts, headache, and URI symptoms, and only one SAE was reported and was not related to exposure to CNTO-1275. The rate and extent of clinical response but not of adverse events were related to the concentration of CNTO-1275 administered. CNTO-1275 was similarly tolerated and demonstrated efficacy at four different SC dosing regimens in a phase II study that further investigated this agent for the treatment of psoriasis in 320 patients who received one of five treatments: (1) one 50 mg SC injection, (2) one 100 mg SC injection, (3) four weekly 50-mg injections, (4) four weekly 100 mg SC injections, or (5) placebo.[202] At the week 12 evaluation, 52% (treatment 1), 59% (treatment 2), 67% (treatment 3), 81% (treatment 4), and 2% (placebo) of patients achieved a PASI-75 response ($p < .001$ vs. placebo). CNTO-1275 is currently in phase III trials for psoriasis (ClinicalTrials.gov, ID NCT00267969, ID NCT00307437) and phase II study for PsA (ClinicalTrials.gov, ID NCT00267956). Another subcutaneous IL-12 monoclonal antibody, ABT-874 (Abbott, Abbott Park, IL), is in phase II study for psoriasis (ClinicalTrials.gov, ID NCT00292396).

Conclusion

Biologics, or biologic therapies, are substances created by scientists from living cells for the treatment or prevention of human diseases. Biologics are approved for the therapy of psoriasis and psoriatic arthritis as well as a number of nondermatologic indications. Biologics include cell adhesion molecule antagonists (alefacept and efalizumab) and cytokine antagonists (etanercept, infliximab and adalimumab). Biologics appear relatively safe, but clinical and laboratory monitoring of safety is recommended at regular intervals, depending on the patient's age, comorbidities, exposures, and other factors. Cytokine (i.e., tumor necrosis factor) antagonists have other potential uses in dermatology, including pyoderma gangrenosum, hidrandenitis suppurativa, and sarcoidosis. Other classes of biologics will be available in the near future. Phase II and III trials are currently ongoing for IL-12/IL-23 targeted therapies.

Acknowledgments. Financial disclosure: Dr. Gottlieb has speakers' bureau memberships with Amgen Inc. and Wyeth Pharmaceuticals; consulting/advisory board agreements with Amgen Inc., Centocor, Inc., Wyeth Pharmaceuticals, Celgene Corp., Bristol Myers Squibb Co., Beiersdorf, Inc., Warner Chilcott, Abbott Labs., Roche, Sankyo, Medarex, Kemia, Celera, TEVA, Actelion, UCB, Novo Nordisk, Almirall, Immune Control, Dermipsor Ltd., Medacorp, DermiPsor, Can-Fite, and Incyte; and research/educational grants from Centocor, Amgen, Wyeth, Immune Control, Celgene, Pharmacare, and Incyte. All income from these activities is paid directly to Dr. Gottlieb's employer. Ms. Berger has no relevant relationships with industry.

References

1. International Nonproprietary Names (INN) for Biological and Biotechnological Substances (A Review). World Health Organization (WHO) Web site. http://www.who.int/medicines/services/inn/BioRevforweb.pdf.
2. Krueger JG. The immunologic basis for the treatment of psoriasis with new biologic agents. J Am Acad Dermatol 2002;46:1–23.
3. Coico R, Sunshine G, Benjamini E. Antibody structure and function. In: Immunology, 5th ed. Hoboken, NJ: John Wiley & Sons, 2003:39–57.
4. Nestle FO, Nickoloff BJ. Dermal dendritic cells are important members of the skin immune system. Adv Exp Med Biol 1995;378:111–6.
5. Wrone-Smith T, Nickoloff BJ. Dermal injection of immunocytes induces psoriasis. J Clin Invest 1996;98:1878–87.
6. Boehncke WH, Zollner TM, Dressel D, Kaufmann R. Induction of psoriasiform inflammation by a bacterial superantigen in the SCID-hu xenogeneic transplantation model. J Cutan Pathol 1997;24:1–7.
7. Gilhar A, David M, Ullmann Y, Berkutski T, Kalish RS. T-lymphocyte dependence of psoriatic pathology in human psoriatic skin grafted to SCID mice. J Invest Dermatol 1997;109:283–8.
8. Hong K, Chu A. Lúdvíksson BR, Berg EL, Ehrhardt RO. IL-12, independently of IFN-gamma, plays a crucial role in the pathogenesis of a murine psoriasis-like skin disorder. J Immunol 1999;162:7480–91.
9. Nickoloff BJ, Wrone-Smith T. Injection of pre-psoriatic skin with CD4+ T cells induces psoriasis. Am J Pathol 1999;155:145–58.
10. Nickoloff BJ, Bonish B, Huang BB, Porcelli SA. Characterization of a T cell line bearing natural killer receptors and capable of creating psoriasis in a SCID mouse model system. J Dermatol Sci 2000;24:212–25.
11. Gilhar A, Ullmann Y, Kerner H, et al. Psoriasis is mediated by a cutaneous defect triggered by activated immunocytes: induction of psoriasis by cells with natural killer receptors. J Invest Dermatol 2002;119:384–91.
12. Boyman O, Hefti HP, Conrad C, Nickoloff BJ, Suter M, Nestle FO. Spontaneous development of psoriasis in a new animal model shows an essential role for resident T cells and tumor necrosis factor-alpha. J Exp Med 2004;199:731–6.
13. Ellis CN, Fradin MS, Messana JM, et al. Cyclosporine for plaque-type psoriasis. Results of a multidose, double-blind trial. New Engl J Med 1991;324:277–84.
14. Gottlieb AB, Grossman RM, Khandke L, et al. Studies of the effect of cyclosporine in psoriasis in vivo: combined effects on activated T lymphocytes and epidermal regenerative maturation. J Invest Dermatol 1992;98:302–9.
15. Gottlieb SL, Gilleaudeau P, Johnson R, et al. Response of psoriasis to a lymphocyte-selective toxin (DAB389IL-2) suggests a primary immune, but not keratinocyte, pathogenic basis. Nat Med 1995;1:442–7.
16. Abrams JR, Lebwohl MG, Guzzo CA, et al. CTLA4Ig-mediated blockade of T-cell costimulation in patients with psoriasis vulgaris. J Clin Invest 1999;103:1243–52.
17. Abrams JR, Kelley SL, Hayes E, et al. Blockade of T lymphocyte costimulation with cytotoxic T

lymphocyte-associated antigen 4–immunoglobulin (CTLA4Ig) reverses the cellular pathology of psoriatic plaques, including the activation of keratinocytes, dendritic cells, and endothelial cells. J Exp Med 2000;192:681–93.

18. Gottlieb AB, Lebwohl M, Totoritis MC, et al. Clinical and histologic response to single-dose treatment of moderate to severe psoriasis with an anti-CD80 monoclonal antibody. J Am Acad Dermatol 2002;47:692–700.

19. Gottlieb AB, Chamian F, Masud S, et al. TNF inhibition rapidly down-regulates multiple proinflammatory pathways in psoriasis plaques. J Immunol 2005;175:2721–9.

20. Marble DJ, Gordon K, Nickoloff B. Localization of TNFα producing cells and reduction in response to TNFα targeted therapy in psoriasis [abstract]. J Invest Dermatol 2006;126:1–156.

21. Kauffman CL, Aria N, Toichi E, et al. A phase I study evaluating the safety, pharmacokinetics, and clinical response of a human IL-12 p40 antibody in subjects with plaque psoriasis. J Invest Dermatol 2004;123:1037–44.

22. Chamian F, Lin S, Novitskaya I, et al. Presence of "inflammatory" dendritic cells in psoriasis vulgaris lesions and modulation by Efalizumab (anti-CD11a) [abstract]. J Invest Dermatol 2004;122:A41.

23. Gottlieb A, Krueger JG, Bright R, et al. Effects of administration of a single dose of a humanized monoclonal antibody to CD11a on the immunobiology and clinical activity of psoriasis. J Am Acad Dermatol 2000;42:428–35.

24. Partsch G, Wagner E, Leeb BF, Broll H, Dunky A, Smolen JS. T cell derived cytokines in psoriatic arthritis synovial fluids. Ann Rheum Dis 1998;57:691–3.

25. Mease PJ, Kivitz AJ, Burch FX, et al. Etanercept treatment of psoriatic arthritis: safety, efficacy, and effect on disease progression. Arthritis Rheum 2004;50:2264–72.

26. Antoni CE, Kavanaugh A, Kirkham B, et al. Sustained benefits of infliximab therapy for dermatologic and articular manifestations of psoriatic arthritis: results from the infliximab multinational psoriatic arthritis controlled trial (IMPACT). Arthritis Rheum 2005;52:1227–36.

27. Antoni C, Krueger GG, de Vlam K, et al. IMPACT 2 Investigators. Infliximab improves signs and symptoms of psoriatic arthritis: results of the IMPACT 2 trial. Ann Rheum Dis 2005;64:1150–7.

28. Gelfand JM, Gladman DD, Mease PJ, et al. Epidemiology of psoriatic arthritis in the population of the United States. J Am Acad Dermatol 2005;53:573–7.

29. Gladman DD. Psoriatic arthritis. Dermatol Ther 2004;17:350–63.

30. Mody E, Husni E, Qureshi A. Diagnosis of arthritis in psoriasis patients presenting with joint pain to a dermatology-rheumatology clinic [abstract]. J Invest Dermatol 2006;126:43.

31. National Psoriasis Foundation (NPF). National Psoriasis Foundation Press Kit for Psoriatic Arthritis Survey, January 2002. http://www.psoriasis.org/files/pdfs/press/papresskit.pdf.

32. Gottlieb AB. Psoriasis: emerging therapeutic strategies. Nat Rev Drug Discov 2005;4:19–34.

33. Gottlieb AB, Kircik L, Eisen D, et al. Use of etanercept for psoriatic arthritis in the dermatology clinic: the experience diagnosing, understanding care, and treatment with etanercept (EDUCATE) study. J Dermatolog Treat [preview article] 2006;1–10. http://journalsonline.tandf.co.uk/openurl.asp?genre=article&id=doi:10.1080/09546630600967166.

34. Callen JP, Krueger GG, Lebwohl M, et al. Summit Planning Group. AAD consensus statement on psoriasis therapies. J Am Acad Dermatol 2003;49:897–9.

35. Nijsten T, Margolis DJ, Feldman SR, Rolstad T, Stern RS. Traditional systemic treatments have not fully met the needs of psoriasis patients: results from a national survey. J Am Acad Dermatol 2005;52:434–44.

36. Mease P, Goffe BS. Diagnosis and treatment of psoriatic arthritis. J Am Acad Dermatol 2005;52:1–19.

37. Krueger GG, Feldman SR, Camisa C, et al. Two considerations for patients with psoriasis and their clinicians: What defines mild, moderate, and severe psoriasis? What constitutes a clinically significant improvement when treating psoriasis? J Am Acad Dermatol 2000;43:281–5.

38. Smith CH, Anstey AV, Barker JNWN, et al. British Association of Dermatologists guidelines for use of biological interventions in psoriasis 2005. Br J Dermatol 2005;153:486–97.

39. Myers W, Christiansen L, Gottlieb AB. Treatment of palmoplantar psoriasis with intramuscular alefacept. J Am Acad Dermatol 2005;53:S127–9.

40. Prossick TA, Belsito DV. Alefacept in the treatment of recalcitrant palmoplantar and erythrodermic psoriasis. Cutis 2006;78:178–80.

41. Weinberg JM. Successful treatment of recalcitrant palmoplantar psoriasis with etanercept. Cutis 2003;72:396–8.

42. Sobell J, Fretzin S. Case studies of efalizumab in hand and foot psoriasis [abstract]. J Am Acad Dermatol 2006;54:AB214.

43. Pearce D, Feldman S, Goffe B. Evaluation of alefacept for the treatment of palmoplantar psoriasis [abstract]. J Am Acad Dermatol 2006;54:AB218.

44. Rivard J, Scherschun L. Treatment of Palmoplantar psoriasis with efalizumab [abstract]. J Am Acad Dermatol 2006;54:AB226.

45. Esposito M, Mazzotta A, de Felice C, Papoutsaki M, Chimenti S. Treatment of erythrodermic psoriasis with etanercept. Br J Dermatol 2006;155:156–9.

46. Weisenseel P, Prinz JC. Sequential use of infliximab and etanercept in generalized pustular psoriasis. Cutis 2006;78:197–9.

47. Trent JT, Kerdel FA. Successful treatment of Von Zumbusch pustular psoriasis with infliximab. J Cutan Med Surg 2004;8:224–8.

48. Benoit S, Toksoy A, Bröcker EB, Gillitzer R, Goebeler M. Treatment of recalcitrant pustular psoriasis with infliximab: effective reduction of chemokine expression. Br J Dermatol 2004;150:1009–12.

49. Schmick K, Grabbe J. Recalcitrant, generalized pustular psoriasis: rapid and lasting therapeutic response to antitumour necrosis factor-α antibody (infliximab). Br J Dermatol 2004;150:367.

50. Newland MR, Weinstein A, Kerdel F. Rapid response to infliximab in severe pustular psoriasis, von Zumbusch type. Int J Dermatol 2002;41:449–52.

51. Gottlieb AB, Lifshitz B, Fu SM, Staiano-Coico L, Wang CY, Carter DM. Expression of HLA-DR molecules by keratinocytes, and presence of Langerhans cells in the dermal infiltrate of active psoriatic plaques. J Exp Med 1986;164:1013–28.

52. Orencia (abatacept) [package insert]. Princeton, NJ: Bristol-Myers Squibb, 2005.

53. Gottlieb AB, Kang S, Linden KG, et al. Evaluation of safety and clinical activity of multiple doses of the anti-CD80 monoclonal antibody, galiximab, in patients with moderate to severe plaque psoriasis. Clin Immunol 2004;111:28–37.

54. Amevive (alefacept) [package insert]. Deerfield, IL: Astellas Pharma US, 2006.

55. Chamian F, Lowes MA, Lin SL, et al. Alefacept reduces infiltrating T cells, activated dendritic cells, and inflammatory genes in psoriasis vulgaris. Proc Natl Acad Sci USA 2005;102:2075–80.

56. da Silva AJ, Brickelmaier M, Majeau GR, et al. Alefacept, an immunomodulatory recombinant LFA-3/IgG1 fusion protein, induces CD16 signaling and CD2/CD16–dependent apoptosis of CD2+ cells. J Immunol 2002;168:4462–71.

57. Cooper JC, Morgan G, Harding S, et al. Alefacept selectively promotes NK cell-mediated deletion of CD45R0+ human T cells. Eur J Immunol 2003;33:666–75.

58. Krueger J, Gilleaudeau P, Kikuchi T, Lee E. Psoriasis-related subpopulations of memory CD4+ and CD8+ T cells are selectively reduced by alefacept [abstract]. J Invest Dermatol 2002;119:345.

59. Goedkoop AY, de Rie MA, Picavet DI, et al. Alefacept therapy reduces the effector T-cell population in lesional psoriatic epidermis. Arch Dermatol Res 2004;295:465–73.

60. Ortonne JP, Lebwohl M, Em Griffiths C. Alefacept-induced decreases in circulating blood lymphocyte counts correlate with clinical response in patients with chronic plaque psoriasis. Eur J Dermatol 2003;13:117–23.

61. Gordon KB, Vaishnaw AK, O'Gorman J, Haney J, Menter A. The Alefacept Clinical Study Group. Treatment of Psoriasis with Alefacept: correlation of clinical improvement with reductions of memory T-cell counts. Arch Dermatol 2003;139:1563–70.

62. Ellis CN, Krueger GG. Alefacept Clinical Study Group. Treatment of chronic plaque psoriasis by selective targeting of memory effector T lymphocytes. N Engl J Med 2001;345:248–55.

63. Lebwohl M, Christophers E, Langley R, Ortonne JP, Roberts J, Griffiths CEM. Alefacept Clinical Study Group. An international, randomized, double-blind, placebo-controlled phase 3 trial of intramuscular alefacept in patients with chronic plaque psoriasis. Arch Dermatol 2003;139:719–27.

64. Gottlieb AB, Casale TB, Frankel E, et al. CD4+ t-cell-directed antibody responses are maintained in patients with psoriasis receiving alefacept: results of a randomized study. J Am Acad Dermatol 2003;49:816–25.

65. Krueger GG, Papp KA, Stough DB, Loven KH, Gulliver WP, Ellis CN. Alefacept Clinical Study Group. A randomized, double-blind, placebo-controlled phase III study evaluating efficacy and tolerability of 2 courses of alefacept in patients with chronic plaque psoriasis. J Am Acad Dermatol 2002;47:821–33.

66. Tan J, Salahuddin K, Malaviya R, Gottieb A. Alefacept induces late-onset apoptosis in infiltrating dermal cells in psoriatic plaques from clinically responsive patients [abstract]. J Am Acad Dermatol 2006;54:AB200.

67. Krueger GG, Ellis CN. Alefacept therapy produces remission for patients with chronic plaque psoriasis. Br J Dermatol 2003;148:784–8.

68. Lowe NJ, Gonzalez J, Bagel J, Caro I, Ellis CN, Menter A. Repeat courses of intravenous alefacept in patients with chronic plaque psoriasis provide consistent safety and efficacy. Int J Dermatol 2003;42:224–30.

69. Gordon KB, Langley RG. Remittive effects of intramuscular alefacept in psoriasis. J Drugs Dermatol 2003;2:624–8.

70. Menter A, Cather JC, Baker D, Farber HF, Lebwohl M, Darif M. The efficacy of multiple courses of alefacept

in patients with moderate to severe chronic plaque psoriasis. J Am Acad Dermatol 2006;54:61–3.

71. Goffe B, Papp K, Gratton D, et al. An integrated analysis of thirteen trials summarizing the long-term safety of alefacept in psoriasis patients who have received up to nine courses of therapy. Clin Ther 2005;27:1912–21.

72. Gottlieb AB, Boehncke WH, Darif M. Safety and efficacy of alefacept in elderly patients and other special populations. J Drugs Dermatol 2005;4:718–24.

73. Thaçi D, Pätzold S, Kaufmann R, Boehncke WH. Treatment of psoriasis with alefacept in patients with hepatitis C infection: a report of two cases. Br J Dermatol 2005;152:1048–50.

74. Kraan MC, van Kuijk AWR, Dinant HJ, et al. Alefacept treatment in psoriatic arthritis: reduction of the effector T cell population in peripheral blood and synovial tissue is associated with improvement of clinical signs of arthritis. Arthritis Rheum 2002;46:2776–84.

75. Mease PJ, Gladman DD, Keystone EC. Alefacept in Psoriatic Arthritis Study Group. Alefacept in combination with methotrexate for the treatment of psoriatic arthritis. Arthritis Rheum 2006;54:1638–45.

76. Raptiva (efalizumab) [package insert]. San Francisco, CA: Genentech, 2005.

77. Gottlieb AB, Miller B, Lowe N, et al. Subcutaneously administered efalizumab (anti-CD11a) improves signs and symptoms of moderate to severe plaque psoriasis. J Cutan Med Surg 2003;7:198–207.

78. Vugmeyster Y, Kikuchi T, Lowes MA, et al. Efalizumab (anti-CD11a)-induced increase in peripheral blood leukocytes in psoriasis patients is preferentially mediated by altered trafficking of memory CD8+ T cells into lesional skin. Clin Immunol 2004;113:38–46.

79. Gottlieb AB, Krueger JG, Wittkowski K, Dedrick R, Walicke PA, Garovoy M. Psoriasis as a model for T-cell-mediated disease: immunobiologic and clinical effects of treatment with multiple doses of efalizumab, an anti-CD11a antibody. Arch Dermatol 2002;138:591–600.

80. Lowes MA, Chamian F, Abello MV, et al. Increase in TNF-α and inducible nitric oxide synthase-expressing dendritic cells in psoriasis and reduction with efalizumab (anti-CD11a). Proc Natl Acad Sci USA 2005;102:19057–62.

81. Joshi A, Bauer R, Kuebler P, et al. An overview of the pharmacokinetics and pharmacodynamics of efalizumab:a monoclonal antibody approved for use in psoriasis. J Clin Pharmacol 2006;46:10–20.

82. Gupta A, Cherman A. Use of efalizumab in special populations [abstract]. J Am Acad Dermatol 2006;54:AB227.

83. Dubertret L, Sterry W, Bos JD, et al. CLEAR Multinational Study Group. CLinical experience acquired with the efalizumab (Raptiva®) (CLEAR) trial in patients with moderate-to-severe plaque psoriasis: results from a phase III international randomized, placebo-controlled trial. Br J Dermatol 2006;155:170–81.

84. Ortonne JP, Shear N, Shumack S, Henninger E. CLEAR Multinational Study Group. Impact of efalizumab on patient-reported outcomes in high-need psoriasis patients: results of the international, randomized, placebo-controlled Phase III Clinical Experience Acquired with Raptiva (CLEAR) trial [NCT00256139]. BMC Dermatol [online] 2005;5:13. http://www.biomedcentral.com/1471–5945/5/13.

85. Carey W, Glazer S, Gottlieb AB, et al. Relapse, rebound, and psoriasis adverse events:an advisory group report. J Am Acad Dermatol 2006;54:S171–81.

86. Gottlieb AB, Hamilton T, Caro I, Kwon P, Compton PG, Leonardi CL. Efalizumab Study Group. Long-term continuous efalizumab therapy in patients with moderate to severe chronic plaque psoriasis: updated results from an ongoing trial. J Am Acad Dermatol 2006;54:S154–63.

87. Gottlieb A, Gordon K, Hamilton T, Leonardi C. Maintenance of efficacy and safety with continuous efalizumab therapy in patients with moderate to severe chronic plaque psoriasis: final phase IIIb study results [abstract]. J Am Acad Dermatol 2005;52:P4.

88. Lebwohl M, Tyring SK, Hamilton TK, et al. Efalizumab Study Group. A novel targeted T-cell modulator, efalizumab, for plaque psoriasis. N Engl J Med 2003;349:2004–13.

89. Menter A, Gordon K, Carey W, et al. Efficacy and safety observed during 24 weeks of efalizumab therapy in patients with moderate to severe plaque psoriasis. Arch Dermatol 2005;141:31–8.

90. Leonardi CL, Papp KA, Gordon KB, et al. Efalizumab Study Group. Extended efalizumab therapy improves chronic plaque psoriasis: results from a randomized phase III trial. J Am Acad Dermatol 2005;52:425–33.

91. Papp KA, Miller B, Gordon KB, et al. Efalizumab Study Group. Efalizumab retreatment in patients with moderate to severe chronic plaque psoriasis. J Am Acad Dermatol 2006;54:S164–70.

92. Gordon KB, Papp KA, Hamilton TK, et al. Efalizumab Study Group. Efalizumab for patients with moderate to severe plaque psoriasis: a randomized controlled trial. JAMA 2003;290:3073–80.

93. Warkentin TE, Kwon P. Immune thrombocytopenia associated with efalizumab therapy for psoriasis. Ann Intern Med 2005;143:761–3.

94. Lowes MA, Turton JA, Krueger JG, Barnetson RS. Psoriasis vulgaris flare during efalizumab therapy

does not preclude future use: a case series. BMC Dermatol [online] 2005;5:9. http://www.biomed-central.com/1471-5945/5/9.

95. Papp KA, Mease PJ, Garovoy MR, Kardatzke D, Leonardi CL. Efalizumab in patients with psoriatic arthritis: results of a phase II, randomized, double-blind, placebo-controlled study. Presented at the 10th International Psoriasis Symposium, June 10–13, 2004, Toronto, Canada; poster 28.

96. Papp K, Hamilton T, Casset-Semanaz F, Curtin F. Safety analysis of efalizumab in the incidence of adverse events for arthropathy: a pooled analysis of 7 clinical trials [abstract]. J Am Acad Dermatol 2006;54:AB 207.

97. Pincelli C, Henninger E, Casset-Semanaz F. Efalizumab therapy and incidence of arthropathy adverse events: a pooled safety analysis from seven clinical trials. Presented at the 15th Congress of the European Academy of Dermatology and Venereology, October 4–8, 2006, Rhodes, Greece.

97a. Myers WA, Najarian D, Gottlieb AB. New onset debilitating arthritis in patients receiving efalizumab. J Dermatolog Treat 2006;17:353–4.

98. Clark GJ, Angel N, Kato M, et al. The role of dendritic cells in the innate immune system. Microbes Infect 2000;2:257–72.

99. Faulkner L, Cooper A, Fantino C, Altmann DM, Sriskandan S. The mechanism of superantigen-mediated toxic shock: not a simple Th1 cytokine storm. J Immunol 2005;175:6870–7.

100. Gottlieb AB. Clinical research helps elucidate the role of tumor necrosis factor-alpha in the pathogenesis of T1–mediated immune disorders: use of targeted immunotherapeutics as pathogenic probes. Lupus 2003;12:190–4.

101. Köck A, Schwarz T, Kirnbauer R, et al. Human keratinocytes are a source for tumor necrosis factor alpha: evidence for synthesis and release upon stimulation with endotoxin or ultraviolet light. J Exp Med 190;172:1609–14.

102. Lizzul PF, Aphale A, Malaviya R, et al. Differential expression of phosphorylated NF-kappaB/RelA in normal and psoriatic epidermis and downregulation of NF-kappaB in response to treatment with etanercept. J Invest Dermatol 2005;124:1275–83.

103. Danning CL, Illei GG, Hitchon C, Greer MR, Boumpas DT, McInnes IB. Macrophage-derived cytokine and nuclear factor kappaB p65 expression in synovial membrane and skin of patients with psoriatic arthritis. Arthritis Rheum 2000;43:1244–56.

104. Papp KA, Tyring S, Lahfa M, et al. Etanercept Psoriasis Study Group. A global phase III randomized controlled trial of etanercept in psoriasis:

safety, efficacy, and effect of dose reduction. Br J Dermatol 2005;152:1304–12.

105. Leonardi CL, Powers JL, Matheson RT, et al. Etanercept Psoriasis Study Group. Etanercept as monotherapy in patients with psoriasis. N Engl J Med 2003;349:2014–22.

106. Gottlieb AB, Gordon KB, Wang A, Zitnik R. Durability of treatment response following withdrawal from etanercept in psoriasis patients. J Invest Dermatol 2004;122:A51–306.

107. Tyring S, Gottlieb A, Papp K, et al. Etanercept and clinical outcomes, fatigue, and depression in psoriasis: double-blind placebo-controlled randomised phase III trial. Lancet 2006;367:29–35.

108. Mease PJ, Goffe BS, Metz J, VanderStoep A, Finck B, Burge DJ. Etanercept in the treatment of psoriatic arthritis and psoriasis: a randomised trial. Lancet 2000;356:385–90.

109. Gottlieb AB, Masud S, Ramamurthi R, et al. Pharmacodynamic and pharmacokinetic response to anti-tumor necrosis factor- monoclonal antibody (infliximab) treatment of moderate to severe psoriasis vulgaris. J Am Acad Dermatol 2003;48:68–75.

110. Chaudhari U, Romano P, Mulcahy LD, Dooley LT, Baker DG, Gottlieb AB. Efficacy and safety of infliximab monotherapy for plaque-type psoriasis: a randomised trial. Lancet 2001;357:1842–7.

111. Gottlieb AB, Evans R, Li S, et al. Infliximab induction therapy for patients with severe plaque-type psoriasis: a randomized, double-blind, placebo-controlled trial. J Am Acad Dermatol 2004;51:534–42.

112. Reich K, Nestle FO, Papp K, et al. EXPRESS study investigators. Infliximab induction and maintenance therapy for moderate-to-severe psoriasis: a phase III, multicentre, double-blind trial. Lancet 2005;366:1367–74.

113. Menter A, Feldman SR, Weinstein GD, et al. A randomized comparison of continuous vs. intermittent infliximab maintenance regimens over 1 year in the treatment of moderate-to-severe plaque psoriasis. J Am Acad Dermatol [online] 2007;56:31. e1–31.e15. Published online September 4, 2006. doi:10.1016/j.jaad.2006.07.017.

114. Mease PJ, Gladman DD, Ritchlin CT, etal. Adalimumab Effectiveness in Psoriatic Arthritis Trial Study Group. Adalimumab for the treatment of patients with moderately to severely active psoriatic arthritis: results of a double-blind, randomized, placebo-controlled trial. Arthritis Rheum 2005;52:3279–89.

115. Enbrel (etanercept) [package insert]. Thousand Oaks, CA: Amgen and Wyeth Pharmaceuticals, Immunex Corp., 2005.

116. Remicade (infliximab) [package insert]. Malvern, PA: Centocor, 2006.

117. Humira (adalimumab) [package insert]. North Chicago, IL: Abbott Laboratories, 2006.

118. Cimzia shows promise in treatment of psoriasis: significant positive results in 12–week phase II trial [press release]. Brussels, Belgium: UCB, July 18, 2006.

119. Malaviya R, Sun Y, Tan JK, et al. Etanercept induces apoptosis of dermal dendritic cells in psoriatic plaques of responding patients. J Am Acad Dermatol 2006;55:590–7.

120. Krueger GG, Elewski B, Papp K, Wang A, Zitnik R, Jahreis A. Patients with psoriasis respond to continuous open-label etanercept treatment after initial incomplete response in a randomized, placebo-controlled trial. J Am Acad Dermatol 2006;54: S112–9.

121. Gordon KB, Gottlieb AB, Leonardi CL, et al. Etanercept Psoriasis Study Group. Clinical response in psoriasis patients discontinued from and then reinitiated on etanercept therapy. J Dermatolog Treat 2006;17:9–17.

122. Moore A, Gordon KB, Kang S, et al. A randomized, open-label trial of continuous versus interrupted etanercept therapy in the treatment of psoriasis. J Am Acad Dermatol 2007;56:598–603.

123. Tyring S, Gordon K, Poulin Y, et al. Long term safety and efficacy of 50 mg of etanercept twice weekly in patients with psoriasis. Arch Dermatol 2007;143:719–26.

124. Mease PJ, Kivitz AJ, Burch FX, et al. Continued inhibition of radiographic progression in patients with psoriatic arthritis following 2 years of treatment with etanercept. J Rheumatol 2006;33: 712–21.

125. de Vlam K, Lories RJU. Efficacy, effectiveness and safety of etanercept in monotherapy for refractory psoriatic arthritis: a 26-week observational study. Rheumatology 2006;45:321–4.

126. Gottlieb AB, Leonardi CL, Goffe BS, et al. Etanercept monotherapy in patients with psoriasis: a summary of safety, based on an integrated multistudy database. J Am Acad Dermatol 2006;54:S92–100.

127. Zeltser R, Valle L, Tanck C, Holyst MM, Ritchlin C, Gaspari AA. Clinical, histological, and immunophenotypic characteristics of injection site reactions associated with etanercept: a recombinant tumor necrosis factor alpha receptor: Fc fusion protein. Arch Dermatol 2001;137:893–9.

128. Myers W, Newman M, Katz B, Gottlieb AB. Ability to develop rhus allergic contact dermatitis in a patient with psoriasis receiving etanercept. J Am Acad Dermatol 2006;55:S127–128.

129. Mease PJ, Ritchlin CT, Martin RW, et al. Pneumococcal vaccine response in psoriatic arthritis patients during treatment with etanercept. J Rheumatol 2004;31:1356–61.

130. Siegfried E, Levy M, Jahreis A, Paller A. Etanercept in children and adolescents with psoriasis [abstract]. J Am Acad Dermatol 2006;54:AB 218.

131. Militello G, Xia A, Stevens SR, Van Voorhees AS. Etanercept for the treatment of psoriasis in the elderly. J Am Acad Dermatol 2006;55:517–9.

132. Khanna M, Shirodkar MA, Gottlieb AB. Etanercept therapy in patients with autoimmunity and hepatitis C. J Dermatol Treat 2003;14:229–32.

133. Magliocco MA, Gottlieb AB. Etanercept therapy for patients with psoriatic arthritis and concurrent hepatitis C virus infection: report of 3 cases. J Am Acad Dermatol 2004;51:580–4.

134. De Simone C, Paradisi A, Capizzi R, Carbone A, Siciliano M, Amerio PL. Etanercept therapy in two patients with psoriasis and concomitant hepatitis C. J Am Acad Dermatol 2006;54:1102–4.

135. Strober B, Gottlieb A, Leonardi C, Papp K. Levels of response of psoriasis patients with different baseline characteristics treated with etanercept [abstract]. J Am Acad Dermatol 2006;54:AB 220.

136. Kavanaugh A, Antoni CE, Gladman D, et al. The Impact Study Group. The infliximab multinational psoriatic arthritis controlled trial (IMPACT): results of radiographic analyses after 1 year. Ann Rheum Dis 2006;65:1038–43.

137. Krüger-Krasagakis S, Galanopoulos VK, Giannikaki L, Stefanidou M, Tosca AD. Programmed cell death of keratinocytes in infliximab-treated plaque-type psoriasis. Br J Dermatol 2006;154:460–6.

138. Markham T, Matthews C, Rogers S, et al. Downregulation of the inhibitor of apoptosis protein survivin in keratinocytes and endothelial cells in psoriasis skin following infliximab therapy. Br J Dermatol 2006;155:1191–6.

139. Markham T, Mullan R, Golden-Mason L, et al. Resolution of endothelial activation and down-regulation of Tie2 receptor in psoriatic skin after infliximab therapy. J Am Acad Dermatol 2006;54:1003–12.

140. Mease P, Gladman D, Ritchlin C, Weinberg M. Clinical efficacy, safety and inhibition of joint destruction of adalimumab in the treatment of moderate to severe psoriatic arthritis: 48-week results of the ADEPT trial [abstract]. J Am Acad Dermatol 2006;54:AB 214.

141. Gordon KB, Langley RG, Leonardi C, et al. Clinical response to adalimumab treatment in patients with moderate to severe psoriasis: double-blind, randomized controlled trial and open-label extension study. J Am Acad Dermatol 2006;55:598–606.

142. Bartelds GM, Wolbink GJ, Stapel S, et al. High levels of human anti-human antibodies to adalimumab in a patient not responding to adalimumab treatment. Ann Rheum Dis 2006;65:1249–50.

143. Gordon KB, Bonish BK, Patel T, Leonardi CL, Nickoloff BJ. The tumor necrosis factor-α inhibitor adalimumab rapidly reverses the decrease in epidermal Langerhans cell density in psoriatic plaques. Br J Dermatol 2005;153:945–53.

144. Katz JA, Antoni C, Keenan GF, Smith DE, Jacobs SJ, Lichtenstein GR. Outcome of pregnancy in women receiving infliximab for the treatment of Crohn's disease and rheumatoid arthritis. Am J Gastroenterol 2004;99:2385–92.

145. Sills ES, Perloe M, Tucker MJ, Kaplan CR, Palermo GD. Successful ovulation induction, conception, and normal delivery after chronic therapy with etanercept: a recombinant fusion anti-cytokine treatment for rheumatoid arthritis. Am J Reprod Immunol 2001;46:366–8.

146. Mishkin DS, Van Deinse W, Becker JM, Farraye FA. Successful use of adalimumab (Humira) for Crohn's disease in pregnancy. Inflamm Bowel Dis 2006;12:827–8.

147. Mahadevan U, Kane S, Sandborn WJ, et al. Intentional infliximab use during pregnancy for induction or maintenance of remission in Crohn's disease. Aliment Pharmacol Ther 2005;21:733–8.

148. Mor A, Bingham CO 3rd, Barisoni L, Lydon E, Belmont HM. Proliferative lupus nephritis and leukocytoclastic vasculitis during treatment with etanercept. J Rheumatol 2005;32:740–3.

149. Chadha T, Hernandez JE. Infliximab-related lupus and associated valvulitis: a case report and review of the literature. Arthritis Rheum 2006;55:163–6.

150. Ali Y, Shah S. Infliximab-induced systemic lupus erythematosus. Ann Intern Med 2002;137:625–6.

151. Cairns AP, Duncan MKJ, Hinder AE, Taggart AJ. New onset systemic lupus erythematosus in a patient receiving etanercept for rheumatoid arthritis. Ann Rheum Dis 2002;61:1031–2.

152. Favalli EG, Sinigaglia L, Varenna M, Arnoldi C. Drug-induced lupus following treatment with infliximab in rheumatoid arthritis. Lupus 2002;11:753–5.

153. Pallotta P, Cianchini G, Ruffelli M, Puddu P. Infliximab-induced lupus-like reaction in a patient with psoriatic arthritis. Rheumatology 2006;45:116–7.

154. Sarzi-Puttini P, Ardizzone S, Manzionna G, et al. Infliximab-induced lupus in Crohn's disease: a case report. Dig Liver Dis 2003;35:814–7.

155. Perez-Garcia C, Maymo J, Lisbona Perez MP, Almirall Bernabe M, Carbonell Abello J. Drug-induced systemic lupus erythematosus in anky-losing spondylitis associated with infliximab. Rheumatology 2006;45:114–6.

156. Shakoor N, Michalska M, Harris CA, Block JA. Drug-induced systemic lupus erythematosus associated with etanercept therapy. Lancet 2002;359:579–80.

157. Carlson E, Rothfield N. Etanercept-induced lupus-like syndrome in a patient with rheumatoid arthritis. Arthritis Rheum 2003;48:1165–6.

158. Benucci M, Li Gobbi F, Fossi F, Manfredi M, Del Rosso A. Drug-induced lupus after treatment with infliximab in rheumatoid arthritis. J Clin Rheumatol 2005;11:47–9.

159. Klapman JB, Ene-Stroescu D, Becker MA, Hanauer SB. A lupus-like syndrome associated with infliximab therapy. Inflamm Bowel Dis 2003;9:176–8.

160. Stratigos AJ, Antoniou C, Stamathioudaki S, Avgerinou G, Tsega A, Katsambas AD. Discoid lupus erythematosus-like eruption induced by infliximab. Clin Exp Dermatol 2004;29:150–3.

161. Brion PH, Mittal-Henkle A, Kalunian KC. Autoimmune skin rashes associated with etanercept for rheumatoid arthritis. Ann Intern Med 1999;131:634.

162. High WA, Muldrow ME, Fitzpatrick JE. Cutaneous lupus erythematosus induced by infliximab. J Am Acad Dermatol [online] 2005;52:E5. Published online March 4, 2005. doi:10.1016/S0190–9622(03)00869–7.

163. Schneider SW, Staender S, Schlüter B, Luger TA, Bonsmann G. Infliximab-induced lupus erythematosus tumidus in a patient with rheumatoid arthritis. Arch Dermatol 2006;142:115–6.

164. Patel T, Gordon KB. Adalimumab: efficacy and safety in psoriasis and rheumatoid arthritis. Dermatol Ther 2004;17:427–31.

165. Bongartz T, Sutton AJ, Sweeting MJ, Buchan I, Matteson EL, Montori V. Anti-TNF antibody therapy in Rheumatoid Arthritis and the risk of serious infections and malignancies:systematic review and meta-analysis of rare harmful effects in randomized controlled trials. JAMA 2006;295:2275–85.

166. Baecklund E, Iliadou A, Askling J, et al. Association of chronic inflammation, not its treatment, with increased lymphoma risk in rheumatoid arthritis. Arthritis Rheum 2006;54:692–701.

167. Gelfand JM, Shin DB, Neimann AL, Wang X, Margolis DJ, Troxel AB. The risk of lymphoma in patients with psoriasis. J Invest Dermatol 2006;126:2194–2201.

168. Okada SK, Siegel JN. Risk of serious infections and malignancies with anti-TNF antibody therapy in rheumatoid arthritis [letter to the editor]. JAMA 2006;296:2201–2.

169. Moreland LW, Weinblatt ME, Keystone EC, et al. Etanercept treatment in adults with established rheumatoid arthritis: 7 years of clinical experience. J Rheumatol 2006;33:854–61.

170. Elewski B, Leonardi C, Gottlieb A, Strober B. Sustained long-term clinical efficacy and safety for up to 2.5 years of etanercept in patients with psoriasis [abstract]. J Am Acad Dermatol 2006;54:AB 225.

171. Chakravarty EF, Michaud K, Wolfe F. Skin cancer, rheumatoid arthritis, and tumor necrosis factor inhibitors. J Rheumatol 2005;32:2130–5.

172. Hubbard VG, Friedmann AC, Goldsmith P. Systemic pyoderma gangrenosum responding to infliximab and adalimumab. Br J Dermatol 2005;152:1059–61.

173. Roy DB, Conte ET, Cohen DJ. The treatment of pyoderma gangrenosum using etanercept. J Am Acad Dermatol 2006;54:S128–34.

174. McGowan JW 4th, Johnson CA, Lynn A. Treatment of pyoderma gangrenosum with etanercept. J Drugs Dermatol 2004;3:441–4.

175. Kaur MR, Lewis HM. Severe recalcitrant pyoderma gangrenosum treated with infliximab. Br J Dermatol 2005;153:689–91.

176. Kouklakis G, Moschos J, Leontiadis GI, et al. Infliximab for treatment of pyoderma gangrenosum associated with clinically inactive Crohn's disease: a case report. Rom J Gastroenterol 2005;14:401–3.

177. Swale VJ, Saha M, Kapur N, Hoffbrand AV, Rustin MHA. Pyoderma gangrenosum outside the context of inflammatory bowel disease treated successfully with infliximab. Clin Exp Dermatol 2005;30:134–6.

178. Stichweh DS, Punaro M, Pascual V. Dramatic improvement of pyoderma gangrenosum with infliximab in a patient with PAPA syndrome. Pediatr Dermatol 2005;22:262–5.

179. Brooklyn TN, Dunnill MGS, Shetty A, et al. Infliximab for the treatment of pyoderma gangrenosum: a randomised, double blind, placebo controlled trial. Gut 2006;55:505–9.

180. Cusack C, Buckley C. Etanercept: effective in the management of hidradenitis suppurativa. Br J Dermatol 2006;154:726–9.

181. Sullivan TP, Welsh E, Kerdel FA, Burdick AE, Kirsner RS. Infliximab for hidradenitis suppurativa. Br J Dermatol 2003;149:1046–9.

182. Rosi YL, Lowe L, Kang S. Treatment of hidradenitis suppurativa with infliximab in a patient with Crohn's disease. J Dermatolog Treat 2005;16:58–61.

183. Adams DR, Gordon KB, Devenyi AG, Ioffreda MD. Severe hidradenitis suppurativa treated with infliximab infusion. Arch Dermatol 2003;139:1540–2.

184. Lebwohl B, Sapadin AN. Infliximab for the treatment of hidradenitis suppurativa. J Am Acad Dermatol 2003;49:S275–6.

185. Katsanos KH, Christodoulou DK, Tsianos EV. Axillary hidradenitis suppurativa successfully treated with infliximab in a Crohn's disease patient. Am J Gastroenterol 2002;97:2155–6.

186. Martinez F, Nos P, Benlloch S, Ponce J. Hidradenitis suppurativa and Crohn's disease: response to treatment with infliximab. Inflamm Bowel Dis 2001;7:323–6.

187. Moul DK, Korman NJ. Severe hidradenitis suppurativa treated with adalimumab. Arch Dermatol 2006;142:1110–2.

188. Scheinfeld N. Treatment of coincident seronegative arthritis and hidradenitis suppurativa with adalimumab. J Am Acad Dermatol 2006;55:163–4.

189. Mallbris L, Ljungberg A, Hedblad MA, Larsson P, Stahle-Backdahl M. Progressive cutaneous sarcoidosis responding to anti-tumor necrosis factor-alpha therapy. J Am Acad Dermatol 2003;48:290–3.

190. Heffernan MP, Anadkat MJ. Recalcitrant cutaneous sarcoidosis responding to infliximab. Arch Dermatol 2005;141:910–1.

191. Haley H, Cantrell W, Smith K. Infliximab therapy for sarcoidosis (lupus pernio). Br J Dermatol 2004;150:146–9.

192. Heffernan MP, Smith DI. Adalimumab for treatment of cutaneous sarcoidosis. Arch Dermatol 2006;142:17–9.

193. Philips MA, Lynch J, Azmi FH. Ulcerative cutaneous sarcoidosis responding to adalimumab. J Am Acad Dermatol 2005;53:917.

194. Tuchinda C, Wong HK. Etanercept for chronic progressive cutaneous sarcoidosis. J Drugs Dermatol 2006;5:538–40.

195. Khanna D, Liebling MR, Louie JS. Etanercept ameliorates sarcoidosis arthritis and skin disease. J Rheumatol 2003;30:1864–7.

196. Piskin G, Tursen U, Sylva-Steenland RMR, Bos JD, Teunissen MBM. Clinical improvement in chronic plaque-type psoriasis lesions after narrow-band UVB therapy is accompanied by a decrease in the expression of INF- inducers—IL-12, IL-18, and IL-23. Exp Dermatol 2004;13:764–72.

197. Tada Y, Asahina A, Takekoshi T, et al. Interleukin 12 production by monocytes from patients with psoriasis and its inhibition by cyclosporin A. Br J Dermatol 2006;154:1180–3.

198. Lee E, Trepicchio WL, Oestreicher JL, et al. Increased expression of interleukin 23 p19 and p40 in lesional skin of patients with psoriasis vulgaris. J Exp Med 2004;199:125–30.

199. Shaker OG, Moustafa W, Essmat S, Abdel-Halim M, El-Komy M. The role of interleukin-12 in the pathogenesis of psoriasis. Clin Biochem 2006;39:119–25.

200. Piskin G, Sylva-Steenland RMR, Bos JD, Teunissen MBM. In vitro and in situ expression of IL-23 by keratinocytes in healthy skin and psoriasis lesions: enhanced expression in psoriatic skin. J Immunol 2006;176:1908–15.
201. Tsunemi Y, Saeki H, Nakamura K, et al. Interleukin-12 p40 gene (IL12B) 3'-untranslated region polymorphism is associated with susceptibility to atopic dermatitis and psoriasis vulgaris. J Dermatol Sci 2002;30:161–6.
202. Krueger GG, Langley R, Leonardi C, Lebwohl M. Results of a phase II study of CNTO 1275 in the treatment of psoriasis [abstract]. J Am Acad Dermatol 2006;54:AB10.

Appendix: Commonly Applied Clinical Trial Endpoints for Psoriasis and PsA[202]

Improvement in psoriasis and PsA can be measured using several clinical scoring systems.

The most commonly used scoring system for skin disease is the Psoriasis Area and Severity Index (PASI). The legs, arms, trunk, and head are each graded for erythema (from 0 to 4), induration (from 0 to 4), and scaliness (from 0 to 4) of lesions, and then the scores are weighted by the amount of body surface area covered by psoriasis on each body part to reach a final PASI score.[202] Total score ranges from 0 to 72. In clinical trials, a responder is someone who achieves a greater than or equal to 75% improvement in PASI score, or a PASI-75 response.[1]

The Physician Global Assessment (PGA) is either a static assessment that estimates global skin disease activity at one point in time or a dynamic assessment of disease activity that considers a patient's improvement from baseline.[2] The static PGA (sPGA or PSGA) is measured on a scale of 0 to 6, where a score of 0 means that a patient is clear of skin disease.[2] The equivalent of a PASI-75 response is a score of 0 (clear) or 1 (almost clear).[1] There is a similar system for subjects to rate their Patient Global Assessment of disease activity.

Common tools used to measure quality of life improvements include the Dermatology Life Quality Index (DLQI) and Medical Outcome Survey Short Form 36 (SF-36).[2] The DLQI is specific to assessing the effects of skin diseases,

and it asks 10 questions regarding symptoms and feelings, daily activities, leisure, work and school, personal relationships, and psoriasis treatments, where each question is graded from 0 to 3 for a total score of 0 to 30.[2] The SF-36 is a general quality of life measurement that is also used in patients with systemic diseases.[2]

In clinical trials, patients with active PsA generally have three or more swollen and tender joints. The American College of Rheumatology (ACR) criteria originally assessed improvement of joint disease in RA patients and have been extended to assess improvement in PsA.[202] The ACR criteria take into account tender joint count (78 joints), swollen joint count (76 joints), patient pain assessment, patient self-assessed disability, patient global assessment, physician global assessment, and acute-phase reactant level in the serum (erythrocyte sedimentation rate [ESR] or C-reactive protein [CRP]).[3] A significant clinical response is ≥20% improvement in the ACR,[1,3] also known as an ACR-20 response, where there is a 20% improvement in tender and swollen joint count as well as in three of the five other components of the criteria.[3]

The Disease Activity Score (DAS) calculates disease activity based on a composite of Ritchie Articular Index (a measurement of joint tenderness), swollen joint count, ESR value, general health, and visual analogue scale (VAS) of joint discomfort.[3] The DAS-28 applies the DAS assessment to 28 joints.[3] Investigators can calculate the mean improvement in disease activity based on this assessment.

The Health Assessment Questionnaire (HAQ) assesses a patient's degree of pain and disability, which is assessed on eight subscales.[3]

The Psoriatic Arthritis Response Criteria (PsARC) measure disease improvement based on a composite of swollen/tender joint counts and assessments of global disease activity.[3]

A medication's effect on radiographic progression of joint disease can be assessed using methods created for rheumatoid arthritis (RA) patients.[3] Investigators examine plain radiographs of the hands (the Sharp method) and the feet (the Van der Heijde modified Sharp method) to grade the joints from 0 to 4 based on abnormalities such as joint space narrowing and bone erosion. The change in these scores over time is a useful measure of disease progression.

29
Topical Immune Response Modifiers: Adjuvants

Annemarie Uliasz and Mark Lebwohl

Key Points

- The topical immune response modifier imiquimod is a low molecular weight heterocycline imidazoquinoline amine.
- Imiquimod stimulates both the innate and the acquired arms of the immune system via induction of T-helper-1 cytokines
- Imiquimod is Food and Drug Administration approved for the treatment of anogenital warts, but is widely used to treat other warts and molluscum contagiosum.
- Nonantiviral uses of imiquimod include actinic keratoses and superficial basal cell carcinomas.

Imiquimod (Aldara™, Graceway Pharmaceuticals), a low-molecular-weight heterocyclic imidazoquinoline amine, is a topical immune modulator that stimulates both the innate and the acquired arms of the immune system. Initially discovered during screening of medications for antiherpes virus activity,[1] imiquimod is Food and Drug Administration (FDA) approved for the treatment of external anogenital warts, superficial basal cell carcinoma, and actinic keratoses. Various case reports and preliminary studies have also suggested imiquimod may be effective in the treatment of a wide range of other infectious, inflammatory, and malignant skin conditions.

Imiquimod offers a noninvasive and tissue-sparing alternative to treatments commonly used for warts or cutaneous tumors such as cryotherapy, electrocautery, surgical excision, laser ablation, trichloroacetic acid, and podofilox. For those individuals who are poor surgical candidates or refuse surgery, or whose anatomic site is not amenable, imiquimod is an effective option. As compared to destructive techniques, imiquimod offers an improved safety profile, as local cytokine production decreases the potential for systemic adverse events. Additionally, imiquimod is less damaging to tissue, resulting in a superior cosmetic outcome. This is especially desirable in treatment of lesions situated in cosmetically sensitive sites including the face, as well as in patients in whom healing from surgical sites is of particular concern. Furthermore, the ease of topical application allows patients to self-treat, which may result in decreased cost and avoidance of multiple clinic visits.

Mechanism of Action

Imiquimod enhances the patient's immune response, stimulating both the innate immune response and the cellular arm of acquired immunity, with resultant antiviral and antitumoral effects.

The innate immune response is stimulated via activation of antigen-presenting cells (APCs) including monocytes, macrophages, and dendritic cells, and the subsequent release of cytokines and chemokines. Imiquimod produces an innate immune response via its action as a Toll-like receptor (TLR) agonist. Toll-like receptors are a family of pattern recognition receptors found on the cell surface of APCs. Specifically, imiquimod binds to TLR-7[2] and TLR-8.[3]

TLR-7 activation by imiquimod triggers a MyD88-dependent signaling cascade.[2] MyD88, a protein that associates with TLRs, acts to recruit

527

protein kinases and transcription factors, resulting in activation of nuclear factor κB (NF-κB). Nuclear factor κB is a transcription factor that, upon activation, migrates to the nucleus and upregulates the production of local proinflammatory cytokines, particularly interferons (IFNs) α, β, and γ, tumor necrosis factor-α (TNF-α), and interleukin-12.[4]

The IFN-α produced by APCs induces CD4[+] T cells to produce the IL-12β2 receptor. The binding of IL-12 to the IL-12β2 receptor induces the secretion of IFN-γ from naive T cells, resulting in a T-helper-1 (Th1) immune response. Conversely, imiquimod suppresses a Th2 immune response by inhibiting IL-4 and IL-5.[5]

Studies have described the effects of imiquimod on Langerhans' cells, the major APCs of the skin.[6] Imiquimod enhances the migration of Langerhans' cells from the skin to regional lymph nodes, potentially enhancing viral and tumoral antigen presentation to naive CD4[+] T cells. This results in differentiation of naive T cells into memory and activated T cells. Upon return to the dermis, the activated T cells produce the Th1 cytokines IFN-α, IFN-γ, and TNF-α. These cytokines are responsible for imiquimod's antiviral and antitumoral effects.

Additionally, imiquimod has been shown to produce apoptosis via circumnavigating mechanisms developed by malignant cells to resist apoptosis signals. One way imiquimod activates apoptosis is via activation of membrane-bound death receptors. For example, imiquimod induces Fas (CD95) receptor (FasR)-mediated apoptosis in basal cell carcinoma cells.[7] Fas, a member of the tumor necrosis receptor family, is a death receptor that mediates apoptosis via CD95 receptor–CD95 ligand (Fas-L) interaction. FasR expression is normally absent on basal cell carcinoma (BCC) cells, allowing tumors to avoid apoptotic signaling. The IFN-α produced by imiquimod induces BCC cells to express FasR.

Another way in which imiquimod induces tumor-selective apoptosis is via the mitochondrial pathway of apoptosis. Imiquimod induces a Bcl-2 –dependent translocation of cytochrome c from the mitochondria to the cytosol.[8,9] This, in turn, leads to activation of caspase-9 and caspase-3 and a subsequent proteolytic cascade, resulting in cell death.

Dosage and Administration

Imiquimod, an off-white, fine crystalline solid, is chemically known as 1-(2-methylpropyl)-1*H*-imidazo[4,5-c]quinolin-4-amine ($C_{14}H_{16}N_4$). The molecular weight of imiquimod is 240.3. Each gram of cream contains 50 mg of imiquimod in an off-white, oil-in-water vanishing base consisting of isostearic acid, cetyl alcohol, stearyl alcohol, white petrolatum, polysorbate 60, sorbitan monostearate, glycerin, xantham gum, purified water, benzyl alcohol, methylparaben, and propylparaben.

Imiquimod cream 5% is supplied in individual 250-mg sachets. One sachet can evenly cover an area of skin up to 386 cm.[2,10] Imiquimod should be applied in a thin layer extending 1 cm beyond the affected area. Imiquimod should be left on the affected area for approximately 8 hours. The frequency of application and duration of therapy depend on the condition being treated.

Safety

Imiquimod is contraindicated in those individuals with hypersensitivity to any of its ingredients. Additionally, it should not be applied in areas of dermatitis, as it has been known to exacerbate inflammatory conditions such as pemphigus, psoriasis, and aphthous ulcers.

Despite case reports of imiquimod use during pregnancy without adverse effects on the fetus, at this time there is insufficient data on the safety of imiquimod in pregnancy to make definitive conclusions.[11] Imiquimod is pregnancy category C. It is unknown if imiquimod is excreted in the breast milk of lactating women.

Application site reactions (erythema, dryness, edema, crusting, weeping, erosion, ulceration, burning, pruritus, and pain) may occur after application of imiquimod cream. Local skin reactions, well tolerated by most patients, are considered a normal and expected part of treatment with imiquimod. The intensity of these reactions tends to increase as dosing frequency increases, and rest periods may be required for some patients. Systemic signs and symptoms such as malaise, nausea, myalgias, fever, and rigors may accompany local inflammatory reactions.

Approved Clinical Uses

External Genital Warts

Anogenital warts, or condyloma acuminata, are a clinical manifestation of human papillomavirus (HPV) infection. The HPV, a nonenveloped double-stranded DNA virus, is classified into more than 100 types, reflecting different oncogenic properties as well as tissue tropism. Anogenital warts are often difficult to eradicate, and most therapies involve lesional destruction. Although lesional destruction results in immediate elimination, these procedures are painful, and recurrence is common, necessitating repeated treatment. Imiquimod, a nondestructive, patient-applied alternative, is unique in that it may be applied by the patient at home, decreasing the number of office visits. More importantly, imiquimod reduces the viral load, thereby decreasing the rate of recurrence.[4]

Imiquimod is FDA approved for the treatment of external anogenital warts in immunocompetent patients over the age of 12 years old. Imiquimod is applied once a day on alternate days (three times per week) until resolution of warts or for up to 16 weeks. Frequency of application may be adjusted according to the local irritation experienced by patients.[12] Those experiencing minimal local irritation may increase the efficacy by increasing the frequency of application, while those experiencing uncomfortable irritation may decrease the frequency of application.

In the treatment of warts, the efficacy of imiquimod is related to reduction of HPV. In a randomized, controlled, molecular study in which tissues were analyzed for HPV DNA and messenger RNA (mRNA) of several cytokines, both a local increase in interferon and a significant reduction in viral load were observed in skin biopsies taken from patients during and following imiquimod treatment.[4] The increased cell-mediated immunity provided by imiquimod results not only in control or reduction of HPV infection, but also in long-term protection from recurrence and reinfection.[4]

Several studies have demonstrated the safety and effectiveness of imiquimod 5% cream for the treatment of external anogenital warts. In a double-blind, placebo-controlled, parallel design study evaluating the safety and efficacy of imiquimod used three times per week for up to 8 weeks,

complete clearance of lesions was observed in 37% of imiquimod-treated subjects.[13]

In another double-blind, placebo-controlled study using imiquimod three times per week for a maximum of 16 weeks, 50% of patients who received imiquimod 5% cream achieved eradication of all treated baseline warts.[14] Of note, 72% of females and 33% of males had complete clearance of warts. The recurrence rate at a 3-month follow-up assessment was determined to be 13%, comparing favorably to physician-administered treatments such as cryotherapy, trichloroacetic acid, and podophyllin.

Similarly, in an international phase III, open-label study evaluating imiquimod 5% cream three times per week for 16 weeks with an additional 16-week period if required, a clearance rate of 53.3% was observed.[15] Of patients who experienced partial clearance in the initial 16-week treatment period, 27.2% reached complete clearance following an additional 16 weeks of treatment. Additionally, patients with recurrence of warts after the initial treatment period achieved a 58.5% clearance rate following reapplication for up to 16 weeks. Again a gender-dependent disparity in results was noted, with 65.4% of women compared to 44.1% of men experiencing complete clearance. This difference was attributed to a higher degree of keratinization of penile skin compared to vulvar skin, the most common sites for genital warts in men and women. Recurrence rates at the end of 3- and 6-month follow-up periods were found to be 8.8% and 23.0%.

Actinic Keratoses

Actinic keratoses (AKs) are precancerous skin lesions frequently occurring on sun-exposed areas of fair-skinned individuals, becoming more prevalent with advanced age. They are precursors to squamous cell carcinoma. Topical therapies are useful alternatives to cryotherapy and excisional surgery for treating areas of diffuse AKs. Furthermore, unlike surgical or ablative treatments, imiquimod possesses the unique capacity to uncover and treat subclinical lesions. Imiquimod is FDA approved for the treatment of facial and scalp AKs in immunocompetent adults. Imiquimod is applied twice weekly for 16 weeks.

Several clinical studies have been performed evaluating the safety and efficacy of imiquimod

5% cream for the treatment of AKs. Persaud and Lebwohl[16] reported the use of topical imiquimod 5% cream for the treatment of AKs on the scalp of three individuals. One subject was treated three times weekly for 4 weeks with nearly complete resolution of AKs accompanied by a marked inflammatory response. Two other subjects treated one half of their scalp with imiquimod, using the other half as comparison. After 8 weeks of two to three times weekly application with frequent rest periods to avoid inflammation, marked reductions in AKs were noted. These patients then continued to use imiquimod cream on both sides of the scalp two times per week for an additional 9 months. Treatment was well tolerated and subsequent reduction in lesions was noted.

Persaud et al.[17] conducted another study in which 22 subjects with at least six bilateral actinic keratoses applied imiquimod or placebo three times a week for 8 weeks. If necessary, a 3-week rest period was allowed, followed by a subsequent reduction in dose frequency. Upon evaluation 8 weeks following treatment, average AK counts were significantly decreased in subjects treated with imiquimod compared to placebo-treated subjects. Of note, 53% of the subjects required rest periods with 18% of the subjects requiring two rest periods.

A randomized, double-blind, vehicle-controlled study was performed in which 25 subjects with AKs on the scalp, forehead, arms, and hands applied imiquimod or placebo three times weekly for 12 weeks.[18] Due to local skin reactions, 48% of the subjects reduced application to twice weekly at week 4 of the study. Clinical and histologic evaluation 2 weeks following the last application showed total resolution of AKs in 84% of those treated with imiquimod. Partial clearance of AKs was seen in 8% of patients treated with imiquimod, while no response was observed in the placebo group. Local skin reactions were tolerated with only one patient requesting a rest period. At a 2-year follow-up evaluation, 20% of subjects in the imiquimod treatment group developed new AKs.[19]

Trials have been performed to identify treatment regimens that optimize efficacy while reducing local skin reactions. An open-label pilot study by Salasche et al.[20] examined imiquimod used in a cycle regimen for the treatment of AKs. Discrete areas containing five to 20 AKs were selected for treatment. Twenty-five patients with 33 treatment areas participated. Imiquimod was applied to the entire treatment area three times a week for 4 weeks followed by a rest period of 4 weeks. If AKs in the treatment area were still present, this cycle was repeated up to three times. Of the 22 patients with 30 treatment areas that completed the study, total clearance of AKs was seen in 46% of the treatment areas after the first cycle and in an additional 36% of the treatment areas after the second cycle. Four patients required rest periods prior to the scheduled 4-week rest period. Of note, AKs continued to clear during the rest periods suggesting that cycle therapy may minimize local reactions while retaining efficacy.

A phase III, randomized, double-blind, parallel group, vehicle-controlled trial involving 286 subjects examined the efficacy and safety of imiquimod versus placebo when applied three times weekly for 16 weeks.[21] Results demonstrated complete clearance in 57.1% of subjects treated with imiquimod as compared to 2.2% of subjects who received vehicle. Partial clearance was seen in 72.1% and 4.3% of subjects in the imiquimod and vehicle groups, respectively.

The results of two other phase III, randomized, double-blind, parallel group, vehicle-controlled trials examined the safety and efficacy of imiquimod applied three times weekly for 16 weeks in the treatment of AKs.[22] Partial and complete clearance rates in subjects in the imiquimod treatment groups were 48.3% and 64.0% as compared to 7.2% and 13.6% in the placebo group.

In comparison to the above studies, which used imiquimod three times weekly, two randomized, double-blind, parallel group, phase III trials involving 436 subjects were conducted evaluating the efficacy and safety of imiquimod applied twice weekly for a duration of 16 weeks in the treatment of facial and scalp AKs.[23] Those treated with imiquimod experienced complete clearance rates of 45.1% compared to 3.2% in the placebo group. Eight weeks posttreatment, the median reduction in baseline lesions was 83%. Furthermore, twice weekly dosing versus three times weekly dosing was associated with fewer local skin reactions, fewer rest periods, and fewer subjects discontinuing treatment due to local skin reactions.

Studies have also demonstrated that imiquimod treatment results in low recurrence rates. One and a half years following the completion of four phase

III studies in which patients applied imiquimod either two or three times weekly for 16 weeks, recurrence rates of approximately 25% (twice weekly application) and 43% (three times weekly application) were noted.[24]

In contrast to other topical treatments for AKs, imiquimod has been shown to be more effective and produce a less severe local skin reaction than 5-fluorouracil (5-FU). A meta-analysis comparing the efficacy of 5-FU and imiquimod in the treatment of AK was performed involving ten studies.[25] Results demonstrated average efficacy rates of 52% for 5-FU and 70% for imiquimod.

Superficial Basal Cell Carcinoma

Arising from the basal layer of the epidermis, BCC is the most common malignancy among Caucasians worldwide.[26] The three most common subtypes are nodular, superficial (sBCC), and morpheaform. Although metastases are rare, BCCs are locally invasive, aggressive, and destructive to the skin and surrounding structures. Treatment is predominantly surgical, consisting of excision, cryosurgery, curettage and electrodesiccation, and Mohs' micrographic surgery. Although surgery offers a high cure rate, imiquimod is an effective alternative and should be considered in cases where patients are poor surgical candidates or cosmetic outcome is a concern.

Imiquimod is FDA approved for the treatment of biopsy-confirmed superficial BCC in immunocompetent adults when surgical methods are less appropriate and when patients may be reliably monitored. Imiquimod is applied five times per week for 6 weeks. Studies have shown that occlusion does not yield a statistically significant effect on the efficacy of imiquimod against BCCs.[27]

Numerous trials evaluating the safety and efficacy of imiquimod 5% cream for the treatment of sBCCs have been performed. A randomized, double-blind pilot study by Beutner et al.[28] involving 35 patients demonstrated the safety and efficacy of imiquimod for the treatment of BCC. The study examined five different treatment regimens, each lasting up to 16 weeks. Outcomes were evaluated clinically and histologically. Of the subjects receiving imiquimod, 83% experienced complete clearing of their lesions. Of note, once-daily dosing was more effective than less frequent dosing. Resolution was

seen in 60% of those treated twice weekly, in 50% of those treated once weekly, and in 9% of those treated with placebo.

A phase II, open-label, randomized trial involving 99 patients reported a clinical and histologic clearance rate of 88% in subjects with superficial BCCs treated with once-daily imiquimod for 6 weeks.[29] Clearance rates for twice-weekly treatment and three-times-weekly treatment were 73% and 70%, respectively. Although patients in a twice-daily regimen arm achieved 100% resolution, the local skin reactions were unacceptable.

Another phase II randomized, double-blind, vehicle-controlled study involving 128 subjects with sBCC examined longer treatment regimens.[30] Subjects received imiquimod or placebo in one of four dosing regimens lasting 12 weeks: twice daily, once daily, five times per week, or three times per week. Clearance rates of 87.1% and 80.8% were observed in those subjects who used imiquimod once daily and five times per week, respectively. Those who treated their tumors three times a week experienced 51.7% clearance, while those in the placebo group displayed a clearance rate of 18.8%. Due to severe local skin reactions in those who used imiquimod twice daily, the safety profile of this regimen was not considered acceptable. Histologic clearance rates for 12 weeks of treatment compared to the clearance rates seen following 6 weeks of treatment in previous studies proved to be similar, suggesting that an additional 6 weeks of treatment may be unnecessary.

Two phase III double-blinded, placebo-controlled studies involving 724 patients with primary sBCC were performed.[31] Subjects with one sBCC were treated with placebo or imiquimod 5% cream once daily either five or seven times per week for 6 weeks. Upon evaluation at 12 weeks posttreatment, 75% of those using imiquimod five times weekly and 73% of those using imiquimod seven times weekly experienced both histologic and clinical clearance compared to 2% to 3% of subjects treated with placebo. As the difference of clearance rates between the two imiquimod dosing regimens was not clinically significant, the authors recommended the five times per week dosing regimen.

Recurrence of sBCCs was evaluated in a follow-up study as part of the above trial in which subjects with no clinical evidence of sBCC following treatment participated. At the 12-week posttreatment assessment, 90% of subjects had no clinical evidence of recurrence. At the 2-year posttreatment assessment, 76% of subjects had no clinical evidence of recurrence.[32]

A long-term open-label study evaluating the clinical recurrence of sBCC after treatment with imiquimod daily for 6 weeks is currently underway.[33] Subjects initially demonstrated a clearance rate of 94%. At 2 years following treatment, 82.0% of the subjects remained clinically clear. In a similar long-term study performed in Europe, subjects used imiquimod once daily five times per week for 6 weeks for the treatment of sBCC. Initial clearance rates were reported to be 90% at 12 weeks posttreatment. Two years following treatment, 79.4% of the subjects remained clinically clear.[34]

Imiquimod has also been found to be beneficial as an adjunct to the surgical removal of BCCs. Use of imiquimod five days per week for 2 to 6 weeks before Mohs' excision of BCC has been reported to significantly reduce the size of the tumor, thereby resulting in a smaller cosmetic defect from the surgery.[35] In addition, a preliminary study in which imiquimod cream was used once daily for 1 month following curettage and electrodesiccation (C&D) of BCC resulted in a reduced frequency of residual tumor as well as an improved cosmetic outcome when compared to C&D alone.[36]

Off-Label Uses

Infectious Conditions

Molluscum Contagiosum

Molluscum contagiosum is a common cutaneous tumor caused by the double-stranded DNA pox virus. Although this infection is often self-limited in immunocompetent patients, patients commonly choose to treat this condition as lesions may be numerous. Current treatment modalities include cryotherapy, curettage, electrodesiccation, and application of trichloroacetic acid or cantharidin. Imiquimod's antiviral and antitumoral properties may offer an effective alternative. Anecdotally, some patients have experienced success with imiquimod, and others have not.

Several case reports have been published demonstrating eradication of molluscum contagiosum in both pediatric and adult populations.[37] In an open-label study involving 15 subjects, imiquimod 5% cream was applied once daily five times per week for 16 weeks. Results demonstrated complete clearance in 80% of the subjects.[38] Furthermore, there are reports of immunosuppressed individuals with molluscum contagiosum responding to imiquimod treatment.[39]

Herpes Simplex Virus 2

Genital herpes is a chronic sexually transmitted infection of the herpes simplex virus 2 (HSV-2). Imiquimod has been reported to be a successful alternative treatment in resistant cases. However, these reports are anecdotal, and there are insufficient data to recommend use of imiquimod for HSV infection.

A case of a 34-year-old, HIV-positive man with herpes simplex II virus infection resistant to acyclovir, famciclovir, and valacyclovir has been reported in which imiquimod 5% cream was used three times in 1 week.[40] Following imiquimod application, the lesions improved with no recurrence at 1 month posttreatment.

Martinez et al.[41] reported the case of a 37-year-old, HIV-positive man with a recurrent anogenital HSV-2 infection despite daily suppressive therapy with acyclovir or valacyclovir. He was treated with imiquimod 5% cream three times the first week and then two times the following week. Two weeks later, the skin lesions improved and HSV-2 detection by culture and polymerase chain reaction (PCR) remained negative. Twelve months posttreatment, during which time the patient did not use suppressive therapy, no recurrence was observed.

Cutaneous Warts

Common warts, caused by HPV types 2, 4, and 7, also appear to respond to imiquimod treatment, but all successful studies until now have been unblinded. An open-label study using imiquimod 5% cream once daily five days per week for up to 16 weeks for the treatment of common warts resulted in complete clearance in 56% of the subjects.[38] After approximately 9 weeks of treatment, wart size was found to be reduced greater than 50%. At a 32-week follow-up evaluation, no recurrence of treated warts was observed.

An open-label trial evaluating the efficacy of imiquimod in the treatment of recalcitrant subungual and periungual warts has been conducted.[42] Salicylic acid was initially applied to the lesions to reduce hyperkeratosis and optimize imiquimod penetration. Imiquimod 5% cream was then applied once per day five times per week for 16 weeks. Results showed that 80% (12/15) of the subjects experienced complete resolution after an average of 3 weeks of treatment.

Further double-blinded, placebo-controlled trials should be done if convincing efficacy is to be established for imiquimod in the treatment of common warts.

Leishmaniasis

Leishmaniasis is a parasitic infection seen in developing countries. It is transmitted to humans through the bite of infected sandflies. Cutaneous leishmaniasis, the most common form of the disease, manifests as skin lesions at the infection site, which may last for months to years. In animal studies, imiquimod was observed to stimulate leishmanicidal activity in macrophages.[43] Imiquimod has also been found to be effective in the treatment of cutaneous leishmaniasis when used in conjunction with meglumine antimonate in patients who have failed to respond to meglumine monotherapy.[44]

Cutaneous Malignancies

Nodular Basal Cell Carcinoma

Compared to sBCC, nodular BCC (nBCC) tends to extend deeper into the dermis. Two multicenter, randomized, dose-response studies were performed evaluating four different dosing regimens for either 6 or 12 weeks.[45] Subjects in the 6-week open-label study were randomized to apply imiquimod once daily for 3 or 7 days per week or twice daily for 3 or 7 days per week. Those in the 12-week placebo-controlled study were randomized to apply imiquimod or vehicle once daily for 3, 5, or 7 days per week or twice daily for 7 days per week. Results demonstrated that dosing once daily 7 days per week resulted in the highest clearance rates: 71% in the 6 week study and 76% in the 12 week study. These results, although statistically significant, do not approach the clearance rates seen in the treatment of sBCC. The difference may be attributable to the fact that nodular tumors tend to be denser and extend deeper into the dermis as compared to superficial tumors.

A more recent open-label study in which 15 subjects with nBCC were treated with imiquimod three times per week for 12 weeks yielded complete clearance in 100% of the subjects.[46]

Basal Cell Nevus Syndrome

Basal cell nevus syndrome is an autosomal dominant disorder that, in addition to various systemic abnormalities, manifests with multiple BCCs. The successful treatment of nevoid basal cell syndrome with imiquimod has been documented. A report of two nonfacial BCCs in a subject with basal nevus syndrome treated with imiquimod 5% cream once daily for 18 weeks resulted in complete clinical and histologic resolution.[47]

Lentigo Maligna and Malignant Melanoma

We consider lentigo maligna an in situ form of malignant melanoma. If left untreated, it may progress to invasive melanoma. An open-label study involving 30 patients with lentigo maligna was conducted in which imiquimod was applied once daily for 3 months. One month following treatment, 93% of subjects experienced complete histologic and clinical clearance.[48] Before imiquimod is routinely used for this condition, longer term follow-up is essential. Our preference is to use imiquimod as an adjunctive therapy following excision of lentigo maligna.

Cases of disseminated metastatic melanoma successfully treated with imiquimod 5% cream have also been reported. A subject with a history of melanoma involving the right knee presented with metastasis to the right lower leg.[49] After the metastases were treated with carbon dioxide laser ablation, new lesions appeared and were subsequently treated with imiquimod 5% cream three times per week. Clinical and histologic clearance was seen after 4 months, and no recurrence was observed after 15 months. However, we are aware of other cases in which recurrence appeared after successful treatment.

Bowen's Disease (Squamous Cell Carcinoma in Situ) and Invasive Squamous Cell Carcinoma

In a phase II, open-label study, imiquimod was applied once daily for 16 weeks for the treatment of Bowen's disease on the legs and shoulders of 15 subjects.[50] Sixteen weeks posttreatment, clearance rates of 93% were observed.

Another randomized, double-blind, placebo-controlled trial involving 31 subjects, revealed that those receiving imiquimod 5% cream daily for 16 weeks resulted in 73% resolution of cutaneous SCC in situ with no relapse during a 9-month follow-up period.[51]

Furthermore, a recent study examined the use of imiquimod 5% cream once daily five times per week for a maximum of 16 weeks in subjects who were unsuitable surgical candidates.[52] Following 8 to 12 weeks of treatment, complete clinical and histologic resolution was observed in four of five Bowen's disease lesions and five of seven invasive SCCs.

Cutaneous T-Cell Lymphoma

Cutaneous T-cell lymphoma manifests as patches or plaques in early stages to tumors and erythroderma in advanced stages. A preliminary open-label pilot study involving six subjects was performed to evaluate the use of imiquimod in the treatment of patch and plaque stage mycosis fungoides when applied three times per week for 12 weeks.[53] Results demonstrated a histologic and clinical response rate of 50%.

Human Immunodeficiency Virus–Related Kaposi's Sarcoma

A case report describes resolution of HIV-related Kaposi's sarcoma following daily application of imiquimod 5% cream for 4 months.[54]

Other Dermatologic Conditions

Keloids and Hypertrophic Scars

Keloids are hypertrophic scars that grow outside of the original borders of an injury. They represent an exaggerated, proliferative healing response. Current treatment includes intralesional corticosteroids, laser therapy, and cryosurgery.

Reports have shown that 24 weeks following the application of postoperative imiquimod 5% cream nightly for 8 weeks to the areas where 13 keloids were excised surgically from 12 patients, none recurred.[55] Another study evaluated the use of imiquimod 5% cream in the prevention of hypertrophic scarring following breast surgery. In this double-blind, randomized, placebo-controlled trial involving 15 subjects, imiquimod was applied over the scar once every 3 to 4 days for 8 weeks. Twenty-four weeks after the surgery, the imiquimod

treated scars were noted to have improved color and elevation when compared to placebo.[56]

Porokeratosis of Mibelli

Porokeratosis of Mibelli is a disorder of epidermal keratinization with potential for malignant transformation. A case of a 77-year old-woman with porokeratosis of Mibelli involving the left shin has been reported.[57] Following application of imiquimod 5% cream to the lesion once a day three times per week for 6 weeks, clinical resolution was observed at a 6-week posttreatment follow-up visit, and no recurrence was seen at a 2-year follow-up visit.

In another case report, a 12-year-old girl with porokeratosis of Mibelli involving her left axilla was treated with imiquimod 5% cream three times per week for 6 weeks.[58] Treatment was well tolerated, and no recurrence was observed 2 years following cessation of treatment.

Infantile Hemangioma

Infantile hemangiomas are benign vascular tumors that present within the first year of life and spontaneously regress over a period of years. Case reports have illustrated success using imiquimod for infantile hemangioma with resolution of lesions after 3 to 5 months.[59]

Granuloma Annulare

Granuloma annulare is a self-limited dermatosis manifesting as confluent papules in an annular configuration often involving the extremities. A case of a 12-year-old girl with granuloma annulare involving the right foot has been reported.[60] After failing to respond to topical superpotent steroids, the lesion was treated with imiquimod 5% cream nightly for 6 weeks. Following 6 weeks of treatment with imiquimod, the lesion had clinically resolved.

The successful use of imiquimod 5% cream in the treatment of granuloma annulare was also documented by Badavanis et al.[61] Four subjects were treated with imiquimod 5% cream once daily from three to seven times per week for up to 12 weeks of treatment. One subject experienced relapse and was treated for an additional 6 weeks with subsequent resolution. All patients remained free of recurrence at 18 months posttreatment.

Conclusion

Imiquimod 5% cream, an immune response modifier, offers a safe and effective alternative to ablative and surgical treatments for external genital
warts, actinic keratoses, and superficial basal cell
carcinomas. Although surgical excision may be
more efficacious in the treatment of skin cancers,
imiquimod may serve as a tissue-sparing, cosmetically appealing, and cost-effective option to those
patients who are poor surgical candidates, who
refuse surgery, or whose anatomic site is not amenable to surgery. As a stimulator of both innate and
acquired immune responses with resultant antiviral
and antitumoral effects, imiquimod demonstrates
potential in the treatment of several other virus-
associated and oncologic cutaneous conditions.

References

1. Miller RL, Gerster JF, Owens ML, Slade HB, Tomai
   MA. Imiquimod applied topically: a novel immune
   response modifier and new class of drug. Int J
   Immunopharmacol 1999;21(1):1–14.
2. Hemmi H, Kaisho T, Takeuchi O, et al. Small antiviral compounds activate immune cells via the TLR7
   MyD88–dependent signaling pathway. Nat Immunol
   2002;3(2):196–200.
3. Jurk M, Heil F, Vollmer J, et al. Human TLR7 or TLR8
   independently confer responsiveness to the antiviral
   compound R-848. Nat Immunol 2002;3(6):499.
4. Tyring SK AI, Stanley MA, et al. A randomized,
   controlled, molecular study of condyloma acuminata
   clearance during treatment with imiquimod. J Infect
   Dis 1998;178:551–555.
5. Wagner TL, Ahonen CL, Couture AM, et al.
   Modulation of TH1 and TH2 cytokine production
   with the immune response modifiers, R-848 and imiquimod. Cell Immunol 10 1999;191(1):10–19.
6. Suzuki H, Wang B, Shivji GM, et al. Imiquimod,
   a topical immune response modifier, induces
   migration of Langerhans cells. J Invest Dermatol
   2000;114(1):135–141.
7. Berman B, Sullivan T, De Araujo T, Nadji M.
   Expression of Fas-receptor on basal cell carcinomas
   after treatment with imiquimod 5% cream or vehicle.
   Br J Dermatol 2003;149(suppl 66):59–61.
8. Schon M, Bong AB, Drewniok C, et al. Tumor-selective induction of apoptosis and the small-molecule
   immune response modifier imiquimod. J Natl Cancer
   Inst 6 2003;95(15):1138–1149.
9. Schon MP, Wienrich BG, Drewniok C, et al. Death receptor-independent apoptosis in malignant melanoma induced
   by the small-molecule immune response modifier imiquimod. J Invest Dermatol 2004;122(5):1266–1276.
10. Berman B, Ricotti CA Jr, Cazzaniga A, Davis SC.
    Determination of the area of skin capable of being
    covered by the application of 250 mg of 5% imiqui-
    mod cream. Dermatol Surg 2004;30(5):784–786.
11. Einarson A, Costei A, Kalra S, Rouleau M, Koren G.
    The use of topical 5% imiquimod during pregnancy:
    a case series. Reprod Toxicol 2006;21(1):1–2.
12. Edwards L. Imiquimod in clinical practice. J Am
    Acad Dermatol 2000;43(1 pt 2):S12–17.
13. Beutner KR, Spruance SL, Hougham AJ, Fox TL,
    Owens ML, Douglas JM Jr. Treatment of genital warts
    with an immune-response modifier (imiquimod).
    J Am Acad Dermatol 1998;38(2 pt 1):230–239.
14. Edwards L, Ferenczy A, Eron L, et al. Self-admin-
    istered topical 5% imiquimod cream for exter-
    nal anogenital warts. HPV Study Group. Human
    PapillomaVirus. Arch Dermatol 1998;134(1):25–30.
15. Garland SM, Sellors JW, Wikstrom A, et al.
    Imiquimod 5% cream is a safe and effective self-
    applied treatment for anogenital warts—results of an
    open-label, multicentre Phase IIIB trial. Int J STD
    AIDS 2001;12(11):722–729.
16. Persaud A, Lebwohl M. Imiquimod cream in the
    treatment of actinic keratoses. J Am Acad Dermatol
    2002;47(4 suppl):S236–239.
17. Persaud AN, Shamuelova E, Sherer D, et al.
    Clinical effect of imiquimod 5% cream in the treat-
    ment of actinic keratosis. J Am Acad Dermatol
    2002;47(4):553–556.
18. Stockfleth E, Meyer T, Benninghoff B, et al. A
    randomized, double-blind, vehicle-controlled
    study to assess 5% imiquimod cream for the treat-
    ment of multiple actinic keratoses. Arch Dermatol
    2002;138(11):1498–1502.
19. Stockfleth E, Christophers E, Benninghoff B, Sterry
    W. Low incidence of new actinic keratoses after
    topical 5% imiquimod cream treatment: a long-term
    follow-up study. Arch Dermatol 2004;140(12):1542.
20. Salasche SJ, Levine N, Morrison L. Cycle therapy
    of actinic keratoses of the face and scalp with 5%
    topical imiquimod cream: An open-label trial. J Am
    Acad Dermatol 2002;47(4):571–577.
21. Szeimies RM, Gerritsen MJ, Gupta G, et al.
    Imiquimod 5% cream for the treatment of actinic
    keratosis: results from a phase III, randomized,
    double-blind, vehicle-controlled, clinical trial with his-
    tology. J Am Acad Dermatol 2004;51(4):547–555.
22. Korman N, Moy R, Ling M, et al. Dosing with 5%
    imiquimod cream 3 times per week for the treat-
    ment of actinic keratosis: results of two phase 3,
    randomized, double-blind, parallel-group, vehicle
    -controlled trials. Arch Dermatol 2005;141(4):
    467–473.

23. Lebwohl M, Dinehart S, Whiting D, et al. Imiquimod 5% cream for the treatment of actinic keratosis: results from two phase III, randomized, double-blind, parallel group, vehicle-controlled trials. J Am Acad Dermatol 2004;50(5):714–721.

24. Lee PK, Harwell WB, Loven KH, et al. Long-term clinical outcomes following treatment of actinic keratosis with imiquimod 5% cream. Dermatol Surg 2005;31(6):659–664.

25. Gupta AK, Davey V, McPhail H. Evaluation of the effectiveness of imiquimod and 5–fluorouracil for the treatment of actinic keratosis: Critical review and meta-analysis of efficacy studies. J Cutan Med Surg 2005;9(5):209–214.

26. Tran H, Chen K, Shumack S. Epidemiology and aetiology of basal cell carcinoma. Br J Dermatol 2003;149(suppl 66):50–52.

27. Sterry W, Ruzicka T, Herrera E, et al. Imiquimod 5% cream for the treatment of superficial and nodular basal cell carcinoma: randomized studies comparing low-frequency dosing with and without occlusion. Br J Dermatol 2002;147(6):1227–1236.

28. Beutner KR, Geisse JK, Helman D, Fox TL, Ginkel A, Owens ML. Therapeutic response of basal cell carcinoma to the immune response modifier imiquimod 5% cream. J Am Acad Dermatol 1999;41(6):1002–1007.

29. Marks R, Gebauer K, Shumack S, et al. Imiquimod 5% cream in the treatment of superficial basal cell carcinoma: results of a multicenter 6-week dose-response trial. J Am Acad Dermatol 2001;44(5):807–813.

30. Geisse JK, Rich P, Pandya A, et al. Imiquimod 5% cream for the treatment of superficial basal cell carcinoma: a double-blind, randomized, vehicle-controlled study. J Am Acad Dermatol 2002;47(3):390–398.

31. Geisse J, Caro I, Lindholm J, Golitz L, Stampone P, Owens M. Imiquimod 5% cream for the treatment of superficial basal cell carcinoma: results from two phase III, randomized, vehicle-controlled studies. J Am Acad Dermatol 2004;50(5):722–733.

32. Pharmaceuticals M. Aldara™ (imiquimod) cream, 5% (package insert). 2005.

33. Quirk C, Gebauer K, Owens M, Stampone P. Two-year interim results from a 5-year study evaluating clinical recurrence of superficial basal cell carcinoma after treatment with imiquimod 5% cream daily for 6 weeks. Australas J Dermatol 2006;47(4):258–265.

34. Gollnick H, Barona CG, Frank RG, et al. Recurrence rate of superficial basal cell carcinoma following successful treatment with imiquimod 5% cream: interim 2-year results from an ongoing 5–year follow-up study in Europe. Eur J Dermatol 2005;15(5):374–381.

35. Torres A, Niemeyer A, Berkes B, et al. 5% imiquimod cream and reflectance-mode confocal microscopy as adjunct modalities to Mohs micrographic surgery for treatment of basal cell carcinoma. Dermatol Surg 2004;30(12 pt 1):1462–1469.

36. Spencer JM. Pilot study of imiquimod 5% cream as adjunctive therapy to curettage and electrodesiccation for nodular basal cell carcinoma. Dermatol Surg 2006;32(1):63–69.

37. Skinner RB, Jr. Treatment of molluscum contagiosum with imiquimod 5% cream. J Am Acad Dermatol 2002;47(4 suppl):S221–224.

38. Hengge UR, Esser S, Schultewolter T, et al. Self-administered topical 5% imiquimod for the treatment of common warts and molluscum contagiosum. Br J Dermatol 2000;143(5):1026–1031.

39. Buckley R, Smith K. Topical imiquimod therapy for chronic giant molluscum contagiosum in a patient with advanced human immunodeficiency virus 1 disease. Arch Dermatol 1999;135(10):1167–1169.

40. Gilbert J, Drehs MM, Weinberg JM. Topical imiquimod for acyclovir-unresponsive herpes simplex virus 2 infection. Arch Dermatol 2001;137(8):1015–1017.

41. Martinez V, Molina JM, Scieux C, Ribaud P, Morfin F. Topical imiquimod for recurrent acyclovir-resistant HSV infection. Am J Med 2006;119(5):e9–11.

42. Micali G, Dall'Oglio F, Nasca MR. An open label evaluation of the efficacy of imiquimod 5% cream in the treatment of recalcitrant subungual and periungual cutaneous warts. J Dermatolog Treat 2003;14(4):233–236.

43. Buates S, Matlashewski G. Treatment of experimental leishmaniasis with the immunomodulators imiquimod and S-28463: efficacy and mode of action. J Infect Dis 1999;179(6):1485–1494.

44. Arevalo I, Ward B, Miller R, et al. Successful treatment of drug-resistant cutaneous leishmaniasis in humans by use of imiquimod, an immunomodulator. Clin Infect Dis 2001;33(11):1847–1851.

45. Shumack S, Robinson J, Kossard S, et al. Efficacy of topical 5% imiquimod cream for the treatment of nodular basal cell carcinoma: comparison of dosing regimens. Arch Dermatol 2002;138(9):1165–1171.

46. Huber A, Huber JD, Skinner RB Jr, Kuwahara RT, Haque R, Amonette RA. Topical imiquimod treatment for nodular basal cell carcinomas: an open-label series. Dermatol Surg 2004;30(3):429–430.

47. Kagy MK, Amonette R. The use of imiquimod 5% cream for the treatment of superficial basal cell carcinomas in a basal cell nevus syndrome patient. Dermatol Surg 2000;26(6):577–578; discussion 578–579.

48. Naylor MF, Crowson N, Kuwahara R, et al. Treatment of lentigo maligna with topical imiquimod. Br J Dermatol 2003;149(suppl 66):66–70.

49. Wolf IH, Smolle J, Binder B, Cerroni L, Richtig E, Kerl H. Topical imiquimod in the treatment of metastatic melanoma to skin. Arch Dermatol 2003;139(3):273–276.

50. Mackenzie-Wood A, Kossard S, de Launey J, Wilkinson B, Owens ML. Imiquimod 5% cream in the treatment of Bowen's disease. J Am Acad Dermatol 2001;44(3):462–470.

51. Patel GK, Goodwin R, Chawla M, et al. Imiquimod 5% cream monotherapy for cutaneous squamous cell carcinoma in situ (Bowen's disease): a randomized, double-blind, placebo-controlled trial. J Am Acad Dermatol 2006;54(6):1025–1032.

52. Peris K, Micantonio T, Fargnoli MC, Lozzi GP, Chimenti S. Imiquimod 5% cream in the treatment of Bowen's disease and invasive squamous cell carcinoma. J Am Acad Dermatol 2006;55(2): 324–327.

53. Deeths MJ, Chapman JT, Dellavalle RP, Zeng C, Aeling JL. Treatment of patch and plaque stage mycosis fungoides with imiquimod 5% cream. J Am Acad Dermatol 2005;52(2):275–280.

54. Rosen T. Limited extent AIDS-related cutaneous Kaposi's sarcoma responsive to imiquimod 5% cream. Int J Dermatol 2006;45(7):854–856.

55. Berman B, Kaufman J. Pilot study of the effect of postoperative imiquimod 5% cream on the recurrence rate of excised keloids. J Am Acad Dermatol 2002;47(4 suppl):S209–211.

56. Zurada JM, Kriegel D, Davis IC. Topical treatments for hypertrophic scars. J Am Acad Dermatol 2006;55(6):1024–1031.

57. Harrison S, Sinclair R. Porokeratosis of Mibelli: successful treatment with topical 5% imiquimod cream. Australas J Dermatol 2003;44(4):281–283.

58. Montes-De-Oca-Sanchez G, Tirado-Sanchez A, Garcia-Ramirez V. Porokeratosis of Mibelli of the axillae: treatment with topical imiquimod. J Dermatol Treat 2006;17(5):319–320.

59. Martinez MI, Sanchez-Carpintero I, North PE, Mihm MC, Jr. Infantile hemangioma: clinical resolution with 5% imiquimod cream. Arch Dermatol 2002;138(7):881–884; discussion 884.

60. Kuwahara RT, Skinner RB Jr. Granuloma annulare resolved with topical application of imiquimod. Pediatr Dermatol 2002;19(4):368–371.

61. Badavanis G, Monastirli A, Pasmatzi E, Tsambaos D. Successful treatment of granuloma annulare with imiquimod cream 5%: a report of four cases. Acta Derm Venereol 2005;85(6):547–548.

30
Topical Immune Response Modifiers: Antiinflammatories

Thomas A. Luger and Martin Steinhoff

Key Points

- New antiinflammatory therapies against atopic dermatitis and other inflammatory skin diseases have become available in recent years.
- Topical calcineurin inhibitors include tacrolimus and pimecrolimus.
- Topical calcineurin inhibitors exert a potent antiinflammatory activity with a low immunosuppressive potential.

In recent years, major findings such as blockade of the calcineurin pathway in T lymphocytes led to the identification of novel targets for the treatment of inflammatory skin diseases. The first systemic specific calcineurin inhibitor (CI) for the treatment of inflammatory skin diseases was cyclosporin A (CsA), which demonstrated efficacy both in psoriasis and atopic dermatitis. Because of its systemic adverse effects and the inability to generate a topical CsA compound, there still exists a need for better immunomodulatory agents.

Later, the calcineurin inhibitor tacrolimus (FK 506) was successfully approved as an efficient topical drug.[1] Recently, another calcineurin inhibitor (pimecrolimus, ASM 981) has been developed and approved for the topical treatment of atopic dermatitis. Both CIs have been shown to function as effective inhibitors of inflammatory responses in the skin. Both appear to target not only T cells but also other inflammatory cells such as mast cells, for example.[2] Since recent reviews have demonstrated the efficacy of modern topical glucocorticoids, this chapter focuses on topical CI, and briefly discusses recent promising developments of topical antiinflammatory agents.[3–12]

Besides CIs, glucocorticoids are widely used topical antiinflammatory agents in dermatology. In recent years, their effects as well as the adverse events have become apparent.[13–17] Because the use of glucocorticosteroids is discussed in Chapter 32, this chapter focuses on the impact of CIs as antiinflammatory agents in dermatology.

Mechanism of Calcineurin Inhibition by Tacrolimus and Pimecrolimus

Tacrolimus and pimecrolimus are ascomycin macrolactam derivatives produced by bacteria. While tacrolimus is a product of *Streptomyces tsukubaensis*, pimecrolimus was generated from *Streptomyces hygroscopicus var. ascomycetus*. Both bind, albeit with different affinity, to a cytosolic immunophilin receptor, defined as FK-binding protein-12 (macrophilin-12).[9] After binding, the macrophilin complex associated with either tacrolimus or pimecrolimus inhibits a calcium-dependent serine-threonine phosphatase, defined as calcineurin. Thereby, dephosphorylation and nuclear translocation of a cytosolic transcription factor, the nuclear factor of activated T-cell protein (NF-ATp) is inhibited.[6,18] Therefore, both tacrolimus and pimecrolimus can be defined as CIs.

In Vitro Effects

Tacrolimus and pimecrolimus inhibit the production of T1 and T2 cytokines such as interleukin-2 (IL-2), IL-4, IL-8, tumor necrosis factor-α (TNF-α), and interferon-γ (IFN-γ) in vitro, and the generation of granulocyte-macrophage colony-stimulating factor (GM-CSF) can be blocked by these compounds. Pimecrolimus is also capable of supporting anti-inflammatory effects on T-helper-2 (Th2) cells by downregulating IL-5 and IL-13 in CD4+ as well as in CD8+ T cells,[19] diminishing the number of CD1+ inflammatory dendritic cells from the epidermis,[19,20] and stimulating apoptosis in skin T cells but not in Langerhans' cells.[20] In mast cells, pimecrolimus inhibits the release of mast cell mediators such as histamine.[1,18,21] In contrast to GC, the topical application of pimecrolimus does not affect the density of epidermal Langerhans' cells,[22] and does not alter the function of dendritic cells with respect to co-stimulatory molecule expression or T-cell proliferation.[23] In keratinocytes or endothelial cells, pimecrolimus does not affect cell adhesion molecule expression.

In contrast to pimecrolimus, tacrolimus modulates certain effects of inflammatory dendritic epidermal cells (IDECs) such as the expression of the high-affinity receptor for IgE (FcεRI).[21,24,25] Tacrolimus also inhibits apoptosis of keratinocytes and T cells, thereby suppressing chemokine secretion by eosinophils and release of inflammatory mediators from mast cells.[20] In contrast to corticosteroids, neither tacrolimus nor pimecrolimus affects fibroblast functions such as collagen synthesis and therefore do not cause skin atrophy. In contrast to GC, pimecrolimus does not impair epidermal barrier function. This may explain why tachyphylaxis has not been observed upon treatment with topical CI.

In Vivo Effects

The in vivo antiinflammatory capacities of tacrolimus and pimecrolimus have been investigated in several animal models of contact dermatitis. Both compounds block the elicitation phase of contact dermatitis, thereby diminishing the inflammatory activity. The in vitro evidence of a significantly lower immunosuppressive potential of pimecrolimus in comparison to tacrolimus has been supported by in vivo animal studies. Here, pimecrolimus, in contrast to tacrolimus, had no effect on the sensitization phase of allergic contact dermatitis and thus apparently does not impair the primary immune response. This has been further supported by a variety of other animal models of immune-mediated diseases. Using a localized rat model of graft-versus-host reaction, pimecrolimus was significantly less effective than tacrolimus. In another rat model of kidney transplantation, pimecrolimus again was less effective in preventing graft rejection when compared to tacrolimus or cyclosporin A. Moreover, upon investigation of the effect on T-helper-cell–assisted B-cell activation in rats, pimecrolimus turned out to be significantly weaker when compared to that of tacrolimus.[24,26,27]

Pharmacokinetic Studies

The question of potential systemic exposure is one major concern in the development of a novel compound for topical application. Therefore, the capacity of pimecrolimus to penetrate into the skin and to permeate through the skin was investigated in vitro using human cadaver skin in comparison to corticosteroids or tacrolimus. Accordingly, the amount of pimecrolimus penetrating into the skin was similar to that of corticosteroids or tacrolimus. However, pimecrolimus was observed to permeate significantly less through skin in comparison to corticosteroids or tacrolimus.[28] Therefore, one may suggest that following the topical application of pimecrolimus, the risk of systemic exposure is low and the ultimate possibility of systemic side effects is most unlikely.[27] This has been supported by several pharmacokinetic studies, which proved that after topical use of pimecrolimus in patients with atopic dermatitis, serum concentrations were equally low regardless of the age, severity of disease, and body area treated. In 99% of the samples tested, concentrations were below 2 ng/mL, which is far below the level of 10 to 15 ng/mL, which is required for a systemic antiinflammatory effect.[29] In contrast to tacrolimus, serum concentrations of pimecrolimus in this range did not cause systemic adverse events as has been shown in several clinical trials.[30,31]

Although the metabolism of pimecrolimus in the skin has not yet been carefully investigated, it might be assumed that it is removed by desquamation. In contrast, serum tacrolimus levels after topical application were detected more frequently following topical application in patients with atopic dermatitis. However, usually these levels were low and transient because circulating tacrolimus was no longer detectable upon improvement of skin barrier function after short-term treatment.[32] The reason for the observed differences between tacrolimus and pimecrolimus, however, is not completely understood. One possible explanation may be the different structure, lipophilicity, as well as content of lipophilic groups of these compounds. Moreover, pimecrolimus in contrast to tacrolimus has a high affinity for epithelial structures such as the skin but a low affinity for lymphoid organs.[27] Pharmacokinetic long-term studies over 1 year have further demonstrated[33] that the blood concentrations of pimecrolimus cream were rather low; moreover, no accumulation was observed and only a minimal increase was detected with increasing body surface area (BSA) during treatment.[33,34] These results suggest that pimecrolimus does not cause any detectable systemic effects during long-term studies.[35,36]

Clinical Studies on Efficacy and Safety of Calcineurin Inhibitors

Both CIs have been developed for the topical treatment of atopic dermatitis and are approved for this indication in many countries around the world. Tacrolimus can be obtained as 0.03% and 0.1% ointment (Protopic®), whereas pimecrolimus is available as a 1% cream (Elidel®). While tacrolimus is approved for the treatment of moderate and severe atopic dermatitis in adults and children ≥2 years old, pimecrolimus cream (1%) is available and approved for mild and moderate cases of atopic dermatitis in adults and children ≥2 years old. In some countries, pimecrolimus has been approved for the therapy of atopic dermatitis regardless of age and severity of the disease.[37–39] For both CIs, several clinical trials verified both compounds to be highly effective for the treatment of atopic dermatitis.[9,24,40]

Meanwhile, topical CIs have been established or reported as alternative therapeutic strategies for skin diseases other than atopic dermatitis. Both tacrolimus ointment and pimecrolimus cream have been documented as successful treatment modalities for rosacea, lichen planus, psoriasis, lichen sclerosus et atrophicans, lupus erythematosus, and many others (reviewed elsewhere[39]).

From an economic point of view, in the long run CIa have been shown to be cost-effective,[41] although at the moment they are more expensive than glucocorticoids.[42] However, as already mentioned, one has to consider age (infants, children, elderly people with skin atrophy), localization (face, groin inframammary area), and severity (large proportions of the skin), for in these cases CIs are superior and safer therapeutic modalities. Thus, a fair calculation between CIs and other drugs such as glucocorticoids (GCs) may be difficult.[41,43,44] More studies are needed to further calculate costs of GC versus CI therapy.

In the first clinical trial of adults with atopic dermatitis, tacrolimus ointment significantly reduced skin lesions and pruritus within 3 weeks of treatment.[45] Subsequently, randomized double-blind controlled studies further defined the efficacy, tolerability, and safety of tacrolimus.[44,46] In adults, 0.1% tacrolimus ointment was as effective as hydrocortisone butyrate 0.1% ointment.[44,47] In children (2 to 15 years), 0.03% ointment was more effective as compared to 1% hydrocortisone acetate ointment,[48] and more effective than a mild topical glucocorticoid ointment.[44] Subsequently, tacrolimus was compared to various topical glucocorticoids. In a meta-analysis of 25 randomized controlled trials, tacrolimus 0.1% ointment was superior to hydrocortisone acetate (1%), hydrocortisone valerate, and hydrocortisone butyrate (0.1%), whereas tacrolimus (0.03%) ointment was as effective as hydrocortisone acetate (1%), but less effective than hydrocortisone butyrate.

After these successful short-term studies revealing efficacy of topical tacrolimus, a multicenter, open-label, noncomparative trial was performed.[49] Within the first week of treatment, most of these patients experienced a significant amelioration of eczema and pruritus. Of note, an increasing improvement was observed until month 3 after treatment. After 12 months, an excellent improvement (≥90%) or clearance of the symptoms was reported in 68.2% of patients. An improvement (≥50%) was noted in 90.9% of the cases.[50] Laboratory parameters did not change significantly during the study period. A burning sensation (47%) usually terminated upon initiation of treatment, and only occasionally caused burning or itching.[50] Importantly, no tachyphylaxis was observed in these patients. The excellent long-term efficacy of tacrolimus ointment for the treatment of atopic dermatitis in children as well as adults was verified in several clinical studies.[51]

By measuring tacrolimus plasma levels in patients treated with tacrolimus ointment it was revealed that in 67.1% of patients tacrolimus plasma levels remained below the level of detection. High levels were found only in 0.4% (≥5 ng/mL) of patients.[52] In patients with Netherton's syndrome, blood concentrations over 20 ng/ml could be detected.[53] Despite these rare cases, systemic exposure after topical application of tacrolimus is very low. In summary, there is no evidence for systemic accumulation resulting in adverse side effects following the long-term treatment with tacrolimus ointment.[54]

The efficacy of pimecrolimus 1% cream for the treatment of atopic dermatitis in adults, children, and infants was verified in several clinical trials.[4,24,39,55–58] Importantly, no significant drug-related adverse events were observed in these studies when applied twice daily. In comparison to both corticosteroids and tacrolimus, the capacity of pimecrolimus to permeate through the skin was significantly lower, indicating a very low risk of systemic exposure following the topical application of pimecrolimus cream.[27] This is also supported by studies with patients suffering from Netherton syndrome.[59,60] Therefore, long-term studies indicate a very low potential of systemic toxicity, immunosuppression, and local or systemic infections for pimecrolimus 1% cream.[61–63]

In children (2 to 17 years) and infants (3 to 23 months) with mild, moderate, or even severe atopic dermatitis, several multicenter clinical trials have further demonstrated,[64] that pimecrolimus 1% cream is highly effective within 8 days for treating both the eczema and the pruritus. No side effects including viral or bacterial infections were reported.[56,65,66] Thus pimecrolimus 1% cream is a safe and effective therapeutic option in children and infants with atopic dermatitis. Of note, significantly more patients in the pimecrolimus group were maintained without glucocorticoid therapy.[65,67]

Due to its efficiency and low profile of adverse events, it is recommended to begin a topical CI therapy at an early stage of atopic dermatitis and probably for other inflammatory skin diseases.[40,68] Under these circumstances, when the disease develops during CI therapy, an intermittent use of other antiinflammatory compounds such as GC will be beneficial.[69] Tacrolimus ointment and pimecrolimus cream may even have a prophylactic effect when used intermittently after an episode of atopic dermatitis when patients still suffer from pruritus (every second to third day). In two clinical trials the efficiency of pimecrolimus was compared to that of glucocorticoids. In a short-term study pimecrolimus was less effective after 3 weeks than betamethasone valerate, although the maximal efficacy of pimecrolimus was not studied in detail. Moreover, in a long-term, double-blind, randomized multicenter clinical trial, the efficacy of pimecrolimus was compared to that of triamcinolone-acetonide 1% cream or 1% hydrocortisone. Although in both groups a significant improvement was observed, less severe side effects were observed in the pimecrolimus group.[70–73]

Effects of Calcineurin Inhibitors on Innate Immunity and Host Defense

The safety and tolerability of tacrolimus ointment has been demonstrated in children and adults with atopic dermatitis. The most common local adverse event was a sensation of burning (in 29.9% of children and 46.8% of adults). Transient itching was noted in some children (23.1%) and adults (25.8%), which was most likely due not to infection but to neuronal activation.[74] The local adverse events were only noted during the first few days of treatment and were mild to moderate.[51] Concerning side effects on skin appendages, the risk of developing folliculitis or acne was increased in a few young adults.[50]

An increased rate of bacterial skin infections could not be observed,[50] and a decreased colonization with Staphylococcus aureus in the eczematous skin lesions was observed,[75] which may be due to a normalization of cutaneous innate immunity after restoration of skin integrity. Atopic dermatitis patients exert an impaired capacity to produce antimicrobial peptides such as defensins and cathelicidins.[76–82] This effect may be due to a predominant T2 immune response in atopic individuals. Moreover, IL-4 and IL-13, which are increased in atopic dermatitis, inhibit the production of antimicrobial peptides.[82]

A slight, nonstatistically significant, increase of local viral infections such as herpes simplex was reported.[11] However, none of these cases caused a therapeutic problem.[83] The idea that pimecrolimus exerts long-term preventive effects in atopic dermatitis was verified by studies showing no relation between pimecrolimus treatment and the occurrence of eczema herpeticatum.[84,85] Moreover, clinical investigations verified that pimecrolimus 1% cream was not associated with a significantly increased risk of the development of fungal, bacterial, or viral skin infections.[61–63]

By using recall antigen tests, no impaired cellular immune response was observed in the skin even after long-term application of tacrolimus 0.1% ointment.[50] Thus, tacrolimus-associated infections may not be regarded as a major risk factor in atopic dermatitis. Moreover, there is no evidence that the capacity to respond to vaccination with an appropriate antibody production is affected after topical pimecrolimus therapy. It does not alter the migratory capacity of antigen-presenting dendritic cells and does not impair the primary immune response.

Despite these studies and reports, cessation of topical application with CI is recommended until total clearance of a viral infection. Surprisingly, the incidence of bacterial infections was found to be decreased during the application of pimecrolimus or tacrolimus. This was most likely due to a normalization of innate defense mechanisms.[82]

Effects of Calcineurin Inhibitors on Pruritus

Calcineurin inhibitors play an important role in the treatment of atopic-induced pruritus.[86] Of note, a significant improvement of pruritus was observed within a few days of treatment using pimecrolimus cream,[63] which has a beneficial effect on the quality of life in patients with atopic dermatitis.[62] Within 1 week of treatment pruritus was significantly decreased in these patients.[87] Thus, pimecrolimus 1% cream is effective for the treatment of mild, moderate, and severe atopic dermatitis in adults as well as children and infants. In randomized multicenter, double-blind studies it was further demonstrated that significantly fewer infants treated with pimecrolimus developed severe flares as compared to controls.[61,63] Itchy lesions that are often resistant to therapy,

such as on the face and neck, also responded well to pimecrolimus therapy.[65] The same adverse events were also observed with tacrolimus in patients with atopic dermatitis, namely burning and a feeling of warmth. These sensations were regarded as mild and transient, lasting only 1 to 3 days.[61–63] This seems to be dependent on a transient release of preformed neuromediators such as substance P (SP) and calcitonin gene–related peptide (CGRP) from primary afferent nerve endings.[74,86,88]

Effects of Calcineurin Inhibitors on Atrophy

The effect of tacrolimus on fibroblast collagen formation was also determined in a double-blind study. Tacrolimus (0.03% and 0.1%), betamethasone valerate, and a vehicle control were compared after 1 week of application for skin thickness and procollagen peptide concentration in suction blister fluids. In contrast to betamethasone valerate, tacrolimus had no effect on procollagen propeptide production and caused no reduction of skin thickness.[89] Thus, the absence of skin atrophy is a major advantage in the treatment of CI.[1,7] In summary, it is well documented that pimecrolimus does not affect collagen synthesis and therefore does not cause skin atrophy in mice or humans.[90]

Risk of Pimecrolimus by Ultraviolet Exposure and in Skin Cancer

The use of systemic immunosuppressants such as cyclosporin A is well known to be associated with an increased risk for the development of ultraviolet (UV)-induced skin cancer such as basal cell carcinoma and squamous cell carcinoma, as well as of the development of actinic keratosis.[91,92] The long-term experience with topical corticosteroids indicates that they might not be applicable for local treatment with immunomodulators. Therefore, it was necessary to analyze the incidence of developing skin cancer after treatment with tacrolimus. The incidence of skin cancer following the use of tacrolimus ointment has remained very low.[93]

In contrast, it is well documented from animal studies that tacrolimus inhibits the development of phorbol ester-(TPA)-induced skin tumors.[94] Tacrolimus also suppresses transforming growth factor-β1 receptor (TGFβ1R) activation,[95] and prevents keratinocyte apoptosis.[96]

Importantly, various animal studies have demonstrated that the topical application of pimecrolimus cream and additional UV-irradiation were not associated with an increased incidence of epidermal or melanocytic skin tumors.[10] Moreover, topical treatment with tacrolimus and pimecrolimus prevents the UV-mediated formation of dimethyl-thymidine dimers, suggesting a protective effect of these compounds against UV exposure. However, future controlled studies are required to further elucidate the role of CI in UV-mediated skin damage. Meanwhile, a preventive strategy using appropriate sunscreens with topical CI treatment is recommended.[10,11,97,98]

The question of tumor formation following long-term treatment with topical tacrolimus cannot be definitively answered at present. Therefore, concomitant UV therapy should be avoided and the patients should be instructed to use UV-protective measures.[10,99]

Comparison of Topical Calcineurin Inhibitors

In a multicenter, randomized study, it was shown that tacrolimus 1% ointment was more effective than pimecrolimus 1% cream in adults and children with moderate/severe atopic dermatitis (AD) and at week 1 with mild AD. Tacrolimus was also superior with respect to itch scores and onset of action while no differences were observed concerning adverse side effects.[100] In summary, the first clinical trials already provided evidence for tacrolimus and pimecrolimus as safe and effective topical compounds for the treatment of AD in adults and children, with improvement both in pruritus as well as eczematous lesions.[46] A recent clinical investigator-blinded trial compared pimecrolimus 1% cream and tacrolimus 0.03% ointment in children. The efficacy of pimecrolimus 1% cream was comparable to that of tacrolimus 0.03% ointment. Pimecrolimus cream was better tolerated, and lesions in the face and neck healed faster after treatment with pimecrolimus cream.[101–103]

However, one has to consider that the vehicle of tacrolimus and pimecrolimus is different: while tacrolimus is approved as an ointment, pimecrolimus is a cream. Therefore, patients with dry skin show a better tolerability of the ointment (tacrolimus), while the cream is predominantly preferred by patients with acute, erosive lesions.

Conclusion

Topical CIs have established a novel, broad, effective, and safe treatment modality for mild to severe subtypes of atopic dermatitis and other inflammatory skin diseases. During the usage of topical tacrolimus or pimecrolimus, respectively, adverse side effects are rare. Topical CIs are the first antiinflammatory compounds that are suitable for effective, long-term treatment of inflammatory skin diseases. Moreover, they also may be used as an early local therapy when the first signs of itching and eczema appear. Perhaps early and effective local therapy using these novel compounds in infants and children may even have a preventive effect.[5,11] Therefore, early therapeutic intervention is recommended when lesions or pruritus occur. However, clinical studies are still required to investigate the course of the chronic skin disease treated with CIs with respect to the frequency and severity of the skin lesion. There is evidence that the quality of life in these patients and their relatives has significantly improved.[5,11]

The availability of tacrolimus ointment and pimecrolimus cream as two different formulations is useful because the different vehicle formulations vary regarding skin dryness, patient age, and severity of the disease. Because of its profile and vehicle pimecrolimus 1% cream can be recommended in infants and children.[27,104]

Thus far, successful treatment with topical CI has been described in atopic dermatitis,[7,10,68,69,72,105,106] seborrheic eczema,[107] steroid-induced perioral dermatitis, steroid-induced rosacea,[108] erythrotelangiectatic as well as papulopustular and edematous rosacea,[109] perianal dermatitis, chronic actinic dermatitis,[110] disseminated granuloma annulare,[111,112] lichen planus,[113] hand eczema, mucous lesions of lichen planus,[114] lichen sclerosus et atrophicans, pyoderma gangrenosum, lupus erythematosus, dermatomyositis, bullous autoimmune diseases, lichen amyloidosus, lichen aureus and chronic actinic dermatitis,[5,11,104,111,115–118] chronic graft-versus-host disease,[119,120] asteatotic eczema,[121] and vitiligo,[122] although UV light may be additionally mandatory.[123,124] In contrast, treatment of alopecia areata in humans with CI was not effective.[123]

The introduction of topical CI as antiinflammatory agents to combat inflammatory skin diseases has already changed our position about the optimal treatment of inflammatory and autoimmune skin diseases. However, the future position of topical CI for the treatment of atopic dermatitis and other inflammatory skin diseases depends on further well-controlled clinical trials.

In the last few years, a huge improvement has been observed for the development of new antiinflammatory therapies against atopic dermatitis and other inflammatory skin diseases by immunomodulatory agents. As new topical compounds, calcineurin-inhibitors or glucocorticoids with less severe adverse events have to be mentioned. Topical CIs such as tacrolimus or pimecrolimus exert a potent antiinflammatory activity with a low immunosuppressive potential. In many controlled clinical trials, tacrolimus ointment as well as pimecrolimus cream have been shown to be highly effective and safe. They are also well tolerated and do not induce skin atrophy in long-term studies. One of the major adverse events observed with CIs is a transient sensation of burning, which ceases within days. UV-protective modalities are recommended during the treatment of topical CI, although side effects such as skin cancer and systemic immunosuppression have not been observed as of yet in controlled clinical studies. In addition to atopic dermatitis topical CI are effective agents for the treatment of many inflammatory skin diseases including perioral dermatitis, seborrheic eczema, and lichen sclerosus et atrophicus. Future studies will have to determine whether early and perhaps prophylactic application of topical CI may prolong or prevent the onset of inflammatory responses in various skin diseases. In recent years, our knowledge about potent topical GCs with fewer side effects has also greatly improved. Long-term studies revealed a low potential of topical GC to induce atrophy as compared to classic GC. Thus, modern topical treatments with topical CI and GC have established an improvement for the treatment of atopic dermatitis. However, other novel specific antiinflammatory therapies are still needed for rapid and safe long-term treatments for atopic dermatitis and other inflammatory or autoimmune skin diseases.

References

1. Gupta AK, Adamiak A, Chow M. Tacrolimus: a review of its use for the management of dermatoses. J Eur Acad Dermatol Venereol 2002;16:100–114.
2. Zuberbier T, Chong SU, Grunow K, et al. The ascomycin macrolactam pimecrolimus (Elidel, SDZ ASM 981) is a potent inhibitor of mediator release from human dermal mast cells and peripheral blood basophils. J Allergy Clin Immunol 2001;108:275–280.
3. Akhavan A, Rudikoff D. The treatment of atopic dermatitis with systemic immunosuppressive agents. Clin Dermatol 2003;21:225–240.
4. Carroll CL, Fleischer AB Jr. Tacrolimus: focusing on atopic dermatitis. Drugs Today (Barc) 2006;42:431–439.
5. Cather JC, Abramovits W, Menter A. Cyclosporine and tacrolimus in dermatology. Dermatol Clin 2001;19:119–137, ix.
6. Gisondi P, Ellis CN, Girolomoni G. Pimecrolimus in dermatology: atopic dermatitis and beyond. Int J Clin Pract 2005;59:969–974.
7. Grassberger M, Steinhoff M, Schneider D, Luger TA. Pimecrolimus—an anti-inflammatory drug targeting the skin. Exp Dermatol 2004;13:721–730.
8. Griffiths CE, Katsambas A, Dijkmans BA, et al. Update on the use of ciclosporin in immune-mediated dermatoses. Br J Dermatol 2006;155(suppl 2):1–16.
9. Paul C, Graeber M, Stuetz A. Ascomycins: promising agents for the treatment of inflammatory skin diseases. Expert Opin Invest Drugs 2000;9:69–77.
10. Ring J, Barker J, Behrendt H, et al. Review of the potential photo-cocarcinogenicity of topical calcineurin inhibitors: position statement of the European Dermatology Forum. J Eur Acad Dermatol Venereol 2005;19:663–671.
11. Tomi NS, Luger TA. The treatment of atopic dermatitis with topical immunomodulators. Clin Dermatol 2003;21:215–224.
12. Wolff K. Pimecrolimus 1% cream for the treatment of atopic dermatitis. Skin Therapy Lett 2005;10:1–6.
13. Donaldson KE, Karp CL, Dunbar MT. Evaluation and treatment of children with ocular rosacea. Cornea 2007;26:42–46.
14. Kirkland R, Pearce DJ, Balkrishnan R, Feldman SR. Critical factors determining the potency of topical corticosteroids. J Dermatol Treat 2006;17:133–135.
15. Schacke H, Rehwinkel H, Asadullah K, Cato AC. Insight into the molecular mechanisms of glucocorticoid receptor action promotes identification of novel ligands with an improved therapeutic index. Exp Dermatol 2006;15:565–573.

16. Schoepe S, Schacke H, May E, Asadullah K. Glucocorticoid therapy-induced skin atrophy. Exp Dermatol 2006;15:406–420.

17. Ventura MT, Calogiuri GF, Muratore L, et al. Cross-reactivity in cell-mediated and IgE-mediated hypersensitivity to glucocorticoids. Curr Pharm Des 2006;12:3383–3391.

18. Grassberger M, Baumruker T, Enz A, et al. A novel anti-inflammatory drug, SDZ ASM 981, for the treatment of skin diseases: in vitro pharmacology. Br J Dermatol 1999;141:264–273.

19. Simon D, Vassina E, Yousefi S, Braathen LR, Simon HU. Inflammatory cell numbers and cytokine expression in atopic dermatitis after topical pimecrolimus treatment. Allergy 2005;60:944–951.

20. Hoetzenecker W, Ecker R, Kopp T, Stuetz A, Stingl G, Elbe-Burger A. Pimecrolimus leads to an apoptosis-induced depletion of T cells but not Langerhans cells in patients with atopic dermatitis. J Allergy Clin Immunol 2005;115:1276–1283.

21. Michel G, Kemeny L, Homey B, Ruzicka T. FK506 in the treatment of inflammatory skin disease: promises and perspectives. Immunol Today 1996;17: 106–108.

22. Meingassner JG, Kowalsky E, Schwendinger H, Elbe-Burger A, Stutz A. Pimecrolimus does not affect Langerhans cells in murine epidermis. Br J Dermatol 2003;149:853–857.

23. Kalthoff FS, Chung J, Musser P, Stuetz A. Pimecrolimus does not affect the differentiation, maturation and function of human monocyte-derived dendritic cells, in contrast to corticosteroids. Clin Exp Immunol 2003;133:350–359.

24. Alomar A, Berth-Jones J, Bos JD, et al. The role of topical calcineurin inhibitors in atopic dermatitis. Br J Dermatol 2004;151(suppl 70):3–27.

25. Hultsch T, Kapp A, Spergel J. Immunomodulation and safety of topical calcineurin inhibitors for the treatment of atopic dermatitis. Dermatology 2005;211:174–187.

26. de Bruin-Weller MS, Bruijnzeel-Koomen CA. [Topical immunomodulators, such as tacrolimus and pimecrolimus, in the treatment of atopic dermatitis]. Ned Tijdschr Geneeskd 2005;149:1096–1100.

27. Stuetz A, Grassberger M, Meingassner JG. Pimecrolimus (Elidel, SDZ ASM 981)—preclinical pharmacologic profile and skin selectivity. Semin Cutan Med Surg 2001;20:233–241.

28. Billich A, Aschauer H, Aszodi A, Stuetz A. Percutaneous absorption of drugs used in atopic eczema: pimecrolimus permeates less through skin than corticosteroids and tacrolimus. Int J Pharm 2004;269:29–35.

29. Van Leent EJ, Ebelin ME, Burtin P, Dorobek B, Spuls PI, Bos JD. Low systemic exposure after repeated topical application of Pimecrolimus (Elidel), SD Z ASM 981) in patients with atopic dermatitis. Dermatology 2002;204:63–68.

30. Gottlieb AB, Griffiths CE, Ho VC, et al. Oral pimecrolimus in the treatment of moderate to severe chronic plaque-type psoriasis: a double-blind, multicentre, randomized, dose-finding trial. Br J Dermatol 2005;152:1219–1227.

31. Marsland AM, Griffiths CE. The macrolide immunosuppressants in dermatology: mechanisms of action. Eur J Dermatol 2002;12:618–622.

32. Kawashima M, Nakagawa H, Ohtsuki M, Tamaki K, Ishibashi Y. Tacrolimus concentrations in blood during topical treatment of atopic dermatitis. Lancet 1996;348:1240–1241.

33. Van Leent EJ, Graber M, Thurston M, Wagenaar A, Spuls PI, Bos JD. Effectiveness of the ascomycin macrolactam SDZ ASM 981 in the topical treatment of atopic dermatitis. Arch Dermatol 1998;134:805–809.

34. Harper J, Green A, Scott G, et al. First experience of topical SDZ ASM 981 in children with atopic dermatitis. Br J Dermatol 2001;144:781–787.

35. Rappersberger K, Komar M, Ebelin ME, et al. Pimecrolimus identifies a common genomic anti-inflammatory profile, is clinically highly effective in psoriasis and is well tolerated. J Invest Dermatol 2002;119:876–887.

36. Wolff K, Caro I, Murell D, Ortonne JP. Safety profile of oral pimecrolimus in atopic eczema and psoriasis: a pooled analysis from two dose-finding studies. J Invest Dermatol 2003;121:1245A.

37. Cohen B. Review of pimecrolimus cream 1% in children for the treatment of mild to moderate atopic dermatitis. Clin Pediatr (Phila) 2007;46:7–15.

38. Hebert AA. Review of pimecrolimus cream 1% for the treatment of mild to moderate atopic dermatitis. Clin Ther 2006;28:1972–1982.

39. Stuetz A, Baumann K, Grassberger M, Wolff K, Meingassner JG. Discovery of topical calcineurin inhibitors and pharmacological profile of pimecrolimus. Int Arch Allergy Immunol 2006;141:199–212.

40. Luger TA, Gollnick H. [Viewpoint of the German Dermatologic Society (DDG) concerning the decision of the American Food and Drug Administration (FDA) on the use of pimecrolimus cream and tacrolimus ointment in the treatment of atopic dermatitis (neurodermatitis)]. J Dtsch Dermatol Ges 2005;3:415–416.

41. Abramovits W, Boguniewicz M, Paller AS, et al. The economics of topical immunomodulators for the treatment of atopic dermatitis. Pharmacoeconomics 2005;23:543–566.

42. Pitt M, Garside R, Stein K. A cost-utility analysis of pimecrolimus vs. topical corticosteroids and

emollients for the treatment of mild and moderate atopic eczema. Br J Dermatol 2006;154:1137–1146.

43. Ellis CN, Drake LA, Prendergast MM, et al. Cost-effectiveness analysis of tacrolimus ointment versus high-potency topical corticosteroids in adults with moderate to severe atopic dermatitis. J Am Acad Dermatol 2003;48:553–563.

44. Garside R, Stein K, Castelnuovo E, et al. The effectiveness and cost-effectiveness of pimecrolimus and tacrolimus for atopic eczema: a systematic review and economic evaluation. Health Technol Assess 2005;9:iii, xi-xiii,1–230.

45. Ruzicka T, Bieber T, Schopf E, et al. A short-term trial of tacrolimus ointment for atopic dermatitis. European Tacrolimus Multicenter Atopic Dermatitis Study Group. N Engl J Med 1997;337:816–821.

46. Hanifin JM, Ling MR, Langley R, Breneman D, Rafal E. Tacrolimus ointment for the treatment of atopic dermatitis in adult patients: part I, efficacy. J Am Acad Dermatol 2001;44:S28–38.

47. Reitamo S, Rustin M, Ruzicka T, et al. Efficacy and safety of tacrolimus ointment compared with that of hydrocortisone butyrate ointment in adult patients with atopic dermatitis. J Allergy Clin Immunol 2002;109:547–555.

48. Reitamo S, Van Leent EJ, Ho V, et al. Efficacy and safety of tacrolimus ointment compared with that of hydrocortisone acetate ointment in children with atopic dermatitis. J Allergy Clin Immunol 2002;109:539–546

49. Hanifin JM, Thurston M, Omoto M, Cherill R, Tofte SJ, Graeber M. The eczema area and severity index (EASI): assessment of reliability in atopic dermatitis. EASI Evaluator Group. Exp Dermatol 2001;10:11–18.

50. Reitamo S, Wollenberg A, Schopf E, et al. Safety and efficacy of 1 year of tacrolimus ointment monotherapy in adults with atopic dermatitis. The European Tacrolimus Ointment Study Group. Arch Dermatol 2000;136:999–1006.

51. Kang S, Lucky AW, Pariser D, Lawrence I, Hanifin JM. Long-term safety and efficacy of tacrolimus ointment for the treatment of atopic dermatitis in children. J Am Acad Dermatol 2001;44:S58–64.

52. Reitamo S. Topical immunomodulators for therapy of atopic dermatitis. In: Bieber T, Leung D, eds. Atopic Dermatits. New York: Marcel Dekker, 2002.

53. Allen A, Siegfried E, Silverman R, et al. Significant absorption of topical tacrolimus in 3 patients with Netherton syndrome. Arch Dermatol 2001;137: 747–750.

54. Drake L, Prendergast M, Maher R, et al. The impact of tacrolimus ointment on health-related quality of life of adult and pediatric patients with atopic dermatitis. J Am Acad Dermatol 2001;44:S65–72.

55. Abels C, Proksch E. [Therapy of atopic dermatitis]. Hautarzt 2006;57:711–723; quiz 724–715.

56. Kaufmann R, Folster-Holst R, Hoger P, et al. Onset of action of pimecrolimus cream 1% in the treatment of atopic eczema in infants. J Allergy Clin Immunol 2004;114:1183–1188.

57. Spergel JM, Leung DY. Safety of topical calcineurin inhibitors in atopic dermatitis: evaluation of the evidence. Curr Allergy Asthma Rep 2006;6:270–274.

58. Thaci D. [Long term management of childhood atopic dermatitis with calcineurin inhibitors]. Hautarzt 2003;54:418–423.

59. Henno A, Choffray A, De La Brassinne M. [Improvement of Netherton syndrome associated erythroderma in two adult sisters through use of topical pimecrolimus]. Ann Dermatol Venereol 2006;133:71–72.

60. Oji V, Beljan G, Beier K, Traupe H, Luger TA. Topical pimecrolimus: a novel therapeutic option for Netherton syndrome. Br J Dermatol 2005;153:1067–1068.

61. Kapp A, Papp K, Bingham A, et al. Long-term management of atopic dermatitis in infants with topical pimecrolimus, a nonsteroid anti-inflammatory drug. J Allergy Clin Immunol 2002;110:277–284.

62. Meurer M, Folster-Holst R, Wozel G, Weidinger G, Junger M, Brautigam M. Pimecrolimus cream in the long-term management of atopic dermatitis in adults: a six-month study. Dermatology 2002;205:271–277.

63. Wahn U, Bos JD, Goodfield M, et al. Efficacy and safety of pimecrolimus cream in the long-term management of atopic dermatitis in children. Pediatrics 2002;110:e2.

64. Breuer K, Werfel T, Kapp A. Safety and efficacy of topical calcineurin inhibitors in the treatment of childhood atopic dermatitis. Am J Clin Dermatol 2005;6:65–77.

65. Eichenfield LF, Lucky AW, Boguniewicz M, et al. Safety and efficacy of pimecrolimus (ASM 981) cream 1% in the treatment of mild and moderate atopic dermatitis in children and adolescents. J Am Acad Dermatol 2002;46:495–504.

66. Leo HL, Bender BG, Leung SB, Tran ZV, Leung DY. Effect of pimecrolimus cream 1% on skin condition and sleep disturbance in children with atopic dermatitis. J Allergy Clin Immunol 2004;114:691–693.

67. Papp K, Staab D, Harper J, et al. Effect of pimecrolimus cream 1% on the long-term course of pediatric atopic dermatitis. Int J Dermatol 2004;43:978–983.

68. Luger TA, Bieber T, Meurer M, et al. [Therapy of atopic eczema with calcineurin inhibitors]. J Dtsch Dermatol Ges 2005;3:385–391.

69. Ellis C, Luger T, Abeck D, et al. International Consensus Conference on Atopic Dermatitis II (ICCAD II): clinical update and current treatment

strategies. Br J Dermatol 2003;148(suppl 63): 3–10.

70. de Prost Y. [The value of topical immunosuppressors in the treatment of atopic dermatitis in children]. Ann Dermatol Venereol 2005;132(Spec. No. 1):1S68–72.

71. Gupta AK, Chow M. Pimecrolimus: a review. J Eur Acad Dermatol Venereol 2003;17:493–503.

72. Thestrup-Pedersen K. Tacrolimus treatment of atopic eczema/dermatitis syndrome. Curr Opin Allergy Clin Immunol 2003;3:359–362.

73. Weinberg JM. Formulary review of therapeutic alternatives for atopic dermatitis: focus on pimecrolimus. J Manag Care Pharm 2005;11:56–64.

74. Stander S, Stander H, Seeliger S, Luger TA, Steinhoff M. Topical pimecrolimus (SDZ ASM 981) and tacrolimus (FK 506) transiently induces neuropeptide release and mast cell degranulation in murine skin. Br J Dermatol 2007;156:1020–1026.

75. Remitz A, Kyllonen H, Granlund H, Reitamo S. Tacrolimus ointment reduces staphylococcal colonization of atopic dermatitis lesions. J Allergy Clin Immunol 2001;107:196–197.

76. Agerberth B, Buentke E, Bergman P, et al. Malassezia sympodialis differently affects the expression of LL-37 in dendritic cells from atopic eczema patients and healthy individuals. Allergy 2006;61:422–430.

77. Fellermann K, Wehkamp J, Stange EF. Antimicrobial peptides in the skin. N Engl J Med 2003;348:361–363; author reply 361–363.

78. Harrison JM, Ramshaw IA. Cytokines, skin, and smallpox-a new link to an antimicrobial Peptide. Immunity 2006;24:245–247.

79. Howell MD, Novak N, Bieber T, et al. Interleukin-10 downregulates anti-microbial peptide expression in atopic dermatitis. J Invest Dermatol 2005;125:738–745.

80. Howell MD, Gallo RL, Boguniewicz M, et al. Cytokine milieu of atopic dermatitis skin subverts the innate immune response to vaccinia virus. Immunity 2006;24:341–348.

81. Howell MD, Wollenberg A, Gallo RL, et al. Cathelicidin deficiency predisposes to eczema herpeticum. J Allergy Clin Immunol 2006;117:836–841.

82. Ong PY, Ohtake T, Brandt C, et al. Endogenous antimicrobial peptides and skin infections in atopic dermatitis. N Engl J Med 2002;347:1151–1160.

83. Lubbe J, Pournaras CC, Saurat JH. Eczema herpeticum during treatment of atopic dermatitis with 0.1% tacrolimus ointment. Dermatology 2000;201:249–251.

84. Papp KA, Breuer K, Meurer M, et al. Long-term treatment of atopic dermatitis with pimecrolimus cream 1% in infants does not interfere with the development of protective antibodies after vaccination. J Am Acad Dermatol 2005;52:247–253.

85. Papp KA, Werfel T, Folster-Holst R, et al. Long-term control of atopic dermatitis with pimecrolimus cream 1% in infants and young children: a two-year study. J Am Acad Dermatol 2005;52:240–246.

86. Stander S, Luger TA. [Antipruritic effects of pimecrolimus and tacrolimus]. Hautarzt 2003;54:413–417.

87. Luger T, Van Leent EJ, Graeber M, et al. SDZ ASM 981: an emerging safe and effective treatment for atopic dermatitis. Br J Dermatol 2001;144:788–794.

88. Stander S, Steinhoff M, Stander H, Luger TA. Morphological evidence of neuropeptide release and mast cell degranulation in tacrolimus and pimecrolimus treated murine skin. J Invest Dermatol 2003;121:912A.

89. Reitamo S, Rissanen J, Remitz A, et al. Tacrolimus ointment does not affect collagen synthesis: results of a single-center randomized trial. J Invest Dermatol 1998;111:396–398.

90. Queille-Roussel C, Paul C, Duteil L, et al. The new topical ascomycin derivative SDZ ASM 981 does not induce skin atrophy when applied to normal skin for 4 weeks: a randomized, double-blind controlled study. Br J Dermatol 2001;144:507–513.

91. Parrish JA. Immunosuppression, skin cancer, and ultraviolet A radiation. N Engl J Med 2005;353: 2712–2713.

92. Yarosh DB, Pena AV, Nay SL, Canning MT, Brown DA. Calcineurin inhibitors decrease DNA repair and apoptosis in human keratinocytes following ultraviolet B irradiation. J Invest Dermatol 2005;125:1020–1025.

93. Soter NA, Fleischer AB Jr, Webster GF, Monroe E, Lawrence I. Tacrolimus ointment for the treatment of atopic dermatitis in adult patients: part II, safety. J Am Acad Dermatol 2001;44:S39–46.

94. Jiang H, Yamamoto S, Nishikawa K, Kato R. Anti-tumor-promoting action of FK506, a potent immunosuppressive agent. Carcinogenesis 1993;14:67–71.

95. Yao D, Dore JJ Jr, Leof EB. FKBP12 is a negative regulator of transforming growth factor-beta receptor internalization. J Biol Chem 2000;275: 13149–13154.

96. Trautmann A, Akdis M, Schmid-Grendelmeier P, et al. Targeting keratinocyte apoptosis in the treatment of atopic dermatitis and allergic contact dermatitis. J Allergy Clin Immunol 2001;108:839–846.

97. Tran C, Luebbe J, Antille C, et al. Calcineurin Inhibitors and skin cancer. J Invest Dermatol 121:1072A.

98. Wooltorton E. Eczema drugs tacrolimus (Protopic) and pimecrolimus (Elidel): cancer concerns. Can Med Assoc J 2003;172:1179–1180.

99. Loser K, Scherer A, Krummen MB, et al. An important role of CD80/CD86–CTLA-4 signaling during photocarcinogenesis in mice. J Immunol 2005;174:5298–5305.

100. Paller AS, Lebwohl M, Fleischer AB Jr, et al. Tacrolimus ointment is more effective than pimecrolimus cream with a similar safety profile in the treatment of atopic dermatitis: results from 3 randomized, comparative studies. J Am Acad Dermatol 2005;52:810–822.

101. Bieber T, Cork M, Ellis C, et al. Consensus statement on the safety profile of topical calcineurin inhibitors. Dermatology 2005;211:77–78.

102. Lubbe J, Friedlander SF, Cribier B, et al. Safety, efficacy, and dosage of 1% pimecrolimus cream for the treatment of atopic dermatitis in daily practice. Am J Clin Dermatol 2006;7:121–131.

103. Simon D, Lubbe J, Wuthrich B, et al. Benefits from the use of a pimecrolimus-based treatment in the management of atopic dermatitis in clinical practice. Analysis of a Swiss cohort. Dermatology 2006;213:313–318.

104. Nghiem P, Pearson G, Langley RG. Tacrolimus and pimecrolimus: from clever prokaryotes to inhibiting calcineurin and treating atopic dermatitis. J Am Acad Dermatol 2002;46:228–241.

105. Luger T. Treatment of immune-mediated skin diseases: future perspectives. Eur J Dermatol 2001;11:343–347.

106. Luger TA, Lahfa M, Folster-Holst R, et al. Long-term safety and tolerability of pimecrolimus cream 1% and topical corticosteroids in adults with moderate to severe atopic dermatitis. J Dermatol Treat 2004;15:169–178.

107. Rallis E, Nasiopoulou A, Kouskoukis C, Koumantaki E. Pimecrolimus cream 1% can be an effective treatment for seborrheic dermatitis of the face and trunk. Drugs Exp Clin Res 2004;30:191–195.

108. Chu CY. The use of 1% pimecrolimus cream for the treatment of steroid-induced rosacea. Br J Dermatol 2005;152:396–399.

109. Crawford KM, Russ B, Bostrom P. Pimecrolimus for treatment of acne rosacea. Skinmed 2005;4:147–150.

110. de Almeida HL Jr, de Oliveira Filho UL. Topical pimecrolimus is an effective treatment for balanitis circinata erosiva. Int J Dermatol 2005;44:888–889.

111. Cyr PR. Diagnosis and management of granuloma annulare. Am Fam Physician 2006;74:1729–1734.

112. Rigopoulos D, Prantsidis A, Christofidou E, Ioannides D, Gregoriou S, Katsambas A. Pimecrolimus 1% cream in the treatment of disseminated granuloma annulare. Br J Dermatol 2005;152:1364–1365.

113. Scheer M, Kawari-Mahmoodi N, Neugebauer J, Kubler AC. [Pimecrolimus (Elidel((R))) for therapy of lichen ruber mucosae.]. Mund Kiefer Gesichtschir 2006;10:403–407.

114. Swift JC, Rees TD, Plemons JM, Hallmon WW, Wright JC. The effectiveness of 1% pimecrolimus cream in the treatment of oral erosive lichen planus. J Periodontol 2005;76:627–635.

115. Graf J, Webb A, Davis J. The use of topical tacrolimus (FK506/Protopic) in cutaneous manifestations of autoimmune diseases. J Clin Rheumatol 2003;9:310–315.

116. Ling MR. Topical tacrolimus and pimecrolimus: future directions. Semin Cutan Med Surg 2001;20:268–274.

117. Mansouri P, Farshi S. Pimecrolimus 1 percent cream in the treatment of psoriasis in a child. Dermatol Online J 2006;12:7.

118. Peyrot I, Sparsa A, Loustaud-Ratti V, et al. [Topical tacrolimus and resistant skin lesions of dermatomyositis]. Rev Med Interne 2006;27:730–735.

119. Conrotto D, Carrozzo M, Ubertalli AV, et al. Dramatic increase of tacrolimus plasma concentration during topical treatment for oral graft-versus-host disease. Transplantation 2006;82:1113–1115.

120. Schmook T, Kraft J, Benninghoff B, et al. Treatment of cutaneous chronic graft-versus-host disease with topical pimecrolimus. Bone Marrow Transplant 2005;36:87–88.

121. Schulz P, Bunselmeyer B, Brautigam M, Luger TA. Pimecrolimus cream 1% is effective in asteatotic eczema: results of a randomized, double-blind, vehicle-controlled study in 40 patients. J Eur Acad Dermatol Venereol 2007;21:90–94.

122. Coskun B, Saral Y, Turgut D. Topical 0.05% clobetasol propionate versus 1% pimecrolimus ointment in vitiligo. Eur J Dermatol 2005;15:88–91.

123. Mehrabi D, Pandya AG. A randomized, placebo-controlled, double-blind trial comparing narrowband UV-B Plus 0.1% tacrolimus ointment with narrowband UV-B plus placebo in the treatment of generalized vitiligo. Arch Dermatol 2006;142:927–929.

124. Ostovari N, Passeron T, Lacour JP, Ortonne JP. Lack of efficacy of tacrolimus in the treatment of vitiligo in the absence of UV-B exposure. Arch Dermatol 2006;142:252–253.

31
Traditional Immune-Modulating Drugs

Stephen E. Wolverton

Key Points

- Traditional immune modulating drugs include calcineurin inhibitors, antimetabolites, and alkylating agents.
- Antimetabolites include purine analogues (e.g., azathioprine and mycophenolate mofetil), and folate antagonists (e.g., methotrexate and dapsone).
- The most widely used systemic calcineurin inhibitor is cyclosporine.
- The most commonly used alkylating agent is cyclophosphamide.

The subject of traditional immune modulating drugs is potentially vast. However, only a small number of these drugs are commonly used by dermatologists. This chapter addresses the key mechanisms of how the majority of inflammatory skin diseases are treated, and discusses six systemic drugs from four drugs groups: (1) calcineurin inhibitors: cyclosporine; (2) antimetabolites/purine analogues: azathioprine and mycophenolate mofetil; (3) antimetabolites/folate antagonists: methotrexate and dapsone; and (4) alkylating agents: cyclophosphamide (Table 31.1). This classification scheme is a reasonable way to categorize the drugs, although it should be noted that several of these drugs have mechanisms of action that differ from the above categories. Furthermore, it is not realistic to discuss all available immune-modulating drugs; several notable drug groups not covered in this chapter include retinoids, antimalarials, and interferons.

The emphasis here is on the primary mechanisms of action, particularly as these mechanisms relate to common indications, significant adverse effects, and drug interactions. The discussion of these indications, adverse effects, and drug interactions is brief, emphasizing those with the greatest clinical relevance for the practicing dermatologist. Chapters and reviews the provide greater detail are cited.

In the past I have divided the above drugs into two broad groups: immunosuppressive and antiinflammatory. But many drugs overlap the categories; methotrexate, for example, has both immunosuppressive and antiinflammatory mechanisms. Thus, considering the drugs discussed as "immune modulating" in a broad sense is a very reasonable approach.

Cyclosporine

Mechanisms of Action[1]

The most established role of CsA in psoriasis and other immune-mediated dermatoses is its effect on T lymphocytes.[2] Calcineurin is a calcium- and calmodulin-dependent enzyme that is of central importance to the T-cell amplification of the immune response, in particular inducing increased levels of interleukin-2 (IL-2) (Fig. 31.1). Cyclosporine inhibits calcineurin, which leads to reduced activity of the transcription factor, nuclear factor of activated T cells 1 (NFAT-1).[3] This transcription factor is important in regulating transcription of a number of cytokine genes, the most significant being IL-2. Because IL-2 causes the

TABLE 31.1. Traditional immune-modulating drugs.

Category	Drug name	Specific enzyme(s) inhibited
Calcineurin inhibitors	Cyclosporine	Calcineurin
Antimetabolites/ purine analogues	Azathioprine	None
	Mycophenolate mofetil	Inosine monophosphate dehydrogenase
Antimetabolites/ folate antagonists	Methotrexate	Dihydrofolate reductase
	Dapsone	Thymidylate synthetase Dihydropteroate synthetase Myeloperoxidase
Alkylating agents	Cyclophosphamide	None

proliferation of activated helper T cells (CD4) and cytotoxic T cells (CD8), impaired IL-2 production leads to a decline in the number of activated CD4 and CD8 cells in the epidermis and dermis.

In addition, cyclosporin A (CsA) inhibits the production of interferon-γ, which in turn downregulates intercellular adhesion molecule 1 (ICAM-1) production. ICAM-1 is expressed on the surface of various cells such as keratinocytes and dermal capillary endothelium, playing an important role in the immune process by affecting trafficking of various inflammatory cells. Finally it is important to note that cyclosporine is a cytochrome P-450 (CYP) 3A4 substrate and inhibitor, explaining many of the numerous potential drug interactions involving cyclosporine.

Clinical Applications of Cyclosporine Mechanisms[1]

Common Indications

1. Psoriasis, atopic dermatitis, refractory urticaria; T-cell inhibition through cyclosporine inhibition of calcineurin and resultant reduced NFAT-1 production.
2. Pyoderma gangrenosum, immunobullous dermatoses (pemphigus and pemphigoid), autoimmune connective tissue diseases (dermatomyositis), and many others; additional dermatoses in which the T cell has a key role in the pathogenesis.

Significant Adverse Effects

1. Renal disease and resultant hypertension; kidney has relatively high levels of calcineurin.

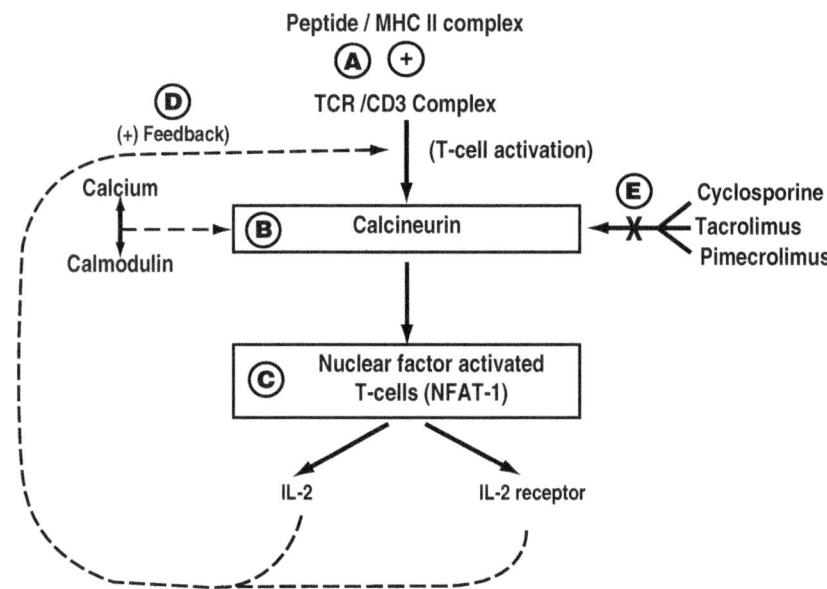

FIG. 31.1. Cyclosporine inhibition of calcineurin. * IL, interleukin; MHC, major histocompatibility complex

2. Neurologic adverse effects (such as tremors, headache, paresthesias); various neurologic cell types likewise with relatively high levels of calcineurin.

Drug Interactions

1. Macrolides (erythromycin > clarithromycin), azole antifungals (ketoconazole > itraconazole); cyclosporine toxicity due to these CYP 3A4 inhibitors.
2. Rifampin (and other "enzyme inducers"); loss of cyclosporine efficacy due to CYP 3A4 inducers.
3. "Statins" such as simvastatin, atorvastatin, lovastatin > rosuvastatin, fluvastatin (best choice pravastatin with no CYP metabolism); cyclosporine CYP 3A4 inhibition increasing the risk of rhabdomyolysis from these statins.
4. Numerous other CYP-based drug interactions (see pertinent table in Lee and Koo[1]).

Azathioprine

Mechanisms of Action[4]

Azathioprine's active metabolites are 6-thioguanine (6-TG) monophosphate and other 6-TG metabolites; these metabolites are structurally very similar to the endogenous purines adenine and guanine.

This structural similarity to the endogenous purines allows these 6-TG metabolites to be incorporated into DNA and RNA, inhibiting purine metabolism and cell division.[5,6] T-cell–mediated function is depressed, and antibody production is diminished in the B cell.[7] Azathioprine also decreases the number of Langerhans' cells (and the ability to present antigens) and other antigen-presenting cells in the skin.[8]

Azathioprine is a prodrug which is rapidly converted to 6-mercaptopurine (6-MP) upon absorption. There are three metabolic pathways which subsequently metabolize 6-MP: (1) hypoxanthine-guanine phosphoribosyltransferase (HGPRT), which leads to formation of the active 6-TG metabolites; (2) thiopurine methyltransferase (TPMT), which leads to inactive metabolites; and (3) xanthine oxidase (XO), which also leads to inactive metabolites (Fig. 31.2).

The degradative pathways TPMT and XO may indirectly alter the levels of 6-TG metabolites in different ways. The TPMT activity is reduced or absent in certain patients with a genetic polymorphism, while XO can be inhibited by drug interactions with azathioprine involving allopurinol.[9,10] The net effect of these clinical scenarios is the risk of significant myelosuppression due to increased 6-TG metabolites. In contrast, patients with high levels of TPMT have relatively low levels of the active 6-TG metabolites and may be therapeutically underdosed with azathioprine.[11,12]

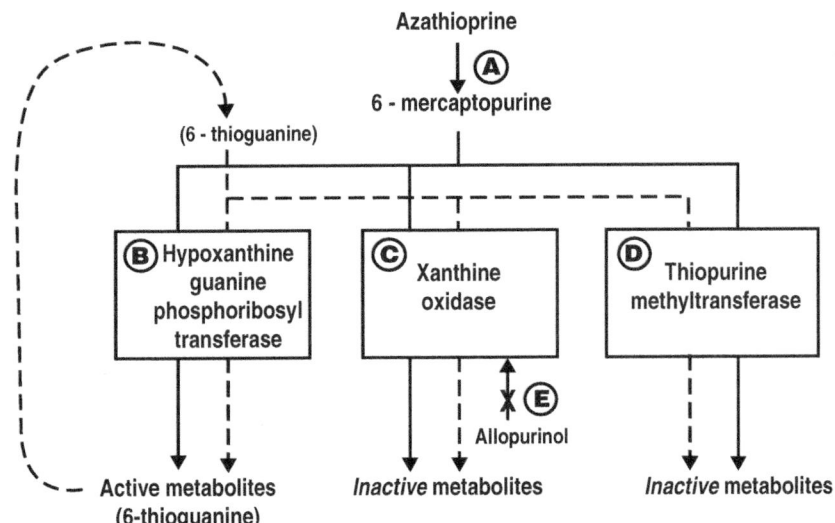

FIG. 31.2. Azathioprine metabolic pathways *

It is important to note that significant variation of TPMT activity is present when comparing different ethnic groups. Genetic testing (genotype) for TPMT is readily available, and can generally at least verify that the patient is a homozygote for high activity (TPMT 1*/1*) or a heterozygote for high activity (TPMT 1*/other allele). Functional assays of thiopurine methyltransferase red blood cell (RBC) activity are also available and widely utilized.[11]

Clinical Applications of Azathioprine Mechanisms[4]

Common Indications

1. Pemphigus and pemphigoid spectrums; azathioprine inhibition of antibody production.
2. Cutaneous vasculitis (refractory), pyoderma gangrenosum, severe atopic dermatitis, chronic actinic dermatitis, sarcoidosis; inhibition of T-cell function.

Significant Adverse Effects

1. Carcinogenicity including non-Hodgkin's B-cell lymphomas (this does not appear to be a significant risk with dermatologic conditions with immunologic etiologies; no doubt is a risk with organ transplantation patients), due to altered immune surveillance resulting from azathioprine immunosuppressive properties.
2. Myelosuppression, especially with genetically decreased TPMT levels, shunting 6-MP increasingly to HGPRT pathway, resulting in increased 6-TG metabolites.
3. Opportunistic infections (theoretically; in reality opportunistic infections are very uncommon with azathioprine use for dermatologic indications), due to altered immune surveillance resulting from T-cell and B-cell effects of azathioprine.
4. Gastrointestinal (GI) adverse effects, such as rapidly dividing cells given that azathioprine a cell-cycle–specific antimetabolite.

Drug Interactions

Allopurinol; XO inhibition by allopurinol shunts increased amounts 6-MP through the HGPRT pathway, leading to increased 6-TG metabolites.

Mycophenolate Mofetil

Mechanisms of Action[13]

Mycophenolate mofetil is rapidly converted to mycophenolic acid (MPA). On systemic absorption, MPA is inactivated by glucuronidation in the liver, and subsequently converted back to its active form by β-glucuronidase within the epidermis and gastrointestinal tract.

Mycophenolic acid has a key role in immune-mediated skin diseases by inhibiting de novo purine synthesis. It is a noncompetitive inhibitor of inosine monophosphate dehydrogenase (Fig. 31.3). Cells relying on de novo purine synthesis, rather than the purine salvage pathway, are preferentially affected. Therefore, the proliferative responses of T lymphocytes and B lymphocytes, which lack the purine salvage pathway, are blocked.[14,15] Virtually all other cell lines in the body can utilize the purine salvage pathway, which lessens the negative effects of this drug on nonimmunologic cells. Mycophenolic acid also leads to decreased levels of immunoglobulins and decreased delayed-type hypersensitivity responses.[16]

Clinical Applications of Mycophenolate Mofetil Mechanisms[13]

Common Indications

1. Pyoderma gangrenosum, psoriasis; relatively selective T-cell inhibition by mycophenolate mofetil.
2. Immunobullous dermatoses (including cicatricial pemphigoid, pemphigus vulgaris, others); relatively selective B-cell inhibition by this drug.

Significant Adverse Effects

1. Gastrointestinal adverse effects; antimetabolite, cell-cycle specific effects on rapidly dividing cells theoretically; however, these cells in the GI tract largely have salvage pathway for purine metabolism.
2. Relatively small number of serious adverse effects; probably the result of the selectivity for the mechanism, with effects primarily on lymphocyte subsets.

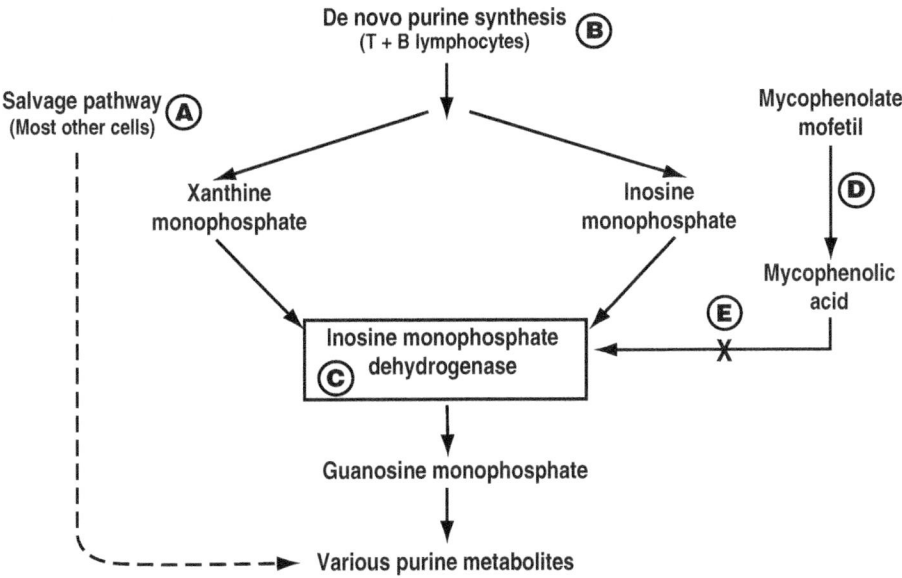

FIG. 31.3. Mycophenolate mofetil inhibition of de novo purine synthesis *

Drug Interactions

Azathioprine, methotrexate, tumor necrosis factor (TNF) inhibitors; pharmacodynamic interaction with potential for increased myelosuppression or opportunistic infections

Methotrexate

Mechanisms of Action[17]

Methotrexate competitively and reversibly binds to dihydrofolate reductase, which prevents the conversion of dihydrofolate to tetrahydrofolate (Fig. 31.4). Tetrahydrofolate is a necessary cofactor in the synthesis of thymidylate and purine nucleotides needed for DNA and RNA synthesis. A partially reversible, competitive inhibition of thymidylate synthetase also occurs within 24 hours after administration of methotrexate. Methotrexate is an antimetabolite specific for the S phase (synthesis, including DNA synthesis) of cell division, with the greatest impact on rapidly dividing cells. Cells of the GI tract and various hematologic cells are rapidly dividing groups of cells that are particularly sensitive to methotrexate inhibition of cell division.

Immunosuppression probably occurs because of inhibition of DNA synthesis in immunologically competent cells. The drug can suppress primary and secondary antibody responses as well.[18,19] There is no significant effect on delayed-type hypersensitivity. An additional effect of MTX is to block migration of activated T cells into various tissues through alteration of various adhesion molecules.[20] The drug's antiinflammatory effects are likely predominantly mediated by local increases in adenosine concentration, which has inherent antiinflammatory properties. This increased adenosine production is the result of complex interactions with aminoimidazole carboxamide ribonucleotide (AICAR) transformylase and ecto-5'-nucleotidase.[21]

Clinical Applications of Methotrexate Mechanisms[17]

Common Indications

1. Psoriasis, related to methotrexate T-cell inhibitory effects.
2. Atopic dermatitis; perhaps T-cell and antiinflammatory effects as well, at least in part due to locally increased adenosine levels.

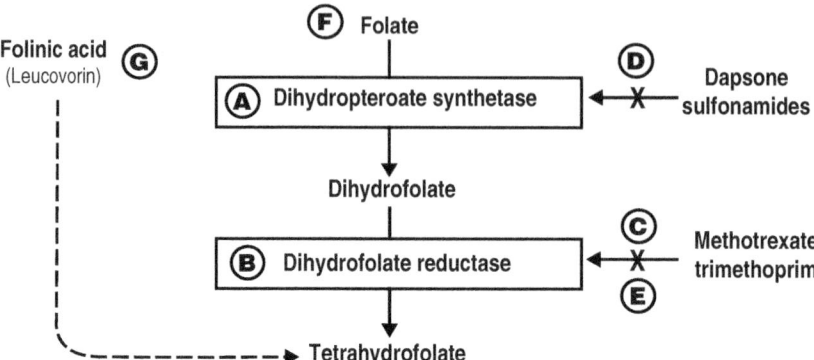

Fig. 31.4. Methotrexate and folate metabolism*

3. Bullous dermatoses (pemphigus and pemphigoid spectrums), autoimmune connective tissue diseases (dermatomyositis, morphea), sarcoidosis; methotrexate has a backup role as steroid-sparing agent due to the drug's immunosuppressive effects.

Significant Adverse Effects

1. Hepatotoxicity; nonimmunologic etiology in the great majority of cases, with methotrexate inducing fatty liver changes (risk further increases with conditions that induce fatty liver such as obesity, diabetes mellitus, excess alcohol).
2. Carcinogenicity; theoretically related to methotrexate immunosuppressive properties (this risk is primarily an issue in rheumatoid arthritis patients; minimal risk if any in psoriasis patients).
3. Gastrointestinal adverse effects such as nausea, related to cell-cycle specific properties as an antimetabolite; this risk is largely reduced by folic acid (folate) supplementation as a competitive antagonist of dihydrofolate reductase (DHFR).
4. Cytopenias such as pancytopenia, agranulocytosis, related to cell-cycle specific properties as an antimetabolite; also largely reduced risk by folic acid (folate) supplementation.

Drug Interactions

1. Trimethoprim, like methotrexate, is a DHFR inhibitor, thus amplifying the effect on this important folate metabolism enzyme.

2. Sulfonamides, dapsone (a sulfone); these drugs are dihydropteroate synthetase inhibitors, magnifying the folate pathway effects of the DHFR inhibitor methotrexate.
3. Alcohol and systemic retinoids, the pharmacodynamic effect being drugs with a risk of liver toxicity as well.

Dapsone

Mechanisms of Action[22]

The antimicrobial activity of dapsone in the treatment of leprosy is the result of inhibition of the folate metabolic pathway, specifically by the inhibition of dihydropteroate synthetase (Fig. 31.4).[23]

In contrast, dapsone inhibits the myeloperoxidase-peroxide-halide–mediated cytotoxic system as a central component of neutrophil respiratory burst (Fig. 31.5). This inhibition likely plays a key role in controlling the degree of neutrophil-induced destruction in cutaneous lesions.[24] The lack of neutrophils in the skin of patients being treated with dapsone suggests that this drug may also affect the chemotaxis of neutrophils. Dapsone inhibits chemotaxis to the chemoattractant N-formyl-methionyl-leucyl-phenylalanine (F-met-leu-phe).[25] The net result of these two effects on neutrophils is the decreased presence of neutrophils (inhibition of chemotaxis) and decreased destructive capacity of neutrophils (inhibition of myeloperoxidase and the resultant respiratory burst) in a wide variety of dermatologic conditions.

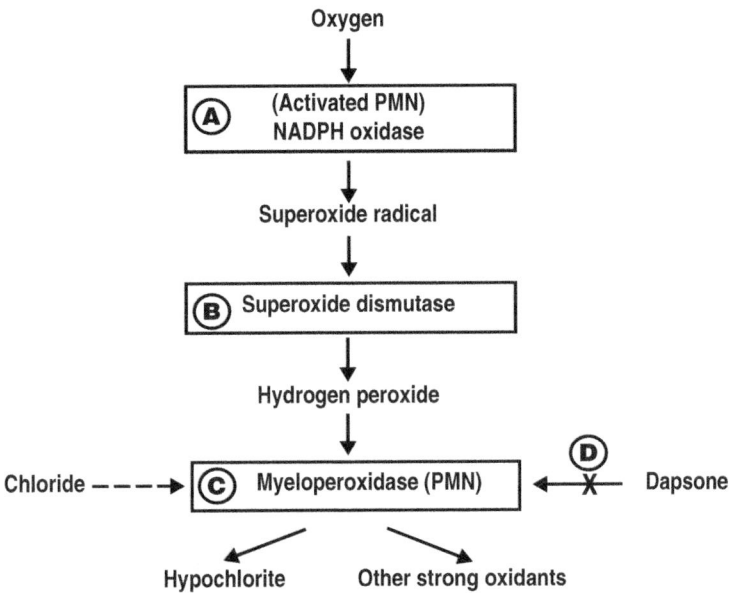

FIG. 31.5. Dapsone and myeloperoxidase oxidative system. * NADPH, reduced nicotinamide adenine dinucleotide phosphate; PMN, polymorphonuclear lymphocytes

The enzyme inhibited by dapsone, myeloperoxidase, is also present in eosinophils and monocytes, with a probable role in respiratory burst-mediated microbial destruction in these cells as well.

Clinical Applications of Dapsone Mechanisms[22]

Common Indications

1. Dermatitis herpetiformis and related conditions such as linear immunoglobulin A (IgA) bullous dermatosis; dapsone effects on neutrophil chemotaxis and respiratory burst mechanism due to myeloperoxidase inhibition.
2. Bullous lupus erythematosus, pyoderma gangrenosum, pemphigoid (bullous, cicatricial), urticarial vasculitis, aphthous stomatitis; also dermatoses with a central role of neutrophils in the disease process; chemotaxis and respiratory burst effects of dapsone.
3. Eosinophilic cellulitis, granuloma faciale; dermatoses with a central role of eosinophils; dapsone myeloperoxidase inhibition in eosinophils as well.
4. Granuloma annulare, granulomatous rosacea; dermatoses with a central role of monocytes and granuloma formation; dapsone myeloperoxidase inhibition in monocytes as well.

5. Infectious diseases such as leprosy, malaria; largely due to dihydropteroate synthetase inhibition.

Significant Adverse Effects

1. Agranulocytosis, mechanism uncertain; however, selectivity for neutrophils (over platelets, red blood cells [RBCs]) likely due at least in part to neutrophil myeloperoxidase inhibition.
2. Hemolysis, not immunologically mediated; instead is related to RBC oxidative stress.
3. Dapsone hypersensitivity syndrome, immunologically mediated, but not directly related to the two primary enzymes dapsone inhibits (myeloperoxidase and dihydropteroate synthetase).

Drug Interactions

1. Trimethoprim, methotrexate; inhibition of dihydrofolate reductase, thus amplifying folate metabolism at two different steps (given dapsone dihydropteroate synthetase inhibition)
2. Sulfonamides; inhibition of dihydropteroate synthetase, theoretically amplifying the effects of dapsone on this enzyme.

Cyclophosphamide

Mechanisms of Action[13]

Systemic cytotoxic agents from the alkylating agents group include cyclophosphamide and chlorambucil. This section discusses the more potent immunosuppressive agent cyclophosphamide. In contrast with the antimetabolites previously discussed, cyclophosphamide is cell-cycle nonspecific. Thus, all cell types can be susceptible to the benefits and adverse effects of this drug. Alkylating agents alter the chemical properties and structure of DNA, regardless of timing in the cell cycle. The highly reactive ethyleneimine intermediate for cyclophosphamide is formed and covalently binds with various nucleophilic centers within DNA. Through their effect on protein synthesis, the alkylating drugs interfere with the production of cytokines, growth factors, adhesion molecules, and other substances required for cell growth and differentiation. As a result, these drugs are often mutagenic.[26]

Cyclophosphamide depresses B-cell function more than T-cell function. The effect on T-cell activity is variable, with greater activity when the drug is given before antigen presentation. In addition, suppressor T cells (CD8) appear to be significantly more affected than helper T cells (CD4).[27]

Three broad primary effects result from alkylation: (1) DNA may cross-link with another nucleophilic residue, (2) there is an abnormal base pairing with thymine, and (3) depurination may occur with resultant chain scission by several different mechanisms. If these mutations overwhelm the DNA repair system, the result is either cell death or mutagenesis and carcinogenesis.[27,28]

Hemorrhagic cystitis and resultant increased risk of bladder carcinoma due to cyclophosphamide are believed to be largely due to local increased concentrations of acrolein metabolites of cyclophosphamide.[29]

Clinical Applications of Cyclophosphamide Drug Mechanisms[13]

Common Indications

1. Cicatricial pemphigoid (sight-threatening), severe pemphigus vulgaris; of the drugs discussed in this chapter, cyclophosphamide is probably the most potent immunosuppressant, and thus can be a definitive treatment of the most serious dermatoses.
2. Systemic vasculitis syndromes (such as Wegener's granulomatosis); similar reasoning as above, although these vasculitis subsets are seldom managed by dermatologists alone.

Significant Adverse Effects

1. Myelogenous leukemias; not an issue with other immunosuppressive agents; probably an issue with cyclophosphamide and other alkylating agents due to the structural alterations of DNA.
2. Bladder carcinoma (typically preceded by hemorrhagic cystitis), due largely to the acrolein metabolites of cyclophosphamide.
3. Myelosuppression; cyclophosphamide is a cell-cycle nonspecific drug, yet still has its greatest effect on rapidly dividing cells.

Drug Interactions

Chlorambucil, methotrexate, azathioprine-induced myelosuppression; pharmacodynamic effect with negatively synergistic impact on myelogenous cell precursors.

Conclusion

Most traditional immune-modulating drugs used by dermatologists fall into four groups: calcineurin inhibitors, antimetabolites/purine analogues, antimetabolites/folate antagonists, and alkylating agents. The systemic calcineurin inhibitor most commonly used by dermatologists is cyclosporine. Purine analogues are represented by azathioprine and mycophenolate mofetil. Methotrexate and dapsone are commonly used folate antagonists. Alkylating agents are represented by cyclophosphamide. All of these drugs have uses in dermatology, but they also have significant side effects and the potential for drug interactions.

References

1. Lee CS, Koo JYM. Cyclosporine. In: Wolverton SE, ed. Comprehensive Dermatologic Drug Therapy, 2nd ed. London: Elsevier, 2007:219–237.

2. Borel JF, Feurer C, Gubler HU. Biological effects of cyclosporin A: a new antilymphocyte agent. Agents Act 1976;6:468–475.

3. Schreiber SL, Crabtree GR. The mechanism of action of cyclosporin and FK506. Immunol Today 1992;13:136–142.

4. Badalamenti SA, Kerdel FA. Azathioprine. In: Wolverton SE, ed. Comprehensive Dermatologic Drug Therapy, 2nd ed. London: Elsevier, 2007:183–195.

5. Anstey VA, Walkelin S, Reynolds NJ. Guidelines for prescribing azathioprine in dermatology. Br J Dermatol 2004;151:1123–1132.

6. Loo TL, Luce JK, Sullivan MP, et al. Clinical pharmacologic observations of 6–mercaptopurine and 6-methylthiopurine ribonucleoside. Clin Pharmacol Ther 1968;9:180–194.

7. Younger IR, Harris DWS, Clover GB. Azathioprine in dermatology. J Am Acad Dermatol 1991;25:281–288.

8. Liu H, Wong C. In vitro immunosuppressive effects of methotrexate and azathioprine on Langerhans cells. Arch Dermatol Res 1997;289:94–97.

9. Weinshilboum RM, Sladek SL. Mercaptopurine pharmacogenetics: monogeneic inheritance of erythrocyte thiopurine methyltransferase activity. Am J Human Gen 1980;32:651–662.

10. Kennedy DM, Hayney M, Lake K. Azathioprine and allopurinol: the price of an avoidable drug interaction. Ann Pharmacother 1996;30:951–954.

11. Snow JL, Gibson LE. A pharmacogenetic basis for the safe and effective use of azathioprine and other thiopurine drugs in dermatologic patients. J Am Acad Dermatol 1995;32:114–116.

12. Wolverton SE. Major adverse effects from systemic drugs: defining the risks. Curr Prob Dermatol 1995;7:1–40.

13. Perlis C, Pan TD, McDonald CJ: Cytotoxic agents. In: Wolverton SE, ed. Comprehensive Dermatologic Drug Therapy, 2nd ed. London: Elsevier, 2007:197–217.

14. Eugui EM, Kirkovitch A, Allison AC. Lymphocyte-selective anti-proliferative and immunosuppressive effects of mycophenolic acid in mice. Scand J Immunol 1991;33:175–183.

15. Eugui EM, Almquist S, Muller CD, et al. Lymphocyte-selective cytostatic and immunosuppressive effects of mycophenolic acid in vitro: Role of deoxyguanosine nucleotide depletion. Scand J Immunol 1991;33:161–173.

16. Schiff MH, Goldblum R, Rees MMC. New DMARD. Mycophenolate mofetil effectively treats refractory rheumatoid arthritis patients for one year. Arthritis Rheum 1991;34:S8.

17. Callen JP, Kulp-Shorten CL, Wolverton SE. Methotrexate. In: Wolverton SE, ed. Comprehensive Dermatologic Drug Therapy, 2nd ed. London: Elsevier, 2007:163–181.

18. Hersh EM, Carbone PP, Wond VG, et al. Inhibition of primary immune response in man by antimetabolites. Cancer Res 1965;25:1997–2001.

19. Mitchells MS, Wade ME, DeCenti RC, et al. Immune suppressive effects of cytosine arabinoside and methotrexate in man. Ann Intern Med 1969;70:535–547.

20. Sigmundsdottir H, Johnston A, Gudjonsson JE, et al. Methotrexate markedly reduces the expression of vascular E-selectin, cutaneous lymphocyte-associated antigen and the numbers of mononuclear leucocytes in psoriatic skin. Exp Dermatol 2004;13:426–434.

21. Chan ESL, Cronstein BN. Molecular action of methotrexate in inflammatory diseases. Arthritis Res 2002;4:266–273.

22. Hall RP, Mickle CP. Dapsone. In: Wolverton SE, ed. Comprehensive Dermatologic Drug Therapy, 2nd ed. London: Elsevier, 2007:239–257.

23. Mancey-Jones B. The mode of action of dapsone in leprosy and other disorders. In: Ryan TJMAC, ed. Essays on Leprosy. Oxford: Alden Press, 1988.

24. Stendahl O, Dahlgren C. The inhibition of polymorphonuclear leukocyte cytotoxicity by dapsone; a possible mechanism in the treatment of dermatitis herpetiformis. J Clin Invest 1977;62:214–220.

25. Harvath L, Yancey KB, Katz SI: Selective inhibition of human neutrophil chemotaxis to N-formyl-methionyl-leucyl-phenylalanine by sulfones. J Immunol 1986;137:1305–1311.

26. McDonald CJ, ed. Immunomodulatory and Cytotoxic Agents in Dermatology. New York: Marcel Dekker, 1997:5–8.

27. Hall AG. Tilby MJ. Mechanisms of action of and modes of resistance to alkylating agents used in the treatment of haematological malignancies. Blood Rev 1992;6:163–173.

28. Calabresi P, Chabner BA. Chemotherapy of neoplastic diseases. In: Goodman LS, Gilman AG, Rall TW, et al., eds. The Pharmacological Basis of Therapeutics. New York: Pergammon Press, 1990:1202–1263.

29. Brock H, Pohl L, Stekar J. Studies of urotoxicity of oxazaphosphorine cytostatics and its prevention. I. Experimental studies on the urotoxicity of alkylating agents. Eur J Cancer Clin Oncol 1981;17:596–607.

32
Topical Corticosteroids

Ulrich R. Hengge

Key Points

- Glucocorticosteroids (GCSs) have antiinflammatory, antiproliferative, and immunosuppressive effects.
- Glucocorticosteroids exert their effects by binding to glucocorticoid receptors (GR) and by modification of transcription of corticosteroid-responsive genes.
- Glucocorticosteroids induce neutrophilia, lymphopenia, eosinopenia, and monocytopenia as well as reduce access of inflammatory cells at the site of active infection.
- To improve the benefit-risk ratio of GCSs, new interventions have been developed, including liposomal GCS, GR agonists, and nitroso-glucocorticoids.
- Drugs that induce the hepatic cytochrome P-450 system accelerate the clearance of GCSs, while other drugs inhibit this system.
- The side effects of GCSs are strictly dose-dependent.
- The vehicle in which the topical steroid is formulated influences the absorption and potency of the drug.

Since Marion Sulzberger introduced glucocorticosteroids (GCSs) in 1951, they have revolutionized clinical medicine.[1] This chapter provides an updated overview of their mode of action, their use in dermatology, and their adverse-effect profile. While systemic GCSs have a long list of indications, topical corticosteroids represent the mainstay for treating inflammatory diseases of the skin. Adverse effects depend on the dose, the duration of treatment, and the preexisting medical conditions. For topical application, the nature of the drug, the vehicle, and the site of application determine the side-effect profile. The most frequent cutaneous adverse effects include atrophy, striae, rosacea, perioral dermatitis, acne, and purpura. With lower frequency, hypertrichosis, pigmentation changes, delayed wound healing, and skin infections as well as contact sensitization are observed. Important systemic adverse effects include musculoskeletal, ophthalmologic, nervous system, metabolic, and cardiovascular manifestations. The main characteristics of GCSs are potent antiinflammatory, antiproliferative, and immunosuppressive effects, which give them a long list of potential indications in medicine. In particular, GCSs are extremely effective in the treatment of many autoimmune and inflammatory diseases.

Synthesis of Glucocorticosteroids

Glucocorticosteroids are produced in the adrenal cortex, which secretes cortisol as well as the weak androgens androstenedione and dehydroepiandrosterone. Normally, cortisol secretion is regulated by hormonal interactions within the hypothalamic-pituitary-adrenal (HPA) axis upon pulse secretion of the hypothalamic corticotropin-releasing hormone (CRH). This prompts the secretion of adrenocorticotropic hormone (ACTH) from the anterior pituitary, which then causes the secretion of cortisol from the adrenal cortex at a daily dose of 20 mg; however, cortisol output may increase by 10 times upon stress.

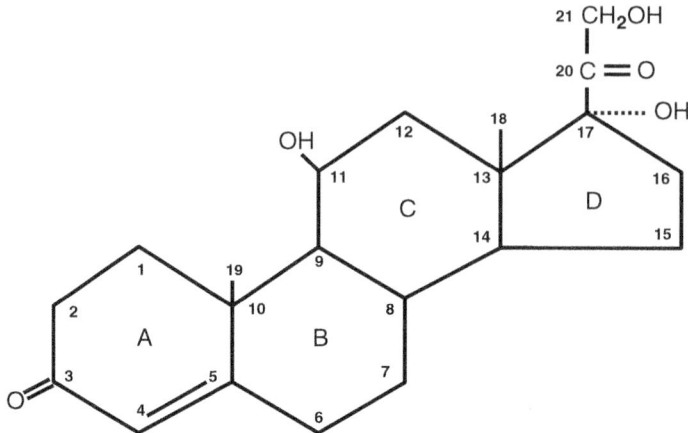

Fig. 32.1. Chemical structure of cortisol. Note the four-ring structure and the hydroxyl group at position 11

Pharmacology

The family of steroids, including GCSs, is based on the four-ring structure of cholesterol, with 3-hexane rings and one pentane ring (Fig. 32.1).[2] Modifications of the basic GCS structure result in agents with variant potency, mineralocorticoid activity, metabolism, and duration of action (Table 32.1). Important for the therapy of patients with hepatic insufficiency is the fact that the ketone group at the 11 position of cortisone must undergo hepatic conversion to a hydroxyl group to produce the active agent hydrocortisone (cortisol). Likewise, prednisone must undergo the same activation by 11-hydroxylation to become the active prednisolone. Therefore, for patients with liver problems, the use of prednisolone is recommended instead of prednisone.

Glucocorticosteroids are absorbed in the jejunum with peak plasma levels occurring within 1 hour. Of note, administration with food does not decrease peak plasma concentrations, but may delay its absorption.

Molecular Mechanism of Action

Glucocorticosteroids exert their effect by binding to glucocorticoid receptors (GRs) and by modification of transcription of corticosteroid-responsive genes. Free GCSs readily diffuse through the plasma membrane to bind to GRs in the cytoplasm, which leads to release of the heat-shock protein (hsp) 90. Upon release of hsp90, two nuclear localization signals are exposed, which allow the nuclear accumulation of the GR complex.

TABLE 32.1. Glucocorticosteroid agents.

Compound	Equivalent glucocortico-steroid dose (mg)	Mineralocorticoid potency (relative)	Duration of activity (h)
Short acting			
Cortisone	25	2 +	8–12
Hydrocortisone	20	2 +	8–12
Intermediate acting			
Prednisone	5	1 +	24–36
Prednisolone	5	1 +	24–36
Methylprednisolone	4	0	24–36
Triamcinolone	4	0	24–36
Long acting			
Dexamethasone	0.60	0	36–54
Betamethasone	0.75	0	36–54

The GR forms a dimer that binds to glucocorticoid response elements within the promoter region of steroid-responsive genes. From this interaction, transrepression or transactivation of regulatory proteins may occur. It has become increasingly clear that many adverse effects of GCS are predominantly caused by transactivation (e.g., diabetes and glaucoma, osteoporosis, skin atrophy, growth retardation, and Cushing syndrome).[3] By contrast, antiinflammatory effects are mostly mediated by transrepression of proinflammatory cytokines or cyclooxygenase-2 (COX-2).[3,4]

The discovery that activation and repression of the GR are genetically separable has fueled intense research on more selective receptor ligands.[5] The precise confirmation that the receptor assumes after ligand binding is determined by the structure of the given binding partner. Upon binding, structural alterations occur that allow interactions of the DNA-binding surface with specific glucocorticoid response elements such as the formation of homodimers and the binding of different co-activators and co-repressors at the ligand-binding domain that induce either activation or repression of gene transcription.[6] In particular, transcriptional repression activity is sensitive to the glucocorticoid-mediated antiinflammatory and antiproliferative effects.[7] Several mechanisms of transcriptional repression such as interactions of the GR with DNA or with nonreceptor protein–protein complexes have been described.[6] Recently, a number of more selective GR ligands have been discovered; they are called selective GR agonists (SEGRAs) or dissociating GCSs.[6] The SEGRAs predominantly induce the desired transrepression effects, whereas transactivation properties are significantly reduced.[3] While some of these compounds have an encouraging side-effect profile, equivalent antiinflammatory efficacy as compared with prednisone and dexamethasone still has to be demonstrated for compounds such as deflazacort.[8]

Effects on Inflammatory Cells

Glucocorticosteroids induce neutrophilia, lymphopenia, eosinopenia, and monocytopenia. They also reduce access of inflammatory cells at the sites of active inflammation. However, important neutrophil functions such as phagocytosis and bactericidal activity remain largely unaffected by pharmacologic doses of GCSs. Transient lymphopenia occurs through redistribution of T lymphocytes to other lymphoid compartments, possibly through a change in adhesion molecule expression.

Potential Indications and Contraindications

The list of potential indications for use of GCS in dermatology is long (Table 32.2). Primary indications are severe forms of eczema and autoimmune diseases, including bullous and collagen vascular diseases. In addition, GCSs are extremely useful drugs in the treatment of graft-versus-host disease.[9] Moreover, a number of cancers such as certain lymphomas and leukemias (e.g., multiple myeloma) respond well to combination therapy that includes GCSs. In these diseases, cancer cells are killed through GCS-mediated induction of apoptosis.

Contraindications include herpesvirus keratitis, active viral infections, invasive mycosis, and allergy to GCSs as well as administration following vaccination. Relative contraindications include hypertension, cardiac insufficiency, peptic ulcers, psychosis, tuberculosis, diabetes, osteoporosis, glaucoma, cataracts, and pregnancy.

Dosing and Administration

Dermatologists most often prescribe GCSs for short periods of time to treat acute dermatoses such as contact dermatitis or different kinds of eczema. The therapeutic principle is to start at a high dose and to reduce the dose upon effect to maintenance dosing below the Cushing equivalent. Many corticoid-sensitive conditions are treated by oral burst therapy followed by a 2- to 3-week tapering course with a drug of intermediate duration of action such as prednisone; typically initial doses are in the range of 40 to 60 mg per day. From a pharmacoeconomic standpoint, GCSs have a very high cost-effectiveness ratio; however, this is hampered by the costs of management of side effects. For example, prednisone is convenient as it is inexpensive and available in many dosages. The drug is usually given as a single dose in the morning rather than

TABLE 32.2. Major indications for systemic GCS use in dermatology.

Inflammatory dermatoses and allergies
   Contact dermatitis (various)
   Atopic dermatitis
   Photodermatitis
   Exfoliative dermatitis
   Erythrodermas
   Urticaria
   Erythema exudativum multiforme
   Stevens-Johnson syndrome
   Erythema nodosum
   Sweet syndrome
Bullous dermatoses
   Pemphigus (all forms)
   Bullous pemphigoid
   Cicatricial pemphigoid
   Linear immunoglobulin A bullous dermatosis
   Epidermolysis bullosa acquisita
   Herpes gestationis
   Erythema multiforme (major/minor)
   Toxic epidermal necrosis
Vasculitis
   Cutaneous (various types)
   Systemic (various types)
Collagen vascular diseases
   Lupus erythematosus (all subsets)
   Dermatomyositis
   Systemic sclerosis
   Mixed connective tissue disease syndrome
   Eosinophilic fasciitis
   Relapsing polychondritis
Neutrophilic dermatoses
   Pyoderma gangrenosum
   Acute febrile neutrophilic dermatosis
   Behçet's disease
Miscellaneous dermatoses
   Sarcoidosis
   Lichen planus
   Polyarteriitis nodosa
   Panniculitis (some types)
   Urticaria/angioedema
   Arthropod bites/stings
   Hemangiomas

dosing being divided over the course of the day in order to minimize HPA axis suppression.

Severe and life-threatening dermatoses such as pemphigus vulgaris or severe drug reaction require higher doses of GCSs to suppress and control the disease. Especially for high-dose treatment, the doses can be separated by 4 to 6 hours to achieve better early control. The next step is to consolidate the drug to a single morning dose, prior to tapering. Alternatively, every-other-day administration may also be used as it has been shown to minimize suppression of the HPA axis. The addition of a steroid-sparing agent (e.g., mycophenolate mofetil or azathioprine) is often necessary for long-term GCS treatment such as for pemphigus vulgaris prior to tapering. Typical tapering is accomplished by 20-mg steps when the initial dose was more than 60 mg per day. Smaller tapers are used for lower initial doses until the physiologic dose range of 7.5 mg per day of prednisone is reached.

Intravenous pulse therapy is used for life-threatening dermatoses using methylprednisolone in doses of 0.5 to 1 g per day for 5 days with a subsequent change to oral therapy. Cardiac conditions due to acute electrolyte shifts and arrhythmias are the most significant complications of a high-dose regimen. Due to the mineralocorticoid activity, potassium substitution may also be necessary.

To minimize corticosteroid side effects associated with GCS use, local application (e.g., inhalation) or fine-tuned dosing regimens have been developed to improve the benefit-risk ratio. One additional progress report includes the development of liposomal GCSs, which selectively accumulate at the site of inflammation.[10] Another current approach to optimize therapy with conventional GCS is to change the timing of glucocorticoid delivery (timed-release capsules) and the combination with 11β-hydroxysteroid dehydrogenase that increases the level and action of endogenous GCSs. For an additional improvement, new drugs such as selective GR agonists or nitroso-glucocorticoids (nitrosteroids) are in development. The nitrosteroids are characterized by an aliphatic or aromatic molecule, which links a conventional GCS derivative with nitric oxide (NO). Representatives of this class are NO-prednisolone and NO-hydrocortisone, which slowly release NO, exerting antiinflammatory effects.[11] The NO effect is synergistic to the effect of prednisolone, leading to an up to 10-fold more potent antiinflammatory response than those of prednisolone alone.[12]

Modes of Application

Glucocorticosteroids can be applied as topical and systemic treatment, but may also be administered locally to the nasal mucosa or be inhaled for the treatment of asthma. Recent studies suggest that inhaled steroids may also exhibit comparable side effects, including growth retardation in children[13] and reduction of bone markers in adolescents.[14] Local injections of triamcinolone are frequently being used to treat keloids. In addition, intraarticular injection represents a local application against rheumatic diseases.

Drug Interactions

As several drugs, such as rifampin, phenytoin, and phenobarbital, induce the hepatic cytochrome P-450 system, the clearance of GCSs may be accelerated in patients taking these medications. Dose-lowering adjustments may be necessary with enzyme inhibitors such as ketoconazole. Estrogens also potentiate the effect of GCS, because the two agents are metabolized similarly and have similar protein-binding characteristics.[15]

The dose of GCS needs to be adjusted in patients with chronic active hepatitis and reduced renal function.[16] Conversely, in patients with hyperthyroidism, the biologic effect of prednisolone is reduced and may require higher doses.

Side Effects

The side effects of GCS are strictly dose-dependent. In addition, some side effects are known to depend on age and sex. In general, the side effects of GCS therapy show different degrees of severity. Table 32.3 contains a list of relevant side effects of GCS.

Musculoskeletal

Osteoporosis

Osteoporosis is the most prevalent of the extremely important and severe musculoskeletal effects of long-term GCS therapy, but can be reduced or prevented with early physician intervention. Osteoporosis develops in 30% to 50% of patients treated with long-term GCS therapy.[17] The typical patients suffer from chronic diseases such as rheumatoid arthritis, chronic destructive pulmonary disease, and asthma, or have had an organ transplantation. Postmenopausal women are especially

TABLE 32.3. Important side effects of glucocorticosteroid therapy.

Musculoskeletal effects
  Osteoporosis
  Osteonecrosis
  Growth retardation
  Myopathy
Ophthalmologic effects
  Cataract
  Glaucoma
  Ocular bacterial, fungal, and viral infections
Nervous system effects
  Euphoria
  Psychosis
  Neuropsychiatric changes (anxiety, insomnia, and emotional lability)
  Pseudotumor cerebri
Metabolic effects
  Hyperglycemia
  Hyperlipidemia
  Weight gain
Cardiovascular effects
  Hypertension
  Atherosclerosis
Infection
Obstetric and gynecologic effects
  Pregnancy and lactation
  Amenorrhea
Gastrointestinal effects
  Nausea and vomiting
  Peptic ulcer disease
Cutaneous effects
  Striae, purpura, telangiectasias, and atrophy
  Cushing syndrome
  Impaired wound healing
Hypothalamic-pituitary-adrenal axis suppression

at a significantly increased risk of fractures.[18] Importantly, the rate of bone loss is highest in the first 6 months of therapy; thereafter, the rate of bone loss is diminished. Upon discontinuation of steroid therapy, patients partly regain bone tissue. Glucocorticosteroid-induced bone loss affects trabecular bone and the cortical rim of vertebrae to a significantly higher degree than cortical bones ("long bones"). This is due to the much higher metabolic turnover rate of trabecular bone. Glucocorticosteroids cause this side effect by reducing intestinal absorption and renal tubular resorption of calcium. The reduced calcium serum concentration causes increased parathormone release that further promotes bone loss (secondary hyperparathyroidism). In addition, GCS can induce decreased gonadal function in both sexes.

The most sensitive technique to diagnose osteoporosis is dual-energy x-ray absorptiometry (DEXA).[19] Bone density studies should be performed every 12 months in patients with long-term corticosteroid therapy. Besides the use of bisphosphonates (alendronate and risedronate) as effective drugs preventing and treating GCS-induced osteoporosis,[20] progress in treating GCS-associated side effects has been limited. There are additional data to support the effectiveness of calcium and vitamin D supplementation in preserving bone mass in patients receiving long-term GCS therapy.[21]

Osteonecrosis

Osteonecrosis (aseptic necrosis) can also result from GCS therapy. It most commonly occurs on the proximal femur or the humeral head. In contrast to osteoporosis, osteonecrosis more frequently affects active patients and is particularly common in men.[22,23]

Growth Retardation

Growth suppression from GCS usually occurs with systemic therapy and may only occasionally be a consequence of extensive treatment with topical or inhaled potent GCS. When GCSs are given under the age of 2 or at puberty,[24] the risk of growth retardation is especially significant. The studied patients were significantly shorter in height, had a significantly greater body mass index, and a higher prevalence of obesity than did the controls.[24] On average, they had received 23 g of GCS for the treatment of nephrotic syndrome. The causes are multifaceted: interference with nitrogen and mineral retention, bone formation, inhibition of mitosis, and collagen synthesis.[25] Treatment of GCS-mediated growth inhibition with growth hormone shows some promise.[26]

Myopathy

There are two forms of myopathy induced by GCS. One form is an acute myopathy seen almost exclusively in patients treated with high-dose intravenous GCS for status asthmaticus. The second form of myopathy is relevant to dermatology and is characterized by progressive symmetric proximal muscle weakness, which is usually painless and begins on the lower extremities after several months of therapy.[27] While the particular mechanism of GCS's effect on muscle mass has not been determined, hypogonadism (e.g., estrogen and testosterone) is likely to be involved, as it is present in many GCS patients. Diagnosis of GCS myopathy may be difficult in some patients, as muscle biopsies usually show nonspecific findings, and electromyographic studies are usually normal in this condition.

Ophthalmologic Effects

Cataract formation upon extended periods of GCS treatment has been described.[28] To detect initial changes, routine eye examinations twice yearly are recommended for all patients treated with long-term systemic GCS.

Open-angle glaucoma may also occur upon GCS treatment, especially in patients with a history of rheumatoid arthritis, type 1 diabetes, or a positive family history for glaucoma.[29] The detection of elevated intraocular pressure is important, as this condition is usually reversible within 1 to 4 weeks, when detected early.

Nervous System Effects

Affective disorders (anxiety, insomnia, euphoria, and emotional lability) are more frequent than confusional or psychotic states. The onset of symptoms is usually within 1 or 2 weeks after starting therapy, especially in patients with a prior history of psychiatric diseases.[27] Importantly, patients with systemic lupus erythematosus, who may suffer from lupus and encephalopathy may be difficult to differentiate from patients with steroid-induced psychosis. Discontinuation of GCS is usually the treatment of choice, rather than starting neuroleptic or antidepressive therapy.

Pseudotumor cerebri, presenting with headache, nausea, vomiting, and papillary edema, is a rare complication of long-term GCS administration and occurs predominantly in boys. It usually occurs when steroids are rapidly tapered or stopped.[27]

Metabolic Effects

The manifestation of hyperglycemia and secondary diabetes is a typical complication of GCS therapy.[30] Relative insulin resistance is produced by decreasing the insulin affinity of cellular receptors and possibly by diminishing postreceptor effects of insulin.[31,32] In addition, GCSs effect insulin-mediated increases in blood flow to muscles and increases in glucose output by increasing the rate-limiting enzyme of gluconeogenesis (i.e., phosphoenolpyruvate carboxy kinase). Therefore, following patients' regular blood glucose levels during continued GCS therapy is important.[33] If needed, insulin is the therapy of choice, as oral antidiabetics often take weeks before the onset of effects.

Hyperlipidemia may be worsened by GCS, especially in patients with diabetes mellitus, obesity, hypothyroidism, or family history of lipid disorders.

Weight gain may occur as a consequence of increased appetite and fluid retention with GCS therapy. Facial, supraclavicular, and posterior cervical fat depots are particularly sensitive to GCS, resulting in the moon face and buffalo humps that are characteristic of long-term GCS treatment. These symptoms severely impact on patients' well-being by negatively affecting their appearance and by predisposing them to obesity-related health issues.

Cardiovascular Effects

Excess GCSs can lead to increased blood pressure as they affect several points of blood pressure regulation. Hypertension may develop as a consequence of the mineralocorticoid activity of exogenous GCS. Usually, the kidney is protected from the effects of excess cortisol through the oxidizing effect of 11β-hydroxysteroid dehydrogenase-2, a tissue-specific enzyme capable of converting cortisol to cortisone. However, aldosterone as well as synthetic steroids with modifications and different positions are not susceptible to this activity and exert a major effect directly on the kidney through both mineralocorticoid receptors and GR, leading to transepithelial sodium transport and sodium reabsorption in the proximal tubule.[34] A similar mode of action may be present in brain, where the 11β-hydroxysteroid dehydrogenase-2 is expressed along with mineralocorticoid receptors in selected areas that are involved in central regulation of salt, water balance, and blood pressure.[35] These processes trigger intravascular and extracellular volume expansion. In addition, a decrease in vasodilatory prostaglandins and prostacyclins has been detected upon GCS therapy,[36] which contributes to hypertension.

Infection

Patients on GCS therapy are at an increased risk for infections, including bacterial, fungal, viral, and protozoal infectious agents. Making the diagnosis is sometimes difficult, as fever and many other signs of inflammation may be masked. Although neutrophilia is induced by GCS, the presence of greater than 6% band forms suggests a coexistent infection.[37] Opportunistic infections such as *Pneumocystis carinii* and *Toxoplasma gondii* may occur in patients on chronic GCS therapy who are not HIV-positive. In addition, reactivation of tuberculosis remains a concern in this patient population.[38] Concomitant isoniazid has been advocated in patients with a positive tuberculin skin test undergoing long-term GCS therapy.

Inhibition of Wound Repair

The inhibition of wound repair results from inhibiting the natural and critical process of inflammation as part of the normal wound-healing process to remove debris and bacteria.[39] Moreover, GCSs inhibit collagen synthesis and collagen cross-linking, and thereby affect structural components of a healing wound.[40]

Obstetric and Gynecologic Effects

Clinical experience in several trials has shown minimal adverse effects in pregnant and lactating women during GCS therapy.[41,42] The American Academy of Pediatrics has determined prednisone to be compatible with breast-feeding, even though there is an excretion in breast milk.[43]

Despite the fact that systemic GCS can cross the placenta to various degrees, there is no proof of the detrimental effect on the developing human brain or on vascular disease such as hypertension and atherosclerosis.[44,45] However, pregnant or lactating women should be monitored for complications such as osteoporosis and glucose intolerance (gestational diabetes).

Gastrointestinal Effects

Nausea and vomiting may occur with oral GCS therapy. These side effects can be minimized if the GCS is taken with food. The association of GCS therapy and peptic ulcer disease remains controversial.[46] In particular, the simultaneous intake of GCSs with nonsteroidal antiinflammatory drugs as well as smoking and alcohol use have to be considered. Concurrent therapy with proton pump blockers is advised in patients with a history of peptic ulcer disease.

Cutaneous Effects

Cutaneous side effects consist of atrophy of the dermis and subcutaneous tissue, striae, rarefaction of elastic tissue (frequently causing corticoid purpura and steroid acne), telangiectasias, and hirsutism. These and other cutaneous side effects are discussed in the section on topical GCS below.

Hypothalamic-Pituitary-Adrenal Axis Suppression

The onset of HPA axis suppression is usually evident within 5 days of high-dose prednisolone therapy, suppressing ACTH and cortisol secretion. With longer treatment duration, clinically important adrenal suppression becomes a concern. Full recovery of adrenals may require up to 1 year in certain cases.[38] In addition, patients with chronic adrenal suppression, including HIV patients, may need GCS supplementation in critical conditions such as perioperative stress or sepsis.

A more common clinical problem than adrenal crisis is the steroid withdrawal syndrome. Patients' symptoms generally include arthralgias, mood swings, headache, lethargy, nausea, and vomiting, and are most frequently noted on rapidly tapering of GCS after extended periods of treatment.[47]

Topical Corticosteroids

Topical corticosteroids (TCSs) have a particular adverse-effect profile, primarily directed at the treated skin area, that occurs regularly with prolonged treatment. The severity depends on the potency of the drug, the vehicle, and the location of its application (Table 32.4). The most frequent adverse effects include atrophy, striae, rosacea, perioral dermatitis, acne, and purpura (Table 32.5). With lower frequency, hypertrichosis, pigmentation changes, delayed wound healing, and exacerbation of skin infections are observed. Of particular interest is the rate of contact sensitization against corticos-

teroids, which is considerably higher than generally believed. Systemic reactions following topical application such as hyperglycemia, glaucoma, and adrenal insufficiency have also been reported, especially in children.

Selection and Characteristics of Topical Glucocorticosteroids

Low- to medium-potency agents are generally used for treating thin, acute, inflammatory skin lesions (e.g., face, intertriginous areas), whereas highly or superpotent agents are often required for treating chronic, hyperkeratotic, or lichenified lesions (e.g., palms and soles) (Table 32.4). Most preparations are applied once or twice daily. More frequent application may be necessary on the palms or soles due to the thick stratum corneum. Every-other-day or weekend-only application may be effective for treating several chronic conditions. Low-potency agents are preferentially used in infants and the elderly. Infants have a high body surface to weight ratio; elderly patients have thin, fragile skin.

The vehicle in which the topical corticosteroid is formulated influences the absorption and potency of the drug.[48] Ointment bases enhance penetration of the drug by their occlusive effect and increase the hydration of the stratum corneum. Creams are preferred for acute and subacute dermatoses; they may be used on moist skin or intertriginous areas.

Marked regional variation in the extent of transcutaneous penetration has been documented.[49] While absorption on the forearm (1%) is poor, the scalp absorbs around 4% and the scrotum up to 35% of applied drug. Consequently, the groin, axillae, neck, and face are more likely to develop local side effects.[50,51] The reasons for this difference in absorption are due to the thickness of the stratum corneum and its lipid composition.[49] For these reasons, the skin of delicate sites such as the eyelids is much more likely to develop side effects of TCS therapy.

Pharmacologic Characteristics of Topical Glucocorticosteroids

Chemical substitution at certain key positions is able to modify the potency of GCS (see Tables 32.1 and 32.4). For example, halogenation at the

TABLE 32.4. Potency of selected topical corticosteroid preparations.

Class 1 (superpotent)	Betamethasone dipropionate ointment, cream 0.05% (Diprolene, Diprosone)
	Clobetasol propionate ointment, cream 0.05% (Temovate, Dermoxin)
	Diflorasone diacetate ointment 0.05% (Florone, Psorcon)
	Halobetasol propionate ointment, cream 0.05% (Ultravate)
Class 2 (potent)	Amcinonide ointment 0.1% (Cyclocort)
	Desoximetasone ointment, cream, gel 0.25% (Topicort, Ibaril)
	Diflorasone diacetate ointment 0.05% (Florone, Maxiflor)
	Fluocinonide ointment, cream, gel 0.05% (Lidex)
	Halcinonide cream 0.1% (Halog)
	Mometasone furoate ointment 0.1% (Elocon, Ecural)
	Triamcinolone acetonide ointment 0.5% (Kenalog)
Class 3 (less potent)	Amcinonide cream, lotion 0.1% (Cyclocort)
	Betamethasone valerate ointment 0.01% (Valisone)
	Diflorasone diacetate cream 0.05% (Florone, Maxiflor)
	Fluticasone propionate ointment 0.005% (Cutivate)
	Fluocortolone 0.25% cream (Ultralan)
	Fluocinonide cream 0.05% (Lidex E cream, Topsyn)
	Halcinonide ointment 0.1% (Halog)
	Triamcinolone acetonide ointment 0.1% (Aristocort A)
	Triamcinolone acetonide cream 0.5% (Aristocort-HP)
Class 4 (mid-strength)	Betamethasone valerate lotion 0.01% (Valisone, Luxiq)
	Desoximetasone cream, gel 0.05% (Topicort-LP)
	Fluocinolone acetonide cream 0.2% (Synalar-HP)
	Fluocinolone acetonide ointment 0.025% (Synalar)
	Flurandrenolide ointment 0.05% (Cordran)
	Halcinonide cream 0.025% (Halog)
	Hydrocortisone valerate ointment 0.2% (Westcort)
	Mometasone furoate cream 0.1% (Elocon, Ecural)
	Triamcinolone acetonide ointment 0.1% (Kenalog)
Class 5 (less mid-strength)	Betamethasone dipropionate lotion 0.05% (Diprosone)
	Betamethasone valerate cream 0.01% (Valisone)
	Fluocinolone acetonide cream 0.025% (Synalar)
	Fluocinolone acetonide oil 0.01% (Derma-Smoothe/FS)
	Flurandrenolide cream 0.05% (Cordran)
	Fluticasone propionate cream 0.05% (Cutivate)
	Hydrocortisone butyrate cream 0.1% (Locoid)
	Hydrocortisone valerate cream 0.2% (Westcort)
	Triamcinolone acetonide lotion 0.1% (Kenalog)
Class 6 (mild)	Alclometasone dipropionate ointment, cream 0.05% (Aclovate)
	Betamethasone valerate lotion 0.05% (Valisone)
	Desonide cream 0.05% (Desowen, Tridesilon)
	Fluocinolone acetonide cream, solution 0.01% (Synalar)
	Prednicarbate 0.1% cream (Dermatop)
	Triamcinolone acetonide cream 0.1% (Aristocort)
Class 7 (least potent)	Dexamethasone cream 0.1% (Decadron phosphate)
	Hydrocortisone 0.5%, 1%, 2.5% (Hytone, others)
	Methylprednisolone 1% (Medrol)
	Topical preparations with flumethasone, prednisolone

570   U.R. Hengge

TABLE 32.5. Adverse effects of topical corticosteroids steroid rebound. steroid, addition, Tachyphylaxis.

Most frequent cutaneous changes
Steroid atrophy
Teleangiectasia
Striae
Purpura
Stellate pseudoscars
Ulceration
Easy bruising
Less frequent cutaneous changes
Steroid acne
Perioral dermatitis
Steroid rosacea
Hirsutism
Hyperpigmentation
Hypopigmentation
Masked microbial infections (tinea incognito)
Aggravation of cutaneous candidiasis, herpes, or Demodex
Reactivation of Kaposi's sarcoma
Granuloma gluteale infantum
Miscellaneous
Steroid rebound, Steroid, addiction, Tachyphylaxis

9-α position enhances the potency by improving activity within the target cell and decreasing breakdown into inactive metabolites.[52] Along the same lines, masking or removing the hydrophilic 17-dihydroxyacetone side chain or the 16-α-hydroxy group increases the molecule's lipophilicity, thus enhancing penetration through the stratum corneum.[52]

The strength of TCS has been classified according to the vasoconstrictor assay, which is based on the extent to which the compound induces cutaneous vasoconstriction ("blanching effect") in normal human subjects (Table 32.4).[53] The vasoconstriction test has been established in 1962 as a rough estimate of the efficacy of TCS.[54,55] It represents a nonspecific and simple in vivo test, since the phenomenon of vasoconstriction is not linked to the receptor-mediated activity of steroids. However, the exact cause of this vasoconstriction remains unknown.[56] Alternatively, the ultraviolet (UV) erythema test measures the inhibitory effects of TCS on an experimentally elicited erythema.[57] The atrophy test is an important addition to the antiinflammatory tests, since it can be used to determine those TCSs that have only a slight antiproliferative effect (atrophogenic potential). Using the Duhring chamber, the corticosteroid to be tested is applied to the same skin area for 3 weeks under occlusion.[58] At this point, the

resulting atrophy and the extent of telangiectasias are evaluated by a defined score.

Under normal conditions, up to 99% of TCSs applied to human skin are removed by rubbing, washing off, and exfoliation, and only about 1% is therapeutically active.[59] However, only this 1% of percutaneously absorbed TCSs can exert systemic adverse effects, while cutaneous adverse effects may also result from the transient presence of TCSs.[60]

Adverse Effects of Topical Glucocorticosteroids

A number of possible adverse effects of TCSs have been reported (see Table 32.5). Principally, systemic GCS can cause the same cutaneous manifestation as TCS.

Atrophy

All TCSs have been shown to cause skin atrophy, albeit to a variable degree.[61,62] Signs of atrophy include telangiectasias (an abnormal dilatation of capillary vessels and arterioles), increased transparency and shininess of the skin, as well as the appearance of striae.[50,63] The factors that influence the degree of skin atrophy include age, body site,

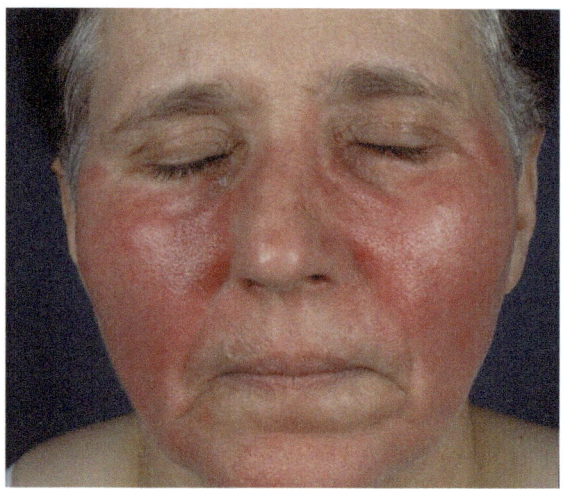

FIG. 32.2. Thickened lichenified skin, severe epidermal atrophy, and erythema following inappropriate use of high-potency corticosteroids on the face and eyelids. Telangiectasias were also present

potency of TCS, and the presence of occlusion. Atrophy has now been recognized as the most common adverse effect of topical corticosteroid therapy (Fig. 32.2).[64] Topical application of corticosteroids can cause atrophy, not only because of the suppressive action on cell proliferation, but also due to inhibition of collagen synthesis.[65] In addition to epidermal and dermal thinning, corticosteroids stimulate human dermal microvascular endothelial cells, leading to the occurrence of telangiectasias.[66]

Striae

Striae (rubrae distensae) are visible linear scars that form in areas of dermal damage, presumably upon mechanical stress (Fig. 32.3).[67] They develop as an initial inflammation and edema in the dermis, followed by the deposition of dermal collagen along the lines of mechanical stress.

Steroid Rosacea

Facial dermatoses are usually steroid-sensitive and do not require potent formulations. The classical history of steroid rosacea begins in a middle-aged woman with intermittent papules and pustules that are initially controlled by steroids of low potency (Fig. 32.4). Subsequently, the lesions reappear, leading to tachyphylaxis and steroid addiction.[68]

Acne

Topical steroids can rapidly induce acneiform eruptions.[69–71] These studies attributed the acnegenic effect to the degradation of the follicular epithelium, resulting in extrusion of the follicular content (Fig. 32.5).

Perioral Dermatitis

Steroid-induced perioral dermatitis was described as a facial eruption in females that was composed of follicular papules and pustules on an erythematous

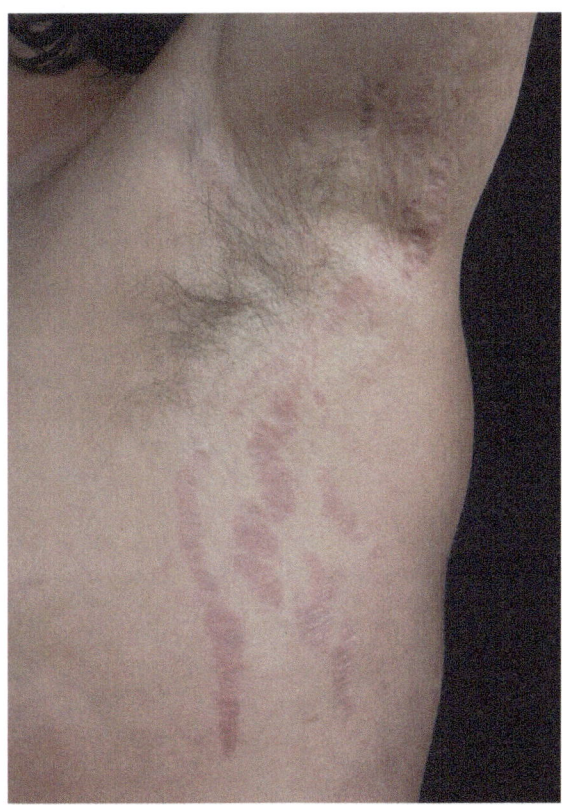

Fig. 32.3. Striae distensae rubrae as a sign of topical corticosteroid (TCS) abuse from treating eczema on the left axilla in a nonobese 27-year-old man

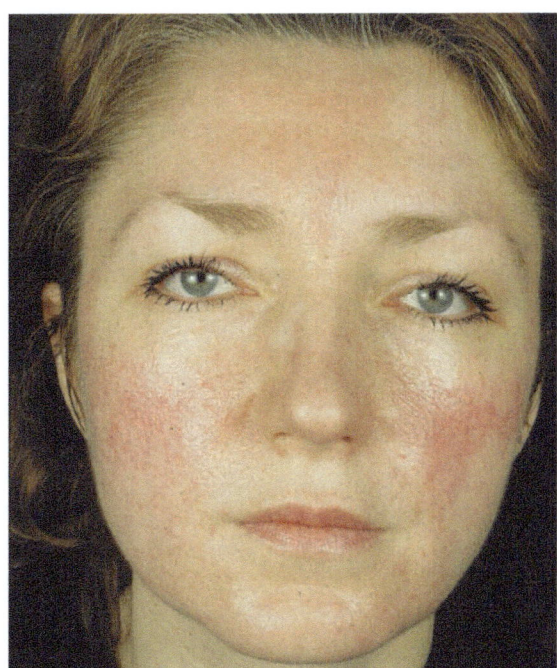

Fig. 32.4. Long-term inadvertent use of TCS for treatment of perioral and cheek dermatitis. Note the prominent telangiectasias

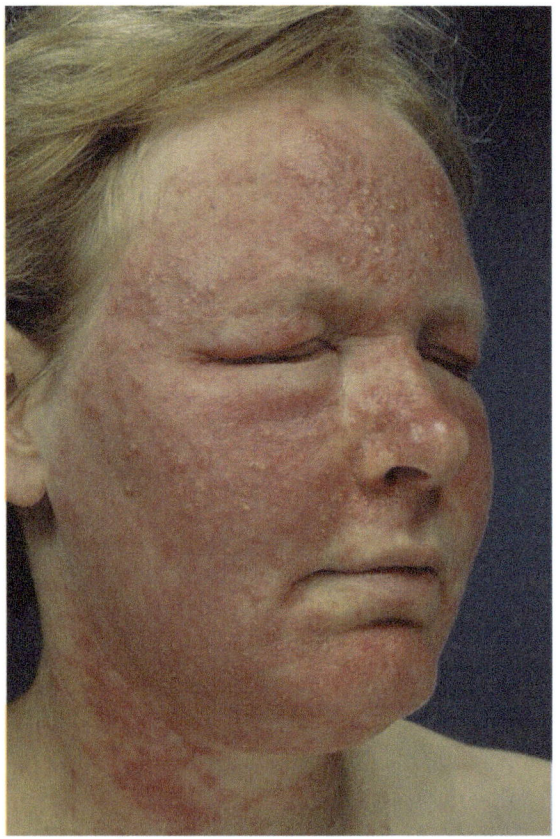

FIG. 32.5. Steroid acne in the face characterized by pustules, erythema, and several open and closed comedones on the forehead. Note the free margins around the vermilion border

background beginning in a perioral distribution with prominent sparing of the skin adjacent to the vermilion border.[72]

Steroid Addiction and Tachyphylaxis

Corticosteroid addiction has been described as an ongoing inadvertent use of potent topical corticosteroids used mostly for inflammatory diseases of the face.[68]

Tachyphylaxis is characterized by decreasing effects of corticosteroids upon continued treatment as revealed by the vasoconstrictor and proliferation inhibition assays. Due to the tissue becoming less sensitive (tachyphylaxis), more potent preparations are frequently being used to achieve comparable effects,[73] yielding more severe side effects.

Hypertrichosis

Steroids promote the growth of vellus hair by an unknown mechanism.[74] Variable degrees of hypertrichosis remain a more common manifestation of systemic corticosteroid use. The darker hair may persist for months after withdrawal of steroids.

Hypopigmentation

Decreased pigmentation after topical use is quite common, though frequently unnoticed. Americans of sub-Saharan African lineage are particularly affected. Most likely, steroids interfere with the synthesis of melanin, leading to patchy areas of hypopigmentation. The lesions are generally reversible upon discontinuation of steroid therapy.

Purpura and Stellate Pseudoscars

Purpura occurs due to severe dermal atrophy and loss of intercellular substance, and blood vessels lose their support and rupture. The resulting fragility of dermal tissue leads to hypopigmented, depressed scars.[75] These stellate pseudoscars develop most frequently over the extremities mostly on severely atrophic, telangiectatic purpuric skin (see Fig. 32.2).

Aggravation of Cutaneous Infections

Mucocutaneous (e.g., skin, nails, mucous membranes) fungal infections are common during treatment with corticosteroids and often occur early in therapy.[76,77] The incidence of skin infections varies, but is probably between 16% and 43%.[76] Infections include tinea versicolor, onychomycosis due to *Trichophyton* and *Candida* species, and dermatophytosis (Fig. 32.6).[76] The term *tinea incognito* serves to describe dermatophyte infections that became unrecognizable because of suppression of inflammation and fungal proliferation.[78]

Granuloma gluteale is a persistent reddish-purple, granulomatous papulonodular eruption occurring on the buttocks, thighs, or inguinal folds in children. It is a well-known consequence of diaper dermatitis that is being treated with corticosteroids.[79]

Delayed Wound Healing

The effects of TCS and systemic GCS on wound healing include keratinocytes (epidermal atrophy,

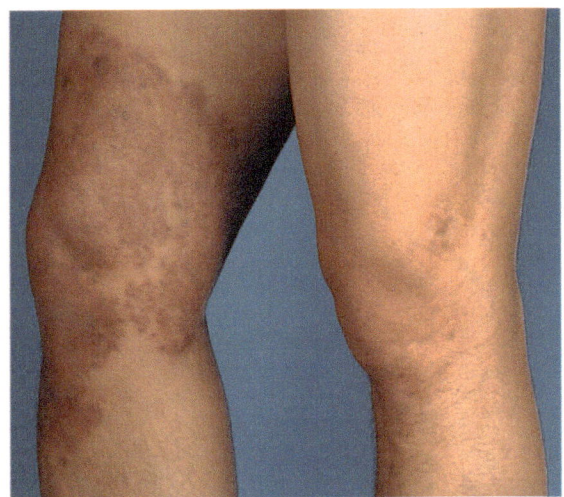

Fig. 32.6. Tinea incognito of the leg. This patient was treated with corticosteroids masking the diagnosis of tinea

delayed reepithelization), fibroblasts (reduced collagen and ground substance resulting in dermal atrophy and striae), vascular connective tissue support (telangiectasias, purpura, easy bruising), and impaired angiogenesis (delayed granulation tissue formation).[38]

Contact Sensitization

Several multicenter studies have been performed addressing contact hypersensitivity to TCS, yielding a prevalence of 0.2% to 6%.[80–83] It seems that nonfluorinated corticosteroids (e.g., hydrocortisone, hydrocortisone-17-butyrate, and budesonide) result in a higher prevalence of corticosteroid allergy in comparison with fluorinated compounds.[84]

Systemic Adverse Effects with Topical Administration

Systemic adverse effects from TCS are relatively infrequent, but may occur. In particular, glaucoma following the use of TCS around the eye has been recognized as a rare but serious problem.[85,86] This is not surprising, if one considers that the penetration of TCS is up to 300 times greater through the eyelid than on other body sites.[49] Topical corticosteroid and systemic GCS therapy have been associated with cataract formation, but systemic GCSs are most often responsible for this complication.[87]

In addition, short-term enhancement of plasma cortisol levels has been detected upon topical application of hydrocortisone.[88] All effective TCSs possess the potential to suppress the HPA axis.[89] Increasing steroid penetration has been shown to increase the potential for HPA suppression especially in children with atopic dermatitis.[90–92] The advent of superpotent derivatives such as clobetasol propionate, betamethasone dipropionate, and diflorasone diacetate have an increased ability to suppress adrenal function. As little as 2 g per day of clobetasol propionate 0.05% cream can cause a decreased morning cortisol after only a few days.[93,94] A recent open-label trial has addressed the potential suppression of the HPA axis using 0.1% fluocinonide cream in pediatric patients with atopic dermatitis with regard to adrenal suppression.[95] In this multicenter, multidosing, open-label trial, 0.1% fluocinonide cream was applied to patients in four different age cohorts, from 3 months to 18 years of age, who suffered from moderate to severe atopic dermatitis in excess of 20% body surface area involvement. No suppression of the HPA axis was observed in any patient treated once daily or in patients younger than 6 years of age. One of 15 (7%) and two of 16 (13%) patients from 3 months to 2 years and 2 to 6 years, respectively, developed HPA axis suppression when receiving twice daily 0.1% fluocinonide treatment to more than 20% of body surface area.[95]

With the majority of patients with HPA suppression demonstrating exclusive laboratory test abnormalities, several cases of severely impaired stress responses have been reported, especially in children following treatment with high potency TCS.[96–98] Recovery from steroid-induced adrenal insufficiency is time-dependent and occurs spontaneously. The administration of TCS has also led to iatrogenic Cushing's syndrome.[99,100] In addition, there is a possibility of retarded growth in children exposed to long-term potent and superpotent topical TCS formulations.[96] For prevention, it has been suggested that less than 50 g per week of potent corticosteroids should be used.[101]

Prevention of Adverse Effects

Guidelines regarding the use of TCS and suggestions were provided to prevent their misuse.[62,102,103] Possible measures to prevent side effects include

TABLE 32.6. Optimal use of topical glucocorticosteroids.

1. Appropriately potent compound to achieve disease control
2. Continuation with a less potent preparation after sufficient response
3. Reduction of frequency of application
4. Continuation of daily application with the weakest effective preparation
5. "Tapering off" treatment upon complete healing
6. Particular care in treating children and the elderly, in particular at certain locations (e.g., scrotum, face and flexures, and around the eyes)

the use of lower potency steroids, the application only in the morning, and alternate-day treatment (reducing tachyphylaxis and avoidance of occlusion) (Table 32.6).[104]

Conclusion

Glucocorticosteroids have antiinflammatory, antiproliferative, and immunosuppressive effects. These effects are exerted by GCS binding to glucocorticoid receptors (GRs) and by modification of transcription of corticosteroid-responsive genes. Neutrophilia, lymphopenia, and eosinopenia are induced by GCSs, which also reduce access of inflammatory cells at the site of active infection. To improve the benefit-risk ratio of GCSs, new interventions have been developed, such as liposomal GCSs, GR agonists, and nitroso-glucocorticosteroids. Some drugs inhibit the P-450 system, reducing clearance of GCSs, while other drugs induce the system, accelerating clearance. The side effects of GCSs are strictly dose-dependent, but the vehicle in which topical steroids are formulated influence the absorption and potency of the drug.

References

1. Sulzberger MB, Witten VH. Effect of topically applied compound F in selected dermatoses. J Invest Dermatol 1952;19:101–2.
2. Feldman SR. The biology and clinical application of systemic corticosteroids. In: Callan JP, ed. Current Problems in Dermatology. St. Louis: Mosby-Year Book, 1992:211–35.
3. Schacke H, Schottelius A, Docke WD, et al. Dissociation of transactivation from transrepression by a selective glucocorticoid receptor agonist leads to separation of therapeutic effects from side effects. Proc Natl Acad Sci USA 2004;101:227–32.
4. Schacke H, Docke WD, Asadullah K. Mechanisms involved in the side effects of glucocorticoids. Pharmacol Ther 2002;96:23–43.
5. Heck S, Bender K, Kullmann M, et al. I kappaB alpha-independent downregulation of NF-kappaB activity by glucocorticoid receptor. EMBO J 1997;16:4698–707.
6. Rosen J, Miner JN. The search for safer glucocorticoid receptor ligands. Endocr Rev 2005;26:452–64.
7. Barnes PJ. Anti-inflammatory actions of glucocorticoids: molecular mechanisms. Clin Sci 1998;94:557–72.
8. Markham A, Bryson HM. Deflazacort. A review of its pharmacological properties and therapeutic efficacy. Drugs 1995;50:317–33.
9. Deeg HJ, Henslee-Downey PJ. Management of acute graft-versus-host disease. Bone Marrow Transplant 1990;6:1–8.
10. Dams ET, Oyen WJ, Boerman OC, et al. 99mTc-PEG liposomes for the scintigraphic detection of infection and inflammation: clinical evaluation. J Nucl Med 2000;41:622–30.
11. Perretti M, Paul-Clark MJ, Mancini L, et al. Generation of innovative anti-inflammatory and anti-arthritic glucocorticoid derivatives that release NO: the nitro-steroids. Dig Liver Dis 2003;35:S41–8.
12. Paul-Clark MJ, Roviezzo F, Flower RJ, et al. Glucocorticoid receptor nitration leads to enhanced anti-inflammatory effects of novel steroid ligands. J Immunol 2003;171:3245–52.
13. Heuck C, Heickendorff L, Wolthers OD. A randomised controlled trial of short term growth and collagen turnover in asthmatics treated with inhaled formoterol and budesonide. Arch Dis Child 2000;83:334–9.
14. Heuck C, Wolthers OD, Hansen M, et al. Short-term growth and collagen turnover in asthmatic adolescents treated with the inhaled glucocorticoid budesonide. Steroids 1997;62:659–64.
15. Frey BM, Frey FJ. The effect of altered prednisolone kinetics in patients with the nephrotic syndrome and in women taking oral contraceptive steroids on human mixed lymphocyte cultures. J Clin Endocrinol Metab 1985;60:361–9.
16. Bergrem H. The influence of uremia on pharmacokinetics and protein binding of prednisolone. Acta Med Scand 1983;213:333–7.
17. Ralston SH. The genetics of osteoporosis. Bone 1999;25:85–6.
18. Lane NE, Lukert B. The science and therapy of glucocorticoid-induced bone loss. Endocrinol Metab Clin North Am 1998;27:465–83.

19. Iqbal MM. Osteoporosis: epidemiology, diagnosis, and treatment. South Med J 2000;93:2–18.

20. Recommendations for the prevention and treatment of glucocorticoid-induced osteoporosis: 2001 update. American College of Rheumatology Ad Hoc Committee on Glucocorticoid-Induced Osteoporosis. Arthritis Rheum. 2001;44:1496–503.

21. Saag KG, Emkey R, Schnitzer TJ, et al. Alendronate for the prevention and treatment of glu-cocorticoid-induced osteoporosis. Glucocorticoid-Induced Osteoporosis Intervention Study Group. N Engl J Med 1998;339: 292–9.

22. Lester RS. Corticosteroids. Clin Dermatol 1989;7: 80–97.

23. Fisher DA. Long-term administration of therapeutic corticosteroids without risk of inducing aseptic necrosis. Int J Dermatol 1998;37:15–7.

24. Leonard MB, Feldman HI, Shults J, et al. Long-term, high-dose glucocorticoids and bone mineral content in childhood glucocorticoid-sensitive nephrotic syndrome. N Engl J Med 2004;351:868–75.

25. Allen DB, Julius JR, Breen TJ, et al. Treatment of glucocorticoid-induced growth suppression with growth hormone. National Cooperative Growth Study. J Clin Endocrinol Metab 1998;83:2824–9.

26. Magiakou MA. Growth in disorders of adrenal hyperfunction. Pediatr Endocrinol Rev 2004;1:S484–9.

27. Lacomis D, Samuels MA. Adverse neurologic effects of glucocorticosteroids. J Gen Intern Med 1991;6:367–77.

28. Limaye SR, Pillai S, Tina LU. Relationship of steroid dose to degree of posterior subcapsular cataracts in nephrotic syndrome. Ann Ophthalmol 1988;20:225–7.

29. Renfro L, Snow JS. Ocular effects of topical and systemic steroids. Dermatol Clin 1992;10:505–12.

30. Ariza-Andraca C, Barile-Fabris LA, Frati-Munari AC, et al. Risk factors for steroid diabetes in rheumatic patients. Arch Med Res 1998;29:259–62.

31. McMahon M, Gerich J, Rizza R. Effects of glucocorticoids on carbohydrate metabolism. Diabetes Metab Rev 1988;4:17–30.

32. Tappy L, Randin D, Vollenweider P, et al. Mechanisms of dexamethasone-induced insulin resistance in healthy humans. J Clin Endocrinol Metab 1994;79:1063–9.

33. Braithwaite SS, Barr WG, Rahman A, et al. Managing diabetes during glucocorticoid therapy. How to avoid metabolic emergencies. Postgrad Med 1998;104:163–76.

34. Brem AS. Insights into glucocorticoid-associated hypertension. Am J Kidney Dis 2001;37:1–10.

35. Roland BL, Li KX, Funder JW. Hybridization histochemical localization of 11 beta-hydroxysteroid dehydrogenase type 2 in rat brain. Endocrinology 1995;136:4697–700.

36. Krakoff LR. Glucocorticoid excess syndromes causing hypertension. Cardiol Clin 1988;6:537–45.

37. Dale DC, Fauci AS, Wolff SM. Alternate-day prednisone. Leukocyte kinetics and susceptibility to infections. N Engl J Med 1974;291:1154–8.

38. Truhan AP, Ahmed AR. Corticosteroids: a review with emphasis on complications of prolonged systemic therapy. Ann Allergy 1989;62:375–91.

39. Anstead GM. Steroids, retinoids, and wound healing. Adv Wound Care 1998;11:277–85.

40. Autio P, Oikarinen A, Melkko J, et al. Systemic glucocorticoids decrease the synthesis of type I and type III collagen in human skin in vivo, whereas isotretinoin treatment has little effect. Br J Dermatol 1994;131:660–3.

41. Esplin MS, Branch DW. Immunosuppressive drugs and pregnancy. Obstet Gynecol Clin North Am 1997;24:601–16.

42. Lacaze-Masmonteil T, Audibert F. Multiple courses of antenatal glucocorticoid treatment and fetal outcome. J Perinat Med 2000;28:185–93.

43. American Academy of Pediatrics Committee on Drugs. The transfer of drugs and other chemicals into human milk. Pediatrics 1994;93:137–50.

44. Edwards LJ, Coulter CL, Symonds ME, et al. Prenatal undernutrition, glucocorticoids and the programming of adult hypertension. Clin Exp Pharmacol Physiol 2001;28:938–41.

45. Rennick GJ. Use of systemic glucocorticosteroids in pregnancy: be alert but not alarmed. Australas J Dermatol 2006;47:34–6.

46. Piper JM, Ray WA, Daugherty JR, et al. Corticosteroid use and peptic ulcer disease: role of nonsteroidal anti-inflammatory drugs. Ann Intern Med 1991;114: 735–40.

47. Dixon RB, Christy NP. On the various forms of corticosteroid withdrawal syndrome. Am J Med 1980;68:224–30.

48. Ayres PJ, Hooper G. Assessment of the skin penetration properties of different carrier vehicles for topically applied cortisol. Br J Dermatol 1978;99:307–17.

49. Feldmann RJ, Maibach HI. Regional variation in percutaneous penetration of 14C cortisol in man. J Invest Dermatol 1967;48:181–3.

50. Hill CJH, Rostenberg A. Adverse effects from topical steroids. Cutis 1978;21:624–8.

51. Lubach D, Bensmann A, Bonemann U. Steroid-induced dermal atrophy: investigations on discontinuous application. Dermatologica 1989;179:67–72.

52. Yohn JJ, Weston WL. Topical glucocorticosteroids. Curr Probl Dermatol 1990;2:31–63.

53. Stoughton RB. Vasoconstrictor assay—specific applications. In: Maibach HI, Surber C, eds. Basel: Karger, 1992:42–53.

54. McKenzie AW, Stoughton RW. Methods for comparing percutaneous absorption of steroids. Arch Dermatol 1962;86:608–10.

55. Kornell RC, Stoughton RB. Correlation of vasoconstrictor assay in clinical activity of psoriasis. Arch Dermatol 1985;121:63–7.

56. Niedner R. Human models. In: Maibach HI, Surber C, eds. Basel: Karger, Basel, 1992:17–25.

57. Sukanto H, Nater JP, Bleumink E. Suppression of ultraviolet erythema by topical corticosteroids. Dermatologica 1980;161:84–8.

58. Frosch PJ, Behrenbeck EM, Frosch K, et al. The Duhring chamber assay for corticosteroid atrophy. Br J Dermatol 1981;104:57–65.

59. Robertson DB, Maibach HI. Topical corticosteroids. Int J Dermatol 1982;21:59–67.

60. Lagos BR, Maibach HI. Frequency of application of topical corticosteroids: an overview. Br J Dermatol 1998;139:763–6.

61. Kirby JD, Munro DD. Steroid-induced atrophy in animal and human models, Br J Dermatol 1976;94: 111–9.

62. Kligman LH, Schwartz E, Lesnik RH, et al. Topical tretinoin prevents corticosteroid-induced atrophy without lessening the anti-inflammatory effect. Curr Probl Dermatol 1993;21:79–88.

63. Epstein NM, Epstein WL, Epstein JH. Atrophic striae in patients with inguinal intertrigo. Arch Dermatol 1963;87:450.

64. Ponec M, De Haas C, Bachra BN, et al. Effects of glucocorticosteroids on cultured human skin fibroblasts. III. Transient inhibition of cell proliferation in the early growth stages and reduced susceptibility in later growth stages. Arch Dermatol Res 1979;265:219–27.

65. Lavker RM, Schechter NM., Lazarus GS. Effects of TCS on human dermis. Br J Dermatol 1986;115: 101–7.

66. Hettmannsperger U, Tenorio S, Orfanos CE, et al. Corticosteroids induce proliferation but do not influence TNF- or IL-1 beta-induced ICAM-1 expression of human dermal microvascular endothelial cells in vitro. Arch Dermatol Res 1993;285:347–51.

67. Ammar NM, Rao B, Schwartz RA, et al. Cutaneous striae. Cutis 2000;65:69–70.

68. Rapaport MJ, Rapaport V. Eyelid dermatitis to red face syndrome to cure: clinical experience in 100 cases. J Am Acad Dermatol 1999;41:435–42.

69. Fulton JE, Kligman AM. Aggravation of acne vulgaris by topical application of corticosteroids under occlusion. Cutis 1968;4:1106.

70. Plewig G, Kligman AM. Induction of acne by topical steroids. Arch Dermatol Forsch 1973;247:29–52.

71. Litt JZ. Steroid-induced rosacea. Am Fam Physician 1993;48:67–71.

72. Mehan R, Ayers S Jr. Perioral dermatitis. Arch Dermatol 1964;89:803.

73. du Vivier A. Tachyphylaxis to topically applied steroids. Arch Dermatol 1976;112:1245–8.

74. Takeda K, Arase S, Takahashi S. Side effects of TCS and their prevention. Drugs 1988;5:15–23.

75. Colomb D. Stellate spontaneous pseudoscars. Senile and presenile forms: especially those forms caused by prolonged corticoid therapy. Arch Dermatol 1972;105:551–4.

76. Aucott JN. Glucocorticoids and infection. Endocrinol Metab Clin North Am 1994;23:655–70.

77. Schwartz RA. Superficial fungal infections. Lancet 2004;364:1173–82.

78. Ive FA, Marks R. Tinea incognito. Br Med J 1968;3:149–52.

79. Hamada T. Granuloma intertriginosum infantum (granuloma glutaeale infantum). Arch Dermatol 1975;111:1072–3.

80. Dooms-Goossens A, Morren M. Results of routine patch testing with corticosteroid series in 2073 patients. Contact Dermatitis 1992;26:182–91.

81. Bircher AJ, Thurlimann W, Hunziker T, et al. Contact hypersensitivity to corticosteroids in routine patch test patients. A multi-centre study of the Swiss Contact Dermatitis Research Group. Dermatology 1995;191:109–14.

82. Lutz ME, el-Azhary RA. Allergic contact dermatitis due to topical application of corticosteroids: review and clinical implications. Mayo Clin Proc 1997;72:1141–4.

83. Isaksson M, Andersen KE, Brandao FM, et al. Patch testing with corticosteroid mixes in Europe. A multicentre study of the EECDRG. Contact Dermatitis 2000;42:27–35.

84. Thomson KF, Wilkinson SM, Powell S, et al. The prevalence of corticosteroid allergy in two U.K. centres: prescribing implications. Br J Dermatol 1999;141:863–6.

85. Cubey RB. Glaucoma following application of corticosteroid to the skin of the eyelids. Br J Dermatol 1976;95:207–8.

86. Zugerman C, Sauders D, Levit F. Glaucoma from topically applied steroids. Arch Dermatol 1976;112:1326.

87. Koda-Kimble MA, Young LL. Applied Therapeutics: The Clinical Use of Drugs, 5th ed. Vancouver, WA: Applied Therapeutics, 1992.

88. Aalto-Korte K, Turpeinen M. Pharmacokinetics of topical hydrocortisone at plasma level after applications once or twice daily in patients with widespread dermatitis. Br J Dermatol 1995;133:259–63.

89. Scoggins RB, Kliman B. Percutaneous absorption of corticosteroids: systemic effects. N Engl J Med 1965;273:831–40.

90. Patel L, Clayton PE, Addison GM, et al. Adrenal function following topical steroid treatment in children with atopic dermatitis. Br J Dermatol 1995;132:950–5.

91. Goodyear HM, Spowart K, Harper JI. "Wet-wrap" dressings for the treatment of atopic eczema in children. Br J Dermatol 1991;125:604.

92. Ellison JA, Patel L, Ray DW, et al. Hypothalamic-pituitary-adrenal function and glucocorticoid sensitivity in atopic dermatitis. Pediatrics 2000;105:794–9.

93. Olsen EA, Cornell RC. Topical clobetasol-17-propionate: review of its clinical efficacy and safety. J Am Acad Dermatol 1986;15:246–55.

94. Ohman EM, Rogers S, Meenan FO, McKenna TJ. Adrenal suppression following low-dose topical clobetasol propionate. J R Soc Med 1987;80:422–4.

95. Schlessinger J, Miller B, Gilbert RD, et al. An open-label adrenal suppression study of 0.1% fluocinonide cream in pediatric patients with atopic dermatitis. Arch Dermatol 2006;142:1568–72.

96. Munro DD. The effect of percutaneously absorbed steroids on hypothalamic-pituitary-adrenal function after intensive use in in-patients. Br J Dermatol 1976; 12:67–76.

97. Weston WL, Sams WM Jr, Morris HG, et al. Morning plasma cortisol levels in infants treated with topical fluorinated glucocorticosteroids Pediatrics 1980;65:103–6.

98. Gilbertson EO, Spellman MC, Piacquadio DJ, et al. Super potent topical corticosteroid use associated with adrenal suppression: clinical considerations. J Am Acad Dermatol 1998;38:318–21.

99. Keipert JA, Kelly R. Temporary Cushing's syndrome from percutaneous absorption of betamethasone 17-valerate. Med J Aust 1971;1:542–4.

100. Himathongkam T, Dasanabhairochana P, Pitchayayothin N, et al. Florid Cushing's syndrome and hirsutism induced by desoximetasone. JAMA 1978;239:430–1.

101. Robertson DB, Maibach HI. Adverse systemic effects of TCS. In: Maibach Hi, Surber C, eds. Basel: Karger, 1992:163–9.

102. Miller JA, Munro DD. TCS: clinical pharmacology and therapeutic use. Drugs 1980;19:119–34.

103. Fusaro RM, Kingsley DN. Topical Glucocorticoids: How they are used and misused. Postgrad Med 1986;79:283–91.

104. von den Harst LC, de Jonge H, Pot F, et al. Comparison of two application schedules for clobetasol 17 propionate. Acta Derm Venereol 1982;62:270–3.

33
Vaccines

Anita Arora, Natalia Mendoza, Anne Marie Tremaine,
and Stephen K. Tyring

Key Points

- Vaccination is ranked as the greatest public health achievement in the last century.
- Universal childhood immunization in the United States has led to a significant decrease in the incidence of several diseases.
- Vaccines may cause adverse reactions but most are mild and well tolerated.
- Many more vaccines are currently in development, and continuing vaccine research provides a promising outlook for prevention of more diseases in the near future
- The future of vaccines includes live-agent vaccines as vectors of other antigens, sequential immunization, and immunization with DNA.

Four criteria are needed for the success of a vaccine-based eradication program: the infection must be limited to humans (no animal reservoir); with viral infections there must be only one or a few strains of the virus, and these strains must have constant antigenic properties; the virus must not persist in the infected host; and the vaccine should be effective.[1] Vaccination as the route to prevention is the best option for controlling the spread of infectious diseases. Immunization can prevent or modify the severity of illness in the individual and interrupt or reduce the transmission of the pathogens to other susceptible people. Through these mechanisms, vaccines against smallpox, polio, measles, and hepatitis B have had an enormous impact on world health over the last 50 years. Vaccination is ranked as the greatest public health achievement in the last century, contributing the most to decreased global morbidity and mortality.[2,3]

There is a still great need for vaccines for many organisms since an inadequate number of antimicrobial drugs are available for the multiple microbes that exist. There are many reasons why it is difficult to produce the many necessary vaccines, including that all microorganisms deploy evasion methods that interfere with effective immune responses; further, for many organisms, it is still unclear which immune responses provide effective protection, particularly in developing vaccines against agents that cause persistent or chronic infections. Persistent or chronic infection, which includes notably the human immunodeficiency virus (HIV), is subject to significant antigenic variation. Most current vaccines are directed against acute infections, when a sublethal dose of the agent is controlled and rapidly cleared by the immune system (Table 33.1).

Control of Infection

Extracellular Infection

Cytokines secreted by CD4+ T-helper-1 (Th1) T cells aid in activating phagocytic cells such as macrophages and thus help in the destruction of the foreign agent in this fashion or complexed with an antibody.

Intracellular Infection

With intracellular infections with viruses, cytotoxic T lymphocytes (CTLs) play a dominant role in controlling and clearing the infection. In addition to its active role in killing infected cells, cytotoxic

TABLE 33.1. Current U.S. vaccines.

Vaccine	Name	Manufacturer	Type	Route
Anthrax	BioThrax	BioPort	Inactivated bacterial	SC
DTaP	Daptacel	Sanofi	Inactivated bacterial	IM
	Infanrix	GSK	Inactivated bacterial	IM
	Tripedia	Sanofi	Inactivated bacterial	IM
DT	Generic	Sanofi	Inactivated bacterial toxoids	IM
DTaP/HiB	TriHIBit	Sanofi	Inactivated bacterial	IM
DTaP/IPV/HiB	Pediarix	GSK	Inactivated bacterial and viral	IM
Haemophilus influenzae type b (Hib)	HibTITER	Wyeth	Inactivated bacterial	IM
	PedvaxHIB	Merck	Inactivated bacterial	IM
	ActHIB	Sanofi	Inactivated bacterial	IM
Hepatitis A	Havrix	GSK	Inactivated viral	IM
	Vaqta	Merck	Inactivated viral	IM
Hepatitis B	Engerix-B	GSK	Inactivated viral (recombinant)	IM
	Recombivax HB	Merck	Inactivated viral (recombinant)	IM
HepA/HepB	Twinrix	GSK	Inactivated viral	IM
HPV	Gardasil	Merck	Inactivated viral (recombinant)	IM
HepB/Hib	Comvax	Merck	Inactivated bacterial and viral	IM
Influenza	Fluarix	GSK	Inactivated viral	IM
	Fluvirin	Chiron	Inactivated viral	IM
	Fluzone	Sanofi	Inactivated viral	IM
	FluMist	Medimmune	Live attenuated viral	Intranasal
Japanese encephalitis	JE-Vax	Sanofi	Inactivated viral	SC
MMR	M-M-R II	Merck	Live attenuated viral	SC
MMRV	ProQuad	Merck	Live attenuated viral	SC
Measles	Attenuvax	Merck	Live attenuated viral	SC
Mumps	Mumpsvax	Merck	Live attenuated viral	SC
Rubella	Meruvax II	Merck	Live attenuated viral	SC
Meningococcal	Menomune	Sanofi	Inactivated bacterial	SC
	Menactra	Sanofi	Inactivated bacterial	IM
Pneumococcal	Pneumovax 23	Merck	Inactivated bacterial	SC or IM
	Prevnar	Wyeth	Inactivated bacterial	IM
Polio	Ipol	Sanofi	Inactivated viral	SC or IM
Rabies	BioRab	BioPort	Inactivated Viral	IM
	Imovax Rabies	Sanofi	Inactivated Viral	IM
	RabAvert	Chiron	Inactivated Viral	IM
Rotavirus	RotaTeq	Merck	Live viral	Oral
Td (tetanus & diphtheria)	Decavac	Sanofi	Inactivated bacterial toxoids	IM
	(Generic)	Massachusetts Biological Labs	Inactivated bacterial toxoids	IM
Tdap (tetanus & diphtheria toxoids/pertussis vaccine	Boostrix	GSK	Inactivated bacterial	IM
	Adacel	Sanofi	Inactivated bacterial	IM
TT (tetanus toxoid)	(Generic)	Sanofi	Inactivated bacterial toxoid	IM
Typhoid	Typhim Vi	Sanofi	Inactivated bacterial	IM
	Vivotif Berna	Sanofi	Live bacterial	IM
Varicella	Varivax	Merck	Live viral	SC
Vaccinia (smallpox)	Dryvax	Wyeth	Live viral	Percutaneous
Yellow fever	YF-Vax	Sanofi	Live viral	SC
Zoster (shingles)	Zostavax	Merck	Live viral	SC

T cells secrete potent cytokines with antiviral and macrophage-activating capabilities, such as interferon-γ (IFN-γ) and tumor necrosis factor-α (TNF-α).[1] With intracellular bacterial infections, the immune response is not as straightforward. Both CD4+ Th1 and CD8+ T cells have an important role in reducing, controlling, and clearing the infection.[4-7]

Regional Immunity

The mucosal surfaces of the human body are far greater in area in comparison to the skin and are well endowed with draining lymphoid tissues, with the exception of the vagina. The main routes of infection are the gut, the rectum, the genitourinary tract, the respiratory tract, and the eye. There is a common mucosal system, so that immunization at one site can result in protection at that and other mucosal areas. For instance, the adenovirus vaccine is administered orally but offers protection against a respiratory infection.[8] In addition, since the female genital tract is devoid of lymph tissue, systemic immunization is necessary to confer protection. Specifically, immunization through the respiratory tract was shown to be superior to other routes in inducing protection in the female genital tract.[7,9-11]

The formation and secretion of secretory immunoglobulin A (sIgA), is the first line of defense in the mucosal immune system; sIgA binds to antigens and their toxins and subsequently aids in prevention of attachment and penetration of the mucosal surface. Cytotoxic T cells have also been shown in the cytobrush specimens from the cervix of HIV-infected women.[12] Thus, protection in mucosal immunity is likely mediated through humoral and cell-mediated mechanisms.

Immunologic Memory

Most organisms are detected and destroyed within hours by defense mechanisms that are not antigen-specific and do not require any prolonged period of induction. This illustrates the mechanism of innate immunity. Only when a pathogen or antigen is able to break this early line of defense will an adaptive immune response ensue, including the production of antigen-specific effector cells, secretion of antibodies by B cells, direct cytotoxic activity

(CTLs), or via the secretion of immunologic mediators and effector molecules such as cytokines and chemokines. Most of the effector cells will die within 10 to 14 days after infection, but some cells survive as highly reactive plasma cells (B cells) or memory cells (B and T cells) to combat subsequent infection. The goal in preventative vaccination is to stimulate the adaptive response in the body with formation of long-lasting antibodies against a specific pathogen and induction of memory cells. The mechanism of how it should be achieved through immunization is less certain, but significant information has been elucidated about immunologic memory thus far.[13-15]

B-Cell Memory

A memory B-cell is one that has undergone immunoglobulin isotype switching and somatic hypermutation.[16] This differentiation process starts late in the primary immune response and takes place in the germinal centers of lymph nodes. Upon reencountering the same pathogen (or antigen in a booster vaccine), the memory cells start dividing at a high rate and differentiate into antibody-secreting plasma cells. Further, memory cells produce antibody of higher average affinity than unprimed B cells; the affinity of that antibody persists to increase during the ongoing secondary and subsequent antibody responses.

T-Cell Memory

After immunization, the number of T cells reactive to a given antigen increases markedly as the majority become effector T cells; then the number falls back to continue at a level significantly (100– to 1000–fold) above the initial frequency. These cells carry cell-surface proteins more characteristic of effector cells than of naive T cells. Both CD4+ and CD8+ T cells can differentiate into two types of memory cells. One type is called effector memory cells because they can quickly mature into effector T cells and secrete large amounts of cytokines such as IFN-γ, interleukin-4 (IL-4), and IL-5 early after re-stimulation. They probably develop from effector T cells and are relatively short-lived.[17] The other type is called central memory cells, and they are long-lived in the absence of antigen and are able to deal with systemic pathogenic infections.

Routes of Vaccination

Most vaccines are currently given by injection, which has two main disadvantages. The first is that injections are painful and expensive, requiring needles, syringes, and a trained injector. Mass vaccination can be arduous through this route. The disadvantage from an immunologic standpoint is that the injection may not be the most effective way of stimulating an appropriate immune response since it is not imitating the route of the majority of the pathogens.

Although the presentation of soluble protein antigens by the oral route often results in tolerance, which is necessary with the large load of food-borne and airborne antigens presented to the gut and respiratory tract, many pathogens that cause significant morbidity and mortality across the world infect mucosal surfaces or enter the body through mucous surfaces. For this reason, several vaccines targeting the mucosal immune response have been and are currently being studied. For instance, there is the Sabin trivalent oral poliovirus vaccine (OPV). Unfortunately due to one case of paralysis, the Centers for Disease Control (CDC) and the American Academy of Pediatrics have recommended that only inactivated polio vaccine (IPV) be used after January 1, 2000.[18] Oral polio vaccines are still being used in areas outside the United States where polio in endemic.[19] In addition, a safe and effective intranasal influenza vaccine has been available for several years.

Due to the significant advances in the technology of immunization, other routes of delivery are being considered. For instance, viral and bacterial antigens have been produced in transgenic plants.[20,21] Plant-based vaccines offer a means to deliver large quantities of a designated antigen in an encapsulated form. This encapsulation appears to protect against rapid and complete degradation of orally administered recombinant proteins. Thus, there is the potential for antigen to be gradually released into the gastrointestinal tract as host tissue is digested. This should theoretically permit an increased proportion of orally administered antigens to reach the effector sites, such as Peyer's patches lining the gastrointestinal tract.[22] A few human vaccine candidates have entered phase I clinical trials. These include diarrheal vaccine candidates targeting enterotoxigenic *Escherichia coli*[23,24] and Norwalk virus[25] and candidates against hepatitis B and rabies.[26,27]

Another route being considered is epicutaneous immunization. In the past few years, it has been elucidated that application of antigen onto bare skin induces potent systemic and mucosal immunity in an antigen-specific manner via Langerhans' and dendritic cells.[28–30] Coadministration of nonspecific adjuvants, such as cholera toxin, is necessary to induce good immune responses. It has recently been demonstrated that a natural adjuvant effect can be achieved by disrupting the stratum corneum prior to topical antigen application; this act stimulates the Langerhans' cells.[28] Epicutaneous immunization also generates active antigen-specific immunity in the gut and particularly augments Th2 responses subsequent to oral antigen[31] and inhalation of antigen.[32] The search for methods of vaccine delivery not requiring a needle and syringe has been influenced by concerns of pandemic disease, bioterrorism, and disease eradication campaigns.[33] Early testing of skin-patch tests is beginning, and past data with epicutaneous influenza vaccine showed that the vaccine was well tolerated by human volunteers.[34]

Vaccine Development

Live-Attenuated Vaccines

Viruses

Live-attenuated viral vaccines are composed of viruses that are traditionally grown in cultured cells. Viruses are typically selected for preferential growth in nonhuman cells, and, in the course of selection, become less capable of growth in human cells. Since these attenuated strains do not replicate well in human hosts, they induce immunity but not disease when given to individuals. There may be a slight possibility that the pathogenic virus can reemerge by a further series of mutations even though attenuated virus strains contain multiple mutations in their genome. Further, attenuated viral vaccines can cause significant damage by inducing viral opportunistic infections in those that are immunodeficient.[35] Live-attenuated viral vaccines are currently in use for smallpox, measles, mumps, rubella, varicella, herpes zoster, polio, influenza (intranasal), yellow fever, and rotavirus.

The vaccines targeting diseases that cause cutaneous manifestations are discussed in this section and throughout the chapter.

Smallpox

Edward Jenner, in 1796, was the first to demonstrate that inoculation of cowpox virus into human skin could lead to protection from subsequent smallpox infection.[36] Jenner named the inoculation substance *vaccine*, based on the Latin word *vacca*, meaning "cow." The vaccines used for smallpox vaccination are derived from vaccinia virus, a species similar to cowpox. The virus that causes smallpox is the variola virus, which belongs to the Poxviridae family and *Orthopoxvirus* genus, which also includes the vaccinia, cowpox, and monkeypox viruses. The smallpox vaccine, consisting of several types of strains of the live attenuated vaccinia virus, has served as the prototype of success of a viral vaccine; it was employed in the eradication of the disease. Prior to immunization, smallpox infection killed hundreds of millions of people unremittingly. The eradication of smallpox has been viewed as one of the greatest achievements in medicine.

Approximately two decades ago, after the complete elimination of smallpox, vaccine production ceased.[37] However, due to the recent concerns about biologic warfare and the use of smallpox as an agent, the danger of this disease has not been eliminated. Thus, renewed interest has been developed in production of the smallpox vaccines. Dryvax (Wyeth) is the currently licensed vaccine used for immunization against smallpox in public health, health-care-response teams, and laboratory workers involved with vaccinia virus research.

Contraindications to the use of this vaccine in the absence of circulating smallpox include allergies to polymyxin B sulfate, streptomycin sulfate, chlortetracycline hydrochloride, and neomycin sulfate. The vaccine should be administered concurrently with antihistamines or glucocorticoids to individuals who have allergic symptoms to the above compounds and have contact with individuals with smallpox. Further, the smallpox vaccine is contraindicated in persons with a history of eczema or atopic dermatitis; in persons who have acute, chronic, or exfoliative skin conditions; in persons who have conditions associated with immunosuppression such as persons infected with human immunodeficiency virus (HIV); in persons who are using topical ocular steroid medications; in persons who are younger than 18 years of age; and in women who are pregnant or intend to become pregnant during the next 4 weeks or who are breast-feeding.[38]

Measles, Mumps, and Rubella

Vaccination for the three classic childhood diseases of measles, mumps, and rubella (MMR) includes live attenuated viruses, and was introduced in the 1960s. The annual reported cases of these infections have declined by more than 98% in the United States and Europe.[39] This decrease in incidence is largely due to the recommendation that all states require a two-dose MMR vaccination prior to children entering school. The two-dose MMR vaccine is advocated to induce immunity in the small percentage of individuals who do not respond to one or more components of the first dose. The most updated recommendations from the CDC are vaccination with the first MMR dose at 12 to 15 months and the second dose at 4 to 6 years of age.[40] Table 33.2 summarizes the childhood immunization schedule for MMR, as well as other vaccines described in this chapter.[41] Immunization evokes a mild subclinical infection that is noncommunicable.

Since the vaccines are composed of live attenuated viruses, they are not recommended for pregnant women or those planning to become pregnant within the next 3 months. The primary concern with pregnant women has been the risk of eliciting the congenital rubella syndrome (CRS). However, a study of 321 women who received the vaccine 3 months prior to or after conception demonstrated no congenital malformations compatible with congenital rubella infection.[42] Another contraindication is a history of anaphylactic hypersensitivity to neomycin. Persons with asymptomatic HIV infection or with mild immunosuppression can get vaccinated with MMR. Further, healthy persons with minor illnesses with or without fever, and those with an allergy to eggs can receive the vaccine as well. The risk of severe anaphylactic shock reaction is exceedingly low in individuals with a history of allergy to eggs.[40] The recommendation is to observe these patients for up to 90 minutes after immunization.[43] Also, despite suggestions that the MMR vaccine has a reported association to autism, studies have proved strong evidence against that hypothesis.[44-46]

TABLE 33.2. Childhood immunization schedule for diseases with cutaneous manifestations.

Dose Vaccine	Dose 1	Dose 2	Dose 3	Dose 4	Dose 5	Boostert
Hepatitis B	Birth	1–2 months of age	6–18 months	X	X	X
Hib	2 months	4 months	12–15 months	X	X	X
MMR	12–15 months	4–6 years	X	X	X	X
Pneumococcal (PCV)	2 months	4 months	6 months	12–15 months	24–59 months[a]	X
Varicella	12–15 months	4–6 years	X	X	X	X
Meningococcal	Single dose[b]	X	X	X	X	X
Hepatitis A	2 doses between 12–23 months[c]		X	X	X	X
Human papillomavirus	Total of 3 doses[d]					

Hib, *Haemophilus influenzae* type B; MMR, measles, mumps, rubella.

[a]This last dose is only needed in high-risk groups. Pneumococcal polysaccharide vaccine (PPV) can be administered to children >24 months of age who are in the high-risk groups.

[b]MPSV4 should be given to patients ages 2 to 10 who have terminal complement deficiency, asplenia, and to other certain high-risk groups. Patients over age 10 can receive either MPSV4 or MCV4. Strongly suggest meningococcal vaccine administration before start of high school or before freshman year of college.

[c]Two doses between 12 and 23 months of age should be given 6 months apart.

[d]In females, a three dose regimen can be initiated starting at age 9. The second dose should occur 2 months after the first dose with the third dose to follow 6 months later.

Source: Adapted from Department of Health and Human Services Centers for Disease Control and Prevention: 2007 Recommended Immunization Schedules for Children in the United States.

Measles

The measles virus is very efficient in transmission, and has been noted to be the most infectious disease of humankind in regard to the minimal number of virions required to elicit infection.[47] Since humans are the only reservoirs for the measles virus, global eradication is a realistic goal. In the U.S., measles is no longer considered an indigenous disease due to universal childhood immunization,[48] and the reported incidence of measles has decreased by >99% since the measles vaccine has become available.

Subsequent to receiving two doses of the vaccine, 95% to 99% of individuals develop serologic evidence of immunity to measles.[49,50] Immunity is viewed as lifelong, and comparable to an acquired infection with the wild-type virus.[51] Rare cases of measles infection have been reported in patients with previously documented postimmunization seroconversion.[52,53]

Adverse effects after measles vaccination are usually mild, and include fever (5% to 15%),[54] transient viral exanthems,[39] and less commonly encephalitis or encephalopathy (less than one per one million vaccinees).[55] Further, a small number of cases have been described of the occurrence of subacute sclerosing panencephalitis (SSPE) in individuals with a history of vaccination but no known history of infection.[56–58] A more detailed review of these cases demonstrated that some cases had unrecognized natural measles infection prior to vaccination, and the SSPE was directly correlated to the infection.[40] Widespread measles immunization has practically eliminated SSPE in the U.S., and the live measles vaccine does not increase the risk of this adverse event.[40]

Mumps

A live attenuated mumps vaccine (Jeryl-Lynn strain) was introduced in 1967 and is prepared in a chick embryo cell culture. Immunization evokes a mild subclinical infection that is noncommunicable. Early clinical efficacy studies have shown that 97% of children and 93% of adults develop serologic evidence of immunity after vaccination[59–61] and serologic and epidemiologic evidence suggests that immunity persists for at least 30 years after immunization.[62–65]

Adverse reactions are usually mild and rare after vaccination, and include low-grade fever, mild parotitis, and viral exanthem. Serious adverse reactions, namely neurologic events are extremely rare and have not been causally associated with the mumps vaccine.[66]

Rubella

The RA 27/3 (rubella abortus 27, explant 3) rubella vaccine is grown in human diploid fibroblast cell culture. It induces a response in more than 97% of recipients.[60,67] Immunity in vaccinated individuals is believed to be lifelong and has been demonstrated to persist for at least 16 years.[68,69]

Adverse events following rubella vaccination include fever, lymphadenopathy, and viral exanthemas, usually between 5 to 12 days after vaccination.[66,70] Arthralgias and arthritis occur more frequently with adult vaccinees, especially women, ranging from 25% to 40% in this population.[71–73] Although no longer common, failure to develop 50% to 60% of immunity to rubella by vaccination leaves women of childbearing age susceptible to developing rubella infection during pregnancy. This causes congenital rubella in children born of mothers who contract rubella during early pregnancy.

Varicella-Zoster Virus

Prior to the prevalent use of varicella vaccine, annual U.S. figures for varicella infection included an estimate of 4 million cases, 11,000 hospitalizations, and 100 deaths.[74] The annual incidence of varicella has decreased significantly since the use of this vaccine. The vaccine, Varivax, developed by Takahashi in 1974 and approved in 1995, is a live attenuated Oka strain vaccine that has been shown to be very safe and effective.[75–77] In May 2006 the Food and Drug Administration (FDA) approved a vaccine 14 times more concentrated than the varicella vaccine against herpes zoster in individuals 60 years age and older.[78] Cell-mediated immunity is increased following vaccination in immunocompetent older adults, and the incidence and severity of herpes zoster[79–83] is reduced. The vaccine lessened the overall incidence of herpes zoster by 51.3% and notably reduced the pain and discomfort by 66.5% among subjects in whom herpes zoster developed. The zoster vaccine had low rates of serious adverse events, which were similar to the placebo vaccine.

Long-term follow-up data of the varicella vaccine depicted protection against chickenpox for at least 17 to 19 years, and, furthermore, all of the subjects vaccinated continue to have persistent antibodies and delayed-type skin reaction to the varicella-zoster antigen.[84] In a double-blind, placebo-controlled study of the Oka vaccine in 914 U.S. children, the varicella vaccine demonstrated an efficacy of 100% at 9 months.[85] Following 7 years of vaccination, 95% of the subjects remained without chickenpox clinically.[86] Additional studies in the U.S. have demonstrated that the Oka vaccine induces humoral and cell-mediated immunity in healthy children,[87–89] with protection for at least 8 years, while other data have suggested effectiveness decreases markedly after 1 year postvaccination.[90] Further, cases series depict that vaccinated individuals have less severe varicella (<50 lesions, no fever, and shorter duration of illness) than those who are unvaccinated.[91,92]

The vaccine is recommended as part of the childhood immunization schedule, and all susceptible children from 12 months of age to 18 years of age should receive the varicella vaccine. The first dose of the Oka vaccine should be administered at 12 to 15 months and the second dose should be given at 4 to 6 years of age.[78] Those over the age of 13 years should receive two doses, 4 to 8 weeks apart, to generate seroconversion rates and antibody responses comparable to those attained in healthy children.[75–77] It is uncertain what the duration of protection is at this time, and the necessity of a booster immunization is unknown. The vaccine is also recommended for susceptible adults, notably those in high-risk situations (e.g., health care personnel); children who have no prior history of chickenpox and are required to be present in school; and immunosuppressed subjects, particularly those with acute lymphocytic leukemia (ALL).[93–95] The varicella-zoster virus (VZV) vaccination is safe for all patients with lymphocyte counts >700/mm^3. Further, recent data suggest that varicella vaccine is >95% effective for prevention of disease and 100% for prevention of moderate or severe disease in susceptible contacts when given within 36 hours of exposure.[96]

A combination vaccine with the live attenuated viruses of MMR and VARIVAX is also available (ProQuad; Merck) and it is administered to individuals 12 months to 12 years of age. Post-licensing studies have shown the combination vaccine to be as effective as separate injections of MMR and Varivax.[97]

Varicella transmission is approximately one-fourth the rate of natural varicella (20% to 25% vs. 87%)[98] if a rash develops in the immunized individual. In children, the incidence of primary varicella is between 18 and 77 per 1 million person years of follow-up.[99] Herpes zoster can later develop from this vaccine type virus or from natural wild-type varicella-zoster virus.[100,101] Although there are reports of herpes zoster in healthy children vaccinees, the incidence is less than that seen in children with prior chickenpox, suggesting the vaccinated children may have a decreased risk for herpes zoster.[92]

The most common side effects from the vaccine include mild tenderness, erythema, induration at the injection site (19.3% to 24.4%), fever (10.2% to 14.7%), and a localized or generalized varicella-like rash (3.8% to 5.5%). The transmission rate of the varicella vaccine virus from a healthy vaccinated individual is low, but may be more likely if a rash appears subsequent to vaccination, particularly in those who are immunocompromised. Vaccinated individuals should avoid close contact with susceptible high-risk individuals for up to 6 weeks. The vaccine is contraindicated in pregnant women or any woman planning to become pregnant within 3 months since the vaccine uses a live attenuated virus and natural varicella can cause fetal harm.[102]

Yellow Fever Virus

A live attenuated vaccine produced from the 17D strain of yellow fever virus is available for subcutaneous administration. It is recommended for travelers to areas where yellow fever is endemic or enzootic, such as tropical parts of South America and Africa. Booster immunizations are required every 10 years. This vaccine is contraindicated in persons allergic to eggs, in pregnant women, in immunocompromised persons, and in children younger than 4 months of age.

Bacteria

The only currently used live-attenuated bacterial vaccine in the U.S. is against the causative agent of typhoid fever, *Salmonella typhi*. This vaccine, given orally, was first developed through chemical mutagenesis in vitro. Protection is conferred by mucosal and serum antibodies as well as cell-mediated immunity.[103] The induction of mucosal antibodies offers protection against infection and disease.[104]

Inactivated Vaccines

Both inactivated viral and bacterial vaccines consist of viruses and bacteria, respectively, treated so that they are unable to replicate. They are less potent in the effector response than the live-attenuated vaccines, and consist of vaccines currently in use against hepatitis A and B, *Haemophilus influenzae* type b (Hib), influenza (intramuscular), Japanese encephalitis, meningococcus, pneumococcus, polio (subcutaneous or intramuscular), rabies, tetanus/diphtheria toxoids, and typhoid fever (intramuscular). Again, in this section, the focus is on the vaccines targeting diseases that cause cutaneous manifestations.

Viruses

Hepatitis A

Both the inactivated and attenuated forms of hepatitis A vaccines have been developed and studied, although only the inactivated vaccine is licensed and available in the U.S. (Havrix and Vaqta). These vaccines are propagated in human diploid fibroblast culture and inactivated by formalin. Immunization typically involves two doses given 6 to 12 months apart in adults and in children aged 1 year and older. Studies of both available vaccines depict excellent safety profiles in addition to comparable immunogenicity and efficacy rates. Overall, 97% to 99% of those vaccinated develop protective levels of antibodies 1 month after the first dose, and 99% to 100% are protected 1 month after second dose.[105–110] Long-term data are limited, but one recent study showed that protection following primary hepatitis A vaccination persists for more than 10 years.[111]

The hepatitis A vaccine is recommended for individuals at least 1 year of age living in or traveling to high endemic areas for hepatitis A. Further, individuals with chronic liver disease due to causes other than hepatitis A, persons engaging in high-risk sexual activity, residents of a community experiencing an outbreak of hepatitis A, and users of illicit injectable drugs are strongly advised to receive hepatitis A vaccination. In addition, in some states and regions, the hepatitis A vaccine is recommended for routine pediatric use.

Adverse effects with hepatitis A vaccination are typically mild, and no serious adverse side effects have been credited to the vaccine in clinical trials.[112] Side effects include soreness at the injection site, headache (14%) and malaise (7%) in adults, and feeding problems (8%) and headache (4%) in children.

Bacteria

Anthrax

Pasteur in 1881 demonstrated the protective efficacy of the first anthrax vaccine when he injected sheep with heat-attenuated *Bacillus anthracis*. In the 1930s, wide use of vaccine composed of attenuated strains markedly decreased the incidence of anthrax in domesticated animals in industrialized countries. The licensed human vaccine, anthrax vaccine adsorbed (AVA), also known as BioThrax since 2002, is a culture supernatant of a toxigenic, nonencapsulated *B. anthracis* strain, V770–NP1–R, derived from the Sterne strain.[113] A vaccine similar to AVA is used in the United Kingdom, produced from culture supernatant-derived human vaccine (PL 1511/0058).[114]

Anthrax vaccinations are recommended for individuals working in the production of *B. anthracis* cultures, those engaged in activities with a high risk of aerosol exposure, individuals in the military, and other groups of persons with a calculable risk.[115] Preexposure vaccinations are currently not recommended for emergency first responders, medical practitioners, and civilians. However, due to the bioterrorist attacks in 2001 and limited supply of anthrax vaccine, supplemental recommendations of the Advisory Committee on Immunization Practices endorse the anthrax vaccine in combination with antimicrobial postexposure prophylaxis (PEP) for unvaccinated persons at risk for inhalational anthrax.[116]

Anthrax vaccine adsorbed has numerous limitations despite being relatively efficacious and safe.[117] The schedule of AVA administration, which consists of subcutaneous injections at 0, 2, and 4 weeks and boosters at 6, 12, and 18 months (with recommended annual boosters to maintain immunity), is probably suboptimal. The enduring protective efficacy in humans is unknown. AVA

contains other cellular elements that aid in the fairly high rate of local and systemic adverse reactions,[117] including injection-site hypersensitivity, edema, pain, headache, arthralgia, asthenia, and pruritus. Approximately 20% of vaccinees develop mild cutaneous reactions such as erythema, edema, and induration. In <1% of recipients, systemic side effects of fever, chills, nausea, and body aches occurred.[118]

Conjugate Vaccines (Fig. 33.1)[1,119]

Many bacteria, including *Neisseria meningitidis* and *Haemophilus* species, have an outer capsule composed of polysaccharides that are species and type specific for particular strains of the bacterium. The goal of vaccination is to generate antibodies against the polysaccharide capsule of the bacteria since the most effective defense against these organisms is opsonization of the polysaccharide coat with antibody. However, children under 2 years of age do not mount a good response against capsular polysaccharide, which is a T-cell–independent antigen. An effective way to overcome this problem is to conjugate bacterial polysaccharide (chemically) to protein carriers, which offer peptides that can be recognized by antigen-specific T cells. Thus, a T-independent response is converted into a T-cell–dependent antipolysaccharide response.[1,35]

Haemophilus Influenzae

In the second generation of Hib vaccines, the polyribosylribitol phosphate (PRP) vaccine has been covalently conjugated with various protein molecules to form the Hib conjugate vaccine. This has resulted in a vaccine that is able to stimulate the immunologic system to produce a T-dependent response, for use in infants.[120] Four different types of the Hib conjugate vaccine have been licensed for use: PRP conjugated to the diphtheria toxoid (PRP-D), PRP conjugated to the outer membrane protein of *Neisseria meningitidis* group B (PRP-OMP), PRP conjugated to tetanus toxoid (PRP-T), and PRP oligosaccharides conjugated to mutant diphtheria toxin CRM (HbOC).[121] Recommended immunization involves three doses of the Hib vaccine given at 2 months, 4 months, and 12 months of age.[41]

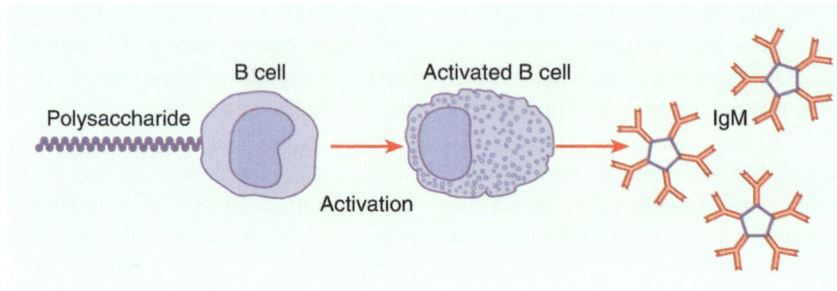

F_{IG}. 33.1. Antibody responses to polysaccharide antigens and polysaccharide–protein conjugates. (A) A polysaccharide antigen binds to an immunoglobulin M (IgM) receptor on the surface of a B cell in lymphoid tissues. Once B cells are activated, they produce and then secrete IgM antibody molecules. The individual Fab segments of the IgM molecule have only a moderate affinity, but because there are 10 such segments, an IgM molecule has a high avidity. (B) In contrast, some polysaccharide–protein conjugates are taken up by dendritic cells, which present peptides from the protein portion of the conjugate to type 2 helper T (Th2) cells. Other conjugate molecules bind to B cells that have IgM receptors specific for the carbohydrate moiety and will undergo endocytosis and be processed by the B cell; the resulting peptides will be expressed with major histocompatibility complex (MHC) class II molecules on the surface of the B cell.

Neisseria Meningitidis

Bacterial meningitis remains a severe threat to global health, with an estimated 500,000 cases worldwide with at least 50,000 deaths and as many cases of neurological damage.[122] *Neisseria meningitidis* is responsible for 60% to 65% of cases of bacterial meningitis, and it is the only bacterium that is able to generate epidemics of meningitis.[123] It is also associated with a petechial eruption or more severe hemorrhagic lesions on the trunk and lower extremities.

The significant determinant of virulence in *N. meningitidis* is the polysaccharide capsule. Among the 13 distinct *N. meningitidis* serogroups that have been defined on the immunohistochemistry of their polysaccharide group, groups A, B, C, W135, and Y account for over 90% of severe meningitis and septicemia. Two meningococcal vaccines, each containing antigens to serogroups A, C, Y, and W-135, are licensed in the U.S. There is currently no vaccine that provides immunity against serogroup B, which accounts for an estimated one third of cases of meningococcal disease.

Over 30 years ago, the first meningococcal polysaccharide vaccine (MPSV4 or Menomune, Sanofi Pasteur), was developed against serogroups A and C among U.S. military recruits.[124–126] It is approved for all ages in which meningococcal vaccine is currently recommended. Further, the vaccine is safe and bestows protection to 90% to 95% of people. However, there are limitations to the vaccine. First, the vaccine offers a short duration of immunity: 1 to 3 years in children younger than 5 years of age[121,127] and 3 to 5 years in adolescents and adults. Second, like other polysaccharide vaccines, this vaccine could not elicit memory T cells, and even after repeated injections, booster responses are low.[128,129] In addition, like other polysaccharide vaccines, this vaccine does not prevent mucosal colonization and hence does not offer herd immunity by breaking up the transmission of *N. meningitidis*.[130,131] For a limited amount of time, this vaccine is a logical option for individuals requiring protection.

The second vaccine, meningococcal conjugate vaccine A, C, Y, and W135 (MCV4 or Menactra, Sanofi Pasteur), was approved in January 2005 for use in individuals 11 to 55 years of age. This conjugate vaccine contains the same antigen as that found in the meningococcal polysaccharide vaccine, but it is conjugated to 48 μg of diphtheria toxoid.[132] What is different regarding this vaccine is that immunity is more durable, and revaccination can generate a rise in antibody level. Although not yet proved, it is suggested that, like other conjugate vaccines, it is likely that this vaccine will offer more durable protection than the polysaccharide vaccine alone and will further reduce nasopharyngeal carriage, allowing herd immunity to occur.

The serogroups A and C vaccines have demonstrated estimated clinical efficacies of >85% among school-aged children and adults and are useful in controlling outbreaks. Serogroups Y and W-135 polysaccharides are safe and immunogenic among adults and children aged >2 years. The advantages of the meningococcal conjugate vaccine have led the Advisory Committee on Immunization Practices (ACIP) of the CDC to extensively widen the recommendations for immunization.[132] If these recommendations are fully effective, the immunization of all children 11 to 19 years of age would be accomplished by 2008.[133]

Both vaccines are currently recommended for use in control of outbreaks as a result of *N. meningitidis* serogroups A, C, Y, and W-135.[132] However, due to its enhanced booster effect, the conjugate vaccine is favored when revaccination is indicated for individuals who have received the meningococcal polysaccharide vaccine before and who remain at higher risk. Long-term follow-up studies are still needed for those that have been immunized with the meningococcal conjugate vaccine to establish if boosters are needed.

FIG. 33.1. (continued) This complex is recognized by the activated Th2 cell, which then secretes interleukin-4 (IL-4), IL-5, and IL-6. These cause the B cell to differentiate and express IgG molecules with polysaccharide specificity. These cells mature in the lymphoid follicles; only cells that express very high affinity IgG molecules become plasma cells and secrete high-affinity IgG that binds strongly to the encapsulated bacteria and mediates opsonic activity and complement-mediated bactericidal activities.[1] A study suggests that the formation of memory B cells is a critical component of protective immunity against infection with *Haemophilus influenzae* type b.[119]

Adjuvants

Purified antigens are not typically immunogenic on their own, and thus most acellular vaccines require adjuvants to enhance their immunogenicity. Alum, the adjuvant most often used, delays the release of an antigen and enhances the generation of antibodies. Most adjuvants are thought to act on antigen-presenting cells, particularly on dendritic cells. Adjuvants manipulate the immune system into reacting as though there were an active infection, and just as different classes of infectious agents elicit different types of immune response, different adjuvants may stimulate different types of response.

Recombinant Subunit Vaccines

Another route to vaccine development is the identification of the T-cell peptide epitopes that stimulate protective T-cell–mediated immunity. T cells recognize their target antigens as small protein fragments or peptides presented by major histocompatibility complex (MHC) molecules at the cell surface, and thus these peptide epitopes, once identified, can then be tried as vaccines. Using peptides has many advantages and some drawbacks.[1] Advantages include that the peptide is chemically defined, stable, and safe and contains only important B-cell and T-cell epitopes. Drawbacks include the complexity in mimicking the conformation of antigen polymers found with many viruses, that B-cell epitopes recognized by neutralizing antibodies are sometimes discontinuous sequences, and the vulnerability of peptides to proteolysis. Several administrations, likely with an adjuvant, may be required. Since 1990, over 100 chemically synthesized short peptide vaccines have been initiated into phase I clinical trials, less than 20 have advanced into phase II, and none has entered phase III clinical trials.[134]

Subunit vaccines have often made use of recombinant-DNA technology. Immunogenicity can be improved and the immune response aimed at induction of both cell-mediated and humoral responses through the formation of aggregates such as immunostimulating complexes, virus-like particles, antigen-coated beads, or lipid-encapsulated antigens under many conditions. Linked peptides are also being tested in the field of subunit vaccines; for instance, aggregates of linked peptides from group A streptococcus as a vaccine against rheumatic fever have demonstrated promising results in animal models.[135,136]

Viruses

Human Papillomavirus

Globally, cervical cancer is the second most common cause of death in women from cancer, after breast cancer, and it is the cause of death of approximately 273,000 women per year.[137] Almost half a million new cases of invasive cervical cancer develop each year, and in the U.S. it was estimated to afflict over 9700 women in 2006.[138] Epidemiologic studies have proved that persistent HPV infection is the main cause of almost all cervical carcinogenesis.[139–141]

Approximately 40 of the 100 HPV genotypes have an affinity for infecting the mucosal epithelium and subsequently causing genital infection. The major types associated with malignancy (16, 18, 31, 33, 45, 52, and 58) and condyloma (6 and 11) are relatively few in number, which has allowed for more focused strategies for immunization against these specific types.[102]

Papillomaviruses are nonenveloped double-stranded DNA viruses with the genome comprised of three regions: the long control region (LCR), the early region (E), and the late region (L). The early region consists of genes *E1* to *E8*, which encode nonstructural proteins. The late regions code for the major (L1) and minor (L2) proteins that compose the viral capsid. The advancement in producing the prophylactic HPV vaccine came from findings that L1 self-assembles into empty capsids, named virus-like particles (VLPs), when it is expressed from eukaryotic vectors such as recombinant vaccinia, baculovirus, and yeast.[142,143] The VLPs do not contain viral DNA and are noninfectious; their similarity to virions offers a neutralizing epitope that subsequently produces an antibody response.

Gardasil® (Merck) is a quadrivalent vaccine that targets HPV types 16, 18, 6, and 11. It is a yeast-expressed vaccine, which was approved by the FDA in 2006 for use in girls and young women of ages 9 to 26 years, and is marketed as a vaccine for prevention of cervical cancer, precancerous genital lesions, and genital warts due to HPV types 6, 11, 16, and 18. Provisional recommendations from

ACIP include giving the second and third dose of the vaccine at months 2 and 6, respectively.[144] In one study involving greater than 12,167 adolescents and women of ages 16 to 23, Gardasil prevented 100% ($n=5301$) of cases of cervical intraepithelial neoplasia (CIN) grades 2 and 3 linked with HPV types 16 and 18 compared to 21 cases in the placebo group ($n=5258$). All subjects elicited 100% antibody responses to the HPV strains 6, 11, and 16, and 99.1% developed strain 18 antibodies. Protection has been observed for at least 36 months following vaccination. Males were also studied in the Gardasil trials, and although 99% antibody response was elicited in this patient population, vaccine efficacy is difficult to study since anogenital cancer is very rare in U.S. males, with the exception of HIV-positive homosexuals. The trial is being extended for several years to investigate if the vaccine is protective in this population.[145,146]

Gardasil has been shown to be generally safe, and well tolerated, with pain, swelling, and erythema at the site of injection being the primary side effects. Females who have an equivocal or abnormal Pap test can receive the quadrivalent vaccine, but data from clinical trials do not suggest that the vaccine will have a therapeutic effect on existing Pap test abnormalities; it would only provide protection against other HPV types not already acquired. Females who are immunocompromised can be vaccinated; however, the immune response may be less than in those who are immunocompetent. Further, those with moderate or severe illness should not be vaccinated until after the illness improves. Provisional contraindications to Gardasil include those with immediate hypersensitivity to yeast or another vaccine component. The Merck vaccine is not recommended for use in pregnancy since data for vaccination during pregnancy is limited, and lactating women cannot receive the vaccine either.[144]

Hepatitis B

The annual incidence of individuals infected with hepatitis B virus (HBV) in the U.S. was estimated to be 200,000 to 300,000 prior to the development of the hepatitis B vaccine.[147] In 1981, a plasma-derived hepatitis B vaccine was licensed in the U.S.; the vaccine was highly effective in inducing immunity, but was associated with several limitations. Large-scale production was not feasible because of the insufficient supply of suitable carrier plasma. Further, despite the chemical treatment of plasma products for safety, there was a small concern regarding the risk of HIV transmission. Both of these issues were resolved with the licensure of the recombinant yeast hepatitis B vaccine (Merck).[148]

This vaccine was the first licensed recombinant viral vaccine prototype as well as the first effective viral vaccine for a sexually transmitted disease. Clinical studies in high-risk homosexual men illustrated three-dose vaccine efficacy of 82% to 93% in preventing acute hepatitis B.[149,150] Approximately 95% of immunocompetent adults develop significant antibody titers following a three-dose hepatitis B vaccination. An estimated 99% of children[151] respond to the vaccination, while only 50% to 70% of those over age 60 develop immunity.[152,153] Factors linked with lower likelihood of seroconversion include immunosuppression, renal failure, prematurity with low birth weight, age older than 40 years, obesity, and smoking.[154–156] In these individuals, annual antibody testing should be completed, and a booster dose administered for those with antibody levels <10 mIU/mL.

Long-term efficacy is expected from the duration of immunity afforded by the hepatitis B vaccine, although few studies are available on this topic.[156] Antibodies levels decline rapidly in the first year following vaccination, and then decline at a slower pace in the following years.[157] The loss of detectable antibodies years after hepatitis B vaccination does not necessarily signify a lack of immunity. Most of the persons vaccinated are protected by immunologic memory in B lymphocytes, which mount an anamnestic response to natural infection.[158] It should be noted, however, that rare cases of hepatitis B infection have been reported in previously vaccinated patients.[159,160] These individuals usually have subclinical disease, and none has developed chronic infection or serious complications.[156]

The immunization regimen includes three doses, given at months 0, 1, and 6. Hepatitis B vaccination is recommended for individuals living in or traveling to areas of high endemicity for hepatitis B, health care personnel, morticians, persons engaging in high-risk sexual activity, persons with chronic liver disease due to causes other than hepatitis B, prisoners, users of illicit injectable drugs, police and fire department personnel who participate in first aid, and all children 0 to 18 years of age. Due to the widespread use of the vaccine in children, a thimerosal-free vaccine was recently approved by the FDA (Merck and GlaxoSmithKline). Thimerosal is a preservative that contains mercury, which has driven the limitation of its use in children.[161]

Adverse effects after hepatitis B vaccination are usually mild and well tolerated. The most common side effects include fatigue (15%), headache (9%), and fever (1% to 9%).[162,163] A postmarketing clinical surveillance of 4.5 million doses of hepatitis B vaccine over 5 years depicted no serious or severe reactions attributable to the vaccine. Reports of a causal relationship between hepatitis B vaccine and a variety of autoimmune diseases have been disproven, and furthermore this vaccine does not increase the risk of multiple sclerosis,[164] nor does it cause a relapse of underlying multiple sclerosis.[165]

In 2001 the FDA licensed a new combination vaccine that protects individuals at least 18 years of age against hepatitis A virus and hepatitis B virus. This vaccine, Twinrix (GlaxoSmithKline), combines two already approved vaccines, Havrix, and Engerix-B, in order for persons at high risk for exposure to both viruses to be immunized against both at the same time and reduce the number of injections needed. This vaccine is administered at months 0, 1, and 6. Data from 11 clinical trials indicate that 99.9% of vaccinees develop seroconversion against hepatitis A virus and 98.5% against hepatitis B surface antigen, with persistence up to 4 years (GlaxoSmithKline Biologics, unpublished data, 2001).

Lyme Disease

Lyme disease is the most common vector-borne human disease in the U.S., with 23,763 cases reported to the CDC in 2002.[166] Since 1982, the annual incidence of Lyme disease has increased more than 25-fold.[167]

Although a recombinant vaccine, Lymerix, for prevention of Lyme disease was approved in 1998, for many reasons including cost, need for frequent revaccinations, and a highly publicized but theoretical risk of precipitating autoimmune arthritis, sales of Lymerix declined rapidly after its initial introduction, and its manufacturer removed the vaccine from the market in 2002.[168,169] As a result, there has been renewed interest in developing new strategies for the reduction of Lyme disease, for instance, the use of oral delivery of an OspA vaccine to reduce carriage of *Borrelia burgdorferi* in its reservoir hosts.[168]

Investigational Vaccines

Live-Agent Vaccines as Vectors of Other Vaccine Antigens

Wide interest exists in the use of vaccines composed of attenuated viruses or bacteria as carriers (vectors) of other antigens. More than 20 different RNA and DNA viruses as well as bacteria are used experimentally as vectors, including poxviruses. All of these strains infect but do not replicate in human cells.[170,171] Since approximately 10% of the large poxvirus genome can be replaced by foreign DNA, genes encoding protective antigens from several different organisms could be placed in a single vaccine strain. This approach allows immunization against several different pathogens at one time, but such a vaccine could not be used twice since the vaccinia vector itself elicits long-lasting immunity that would neutralize its effectiveness on a second dose. Further, live-attenuated strains of *Salmonella* have been used as vectors of tetanus toxoid, *Listeria monocytogenes*, *Bacillus anthracis*, *Leishmania major*, *Yersinia pestis*, and *Schistosoma mansion* to provide mucosal response due its oral administration.[1,35]

Immunization with DNA

Vaccination with DNA is one of the most promising novel immunization techniques against pathogens in which conventional vaccination regimens have failed. A DNA plasmid encoding a desired protein is injected into the muscle or skin of an animal, where it subsequently enters host cells and directs the synthesis of its polypeptide antigen. Once the plasmid antigen is processed and presented by transected host cells, a cellular and humoral immune response against the antigen is elicited. The DNA vector is bacterial-derived and outfitted with eukaryotic or viral promoter/

enhancer transcription elements that direct the high-efficiency transcription of the plasmid-antigen within the nucleus of the host cell. The most common way of administering DNA vaccines has been parenterally, but noninvasive routes of delivery involving the topical application of pure DNA plasmid to skin or mucosa have been illustrated (Fig. 33.2).[1,172]

This approach has many potential advantages, including low cost, stability, and inability to return into virulence. A possible disadvantage would be integration of the DNA into the genome of the host cell, leading to transformation or tumorigenic events, but such occurrences have not yet been observed.[1]

Sequential Immunization

There are also a group of pathogens that do not respond to the vaccine approaches described thus far. These pathogens include HIV, *Mycobacterium tuberculosis*, and the malaria parasite, all which traditionally evade the humoral response elicited by traditional vaccines.[173] Thus, over the past few years there has been a drive to generate vaccines targeting the cell-mediated immune system for

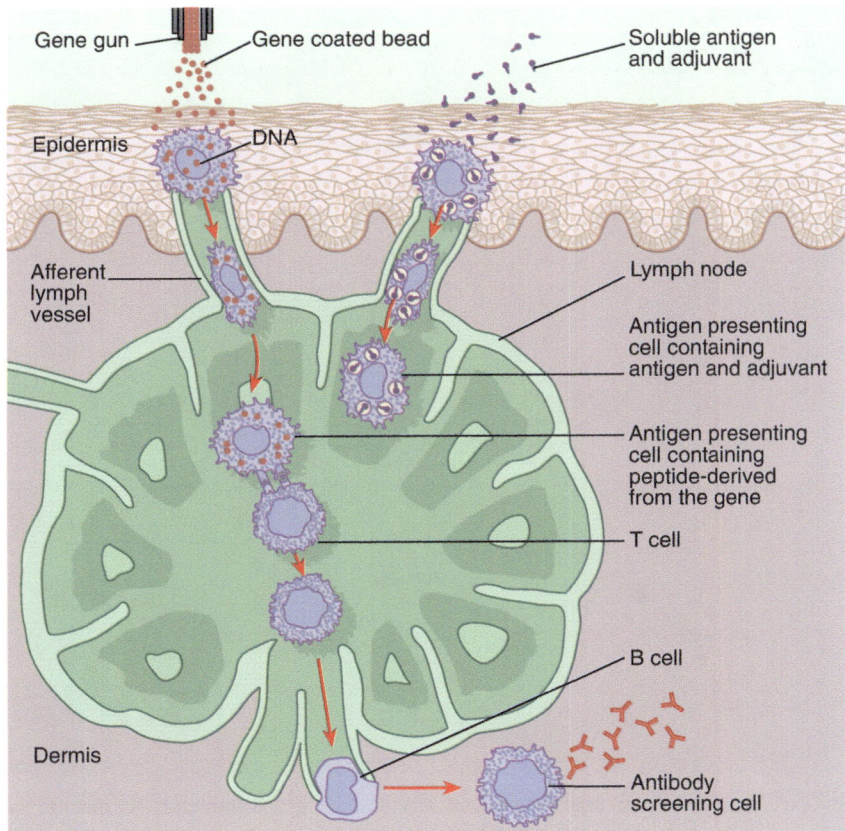

FIG. 33.2. Activation of helper T cells after the application of antigen-coated beads with the aid of a "gene gun" or the application of soluble antigen to the skin as an alternative to vaccination with a needle. A gene gun is used ballistically to accelerate the transdermal passage of microscopic gold beads coated with DNA plasmids (about 600 copies per bead) through the stratum corneum into the epidermis, where some are taken up by resident dendritic (Langerhans') cells. Alternatively, a soluble antigen together with an adjuvant, usually cholera toxin, is applied to the skin (transcutaneous immunization). Some antigen reaches the epidermis and also undergoes endocytosis by Langerhans' cells. During migration to the draining lymph node through the afferent lymphatics, these cells mature and express receptors for chemokines. The foreign DNA is expressed, and the antigens are degraded, some of which bind to MHC antigens. These activated T cells can interact with an activated B cell to induce a humoral response.[1] (Copyright © 2001 Massachusetts Medical Society. All rights reserved.)

these and related pathogens. With the advent of vaccines, repeated administration with the same vaccine (homologous boosting) has proven to be very effective for boosting humoral response. However, this approach is not effective at boosting cellular immunity since prior immunity to the vector appears to impair robust antigen presentation and the generation of appropriate inflammatory signals. One approach to evade this problem has been to sequentially administrate vaccine, usually weeks apart, using different antigen-delivery systems (heterolo-

gous boosting). This method is referred to as prime-boosting, and is very effective at generating high levels of T-cell memory (Fig. 33.3).[174] Although many of the initial studies were to develop a vaccine to control malaria, this method of vaccine development was applied to a variety of other pathogens.[175]

Much advancement has been made in vector design and progress, and several vectors have proven to be effective, which include replication-defective adenoviruses, fowlpox viruses, vaccinia virus, influenza virus, Sendai virus, and naked

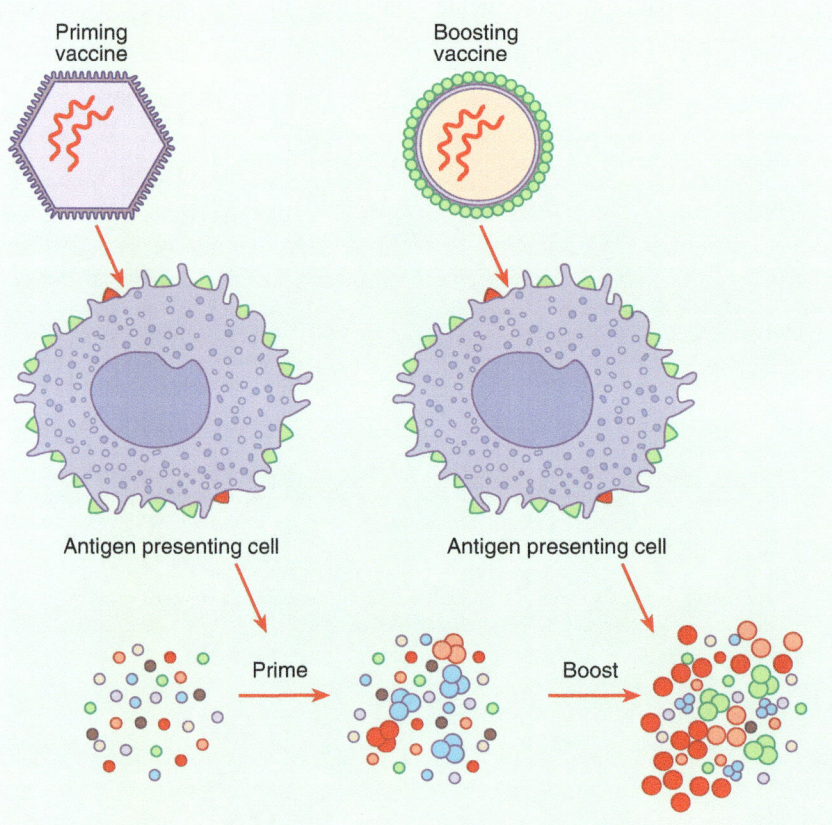

FIG. 33.3. Prime–boost vaccination strategies synergistically amplify T-cell immunity to specific antigens. Priming with the first vaccine results in the presentation of both the target antigen (red triangles) and vector antigens (blue triangles) on antigen-presenting cells (APCs). The APCs then stimulate naive T cells in the lymph nodes and drive the expansion of both target-specific T cells (red cells, high-avidity cells are indicated by the darker red) and vector-specific T cells (blue cells). Subsequent boosting with a second vaccine results in the re-presentation of the target antigen (red triangles) and antigens from the second vector (green triangles) on APCs. These APCs then drive the expansion of target-specific memory T cells (red cells) and vector-specific naive T cells (green cells). This results in both a synergistic expansion of the T cell specific for the target antigen and selection of T cells that have greater avidity for the antigen. The situation with priming and boosting vectors that induce strong T-cell responses to themselves, as well as the target antigens, is shown. However, it should be noted that many vectors, such as DNA and some of the popular replication-defective viral vectors, induce little or no response to the vectors themselves. This is probably a key issue underlying their efficacy. (From Woodland DL. Jump-starting the immune system: prime–boosting comes of age. Trends Immunol 2004;5:98–104. Copyright 2004, with permission from Elsevier.)

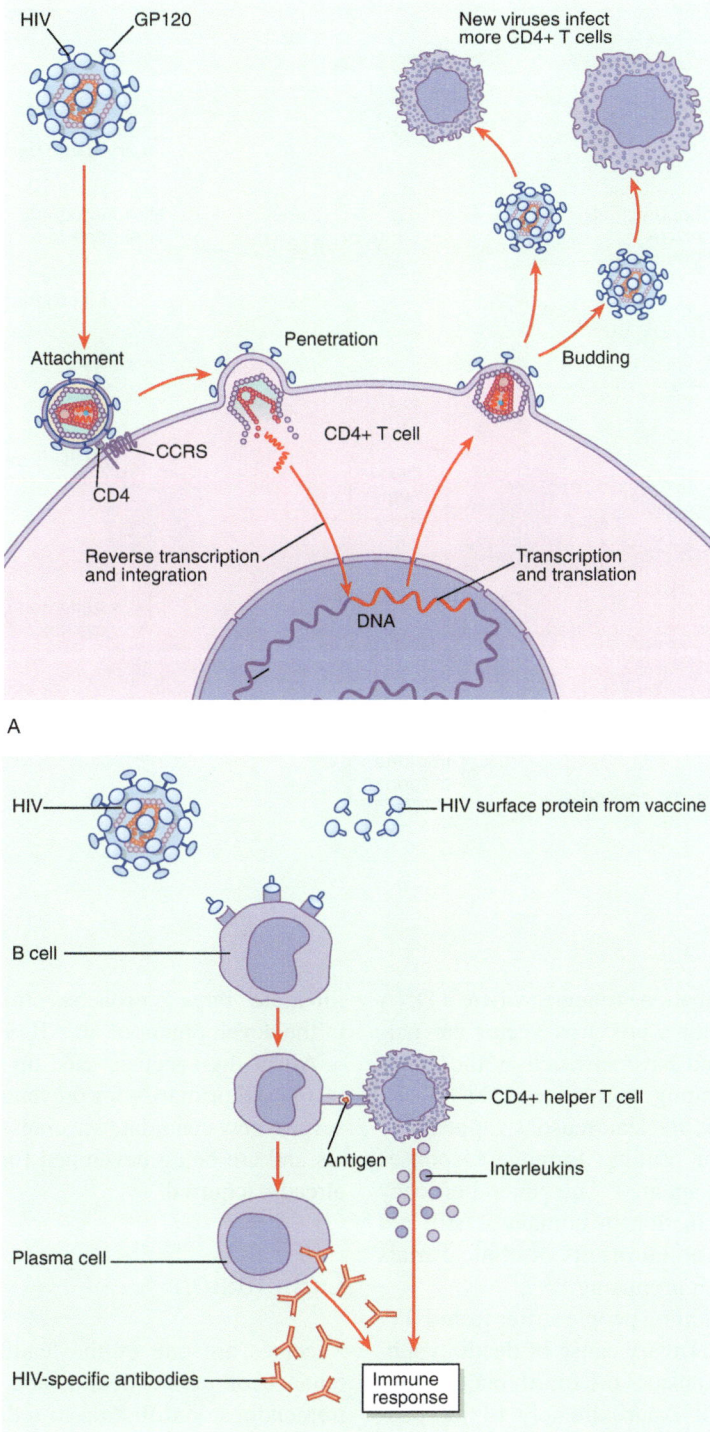

FIG. 33.4. Approaches to HIV-vaccine development. The mechanism of normal HIV infection is shown (A), along with the mechanisms of three types of potential vaccines: a subunit vaccine containing a synthetic protein from the CD4–binding site on the envelope of the virus (B), a naked DNA vaccine, and a recombinant vaccine with a bacterial or viral vector (C).[185] (Copyright © 2005 Massachusetts Medical Society. All rights reserved.)

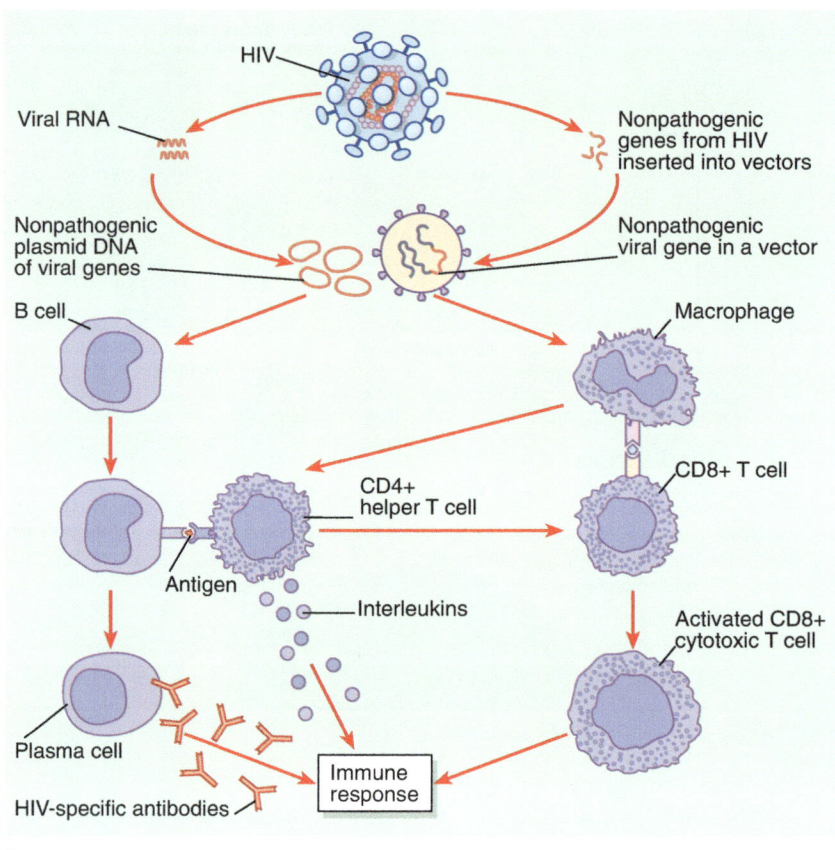

C

FIG. 33.4. (continued)

DNA.[174,176–180] Vaccination strategies where a DNA prime is boosted with a poxvirus vector are particularly effective and have surfaced as the major approach for generating protective CD8[+] T-cell immunity. DNA, for unclear reasons, appears to be more effective at priming immune responses versus as a boosting agent.[181] The general efficacy of prime-boost vaccination in humans is still not yet determined; the initial results of clinical trials in progress have been promising.[182,183]

Currently over 4 million people suffer from HIV/AIDS, which is the primary cause of death in sub-Saharan Africa and ranks as the fourth major cause of death in the world. Approximately 14,000 people/day (5 million persons/year, including 600,000 children less than 15 years of age) become infected with HIV, with more than 95% of them residing in nonindustrialized countries.[184] The production of a safe, effective, easily administered and affordable AIDS vaccine is greatly needed. Figure 33.4[185]

illustrates three approaches currently being studied in the development of an AIDS vaccine.

All of the vaccines used up to the 20th century were used primarily for prevention. In recent years, several new candidate vaccines have undergone trials and are being developed for infections that are already acquired.

Conclusion

Vaccines are one of the leading tools for maintenance of public health, and they have made a tremendous contribution to reducing the incidence of numerous diseases. While there has been much success with immunization, there are still many diseases uncontrolled by vaccination, and there are still challenges regarding implementing vaccine programs and dispelling fears about immunization side effects. Most associations between vaccines and adverse events are not demonstrated to be causal. Nevertheless, suspected relationships between vaccines and adverse events need to be reported to the Vaccine Adverse Event Reporting System (telephone 800–822–7967) in order to maintain an excellent safety record of vaccines.

Approximately 200 years of research have allowed us to direct the immune system for the gain of the people, and to have a clearer comprehension of microbial pathogenesis and host responses. From the continual presence of experimental and clinical trials, we can expect to see safe and effective vaccines for numerous infectious diseases in the future.

References

1. Ada G. Vaccines and vaccination. N Engl J Med 2001;345(14):1042–53.
2. CDC. Achievements in public health, 1900–1999: impact of vaccines universally recommended for children—United States, 1990–1998. MMWR Morb Mortal Wkly Rep 1999;48:243–8.
3. CDC. Ten great public health achievement: United States, 1900–1999. MMWR Morb Moral Wkly Rep 1999;48:241–3.
4. Sprent J, Webb SR. Function and specificity of T cell subsets in the mouse. Adv Immunol 1987;41: 39–133.
5. Delves PJ, Roitt IM. The immune system. First of two parts. N Engl J Med 2000;343(1):37–49.
6. Croft M, Carter L, Swain SL, Dutton RW. Generation of polarized antigen-specific CD8 effector populations: reciprocal action of interleukin (IL)-4 and IL-12 in promoting type 2 versus type 1 cytokine profiles. J Exp Med 1994;180(5):1715–28.
7. Ada G. The Immunology of Vaccination. In: Plotkin SA, Orenstein WA, eds. Vaccines, 4th ed. Philadelphia: WB Saunders, 2004:31–46.
8. Gaydos CA, Gaydos JC. Adenovirus vaccines. In: Plotkin SA, Orenstein WA, ed. Vaccines. Philadelphia: WB Saunders, 1999:609–18.
9. Mestecky J, Moldoveanu Z, Russell MW. Immunologic uniqueness of the genital tract: challenge for vaccine development. Am J Reprod Immunol 2005;53(5): 208–14.
10. Dupuy C, Buzoni-Gatel D, Touze A, Bout D, Coursaget P. Nasal immunization of mice with human papillomavirus type 16 (HPV-16) virus-like particles or with the HPV-16 L1 gene elicits specific cytotoxic T lymphocytes in vaginal draining lymph nodes. J Virol 1999;73(11):9063–71.
11. Milligan GN, Dudley-McClain KL, Chu CF, Young CG. Efficacy of genital T cell responses to herpes simplex virus type 2 resulting from immunization of the nasal mucosa. Virology 2004;318(2):507–15.
12. Musey L, Hu Y, Eckert L, Christensen M, Karchmer T, McElrath MJ. HIV-1 induces cytotoxic T lymphocytes in the cervix of infected women. J Exp Med 1997;185(2):293–303.
13. Ahmed R, Gray D. Immunological memory and protective immunity: understanding their relation. Science 1996;272(5258):54–60.
14. Zinkernagel RM. On differences between immunity and immunological memory. Curr Opin Immunol 2002;14(4):523–36.
15. Storni T, Kundig TM, Senti G, Johansen P. Immunity in response to particulate antigen-delivery systems. Adv Drug Deliv Rev 2005;57(3):333–55.
16. Gray D, Siepmann K, Wohlleben G. CD40 ligation in B cell activation, isotype switching and memory development. Semin Immunol 1994;6(5):303–10.
17. Sallusto F, Lenig D, Forster R, Lipp M, Lanzavecchia A. Two subsets of memory T lymphocytes with distinct homing potentials and effector functions. Nature 1999;401(6754):708–12.
18. Levin A. Vaccines today. Ann Intern Med 2000;133(8):661–4.
19. Aylward RB. Eradicating polio: today's challenges and tomorrow's legacy. Ann Trop Med Parasitol 2006;100(5–6):401–13.
20. Yusibov V, Shivprasad S, Turpen TH, Dawson W, Koprowski H. Plant viral vectors based on tobamoviruses. Curr Top Microbiol Immunol 1999;240:81–94.
21. Plant biotechnology: new products and applications. In: Hammond J MP, Yusibov V, eds, ed. Current Topics in Microbiology and Immunology. London: Springer-Verlag, 1999:1–196.
22. Streatfield SJ. Mucosal immunization using recombinant plant-based oral vaccines. Methods (San Diego, CA) 2006;38(2):150–7.
23. Tacket CO, Pasetti MF, Edelman R, Howard JA, Streatfield S. Immunogenicity of recombinant LT-B delivered orally to humans in transgenic corn. Vaccine 2004;22(31–32):4385–9.
24. Tacket CO, Mason HS, Losonsky G, Clements JD, Levine MM, Arntzen CJ. Immunogenicity in humans of a recombinant bacterial antigen delivered in a transgenic potato. Nature Med 1998;4(5):607–9.
25. Tacket CO, Mason HS, Losonsky G, Estes MK, Levine MM, Arntzen CJ. Human immune responses to a novel Norwalk virus vaccine delivered in transgenic potatoes. J Infect Dis 2000;182(1):302–5.
26. Thanavala Y, Mahoney M, Pal S, et al. Immunogenicity in humans of an edible vaccine for hepatitis B. Proc Natl Acad Sci USA 2005;102(9):3378–82.
27. Kapusta J, Modelska A, Figlerowicz M, et al. A plant-derived edible vaccine against hepatitis B virus. FASEB J 1999;13(13):1796–9.

28. Strid J, Hourihane J, Kimber I, Callard R, Strobel S. Disruption of the stratum corneum allows potent epicutaneous immunization with protein antigens resulting in a dominant systemic Th2 response. Eur J Immunol 2004;34(8):2100–9.

29. Herrick CA, Xu L, McKenzie AN, Tigelaar RE, Bottomly K. IL-13 is necessary, not simply sufficient, for epicutaneously induced Th2 responses to soluble protein antigen. J Immunol 2003;170(5):2488–95.

30. Wang LF, Lin JY, Hsieh KH, Lin RH. Epicutaneous exposure of protein antigen induces a predominant Th2–like response with high IgE production in mice. J Immunol 1996;156(11):4077–82.

31. Strid J, Hourihane J, Kimber I, Callard R, Strobel S. Epicutaneous exposure to peanut protein prevents oral tolerance and enhances allergic sensitization. Clin Exp Allergy 2005;35(6):757–66.

32. Spergel JM, Mizoguchi E, Brewer JP, Martin TR, Bhan AK, Geha RS. Epicutaneous sensitization with protein antigen induces localized allergic dermatitis and hyperresponsiveness to methacholine after single exposure to aerosolized antigen in mice. J Clin Invest 1998;101(8):1614–22.

33. Giudice EL, Campbell JD. Needle-free vaccine delivery. Adv Drug Deliv Rev 2006;58(1):68–89.

34. Van Kampen KR, Shi Z, Gao P, et al. Safety and immunogenicity of adenovirus-vectored nasal and epicutaneous influenza vaccines in humans. Vaccine 2005;23(8):1029–36.

35. Fikrig E, Insel R, Knight A, Lolis E, Pawelec G, Vitetta E. Manipulation of the immune response. In: Janeway CA, Travers P, Walport M, Schlomchik MJ, eds. ImmunoBiology, 6th ed. New York: Garland Science, 2005:613–61.

36. Henderson D, Moss, B. Smallpox and vaccinia. In: Plotkin SA, Orenstein WA, eds. Vaccines, 3rd ed. Philadelphia: WB Saunders, 1999:74–97.

37. Is smallpox history? Lancet 1999;353:1539.

38. Cono J, Casey CG, Bell DM. Smallpox vaccination and adverse reactions. Guidance for clinicians. MMWR Recomm Rep 2003;52(RR-4):1–28.

39. Wharton M, Cochi SL, Williams WW. Measles, mumps, and rubella vaccines. Infect Dis Clin North America 1990;4(1):47–73.

40. Watson JC, Hadler SC, Dykewicz CA, Reef S, Phillips L. Measles, mumps, and rubella–vaccine use and strategies for elimination of measles, rubella, and congenital rubella syndrome and control of mumps: recommendations of the Advisory Committee on Immunization Practices (ACIP). MMWR Recomm Rep 1998;47(RR-8):1–57.

41. The recommended immunization schedule for persons aged 0–18 years—United States 2007. CDC website: http://www.cdc.gov/vaccines/recs/schedules/child-schedule.htm.

42. Preblud SR. Some current issues relating to rubella vaccine. JAMA 1985;254(2):253–6.

43. James JM, Burks AW, Roberson PK, Sampson HA. Safe administration of the measles vaccine to children allergic to eggs. N Engl J Med 1995;332(19):1262–6.

44. Dales L, Hammer SJ, Smith NJ. Time trends in autism and in MMR immunization coverage in California. JAMA 2001;285(9):1183–5.

45. Kaye JA, del Mar Melero-Montes M, Jick H. Mumps, measles, and rubella vaccine and the incidence of autism recorded by general practitioners: a time trend analysis. BMJ (Clin Res Ed) 2001;322(7284):460–3.

46. Madsen KM, Hviid A, Vestergaard M, et al. A population-based study of measles, mumps, and rubella vaccination and autism. N Engl J Med 2002;347(19):1477–82.

47. Gellin BG, Katz SL. Putting a stop to a serial killer: measles. J Infect Dis 1994;170(suppl 1):S1–2.

48. Measles—United States, 1999. MMWR 2000;49(25):557–60.

49. Watson JC, Pearson JA, Markowitz LE, et al. An evaluation of measles revaccination among school-entry-aged children. Pediatrics 1996;97(5):613–8.

50. Davis RM, Whitman ED, Orenstein WA, Preblud SR, Markowitz LE, Hinman AR. A persistent outbreak of measles despite appropriate prevention and control measures. Am J Epidemiol 1987;126(3):438–49.

51. Krugman S. Further-attenuated measles vaccine: characteristics and use. Rev Infect Dis 1983;5(3):477–81.

52. Mathias RG, Meekison WG, Arcand TA, Schechter MT. The role of secondary vaccine failures in measles outbreaks. Am J Public Health 1989;79(4):475–8.

53. Reyes MA, de Borrero MF, Roa J, Bergonzoli G, Saravia NG. Measles vaccine failure after documented seroconversion. Pediatr Infect Dis J 1987;6(9):848–51.

54. Peltola H, Heinonen OP. Frequency of true adverse reactions to measles-mumps-rubella vaccine. A double-blind placebo-controlled trial in twins. Lancet 1986;1(8487):939–42.

55. Measles—United States, 1988. MMWR 1989;38(35):601–5.

56. Modlin JF, Jabbour JT, Witte JJ, Halsey NA. Epidemiologic studies of measles, measles vaccine, and subacute sclerosing panencephalitis. Pediatrics 1977;59(4):505–12.

57. Subacute sclerosing panencephalitis surveillance—United States. MMWR 1982;31(43):585–8.

58. Dyken PR. Subacute sclerosing panencephalitis. Current status. Neurol Clin 1985;3(1):179–96.

59. Hilleman MR, Buynak EB, Weibel RE, Stokes J Jr. Live, attenuated mumps-virus vaccine. N Engl J Med 1968;278(5):227–32.

60. Weibel RE, Stokes J Jr, Buynak EB, Whitman JE Jr, Hilleman MR. Live attenuated mumps-virus vaccine. 3. Clinical and serologic aspects in a field evaluation. N Engl J Med 1967;276(5):245–51.

61. Sugg WC, Finger JA, Levine RH, Pagano JS. Field evaluation of live virus mumps vaccine. J Pediatr 1968;72(4):461–6.

62. Chang TW, DesRosiers S, Weinstein L. Clinical and serologic studies of an outbreak of rubella in a vaccinated population. N Engl J Med 1970;283(5):246–8.

63. van Loon FP, Holmes SJ, Sirotkin BI, et al. Mumps surveillance–United States, 1988–1993. MMWR CDC Surveill Summ 1995;44(3):1–14.

64. Hersh BS, Fine PE, Kent WK, et al. Mumps outbreak in a highly vaccinated population. J Pediatr 1991;119(2):187–93.

65. Weibel RE, Buynak EB, McLean AA, Hilleman MR. Persistence of antibody after administration of monovalent and combined live attenuated measles, mumps, and rubella virus vaccines. Pediatrics 1978;61(1):5–11.

66. Bakshi SS, Cooper LZ. Rubella and mumps vaccines. Pediatr Clin North America 1990;37(3):651–68.

67. Hilleman MR, Weibel RE, Buynak EB, Stokes J Jr, Whitman JE Jr. Live attenuated mumps-virus vaccine. IV. Protective efficacy as measured in a field evaluation. N Engl J Med 1967;276(5):252–8.

68. Chu SY, Bernier RH, Stewart JA, et al. Rubella antibody persistence after immunization. Sixteen-year follow-up in the Hawaiian Islands. JAMA 1988;259(21):3133–6.

69. O'Shea S, Best JM, Banatvala JE, Marshall WC, Dudgeon JA. Rubella vaccination: persistence of antibodies for up to 16 years. Br Med J (Clin Res Ed) 1982;285(6337):253–5.

70. Kimberlin DW. Rubella immunization. Pediatr Ann 1997;26(6):366–70.

71. Freestone DS, Prydie J, Smith SG, Laurence G. Vaccination of adults with Wistar RA 27/3 rubella vaccine. J Hyg 1971;69(3):471–7.

72. Polk BF, Modlin JF, White JA, DeGirolami PC. A controlled comparison of joint reactions among women receiving one of two rubella vaccines. Am J Epidemiol 1982;115(1):19–25.

73. Preblud SR, Serdula MK, Frank JA Jr, Brandling-Bennett AD, Hinman AR. Rubella vaccination in the United States: a ten-year review. Epidemiol Rev 1980;2:171–94.

74. Prevention of varicella. Update recommendations of the Advisory Committee on Immunization Practices (ACIP). MMWR Recomm Rep 1999;48(RR-6):1–5.

75. Arvin AM. Varicella vaccine—the first six years. N Engl J Med 2001;344(13):1007–9.

76. Vazquez M, LaRussa PS, Gershon AA, Steinberg SP, Freudigman K, Shapiro ED. The effectiveness of the varicella vaccine in clinical practice. N Engl J Med 2001;344(13):955–60.

77. Wise RP, Salive ME, Braun MM, et al. Postlicensure safety surveillance for varicella vaccine. JAMA 2000;284(10):1271–9.

78. http://www.cdc.gov/nip/vaccine/varicella/varicella_acip_recs_prov_june_2006.pdf.

79. Levin MJ, Murray M, Rotbart HA, Zerbe GO, White CJ, Hayward AR. Immune response of elderly individuals to a live attenuated varicella vaccine. J Infect Dis 1992;166(2):253–9.

80. Oxman MN. Immunization to reduce the frequency and severity of herpes zoster and its complications. Neurology 1995;45(12 suppl 8):S41–6.

81. Levin MJ, Barber D, Goldblatt E, et al. Use of a live attenuated varicella vaccine to boost varicella-specific immune responses in seropositive people 55 years of age and older: duration of booster effect. J Infect Dis 1998;178(suppl 1):S109–12.

82. Levin MJ, Smith JG, Kaufhold RM, et al. Decline in varicella-zoster virus (VZV)-specific cell-mediated immunity with increasing age and boosting with a high-dose VZV vaccine. J Infect Dis 2003;188(9):1336–44.

83. Trannoy E, Berger R, Hollander G, et al. Vaccination of immunocompetent elderly subjects with a live attenuated Oka strain of varicella zoster virus: a randomized, controlled, dose-response trial. Vaccine 2000;18(16):1700–6.

84. Asano Y, Suga S, Yoshikawa T, et al. Experience and reason: twenty-year follow-up of protective immunity of the Oka strain live varicella vaccine. Pediatrics 1994;94(4 pt 1):524–6.

85. Weibel RE, Neff BJ, Kuter BJ, et al. Live attenuated varicella virus vaccine. Efficacy trial in healthy children. N Engl J Med 1984;310(22):1409–15.

86. Kuter BJ, Weibel RE, Guess HA, et al. Oka/Merck varicella vaccine in healthy children: final report of a 2-year efficacy study and 7–year follow-up studies. Vaccine 1991;9(9):643–7.

87. Watson B, Boardman C, Laufer D, et al. Humoral and cell-mediated immune responses in healthy children after one or two doses of varicella vaccine. Clin Infect Dis 1995;20(2):316–9.

88. Watson B, Keller PM, Ellis RW, Starr SE. Cell-mediated immune responses after immunization of healthy seronegative children with varicella vaccine: kinetics and specificity. J Infect Dis 1990;162(4):794–9.

89. White CJ, Kuter BJ, Hildebrand CS, et al. Varicella vaccine (VARIVAX) in healthy children and adolescents: results from clinical trials, 1987 to 1989. Pediatrics 1991;87(5):604–10.

90. Watson B, Gupta R, Randall T, Starr S. Persistence of cell-mediated and humoral immune responses

in healthy children immunized with live attenuated varicella vaccine. J Infect Dis 1994;169(1):197–9.

91. Watson BM, Piercy SA, Plotkin SA, Starr SE. Modified chickenpox in children immunized with the Oka/Merck varicella vaccine. Pediatrics 1993;91(1):17–22.

92. White CJ. Clinical trials of varicella vaccine in healthy children. Infect Dis Clin North Am 1996;10(3):595–608.

93. Gershon AA, Steinberg SP, Gelb L, et al. Live attenuated varicella vaccine. Efficacy for children with leukemia in remission. JAMA 1984;252(3):355–62.

94. Hardy I, Gershon AA, Steinberg SP, LaRussa P. The incidence of zoster after immunization with live attenuated varicella vaccine. A study in children with leukemia. Varicella Vaccine Collaborative Study Group. N Engl J Med 1991;325(22):1545–50.

95. Heller L, Berglund G, Ahstrom L, Hellstrand K, Wahren B. Early results of a trial of the Oka-strain varicella vaccine in children with leukaemia or other malignancies in Sweden. Postgrad Med J 1985;61(suppl 4):79–83.

96. Watson B, Seward J, Yang A, et al. Postexposure effectiveness of varicella vaccine. Pediatrics 2000;105(1 Pt 1):84–8.

97. Knuf M, Habermehl P, Zepp F, et al. Immunogenicity and safety of two doses of tetravalent measles-mumps-rubella-varicella vaccine in healthy children. Pediatr Infect Dis J 2006;25(1):12–8.

98. Tsolia M, Gershon AA, Steinberg SP, Gelb L. Live attenuated varicella vaccine: evidence that the virus is attenuated and the importance of skin lesions in transmission of varicella-zoster virus. National Institute of Allergy and Infectious Diseases Varicella Vaccine Collaborative Study Group. J Pediatr 1990;116(2):184–9.

99. Guess HA, Broughton DD, Melton LJ 3rd, Kurland LT. Epidemiology of herpes zoster in children and adolescents: a population-based study. Pediatrics 1985;76(4):512–7.

100. Gelb LD, Dohner DE, Gershon AA, et al. Molecular epidemiology of live, attenuated varicella virus vaccine in children with leukemia and in normal adults. J Infect Dis 1987;155(4):633–40.

101. Hammerschlag MR, Gershon AA, Steinberg SP, Clarke L, Gelb LD. Herpes zoster in an adult recipient of live attenuated varicella vaccine. J Infect Dis 1989;160(3):535–7.

102. Wu JJ, Huang DB, Pang KR, Tyring SK. Vaccines and immunotherapies for the prevention of infectious diseases having cutaneous manifestations. J Am Acad Dermatol 2004;50(4):495–528;quiz 9–32.

103. Salerno-Goncalves R, Pasetti MF, Sztein MB. Characterization of CD8(+) effector T cell responses in volunteers immunized with Salmonella enterica serovar Typhi strain Ty21a typhoid vaccine. J Immunol 2002;169(4):2196–203.

104. Dietrich G, Griot-Wenk M, Metcalfe IC, Lang AB, Viret JF. Experience with registered mucosal vaccines. Vaccine 2003;21(7–8):678–83.

105. Balcarek KB, Bagley MR, Pass RF, Schiff ER, Krause DS. Safety and immunogenicity of an inactivated hepatitis A vaccine in preschool children. J Infect Dis 1995;171(suppl 1):S70–2.

106. Clemens R, Safary A, Hepburn A, Roche C, Stanbury WJ, Andre FE. Clinical experience with an inactivated hepatitis A vaccine. J Infect Dis 1995;171(suppl 1):S44–9.

107. Horng YC, Chang MH, Lee CY, Safary A, Andre FE, Chen DS. Safety and immunogenicity of hepatitis A vaccine in healthy children. Pediatr Infect Dis J 1993;12(5):359–62.

108. Westblom TU, Gudipati S, DeRousse C, Midkiff BR, Belshe RB. Safety and immunogenicity of an inactivated hepatitis A vaccine: effect of dose and vaccination schedule. J Infect Dis 1994;169(5):996–1001.

109. Block SL, Hedrick JA, Tyler RD, et al. Safety, tolerability and immunogenicity of a formalin-inactivated hepatitis A vaccine (VAQTA) in rural Kentucky children. Pediatr Infect Dis J 1993;12(12):976–80.

110. Werzberger A, Mensch B, Kuter B, et al. A controlled trial of a formalin-inactivated hepatitis A vaccine in healthy children. N Engl J Med 1992;327(7):453–7.

111. Rendi-Wagner P, Korinek M, Winkler B, Kundi M, Kollaritsch H, Wiedermann U. Persistence of seroprotection 10 years after primary hepatitis A vaccination in an unselected study population. Vaccine 2006;25(5):927–31.

112. Innis BL, Snitbhan R, Kunasol P, et al. Protection against hepatitis A by an inactivated vaccine. JAMA 1994;271(17):1328–34.

113. Puziss M, Manning LC, Lynch JW, Barclaye, Abelow I, Wright GG. Large-scale production of protective antigen of Bacillus anthracis in anaerobic cultures. Appl Microbiol 1963;11:330–4.

114. Hambleton P, Carman JA, Melling J. Anthrax: the disease in relation to vaccines. Vaccine 1984;2(2):125–32.

115. CDC. Biosafety in Microbiological and Biomedical Laboratories, 4th ed. Washington, DC: US Department of Health and Human Services, 2000:88–9.

116. Use of anthrax vaccine in response to terrorism: supplemental recommendations of the Advisory Committee on Immunization Practices. MMWR 2002;51(45):1024–6.

117. Is it safe? Does it work? In: Joellenbeck LM, Zwanziger LL, Durch JS, Strom BL, eds. The

Anthrax Vaccine. Washington, DC: National Academy Press, 2002:265.

118. Brachman PR, Burger ES, Mc CL, Oberheim WA. The clinical, anatomical and mechanical analysis of the tibialis anticus muscle and its tendon. J Am Podiatr Assoc 1962;52:185–97.

119. Lucas AH, Granoff DM. Imperfect memory and the development of Haemophilus influenzae type B disease. Pediatr Infect Dis J 2001;20(3):235–9.

120. Nascimento-Carvalho CM, de Andrade AL. Haemophilus influenzae type b vaccination: long-term protection. J Pediatria 2006;82(3 suppl): S109–14.

121. Reingold AL, Broome CV, Hightower AW, et al. Age-specific differences in duration of clinical protection after vaccination with meningococcal polysaccharide A vaccine. Lancet 1985;2(8447):114–8.

122. Jones C. Vaccines based on the cell surface carbohydrates of pathogenic bacteria. Anais da Academia Brasileira de Ciencias 2005;77(2):293–324.

123. Girard MP, Preziosi MP, Aguado MT, Kieny MP. A review of vaccine research and development: meningococcal disease. Vaccine 2006;24(22):4692–700.

124. Gotschlich EC, Goldschneider I, Artenstein MS. Human immunity to the meningococcus. IV. Immunogenicity of group A and group C meningococcal polysaccharides in human volunteers. J Exp Med 1969;129(6):1367–84.

125. Artenstein MS, Gold R, Zimmerly JG, Wyle FA, Schneider H, Harkins C. Prevention of meningococcal disease by group C polysaccharide vaccine. N Engl J Med 1970;282(8):417–20.

126. Liu TY, Gotschlich EC, Jonssen EK, Wysocki JR. Studies on the meningococcal polysaccharides. I. Composition and chemical properties of the group A polysaccharide. J Biol Chem 1971;246(9): 2849–58.

127. Lepow ML, Goldschneider I, Gold R, Randolph M, Gotschlich EC. Persistence of antibody following immunization of children with groups A and C meningococcal polysaccharide vaccines. Pediatrics 1977;60(5):673–80.

128. Borrow R, Joseph H, Andrews N, et al. Reduced antibody response to revaccination with meningococcal serogroup A polysaccharide vaccine in adults. Vaccine 2000;19(9–10):1129–32.

129. MacLennan J, Obaro S, Deeks J, et al. Immune response to revaccination with meningococcal A and C polysaccharides in Gambian children following repeated immunisation during early childhood. Vaccine 1999;17(23–24):3086–93.

130. Hassan-King MK, Wall RA, Greenwood BM. Meningococcal carriage, meningococcal disease and vaccination. J Infect 1988;16(1):55–9.

131. Moore PS, Harrison LH, Telzak EE, Ajello GW, Broome CV. Group A meningococcal carriage in travelers returning from Saudi Arabia. JAMA 1988;260(18):2686–9.

132. Bilukha OO, Rosenstein N. Prevention and control of meningococcal disease. Recommendations of the Advisory Committee on Immunization Practices (ACIP). MMWR Recomm Rep 2005;54(RR-7):1–21.

133. Gardner P. Clinical practice. Prevention of meningococcal disease. N Engl J Med 2006;355(14):1466–73.

134. Hans D, Young PR, Fairlie DP. Current status of short synthetic peptides as vaccines. Medicinal Chem (Shariqah, United Arab Emirates) 2006;2(6):627–46.

135. Olive C, Batzloff M, Horvath A, et al. Potential of lipid core peptide technology as a novel self-adjuvanting vaccine delivery system for multiple different synthetic peptide immunogens. Infect Immun 2003;71(5):2373–83.

136. Olive C, Sun HK, Ho MF, et al. Intranasal administration is an effective mucosal vaccine delivery route for self-adjuvanting lipid core peptides targeting the group a streptococcal m protein. J Infect Dis 2006;194(3):316–24.

137. Ferlay J, Bray F, Pisani P, Parkin DM, GLOBOCAN 2002: Cancer Incidence, Mortality and Prevalence Worldwide. Lyon: IARC Press, 2004.

138. American Cancer Society. Cancer Facts and Figures 2006.

139. Bosch FX, Lorincz A, Munoz N, Meijer CJ, Shah KV. The causal relation between human papillomavirus and cervical cancer. J Clin Pathol 2002;55(4):244–65.

140. zur Hausen H. Papillomaviruses and cancer: from basic studies to clinical application. Nature Rev 2002;2(5):342–50.

141. Walboomers JM, Jacobs MV, Manos MM, et al. Human papillomavirus is a necessary cause of invasive cervical cancer worldwide. J Pathol 1999;189(1):12–9.

142. Kirnbauer R, Booy F, Cheng N, Lowy DR, Schiller JT. Papillomavirus L1 major capsid protein self-assembles into virus-like particles that are highly immunogenic. Proc Natl Acad Sci USA 1992;89(24):12180–4.

143. Neeper MP, Hofmann KJ, Jansen KU. Expression of the major capsid protein of human papillomavirus type 11 in Saccharomyces cerevisae. Gene 1996;180(1–2):1–6.

144. http://www.cdc.gov/std/hpv/default.htm.

145. Harper DM, Franco EL, Wheeler CM, et al. Sustained efficacy up to 4.5 years of a bivalent L1 virus-like particle vaccine against human papillomavirus types 16 and 18: follow-up from a randomised control trial. Lancet 2006;367(9518):1247–55.

146. Graham J. FDA panel backs key STD vaccine. Chicago Tribune 2006; May 18.

147. Armstrong GL, Mast EE, Wojczynski M, Margolis HS. Childhood hepatitis B virus infections in the United States before hepatitis B immunization. Pediatrics 2001;108(5):1123–8.

148. Douglas RG Jr. The heritage of hepatitis B vaccine. JAMA 1996;276(22):1796–8.

149. Szmuness W, Stevens CE, Harley EJ, et al. Hepatitis B vaccine: demonstration of efficacy in a controlled clinical trial in a high-risk population in the United States. N Engl J Med 1980;303(15):833–41.

150. Francis DP, Hadler SC, Thompson SE, et al. The prevention of hepatitis B with vaccine. Report of the centers for disease control multi-center efficacy trial among homosexual men. Ann Intern Med 1982;97(3):362–6.

151. Katkov WN, Dienstag JL. Hepatitis vaccines. Gastroenterol Clin North Am 1995;24(1):147–59.

152. Denis F, Mounier M, Hessel L, et al. Hepatitis-B vaccination in the elderly. J Infect Dis 1984;149(6):1019.

153. Heyward WL, Bender TR, McMahon BJ, et al. The control of hepatitis B virus infection with vaccine in Yupik Eskimos. Demonstration of safety, immunogenicity, and efficacy under field conditions. Am J Epidemiol 1985;121(6):914–23.

154. Roome AJ, Walsh SJ, Cartter ML, Hadler JL. Hepatitis B vaccine responsiveness in Connecticut public safety personnel. JAMA 1993;270(24):2931–4.

155. Wood RC, MacDonald KL, White KE, Hedberg CW, Hanson M, Osterholm MT. Risk factors for lack of detectable antibody following hepatitis B vaccination of Minnesota health care workers. JAMA 1993;270(24):2935–9.

156. Zimmerman RK, Ruben FL, Ahwesh ER. Hepatitis B virus infection, hepatitis B vaccine, and hepatitis B immune globulin. J Family Pract 1997;45(4):295–315; quiz 7–8.

157. Jilg W, Schmidt M, Deinhardt F. Persistence of specific antibodies after hepatitis B vaccination. J Hepatol 1988;6(2):201–7.

158. Stevens CE, Taylor FE, Tong MJ. Hepatitis B Vaccine: An Overview. New York: Grune and Stratton, 1984.

159. Hadler SC, Erben JJ, Matthews D, Starko K, Francis DP, Maynard JE. Effect of immunoglobulin on hepatitis A in day-care centers. JAMA 1983;249(1):48–53.

160. Stevens CE, Toy PT, Taylor PE, Lee T, Yip HY. Prospects for control of hepatitis B virus infection: implications of childhood vaccination and long-term protection. Pediatrics 1992;90(1 pt 2):170–3.

161. Availability of hepatitis B vaccine that does not contain thimerosal as a preservative. MMWR 1999;48(35):780–2.

162. Andre FE, Safary A. Summary of clinical findings on Engerix-B, a genetically engineered yeast derived hepatitis B vaccine. Postgrad Med J 1987;63(suppl 2):169–77.

163. CDC. Update: vaccine side effects, adverse reactions, contraindications and precautions-recommendations of the Advisory Committee on Immunization Practices (ACIP). MMWR Morb Mortal Wkly Rep 1996;45:1–35.

164. Ascherio A, Zhang SM, Hernan MA, et al. Hepatitis B vaccination and the risk of multiple sclerosis. N Engl J Med 2001;344(5):327–32.

165. Confavreux C, Suissa S, Saddier P, Bourdes V, Vukusic S. Vaccinations and the risk of relapse in multiple sclerosis. Vaccines in Multiple Sclerosis Study Group. N Engl J Med 2001;344(5):319–26.

166. Summary of notifiable diseases—United States, 2000. MMWR 2002;49(53):i-xxii, 1–100.

167. Recommendations for the use of Lyme disease vaccine. Recommendations of the Advisory Committee on Immunization Practices (ACIP). MMWR Recomm Rep 1999;48(RR-7):1–17, 21–5.

168. Scheckelhoff MR, Telford SR, Hu LT. Protective efficacy of an oral vaccine to reduce carriage of Borrelia burgdorferi (strain N40) in mouse and tick reservoirs. Vaccine 2006;24(11):1949–57.

169. Hitt E. Poor sales trigger vaccine withdrawal. Nature Med 2002;8(4):311–2.

170. Kent SJ, Zhao A, Best SJ, Chandler JD, Boyle DB, Ramshaw IA. Enhanced T-cell immunogenicity and protective efficacy of a human immunodeficiency virus type 1 vaccine regimen consisting of consecutive priming with DNA and boosting with recombinant fowlpox virus. J Virol 1998;72(12):10180–8.

171. Robinson HL, Montefiori DC, Johnson RP, et al. Neutralizing antibody-independent containment of immunodeficiency virus challenges by DNA priming and recombinant pox virus booster immunizations. Nature Med 1999;5(5):526–34.

172. Shedlock DJ, Weiner DB. DNA vaccination: antigen presentation and the induction of immunity. J Leuk Biol 2000;68(6):793–806.

173. Seder RA, Hill AV. Vaccines against intracellular infections requiring cellular immunity. Nature 2000;406(6797):793–8.

174. Ramshaw IA, Ramsay AJ. The prime-boost strategy: exciting prospects for improved vaccination. Immunology today 2000;21(4):163–5.

175. Newman MJ. Heterologous prime-boost vaccination strategies for HIV-1: augmenting cellular immune responses. Curr Opin Invest Drugs 2002;3(3):374–8.

176. McShane H. Prime-boost immunization strategies for infectious diseases. Curr Opin Mol Ther 2002;4(1):23–7.

177. Takeda A, Igarashi H, Nakamura H, et al. Protective efficacy of an AIDS vaccine, a single DNA priming followed by a single booster with a recombinant replication-defective Sendai virus vector, in a macaque AIDS model. J Virol 2003;77(17):9710–5.

178. Nakaya Y, Zheng H, Garcia-Sastre A. Enhanced cellular immune responses to SIV Gag by immunization with influenza and vaccinia virus recombinants. Vaccine 2003;21(17–18):2097–106.

179. Barouch DH, McKay PF, Sumida SM, et al. Plasmid chemokines and colony-stimulating factors enhance the immunogenicity of DNA priming-viral vector boosting human immunodeficiency virus type 1 vaccines. J Virol 2003;77(16):8729–35.

180. Gherardi MM, Najera JL, Perez-Jimenez E, Guerra S, Garcia-Sastre A, Esteban M. Prime-boost immunization schedules based on influenza virus and vaccinia virus vectors potentiate cellular immune responses against human immunodeficiency virus Env protein systemically and in the genitorectal draining lymph nodes. J Virol 2003;77(12):7048–57.

181. Woodland DL. Jump-starting the immune system: prime-boosting comes of age. Trends Immunol 2004;25(2):98–104.

182. McNeil JG, Johnston MI, Birx DL, Tramont EC. Policy rebuttal. HIV vaccine trial justified. Science 2004;303(5660):961.

183. Moorthy VS, McConkey S, Roberts M, et al. Safety of DNA and modified vaccinia virus Ankara vaccines against liver-stage P. falciparum malaria in non-immune volunteers. Vaccine 2003;21(17–18):1995–2002.

184. Joint United Nations Programme on HIV/AIDS (UNAIDS). Report on the global AIDS epidemic, Geneva Switzerland, December 2005.

185. Markel H. The search for effective HIV vaccines. N Engl J Med 2005;353(8):753–7.

34
Intravenous Immunoglobulins

Doerte Bittner and Alexander Enk

Key Points

- Intravenous immunoglobulin (IVIG) is a blood product derivative that is derived from purified human plasma, of which the final product is polyclonal immunoglobulin G, with trace amounts of other immunoglobulins and albumin.
- The mechanism of action of IVIG is complex and has not been fully elucidated.
- Intravenous immunoglobulin has been used successfully to treat a number of dermatologic conditions, such as pemphigus vulgaris, bullous pemphigoid, dermatomyositis, vasculitis toxic epidermal necrolysis, and epidermolysis bullosa acquisita.
- This drug is expensive, and has not been thoroughly studied in controlled clinical trials. Most of the clinical evidence for the use of IVIG is predominantly anecdotal.

Intravenous immunoglobulins (IVIGs) have been used for more than 25 years in diseases with primary or secondary immunodeficiencies, autoimmune disorders, and certain infectious states, and is still offering new hope for the treatment of many severe dermatologic diseases. The ability of IVIG to treat immunologically diverse disorders effectively, coupled with its excellent safety profile, has led clinicians to use the drug more liberally. Thus, even in diseases for which clinical data are insufficient and not evidence-based, and in patients with coexisting conditions, IVIG has become a viable option.

Between 3000 and 10,000 donors contribute to each batch of IVIG blood product derivative; IVIG is manufactured from the sterilized, purified human plasma. The final IVIG preparation is primarily composed of polyclonal immunoglobulin G (IgG), with trace amounts of IgA, IgM, and albumin. There is, however, a significant variation between each batch, related to the concentration of a particular antibody.[1] The half-life on infused IVIG is approximately 3 weeks. For antibody deficiencies, IVIG is used at a replacement dose of 200 to 400 mg/kg body weight three times a week. In contrast, high-dose IVIG, given most frequently at 2 g/kg body weight/month, is used as a immunomodulatory agent.[2]

Intravenous immunoglobulin's mechanism of therapeutic action is complex and has not been fully elucidated.

Reduction of circulating antibodies via anti-idiotype antibodies,[3] neutralization of toxins that trigger autoantibody production,[4] modulation of serum levels of proinflammatory cytokines,[5] functional blockade of the Fc receptors,[6] induction of leucocyte apoptosis,[7,8] and an array of antiapoptotic effects, are just some of its many biologic effects. In addition to inactivation of lytically active Fas ligand (Fas-L) in patients serum, IVIG has also been shown to protect target cells from apoptosis by upregulating Bcl-2 expressions, to interfere with the tumor necrosis factor-α (TNF-α) and interferon signaling pathways,[9] to attenuate T-cell and dendritic-cell stimulation[10,11] with reduced T-cell adhesion to extracellular matrix,[12] and to increase sensitivity to corticosteroid action by increasing glucocorticoid affinity.[13]

Safety

Adverse reactions caused by immunoglobulin therapy occur in up to 15% of infusions. The most common side effects occur within 30 to 60 minutes into the infusion and include headache, flushing, malaise, chest tightness, fever, chills, myalgia, fatigue, dyspnea, back pain, nausea, vomiting, diarrhea, blood pressure changes, and tachycardia. These are caused by activation of the complement cascade by aggregation of immunoglobulin. The symptoms are usually mild and self-limiting and can easily be managed by slowing or temporarily discontinuing the infusion. If symptoms are anticipated, the patient may be premedicated with antihistamines, analgesics, or even low-dose intravenous steroids.

To avoid these side effects, stabilizing agents, such as sucrose, maltose, dextrose, and glycine, are used in conjunction with immunoglobulin. Erythema, pain, phlebitis, and eczematous dermatitis may also occur at the infusion site.[14]

One of the most serious and potentially lethal toxicities of IVIG therapy is acute renal failure. Of reported renal adverse events in the United States, 69% have been associated with products containing the highest concentrations of sucrose.[15,16] The mechanism thought to underlie the development of renal failure (osmotic nephrosis) with sucrose results from proximal convoluted tubular cell swelling causing tubular luminal swelling.[17] More than half of patients who develop acute renal failure following IVIG administration are older than 65 years, or have preexisting renal insufficiency, diabetes mellitus, volume depletion, or paraproteinemia, or use nephrotoxic drugs.[18]

Other serious and potentially fatal side effects are stroke, myocardial infarction (MI), and other thrombotic complications. Risk of acute MI seems to increase with the use of high-dose IVIG and in older individuals, especially those with at least one cardiovascular risk factor, such as ischemic heart disease, hypertension, or hypercholesterolemia. Risk of stroke is associated with preexisting thrombogenic risk factors. Stroke and MI occur during the IVIG infusion, although they were also observed within 1 to 8 days following IVIG infusion.[19] Arterial thrombosis seems to occur early after IVIG administration (49% within 4 hours, 77% within 24 hours) and is associated with advanced age and atherosclerotic vascular disease;

venous thrombosis seems to occur later (in 54% more than 24 hours after IVIG administration), and is associated with factors contributing to venous stasis such as obesity and immobility.[20]

Anaphylaxis has been reported in IgA-deficient patients with anti-IgA antibodies. As most IVIG preparations contain trace amounts of IgA, administration of IVIG may result in antigen-antibody complex formation.

Aseptic meningitis, often presenting with headache and only photophobia, has also been described as a rare complication.[21] It occurs mainly in children [especially children with idiopathic thrombogenic purpura (ITP)] 48 to 72 hours after the IVIG infusion and can be prevented with nonsteroidal antirheumatic drugs. The symptoms resolve completely and do not return with subsequent infusions. More common in patients with a history of migraines, aseptic meningitis may last several days.

Other late and infrequent adverse effects include neutropenia, autoimmune hemolytic anemia, and, uncommonly, arthritis. Pseudohyponatremia following IVIG is important to be recognized.

To prevent side effects, high-risk patients have to be identified. Thus, it is vitally important that a thorough and comprehensive medical evaluation be performed on every patient who is being evaluated for potential IVIG therapy. The clinician should consider other nephrotoxic medications, preexisting renal function, advanced age, diabetes mellitus, hypertension and hyperviscosity, previous thromboembolic diseases, being bedridden, diabetes mellitus, hypertension, dyslipidemia, and dehydration. The evaluation should include a hematologic screen including complete blood cell counts and liver function and renal function studies prior to starting IVIG therapy. Immunoglobulin levels are measured to exclude IgA deficiency. In the absence of IgA, or in the presence of low IgA, anti-IgA titers are ordered to minimize the risk of anaphylaxis. Screening for rheumatoid factor and cryoglobulins is recommended as these patients are at an increased risk of acute renal failure. For medicolegal reasons, baseline testing for hepatitis B and C and the human immunodeficiency virus is advisable.

In patients at risk of renal failure, thromboembolic events, or aseptic meningitis, administration of a non–sucrose-containing IVIG product after accomplishing hydration, in a low concentration and a slow infusion rate while supervising urine output and kidney function, is recommended.[22,23] Patients with a background of IgA deficiency should ideally be treated with a preparation containing low levels of IgA.

In general, patients should be monitored closely for these types of adverse events during the whole period of IVIG therapy, as thrombotic manifestations occurred in patients who had received multiple IVIG infusions without exhibiting complications.[24]

Clinical Use in Dermatologic Diseases

Because the diseases treated with IVIG are rare, most support for use of this drug is provided by case reports or small clinical trials; there are few controlled randomized trials. Regardless, IVIG has proven to be extremely efficacious, and thus has become the standard of care for a wide variety of clinical syndromes, even outside the realm of immunology.

Autoimmune Mucocutaneous Blistering Diseases

Autoimmune mucocutaneous blistering diseases are a group of rare, potentially fatal, diseases that affect the mucous membranes and the skin. The clinical presentation, the course, and the prognosis are significantly variable. The immunopathology is well characterized, and the target antigens to which the autoantibodies are directed have been studied by various investigators. A significant majority of the patients respond to conventional therapy, which consists of high-dose long-term systemic corticosteroids and immunosuppressive agents.

In pemphigus vulgaris where loss of the normal cell-to-cell adhesion within the stratified epithelium (acantholysis) occurs as a result of circulating IgG autoantibodies to desmoglein 3, IVIG is an effective treatment (Figs. 34.1 and 34.2). Severe pemphigus is conventionally treated with high-dose oral prednisone, usually in combination with an immunosuppressive agent. Some patients experience significant side effects, which are sometimes fatal,

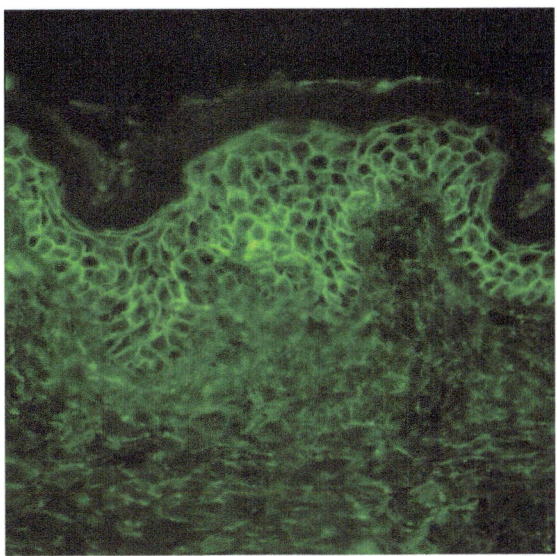

FIG. 34.1. Pemphigus vulgaris. Flaccid, easily rupured vesicles and bullae on normal-appearing skin

from prolonged immunosuppression. Intravenous immunoglobulin seems to be an effective treatment alternative by selectively decreasing circulating concentrations of pathogenic pemphigus antibodies. Serum concentrations of the specific antibodies have been reported to decrease by more than half within 1 to 2 weeks of initiation of IVIG.[25] The autoantibody titers to desmoglein 3 and 1, as measured by enzyme-linked immunosorbent assay (ELISA), can be used to monitor the serologic response to treatment in pemphigus vulgaris[26] and pemphigus

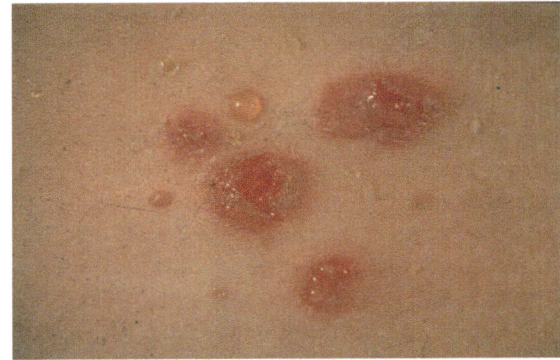

FIG. 34.2. Pemphigus vulgaris. Direct immunofluorescence staining reveals IgG and often C3 deposits in lesional and paralesional skin

foliaceus patients.[27] The autoantibody titers to components of the basement membrane zone (Ag1 and Ag2) are used to monitor the response in bullous pemphigoid.[28]

As a monotherapy, IVIG rapidly controls disease activity in many patients suffering of pemphigus vulgaris, pemphigus foliaceus, or bullous pemphigoid within 1 to 2 weeks. This even holds true in cases previously unresponsive to high doses of systemic steroids.[3,29] In cases of childhood and juvenile pemphigus, IVIG can delay the need for administration of immunosuppressive drugs with the potential of serious adverse effects.[30] Despite that, IVIG cannot be recommended as a monotherapy.

Studies have shown IVIG to be a powerful adjuvant steroid-sparing medication in pemphigus vulgaris[31] and pemphigus foliaceus.[32] As a disease-modifying drug, IVIG supports the effects of cytotoxic drugs, such as cyclophosphamide, azathioprine, mycophenolate, or rituximab, and vice versa.[25,33,34] An associated aggressive topical therapy can be supportive in all these treatment strategies.

According to most studies, the currently recommended dose of immunoglobulins is 2 g/kg body weight per cycle, infused over 2 to 5 days.[35] However, clinical improvement has been noted with lower doses.[36] As the half-life of IVIG ranges from 3 to 5 weeks, the infusions are given monthly until there is effective disease control. Although results are usually seen within weeks, sometimes more cycles have to be given until the first improvement appears. If there is no improvement after more than six cycles, IVIG therapy can be stopped. With attained disease remission, it is possible in many cases to reduce the cycle frequency by increasing the intervals between infusions from 4 to 6, 8, and 10 weeks[36]; it is questionable if the interval can be extended to 12, 14, and 16 weeks. If the patient is on multiple drugs, the drugs should be tapered one at a time. Because of the correlation between serum intercellular antibody concentrations and disease activity, tapering should proceed more slowly if the concentration of these antibodies does not continue to fall. As IVIG produces a lasting and long-term clinical remission, rather than a temporary arrest of the disease, the IVIG infusions can finally be discontinued after 12 cycles. Long-term therapy is not required.

The current recommended guidelines for IVIG are as follows: for failure of conventional therapy, prescribe prednisolone 2 g/kg body weight/day

plus azathioprine or mycophenolate mofetil or cyclophosphamide. For uncontrolled, rapid debilitating disease, relative or absolute contraindications to the use of high-dose long-term systemic corticosteroid therapy include osteoporosis, aseptic hip necrosis, or infections, and significant adverse effects are possible from conventional therapy.

A number of case series or anecdotal evidence have found IVIG also effective in the treatment of mucous membrane pemphigoid, herpes gestations, and epidermolysis bullosa acquisita.

Dermatomyositis

Dermatomyositis is characterized by muscle weakness and muscle inflammatory infiltrates (Fig. 34.3). High-dose corticotherapy (1 mg/kg/day of prednisone) constitutes the first-line treatment and is active in more that 70% of dermatomyositis. In the case of primary or secondary resistance to, intolerance of, or dependence on corticosteroids (or other immunosuppressants) and in children, IVIGs are an established treatment modality. The IVIGs improve skin and

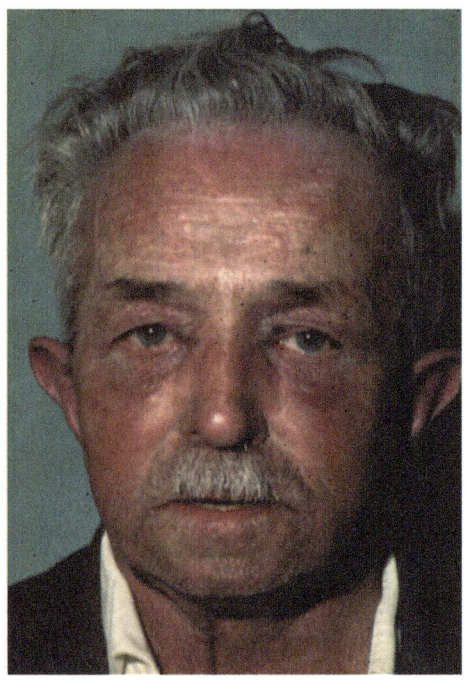

FIG. 34.3. Dermatomyositis. Heliotrop erythema of upper eyelids and edema of the lower eyelids, with erythema extending to the scalp and the entire face

muscle manifestations of (corticoresistant) dermatomyositis, with the first results occurring after 2 to 8 weeks.[37,38] In the complement-dependent microangiopathy of dermatomyositis, IVIG works by inactivating immune complexes and selectively attenuating complement amplification.[39] The data justify the use of IVIG early in the course of the disease, regardless of the type (idiopathic, paraneoplastic, or juvenile). In serious cases, IVIG can even be used as a first-line treatment; however, a long-term IVIG monotherapy has not been shown to be effective.

As in bullous autoimmune diseases, IVIGs are given monthly at doses of 2 g/kg body weight/cycle on 2 to 5 consecutive days, initially every 4 weeks for 3 to 6 months. If no improvement is seen 6 months into the treatment, the infusions can be stopped. With good response to the treatment, the intervals can be stretched to 6 weeks. After 12 cycles a treatment pause can be attempted. Unlike the pemphigus group, antibodies and creatinine kinase are not correlating with disease activity and therefore are not helpful in managing the disease. In some cases the serum concentration of soluble interleukin-2 (IL-2) receptors or C-reactive protein (CRP) gives hints of the inflammatory activity. Magnetic resonance imaging (MRI) scans are helpful but costly tools in evaluation of disease activity. For these reasons, the clinical picture is essential in evaluating the treatment success; under IVIG and simultaneous, careful reduction of steroids, the erythema and Gottron's papules should fade.

Vasculitis

Vasculitis is characterized by a systemic inflammation of blood vessels in the skin and in internal organs. Frequently presenting symptoms include diffuse arthralgias, myalgias, fever, malaise, and weight loss, but also signs of multiorgan damage (such as proteinuria, chest pain, abdominal pain, or neurologic complaints) accompany the course of the disease. Clinically, skin involvement is characteristic, manifested by erythema, purpura, ulcerations, and necrosis. Typical lab findings include increased sedimentation rate, anemia, and decreased albumin. In about 50% of primary vasculitis, specific autoantibodies, antineutrophil cytoplasmic antibodies (ANCAs), are seen. These cytoplasmic and perinuclear ANCAs not only are serologic markers for vasculitic disorders, but also

are thought to be directly involved in the pathogenesis of necrotizing vascular injury. In vitro, both perinuclear and cytoplasmic ANCAs are capable of causing cytokine-primed neutrophils to undergo degranulation and respiratory burst, releasing toxic oxygen species and lytic enzymes. A massive release of cytokines such as IL-1, tumor necrosis factor-α (TNF-α), and interferon-γ (INF-γ) leads to upregulation of adhesion molecules endothelial leukocyte adhesion molecule (ELAM-1) and intercellular adhesion molecule 1 (ICAM-1), a first step in the endothelial inflammation cascade. Antiidiotype antibodies, which inhibit ANCAs in vitro, are found in pooled human gammaglobulin preparations. Intravenous immunoglobulin infusions in vivo have produced dramatic improvements in the necrotizing vascular injury produced by ANCAs, and a rapid reduction in these autoantibody levels is seen postintravenous immunoglobulin infusion in most patients. Intravenous immunoglobulin was also found to inhibit the TNF-α– and IL-1–induced proliferation of endothelial cells and to impede their expression of adhesion molecules, chemokines, and proinflammatory molecules.

When the mainstay of treatment fails (high-dose glucocorticoids and adjuvant immunosuppressants such as cyclophosphamide or azathioprine, given over weeks to months), IVIG is a potential alternative or adjunctive treatment for ANCA-associated systemic vasculitis, with less toxicity than the conventional immunosuppressive agents. Intravenous immunoglobulin treatment was found beneficial in several vasculitic disorders including systemic and organ-specific diseases.[40–43] Its use early in the course of the disease may help effectively stop apoptotic cell death and limit the degree of damage, especially in serious forms like hemorrhagic-necrotizing vasculitis or in massive necrosis of Wegener's disease. Therefore, the use of IVIG may be justified as a first-line agent in systemic vasculitis.[44] Repeated courses of IVIG in 4-week intervals are necessary before the success of therapy can be completely evaluated. As mentioned earlier, the intervals may be stretched if clinical responses justify it.

Kawasaki's disease is an acute febrile, systemic vasculitic syndrome of an unknown etiology that primarily occurs in children younger than 5 years of age. It is one of the most common causes of acquired coronary artery disease in the developed world. An IVIG dose of 2 g/kg body weight is already an established treatment that is given as a single-dose treatment within 10 days of the onset of symptoms. There are recent studies suggesting that doses of only 1 mg/kg body weight might work just as well.[45]

Toxic Epidermal Necrolysis

Toxic epidermal necrolysis (TEN) is another acute dermatologic disease, the presentation of which may constitute a true life-threatening emergency. The disorder is characterized by separation of the epidermis from the dermis with involvement of more than 30% of the cutaneous surface. Commonly, the mucous membranes are also involved. The transcutaneous fluid loss is large and is associated with electrolyte abnormalities that require intensive care treatment. Bacterial colonization is common and associated with sepsis. No specific treatment exists to date and the mortality rate for TEN approaches 40%.

Toxic epidermal necrolysis is mediated by overexpression of Fas-ligand, which induces apoptosis in foreign antigens expressing keratinocytes and extensive dermal/epidermal separation. This Fas-mediated keratinocyte apoptosis can be inhibited in vitro by antagonistic monoclonal antibodies to Fas and by IVIGs, which have been shown to contain natural anti-Fas antibodies. Over the last 6 years, numerous retrospective reviews, case reports, and noncontrolled clinical studies have analyzed the therapeutic effect of IVIG in TEN and Stevens-Johnson syndrome. Most studies report improvement in arresting disease progression and reduction in time to skin healing. Because of variations among studies, the findings cannot be optimally compared. In general, mortality varied from 0% to 12% in the many studies that supported the use of IVIG,[46–48] and 25% to 41.7% in those that did not demonstrate a beneficial effect.[49] In the latter, doses of 2 g/kg were used and most deaths occurred in elderly patients who had preexisting renal insufficiency. Taken together, the evidence suggests a potential benefit from a single cycle of 2 g/kg of IVIG with the possibility of some further improvement at higher doses on subgroup analysis.[50] Also mortality seems to be reduced when using doses of 3 g/kg body weight/cycle in the treatment of

TEN.[51] Importantly, also children with severe cutaneous drug reactions can be safely and effectively treated with IVIG.[52] In studies, the dosing regimen for these very young patients was 0.5 g/kg per day, the average total dose was 2.2 g/kg over 3 to 4 consecutive days.

Given the potentially fatal nature of TEN and the ethical issues involved, a randomized controlled trial will most likely never be performed.

Systemic Lupus Erythematosus

Systemic lupus erythematosus (SLE) is a multisystem autoimmune disease with diverse manifestations. Several case reports and series support a beneficial role of IVIG in SLE, both as salvage immunotherapy and in control of disease activity in general or amelioration of classic disease manifestations.[53–56] The response rate to IVIG therapy ranges from 33% to 100%. A broad spectrum of clinical manifestations, such as refractory thrombocytopenia, pancytopenia, central nervous system involvement, and secondary antiphospholipid syndrome were reported to be successfully controlled by IVIG. The beneficial effects of IVIG on overall disease activity are usually prompt, with marked improvement within a few days, but they are often of limited duration. Clinical response can be maintained by continuous monthly IVIG infusions.

Lupus nephritis is one of the most serious manifestations of SLE that usually arises within 5 years of diagnosis. Pathogenic immune complexes initiate an inflammatory response by activating the complement cascade and recruiting inflammatory cells. Morbidity is related to the renal disease itself, as well as to immunosuppressive treatment-related complications and comorbidities. There are encouraging reports on the efficacy of IVIG in lupus nephritis resistant to conventional therapy. In most cases proteinuria, nephrotic syndrome, and values of creatinine clearance were improved,[57] but the exact success rate and clinical indications remain undetermined.

Although some studies showed no change in antinuclear antibody (ANA) titers and complement levels under IVIG infusions,[58] in most studies IVIG therapy led to decreased ANA levels and immune complexes and increased hemoglobin and C3/C4 levels.[59] One study suggested a tendency toward a better response of patients with abnormal baseline levels of complement and SS-A/SS-B antibodies before the IVIG courses.[59]

At present, IVIG in SLE is indicated either in severe cases nonresponsive to other therapeutic modalities, or when SLE can be controlled only with high-dose steroids. In such patients, IVIG becomes a useful steroid-sparing agent. However, this needs to be confirmed in double-blind, placebo-controlled studies.

Atopic Dermatitis

Atopic dermatitis generally responds to topical therapy; however, small numbers of patients have severe resistant disease despite second-line therapies. High-dose IVIG is inhibiting T-cell–mediated, Fas-induced keratinocyte apoptosis,[60] and has been suggested to be of benefit in a small number of uncontrolled trials and case reports,[50] although some trials did not find a clinically significant improvement. If the trials are taken together, an improvement was observed in 61% of atopic dermatitis patients treated with IVIG. Adults appeared less likely to respond than children, and the duration of response was also more prolonged in children. Adjunctive therapy in adults was more effective than monotherapy, whereas monotherapy was effective in 90% of children. The indications for IVIG in atopic dermatitis should be further assessed using double-blind placebo-controlled trials.

There are only a few case reports or trials of the use of IVIG (2 g/kg body weight) in therapy-resistant systemic sclerosis,[61] mixed connective tissue disease,[62] scleromyxedema,[63,64] psoriasis,[65] psoriasis arthritis,[66] pyoderma gangrenosum,[67] and chronic urticaria.[68] Although results sound promising, the current data are insufficient to recommend the routine administration of IVIG in these patients.

Conclusion

Off-label uses for high-dose IVIG are becoming increasingly common in dermatology.[69] Intravenous immunoglobulins are extremely well tolerated, but their use must be carefully weighed in light of their human biologic origin, the logistic problems associated with their administration, and their high cost of at least $10,000 per treatment cycle. Although IVIG is a very expensive drug, studies have shown that the mean total cost of IVIG therapy is statistically significantly less than that of conventional therapy during the entire course of the disease and on an annual basis. Normally none of the IVIG-treated patients require additional physician visits, laboratory tests, or hospitalizations specifically related to IVIG therapy.[35] Intravenous immunoglobulin also helps prevent long-term side effects of immunosuppressant drugs such as osteoporosis, diabetes mellitus, infections, and alveolitis. On the other hand, IVIG causes side effects such as meningitis, thrombotic events, and kidney failure.

Controlled, double-blind, long-term clinical trials and a better understanding of the complex immunomodulating mechanism of IVIG are required to ultimately optimize dose, frequency, duration, and mode of IVIG administration as well as efficacy, pharmacoeconomics, and adjunctive therapies. However, the use of expensive IVIG should be based not only on clinical data, but also, and especially, on the biologic rationale for its use.

Intravenous immunoglobulin is finding increasing use in dermatology to treat a variety of inflammatory conditions, many, but not all, of which are autoantibody mediated. In general, this treatment is safe and well tolerated. Its mechanisms of actions are complex, and not fully understood. It involves antiidiotype antibodies, catabolism of autoantibodies, blockade of Fc receptors, and inactivation of Fas ligand. Because of the expense and risks of using this agent, it should be used judiciously under very specific circumstances. This treatment frequently plays an important role in the management of severe, recalcitrant skin diseases, frequently in the setting of combination treatment with other immunosuppressive or immune modulating agents.

References

1. Lamari F, Anastassiou ED, Tsegenidis T, et al. An enzyme immunoassay to determine the levels of specific antibodies toward bacterial surface antigens in human immunoglobulin preparations and blood serum. J Pharm Biomed Anal 1999;20:913–920.

2. Jolles S, Sewell WAC, Misbah SA. Clinical uses of intravenous immunoglobulin. Clin Exp Immunol 2005;142(1):1–11.

3. Bystryn JC, Jiao D, Natow S. Treatment of pemphigus with intravenous immunoglobulin. J Am Acad Dermatol 2002;47:358–363.

4. Norrby-Teglund A, Low DE, McGeer A, et al. (1997) Superantigenic activity produced by group A streptococcal isolates is neutralized by plasma from IVIG-treated streptococcal toxic shock syndrome patients. Adv Exp Med Biol 1997;418:563–566.

5. Bhol KC, Desai A, Kumari S. Pemphigus vulgaris: the role of IL-1 and IL-1 receptor antagonist in pathogenesis and effects of intravenous immunoglobulin on their production. Clin Immunol 2001;100:172–180.

6. Kaneko Y, Nimmerjahn F, Ravetch JV. Anti-inflammatory activity of immunoglobulin G resulting from Fc sialylation. Science 2006;313(5787):670–673.

7. Takeshita S, Tsujimoto H, Nakatani K. Intravenous immunoglobulin preparations promote apoptosis in lipopolysaccharide-stimulated neutrophils via an oxygen-dependent pathway in vitro. APMIS 2005;113(4):269–277.

8. Prasad NK, Papoff G, Zeuner A, et al. (1998) Therapeutic preparations of normal polyspecific IgG (IVIG) induce apoptosis in human lymphocytes and monocytes: a novel mechanism of action of IVIG involving the Fas apoptotic pathway. J Immunol 1998;161:3781–3790.

9. Crow AR, Song S, Semple JW, et al. A role for IL-1 receptor antagonist or other cytokines in the acute therapeutic effects of IVIG? Blood 2007;109(1):155–158.

10. Tha-In T, Metselaar HJ, Tilanus HW. Superior immunomodulatory effects of intravenous immunoglobulins on human T-cells and dendritic cells: comparison to calcineurin inhibitors. Transplantation 2006;81(12):1725–34.

11. Bayry J, Lacroix-Desmazes S, Delignat S. Intravenous immunoglobulin abrogates dendritic cell differentiation induced by interferon-alpha present in serum from patients with systemic lupus erythematosus. Arthritis Rheum 2003;48(12):3497–3502.

12. Jerzak M, Rechberger T, Gorski A. Intravenous immunoglobulin therapy influences T cell adhesion to extracellular matrix in women with a history of recurrent spontaneous abortions. Am J Reprod Immunol 2000;44(6):336–341.

13. Spahn JD, Leung DY, Chan MT, et al. Mechanisms of glucocorticoid reduction in asthmatic subjects treated with intravenous immunoglobulin. J Allergy Clin Immunol 1999;103:421–426.

14. Jolles S, Hughes J, Withaker S. Dermatological uses of high-dose intravenous immunoglobulin. Arch Dermatol 1999;134(1):80–86.

15. Epstein JS, Zoon KC. Letter to healthcare providers. Important drug warning: immune globulin intravenous (human). U.S. Food and Drug Administration, Center for Biologics Evaluation and Research. www.fda.gov/cber/ltr/igiv111398.htm. 2004.

16. Zhang R, Szerlip HM. Reemergence of sucrose nephropathy: acute renal failure caused by high-dose intravenous globulin therapy. South Med J 2000;93(9):901–904.

17. Shah S, Vervan M. Use of i.v. immune globulin and occurrence of associated acute renal failure and thrombosis. Am J Health Syst Pharm 2005;62(7):720–725.

18. Orbach H, Katz U, Sherer Y, et al. Intravenous immunoglobulin: adverse effects and safe administration. Clin Rev Allergy Immunol 2005;29(3):173–184.

19. Marie I, Maurey G, Herve F, et al. Intravenous immunoglobulin-associated arterial and venous thrombosis; report of a series and review of literature. Br J Dermatol 2006;155(4):714–721.

20. Paran D, Herishanu Y, Elkayam O, et al. Venous and arterial thrombosis following administration of intravenous immunoglobulins. Blood Coagul Fibrinolysis 2005;16(5):313–318.

21. Lafferty TE, DeHoratius RJ, Smith JB. Aseptic meningitis as a side effect of intravenous immune gammaglobulin. J Rheumatol 1997;24(12):2491–2492.

22. Chapman SA, Gilkerson KL, Davin TD, et al. Acute renal failure and intravenous immune globulin: occurs with sucrose-stabilized, but not with D-sorbitol-stabilized, formulation. Ann Pharmacother 2004;38(12):2059–2067.

23. Pierce LR, Jain N. Risks associated with the use of intravenous immunoglobulin. Transfus Med Rev 2003;17:241–251.

24. Alexandrescu DT, Dutcher JP, Hughes JT, et al. Strokes after intravenous gamma globulin: thrombotic phenomenon in patients with risk factors or just coincidence? Am J Hematol 2005;78(3):216–220.

25. Brystryn JC, Jiao D. IVIG selectively and rapidly decreases circulating autoantibodies in pemphigus vulgaris. Autoimmunity 2006;39:601–607.

26. Sami N, Bhol KC, Ahmed RA. Influence of intravenous immunoglobulin therapy on autoantibody titers to desmoglein 3 and desmoglein 1 in pemphigus vulgaris. Eur J Dermatol 2003;13(4):377–381.

27. Sami N, Bhol KG, Ahmed AR. Influence of IVIG therapy on autoantibody titers to desmoglein 1 in patients with pemphigus foliaceus. Clin Immunol 2002;105(2):192–198.

28. Sami N, Ali S, Bhol KG, et al. Influence of intravenous immunoglobulin therapy on autoantibody titres to BP Ag1 and BP Ag2 in patients with bullous pemphigoid. J Eur Acad Dermatol Venereol 2003;17(6):641–645.

29. Ahmed AR. Intravenous immunoglobulin therapy for patients with bullous pemphigoid unresponsive to conventional immunosuppressive treatment. J Am Acad Dermatol 2001;45(6):825–835.

30. Szep Z, Danilla T, Buchvald D. Treatment of juvenile pemphigus vulgaris with intravenous immunoglobulins. Cas Lek Cesk 2005;144(109):700–703.

31. Mittmann N, Chan B, Knowles S, et al. Effect of intravenous immunoglobulin on prednisone dose in patients with pemphigus vulgaris. J Cutan Med Surg 2006;10(5):222–227.

32. Sami N, Quereshi A, Ahmed AR. Steroid sparing effect of intravenous immunoglobulin therapy in patients with pemphigus foliaceus. Eur J Dermatol 2002;12(2):174–178.

33. Ahmed AR, Spigelman Z, Cavacini LA, et al. Treatment of pemphigus vulgaris with rituximab ad intravenous immune globulin. N Engl J Med 2006;355(17):1772–1779.

34. Levy A, Doutre MS, Lesage FX, et al. Treatment of pemphigus with intravenous immunoglobulin. Ann Dermatol Venereol 2004;131(11):957–961.

35. Daoud YJ, Amin KG. Comparison of cost of immune globulin intravenous therapy to conventional immunosuppressive therapy in treating patients with autoimmune mucocutaneous blistering diseases. Int Immunopharmacol 2006;6(4):600–606.

36. Ahmed AR, Dahl MV. Consensus statement on the use of intravenous immunoglobulin therapy of autoimmune mucocutaneous blistering diseases. Arch Dermatol 2003;139(8):1051–1059.

37. Dalakas MC. The role of high-dose immune globulin intravenous in the treatment of dermatomyositis. Int Immunopharmacol 2006;6(4):550–556.

38. Gottfried I, Seeber A, Anegg B, et al. High dose intravenous immunoglobulin (IVIG) in dermatomyositis: clinical responses and effect on sIL-2R levels. Eur J Dermatol 2000;10(1):29–35.

39. Basta M, Van Goor F, Luccioli S. F(ab)¹2–mediated neutralization of C3a and C5a anaphylatoxins: a novel effector function of immunoglobulins. Nat Med 2003;9(4):431–438.

40. Jayne DR, Chapel H, Adu D, et al. Intravenous immunoglobulin for ANCA-associated systemic vasculitis with persistent disease activity. Q J Med 2000;93(7):433–439.

41. Jayne DR, Davies MJ,Fox CJ, et al. Treatment of systemic vasculitis with pooled intravenous immunoglobulin. Lancet 1991;337(8750):1137–1139.

42. Richter C, Schnabel A, Csernok E, et al. Treatment of anti-neutrophil cytoplasmic antibody (ANCA)-associated systemic vasculitis with high-dose intravenous immunoglobulin. Clin Exp Immunol 1995;101(1):2–7.

43. Jayne DR, Lockwood CM. Pooled intravenous immunoglobulin in the management of systemic vasculitis. Adv Exp Med Biol 1993;336:469–472.

44. Jayne DR, Lockwood CM. Intravenous immunoglobulin as a sole therapy for systemic vasculitis. Br J Rheumatol 1996;35(11):1150–1153.

45. Sakata K, Hamaoka K, Ozawa SI, et al. A randomized prospective study on the use of 2 g-IVIG or 1 g-IVIG as therapy for Kawasaki disease. Eur J Pediatr 2007;166:565–571.

46. Prins C, Kerdel FA, Padilla RS, et al. TEN-IVIG Study Group Treatment of toxic epidermal necrolysis with high-dose intravenous immunoglobulins: multicenter retrospective analysis of 48 consecutive cases. Arch Dermatol 2003;139(1):85–86.

47. Trent JT, Kerdel FA. Intravenous immunoglobulin for the treatment of toxic epidermal necrolysis. Arch Dermatol 2003;139(1):85–86.

48. Viard I, Wehrli P, Bullani R, et al. (1998) Inhibition of toxic epidermal necrolysis by blockade of CD95 with human intravenous immunoglobulin. Science 1998;282(5388):490–493.

49. Bachot N, Revuz J, Roujeau JC. Intravenous immunoglobulin treatment for Stevens-Johnson syndrome and toxic epidermal necrolysis: a prospective noncomparative study showing no benefit on mortality or progression. Arch Dermatol 2003;139(1):33–36.

50. Jolles S, Sewell C, Webster D, et al. Adjunctive high-dose intravenous immunoglobulin treatment for resistant atopic dermatitis: efficacy and effects on intracellular cytokine levels and CD4 counts. Acta Derm Venereol 2003;83(6)433–437.

51. French LE. Toxic epidermal necrolysis and Stevens Johnson syndrome: our current understanding. Allerg Int 2006;55(1):9–16.

52. Metry DW, Jung P, Levy ML. Use of intravenous immunoglobulin in children with Stevens-Johnson syndrome and toxic epidermal necrolysis: seven cases and review of literature. Pediatrics 2003;112(6 pt 1):1430–1436.

53. Levy Y, Sherer Y, George J, et al. Intravenous immunoglobulin treatment of lupus nephritis. Semin Arthritis Rheum 2000;29(5):321–327.

54. Levy Y, Sherer Y, Ahmed A, et al. A study of 20 SLE patients with intravenous immunoglobulin—clinical and serologic response. Lupus 1999;8(9):705–712.

55. Sherer Y, Shoenfeld Y. Intravenous immunoglobulin for immunomodulation of systemic lupus erythematosus. Autoimmun Rev 2006;5(2):153–155.

56. Boletis JN, Ioannidis JP, Boki KA, et al. Intravenous immunoglobulin compared with cyclophosphamide for proliferative lupus nephritis. Lancet 1999;354(9178):569–570.

57. Orbach H, Tishler M, Shoenfeld Y. Intravenous immunoglobulin and the kidney—a two-edged sword. Semin Arthritis Rheum 2004;34(3):593–601.

58. Schroeder JO, Zeuner RA, Euler HH, et al. (1996) High dose intravenous immunoglobulins in systemic lupus erythematosus: clinical and serological results of a pilot study. J Rheumatol 1996;23(1):71–75.

59. Francioni C, Galeazzi M, Fioravanti A, et al. (1994) Long-term i.v. IG treatment in systemic lupus erythematosus. Clin Exp Rheumatol 1994;12(2):163–168.

60. Trautmann A, Akdis M, Schmid-Grendelmeier P, et al. Targeting keratinocyte apoptosis in the treatment of atopic dermatitis and allergic contact dermatitis. J Allergy Clin Immunol 2001;108(5):839–846.

61. Levy Y, Amital H, Langevitz P, et al. Intravenous immunoglobulin modulates cutaneous involvement and reduces skin fibrosis in systemic sclerosis: an open-label study. Arthritis Rheum 2004;50(3):1005–1007.

62. Ulmer A, Kotter I, Pfaff A, et al. Efficacy of pulsed intravenous immunoglobulin therapy in mixed connective tissue disease. J Am Acad Dermatol 2002;46(1):123–127.

63. Majeski C, Taher M, Grewal P, et al. Combination oral prednisone and intravenous immunoglobulin in the treatment of scleromyxedema. J Cutan Med Surg 2005;9(3):99–104.

64. Kulczycki A, Nelson M, Eisen A, et al. Skleromyxoedema: treatment of cutaneous and systemic manifestations with high-dose intravenous immunoglobulin. Br J Dermatol 2003;149(6):1276–1281.

65. Taguchi Y, Takashima S, Yoshida S, et al. Psoriasis improved by intravenous immunoglobulin therapy. Intern Med 2006;45(14):879–880.

66. Gurmin V, Mediwake R, Fernando M, et al. Psoriasis: response to high-dose intravenous immunoglobulin in three patients. Br J Dermatol 2002;147(3):554–557.

67. Meyer N, Ferraro V, Mignard MH, et al. Pyoderma gangrenosum treated with high-dose intravenous immunoglobulins: two cases and review of the literature. Clin Drug Invest 2006;26(9):541–546.

68. Kroiss M, Vogt T, Landthaler M, et al. The effectiveness of low-dose intravenous immunoglobulin in chronic urticaria. Acta Derm Venereol 2000;80(3):225.

69. Rutter A, Luger TA. Intravenous immunoglobulin: an emerging treatment for immune-mediated skin diseases. Curr Opin Invest Drugs 2000;3(5):713–719.

Section IV
Autoimmunity, Immunodeficiency, and Immune – Associated Dermatoses

35
Novel Approach to the Evaluation of Primary Immunodeficiencies

Clemens Esche and Bernard A. Cohen

Key Points

- Primary immunodeficiency diseases usually manifest early in infancy and childhood, but some manifest later in life.
- The skin and the gastrointestinal (GI) and sinopulmonary tracts are major sites of involvement, since they interface with the environment.
- These diseases are a result of heritable genetic defects that are usually recessive conditions, and frequently located on the X chromosome, hence a male predominance.
- Clinical manifestations are recurrent and severe deep infections in the skin or GI or sinopulmonary tract that require intravenous antibiotics, as well as infections with opportunistic organisms (for example, *Giardia lamblia*).
- The major causes of the primary immunodeficiency diseases include B-lymphocyte disorders, T-lymphocyte disorders, combined B- and T-cell disorders, as well as unconventional disorders such as interleukin-1 receptor–associated kinase 4 (IRAK-4) deficiency and warts, hypogammaglobulinemia, immunodeficiency, and myelokathexis (WHIM) syndrome (*CXCR4* deficiency).
- Early diagnosis is critical to effectively manage these conditions in the afflicted patients and to identify disease gene carriers for genetic counseling.

Although most primary immunodeficiencies (PIDs) manifest early in infancy and childhood, some may escape detection until later in life. It has been estimated that there are over 500,000 affected patients in the United States, and more than 120 different PIDs have been discovered.[1] Moreover, 20 new disorders have been described in the last 4 years since the most recent update by the International Union of Immunological Societies Committee.[2]

This chapter outlines a practical approach to clinical diagnosis, and discusses state-of-the-art genetic markers, diagnostic tools, and treatment of primary immunodeficiency disorders.

Recognizing Immune Deficiencies

The genetic defect in many of these conditions has been identified. Most are recessive and located on the X chromosome. As a consequence, the majority of PIDs are diagnosed in infancy. There is a 5:1 predominance of males to females. In contrast, there is a slight female predominance in those patients diagnosed as adults.

The diagnosis of PID may be delayed when the practitioner fails to recognize early clinical markers. The gastrointestinal (GI) tract, sinopulmonary tract, and the skin are the principal sites of environment–host interactions, and these organs systems are associated with many of the initial presenting symptoms. A list of warning signs has been developed by the Jeffrey Model Foundation and the Immune Deficiency Foundation and is available at http://www.info4pi.org/patienttopatient/index.cfm?section=patienttopatient&content=warningsigns. The list includes the following signs (Table 35.1): eight or more otitis media infections per year, two or more serious sinus infections per year, two or more pneumonias per year, recurrent deep infections or

TABLE 35.1. Ten warning signs of primary immunodeficiency.

1. Eight or more ear infections within 1 year
2. Two or more serious sinus infections within 1 year
3. Two or more months on antibiotics with little effect
4. Two or more pneumonias within 1 year
5. Failure of an infant to gain weight or grow normally
6. Recurrent, deep skin or organ abscesses
7. Persistent thrush in mouth or elsewhere on skin, after age 1
8. Need for intravenous antibiotics to clear infections
9. Two or more deep-seated infections
10. A family history of primary immunodeficiency

TABLE 35.2. Clinical syndromes of mucocutaneous candidiasis.

Chronic oral candidiasis
Iron deficiency
HIV infection
Denture stomatitis
Inhaled corticosteroid use
Familial chronic mucocutaneous candidiasis
Autoimmune polyendocrinopathy-candidiasis-ectodermal dystrophy
Chronic localized candidiasis
Chronic mucocutaneous candidiasis with thymoma
Candidiasis with chronic keratitis
Candidiasis with the hyper-IgE syndrome

infections in unusual areas (e.g., muscle, liver), the need for intravenous antibiotics to clear infections, infections with an opportunistic organism (e.g., *Pneumocystis carinii, Giardia*), and persistent thrush in patients older than 1 year of age.

Classification of Primary Immunodeficiencies

Classically, PIDs are classified into B-lymphocyte (constituting 70% of all PIDs), T-lymphocyte (20%), combined B-cell and T-cell (less than 1%), natural killer (NK)-cell (less than 1%), phagocyte (9%), and complement deficiencies (less than 1%). However, many PIDs affect multiple cell lineages (e.g., severe combined immunodeficiencies [SCIDs] and Wiskott-Aldrich syndrome). In addition, some immune defects affect multiple functional component of the immune system (e.g., the hyperimmunoglobulin E syndrome combines susceptibility to infections and atopy).

A new classification based on clinical findings at the bedside, such as specific infections, allergies, and autoimmune phenomena, rather than laboratory-based immunologic parameters, was recently proposed.[2] The authors suggested the addition of a group of unconventional disorders defined by susceptibility to specific infections in otherwise healthy individuals (Table 35.2). Examples of this concept include interleukin-1 (IL-1) receptor–associated kinase 4 (IRAK-4) deficiency, which causes susceptibility to pneumococcal infections, and the warts, hypogammaglobulinemia, immunodeficiency, and myelokathesis (WHIM) syndrome, which is caused by mutations in the *CXCR4* gene that induce susceptibility to herpes viruses.

Primarily Antibody Production (B-Cell) Deficiencies

Defects in B-cell function resulting in antibody deficiency represent the most common (70%) type of PIDs in humans. Often symptoms do not appear until the latter part of the first year of life when passively acquired immunoglobulin G (IgG) from the mother drops below protective levels. Encapsulated bacteria (*Haemophilus, Pneumococcus, Streptococcus*), parasites (*Giardia*), and enteroviruses along with papillomaviruses pose the most serious risk of infection. Children often present with poor growth, recurrent sinopulmonary infections, and GI malabsorption resulting from chronic and recurrent GI infections.[3] Autoimmunity (hemolytic anemia, thrombocytopenia, neutropenia) may be caused by the inappropriate production of self-reactive immunoglobulins. Infections with fungal pathogens do not usually occur.

Evaluation of a patient with a suspected humoral defect should include quantitative immunoglobulin levels (IgA, IgE, IgM, IgG). However, normal results do not rule out a B-cell defect. Assessment of protective vaccine titers (tetanus, diphtheria, pneumococcal) can be used after the primary immunization series has been completed (6 months to 6 years). Patients with low titers should be revaccinated and tested for vaccine titer levels 3 to 4 weeks later. Selective use of antibiotics and regular intravenous immunoglobulin (IVIG) infusions decrease the risk of acute and chronic infections and facilitate normal growth.

X-linked (Bruton) Agammaglobulinemia

The most common defect in early B-cell development is X-linked agammaglobulinemia (XLA), also known as congenital agammaglobulinemia.[4] First described by Bruton, XLA is considered a prototype PID because the clinical and laboratory findings are distinctive. It originates from a block in B-cell differentiation, resulting in severely decreased numbers of B lymphocytes and an almost complete lack of plasma cells as well as negligible or very low immunoglobulin levels of all isotypes. Cellular immunity remains unaffected.

Carrier Testing

Only about 50% of patients with XLA have a family history of immunodeficiency. If a mutation has been identified in a particular family, mutation analysis is the most reliable option.[5] X-linked agammaglobulinemia–causing mutations are available in a database at http://bioinf.uta.fi/BTKbase. When a mutation in the Bruton tyrosine kinase *(Btk)* encoding gene has been identified in a male with sporadic XLA, the mother is a carrier of that mutation 80% to 85% of the time, while the maternal grandmother is a carrier <20% of the time. Female carriers are healthy but display nonrandom X-chromosome inactivation in their B cells. Therefore, when a mutation in *Btk* has not been identified, or when critical family members are not available for linkage studies, X-chromosome–inactivation analysis can be used to provide carrier detection for females at risk of being carriers.

Prenatal Diagnosis

Male infants can be diagnosed when the mother has been recognized as a carrier. Chorionic villus sampling (CVS) can be performed early in pregnancy, and DNA analysis can be used when the exact mutation has been determined for the family. Amniocentesis can be performed later in gestation. Collection of fetal lymphocytes through in utero umbilical cord sampling can be used to enumerate CD19+ B cells and mature T cells by fluorescence-activated cell sorting (FACS), but this procedure poses some risk to the fetus (ranging from <1% to 5%). At birth, cord blood can be sent for FACS analysis of lymphocyte populations. Quantitative IgG levels are not useful; cord and fetal levels largely measure maternal IgG transported across the placenta.

Key Features

Patients are generally healthy in the newborn period due to transplacentally acquired maternal IgG. Recurrent infections due to encapsulated bacteria including *Streptococcus pneumonia, Staphylococcus aureus, Haemophilus influenzae,* and *Neisseria meningitides* typically start to develop in the second half of the first year of life, particularly sinopulmonary tract infections (60% of patients), gastroenteritis (35%), pyoderma (25%), arthritis (20%), meningitis-encephalitis (16%), conjunctivitis (8%), septicemia (10%), and osteomyelitis (3%). The most reliable finding on physical examination is the paucity of lymphoid tissue (adenoids, lymph nodes, spleen). In patients without a family history of immunodeficiency, the mean age at diagnosis is 3 years. Because cellular immunity is intact, patients do not appear to have an unusual susceptibility to most viral, fungal, and mycobacterial infections. Specifically, varicella, cytomegalovirus (CMV), respiratory syncytial virus (RSV), parainfluenza, and rotavirus are rarely a problem. Exceptions to this include viral hepatitis and chronic enteroviral encephalitis. Patients typically do not have failure to thrive unless they develop bronchiectasis or persistent enteroviral disease.

Differential Diagnosis

The differential diagnosis includes acrodermatitis enteropathica, ataxia teleangiectasia, atopic dermatitis, avitaminosis A, and SCID.

Workup

The most specific and most reliable laboratory finding is the profound decrease in B-cell numbers in the circulation. In the normal individual, 5% to 20% of the peripheral blood lymphocytes express CD19, while in patients with XLA the mean percentage of B cells is 0.1%. The diagnosis of XLA should be considered in any patient who has hypogammaglobulinemia and <2% CD19+ B cells in the circulation, particularly if the onset of recurrent infections occurred in the first few years of life.

Management

Symptoms usually improve or even resolve with antibiotics and immunoglobulin replacement (IVIG) therapy.

Prognosis

In the 1950s and 1960s, the majority of patients died of infections in early childhood. In the 1970s, a significant proportion of patients died of chronic enteroviral infections or progressive pulmonary disease before they reached adulthood. Today, the majority of patients pass into adulthood with few significant problems. Chronic sinopulmonary bacterial infections and enteroviral GI infections pose the greatest threats to survival, particularly when the diagnosed is delayed.

Selective IgA Immunodeficiency

Patients are usually diagnosed based on the laboratory measurement of serum IgA concentration. The clinical presentation is not necessarily taken into consideration. The consensus of the Pan-American Group for Immunodeficiency (PAGID) and the European Society for Immunodeficiency (ESID) is that a definitive diagnosis of selective IgA deficiency can be made in a male or female patient more than 4 years of age who has a serum IgA of less than 7 mg/dL (0.07 g/L), but normal serum IgG and IgM, in whom other causes of hypogammaglobulinemia have been excluded. By their definition, these patients have a normal IgG antibody response to vaccination.[6]

Management

Most patients can be managed with prophylactic or periodic antibiotics, but a few may benefit from immunoglobulin therapy, regardless of whether an associated IgG functional defect can be demonstrated.

Common Variable Immunodeficiency

Common variable immunodeficiency (CVID), also called acquired hypogammaglobulinemia, adult-onset hypogammaglobulinemia, or dysgammaglobulinemia, is the most prevalent human PID requiring medical attention. It is characterized by generalized defective antibody production and recurrent sinopulmonary bacterial infections. The word *variable* in CVID denotes variability in the age of presentation (it occurs in early childhood, adolescence, or young adulthood) and variability in the degree and type of hypogammaglobulinemia.

Rather than a distinct disease, CVID represents a group of disorders with disturbances of the adaptive as well as innate immune system.[7] Patients present with heterogeneous clinical features and myriad immunologic abnormalities that most commonly affect them during the second and third decade. Patients are predisposed to malignancy, especially lymphoma, as well as various autoimmune diseases.

The underlying molecular mechanisms that lead to CVID remain elusive in 90% of cases.[7] However, in the last 2 years, the first genetic defects underlying common variable immunodeficiency, including *ICOS, TACI, BAFF-R* and *CD19*, have been identified. An analysis of dendritic cells has demonstrated alterations in a majority of patients in addition to the disturbed T and B-cell function.[7] Investigators have also suggested that several changes in the adaptive immune system might be secondary to chronic inflammation resulting in HHV8 infection in a subgroup of CVID patients with granulomatous disease, autoimmune phenomena, and T-cell dysfunction.

Prevalence

The prevalence is 1 in 25,000 newborns.

Key Features

Recurrent infections and deficiencies of IgA and IgG are present in most patients, and IgM deficiency is present in half. A quarter of patients develop autoimmune disorders, and a quarter have chronic gastrointestinal disturbances. There is also an increased risk of malignancy.

Management

Prophylactic intravenous or subcutaneous immunoglobulin replacement provides effective treatment for most patients. Minimum trough serum levels of over 5 to 7 g/L are recommended. In a small study of 24 patients, a trough level of 6 g/L helped reduce the rate of bacterial infections and prevent progression of chronic pulmonary disease measured by pulmonary function test and HRCT[7] in most patients.

Prognosis

The occurrence of granulomatous inflammation is associated with a worse prognosis compared with common variable immunodeficiency patients without granuloma. CVID patients with hepatitis C have a very poor prognosis.

Primarily Cellular (T Cell) Deficiencies

Cellular deficiency disorders account for 5% to 10% of primary immunodeficiencies. Genetic defects in T-cell function lead to susceptibility to infections by certain organisms (*Mycobacterium, Pneumocystis, Candida*, Epstein-Barr virus [EBV], CMV, varicella-zoster virus) and a num-ber of other clinical disorders with life-threatening complications. T-cell–deficient infants are occasionally born with graft-versus-host disease resulting from incidental transfer of competent maternal T lymphocytes in utero by placental–fetal bleeds.

Although it is tempting to classify primarily cellular deficiencies as isolated T-cell disorders, B-cell function and antibody production are also often impaired when T-cell function is severely impaired. For clinical purposes, cellular PIDs are usually defined based on defective T-cell or NK-cell function with intact or largely intact humoral immunity. The PIDs resulting from defects in phagocyte dysfunction are reviewed separately.

Most of these disorders can be diagnosed by screening for lymphopenia or for T-cell deficiency in cord blood at birth. Clinical evaluation should include a complete blood count with differential, lymphocyte subsets obtained by flow cytometry, vaccine titers (tetanus, diphtheria, pneumococcal),quantitative immunoglobulin levels (IgA, IgE, IgM, IgG), and T-cell proliferation assays. Skin testing (*Candida*, purified protein derivative [PPD]) allows determination of the ability of T cells to respond to foreign antigen. Therapeutic options are limited; bone marrow transplantation is the treatment of choice.[8]

DiGeorge Syndrome

DiGeorge syndrome (DGS), also known as Di-George sequence, velocardiofacial syndrome, conotruncal anomalies face syndrome, Cayler syndrome, Sedlackova syndrome, and 22q11 deletion syndrome, is caused by a microdeletion of chromosome 22 at the q11.2 band. These various terms applied to patients with 22q11.2 deletions merely represent nosologic differences rather than different diagnoses. In an effort to unify the rapidly expanding number of conditions found to be caused by chromosome 22q11 deletions, Wilson et al.[9] proposed the acronym CATCH22 for *c*onotruncal heart defect, *a*bnormal face, *T*-cell deficiency, *c*lefting, and *h*ypocalcemia).

Deletion 22q11.2 is among the most clinically variable syndromes, with a phenotypic spectrum of more than 180 features (see Table I in Robin and Shprintzen[10]). Newborns are diagnosed when they present with a major malformation or medical complication such as congenital heart disease, hypocalcemia, and occasionally overt cleft palate.

Inheritance

Most cases are sporadic, but a few familial cases suggest possible autosomal-dominant inheritance.

Prevalence

The prevalence is 1 in 2000 newborns.

Key Features

The key features include a conotruncal cardiac defect (74%), hypoparathyroidism (50–60%), a thymic defect (77%), velopharyngeal dysfunction with or without cleft palate, dysmorphic face including low-set ears, telecanthus with short palpebral fissures, a square nasal tip, a short philtrum and a relatively small mouth with thin lips, impaired development, and immunodeficiency resulting from thymic hypoplasia. Infections are not a common presenting manifestation. Dermatologic features include abundant scalp hair and thin-appearing skin (venous patterns easily visible). Patients with complete Di George syndrome (less than 1% of patients) demonstrate an extrinsic defect resulting in a lack of T cells because of impaired thymic development. They display a clinical syndrome resembling that of patients with SCID, who lack T cells because of an intrinsic defect.

Workup

Fluorescence in-situ hybridization (FISH) has been instrumental in identifying patients who are deleted at 22q11.2. Since FISH has become available, the number of patients diagnosed has increased dramatically.[10]

Management

An early diagnosis of complete DGS is important to ensure the best treatment. The results of thymus and hematopoietic stem cell transplantations are currently being evaluated.

Prognosis

The prognosis is variable, ranging from neonatal death to a normal life span.

Wiskott-Aldrich Syndrome

The Wiskott-Aldrich syndrome (WAS) is characterized by immune dysregulation and microthrombocytopenia. In its less severe form, known as X-linked thrombocytopenia (XLT), mutations in the same gene produce the characteristic platelet abnormality but minimal immunologic disturbance. However, the natural history of XLT is less well defined than for WAS, and for some patients immune dysregulation may develop over time. Many patients with XLT are also probably undiagnosed, or misdiagnosed as chronic idiopathic thrombocytopenia (ITP).[11]

Inheritance

The inheritance is X-linked recessive.

Carrier Testing

If the specific WAS gene mutation is identified in an affected child, that child's mother can then be tested to confirm that she carries the gene. Other members of the mother's family may also want to consider testing to find out if they carry the same mutation.

Prenatal Diagnosis

In families where there has been one child born with WAS, prenatal testing should be offered in subsequent pregnancies. There is a 50% chance with each subsequent pregnancy that the mother, who is a carrier, will transmit the abnormal copy of the gene to her baby. The key is to first identify the particular WAS gene mutation in the child with WAS. Then, early in a pregnancy, cells can be obtained from the developing fetus by chorionic villus sampling or amniocentesis, and checked for the same mutation.

Key Features

The classic triad is eczema, thrombocytopenia, and draining ears (recurrent infection). Because of the wide spectrum of findings, the diagnosis should be considered in any boy presenting with unusual bleeding or bruises, congenital or early-onset thrombocytopenia, and small platelets. Patients also exhibit increased susceptibility to autoimmune disorders and cancer.

Differential Diagnosis

The differential diagnosis includes atopic dermatitis, SCID, hyper-IgE-syndrome, and chronic granulomatous disease.

Workup

The workup entals a complete blood count (CBC) with differential, platelets, and mean platelet volume.

Management

Supportive treatment includes platelet transfusions, intravenous gammaglobulin, and antibiotic prophylaxis to prevent otitis media or pneumonia and sometimes splenectomy for severe thrombocytopenia. Curative therapy with bone marrow or stem cell transplantation is the treatment of choice.

The first clinical trial is underway to assess the safety and efficacy of transplanting autologous WASP-reconstituted (WASP = Wiskott Aldrich associated protein) hematopoietic stem cells.[12]

Prognosis

The prognosis has improved due to antibiotic therapy, IVIG, and bone marrow transplantation. However, because T-cell function declines over time, WAS is considered a progressive disorder and without bone marrow transplantation males usually die in their early 20s from an overwhelming infection or a malignancy.

Ataxia-Telangiectasia (Louis-Bar Syndrome)

Ataxia-telangiectasia (AT) is a systemic autosomal recessive condition caused by mutations in the ataxia-teleangiectasia mutated *(ATM)* gene on 11q22–23. Immunodeficiency causes frequent sinopulmonary infections that, combined with recurrent aspiration, lead to chronic lung disease.[13] The incidence of infections is variable, with some individuals having no higher incidence than unaffected siblings, whereas others succumb to progressive respiratory infection, usually because of severe defects in both humoral and cellular immunity. Epidemiologic and molecular studies have finally provided conclusive evidence that *ATM* mutations that cause ataxia-telangiectasia are breast cancer susceptibility alleles.

Inheritance

The inheritance is autosomal recessive.

Prevalence

The prevalence is 1 in 40,000 to 1 in 50,000 newborns.

Carrier Testing

Testing entails doing a mutation analysis.

Prenatal Diagnosis

Diagnosis entails doing a mutation analysis.

Key Features

There is clinical heterogeneity within the disorder ranging from the classic form with onset in infancy and steady progression of symptoms, to milder forms where progression may be slower or onset may be later.[14] Most patients develop ataxia by age 2, and involvement of both upper and lower limbs results in the need for a wheelchair for mobility by adolescence. Speech and eye movement are also affected. Other features include t(7;14)

translocations, immunodeficiency, a high serum α-fetoprotein concentration, growth retardation, telangiectasia (most noticeably on the bulbar conjunctiva), and a high risk of developing a lymphoid tumor. Patients also show an increased sensitivity to ionizing radiation. Dermatologic features include café-au-lait macules and a progeric facies with decreased subcutaneous fat.

Differential Diagnosis

The differential diagnosis includes Hartnup disease, Cockayne syndrome, De Sanctis-Cacchione syndrome, Friedreich ataxia, Rendu-Osler-Weber disease, and Bloom syndrome.

Workup

T-suppressor cells are increased while T-helper cells are decreased. α-Fetoprotein is elevated, and IgA, IgG2, and IgE are decreased or absent.

Diagnosis

Diagnosis is suspected in young children who show signs of cerebellar ataxia, oculomotor apraxia, and telangiectasias of the conjunctivae. Magnetic resonance imaging (MRI) examination shows cerebellum atrophy. Other tests that may support the diagnosis include elevated serum α-fetoprotein (above 10 ng/mL in more than 90% of patients), cytogenetic analysis (7:14 translocation (t[7;14][q11;q32]) in 5% to 15% of affected individuals), and colony in vitro assay (irradiation of colony formation of lymphoblastoid cells). The colony in vitro assay is a very sensitive test, but takes approximately 3 months for results, and is available only in specialized centers.

The diagnosis of AT can be confirmed by identification of both *ATM* mutations. In practice, the size of the *ATM* coding sequence and the absence of common mutations can make this a lengthy and sometimes uncertain procedure. In contrast, the presence of increased chromosomal radiosensitivity can be established quickly as can the total absence (in most cases) or the greatly reduced expression of the ATM protein in a lymphoblastoid cell line made from the patient's lymphocytes. Finally, the kinase activity of any residual ATM protein can be assayed in cases where an unusual presentation is seen.

Management

Management is supportive. Sun avoidance and sunscreen may help prevent progeric changes.

Prognosis

Most patients are confined to a wheelchair by 10 years of age. Premature death is secondary to lymphoreticular malignancy or infection in the second decade of life. Support groups are available at http://www.atcp.org/, http://www.ataxia.org/, and http://www.rarediseases.org/.

Combined Antibody (B Cell) and Cellular (T Cell) Immunodeficiencies

These conditions account for 20% to 25% of primary immune deficiencies. Combined immunodeficiencies can be further divided into combined immunodeficiencies (CIDs) and severe combined immunodeficiencies (SCIDs); patients with the latter develop severe life-threatening complications. Lymphopenia in neonates and infants should prompt a laboratory evaluation for this group of disorders.[15] It is critical to make the diagnosis before patients acquire a severe infection or receive live attenuated viral vaccines (measles, mumps, rubella, varicella, bacillus Calmette-Guérin [BCG]), which could be lethal.

Severe Combined Immunodeficiency

Severe combined immunodeficiencies represent an expanding group of PIDs many with known molecular defects. As the name suggests, SCIDs display the most severe cellular immune dysfunction, sometimes with complete absence of functional lymphocytes since it is combined with severe humoral defects, too.

Inheritance

The inheritance is X-linked recessive (most common); γ-chain IL-r receptor gene, autosomal recessive; adenosine deaminase gene (20% of cases), autosomal recessive; or Janus kinase 3 gene.

Mutations in nine different genes have been found to cause SCID in humans. The products of three of the genes—*IL-2RG, Jak3,* and *IL-7Rα*—are components of cytokine receptors, and the products of three more—*RAG1, RAG2,* and *Artemis*—are essential for effecting antigen receptor gene rearrangement. Additionally, a deficiency of CD3δ, a component of the T-cell antigen receptor, results in a near absence of circulating mature CD3+ T cells and a complete lack of γ/δ T cells. Adenosine deaminase deficiency results in toxic accumulations of metabolites that cause T-cell apoptosis. Finally, a deficiency of CD45, a critical regulator of signaling thresholds in immune cells, also causes SCID.

Severe combined immunodeficiency can result from mutations in multiple genes that encode components of the immune system. Three such components are cytokine receptor chains or signaling molecules; five are needed for antigen receptor development; one is adenosine deaminase—a purine salvage pathway enzyme; and the last is a phosphatase, CD45.

Prenatal Diagnosis

Diagnosis entails DNA analysis if gene defect known, or adenine deaminase (ADA) assay in cultured amniocytes (in ADA deficiency only).

Key Features

Affected infants begin to have problems with oral moniliasis, diarrhea, and failure to thrive in the first few months of life.[16] Although the diagnosis of SCID can be made much earlier, it is frequently not made until serious infections develop, with the average age at referral for immune testing being approximately 6 months. Persistent infections with opportunistic organisms, such as *Candida albicans, P. carinii,* varicella, adenovirus, RSV, parainfluenza 3, CMV, EBV, and BCG, lead to death. These infants also lack the ability to reject allografts, leaving them at risk for fatal graft versus host disease. This condition is uniformly fatal in the first 2 years of life unless immune reconstitution can be accomplished. Recognition of the characteristic lymphopenia can result in early diagnosis sometimes at birth.

Differential Diagnosis

The differential diagnosis includes AIDS, hyper-IgE-syndrome, histiocytosis, and Omenn's syndrome.

Workup

Nearly all cases could be diagnosed at birth if routine blood counts and manual differentials were done and flow cytometry and T-cell function studies were performed when lymphocyte counts are below the newborn normal range (2000–11,000/mm³).

Management

Severe combined immunodeficiency is a pediatric emergency. If the diagnosis is made at birth or shortly thereafter, definitive therapy in the form of human leukocyte antigen (HLA)-identical or haploidentical allogeneic bone marrow stem cell transplantation can result in a survival rate as high as 97%, regardless of the molecular type of SCID. However, if the diagnosis is made later, serious infections develop for which antibiotics are minimally effective, and the survival rate is much lower. Unfortunately, allogeneic stem cell transplantation is not without risk in these children, because many recipients experience incomplete B-cell or NK-cell immune reconstitution. Gene therapy, which has been successfully performed in a few patients,[16] results in more complete immune reconstitution. However, gene therapy cannot be performed unless the abnormal gene for a specific patient is known.

Prognosis

The disorder is fatal in infants who are untreated. Bone marrow transplantation is successful in at least 75%. If infants are treated in the first month, before the onset of severe infections, survival may be 97%.

Griscelli Syndrome

Griscelli syndrome (GS) is characterized by pigmentary dilution of the skin and the hair (silver hair), the presence of large clumps of pigment in hair shafts, and an accumulation of melanosomes in melanocytes. The associated immunodeficiency often involves impaired NK-cell activity, absent delayed-type hypersensitivity, and a poor cell proliferation response to antigenic challenge.

Inheritance

The inheritance is autosomal recessive.

Prevalence

The prevalence is rare, as less than 60 cases have been reported.

Prenatal Diagnosis

Prenatal diagnosis can be performed by light microscopic examination of hair from fetal scalp biopsy specimens, or by molecular genetic studies of fetal DNA, if the mutation is known.

Key Features

Key features include pigmentary dilution of skin, pyogenic skin infections, silver-gray hair, neutropenia, and thrombocytopenia.

Patients with GS type 1 have silvery gray hair, light-colored skin, early-onset severe psychomotor retardation, and normal immune status. Type 1 is caused by a mutation in the myosin Va *(MYO5A)* gene located on chromosome 15q21, which regulates organelle transport in both melanocytes and neuronal cells.[17]

Patients with GS type 2 (originally described as partial albinism with immunodeficiency) have silvery gray hair, frequent pyogenic infections of skin and internal organs, hemophagocytic lymphohistiocytosis with accelerated phases, and variable neurologic defects in the absence of primary neurologic disease. Type 2 is caused by mutation in the Rab27a *(RAB27A)* gene located on chromosome 15q21, less than 1.6cM from the *MYO5A* gene.[17]

Patients with GS type 3, which entails restricted expression of the disease, have hypopigmentation in the hair and skin. The nervous and immune systems do not show any abnormality. Two cases of this type have been reported. In the first case, a mutation was found in the gene located on chromosome 2q37.3 that encodes melanophilin, which is a member of the Rab effector family. The second case was caused by an F-exon deletion in the *MYO5A* gene.[17]

Differential Diagnosis

The differential diagnosis includes Chediak-Higashi syndrome, Elejalde syndrome, chronic granulomatous disease, and oculocutaneous albinism type II.

Workup

Workup involves examination of the hair, which shows uneven clumps of melanin in the medulla of the hair shaft on light microscopy, and a CBC, which shows absent cytoplasmic inclusion bodies in neutrophils.

Management

In patients with GS type 1, there is no definitive cure, and the outcome is guarded as it depends on the severity of neurologic manifestations.[17] Patients should receive supportive care for primary neurologic symptoms such as hypotonia and developmental delay, and seizures should be controlled adequately when present. Patients with GS type 2 have a grave prognosis, as type 2 proves fatal unless bone marrow transplantation is carried out as early as possible. High-dose systemic steroids and other immunosuppressives can delay the hyperactivation of lymphocytes and macrophages, and reduce symptoms attributable to organ infiltration. These drugs can be used as a palliative therapy or to induce remission until bone marrow transplantation is carried out. Patients with GS type 3, which does not pose a threat to those affected, need no active intervention.

Prognosis

Accelerated phases of uncontrolled lymphocyte and macrophage activation with lymphohistiocytic infiltration of the central nervous system lead to death, unless early bone marrow transplantation can be performed.

Bloom Syndrome

Bloom syndrome is a condition of intrauterine and postnatal growth failure, facial erythema, immunodeficiency, male sterility, and early malignancies. It displays one of the strongest known correlations between chromosomal instability and an increased risk of malignancy at an early age, specifically leukemia and lymphoma. Carcinomas of the larynx, lung, esophagus, colon, cervix, and breast develop in adults. Approximately one-third of individuals with Bloom syndrome are of Jewish descent.

Inheritance

The inheritance is autosomal recessive.

Carrier Testing

A carrier screening requires a sample of blood. The tests can determine whether or not a gene change is present in the gene for Bloom syndrome. It is possible to detect the specific gene change that is seen in Ashkenazi Jews with Bloom syndrome. The test is not as accurate for individuals who are from other ethnic background.

Prenatal Diagnosis

Chorionic villus sampling or amniocentesis can be performed early in the pregnancy.

Key Features

Key features include proportional dwarfism, immune deficiency, and a greatly enhanced risk for most cancers. The elevated cancer risk is manifested by increased and early appearance of leukemias, lymphomas, rare tumors, and carcinomas, with a mean age of onset of 25 years. Skin features include photodistributed erythema with telangiectasias in butterfly distribution on nose and cheeks, cheilitis, and café-au-lait macules.

Differential Diagnosis

The differential diagnosis includes Cockayne syndrome, Rothmund-Thomson syndrome, lupus erythematosus, and erythropoietic protoporphyria.

Workup

The workup entails doing a DNA analysis, chromosome analysis, and immunoglobulin levels.

Management

Management includes carcinoma surveillance, short stature management, sun protection, and antibiotics.

Prognosis

There is an increased risk of premature death in the second to third decade due to malignancy.

Additional information on Bloom syndrome is available at the Bloom's Syndrome Registry (contact James L. German III, MD, Professor, Departments of Pediatrics and Microbiology, Cornell University Medical College, 1300 York

Avenue, New York, NY 10021; telephone: 212-746-3956).

Defective Phagocyte Function

Neutrophils and monocytes are part of the innate immune system and are critical in initiating immune responses to bacterial infections. Therefore, patients with neutrophil defects present with a history of recurrent abscesses, abscesses in unusual areas (liver, muscle, abdominal cavity), recurrent oral ulcers, pneumonias, poor wound healing, or delayed umbilical cord separation.[15] The initial evaluation of patients suspected of having a neutrophil defect is the CBC with a manual differential. Although the presence of a normal absolute neutrophil count is encouraging, it does not rule out a functional defect. Kostmann's syndrome is a rare congenital disorder of neutrophil production due to impairment of myeloid differentiation in the bone marrow, with the neutrophil count being characteristically less than 500×10^3 cells/L. Severe persistent neutropenia results in an increased susceptibility to frequent bacterial infections. The condition can be treated with recombinant human granulocyte colony-stimulating factor (G-CSF).

Chronic Granulomatous Disease

Chronic granulomatous disease (CGD) is a primary immunodeficiency disorder caused by inherited defects in the reduced nicotinamide adenine dinucleotide phosphate (NADPH) oxidase complex. This enzyme complex is used by phagocytic cells to generate microbicidal superoxide and its metabolites hydrogen peroxide, hydroxyl anion, and hypohalous acid. As a consequence, patients are susceptible to recurrent life-threatening pyogenic infections, particularly those caused by catalase-positive bacteria and fungi. In addition, CGD patients often have poor wound healing and chronic inflammation, leading to granuloma formation.

Inheritance

The inheritance is X-linked recessive in 70%, and autosomal recessive in 30%.

Carrier Testing

The nitroblue tetrazolium (NBT) test is useful in identifying carrier female relatives of male CGD patients in whom peripheral leukocytes consist of two cell populations, only one of which reduces NBT. The proportion of NBT-positive leukocytes varies among individual female carriers, consistent with random inactivation of the X chromosome.

Prenatal Diagnosis

Prenatal diagnosis can be done by analysis of neonatal neutrophil oxidant production from umbilical vein samples obtained by fetoscopy. This can be performed well only into the second trimester, which puts the fetus at substantial fetal. Oxidant production from amniocytes is unreliable. Alternatively, DNA can be analyzed from amniocytes or chorionic villus samples. Intrageneic restriction fragment length polymorphisms (RFLPs) have been identified in the *gp91phox* and *p67phox* genes. Recently, investigators identified highly polymorphic (CA/GT)n repeats at two locations in the *gp91phox* gene that are promising tools for prenatal diagnosis. When specific mutations within a family are known, direct sequencing of fetal DNA should be performed.[18]

Key Features

Pneumonia is the most common infection (79% of patients, most commonly *Aspergillus*), followed by suppurative adenitis (53% of patients, most commonly *Staphylococcus*), subcutaneous abscess (42% of patients, most commonly *Staphylococcus*), liver abscess (27% of patients, most commonly *Staphylococcus*), osteomyelitis (25% of patients, most commonly *Serratia*), and sepsis (18% of patients, most commonly *Salmonella*).[19]

Differential Diagnosis

The differential diagnosis includes hyper-IgE syndrome, SCID, and Chediak-Higashi syndrome.

Workup

The workup entails NBT reduction assay, immunoblot of defective NADPH enzymes, immunoglobulin levels, and CBC.

Management

Outpatient management relies on the use of prophylactic antibiotics and interferon-γ. When infection is suspected, aggressive effort to obtain culture material is required. Treatment of infections involves prolonged use of systemic antibiotics, surgical debridement when feasible, and, in severe infections, use of granulocyte transfusions. Gene therapy holds great promise as an alternative treatment for patients without suitable marrow donors or where bone marrow transplantation is not a viable option.

Prognosis

There is a variable life span depending on control of infections. Most patients have a normal life span but a poor quality of life.

Chediak-Higashi Syndrome

Chediak–Higashi syndrome (CHS) is characterized by oculocutaneous albinism, recurrent infections, microscopic finding of large granules in hematopoietic and other cells, bleeding diathesis, and neurologic abnormalities. Pathologic mutations in the lysosomal trafficking regulator gene localized to human chromosome 1q42–q43 are responsible for development of CHS.

Inheritance

The inheritance is autosomal recessive.

Key Features

Chediak–Higashi syndrome is characterized by partial oculocutaneous albinism, frequent pyogenic infections, the presence of abnormal granules in the granulocytes of blood and bone marrow, and an accelerated lymphohistiocytic phase. The condition is typically detected around the age of 5 years, and the patients are affected by frequent and severe pyogenic infections of the skin, lung, and respiratory tract, secondary to abnormal neutrophil function. Approximately 80% of patients undergo an accelerated phase, which is characterized by a lymphohistiocytic lymphoma-like infiltration of multiple organs, associated with anemia, bleeding disorders, hepatosplenomegaly, fever, jaundice, and neurologic changes leading to death.

Differential Diagnosis

The differential diagnosis includes oculocutaneous albinism type II, Hermansky-Pudlak syndrome, chronic granulomatous disease, Griscelli syndrome, and Elejalde syndrome.

Workup

The hallmark of this disorder is the occurrence of giant granules in the granulocytes and their precursors and can be easily diagnosed by examining the peripheral blood smear.

Management

Management is interdisciplinary, and entails bone marrow transplant, chemotherapy, high-dose ascorbic acid, antibiotics, and sun protection.

Prognosis

The few patients who live to adulthood develop progressive neurologic dysfunction.

Support Group

Support groups are available at http://www.chediak-higashi.org/ and http://www.ipopi.org/.

Complement Deficiency

Defects in the complement system account for less than 2% of the known patients who have PIDs. Genetic defects have been described for almost all complement components. Defects in the early components of the classic pathway manifest primarily as immune-complex disease. Defects in the early components of the alternative pathway or in the membrane attack components lead to increased susceptibility to infections with pyogenic bacteria and *Neisseria*. Screening for most complement defects is accomplished by performing a total hemolytic complement (CH_{50}) assay. C3 and C4 should also be measured if the CH_{50} assay is abnormal, because levels of these proteins can help define the pathway in which the complement defect is located.

Defects of Unknown Origin

Hyper-IgE (Job's) Syndrome

Based on the biblical character Job, who was afflicted with extensive furuncles, the original report of this condition described two patients with staphylococcal skin abscesses that failed to demonstrate normal erythema and warmth, and hence were called "cold abscesses." The clinical triad of high serum levels of IgE (>2000 IU/mL), recurring staphylococcal skin abscesses, and pneumonia with pneumatocele formation occurs in 77% of patients.

Inheritance

The inheritance in most cases is sporadic. Autosomal-dominant and autosomal-recessive inheritance have been reported.

Key Features

The immune phenotype of hyper-IgE syndrome is characterized by recurrent staphylococcal infections of the skin and lungs, pneumatocele formation, eczema, candidiasis, eosinophilia, and elevated levels of IgE. Nonimmunologic features include, in decreasing frequency, characteristic facial appearance, scoliosis, retained primary dentition, joint hyperextensibility, recurrent bone fractures after minimal trauma, and craniosynostosis.

Differential Diagnosis

The differential diagnosis includes atopic dermatitis and eosinophilic pustular folliculitis.

Workup

The workup shows extreme elevation of serum IgE (>2000 IU/mL), and serum eosinophil counts are more than two standard deviations above the normal range.

Management

Because the primary defect is unknown, no definitive therapy is available. The most successful regimen is lifelong prophylactic antistaphylococcal and antifungal therapy. Immunoglobulin substitution is not indicated unless an impaired antibody response is observed. Surgical drainage of abscesses may be indicated.

Prognosis

If the condition is recognized early in life and the patient is kept on chronic antistaphylococcal antibiotic therapy, the prognosis is good.

Support Group

Support groups are available at http://www.ipopi.org/ and http://www.primaryimmune.org/.

Chronic Mucocutaneous Candidiasis

This is a spectrum of disorders in which patients have persistent or recurrent infections of the skin, nails, and mucous membranes caused by *C. albicans*.[20] Several clinical syndromes have been defined (Table 35.2).

Inheritance

The majority of childhood cases have an autosomal recessive mode of inheritance, but autosomal dominant inheritance is also recognized, and some cases are sporadic.

Key Features

Childhood chronic mucocutaneous candidiasis (CMC) usually starts early, presenting with persistent *Candida* infection of the diaper area and mouth. The infection usually spreads to involve the nails, scalp, extremities, and other areas of the skin. Most of these patients go on to develop autoimmune endocrinopathies as part of the autoimmune polyendocrinopathy syndrome type 1 (APS1),[21] recently coined autoimmune polyendocrinopathy candidiasis ectodermal dystrophy (APECED). This is characterized by hypoparathyroidism, adrenal or gonadal failure, and, less frequently, insulindependent diabetes mellitus or hypothyroidism. Malabsorption, gastric cell atrophy, or autoimmune hepatitis is seen in about a third of these patients. Dental enamel dysplasia, keratopathy, alopecia, or vitiligo is often present. Another form of childhood-onset CMC has been recognized for years, although it was only recently proposed as a distinct syndrome. These patients typically have an autosomal dominant mode of inheritance and present with or without isolated hypothyroidism but are spared other endocrinopathies. It is not clear whether this may be a subtype of APS1/APECED or a separate disease entity.

Differential Diagnosis

The differential diagnosis includes DiGeorge syndrome and SCID.

Workup

Because CMC often takes several years to develop, the diagnosis can be difficult initially, especially when only one of the typical APS1 manifestations is present. Increased awareness of the condition combined with analysis of specific autoantibodies, particularly neutralization antibodies against type I interferons, and follow-up by mutational analysis of the *AIRE* gene, should help diagnose this rare condition earlier.

Management

Management entails systemic antifungals; most patients relapse upon cessation of therapy.

Prognosis

The prognosis is good.

Support Group

Support groups are available at http://www.ipopi. org/ and http://www.primaryimmune.org/.

Nonconventional Primary Immunodeficiencies

Inborn defects in Toll-like receptor signaling are recently described primary immunodeficiencies that predispose affected children to life-threatening infections. Patients with interleukin-1 receptor-associated kinase-4 deficiency are prone to invasive pneumococcal disease, and patients with UNC-93B deficiency are prone to herpes simplex virus encephalitis. These genetic disorders are underdiagnosed, partly because diagnosis currently requires expensive and time-consuming techniques available at only a few specialized centers worldwide.

Interleukin-1 Receptor-Associated Kinase-4 Deficiency

Picard et al.[22] described three unrelated children with recurrent infections and poor inflammatory response in whom extracellular, pyogenic bacteria were the only microorganisms responsible for infection. Gram-positive *Streptococcus pneumoniae* and *Staphylococcus aureus* were the most frequently found and were the only pathogens identified in two patients. Infections began early in life but became less frequent with age, and the patients were well with no treatment at ages 6, 11, and 7 years. All known primary immunodeficiencies were excluded. In particular, the patients had normal serum antibody titers against protein and polysaccharide antigens, including those from *S. pneumoniae*. In a follow-up of the patients reported by Picard et al., Day et al.[23] found that two continued to do well, but one, an 8-year-old girl, was unable to sustain antibody responses to polysaccharide or protein antigens or to a neoantigen-bacteriophage. She continued to have recurring bacterial and fungal infections, eventually requiring IVIG therapy. They recommended testing for IRAK-4 deficiency in patients with recurrent bacterial and fungal infections without sustained antibody response to immunization.

UNC-93B Deficiency

The recent observation of human UNC-93B deficiency in two children with sporadic herpes simplex encephalitis indicates that the presence of monogenic disorders may predispose patients specifically to a single infectious agent without affecting host defense against many other pathogens.[24] Peripheral blood mononuclear cells from these patients produced reduced amounts of type I and type II interferons in response to herpes simples virus type 1 stimulation but not in response to ten other viruses, thus highlighting the presence of specific susceptibility defects. The specificity of defects, such as UNC-93B, for a single pathogen that manifests as sporadic events in otherwise healthy individuals makes their identification highly challenging. Whereas studies such as these have several important therapeutic implications, further studies are needed to confirm the validity of these markers as prognostic indicators for oncolytic viral therapy.

Conclusion

Early recognition and diagnosis is vital since it alters the course of many primary immunodeficiencies. As a consequence it is critical that the primary care provider consider these disorders when a patient presents with increased numbers of cutaneous and sinopulmonary infections, infections caused by unusual organisms, or persistence of difficult-to-treat infections.

References

1. Notarangelo L, Casanova JL, Fischer A, et al. Primary immunodeficiency diseases: an update. J Allergy Clin Immunol 2004;114(3):677–87.
2. Casanova JL, Fieschi C, Bustamante J, et al. From idiopathic infectious diseases to novel primary immunodeficiencies. J Allergy Clin Immunol 2005;116:426–30.
3. Ballow M. Primary immunodeficiency disorders: antibody deficiency. J Allergy Clin Immunol 2002;109:581–91.
4. Conley ME, Rohrer J, Minegishi Y. X-linked Agammaglobulinemia. Clin Rev Allergy Immunol 2000;19(2):183–204.
5. Valiaho J, Smith CIE, Vihinen M. BTKbase: the mutation database for X-linked agammaglobulinemia. Hum Mutat 2006;27(12):1209–17.
6. Latiff AHA, Kerr MA. The clinical significance of immunoglobulin A deficiency. Ann Clin Biochem 2007;44:131–139.
7. Goldacker S, Warnatz K. Tackling the heterogeneity of CVID. Curr Opin Allergy Clin Immunol 2005;5(6):504–9.
8. Kumar A, Teuber SS, Gershwin ME. Current perspectives on primary immunodeficiency diseases. Clin Dev Immunol 2006;13(2–4):223–259.
9. Wilson DI, Burn J, Scambler P, Goodship J. DiGeorge syndrome: part of CATCH22. J Med Genet 1993;30(10):852–6.
10. Robin NH, Shprintzen. Defining the clinical spectrum of deletion 22q11.2. J Pediatr 2005;147(1):90–6.
11. Thrasher AJ, Kinnon C. The Wiskott-Aldrich syndrome. Clin Exp Immunol 2000;120(1):2–9.
12. Boztug K, Dewey RA, Klein C. Development of hematopoietic stem cell gene therapy for Wiskott-Aldrich syndrome. Curr Opin Mol Ther 2006;8(5):390–5.
13. Lefton-Greif MA, Crawford TO, Winkelstein JA, et al. Oropharyngeal dysphagia and aspiration in patients with ataxia-teleangiectasia. J Pediatr 2000;136:225–31.
14. Nowak-Wegrzyn A, Crawford TO, Winkelstein JA, et al. Immunodeficiency and infections in ataxia-telangiectasia. J Pediatr 2004;144(4):505–11.
15. Verbsky JW, Grossman WJ. Cellular and genetic basis of primary immune deficiencies. Pediatr Clin North Am 2006;53:649–684.
16. Fischer A. Severe combined immunodeficiencies (SCID). Clin Exp Immunol 2000;122(2):143–9.
17. Malhotra AK, Bhaskar G, Nanda M, et al. Griscelli syndrome. J Am Acad Dermatol 2006;55(2):337–40.
18. Segal BH, Leto TL, Gallin JI, Malech HL, Holland SM. Genetic, biochemical, and clinical features of chronic granulomatous disease. Medicine (Baltimore) 2000;79(3):170–200.
19. Winkelstein JA, Marino MC, Lederman HM, et al. Chronic granulomatous disease. Report on a national registry of 368 patients. Medicine (Baltimore) 2006;85(4):193–202.
20. Kirkpatrick CH. Chronic Mucocutaneous Candidiasis. Pediatr Infect Dis J 2001;20:197–206.
21. Betterle C, Greggio NA, Volpato M. Clinical review 93: Autoimmune polyglandular syndrome type 1. J Clin Endocrinol Metab 1998;83(4):1049–55.
22. Picard C, Puel A, Bonnet M, et al. Pyogenic bacterial infections in humans with IRAK-4 deficiency. Science 2003;299(5615):2076–9.
23. Day N, Tangsinmankong N, Ochs H, et al. Interleukin receptor-associated kinase (IRAK-4) deficiency associated with bacterial infections and failure to sustain antibody responses. J Pediatr 2004;144(4):524–6.
24. Casrouge A, Zhang SY, Eidenschenk C, et al. Herpes simplex virus encephalitis in human UNC-93B deficiency. Science 2006;314(5797):308–12.

36
Iatrogenic Immunodeficiency and Skin Disease

Brenda L. Bartlett and Jennifer Z. Cooper

Key Points

- The number of living organ transplant recipients (OTRs) continues to grow due to an increased number of transplants performed and a longer patient and graft survival time, thereby increasing the number of patients on immunosuppression.
- The immunosuppression required to maintain allografts leads to a significantly increased rate of both internal and cutaneous malignancies, with skin cancer being the most common.
- The skin cancer seen in immunosuppressed patients, primarily nonmelanoma skin cancer (NMSC), occurs earlier and behaves more aggressively than does NMSC in the general population.
- Of the various types of skin cancers seen in OTR, squamous cell carcinoma (SCC) is the leading cause of mortality.
- It is important to be aware of the associated risk factors so that OTRs who are at increased risk can be identified and followed even more closely by dermatologists and the transplant physicians.
- Immunosuppressive drugs accelerate the development of skin cancer by being directly carcinogenic and by creating a state of compromised immune surveillance.
- Human papillomavirus infection has been recognized as a putative risk factor in NMSC of OTR.

As the number of organ transplant recipients (OTRs) continues to increase, so too, does the need for a thorough understanding of these patients and the complications they are likely to encounter. The number of living OTRs continues to grow due to an increased number of transplants performed and a longer patient and graft survival time. As of 2004, there are an estimated 168,000 living OTRs in the United States. The number of organ transplants grows annually, with approximately 26,500 performed in 2004, nearly 6% more than 2003.[1] Kidney transplants account for the majority of these, followed by liver transplants. Heart and lung are the next two most commonly transplanted organs.[2] The immunosuppression required to maintain these allografts leads to a significantly increased rate of both internal and cutaneous malignancies, with skin cancer being the most common.[3] It is therefore likely that dermatologists will be caring for an increasing number of organ transplant recipients.

Types of Skin Cancer

Skin cancer is the most common malignancy for which OTRs are at risk.[4] They are at particularly increased risk of nonmelanoma skin cancers (NMSCs) with a rate of 50 times that in the general population.[5] Compared to immunocompetent individuals, transplant recipients are 15 years younger at the time of NMSC diagnosis.[6] Comparable results from various studies show that NMSC is diagnosed in 15% to 43% of OTRs 10 years post-transplantation.[7] These NMSCs occur earlier and behave more aggressively compared to NMSCs in the general population. The lesions are frequently multiple, have a more rapid rate of growth, and have an increased rate of recurrence and metastasis than seen in nontransplant patients.[8]

In the general population, basal cell carcinomas (BCCs) occur approximately four times more frequently than squamous cell carcinomas (SCCs), but this ratio of BCC to SCC is reversed in OTRs.[8] In addition to increased rates of NMSCs, studies have also found an increased risk of malignant melanoma, particularly in the pediatric population.[9] The Kaposi's sarcoma incidence is increased by 84-fold in transplant recipients compared to the general population.[10] Merkel cell carcinoma, a rare neuroendocrine skin cancer, has also been found more commonly in OTRs and is more aggressive than in the general population.[11] Of the various types of skin cancers seen in OTRs, SCC is the leading cause of mortality. Data from the Cincinnati Tumor Registry shows that 63% of deaths of OTRs who died from skin malignancies were due to SCC.[12]

Risk Factors

Several risk factors have been identified to help determine which patients are most likely to develop skin cancer posttransplantation. One clear contributor to the development of NMSCs in both the general population and OTRs is ultraviolet radiation (UVR).[13] This is supported by the tendency of lesions to develop in sun-exposed areas and by the increased risk of NMSC in OTRs reported in parts of the world with high levels of sun exposure.[14] The role of UVR as a risk factor is also supported by the fact that recipients with Fitzpatrick skin types I, II, or III have been shown to be at increased risk, which is true of the nontransplant population as well.[15,16] Additionally, older patients are more likely to develop skin cancer, which is in part attributed to greater cumulative sun exposure prior to transplantation.[17,18]

Ultraviolet radiation acts as both an initiator and a promoter of skin cancer. It is directly mutagenic to epidermal keratinocytes but also has local immunosuppressive effects by reducing the number of Langerhans' cells, thus impairing antigen presentation and recognition.[19,20]

Another well-recognized important risk factor for NMSC is immunosuppression. An increasing number of patients are on long-term immunosuppression due to the increased number of organ transplants and the increasing survival of both the organs and their recipients. The duration and intensity of immunosuppression are directly related to the degree of cancer risk.[21] It is thought that immunosuppressive drugs accelerate the development of skin cancer by being directly carcinogenic and by creating a state of compromised immune surveillance.[22–25] Cutaneous tumors tend to appear 3 to 7 years after the onset of chronic immunosuppressive therapy.[26] The various immunosuppressive agents have different mechanisms of action, which will be discussed later in this chapter.

Differences in skin cancer incidence have also been reported depending on the type of organ transplantation, with heart transplantation having a greater risk than kidney transplantation.[27] Liver transplant recipients have a less significant risk than kidney recipients.[26] The relative differences in risk may be due to a varying level of immunosuppression required to maintain each organ type.[28] In kidney transplant recipients, an effect of pretransplant end-organ disease has been identified. The incidence of NMSC was increased in patients who received a transplant for polycystic kidney disease and decreased in patients with diabetic nephropathy as the primary cause of renal failure. This is hypothesized to be due to the poor immunosuppressive drug absorption seen in diabetics due to gastroparesis and autonomic neuropathy.[29]

It is important to be aware of these risk factors so that OTRs who are at increased risk can be identified and followed even more closely by dermatologists and the transplant physicians. Knowledge and identification of these risk factors both before and after transplantation is vital to determining the appropriate level of follow-up. In addition, discussion of these risk factors with the patients may encourage them to practice safer sun-exposure habits and contact a physician earlier should they have a lesion of concern.

Human Papillomavirus and Its Role in Skin Cancer in Organ Transplant Recipients

It is known that OTRs have an increased incidence of both viral warts and NMSCs posttransplantation.[30] Identification of human papillomavirus (HPV) within these lesions suggests that HPV is pathogenic to the development of skin cancer in transplant recipients. Up to 90% of transplant recipients have HPV-induced warts. Although considered benign lesions in immunocompetent individuals, warts in transplant patients have been shown both clinically and histologically to progress into dysplastic lesions and invasive SCC.[31] This implies that warts may be of different prognostic significance for OTRs.[32]

An increasing number of HPV viral types are being identified in skin lesions of OTRs. This is mostly attributed to the improved methods of detection of the virus using polymerase chain reaction (PCR) with degenerate primers instead of consensus primers.[32,33]

Studies show that among the numerous HPV types that have been isolated from SCC of OTRs, there is a predominance of HPV types 5 and 8.[32] Of note, these two types were also found to predominate in SCCs of patients with epidermodysplasia verruciformis (EV), which is a rare inherited disorder characterized by widespread warts and associated with a deficiency of cellular immunity. Approximately 30% of EV patients develop skin cancers. A diverse range of HPV types have been identified in these lesions, which is now referred to as the EV-HPV type supergroup and includes types 5 and 8.[33]

Studies have detected HPV DNA more frequently in SCCs of OTRs compared with SCCs of nonimmunosuppressed individuals. In contrast, OTRs and nonimmunosuppressed individuals had similar rates of detection of HPV DNA in BCCs.[32,34] The prevalence of HPV in BCCs of OTRs and immunocompetent individuals has varied in several studies,[35,36] whereas it was a common finding of all related studies that among immunosuppressed patients, HPV DNA was more frequently detected in SCC than BCC. This indicates that HPV infection is more closely associated with SCC rather than BCC development.

The extent to which HPV plays a role in NMSC development in transplant patients is still unclear. In addition to SCCs, HPV viral DNA has also been identified in benign tumors, in the normal skin of immunocompetent individuals, and in the normal skin of OTRs.[37] Immunosuppression may lead to a chronic state of HPV infection in these patients but is not alone sufficient to cause tumorigenesis. It is thought that a cofactor such as UVR may be necessary for induction of dysplastic change.[38,39]

One factor that might argue against the theory of HPV infection as a direct risk factor is the relatively low viral load found in skin cancers. Although a slightly higher amount of viral DNA was found in skin cancers of OTRs compared to immunocompetent individuals, the level of viral DNA was still far lower than that seen in genital and cutaneous warts.[32] Additionally, long-standing warts in transplant recipients do not inevitably progress to skin cancers. Despite the strong association between the number of HPV-induced warts and the development of skin cancer, studies have shown an equally high prevalence of EV-HPV DNA in keratotic skin lesions in transplant recipients both with and without cancer. The detection rate and spectrum of HPV infection between these same two groups in hyperkeratotic papillomas, actinic keratoses, and SCCs was similar.[39]

Human papillomavirus and its role in cervical cancer has been well established.[40] It is generally accepted that integration of the viral genome into the host genome confers increased aggressiveness.[41] One study analyzed 181 specimens ranging in severity from condyloma to invasive cervical carcinoma. Only 3% of biopsy specimens of cervical intraepithelial neoplasia showed integrated HPV DNA. In contrast, 81% of cervical carcinomas ($p < .001$) showed integrated HPV DNA. All HPV-18–containing carcinomas had integrated HPV DNA, which may be related to its greater transforming efficiency in vitro and its reported clinical association with more aggressive cervical cancers.[42] Studies have also shown that HPV-16 DNA is not always present in the integrated form in tumors, suggesting that integration and subsequent inactivation of the transcriptional regulator E2 are not essential steps for the development of HPV-16–associated carcinoma.[43] Further studies specifically addressing the relative risk of episomal versus integrated viral DNA in the cutaneous malignancies of OTRs would be of interest.

The recognition of HPV infection as a putative risk factor in NMSCs of OTRs has led to the investigation of synthetic immune response modifiers such as imiquimod as possible treatment of these lesions. A randomized, blinded, placebo-controlled study that looked at the safety and efficacy of 5% imiquimod cream showed it to be a safe treatment in OTRs on skin areas up to $60\,cm^2$. The study showed imiquimod 5% cream may decrease cutaneous dysplasia and the frequency of squamous tumors developing in high-risk patients. Of significance, renal graft function, assessed via serum creatinine measurement, was unaffected. Despite the promising effects of this drug, larger confirmatory studies are still necessary.[44,45]

Immunosuppressive Agents Used in Organ Transplant Recipients

The use of systemic immunosuppressive agents in organ transplant recipients is a well-established risk factor for the development of NMSC. Multiple immunosuppressive agents exist and more are continuing to be developed. The impact of each agent in the development of NMSC is difficult to discern since more than one agent is usually used in each OTR. Intervening factors such as UVR exposure, skin type, and HPV burden, among others, exist, which further cloud the situation. The various immunosuppressive agents may contribute to NMSC development by two mechanisms: impairment of immune surveillance and direct carcinogenesis.[22–25] Studies show conflicting results indicating which agents seem to carry the greatest risk. However, there is a consensus that the dose and duration of immunosuppression are more important as risk factors than any one agent in particular.[21] This is supported by the fact that increased incidence of NMSC is seen in patients on normal-dose immunosuppression compared to low-dose immunosuppression.[46] Additionally, patients receiving a triple regimen are at higher risk of NMSC development than those on double regimens.[47] Finally, reduction of immunosuppressant doses has been shown to be a reasonable adjuvant therapeutic strategy in OTRs with multiple or high-risk skin malignancies.[48]

Various trends in the use of the different immunosuppressants have developed over time. The Organ Procurement and Transplantation Network and Scientific Registry of Transplant Recipients Annual Report (OPTN/SRTR) has divided the use of immunosuppressants into several "eras" (Table 36.1).[49] During the experimental era (1954–1962) prednisone was the only available agent and the only routine transplants performed were those of kidneys of identical twins. The azathioprine era (1962–1983) began with the development of azathioprine (AZA) as an adjunct to prednisone and allowed for cadaveric renal transplants. The Food and Drug Administration (FDA) approval of cyclosporin A (CsA) in 1983 led to the cyclosporine era lasting until the early 1990s. The use of CsA led to increased graft survival and routine extrarenal organ transplantation. The modern era (1990s to present) has seen the development of new immunosuppressive agents with even greater survival rates.

Immunosuppressive agents can be divided into induction agents and maintenance agents. Induction agents are antibodies given perioperatively to induce tolerance to the graft by depleting host T-cell activity. Newer agents, basiliximab and daclizumab, rabbit antithymocyte globulin and anti–interleukin-2 receptor antibodies, respectively, are used in the majority of inductions.[50] Maintenance immunosuppressives can be classified as antimetabolites, calcineurin inhibitors, and rapamycin, each of which has different mechanisms of action, allowing for synergistic effects when used in combination.

Azathioprine acts as an antimetabolite. It is a purine analogue that blocks B- and T-cell proliferation through the inhibition of purine synthesis and metabolism. Adverse effects of AZA such as bone marrow suppression and hepatitis result from

TABLE 36.1. Immunosuppressants and organ transplantation.

Immunosuppressant era	Time period	Agent(s) used	Organs transplanted
Experimental era	1954–1962	Prednisone alone	Kidneys of identical twins
Azathioprine era	1962–1983	Prednisone and azathioprine	Cadaveric kidneys
Cyclosporine era	1983–1990	Cyclosporine	Extrarenal transplants
Modern era	1990–present	Tacrolimus and sirolimus	Extrarenal transplants with increased organ survival

Source: Helderman et al.[49]

its broad inhibition of purine synthesis.[50] Another antimetabolite, mycophenolate mofetil (MMF), is a prodrug that is metabolized into the active compound mycophenolic acid, which inhibits de novo purine biosynthesis. Mycophenolate mofetil, approved in 1995 for use in renal transplant recipients, is now being used widely in place of AZA.[51] In addition to bone marrow suppression, MMF also causes gastrointestinal distress. Improved gastrointestinal tolerability has been shown with the use of an enteric-coated formulation in stable renal transplant recipients.[52]

Cyclosporin A, a calcineurin inhibitor, blocks activation of T cells by preventing the expression of cytokine interleukin-2 (IL-2). It binds to cytoplasmic nuclear factor of activated T cells (NFAT), a family of transcription factors, thereby preventing transcription of growth factors such as IL-2.[50] Cyclosporin A is also known to enhance the expression of transforming growth factor-β (TGF-β), which is also known to inhibit IL-2–stimulated T-cell proliferation and generation of cytotoxic T lymphocytes.[51] The carcinogenic effect of CsA has been shown in a study where patients treated with corticosteroids, AZA, and CsA had a threefold increase in the risk of skin cancer when compared to patients on corticosteroids and AZA alone.[10] Other studies have found that lesions occur earlier in CsA-treated patients.[10,47] Cyclosporin A may have a direct cellular effect that promotes the progression of cancer independently from its effects on host immune cells. An ex vivo study showed that CsA-treated adenocarcinoma cells transformed noninvasive cells to invasive cells with pseudopodia and increased cell motility.[22] These changes were dose-dependent and reversible. Monoclonal antibodies directed against TGF-β prevented these changes, indicating that CsA-induced TGF-β production as a mechanism.

Tacrolimus (TAC), another calcineurin inhibitor, binds the cytoplasmic protein, FK-binding protein (FKBP), and prevents production of IL-2 by inhibiting phosphatase activity of calcineurin. TAC is 100 times more potent than CsA,[53] and, in addition to nephrotoxicity, its side effects include glucose intolerance and reversible alopecia.[51] Tacrolimus has been shown in vitro to promote tumor growth in human hepatoma cells.[54] It has been suggested that tacrolimus may be less oncogenic than CsA based on a lower prevalence of enhanced TGF-β transcription.[55]

Sirolimus, also known as rapamycin, is a relatively new antitumor agent, which shows promise in decreasing the risk of NMSC in OTRs. The cellular target of sirolimus, mTOR or mammalian target of rapamycin, is considered a member of the phosphatidylinositol-3-kinase (PI3K) family.[56] Sirolimus binds the intracellular protein FK-binding protein-12 (FKBP12), forming a high-affinity complex that in turn binds mTOR. The binding of mTOR, also called FRAP (FKBP-rapamycin associated protein), ultimately results in cell cycle arrest at the G1/S phase through the dephosphorylation and inactivation of p70 ribosomal protein S6 kinase.[57] Consequently, this leads to the inhibition of interleukin-stimulated lymphocyte division and antibody production.[51] More specifically, sirolimus inhibits the response to interleukin-2 (IL-2), thereby blocking activation of T and B cells.[52]

Sirolimus has been shown to have antineoplastic properties in both in vitro and in vivo studies.[58,59] Studies have shown a decrease in metastatic area in mice treated with rapamycin and an increase in tumoral area in mice treated with CsA. The decrease in tumor growth in mice treated with rapamycin is attributed to a decrease in neovascularization, whereas the increase in tumor growth in CsA-treated mice was associated with extensive neovascularization. Sirolimus has been shown to inhibit vascular endothelial growth factor (VEGF) both in vitro and in vivo.[59] Another study using a human renal cell cancer pulmonary metastasis model showed sirolimus reduced, whereas CsA increased, the number of pulmonary metastases. Circulating levels of VEGF and TGF-β were found to be lower in rapamycin-treated mice than in controls or CsA-treated mice.[60]

Despite the relatively recent introduction of sirolimus, its use as an immunosuppressive agent in OTRs has been studied. The incidence of skin cancer in sirolimus-treated OTRs was assessed at 2 years posttransplantation and comprised 1981 patients from five multicenter studies. All patients received CsA and corticosteroids and had varying combinations of sirolimus (SRL), AZA, or placebo.[61] The study showed that patients receiving SRL immunotherapy without CsA have a lower incidence of malignancy than patients receiving both SRL and CsA. However the patients on combination therapy showed significantly lower incidence of skin cancer compared to CsA and placebo. The study also found that use of SRL concentration-controlled immunotherapy and early elimination of CsA resulted in significantly lower rates of malignancy.

Sirolimus is well tolerated and has the advantage of less nephrotoxicity and hypertension compared to calcineurin inhibitors. Side effects of sirolimus include hyperlipidemia, thrombocytopenia, leucopenia, and anemia.[62] Although sirolimus, as well as preliminary data of its derivative CCI-779 (everolimus) look promising, it is important to recognize that further studies are needed to assess its effects due to the relatively new development of the drug and the latency of onset of NMSC in OTRs.

Human Leukocyte Antigen Subtypes and Nonmelanoma Skin Cancer

Recipient human leukocyte antigen (HLA) type has been suggested as a possible risk factor for NMSC in OTRs. Several theories on how HLA type may play a role in increasing the risk of NMSC exist. Several studies investigating HLA types and the risk of NMSC in OTRs have been done, with conflicting results.[63] Two of the largest studies have found HLA-A11 to increase the posttransplant risk of NMSC.[63,64] Of these two studies, one was able to successfully identify a subset of Caucasian renal transplant recipients in a northern climate who were at increased risk at both short- and long-term follow-up after transplantation. This increased risk associated with HLA-A11 is only conferred in patients with lighter, sun-sensitive skin.[63] This study suggests a role for more aggressive monitoring in patients with HLA-A11 type. Further studies need to be conducted to confirm these findings and perhaps identify other HLA types that may have significance to OTRs and their risk of NMSC.

Treatment and Follow-Up Recommendations of Nonmelanoma Skin Cancer in Organ Transplant Recipients

Management of OTRs is challenging for dermatologists due to the chronic immunosuppression and progressively increasing risk of NMSC.

The American Society of Transplantation (AST) recommends that patients perform monthly skin self-examinations and have their skin examined by a physician annually.[65] A survey that weighed the advantages and disadvantages of various clinical settings of OTRs concluded that regardless of the clinical design, certain principles are key to providing the best care.[66] The survey stressed the importance of close communication with the transplant team, education of other care providers regarding OTRs' unique dermatologic concerns, patient education as a key to prevention, and close follow-up determined by the risk of skin cancer.

The International Transplant-Skin Cancer Collaborative (ITSCC) has combined data from many studies to develop useful clinical guidelines for the treatment of skin cancer in OTRs.[67] Precancerous lesions such as warts and actinic keratoses should be recognized and treated early to reduce the viral burden and the extent of intraepithelial neoplasia (Figs. 36.1 to 36.3). Treatment of precancerous lesions includes cryosurgery, topical 5-fluorouracil, topical imiquimod, and curettage with electrodesiccation (ED&C). Topical and systemic retinoids may be used as chemoprevention of skin cancer but are only effective while the retinoid is being used.[68,69]

Less aggressive SCC can be managed with destructive modalities such as ED&C or cryosurgery, or they can be excised with Mohs' micro-

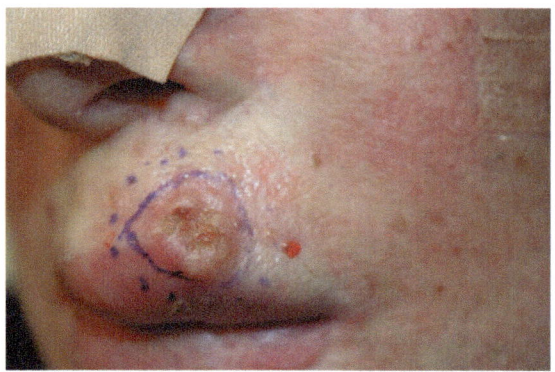

FIG. 36.1. A 58-year-old heart transplant patient who was previously treated with radiation to the circumoral area for multiple cutaneous squamous cell carcinomas. This is a recurrent moderately differentiated squamous cell carcinoma within the radiation field

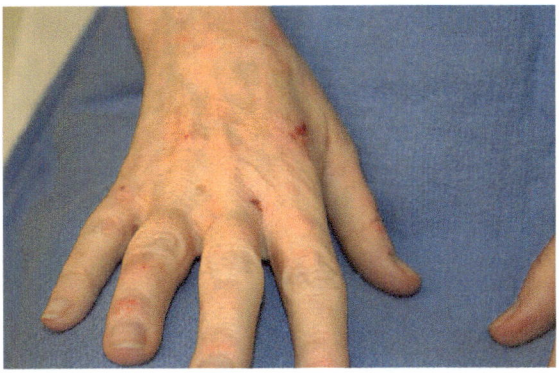

FIG. 36.2. A 58-year-old heart transplant patient with multiple actinic keratoses of the dorsal hands

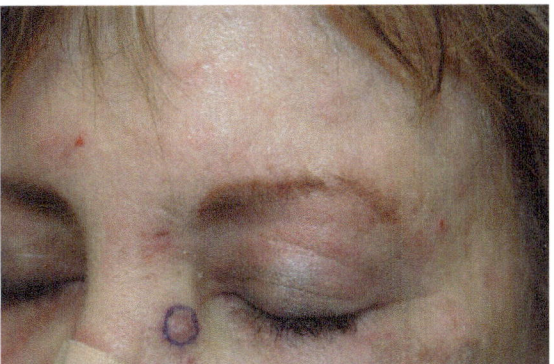

FIG. 36.3. A 58-year-old heart transplant patient with multiple actinic keratoses of the forehead and a lesion on the left nasal sidewall that was biopsied to reveal well-differentiated squamous cell carcinoma

graphic surgery or excision with postoperative margin assessment (Table 36.2).

Aggressive SCC should be removed completely using excisional techniques including Mohs, excision with intraoperative frozen section control, or excision with postoperative margin assessment. Additional modalities may be useful in some instances. Radiation therapy may be considered as adjunctive therapy or as a primary modality for inoperable tumors (Fig. 36.1). Although not routinely used, small studies are beginning to support the role of sentinel lymph node biopsy (SLNB) in the evaluation of high-risk NMSC.[70]

Chemoprophylaxis with oral retinoids such as acitretin has been shown to be effective in reducing the rate of development of premalignant and malignant lesions in OTR.[69,71] This effect is only exhibited while the patient is actively taking the retinoid. After cessation of the drug, the rate of development of lesions returns to baseline or may even exceed the prior rate of development. Retinoids have several side effects that are often very difficult for patients to tolerate on a long-term basis. These side effects include dry skin, dry lips, significant hair loss, pruritus, and arthralgias.[69] Areas of multiple SCC, such as the dorsum of the hand, have been successfully treated with excision and split-thickness skin grafting. Although the grafted area remains lesion-free for an extended period, this procedure has significant morbidity and requires an extensive recovery.[72,73] In cases of life-threatening

TABLE 36.2. Cutaneous squamous cell carcinomas in organ transplant recipients.

Characteristic	Less aggressive SCC	More aggressive SCC
Size:		
Mask areas of face,* genitals, hands, feet	<0.6 cm	≥0.6 cm
Cheeks, forehead, neck, scalp	<1.0 cm	≥1.0 cm
Trunk and extremities	<2.0 cm	≥2.0 cm
Rate of growth	Static or slow-growing	Rapid
Ulceration	No	Yes
Clinical margins	Distinct, well defined	Indistinct
Satellite lesions	No	Yes
Neurotropism	Absent	Present
Histology:		
Invasiveness	In situ/invasion limited to papillary dermis	Deep extension into subcutaneous fat
Perivascular or intravascular invasion	No	Yes
Differentiation	Well-differentiated	Poorly differentiated

*Mask area includes central face, eyelids, eyebrows, periorbital, nose, lips, chin, mandible, pre- and postauricular areas, temple, ear.
Source: Christenson et al.[66]

skin cancers, reduction of immunosuppression may be considered. Studies have shown that renal transplant recipients with very aggressive SCC have an improved prognosis following dose reduction compared to those whose immunosuppression was left unchanged.[74] It has also been shown that graft function may continue despite reduction of immunosuppression.[75,76] It is important when considering reduction of immunosuppressive therapy that it is done in consultation with the transplant physician. If the need to reduce the level of immunosuppression is warranted, transplant physicians often prefer to lower the dose of AZA first, as CsA confers better allograft survival.[77]

Conclusion

Skin cancer in OTRs is a continuing problem as the number of living OTRs grows due to an increasing number of transplants performed and longer patient and graft survival time. This, in turn, has led to a growing number of patients on chronic immunosuppression. Chronic immunosuppression, along with other risk factors, places these patients at higher risk of developing malignancies, the most common being cutaneous malignancies. It is hoped that further investigation of these risk factors and the identification of others will lead to improved prevention, management, and treatment of these patients. In addition, it is hoped that further investigation of current immunosuppressive regimens and the development of new immunosuppressive agents will lead to decreased morbidity and mortality, particularly from cutaneous malignancies.

Management of these patients requires a multifaceted approach involving the transplant team, dermatologists, other care providers and the patients. It is important as dermatologists to make all those involved in the care of these patients aware of their unique dermatologic concerns. Treatment and follow-up may then be determined on an individual basis based on the patient's risk factors and the relative risk of the skin cancer.

References

1. Health Resources and Services Administration, Healthcare Systems Bureau, Division of Transplantation, by the Organ Procurement and Transplantation Network contractor, the United Network for Organ Sharing (UNOS), and the Scientific Registry of Transplant Recipients contractor, the University Renal Research and Education Association (URREA) 2005, OPTN/SRTR Annual Report, Transplant by Organ and Donor Type 1995–2004 Table 1.7, http://www. ustransplant.org/annual_reports/current/107_dh.htm (July 20, 2006).
2. 2004 Annual Report of the U.S. Organ Procurement and Transplantation Network and the Scientific Registry of Transplant Recipients: Transplant Data 1994–2003. Department of Health and Human Services, Health Resources and Services Administration, Healthcare Systems Bureau, Division of Transplantation, Rockville, MD; United Network for Organ Sharing, Richmond, VA; University Renal Research and Education Association, Ann Arbor, MI.
3. Randle H. The historical link between solid-organ transplantation, immunosuppression, and skin cancer. Derm Surg 2004;30:595–597.
4. Agraharkar ML, Cinclair RD, Kuo YF, et al. Risk of malignancy with long-term immunosuppression in renal transplant recipients. Kidney Int 2004;66:383–389.
5. Moloney FJ, Comber H, O'Lorcain P, et al. A population-based study of skin cancer incidence and prevalence in renal transplant recipients. Br J Dermatol 2006;154:498–504.
6. Harwood C, Proby C, McGregor J, et al. Clinicopathologic features of skin cancer in organ transplant recipients: a retrospective case-control series. J Am Acad Dermatol 2006;54(2):290–300.
7. Lindelhof B, et al. Incidence of skin cancer in 5356 patients following organ transplantation. Br J Dermatol 2000;143:523–519.
8. Euvrard S, Kanitakis J, Claudy A. Skin cancers after organ transplantation. N Engl J Med 2003;345:1681–91.
9. Euvrard S, Kanitakis J, Cochat P, et al. Skin cancers following pediatric organ transplantation. Derm Surg 2004;30:616–621.
10. Jensen P, Hansen S, Moller B, et al. Skin cancer in kidney and heart transplant recipients and different long-term immunosuppressive therapy regimens. J Am Acad Dermatol 1999;40:177–186.
11. Penn I, First MR. Merkel's Cell carcinoma in organ transplant recipients: report of 14 cases. Transplantation 1999;68:1717–1721.
12. Penn I. Neoplastic consequences of transplantation and chemotherapy. Cancer Detect Prev 1987;S1:149–157.
13. Rosso S, Zanetti R, Martinez C, et al. The multicentre south European study "Helios," II: different sun exposure patterns in the aetiology of basal cell and squamous cell carcinomas of the skin. Br J Cancer 1996;166:72–74.

14. Ong C, Keogh A, Kossard S, et al. Skin cancer in Australian heart transplant recipients. J Am Acad Dermatol 1999;40(1):27–34.

15. Espana A, Martinez-Gonzalez MA, Garcia-Granero M, et al. A prospective study of incident nonmelanoma skin cancer in heart transplant recipients. J Invest Dermatol 2000;115:1158–60.

16. Bavnick JN, De Boer A, Vermeer BJ, et al. Sunlight, keratotic skin lesions, and skin cancer in renal transplant recipients. Br J Dermatol 1993;129:242–249.

17. Ramsay HM, Fryer AA, Reece S, et al. Clinical risk factors associated with nonmelanoma skin cancer in renal transplant recipients. Am J Kidney Dis 2000;36:167–176.

18. Webb MC, Compton F, Andrews PA, et al. Skin tumours posttransplantation: a retrospective analysis of 28 years' experience at a single centre. Transplant Proc 1997;29:828–830.

19. Kripke ML. Ultraviolet radiation and immunology: something new under the sun—presidential address. Cancer Res 1994;54:6102–5.

20. Parrish JA. Ultraviolet radiation affects the immune system. Pediatrics 1983;71:129–133.

21. Jensen P, et al. Are renal transplant recipients on CsA-based immunosuppressive regimens more likely to develop skin cancer than those on azathioprine and prednisolone? Transplant Proc 1999;31(1–2):1120.

22. Hojo M, Morimoto T, Maluccio M, et al. Cyclosporine induces cancer progression by a cell-autonomous mechanism. Nature 1999;397:530–534

23. Kelly GE, Meikle W, Sheil AG. Effects of immunosuppressive therapy on the induction of skin tumors by ultraviolet irradiation in hairless mice. Transplantation 1987;44:429–434.

24. Servilla KS, Burnham DK, Daynes RA. Ability of cyclosporine to promote the growth of transplanted ultraviolet radiation-induced tumors in mice. Transplantation 1987;44:291–295.

25. Boyle J, MacKie RM, Briggs JD, et al. Cancer, warts, and sunshine in renal transplant patients. A case-control study. Lancet 1984;1:702–705.

26. Penn I. Posttransplantation de novo tumors in liver allograft recipients. Liver Transpl Surg 1996;2:52–59.

27. Gjersvik P, Hansen S, Moller B, et al. Are heart transplant recipients more likely to develop skin cancer than kidney transplant recipients? Transpl Int 2000;13(suppl 1):S380–381.

28. Euvrard S, Kanitakis J, Pouteil-Noble C, et al. Comparative epidemiologic study of premalignant and malignant epithelial cutaneous lesions developing after kidney and heart transplantation. J Am Acad Dermatol 1995;33:222–229.

29. Otley C, Cherikh W, Salasche S, et al. Skin cancer in organ transplant recipients: effect of pre-transplant end-organ disease. J Am Acad Dermatol 2005;53:783–790.

30. Kuijken I, Bouwes Bavnick J. Skin Cancer risk associated with immunosuppressive therapy in organ transplant recipients. BioDrugs 2000;14:319–329.

31. Blessing K, McLaren KM, Benton EC, et al. Histopathology of skin lesions in renal allograft recipients: an assessment of viral features and dysplasia. Histopathology 1989;14:129–139.

32. Stockfleth E, Nindl I, Sterry W, et al. Human Papillomaviruses in transplant-associated skin cancers. Am Soc Derm Surg 2004;30:604–609.

33. McGregor JM, Proby CM. The role of papillomaviruses in human non-melanoma skin cancer. Skin Cancer 1996;26:219–236.

34. Berkhout RJ, Bouwes Bavnick JN, ter Schegget J. Persistence of human papillomavirus DNA in benign and (pre)malignant skin lesions from renal transplant recipients. J Clin Microbiol 2000;38(6):207–96.

35. Harwood CA, Surentheran T, McGregor JM, et al. Human papillomavirus infection and nonmelanoma skin cancer in immunosuppressed and immunocompetent individuals. J Med Virol 2000;61:289–297.

36. Berkhout RJM, Bouwes Bavnick JN, ter Schegget J. Persistence of human papillomavirus DNA in benign and (pre)malignant skin lesions from renal transplant recipients. J Clin Microbiol 2000;38:2087–2096.

37. Shamanin V, zur Hausen H, Lavergne D, et al. Human papillomavirus infections in nonmelanoma skin cancers in renal transplant recipients and non-immunosuppressed patients. J Natl Cancer Inst 1996;88:802–821.

38. Leigh IM, Glover MT. Cutaneous warts and tumours in immunosuppressed patients. J R Soc Med 1995;88:61–62.

39. Bouwes Bavnick JN, Feltkamp M, Strujik L, et al. Human papillomavirus infection and skin cancer risk in organ transplant recipients. J Invest Dermatol Symp Proc 2001;6(3):207–11.

40. Bosch FX, Sanjosé S. Human papillomavirus and cervical cancer: burden and assessment of causality. J Natl Cancer Inst Monogr 2003;31:3–13.

41. Wang SS, Hildesheim A. Viral and host factors in human papillomavirus persistence and progression. J Natl Cancer Inst Monogr 2003;31:35–40

42. Cullen AP, Reid R, Campion M, Lörincz AT. Analysis of the physical state of different human papillomavirus DNAs in intraepithelial and invasive cervical neoplasm. J Virol 1991;65:606–612.

43. Pirami L, Giache V, Becciolini A. Analysis of HPV16, 18, 31, and 35 DNA in pre-invasive and

invasive lesions of the uterine cervix. J Clin Pathol 1997;50:600–604

44. Otley C, Berg D, et al. Reduction of immunosuppression for transplant-associated skin cancer: expert consensus survey. Br J Dermatol 2006;154:395–400.

45. Kovach B, Stasko T. Use of topical immunomodulators in organ transplant recipients. Dermatol Ther 2005;18:19–27.

46. Dantal J, Hourmant M, Cantorovich D, et al. Effect of long-term immunosuppression in kidney graft recipients on cancer incidence: a randomized comparison of two cyclosporin regimens. Lancet 1998;351:623–628.

47. Glover M, Deeks J, Raftery M, et al. Immunosuppression and risk of nonmelanoma skin cancer in renal transplant recipients. Lancet 1997;349(9049):398.

48. Otley C, Maragh S. Reduction of immunosuppression for transplant-associated skin cancer: rationale and evidence of efficacy. Dermatol Surg 2005;31: 163–168.

49. Helderman J, et al. 2002 Annual Report of the U.S Scientific Registry of Transplant Recipients and the Organ Procurement and Transplantation Network: Transplant Data Chapter IV Immunosuppression: Practice and Trends 2002. Rockville, MD and Richmond, VA: HHS/HRSA/OSP/DOT and UNOS, 2002.

50. Durando C, Reichel J. The relative effects of different systemic immunosuppressives on skin cancer development in organ transplant patients. Dermatologic Therapy 2005;18:1–11.

51. Euvrard S, Ulrich C, Lefrancois N. Immunosuppressants and skin cancer in transplant patients: focus on rapamycin. Dermatol Surg 2004;30:628–633.

52. Sirolimus. Wikipedia, the free encyclopedia. http://www.reference.com/browse/wiki/Sirolimus.

53. Massari P, Duro-Garcia V, Giron F, et al. Safety assessment of the conversion from mycophenolate mofetil to enteric-coated mycophenolate sodium in stable renal transplant recipients. Transplant Proc 2005;37:916–919.

54. Ochiai T, Nakajima M, et al. Effect of a new immunosuppressive agent, FK506, on heterotopic cardiac allotransplantation in the rat. Transplant Proc 1987;19(1 pt 2):1284–1286.

55. Schumacher G, Oidtmann M, Rosewicz S, et al. Sirolimus inhibits growth of human hepatoma cells in contrast to tacrolimus which promotes cell growth. Transplant Proc 2002;34:1392–1393.

56. Fung J, Kwak E, Kusne S, et al. De novo malignancies after liver transplantation: a major cause of late death. Liver Transplant 2001;7:S109–118.

57. Sehgal SN, Molnar-Kimber K, Ocain TD, et al. Rapamycin: a novel immunosuppressive macrolide. Med Res Rev 1994;14:1–22.

58. Huang S, Houghton PJ. Inhibitors of mammalian target of rapamycin as novel antitumor agents: from bench to clinic. Curr Opin Invest Drugs 2002;3:295–304.

59. Huang S, Houghton PJ, Guba M, et al. Rapamycin inhibits primary and metastatic tumor growth by antiangiogenesis: involvement of vascular endothelial growth factor. Nat Med 2002;8:128–135.

60. Luan FL, Ding R, Sharma VK, et al. Rapamycin is an effective inhibitor of human renal cancer metastasis. Kidney Int 2003;63:917–926.

61. Matthew T, Kreis H, Friend P. Two-year incidence of malignancy in sirolimus-treated renal transplant recipients: results from five multicenter studies. Clin Transplant 2004;18:446–449.

62. Morelson E, Kreis H. Sirolimus therapy without calcineurin inhibitors: Necker Hospital five year experience. Transplant Proc 2003;35:52S–7S.

63. Bock A, Bliss R, Matas A, Little J. Human leukocyte antigen type as a risk factor for nonmelanomatous skin cancer in patients after renal transplantation. Transplantation 2004;78:775–778.

64. Bouwes Bavinck JN, Claas FH, Hardie DR, et al. Relation between HLA antigens and skin cancer in renal transplant recipients in Queensland, Australia. J Invest Dermatol 1997;108(5):708–710.

65. Kasiske BL, Vasquez MA, Harmon WE, et al. Recommendations for the outpatient surveillance of renal transplant recipients. J Am Soc Nephrol 2000;11:S1–S86.

66. Christenson L, et al. Specialty clinics for the dermatologic care of solid-organ transplant recipients. Derm Surg 2004;30:598–603.

67. Stasko T, Brown M, Carucci J, et al. Guidelines for the management of squamous cell carcinoma in organ transplant recipients. Derm Surg 2004;30:642–650.

68. Euvrard S, Verschoore M, Teraine J, et al. Topical retinoids for warts and keratosis in transplant recipients. Lancet 1992;340:48.

69. De Graaf YGL, Euvrard S, Bouwes Bavinck JN. Systemic and topical retinoids in the management of skin cancer in organ transplant recipients. Derm Surg 2004;30:656–661.

70. Altinyollar H, Berberoglu U, Celen O. Lymphatic mapping and sentinel lymph node biopsy in squamous cell carcinoma of the lower lip. Eur J Surg Oncol 2002;28:72–74.

71. Yuan ZF, Davis A, MacDonald K, et al. Use of acetretin for the skin complications in organ transplant recipients. Lancet 1991;338:1407.

72. Scholtens RE, van Zuuren EJ, Posma AN. Treatment of recurrent squamous cell carcinoma of the hand in immunosuppressed patients. J Hand Surg Am 1995;20:73–76.

73. van Zuuren EJ, Posma AN, Scholtens RE, et al. Resurfacing the back of the hand as treatment and prevention of multiple skin cancers in kidney

transplant recipients. J Am Acad Dermatol 1994;31: 760–764.

74. Moloney FJ, Kelly PO, Kay EW, et al. Maintenance versus reduction of immunosuppression in renal transplant recipients with aggressive squamous cell carcinoma. Derm Surg 2004;30:674–678.

75. Mazariegos GV, Reyes J, Marino I, et al. Risks and benefits of weaning of immunosuppression in liver transplant recipients: long-term follow-up. Transplant Proc 1997;29:1174–1177.

76. Mazariegos GV, Reyes J, Marino I, et al. Weaning of immunosuppression in liver transplant recipients. Transplantation 1997;63:243–249.

77. Berg D, Otley C. Skin cancer in organ transplant recipients: Epidemiology, pathogenesis, and management. J Am Acad Dermatol 2002;47:1–17.

37
Granulomatosis

Kurt Q. Lu

Key Points

- Interferon-γ (IFN-γ) is a critical cytokine in formation of multinucleated giant cells (MGCs).
- Macrophage fusion receptor (MFR) and its ligand CD47 have been implicated in facilitating cell fusion and cell-to-cell recognition in specialized multinucleated giant cells, for example, osteoclasts and foreign body giant cells.
- There appear to be genetic susceptibility factors for development of sarcoidosis.
- The involved cytokines in granuloma formation are of the T-helper-1 (Th1) phenotype.
- Sarcoidosis patients have a high number of T-regulatory cells.
- Polymorphisms of *CARD15/NOD2* have been associated with Crohn's disease.
- Citrullination, a posttranslation modification process, has been demonstrated to increase peptide and major histocompatibility complex (MHC) affinity, suggesting it can modulate immune responses.

The disease entities in the group of granulomatous disorders share some histologic commonalities; however, the etiology of most remains largely unknown. In *Clinical Immunodermatology*, the forerunner of this book, Mark Dahl[1] offered a schematic by which to classify granulomatous inflammation based on appearance, precipitating factors, and degree of lymphocytic infiltration (nonimmunologic vs. immunologic) but warned that the distinctions are more apparent than real. More than a decade later, the caveat holds true. Granulomatosus represents a distinctive reactive process in the spectrum of inflammation where the histiocyte is the

key involved cell. A granuloma is a focal collection of activated and modified histiocytes, sometimes epithelioid in appearance, usually surrounded by a rim of leukocytes.[2] While histiocytes are now firmly established as monocyte/macrophage-derived cells based on surface immunohistochemical markers, past reliance solely on cell morphology has led to confusion, as numerous diverse, reactive, and neoplastic cell populations can aggregate in the cutaneous microenvironment resembling histiocytes, commonly referred as histiocytoid.

Conceptually, the etiology of granulomatosus is thought of as an immune defense and reactive process. This is exemplified by various prototypic diseases such as tuberculosis and leprosy, representing infectious granulomas, and common conditions such as ruptured keratin cysts and suture granulomas, representing endogenous and exogenous foreign-body reactions, respectively. Either undiscovered or undetectable by current investigative modalities, several granulomatous entities, such as sarcoidosis and the group of necrobiotic granulomas, do not consistently demonstrate the presence of either infectious or foreign-body material.

Another classification categorized granulomas distinguishes as immunologic or nonimmunologic.[1] While both classifications involve macrophage activation admixed with leukocytes at the initiation of granuloma formation, the persistence of lymphocytes within the lesion are features of immunologic granulomas. In general, nonimmunologic granulomas involve the introduction of large amounts of insoluble material while immunologic granulomas may result from introduction of a small amount of substances (Fig. 37.1). These

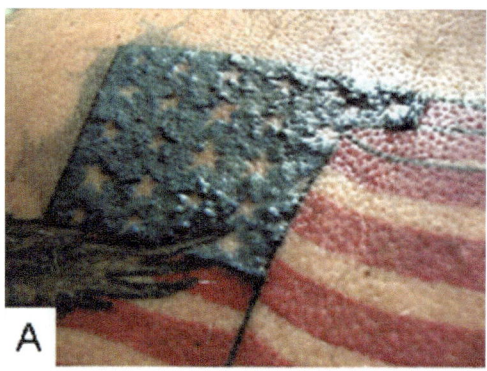
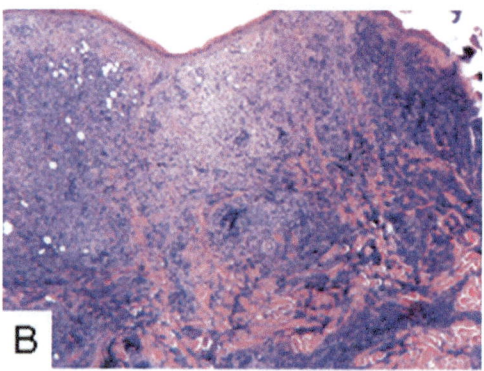
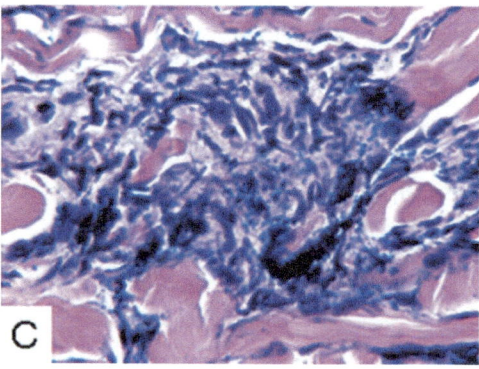

FIG. 37.1. Local hypersensitivity reaction to tattoo pigment. (A) Plaque and nodular reaction to decorative blue tattoo. (B) Scanning magnification shows a dense deep infiltrate of predominantly mononuclear cells with scattered giant cell throughout all levels of dermis. (C) High-power magnification shows presence of fine blue/green pigment (Courtesy of A. Gilliam, MD, and M. Smith, MD.)

substances range from pathogenic stimuli, such as bacteria, fungi, mycobacteria, and certain virus and molds, to chemical initiators. Still, even within the

immunologic scheme, sarcoidosis and the necrobiotic granulomas cannot be neatly classified.

Role of Monocytes and Macrophages

Some insight into the clinical spectrum of granulomatous diseases may be gained by examining the characteristics and function of the histiocyte or monocytes/macrophages (Mo/Macs). Mo/Macs are often regarded as the primary phagocytic population of the innate immune system with some antigen-presenting capabilities. However, they express several classes of receptors and are able to produce a cadre of enzymatic and metabolic mediators, suggesting a broader ro le than microbial surveillance.[3]

In its innate immunity role the Mo/Macs bear multiple cell-surface molecules that mediate diverse pathogen recognition and processing as well as those that mediate recruitment and trafficking of inflammatory cells to the site of infection, such as toll-like receptors (TLRs) and chemokine receptors, respectively.[4,5] A cornerstone feature of the Mo/Macs is their dynamic modification in response to acute inflammation or infection. They display high cellular plasticity and are driven by local microanatomic and systemic environmental factors.[6,7] Resting monocytes comprise 2% to 10% of peripheral blood leukocytes and can be marginated in response to chemotactic factors released as a result of systemic events. The cells can infiltrate most tissue where they transform into activated macrophages. Additionally, various organs have resident tissue-specific differentiated Mo/Macs, mostly myeloid in origin, comprising a network called the mononuclear phagocyte system.[8]

Mo/Macs also occupy a unique niche in the inflammatory response. One bystander effect of inflammation is apoptosis, requiring swift and efficient engulfment without inciting further inflammation or allowing leakage of potentially immunogenic material.[9] It has recently been shown that macrophages use distinct processes to clear apoptotic cells vs. necrotic cells by a "zipper-like" phagocytosis vs. macropinocytosis, respectively.[10] Mo/Macs express and utilize various receptors including scavenger receptors, complement receptors, and integrins to recognize apoptotic bodies and mediate removal to control potential inflammatory responses.[11] Hence, Mo/Macs are slowly being recognized as having a more sophisticated role in inflammation.

Multinucleated Giant Cells

In the face of infection, the presence of Mo/Macs may signal both a reactive, protective process, and a homeostatic, restorative process. As fusion and aggregation ensue, macrophages and monocytes form histologically striking structures such as multinucleated giant cells (MGCs) and granulomas, respectively (Fig. 37.2).[12] The process resulting in formation of these structures remains poorly understood. Mo/Macs can be stimulated to generate MGCs in vitro by the addition of various cytokines and conditioned medias.[13] Interferon-γ (IFN-γ) has been identified as a critical cytokine in MGC formation.[14] In specialized

MGCs such as osteoclasts and foreign body giant cells, the macrophage fusion receptor (MFR) and its ligand CD47 have been implicated to facilitate cell fusion and cell-to-cell recognition.[15] The latter is important for cell-cell reciprocity, allowing multinucleation rather than activation of intracellular degradative processes in the newly fused cell. Recently, a molecule called DC specific transmembrane protein (DC-STAMP) was shown to be required for fusion of Mo/Macs into giant cells.[16] The ligand for DC-STAMP is currently unknown. However, its structural similarity to chemokine receptors suggests the possibility that the ligand may be a soluble chemokine. Chemokines such as CCL2 have already been

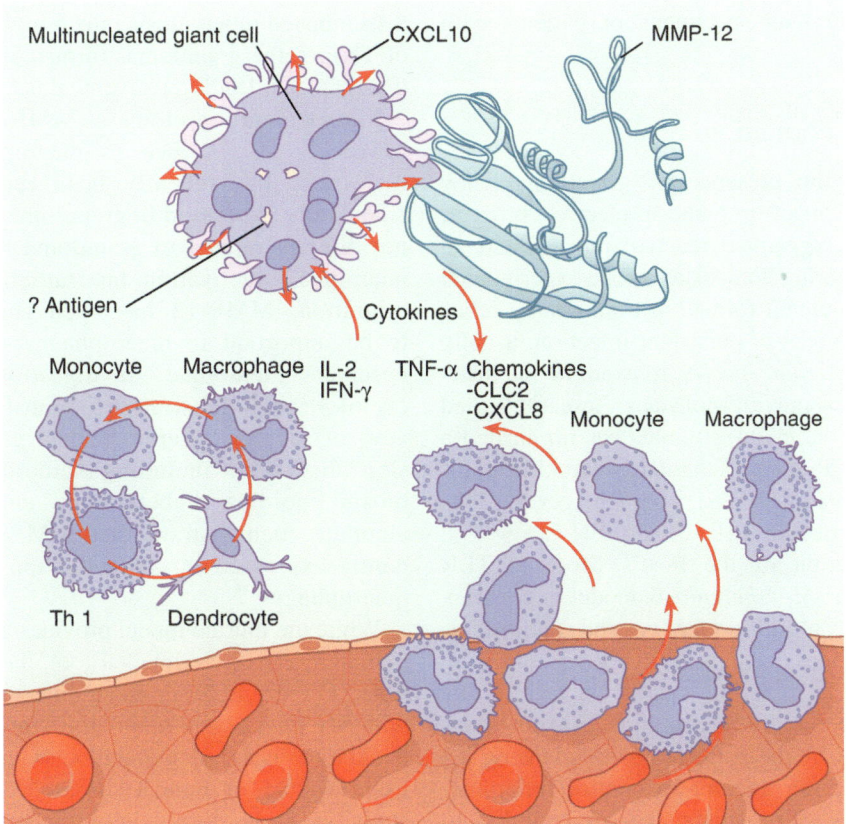

FIG. 37.2. Schematic for granuloma formation. Monocyte/macrophage (Mo/Mac) interaction with an antigen provokes an inflammatory response. Under influence of various cytokines and chemokines, some Mo/Macs undergo cell fusion to form multinucleated giant cells (MGCs). Once formed, MGCs secrete steady-state chemokines, attracting more Mo/Macs. Other activated Mo/Macs enlarge and differentiate into epithelioid histiocytes. Aggregation results in granulomas. Activation by tumor necrosis factor-α (TNF-α) and interferon-γ (IFN-γ) is important in granuloma formation and maintenance

shown to play a role in foreign body giant cell formation.[17]

Recently, it was demonstrated that during cell differentiation into MGCs, high amounts of chemokines were induced in Mo/Macs.[18] However, once the MGC was fully differentiated, the expression of the chemokines such CCL2 and CXCL10 became constitutive and could not be further upregulated by exposure to *Mycobacterium tuberculosis*. This suggests two distinct phases in MGC formation. First, in acute infection, the development of MGCs induces rapid recruitment of Mo/Macs via chemokine release. Second, the differentiated MGC stimulates a steady influx of Mo/Macs, presumably toward the development of granulomas, via a steady state of chemokine gradient. The connection between granulomatous infection and chemokines is supported by reports showing high amounts of chemokines in lung specimens of patients with tuberculosis.[19,20]

Granuloma Formation

Functionally, the presence of granulomas may represent an intact immune protective process, possibly an exaggerated reactive process and an attempt at restoring homeostasis. The experimental model of granuloma formation traditionally relies on a murine model of persistent infection, usually with *Mycobacterium species*, to examine the interaction of pathogen with Mo/Macs. Research aimed at unraveling the inciting signals has implicated a role for TLRs, the proinflammatory cytokine tumor necrosis factor-α (TNF-α), and T-helper 1 (Th1) cytokines interleukin-2 (IL-2) and IFN-γ.[21,22]

The elicitation of the host's Mo/Mac TLR response in the *M. tuberculosis* model is complex because both proinflammatory and antiinflammatory cytokines have been reported following *M. tuberculosis* exposure.[23] It is unclear if this dichotomy represents an immune evasion strategy employed by the pathogen or a balancing act by the host in an attempt to control inflammatory responses. Surprisingly, the susceptibility to *M. tuberculosis* was low in numerous TLR knockout (TLR2, TLR4, and TLR6) mouse models. However, the myeloid differentiation factor 88 (MyD88) knockout mice displayed high susceptibility to disease,[24,25] thus demonstrating the importance of TLRs in host defense against mycobacteria

since MyD88 functions as an adaptor molecule used by many TLRs following ligand activation. Studies using mycobacteria and other pathogens have demonstrated the importance of MyD88 in granuloma formation via IFN-γ induction.[26,27]

More than a decade earlier, Flynn and colleagues reported that IFN-γ knockout mice infected with *M. tuberculosis* develop disseminated tuberculosis. They demonstrated that disease susceptibility followed granuloma necrosis due to lack of macrophage activating signals needed for granuloma maintenance.[28,29] It is now known that intact Th1 adaptive responses are important in the production of cytokines to form adequate granulomatous immune responses. Th1 cells play a role in both the formation and maintenance of granulomas by inducing and sustaining Mo/Mac recruitment. Similarly, mice deficient in TNF-α succumb to disseminated tuberculosis infection. In the absence of TNF-α, the granulomas formed are structurally disorganized, leading to eventual necrosis.[30,31]

Matrix metalloproteinase (MMP), specifically MMP-12, also known as macrophage metalloelastase, has recently been reported to be abundantly expressed in granulomas.[32] Although not directly related to granuloma formation via macrophage activation but rather macrophage migration, MMP-12 has been shown in vivo to be important in macrophage penetration of basement membrane via digestion of a variety of stromal substrates.[33,34] Furthermore, surveys of several different human granulomatous skin disorders, including sarcoidosis, necrobiosis lipoidica diabeticorum, and granuloma annulare, demonstrate that MMP-12 is abundantly expressed in colocalization with CD68+ macrophages.[35]

While the murine model provides a useful mammalian in vivo experimental tool, there are limitations. For example, cross-strain murine infection with *Mycobacterium tuberculosis* produces multibacillary noncaseating granulomas, contrasting the usual course in human disease.[36] Furthermore, study of early events in granuloma formation, namely Mo/Mac recruitment, modification, and aggregation, is limited by static ex vivo histologic examination of tissue in this model.

Recent development of nonmammalian granuloma models have helped broadened our understanding of granuloma formation. This is possible through examination of host interaction with *Mycobacterium marinum* in species phylogenetically distinct from humans such as *Dictyostelium, Drosophila*, and zebrafish.[37] While extrapolation into human disease pathogenesis may not be immediately apparent, the observations suggest that pathogen recognition via pathogen-associated molecule patterns (PAMPs) and macrophage aggregation may be evolutionary conserved processes. The *Dictyostelium* is a single-cell ameba that has similarities to the phagocytic histiocyte. *Drosophila* is an already-known model of innate immunity. Taking advantage of the physical transparency of zebrafish embryos, researchers have directly visualized migration and aggregation of macrophages, hallmarks of granulomas, following infection with *M. marinum*.[38] Furthermore, at the embryonic stage, zebrafish lack circulating lymphocytes, which suggests that granuloma formation can be initiated in the absence of an adaptive immune contribution.

Granulomatous Disease

Except for infectious and foreign body granulomatosus, the factors determining the noninfectious granulomatous diseases are largely unknown. Granulomas formed by foreign body reactions may not be a diagnostic dilemma in the appropriate clinical setting. For noninfectious granulomatosus, recognition of the reaction patterns and the cellular mediators is useful for classifying the clinical entities that ultimately may provide a better understanding the etiopathogenesis (Fig. 37.3). While the group of diseases involves infiltration and aggregation of immune cells, this does not necessitate that the disorder be immunologically mediated. Histiocytic aggregation may be seen in reactive processes.

Sarcoidosis is slowly being unraveled. It is the most studied nontuberculid granulomatous disease because of its affect on multiple organ systems and associated mortality and morbidity. Understanding the underlying molecular and cellular processes

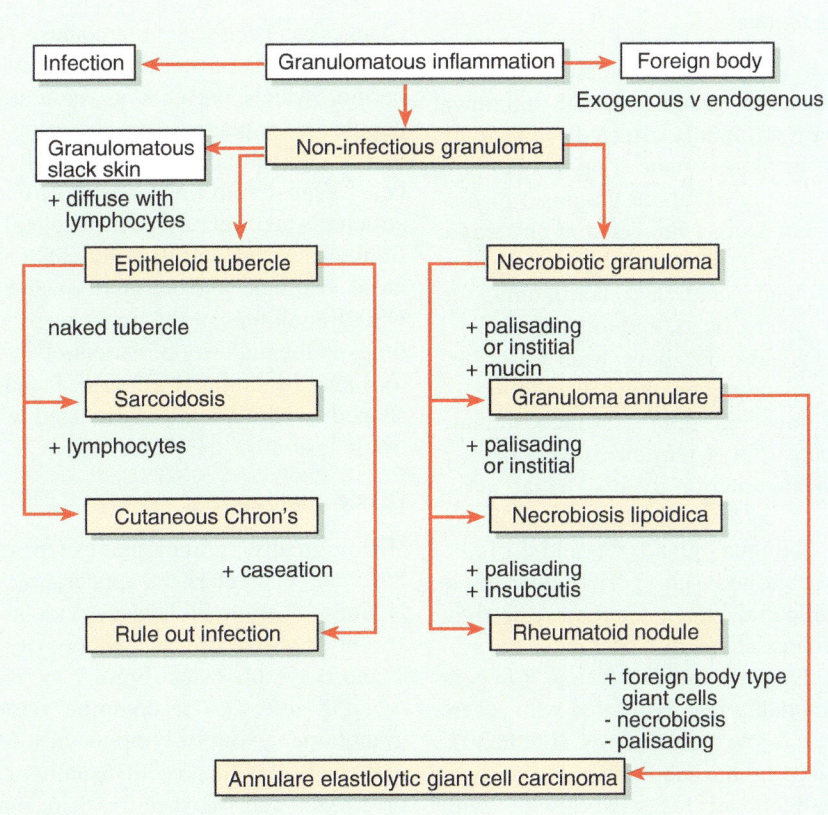

FIG. 37.3. An approach to the histologic diagnosis of granulomas

of this prototypic granulomatous disease may help elucidate pathogenesis of other noninfectious granulomatous disorders.

Other diseases include cutaneous Crohn's, which is a spectrum of cutaneous manifestations associated with the inflammatory gastrointestinal disease, not all of which are granulomatous. The group of necrobiotic granulomas, including granuloma annulare, necrobiosis lipoidica, and rheumatoid nodule, share some common histologic features but no consistent correlations with a single underlying systemic disease. Except for vasculitis and potential ulceration in the latter entity, the cutaneous conditions are largely benign. Annular elastolytic giant cell granuloma is a rare disease that is considered by some to be a variant of granuloma annulare, but with histologically distinct features. Similarly, it has a fairly benign course and may be self-limiting.

Noninfectious Epithelioid Granulomas

Sarcoidosis

Clinical Manifestations

Sarcoidosis is a multisystem disease characterized by noncaseating granulomas of unknown etiology.[39] The organ mainly affected is the lung. Involvement of the skin is seen in up to one third of patients and usually occurs at the onset of disease; however, skin lesions can occur at any stage. Other organs affected include the liver, spleen, eyes, kidneys, glands, and, less commonly, the central nervous system, heart, and musculoskeletal system. Several syndromes have been described in sarcoidosis depending on the constellation of symptoms and involved organs, which include Heerfordt-Waldenström syndrome (fever, parotid gland enlargement, anterior uveitis, facial nerve palsy); Mikulicz's syndrome (parotid, submandibular, lacrimal, and sublingual glands)[40]; and Lofgren syndrome (erythema nodosum, periarticular ankle inflammation, bilateral hilar adenopathy, or right paratracheal lymphadenopathy). The latter is associated with a benign self-remitting course.[41] In general, while the mortality rate associated with severe pulmonary disease is low in sarcoidosis, 10% to 30% of patients develop chronic debilitating disease.

Sarcoidosis affects all races worldwide with varying incidence. In the United States, African Americans have a 3.8-fold increased risk compared to whites, affecting women more than men.[42] The cutaneous manifestation of sarcoidosis is diverse. Several studies have established that the skin disease does not correlate with prognosis or the extent of visceral involvement.[42,43] However, there is correlation of erythema nodosum, usually a self-limiting condition seen most frequently in young women on initial presentation, with acute disease, and large plaques with chronic disease.[42,44,45] A recent retrospective analysis of a small cohort of patients with the subcutaneous form of sarcoidosis suggests that this variant may be a subset associated with systemic disease.[46]

Skin manifestations include nonpainful reddish-brown papules and plaques often symmetrically involving the face, lips, neck, trunk, or upper extremities.[47] Other cutaneous manifestations of sarcoidosis include nodules usually on the trunk and extremities. Lesions may have an ichthyosiform, annular, angiolupoid (large telangiectatic), or psoriasiform appearance. Atrophy can be seen in plaque lesions. Scalp lesions have varying amounts of scale and may result in alopecia. Various nonspecific nail and mucosal changes can been seen in sarcoidosis patients.

Another manifestation of sarcoidosis is lupus pernio, which presents as indurated violaceous papules and plaques on the nose, cheeks, and ears.[48] Ulceration can be seen in these lesions and is associated with involvement of underlying bone structures as well as other skeletal radiographic findings. Nasal alar lesions can extend into the nasal vestibule and nasal floor and is associated with granulomas in the upper respiratory tract and lungs in the majority of patients.[49,50] The digits and toes may be similarly affected, leading to sausage-shaped swelling, and is associated with underlying cystic lesions of the phalanges.[51]

Histopathology

Histologically, granulomas seen in sarcoidosis have the characteristic appearance of focal collections of epithelioid histiocytes associated with absent or sparse ring of lymphocytes composed of T and B lymphocytes (Fig. 37.4). The term *naked tubercle* refers to a common observation of a granuloma devoid of lymphocytes. Multinucleated giant cells may be present, usually of the Langhans type. Although not specific, there may be asteroid and Schaumann bodies. There is typically no central caseation; however, there may be changes

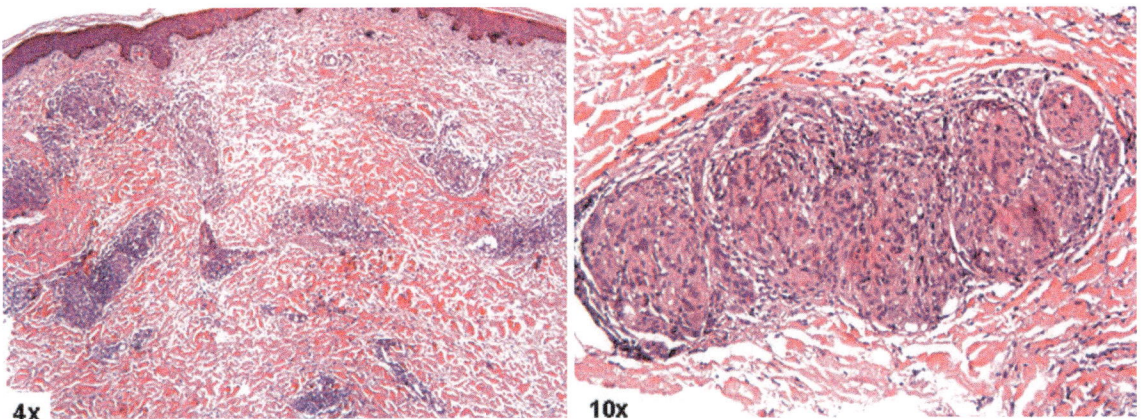

FIG. 37.4. Histology of sarcoidosis. Scanning magnification shows noncaseating granulomas with sparse inflammatory infiltrates in the upper and middle reticular dermis. The higher power magnification is of sarcoid tubercle. (Courtesy of A. Gilliam, MD.)

secondary to deposition of immunoglobulins, complement, and fibrinogen. The presence of caseation should prompt a search for infectious causes.

Both TNF-α and IFN-γ have been associated with granuloma formation.[52,53] It is known that prolonged activation by these cytokines usually leads to apoptosis. However, the characteristic granulomas in sarcoidosis patients are noncaseating. It is unclear why there is the absence of apoptosis in the sarcoid granulomas. Studies have found upregulated expression of an IFN-γ–induced antiapoptotic molecule p21Waf1, a cdk inhibitor, in sarcoidosis patients.[54]

Pathogenesis

Numerous hypotheses have been put forth on the etiology of sarcoidosis, including infectious, autoimmune, and environmental. The etiology and pathogenesis of sarcoidosis is complicated by highly varied disease presentation ranging from single-organ to multisystem involvement, the lack of specific symptomatology, and the waxing and waning nature of the disease. Both the clinical and tissue diagnosis of the disease require exclusion of other conditions such as mycobacterial or deep fungal infections, Wegener's granulomatosus, cancer, and environmental exposures.

A historic test for the diagnosis of sarcoidosis is the Kveim-Siltzbach skin test,[55–57] which was performed by injecting a suspension of sarcoid spleen material intradermally into the skin of a suspected sarcoid patient. The formation of a noncaseating granuloma observed histologically 4 weeks later at the site of injection indicates a positive test. Studies of T cells at the Kveim-Siltzbach reaction sites have demonstrated an oligoclonal population of αβ+ CD4+ T cells, which argues for sarcoidosis as an antigen-driven disease.[58] This is supported by findings of similar oligoclonality, with a dominant V beta bias, in sarcoid lung T cells.[59]

Infectious Etiology. Despite investigations of viral and mycobacterial causes of sarcoidosis, no consistency has been found. Human herpesvirus 8 (HHV-8) was postulated to be associated with sarcoidosis but has been met with many reports of negative findings in sarcoidosis patients worldwide.[60–63] Mycobacterial DNA sequences have been found in various tissues in some sarcoidosis patients, while others report negative findings.[64–67] However, to date no mycobacteria have been successfully cultured.[68]

Recent reports identified mycobacterial catalase-peroxidase (mKatG) as a potential pathogenic antigen in sarcoidosis.[58] Additionally, IgG antibodies to mKatG could be detected in the sera in half the sarcoidosis patients examined. However, the studies were conducted in a small cohort of patients.

Environmental Exposure. Evidence of the role of environmental exposure in the pathogenesis of sarcoidosis comes from reports of a higher incidence of disease in certain occupations, such as firefighters and aircraft carrier personnel.[69,70] Additionally, disease clusters indirectly implicate an environmental etiology.[71] In a recent multicenter case-control study, researchers did not find a single proximate cause. However they reported positive associations with insecticides, an agricultural environment, and microbial bioaerosols such as mold and mildew.[72] Interestingly, a negative association with cigarette smoking was found in the study, consistent with previous reports.[73,74]

Genetic Susceptibility. Numerous searches for genetic susceptibility factors have not yielded consistent results. Several reports have reported disease susceptibility with human leukocyte antigen (HLA) 1, B8, DRB1, and DRB3 alleles.[75] A recent comprehensive review by Ianuzzi and Rybicki[75] discusses the evidence for candidate genes including complement receptor-1 *(CR1)*, heat shock protein A1L *(HSPA1L)*, and genome scans in the genetics of sarcoidosis.

CARD15/NOD2 has been linked to Blau syndrome, a granulomatous disease affecting the eyes, joints, and skin.[76] *CARD15*, expressed by mononuclear phagocytes, encodes *NOD2*, which recognizes a component of bacterial peptidoglycan.[77] The gene has also been associated with inflammatory bowel disease.[78] One report found an association of mutations in *CARD15/NOD2* with early-onset childhood sarcoidosis, a distinct type of sarcoidosis in children younger than 4 years of age characterized by eye, joint, and skin involvement.[79] However, attempts to find an association of *CARD15/NOD2* in adult sarcoidosis have demonstrated no relationship.[75]

Despite several proposals of correlative serum markers, including serum amyloid A and C-reactive protein, no consistent correlations have been demonstrated. Even serum angiotensin-converting enzyme (ACE), initially promising, has not been a consistent marker of disease activity.[80,81] Other markers currently being examined include macrophage inflammatory protein 1 (MIP-1) and vascular endothelial growth factor (VEGF).[82,83]

There are reports of sibling discordance, but also reports finding increased disease relative risk in families.[84,85] No definitive HLA genes have been uniquely established in African-American sarcoidosis patients, a group identified to have a 3.8 times increased annual incidence in the United States. However, recent linkage studies suggest that more than one gene may be involved in disease susceptibility in African Americans.[86]

Immune Regulation. There are numerous lines of research indicating that the involved lymphocytes are of the Th1 phenotype, producing cytokines such as IL-2, IFN-γ, and enhanced TNF-α.[87,88] Findings of hypergammaglobulinemia in sarcoidosis patients led to the question of B-cell involvement in disease pathogenesis. It is now believed that the hypergammaglobulinemia is secondary to IL-2 and IFN-γ stimulation of B cells.[89,90] However, adding to the puzzle of sarcoidosis is that despite activation of networks of proinflammatory cytokines and robust recruitment of cells, there is often an associated state of either complete or partial anergy.[91,92] This is demonstrated by a lack of response to the tuberculin skin test or decreased sensitization to agents such as the contact sensitizer dinitrochlorobenzene (DNCB) seen in up to two thirds of sarcoidosis patients. Explanations offered for the observation of decreased delayed-type hypersensitivity was due to peripheral lymphopenia from sequestering and compartmentalization of T cells into granulomas. However, recent data suggest that sarcoidosis patients have an unusually high number of innate T regulatory (T_{reg}) cells, with constitutive CD25[bright]/CD4[+] cells, both in the peripheral circulation and at the periphery of granulomas.[93] T_{reg}s from sarcoidosis patients demonstrated similar capabilities of suppressing responder cell proliferation as compared to controls. However, the T_{reg}s from sarcoidosis patients inhibited IL-2 but not TNF-α or IFN-γ production by responder cells as compared to normal controls in which all three cytokines were completely inhibited. Since TNF-α is associated with sarcoidosis and granuloma formation, these findings may explain the concurrence of cell activation with a global state of anergy.

It is known that 8% to 21% of patients with common variable immunodeficiency (CVID) develop a granulomatous disease resembling sarcoidosis.[94] Since CVID is not a single entity but rather a heterogeneous syndrome, a retrospective study correlating patients with granulomatous disease and specific immunologic derangement may provide some clues in the pathogenesis of sarcoidosis. Some CVID patients develop hyperproliferation of CD4[+] cells, yet some have increased apoptosis of CD4[+] cells. Sixty percent of patients have a diminished response to T-cell receptor stimulation and expression of CD25, the receptors for IL-2.

Treatment

There are numerous anecdotal and a few case series that discuss the treatment of sarcoidosis. But clinical trials are even fewer. The mainstay sarcoidosis therapy includes all preparations of corticosteroids. Nonconventional therapies include antimalarials, methotrexate, and thalidomide.[95] Biologics aimed at antagonizing TNF-α are currently being studied.[95]

Cutaneous Crohn's Disease

Crohn's disease is characterized by segmental granulomatous inflammation of the intestinal tract. Cutaneous manifestation of the disease occurs in 14% to 44% of patients including pyoderma gangrenosum, erythema nodosum, contiguous oral and perianal disease, and "metastatic" Crohn's disease.[96] The latter is a rare entity that denotes a cutaneous lesion distant from extension or fistula formation from oral, anal, or ostomy sites.

The clinical spectrum of cutaneous manifestation of Crohn's disease is wide and has inconsistent correlation with internal disease activity. Classically, the extragenital skin lesions are dusky erythematous plaques that may develop into ulcers. Histopathologic examination reveals a sarcoid-like epithelial granuloma; however, necrobiosis has been reported.[97,98] Unlike sarcoidosis, there are surrounding lymphocytes.

In a recent retrospective study of 33 cases examining the histologic spectrum of skin lesions in patients with active gastrointestinal disease, the authors found diverse reaction patterns including palisading granulomatous dermatitis, folliculocentric vasculopathy, neutrophilic dermatoses, suppurative and granulomatous panniculitis, nonfolliculocentric vasculopathy, lichenoid granulomatous dermatitis, psoriasis, and epithelioid granulomata.[99] Only one case of "classic" metastatic epithelioid granulomata was observed. To elucidate the etiology of cutaneous Crohn's, the authors further examined the gastrointestinal and corresponding skin specimens for bacterial 16s rRNA. They report no bacterial 16S rRNA, examined by in situ reverse-transcriptase polymerase chain reaction (RT-PCR), in skin lesions while being present in gastrointestinal biopsies, suggesting that bacterial dissemination may not be involved in cutaneous lesions. However, reactivity to bacterial products may play a role in the cutaneous manifestation of Crohn's.

As discussed earlier, polymorphisms in *CARD15/NOD2* have been associated with Crohn's disease.[100] However, the mechanism leading to predisposition of disease is unclear. One hypothesis is that mutation in *CARD15* leads to a defect in the acute inflammatory response to intestinal bacteria, leading to the allowance of materials to breach the gut barrier. The subsequent response to the bacterial products leads to a granulomatous reaction.[101]

Necrobiotic Granuloma

The group of necrobiotic granulomas consists of granuloma annulare (GA), necrobiosis lipoidica diabeticorum (NLD), and rheumatoid nodules. The etiology of the diseases is unknown. The common histologic reaction pattern is palisading granulomas with areas of altered or degenerated connective tissue. Variations such as interstitial granulomatous inflammation can be seen in GA and NLD.

Granuloma Annulare

Granuloma annulare is a benign disorder limited to the skin. There have been many proposed inciting factors such as trauma, insect bites, and viral infection. The association with systemic disease such as diabetes mellitus has been inconsistent. Atypical variants of GA have been described in patients with HIV/AIDS and lymphoma.[102,103] The localized variant is most commonly seen, occurring as annular or arcuate plaques on the hands and arms.[104] It can also involve the extremities and trunk. Other variants described include the generalized, perforating, subcutaneous, and patch form of the disease. On pathology, the recognizable pattern is of palisaded epithelioid histiocytes with a central acellular area of pallor, increased mucin, and altered collagen and elastic fibers (Fig. 37.5A). However, the most common pattern is the infiltrative or interstitial pattern where histiocytes are interspersed between collagen with subtle alteration of the fibers.

The entity annular elastolytic giant cell granuloma is regarded by some as a variant of GA. Lesions are also asymptomatic. On pathology there are foreign-body–type giant cells without a palisading granulomatous inflammation (Fig. 37.5B). There is usually no altered collagen. An elastin stain should show loss of elastic fibers in granulomatous areas.

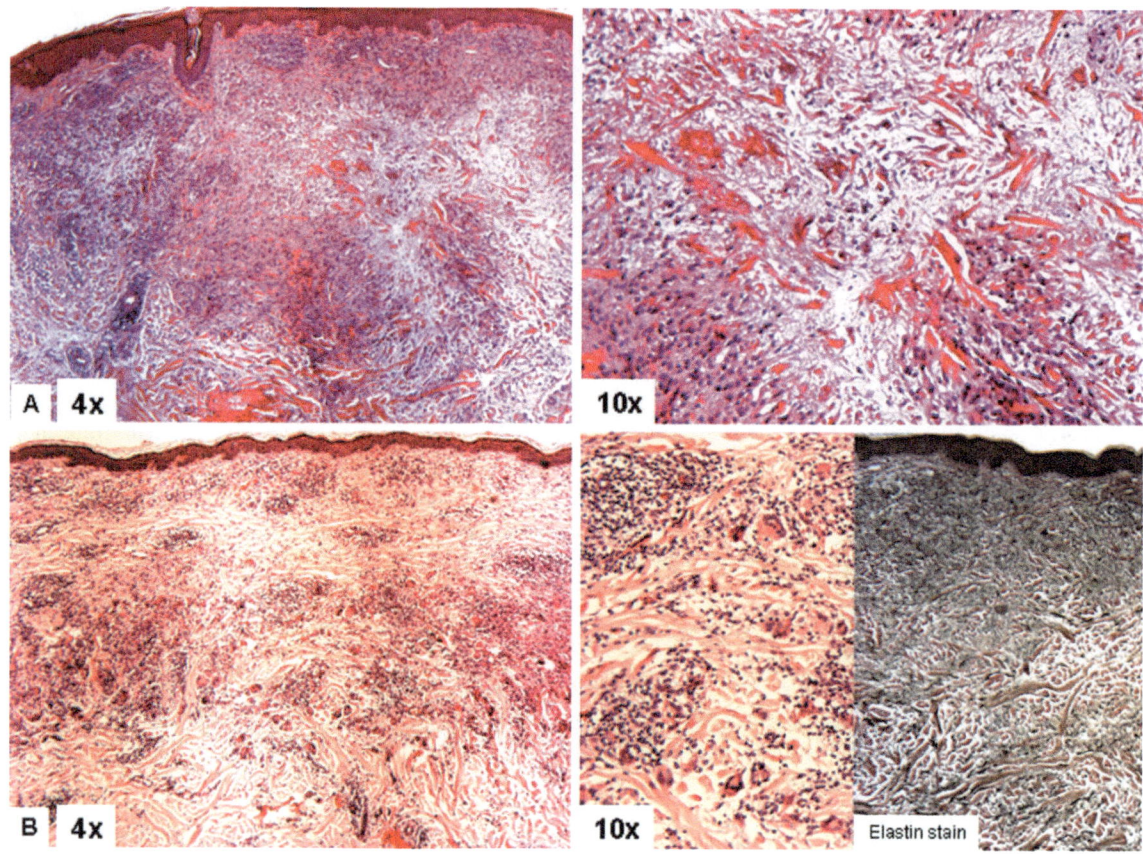

FIG. 37.5. Histology of granuloma annulare (GA) and annular elastolytic giant cell granuloma (AEGCG). (A) Scanning and high-power magnification show palisaded granulomas with abundant mucinous stroma. (B) Scanning and high-power magnification show sun damaged skin with numerous giant cells containing fragmented elastic fibers. (Courtesy of A. Gilliam, MD.)

Rheumatoid Nodules

Rheumatoid nodules can be seen in the clinical setting of adult-type polyarticular rheumatoid arthritis and is a rare feature of rheumatic fever.[105] The history and the context of presentation aid in the diagnosis. The etiology of rheumatoid arthritis (RA) remains unknown. Disease susceptibility is strongly associated with class II region genes, *HLA-DR-RB1*.[106–108]

There is high suspicion that RA is mediated by autoantibodies, specifically by a group that recognizes citrullinated proteins, including the antiperinuclear factor, antikeratin antibodies, and antifilaggrin antibodies.[109] These antibodies are commonly found in the sera and synovial fluid of RA patients.[110] In a small study of 26 patients,

citrullinated proteins were observed in 70% of the rheumatoid nodules.[111]

Citrullination, a posttranslation modification process, has been demonstrated to increase peptide and major histocompatibility complex (MHC) affinity, suggesting that it can modulate immune responses.[112] The enzyme mediating citrullination is peptidylarginine deaminase, found in inflammatory cells including neutrophils, monocytes, and macrophages.[113] Hence, it is tempting to speculate a relation of the Mo/Macs and granulomatous reaction in the skin with citrullination as a potential source of "autoantigens." Recently, T cells recognizing the specific modification of antigens by citrullination was described.[114] It remains to be determined if they are the pathogenic mediators of RA.

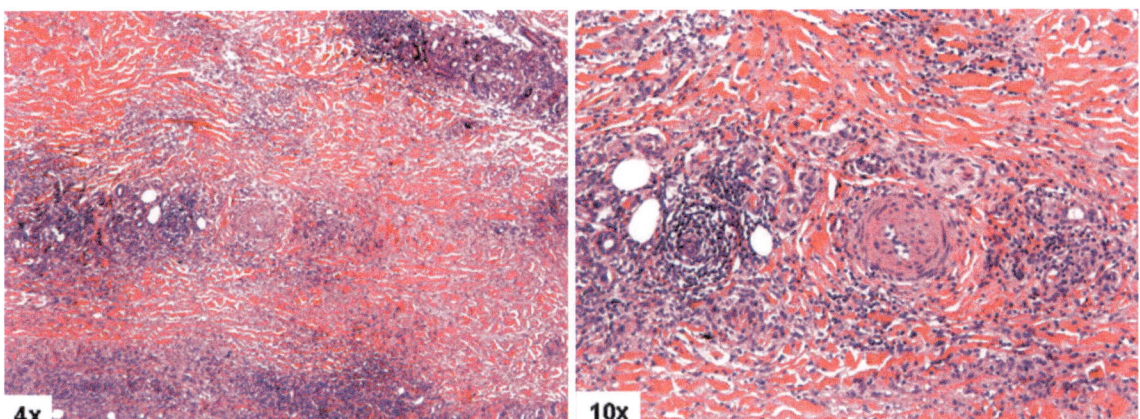

FIG. 37.6. Histology of necrobiosis lipoidica diabeticorum. Scanning magnification shows "layer-cake" architecture of inflammatory granulomas alternating with dense fibrosis. High-power magnification shows a angiocentric granulomatous infiltrate. (Courtesy of A. Gilliam, MD.)

Necrobiosis Lipoidica diabeticorum

Necrobiosis lipoidica diabeticorum was originally described in patients with diabetes, but the demonstration of nondiabetic patients with the condition has led to reconsideration of its name. The disease has a characteristic presentation of asymptomatic yellow-brown plaques involving the pretibial areas. The lesions over time become atrophic with development of telangiectasias. Ulceration can develop; however, the disease is generally benign. On pathology, the "cake layers" of granulomatous inflammation and parallel degenerated collagen is typically seen (Fig. 37.6). The pattern can be palisaded or interstitial.

The etiology of NLD is unknown. Thirty years ago Ullman and Dahl[115] suggested that the disease may be secondary to vasculitis based on findings of immunoglobulin M (IgM) and complement C3 deposition in blood vessels of affected skin. Recently, NLD skin sections were shown to stain for gli-1, a transcription factor in the hedgehog signaling pathway. The significance remains to be seen.

Conclusion

Traditionally, Mo/Macs are simply thought of as phagocytes. Hence that frame of reference prompted investigations with the goal of identifying causal pathogens in granulomatous diseases.

Macrophages are very plastic cells found in most tissues and are responsive to their microenvironment. New understanding of the diverse homeostatic and regulatory functions of the histiocytes (Mo/Macs) should broaden our understanding of this inflammatory response.

Furthermore, diseases with overactive and chronic persistence of Mo/Mac and granulomatous inflammation can be the potential target of liposomes, specific uptake by Mo/Mac, or via targeting their unique receptors such as anti-FcγRII receptor (CD32). However, the degree to which macrophages play a role in promoting lesions and their persistence is not fully understood in some of these diseases. Agents that limit Mo/Mac response may play an important role in understanding the pathophysiology of these dermatoses.

References

1. Dahl M. Clinical Immunodermatology, 3rd ed. St. Louis: Mosby, 1996.
2. Kumar V, Abbas A, Fausto N, eds. Robbins & Cotran Pathologic Basis of Disease. Philadelphia: Elsevier Saunders, 2005:82-83.
3. Lu K, McCormick T, Gillam A, Kang K, Cooper K. Monocytes and macrophages in human skin. In: Bos JD, ed. Skin Immune System, 3rd ed. Boca Raton, FL: CRC Press, 2005.
4. Pluddemann A, Mukhopadhyay S, Gordon S. The interaction of macrophage receptors with bacterial ligands. Expert Rev Mol Med 2006;8:1–25.

5. Akira S, Takeda K, Kaisho T. Toll-like receptors: critical proteins linking innate and acquired immunity. Nat Immunol 2001;2:675–80.

6. Stout RD, Suttles J. Functional plasticity of macrophages: reversible adaptation to changing microenvironments. J Leukoc Biol 2004;76:509–13.

7. Fogg DK, Sibon C, Miled C, et al. A clonogenic bone marrow progenitor specific for macrophages and dendritic cells. Science 2006;311:83–7.

8. Hume DA. The mononuclear phagocyte system. Curr Opin Immunol 2006;18:49–53.

9. Henson PM, Hume DA. Apoptotic cell removal in development and tissue homeostasis. Trends Immunol 2006;27:244–50.

10. Krysko DV, Denecker G, Festjens N, et al. Macrophages use different internalization mechanisms to clear apoptotic and necrotic cells. Cell Death Differ 2006;13:2011–22.

11. Krysko DV, D'Herde K, Vandenabeele P. Clearance of apoptotic and necrotic cells and its immunological consequences. Apoptosis 2006;11:1709–26.

12. Anderson JM. Multinucleated giant cells. Curr Opin Hematol 2000;7:40–7.

13. Gasser A, Most J. Generation of multinucleated giant cells in vitro by culture of human monocytes with Mycobacterium bovis BCG in combination with cytokine-containing supernatants. Infect Immun 1999;67:395–402.

14. Weinberg JB, Hobbs MM, Misukonis MA. Recomhuman gamma-interferon induces human monocyte polykaryon formation. Proc Natl Acad Sci USA 1984;81:4554–7.

15. Vignery A. Macrophage fusion: the making of osteoclasts and giant cells. J Exp Med 2005;202:337–40.

16. Yagi M, Miyamoto T, Sawatani Y, et al. DC-STAMP is essential for cell-cell fusion in osteoclasts and foreign body giant cells. J Exp Med 2005;202:345–51.

17. Kyriakides TR, Foster MJ, Keeney GE, et al. The CC chemokine ligand, CCL2/MCP1, participates in macrophage fusion and foreign body giant cell formation. Am J Pathol 2004;165:2157–66.

18. Zhu XW, Friedland JS. Multinucleate giant cells and the control of chemokine secretion in response to Mycobacterium tuberculosis. Clin Immunol 2006;120:10–20.

19. Sadek MI, Sada E, Toossi Z, Schwander SK, Rich EA. Chemokines induced by infection of mononuclear phagocytes with mycobacteria and present in lung alveoli during active pulmonary tuberculosis. Am J Respir Cell Mol Biol 1998;19:513–21.

20. Kurashima K, Mukaida N, Fujimura M, et al. Elevated chemokine levels in bronchoalveolar lavage fluid of tuberculosis patients. Am J Respir Crit Care Med 1997;155:1474–7.

21. Algood HM, Chan J, Flynn JL. Chemokines and tuberculosis. Cytokine Growth Factor Rev 2003;14:467–77.

22. Bergeron A, Bonay M, Kambouchner M, et al. Cytokine patterns in tuberculous and sarcoid granulomas: correlations with histopathologic features of the granulomatous response. J Immunol 1997;159:3034–43.

23. Salgame P. Host innate and Th1 responses and the bacterial factors that control Mycobacterium tuberculosis infection. Curr Opin Immunol 2005;17:374–80.

24. Feng CG, Scanga CA, Collazo-Custodio CM, et al. Mice lacking myeloid differentiation factor 88 display profound defects in host resistance and immune responses to Mycobacterium avium infection not exhibited by Toll-like receptor 2 (TLR2)- and TLR4-deficient animals. J Immunol 2003;171:4758–64.

25. Scanga CA, Bafica A, Feng CG, Cheever AW, Hieny S, Sher A. MyD88-deficient mice display a profound loss in resistance to Mycobacterium tuberculosis associated with partially impaired Th1 cytokine and nitric oxide synthase 2 expression. Infect Immun 2004;72:2400–4.

26. Layland LE, Wagner H, da Costa CU. Lack of antigen-specific Th1 response alters granuloma formation and composition in Schistosoma mansoni-infected MyD88-/- mice. Eur J Immunol 2005;35:3248–57.

27. Bulut Y, Michelsen KS, Hayrapetian L, et al. Mycobacterium tuberculosis heat shock proteins use diverse Toll-like receptor pathways to activate proinflammatory signals. J Biol Chem 2005;280:20961–7.

28. Cooper AM, Dalton DK, Stewart TA, Griffin JP, Russell DG, Orme IM. Disseminated tuberculosis in interferon gamma gene-disrupted mice. J Exp Med 1993;178:2243–7.

29. Flynn JL, Chan J, Triebold KJ, Dalton DK, Stewart TA, Bloom BR. An essential role for interferon gamma in resistance to Mycobacterium tuberculosis infection. J Exp Med 1993;178:2249–54.

30. Bean AG, Roach DR, Briscoe H, et al. Structural deficiencies in granuloma formation in TNF gene-targeted mice underlie the heightened susceptibility to aerosol Mycobacterium tuberculosis infection, which is not compensated for by lymphotoxin. J Immunol 1999;162:3504–11.

31. Flynn JL, Goldstein MM, Chan J, et al. Tumor necrosis factor-alpha is required in the protective immune response against Mycobacterium tuberculosis in mice. Immunity 1995;2:561–72.

32. Kahnert A, Seiler P, Stein M, et al. Alternative activation deprives macrophages of a coordinated defense program to Mycobacterium tuberculosis. Eur J Immunol 2006;36:631–47.

33. Gronski TJ Jr, Martin RL, Kobayashi DK, et al. Hydrolysis of a broad spectrum of extracellular

matrix proteins by human macrophage elastase. J Biol Chem 1997;272:12189–94.

34. Shipley JM, Wesselschmidt RL, Kobayashi DK, Ley TJ, Shapiro SD. Metalloelastase is required for macrophage-mediated proteolysis and matrix invasion in mice. Proc Natl Acad Sci USA 1996;93:3942–6.

35. Vaalamo M, Kariniemi AL, Shapiro SD, Saarialho-Kere U. Enhanced expression of human metalloelastase (MMP-12) in cutaneous granulomas and macrophage migration. J Invest Dermatol 1999;112:499–505.

36. Orme IM. The mouse as a useful model of tuberculosis. Tuberculosis (Edinb) 2003;83:112–5.

37. Pozos TC, Ramakrishnan L. New models for the study of Mycobacterium-host interactions. Curr Opin Immunol 2004;16:499–505.

38. Davis JM, Clay H, Lewis JL, Ghori N, Herbomel P, Ramakrishnan L. Real-time visualization of mycobacterium-macrophage interactions leading to initiation of granuloma formation in zebrafish embryos. Immunity 2002;17:693–702.

39. Newman LS, Rose CS, Maier LA. Sarcoidosis. N Engl J Med 1997;336:1224–34.

40. Braverman I. In: Freedberg I, Eisen A, Wolff K, Austen K, Goldsmith L, Katz S, eds. Sarcoidosis. Fitzpatrick's Dermatology in General Medicine, 6th ed. New York: McGraw-Hill, 2003:1781.

41. Mana J, Gomez-Vaquero C, Montero A, et al. Lofgren's syndrome revisited: a study of 186 patients. Am J Med 1999;107:240–5.

42. Veien NK, Stahl D, Brodthagen H. Cutaneous sarcoidosis in Caucasians. J Am Acad Dermatol 1987;16:534–40.

43. Hanno R, Needelman A, Eiferman RA, Callen JP. Cutaneous sarcoidal granulomas and the development of systemic sarcoidosis. Arch Dermatol 1981;117:203–7.

44. Mana J, Marcoval J, Graells J, Salazar A, Peyri J, Pujol R. Cutaneous involvement in sarcoidosis. Relationship to systemic disease. Arch Dermatol 1997;133:882–8.

45. Yanardag H, Pamuk ON, Karayel T. Cutaneous involvement in sarcoidosis: analysis of the features in 170 patients. Respir Med 2003;97:978–82.

46. Ahmed I, Harshad SR. Subcutaneous sarcoidosis: is it a specific subset of cutaneous sarcoidosis frequently associated with systemic disease? J Am Acad Dermatol 2006;54:55–60.

47. Mangas C, Fernandez-Figueras MT, Fite E, Fernandez-Chico N, Sabat M, Ferrandiz C. Clinical spectrum and histological analysis of 32 cases of specific cutaneous sarcoidosis. J Cutan Pathol 2006;33:772–7.

48. James DG. Sarcoidosis: milestones to the millennium. Sarcoidosis Vasc Diffuse Lung Dis 1999;16:174–82.

49. Neville E, Mills RG, Jash DK, Mackinnon DM, Carstairs LS, James DG. Sarcoidosis of the upper respiratory tract and its association with lupus pernio. Thorax 1976;31:660–4.

50. Aubart FC, Ouayoun M, Brauner M, et al. Sinonasal involvement in sarcoidosis: a case-control study of 20 patients. Medicine (Baltimore) 2006;85:365–71.

51. Yanardag H, Pamuk ON. Bone cysts in sarcoidosis: what is their clinical significance? Rheumatol Int 2004;24:294–6.

52. Kindler V, Sappino AP, Grau GE, Piguet PF, Vassalli P. The inducing role of tumor necrosis factor in the development of bactericidal granulomas during BCG infection. Cell 1989;56:731–40.

53. Agostini C, Semenzato G. Cytokines in sarcoidosis. Semin Respir Infect 1998;13:184–96.

54. Xaus J, Besalduch N, Comalada M, et al. High expression of p21 Waf1 in sarcoid granulomas: a putative role for long-lasting inflammation. J Leukoc Biol 2003;74:295–301.

55. Teirstein AS. The Kveim-Siltzbach test. Clin Dermatol 1986;4:154–64.

56. James DG, Williams WJ. Kveim-Siltzbach test revisited. Sarcoidosis 1991;8:6–9.

57. Siltzbach LE. The Kveim test in sarcoidosis. A study of 750 patients. JAMA 1961;178:476–82.

58. Song Z, Marzilli L, Greenlee BM, et al. Mycobacterial catalase-peroxidase is a tissue antigen and target of the adaptive immune response in systemic sarcoidosis. J Exp Med 2005;201:755–67.

59. Moller DR, Konishi K, Kirby M, Balbi B, Crystal RG. Bias toward use of a specific T cell receptor beta-chain variable region in a subgroup of individuals with sarcoidosis. J Clin Invest 1988;82:1183–91.

60. Di Alberti L, Piattelli A, Artese L, et al. Human herpesvirus 8 variants in sarcoid tissues. Lancet 1997;350:1655–61.

61. Belec L, Mohamed AS, Lechapt-Zalcman E, Authier FJ, Lange F, Gherardi RK. Lack of HHV-8 DNA sequences in sarcoid tissues of French patients. Chest 1998;114:948–9.

62. Maeda H, Niimi T, Sato S, et al. Human herpesvirus 8 is not associated with sarcoidosis in Japanese patients. Chest 2000;118:923–7.

63. Knoell KA, Hendrix JD, Jr., Stoler MH, Patterson JW, Montes CM. Absence of human herpesvirus 8 in sarcoidosis and Crohn disease granulomas. Arch Dermatol 2005;141:909–10.

64. Saboor SA, Johnson NM, McFadden J. Detection of mycobacterial DNA in sarcoidosis and tuberculosis with polymerase chain reaction. Lancet 1992;339:1012–5.

65. Ikonomopoulos JA, Gorgoulis VG, Zacharatos PV, et al. Multiplex polymerase chain reaction for the

detection of mycobacterial DNA in cases of tuberculosis and sarcoidosis. Mod Pathol 1999;12:854–62.

66. Eishi Y, Suga M, Ishige I, et al. Quantitative analysis of mycobacterial and propionibacterial DNA in lymph nodes of Japanese and European patients with sarcoidosis. J Clin Microbiol 2002;40:198–204.

67. Marcoval J, Benitez MA, Alcaide F, Mana J. Absence of ribosomal RNA of Mycobacterium tuberculosis complex in sarcoidosis. Arch Dermatol 2005;141:57–9.

68. Milman N, Lisby G, Friis S, Kemp L. Prolonged culture for mycobacteria in mediastinal lymph nodes from patients with pulmonary sarcoidosis. A negative study. Sarcoidosis Vasc Diffuse Lung Dis 2004;21:25–8.

69. Prezant DJ, Dhala A, Goldstein A, et al. The incidence, prevalence, and severity of sarcoidosis in New York City firefighters. Chest 1999;116:1183–93.

70. Sarcoidosis among U.S. Navy enlisted me, 1965–1993. MMWR Morb Mortal Wkly Rep 1997;46:539–43.

71. Parkes SA, Baker SB, Bourdillon RE, Murray CR, Rakshit M. Epidemiology of sarcoidosis in the Isle of Man—1: a case controlled study. Thorax 1987;42:420–6.

72. Newman LS, Rose CS, Bresnitz EA, et al. A case control etiologic study of sarcoidosis: environmental and occupational risk factors. Am J Respir Crit Care Med 2004;170:1324–30.

73. Valeyre D, Soler P, Clerici C, et al. Smoking and pulmonary sarcoidosis: effect of cigarette smoking on prevalence, clinical manifestations, alveolitis, and evolution of the disease. Thorax 1988;43:516–24.

74. Douglas JG, Middleton WG, Gaddie J, et al. Sarcoidosis: a disorder commoner in non-smokers? Thorax 1986;41:787–91.

75. Ianuzzi MC, Rybicki BA. Genetics of sarcoidosis: candidate genes and genome scans. Proc Am Thorac Soc 2007;4:108–16.

76. Miceli-Richard C, Lesage S, Rybojad M, et al. CARD15 mutations in Blau syndrome. Nat Genet 2001;29:19–20.

77. Inohara N, Ogura Y, Fontalba A, et al. Host recognition of bacterial muramyl dipeptide mediated through NOD2. Implications for Crohn's disease. J Biol Chem 2003;278:5509–12.

78. Hugot JP, Chamaillard M, Zouali H, et al. Association of NOD2 leucine-rich repeat variants with susceptibility to Crohn's disease. Nature 2001;411:599–603.

79. Kanazawa N, Okafuji I, Kambe N, et al. Early-onset sarcoidosis and CARD15 mutations with constitutive nuclear factor-kappaB activation: common genetic etiology with Blau syndrome. Blood 2005;105:1195–7.

80. Rybicki BA, Maliarik MJ, Poisson LM, Iannuzzi MC. Sarcoidosis and granuloma genes: a family-based study in African-Americans. Eur Respir J 2004;24:251–7.

81. Thomas KW, Hunninghake GW. Sarcoidosis. JAMA 2003;289:3300–3.

82. Capelli A, Di Stefano A, Lusuardi M, Gnemmi I, Donner CF. Increased macrophage inflammatory protein-1alpha and macrophage inflammatory protein-1beta levels in bronchoalveolar lavage fluid of patients affected by different stages of pulmonary sarcoidosis. Am J Respir Crit Care Med 2002;165:236–41.

83. Morohashi K, Takada T, Omori K, Suzuki E, Gejyo F. Vascular endothelial growth factor gene polymorphisms in Japanese patients with sarcoidosis. Chest 2003;123:1520–6.

84. Rybicki BA, Hirst K, Iyengar SK, et al. A sarcoidosis genetic linkage consortium: the sarcoidosis genetic analysis (SAGA) study. Sarcoidosis Vasc Diffuse Lung Dis 2005;22:115–22.

85. Judson MA, Hirst K, Iyengar SK, et al. Comparison of sarcoidosis phenotypes among affected African-American siblings. Chest 2006;130:855–62.

86. Iannuzzi MC, Iyengar SK, Gray-McGuire C, et al. Genome-wide search for sarcoidosis susceptibility genes in African Americans. Genes Immun 2005;6:509–18.

87. Moller DR. Cells and cytokines involved in the pathogenesis of sarcoidosis. Sarcoidosis Vasc Diffuse Lung Dis 1999;16:24–31.

88. Robinson BW, McLemore TL, Crystal RG. Gamma interferon is spontaneously released by alveolar macrophages and lung T lymphocytes in patients with pulmonary sarcoidosis. J Clin Invest 1985;75:1488–95.

89. Tannenbaum H, Rocklin RE, Schur PH, Sheffer AL. Immune function in sarcoidosis. Studies on delayed hypersensitivity, B and T lymphocytes, serum immunoglobulins and serum complement components. Clin Exp Immunol 1976;26:511–9.

90. Kataria YP, Holter JF. Immunology of sarcoidosis. Clin Chest Med 1997;18:719–39.

91. Cosemans J, Louwagie AC. Tuberculin and DNCB skin tests and in vitro lymphocyte transformation in patients with sarcoidosis. Acta Clin Belg 1979;34:353–9.

92. Morell F, Levy G, Orriols R, Ferrer J, De Gracia J, Sampol G. Delayed cutaneous hypersensitivity tests and lymphopenia as activity markers in sarcoidosis. Chest 2002;121:1239–44.

93. Miyara M, Amoura Z, Parizot C, et al. The immune paradox of sarcoidosis and regulatory T cells. J Exp Med 2006;203:359–70.

94. Knight AK, Cunningham-Rundles C. Inflammatory and autoimmune complications of common variable immune deficiency. Autoimmun Rev 2006;5:156–9.

95. Baughman RP, Lower EE. Newer therapies for cutaneous sarcoidosis: the role of thalidomide and other agents. Am J Clin Dermatol 2004;5:385–94.

96. Burgdorf W. Cutaneous manifestations of Crohn's disease. J Am Acad Dermatol 1981;5:689–95.

97. Witkowski JA, Parish LC, Lewis JE. Crohn's disease—non-caseating granulomas on the legs. Acta Derm Venereol 1977;57:181–3.

98. Hackzell-Bradley M, Hedblad MA, Stephansson EA. Metastatic Crohn's disease. Report of 3 cases with special reference to histopathologic findings. Arch Dermatol 1996;132:928–32.

99. Crowson AN, Nuovo GJ, Mihm MC, Jr., Magro C. Cutaneous manifestations of Crohn's disease, its spectrum, and its pathogenesis: intracellular consensus bacterial 16S rRNA is associated with the gastrointestinal but not the cutaneous manifestations of Crohn's disease. Hum Pathol 2003;34:1185–92.

100. Ogura Y, Bonen DK, Inohara N, et al. A frameshift mutation in NOD2 associated with susceptibility to Crohn's disease. Nature 2001;411:603–6.

101. Marks DJ, Harbord MW, MacAllister R, et al. Defective acute inflammation in Crohn's disease: a clinical investigation. Lancet 2006;367:668–78.

102. Toro JR, Chu P, Yen TS, LeBoit PE. Granuloma annulare and human immunodeficiency virus infection. Arch Dermatol 1999;135:1341–6.

103. Li A, Hogan DJ, Sanusi ID, Smoller BR. Granuloma annulare and malignant neoplasms. Am J Dermatopathol 2003;25:113–6.

104. Muhlbauer JE. Granuloma annulare. J Am Acad Dermatol 1980;3:217–30.

105. Stollerman GH. Rheumatic fever. Lancet 1997;349:935–42.

106. Liu SC, Chang TY, Lee YJ, et al. Influence of HLA-DRB1 genes and the shared epitope on genetic susceptibility to rheumatoid arthritis in Taiwanese. J Rheumatol 2007.

107. Wordsworth BP, Lanchbury JS, Sakkas LI, Welsh KI, Panayi GS, Bell JI. HLA-DR4 subtype frequencies in rheumatoid arthritis indicate that DRB1 is the major susceptibility locus within the HLA class II region. Proc Natl Acad Sci USA 1989;86:10049–53.

108. Moreno I, Valenzuela A, Garcia A, Yelamos J, Sanchez B, Hernanz W. Association of the shared epitope with radiological severity of rheumatoid arthritis. J Rheumatol 1996;23:6–9.

109. De Rycke L, Peene I, Hoffman IE, et al. Rheumatoid factor and anticitrullinated protein antibodies in rheumatoid arthritis: diagnostic value, associations with radiological progression rate, and extra-articular manifestations. Ann Rheum Dis 2004;63:1587–93.

110. Schellekens GA, Visser H, de Jong BA, et al. The diagnostic properties of rheumatoid arthritis antibodies recognizing a cyclic citrullinated peptide. Arthritis Rheum 2000;43:155–63.

111. Bongartz T, Cantaert T, Atkins SR, et al. Citrullination in extra-articular manifestations of rheumatoid arthritis. Rheumatology (Oxford) 2007;46:70–5.

112. Hill JA, Southwood S, Sette A, Jevnikar AM, Bell DA, Cairns E. Cutting edge: the conversion of arginine to citrulline allows for a high-affinity peptide interaction with the rheumatoid arthritis-associated HLA-DRB1*0401 MHC class II molecule. J Immunol 2003;171:538–41.

113. Vossenaar ER, Radstake TR, van der Heijden A, et al. Expression and activity of citrullinating peptidylarginine deiminase enzymes in monocytes and macrophages. Ann Rheum Dis 2004;63:373–81.

114. Ireland J, Herzog J, Unanue ER. Cutting edge: unique T cells that recognize citrullinated peptides are a feature of protein immunization. J Immunol 2006;177:1421–5.

115. Ullman S, Dahl MV. Necrobiosis lipoidica. An immunofluorescence study. Arch Dermatol 1977;113:1671–3.

38
Vitiligo Vulgaris

James J. Nordlund, I. Caroline Le Poole, and Raymond E. Boissy

Key Points

- Vitiligo vulgaris is defined as an idiopathic, acquired type of leukoderma manifested by depigmentation of the epidermis resulting from destruction of melanocytes.
- Vitiligo usually affects interfollicular melanocytes and spares follicular melanocytes, but both types can be destroyed in severe cases.
- Early vitiligo results in hypopigmentation, that is, tri- or pentachrome vitiligo, but advanced vitiligo causes depigmentation.
- In vitiligo certain sets of genes render the melanocyte fragile and susceptible to undergoing apoptosis.
- The genetic basis for vitiligo is multifactorial.
- Medical therapies for vitiligo involve ultraviolet radiation or topical medications, for example, steroids or immunomodulators.
- Surgical treatment for vitiligo involves grafting of autologous skin.

Vitiligo vulgaris is a common disorder described in ancient texts from many civilizations.[1] Vitiligo, like many other cutaneous disorders, is not fatal and causes no biologic disabilities. However, it does cause significant morbidity from the disfigurement.[2–8] The earliest peoples found ways to treat loss of skin color with a variety of plants[9] and potions[10] because of the detrimental impact of depigmentation on people, especially those with darker skin color. In addition the depigmented skin has altered physiologic responses.[11,12] The alteration in function is understandable in light of the complex interactions of the three main cells of the epidermis: keratinocytes, Langerhans' cells, and melanocytes.[13] Vitiligo is an important disorder to study and understand for all the insights it can give us into the complexities of the epidermis.[14,15]

Definition and Some Enigmas About Vitiligo

Vitiligo vulgaris is defined as an idiopathic, acquired type of leukoderma manifested by depigmentation of the epidermis resulting from destruction of melanocytes.[16] Usually vitiligo affects interfollicular melanocytes and spares follicular melanocytes, although in some patients both types of melanocytes are destroyed. When the destruction of melanocytes begins, the skin can be hypopigmented (i.e., partial loss of melanocytes) called tri- or pentachrome vitiligo.[17,18] As vitiligo progresses, it causes depigmentation or total loss of melanocytes. Clinically the depigmentation can be focal, unilateral/segmental, or bilateral and widespread. The macules can be small or coalesce into large areas of white skin. Occasionally the entire integument is depigmented or almost depigmented. This advanced stage is called total vitiligo. The epidermis is normal in all respects except for loss of pigmentation.

One persisting enigma about vitiligo is whether it is purely a skin disorder or a disorder of the pigmentary system scattered throughout the body. (For review of the pigmentary system, see Nordlund et al.[19]) There are pigment cells in eyes, within the choroid and in the retinal pigment epithelium.[20]

There are other pigment cells in the ears[20] and in the leptomeninges overlying the medulla oblongata.[21] Results of some studies indicate the pigment cells of the eyes in humans with vitiligo and in a mouse and chicken vitiligo model can be involved, at least subclinically.[22–30] The Vogt-Koyanagi-Harada and Alezzandrini syndromes might be manifestations of vitiligo with clinically apparent eye involvement.[23,31–34] Although there is no consensus on this point, these authors propose that vitiligo is a systemic disorder of all melanocytes extant in any organ.

A second question relates to whether vitiligo vulgaris and chemical leukoderma are the same or different disorders. It is clear that some chemicals such as monobenzone can induce depigmentation and destruction of melanocytes in some individuals.[35–38] There are many phenolic chemicals in foods, beverages, and plants that might be melanocytotoxic and cause leukoderma. One might postulate that all vitiligo is a manifestation of chemical depigmentation, but the source of the inciting chemical is unknown. At this time, there is no way to determine whether vitiligo and chemical leukoderma are the same or different disorders (see Chemical Melanocytotoxins, below).

A third issue relates to halo nevi. These are moles or nevocellular nevi composed of melanocytes that acquired a depigmented halo.[39] The mole typically involutes and disappears and the white patch repigments. It has been suggested halo nevi are a type of vitiligo.[28,40] However, halo nevi are common in younger individuals, as many as a third of younger individuals having one or more halo nevi.[41] There are individuals with 10 or more halo nevi. Depigmentation in these individuals is limited to the skin around the nevus. Almost invariably the skin regains its normal color and the white spots disappear. There is no progressive or widespread depigmentation. On reconsideration,[28] it seems more likely that halo nevi are a phenomenon unrelated to vitiligo.[39]

A fourth issue involves follicular melanocytes. It has been suggested that the premature graying or whitening of the hair is a form of vitiligo.[27,42] There are families in which the parents and siblings acquire totally white hair at an early age, before the age of 40 years or earlier. These individuals have no pigmentary changes in the skin. It is now clear that white hair is a manifestation of loss of melanocytes from the outer root sheath and bulge area as well as from the hair bulb.[43,44] The loss of melanocytes occurs naturally as a function of age, although it probably has a genetic origin. Follicular melanocytes have a different morphology and different surface antigens compared to interfollicular melanocytes. It seems unlikely that early whitening of hair represents destruction of the follicular melanocytes by a process that is identical to that which destroys interfollicular melanocytes in vitiligo. However, until the mechanisms for vitiligo and whitening of hair are identified, this remains an unresolved question.

A fifth enigma relates to the depigmentation associated with melanoma. It is well recognized that metastatic melanoma is associated with depigmentation.[39,45–53] The depigmentation typically is located on the chest, shoulders, and upper part of the back.[39] The distribution is markedly different from that of classic vitiligo vulgaris, which typically spares the back. It seems that this type of depigmentation is associated with a prolonged survival in those with metastatic melanoma,[53] a notoriously progressive disease. Various forms of immunotherapy using killed melanoma cells or extracts prepared for treatment of those with metastatic melanoma produce depigmentation in the recipients.[54–61] It appears there are either anti–melanocyte/melanoma antibodies, cytotoxic T cells, or both induced by the immunization with the vaccines (see Role of Melanocytes Within the Skin Immune System, below). Immunization with melanoma cells probably induces a direct attack against the melanocytes causing necrosis of the cell. In vitiligo it has been suggested the melanocyte destruction occurs by apoptosis.[38] It might be that depigmentation associated with melanoma is similar, but not identical, to that of vitiligo vulgaris.

Thus vitiligo is a form of depigmentation caused by destruction of melanocytes and seems to involve melanocytes in all parts of the pigment system—skin, eyes, ears, and possibly meninges. The etiology is unknown but seems to have a genetic basis, as discussed later. How similar its cause is to the processes involved in other forms of depigmentation such as chemical leukoderma and depigmentation of metastatic melanoma is uncertain.

General Characteristics of Vitiligo

Vitiligo vulgaris in its various forms has been observed in all regions of the world. It is thought that vitiligo affects all ethnic groups with the same frequency, about 0.5%, or 1 per 200 individuals.[62–65] Those with darker skin color have a more obvious cosmetic defect than those of European ancestry with very light complexions. Even those with the lightest skin are distressed to some degree by the loss of color, but the social implications are less for them. Vitiligo is a young person's disorder. It begins before the age of 20 years in about half of those afflicted and by age of 40 years in 95% of patients.[66]

After its onset, vitiligo can exhibit various degrees of hypopigmentation until all the melanocytes are destroyed. At that point the skin is white. The partial loss of color has been called trichrome or even pentachrome vitiligo.[17,18,67] It is important to emphasize that the melanocytes are destroyed and not merely functionally abnormal (see Immunohistology of Vitiligo Skin, below). Were the melanocytes present, treatment options would be more numerous and there would be no need for a melanocyte reservoir[68,69] as a prerequisite for success with medical therapies. Surgical grafting techniques would be unnecessary.

Rarely as vitiligo begins or spreads, it can produce clinical signs of inflammation such as erythema and scaling.[33,70] This phenomenon is called inflammatory vitiligo. The epidermis is otherwise normal. Depigmented epidermis showing signs of atrophy, injury, inflammation, or other processes typically is a manifestation of some other disorder affecting the skin.

Vitiligo, as with other skin disorders, exhibits the isomorphic response, also called the Koebner phenomenon. Minor injuries to the epidermis can result in depigmentation at the site of injury. Scratches, abrasions, surgical scars, burns of any type, or cosmetic procedures such as dermabrasions can spread the depigmentation.[71–73] The normal appearing skin of a patient with vitiligo is not truly normal. Histologic studies show that the normal-appearing skin has subtle morphologic aberrations (see Electron Microscopy and Apoptosis, below).[74] Minor injuries amplify the trivial abnormalities into destruction of melanocytes.

Types of Vitiligo

There are three types of vitiligo: focal, unilateral (segmental), and bilateral (generalized). They all are characterized by depigmentation. Each has a unique clinical course and response to therapy.

Focal Vitiligo

Focal vitiligo is defined as depigmentation confined to a few macules scattered randomly on the integument (Fig. 38.1). It has two possible outcomes. For some fortunate individuals, the depigmentation remains localized to these few spots—a limited form of vitiligo. These individuals respond to either medical or, at times, surgical treatments as described later. For those less fortunate, focal vitiligo can be the presenting manifestation for generalized vitiligo. Then it tends to be progressive over the years, causing significant cosmetic problems.

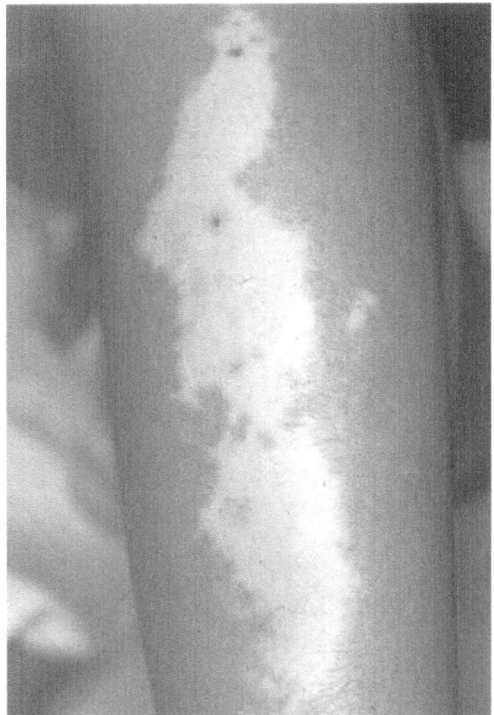

FIG. 38.1. Tibial surface of a woman who developed depigmentation spontaneously as a teenager. It remained localized until her adult years. The area was repigmented with surgical grafting because all hair in the area was white

Unilateral (Segmental) Vitiligo

The second type is unilateral vitiligo more commonly labeled segmental vitiligo (Fig. 38.2). The term *segmental vitiligo* has misleading connotations. Many observers equate segmental with dermatomal. Unilateral vitiligo is almost never distributed in a pattern consistent with one or several dermatomes. Rather the patterns of depigmentation involve small to larger areas of skin on one side of the body. The patterns are repetitious from patient to patient.[75,76] Often the patterns of unilateral vitiligo resemble those seen in nevus depigmentosus, suggesting that melanocytes during embryogenesis have specific developmental patterns. Unilateral vitiligo does not follow Blaschko's lines.

The clinical course of segmental vitiligo is different from that of generalized vitiligo. Unilateral, segmental vitiligo seems to affect children more often than adults.[77] After onset, the depigmentation spreads for 1 to 2 years only within the involved segment. The activity of the disease then stops. There are very rare patients with unilateral vitiligo who later develop bilateral vitiligo.

If the white skin is located on the trunk or covered skin, the cosmetic defect is minimal or at least can be covered by clothing. Typically generalized vitiligo vulgaris affects only interfollicular melanocytes and the hairs remain pigmented. In contrast, in about half of those with unilateral vitiligo, both interfollicular and follicular melanocytes are destroyed. The hairs within the patch are white, an indication that the melanocyte reservoir has been destroyed. The loss of the follicular melanocytes has critical implications for response to medical or surgical therapies as discussed later. Because of the limited progression of unilateral vitiligo, it tends to be easier to treat successfully and permanently.

Acrofacial and Generalized Vitiligo

The third type of vitiligo is the most common (Fig. 38.3). It is a generalized form that begins typically on the fingers and the feet, and around the mouth and eyes.[12,78] At this stage it is called acrofacial vitiligo. Typically it spreads to involve the arms, neck, chest, genitalia, knees, and legs. It often spares the back or involves only a small area over the sacral spines. This type of vitiligo can begin at any age and is seen in young children ages 3 or 4 years, teenagers, young adults, or mature adults. It begins occasionally in later life, as late as 70 years.

After onset, the disorder progresses slowly and intermittently for many years. It spreads to affect large areas on the face, neck, dorsal and ventral forearms, axillae, inner thighs, and knees. The patient can be severely disfigured. Occasionally it affects the entire integument, in which case it is called total vitiligo. In one sense total vitiligo is a desirable end point. The disfigurement is caused by the skin having two or more skin colors. Patients with total vitiligo have only one color—white. Having one color is usually better than having two or more. At times therapy is directed at spreading the vitiligo by removal of residual normal color

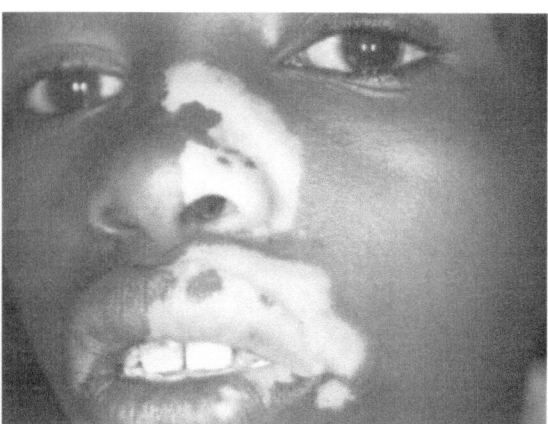

FIG. 38.2. Unilateral vitiligo in an African boy. Note the pattern does not correspond to a dermatome

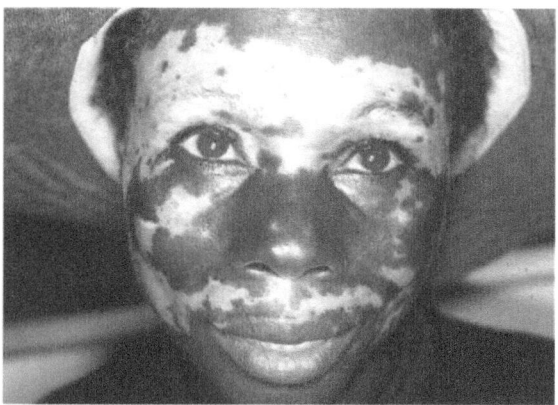

FIG. 38.3. Typical appearance of a man with generalized vitiligo affecting the skin around the eyes, nares, and mouth, and the chest and hands

(see Medical Therapies, below). Rarely the depigmentation spontaneously spreads so rapidly that within months or a year virtually the entire integument and all body hair turn white.

The bilateral type of vitiligo is most difficult to treat for several reasons. First, it affects glabrous skin, which is epidermis that is devoid of hair follicles such as the dorsum of the fingers, the ventral surface of the wrist, the lips, the genitalia, and the feet. Such skin has no melanocyte reservoir for repigmentation. This skin cannot respond to medical treatment and remains visible and depigmented for the entire life of the individual.

Second, generalized vitiligo can become quiescent and respond well to medical therapies. However, at later times it reactivates and the repigmented skin loses its color. The loss of pigment a second or third time is disheartening for the patients, especially those who are teenagers or young adults at a critical time in their social development.

Functional Alterations in Depigmented Skin

The epidermis has three main cell types and smaller populations of other cells such as Merkel cells and indeterminate cells. The melanocyte interacts with the keratinocytes and Langerhans' cells in many ways.[13] It seems that loss of the melanocyte does have implications for the function of the epidermis.[11]

Skin Cancer

Melanomas cannot arise in skin depigmented by vitiligo because melanomas are cancers of melanocytes. Individuals with vitiligo can get melanomas in their normal-appearing skin.[53] It is not known whether patients with vitiligo are more or less susceptible to development of melanoma. In contrast, patients with vitiligo can develop nonmelanoma skin cancer.[12,79] However, this seems to be a rare event, with very few such cancers having been reported.[12,80,81] There have been several studies on the prevalence of sun damage in depigmented skin. The incidence and degree of sun damage are also less in depigmented skin even in those who have had intense exposure either to natural sunlight or

have been treated with psoralen plus ultraviolet A (PUVA), a recognized carcinogen.[80–84] In contrast albinos, in particular those with oculocutaneous albinism type 2, have a high incidence of nonmelanoma skin cancer, mostly squamous cell carcinomas and a few basal cell carcinomas.[85–89] Melanomas are rare in albinos, although a few have been reported.[89–92] It is not clear why the depigmented skin of vitiligo is resistant to malignant transformation or even actinic damage. There are no reports on PubMed of patients with piebaldism developing nonmelanoma skin cancer. The mechanisms by which vitiliginous or albino skin have altered susceptibility to various types of skin cancer is not known.

Alterations in the Immune and Inflammatory Response

Several investigators have studied the response of depigmented skin to irritants such as anthralin.[93,94] It was noted that there were more granulocytes and monocytes in depigmented skin than in normal-appearing skin.[94] This suggests that loss of the melanocyte alters the response of the skin to irritants.

Alterations in cutaneous reactivity to contact allergens in depigmented skin has been noted in mice many years ago.[95] A mouse model for vitiligo was later identified.[96] These mice have a mutation in the *MITF* gene[97] called a mi^{vit}/mi^{vit} mutation. They are born with an almost black pelage and a piebald band on their thorax. As their fur advances through the stages of molting, the fur and epidermis become progressively more white. The cause is a loss of melanocytes within the epidermis and hair follicles.[26] The number of Langerhans' cells remains constant.[98] These mice lose their response to contact allergens such as dinitrofluorobenzene (DNFB) as their skin depigments. However, they retain their ability to respond to antigens injected into the dermis.[99] In vitro the Langerhans' cells exhibited normal functionality. These animals have a highly muted ability to express intercellular adhesion molecule 1 (ICAM-1).[100] The loss of epidermal immune responsiveness with maintenance of dermal immune reactivity supports the concept that melanocytes are involved in the epidermal immune response (see Role of Melanocytes Within the Skin Immune System, below).

Monobenzone is a medication used to depigment individuals with vitiligo too extensive to repigment.[37] It has been observed that some individuals with vitiligo develop a contact allergy to this molecule. Of interest, an inflammatory dermatitis is exhibited only in the pigmented, normal-appearing skin.[101] There have been several studies done to measure the contact reactivity of depigmented skin in human subjects with vitiligo.[102,103] In both of these studies the reaction to DNFB was muted in depigmented skin, although reactivity to candida antigens injected into the dermis was normal. The investigators found the number of Langerhans' cells were normal. These findings are similar to those observed in the vitiligo mouse model. The results suggest that either the Langerhans' cells are functionally abnormal in depigmented skin or that the melanocytes are involved in allergic reactions. In the vitiligo mice Langerhans' cells function normally.[100] It seems likely that melanocytes interacting with Langerhans' cells are involved in cutaneous immunity (see Role of Melanocytes Within the Skin Immune System, below).[13]

Various inflammatory conditions such as lichen planus and psoriasis affecting individuals with vitiligo can spare the depigmented skin or at other times affect it exclusively.[11,104–122] Dermatitis herpetiformis has been associated with vitiligo[123–128] and was noted to preferentially affect the depigmented skin.

Clinical Studies on the Epidemiology of Vitiligo and Familial Patterns of Inheritance

Vitiligo affects individuals of all ethnic backgrounds. It is commonly thought to affect about 1% to 2% of the population.[65] However, this is probably a significant overestimate, and the prevalence is more likely to be about 0.5%, or 1 per 200 individuals.[62,64,129] The prevalence in small localities can be much higher, as high as 8%.[130] The prevalence is higher in older populations because the onset typically is during childhood or early adulthood, before the age of 40 years. Although more women than men consult physicians about their vitiligo, vitiligo seems to affect males and females equally.[131,132]

Vitiligo aggregates within families. Its patterns of distribution within a kinship are not consistent with a single gene disorder whether that be autosomal dominant or recessive. Rather, vitiligo seems to exhibit multilocus recessivity, possibly involving three different genes.[131–133] Thus within the primary kinship the prevalence of vitiligo averages about 7%, or 1 in 14, a significant increase over the population at large. A number of genes that seem to be involved in causing vitiligo have been identified (see Genetic Basis for Vitiligo, below).

Therapy for Vitiligo

The Importance of the Melanocyte Reservoir

The depigmentation characteristic of vitiligo is a result of the destruction of melanocytes.[16] To regain pigmentation, it is necessary to replace the melanocytes from a reservoir. Melanocytes within the outer root sheath or bulge area of the hair follicle are the major reservoir.[68,69,134,135] Skin responding to therapy exhibits freckles emanating from the follicular orifices.[12] Glabrous (smooth, hairless) skin or depigmented skin with white hairs cannot repigment with medical therapies because they lack a reservoir from which melanocytes can repopulate the depigmented skin. The dorsum of the fingers, the ventral surface of the wrists, the feet, the toes, the lower ankles, the genitalia, and the lips are glabrous. Such skin must have the reservoir replaced by surgical grafting.[136,137] Segmental vitiligo causes destruction of follicular melanocytes in about 50% of those affected. These areas also must be treated with grafting. Because it has a limited time course, individuals with localized or unilateral vitiligo are excellent candidates for surgical grafting.[138,139]

Medical Therapies

Medical therapies have two components: ultraviolet radiation and one of various topical medications. Ultraviolet radiation is the most potent stimulant of melanocyte proliferation. The best available source is natural sunlight. Artificial lights are commonly used to control the dose of light the patient receives to avoid burning and causing the isomorphic response. The causes of vitiligo are not known. There are two popular hypotheses: an intrinsic melanocyte defect and an external immune attack. These are not mutually exclusive theories.[140] All of the treatments employed alter and suppress immunity, and their value in reversing an immune mechanism is apparent. It is less clear how they might be effective if there is an intrinsic melanocyte defect.

Psoralen plus ultraviolet A has been the traditional source of ultraviolet radiation.[141–147] It is effective in many patients. In recent years the recognition that PUVA is followed by development of various skin cancers including melanomas has made it a less popular treatment.[79,80,148–150] More recently narrow band UVB (spectrum of 310 to 314 nm) has become popular and is thought to be as effective as PUVA.[151–160] It can be delivered either by laser or fluorescent bulbs. Narrow-band UVB does not require a photosensitizing medication such as psoralen. Thus it is cheaper and easier to deliver.

Topical medications are usually combined with phototherapy for optimal results.[159] Topical therapies include topical steroids, immunomodulators such as tacrolimus* (Protopic) or pimecrolimus* (Elidel), and vitamin D* analogues. Other topical agents have been proposed but have not been shown to be effective.[161,162]

Topical steroids* are especially useful.[163,164] They can be used safely for children and adults.[165–168] Often they are combined with other medications such as tacrolimus* or pimecrolimus*.[169–177] Steroids have been combined with analogues of vitamin D (Dovonex)* with success.[178,179] (For detailed information about treatment, see Nordlund and Ortonne[12] and Hann and Nordlund.[180]) Unilateral vitiligo is a self-limiting disorder, and patients usually are successfully treated by either medical or surgical treatments. In contrast, bilateral generalized vitiligo tends to progress over time. Patients who regain some or much pigmentation often lose it at a later time.

Some patients have very widespread vitiligo that is not amenable to repigmentation. For these patients, removal of the remaining pigmentation by applications of monobenzone (Benoquin) is the treatment of choice. It takes a long time, up to a year to two, but patients achieve a single color and invariably are delighted with the final results.[37,101,164,181]

*This drug has not been approved for this purpose by the Food and Drug Administration at the time of publication.

Surgical Therapies for Vitiligo

Grafting of autologous skin is an excellent therapy for those with focal, unilateral, or quiescent bilateral vitiligo. There are many techniques by which melanocytes can be transferred from one site to another. The number of individuals for whom grafting is indicated is small.[71–73,139,182–187] For a review of surgical techniques, see Halder and Nordlund[137] and Hann and Nordlund.[180]

Histologic Studies

Routine Studies

Many studies have been done on skin from patients with vitiligo. Specimens from the depigmented, normal-appearing and border skin have been studied with a variety of techniques for light and electron microscopy.[74,188–200] The original studies were done on tissues stained with hematoxylin and eosin. The depigmented and normal-appearing skin show few pathologic changes. There is a sprinkling of lymphocytes at the border of the lesions.[190,194] Subsequent studies were done with melanin stains, usually the Fontana Masson technique. The depigmented skin was devoid of both melanin and basilar dendritic cells containing melanin, an observation suggesting loss of all melanocytes. The border skin had partial loss of melanin. Subsequently dopa oxidase stains were done. Dopa oxidase is specific for cells that are synthesizing melanin. None or very few were found in the depigmented skin.[201] Other histochemical stains have been used to distinguish the melanocytes from Langerhans' cells. The conclusion of all of these studies was that the melanocytes were absent from depigmented skin.

Other physiologic data support this conclusion very strongly. It is possible to culture melanocytes from individuals with vitiligo.[202] Attempts to culture melanocytes from depigmented vitiliginous skin have failed, an indication the melanocytes were not present (R. Boissy, personal communication). Therapy of vitiliginous skin provides additional support for this concept of melanocyte destruction. Depigmented glabrous skin or depigmented skin with white hair does not respond to medical therapies but responds readily to surgical transplantation (see The Importance of the Melanocyte Reservoir, above).[12] The observations confirm that melanocytes are absent from the depigmented skin.

Immunohistology of Vitiligo Skin

In recent years, more advanced studies have been done using immunostaining to document the face of melanocytes and to identify the sparse infiltrating cells found at the border of depigmented and normal-appearing skin. Loss of melanocytes in lesional skin is supported by immunostaining of skin cryosections using antibodies reactive in part with markers independent of melanin synthesis.[203] Melanocytes normally express high levels of the antiapoptotic molecule Bcl-2. Depigmented skin shows a few cells or no cells with Bcl-2, thereby confirming that there is an absence of melanocytes.[204]

There are a number of mechanisms whereby melanocytes can be removed or destroyed, leaving the skin depigmented. In perilesional areas some vitiligo melanocytes lose attachment to the basement membrane and disappear in the course of epidermal renewal.[205] The presence of excessive amounts of tenascin in lesional skin can interfere with effective melanocyte adhesion.[206] Vitiligo melanocytes are not intrinsically adhesion-impaired,[206] but they exhibit an aberrant morphology in perilesional areas of vitiligo skin.[207] It appears that melanocytes are destroyed in situ.

Reduced perilesional melanocyte viability is observed only in expanding lesions. Although melanocytes are very resilient to apoptosis, stress-inducing factors with a selective effect on melanocytes, including exposure to phenols or UV overexposure, can induce melanocyte apoptosis or necrosis within the affected areas.[38,208] Melanocytes apparently are selectively more susceptible to stress-induced destruction. In contrast, the rapid turnover of keratinocytes, the migratory capacity of Langerhans' cells, and the location of fibroblasts deeper in the dermis protect these cells in times of stress.

There are other histologic changes within the epidermis associated with progressive depigmentation. Merkel cells are absent in the depigmented skin from patients with vitiligo.[200,209] It is not clear what impact this defect has on the functional capabilities of epidermis. During active depigmentation, patients often report an itchy sensation, suggesting release of histamine by mast cells and the presence of an inflammatory infiltrate (unpublished observation).[210] Schwann cells have a thickened basement membrane,[211,212] a morphologic indication of nerve regeneration. There is an increased quantity of neuropeptide Y in lesional vitiliginous skin, suggesting that aberrant innervation of the skin is involved in melanocyte injury.[213]

Traumatized melanocytes are an easy target for the innate as well as the specific immune response. In perilesional and lesional vitiligo skin there is a reduced expression of molecules that can protect basal epidermal cells from complement activation, namely CD59, decay accelerating factor (DAF), and membrane cofactor protein (MCP).[214] Expression of these molecules was shown to protect cultured melanocytes from complement-mediated damage.[215] Heterogeneous abnormalities of the *C4B* gene encoding the fourth component of complement have been described in vitiligo patients, further supporting the concept that vitiligo is associated with abnormalities in the complement system.[216] In the absence of adequate protection, melanocytes binding antibodies or complement are increasingly vulnerable to necrotic or apoptotic cell death, generating a pool of antigen to be processed by infiltrating dermal dendritic cells and epidermal Langerhans' cells. In this respect it is of interest that Langerhans' cells frequently line up at the basement membrane in lesional vitiligo skin, seemingly replacing dying melanocytes.[217,218] The physiology of Langerhans' cells and other dendritic cell subsets within the vitiligo skin microenvironment has not been studied extensively, although the expression of tumor necrosis factor (TNF)-related apoptosis induced by infiltrating dendritic cells suggests that dendritic cells may induce apoptosis in epidermal cells actively expressing TNF-related apoptosis-inducing ligand (TRAIL) receptors, as observed for melanocytes in perilesional skin.[219]

In most cases of vitiligo, inflammation is not clinically manifest, but approximately 3% of patients display "inflammatory vitiligo" where expanding lesions are surrounded by a narrow, elevated red margin.[197] Given the sparse distribution of melanocytes throughout the epidermis, it is not surprising that in vitiligo, inflammation is less extensive than, for example, in psoriasis, where an abundance of keratinocytes rather than sparse melanocytes are the prime target of the inflammatory response. The composition of cellular infiltrates in vitiligo skin was initially analyzed in patients with inflammatory vitiligo. Similar infiltrates are observed in patients with noninflammatory, progressive generalized vitiligo.[198,220,221] The consistent presence of macrophages, dendritic cells and CD4+ as well CD8+ T cells in perilesional skin of patients with progressive disease, as illustrated in Fig. 38.4, provides us with an explanation for the centrifugal expansion of lesions away from the site of original trauma through an ongoing immune response targeting epidermal melanocytes.[222] Increased expression of interferon-γ (IFN-γ)-responsive human leukocyte antigen (HLA)-DR and ICAM-1, and reduced expression of ganglioside D3 (CDw60) molecules in expanding, perilesional skin sites suggest that depigmentation involves expression of type 1 cytokines.[223,224] In part, melanocyte expression of HLA-DR and ICAM-1 may be induced by patient IgG antimelanocyte antibodies.[225] Since immune infiltrates interfere with the graft taking, patients with active disease are not eligible for surgical repigmentation. Thus it is important to recognize a fundamental difference between patients with active and those with stable disease.[226] Overall, combined immunohistologic data point to the involvement of a specific, cell-mediated immune response in progressive depigmentation as discussed elsewhere in this chapter.

Electron Microscopy and Apoptosis

That melanocytes are absent from the epidermis of lesional vitiligo skin has been confirmed by several investigators by ultrastructural analysis using electron microscopy.[48,74,217,227–229] Neither melanocytes nor undefined clear cells possibly representing dedifferentiated melanocytes have been observed in the stratum basale of lesional skin. In contrast, basal epithelial cells attached to the basement membrane at the dermal-epidermal junction are exclusively of the keratinocyte lineage, indicating that the melanocyte population was removed from the vitiligo lesion.

Significant observations have been made at the marginal area between the vitiligo lesion and the adjacent normally pigmented skin that indicate a mechanism for the removal of the melanocyte from the vitiligo lesion. In these areas, melanocytes can be markedly reduced in number and morphologically

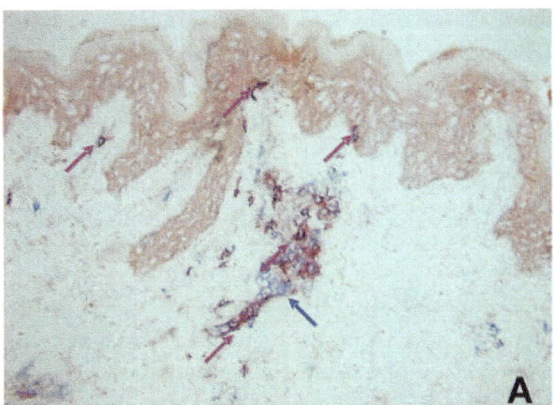

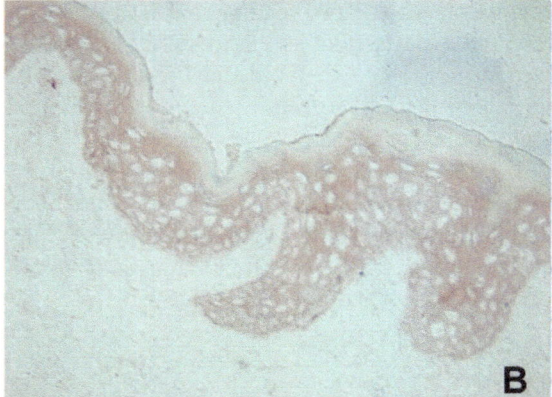

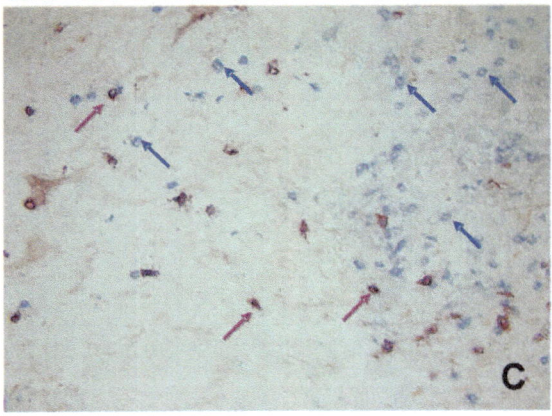

FIG. 38.4. Tissue infiltration by T lymphocytes. Immunologic double staining to detect CD8+ T cells in red and CD3+ T cells in blue. In these images cytotoxic T cells are purple (CD3+CD8+), whereas helper and suppressor T cells are blue (CD3+CD8−). (A) Perilesional skin from vitiligo patient with active disease. (B) Same biopsy away from the margin. (C) Melanoma tumor. Note increased proportion of CD8+ versus CD4+ T cells (purple versus blue arrows) in depigmenting vitiligo skin

aberrant.[191,193,203,227,230,231] Specifically, these melanocytes exhibit larger cell bodies with more elaborate dendricity. In addition, peripheral melanocytes can display morphologic characteristics of apoptosis as opposed to necrosis.[201] These characteristics consist of cellular shrinkage, increased nuclear heterochromatin, and cellular fragmentation (Fig. 38.5). Apoptosis is a process of programmed cell death that prevents damaged/dying cells from instigating an immune response.[232,233] Ultimately, apoptosis results in the generation of apoptotic cell bodies from the cellular fragments that are removed without stimulating a cellular or humoral immune response. However, macrophages are rarely observed at the edge of a vitiligo lesion.[191,231] It has been demonstrated that keratinocytes themselves are avidly phagocytic cells[234,235] and theoretically could effectively phagocytose fragmented apoptotic vitiligo melanocytes and carry the debris with them as they migrate to the stratum corneum where they are desquamated. These morphologic observations suggest that melanocytes can be removed from the epidermis via an apoptotic mechanism.[38]

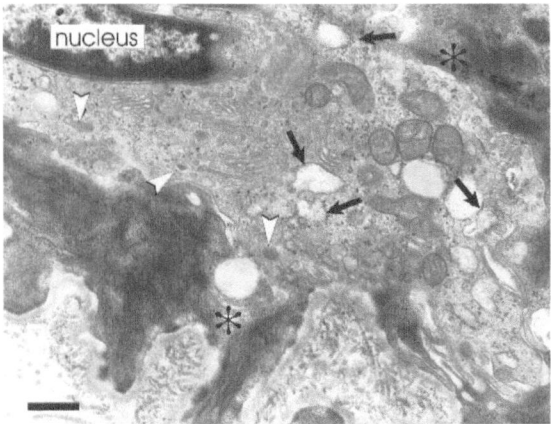

FIG. 38.5. Electron micrograph of the dermal/epidermal junction of pigmented skin biopsied immediately adjacent to a vitiligo lesion from a patient with vitiligo demonstrating melanocytes containing melanosomes (white arrowheads), dilated profiles of the rough endoplasmic reticulum (arrows), and a nucleus with a significant amount of heterochromatin plus neighboring keratinocytes with peripherally localized granular material (asterisks) within the cytoplasm. Bar = 2.0 μm

Keratinocyte aberrations have been demonstrated in the edge of the vitiligo lesion, suggesting that this cell type may also be affected in vitiligo. Vacuolar degeneration of keratinocytes and the appearance of extracellular granular material (EGM) resembling ribosomes between the melanocytes and the keratinocytes, as well as between the keratinocytes themselves, have been demonstrated.[74] The initial morphologic hallmarks of apoptosis within melanocytes and the extracellular granular material have been noted up to 15 cm from a lesion.[74,201] In addition, dilated profiles of the rough endoplasmic reticulum have been noted in melanocytes within the pigment skin near a lesion.[236] These dilated profiles indicate cellular dysfunction that may result from impairment in the translation of products from mutant genes or the onset of apoptosis (Fig. 38.5).

Apoptosis is a genetically regulated process that allows challenged or terminally stressed cells to undergo death in a controlled and regimented manner.[237] Special enzymes, cysteine proteases, also called caspases, that cleave cellular proteins plus protein members of the Bcl-2 family of pro- and antiapoptotic regulators all participate to control this specialized process. Mechanisms that can induce a cell to undergo apoptosis may be multiple. Cellular stress can alter the normal electrical charge across the mitochondrial membrane resulting in loss of permeability and the release of cytochrome C to activate the caspase enzyme cascade.[238] Immune signals can also induce cell to undergo apoptosis.[239] Cytokines, such as IFN-γ, TNF-α, and interleukin-1 (IL-1) can initiate apoptosis. These cytokines can be stimulated to be released from keratinocytes, melanocytes, and lymphocytes. Activated lymphocytes have other mechanisms for inducing apoptosis, such as the release of perforin and granzymes or triggering of the CD95 receptor on target cells. Induction of apoptosis via a heightened autoimmune response, as proposed for a subset of patients with vitiligo, may be the mechanism underlying melanocyte destruction in this form of vitiligo. Evidence that vitiligo melanocytes are prone to developing apoptosis comes from studies on the etiology of contact/occupational vitiligo (see Chemical Melanocytotoxins, below).

The Pathogenesis of Vitiligo

Chemical Melanocytotoxins

The etiology of vitiligo is complex.[42,140,180,240,241] The current dogma suggests that certain sets of genes render the melanocyte fragile and susceptible to undergoing apoptosis that in turn predisposes individuals to developing vitiligo.[131,242] A precipitating event/factor must initiate programmed cell death. Some proposed precipitating factors are sunburn, skin injury, and exposure to cytotoxic compounds. Common among these factors is their ability to stimulate melanin synthesis. Melanocyte-stimulating hormone induced by UV overexposure,[243] and cytokines produced during emotional stress or physical trauma (e.g., nerve growth factor, neurotrophins, adrenocorticotropic hormone [ACTH], endorphins, etc.)[244–247] can all trigger melanin synthesis by melanocytes. During the biochemical synthesis of melanin, specific quinones (e.g., DOPAquinone) and indoles (e.g., dihydroxyindoles) are generated as intermediates. These melanin intermediates can be cytotoxic to the melanocyte itself if aberrantly expressed.[248,249] Quinones and indoles can readily generate oxidative stress.[250–252] If abundant within the cell, these compounds can oxidize, either enzymatically or spontaneously,[250] and produce reactive oxygen species (ROSs),[252] which are hazardous to the cells initially causing lipid peroxidation, etc.[253] but ultimately inducing apoptosis.[254] Therefore, it is conceivable that in the genetically susceptible vitiligo melanocyte, elevated oxidative stress resulting from the generation of melanin intermediates exceeds the tolerable threshold for these sensitive cells, thereby inducing apoptosis.

The hypothesis that quinone/indole intermediates generate oxidative stress in the genetically susceptible melanocyte arose from our previous work on a distinctive form of vitiligo—contact/occupational vitiligo.[42,240,255] This type of depigmentation is distinguishable from vitiligo in that its onset correlates with exposure to certain environmental chemicals. These toxins are aromatic or aliphatic derivatives of phenols and catechols (e.g., monobenzyl ether of hydroquinone, 4-tert-butylphenol [4-TBP], etc.). The cutaneous depigmentation begins at the site of chemical contact but eventually extends further or occurs at unexposed sites. In some individuals the depigmentation develops into progressive, generalized vitiligo.[36] Monobenzyl ether of hydroquinone in a 20% concentration is a medication available by prescription that is used for depigmenting patients with vitiligo too extensive to regain color. Interestingly, these creams are not toxic to melanocytes from all individuals. Even at high dosages only a subset of patients depigment in response to application. In contrast, patients with vitiligo depigment more readily in response to application of the medication. This suggests that these agents are not simple poisons for melanocytes but are injurious to only those genetically susceptible (i.e., vitiligo).

Tyrosine is the substrate for tyrosinase that initiates the biochemical pathway for melanin synthesis.[42] Phenols and catechols are structurally similar to tyrosine. It was originally proposed that phenols and catechols compete with tyrosine for hydroxylation by tyrosinase,[249,256,257] generating semiquinone free radicals that induce cell death.[258–261] However, tyrosinase does not mediate the cytotoxicity of 4-TBP.[262] Since 4-TBP is more cytotoxic to melanocytes than to keratinocytes or to dermal fibroblasts,[219,262] a melanocyte-specific process must underlie its cytotoxic effects. Another melanocyte-specific enzyme, tyrosinase-related protein 1 (Tyrp1), may mediate the action of phenol/catechol derivatives such as 4-TBP.[263] Tyrp1 is the most abundant melanocyte specific protein[264] that exhibits 5,6-dihydroxyindole-2-carboxylic acid (DHICA) oxidase activity in murine[265] but not human[266] melanocytes. In human melanogenesis, Tyrp1 exhibits efficient tyrosine hydroxylase activity that putatively primes the onset of melanogenesis.[267,268] It is possible that Tyrp1 catalyzes the conversion of phenols and catechols into intermediates that induce oxidative stress, thus mediating cytotoxicity. Expression of Tyrp1 may be upregulated either genetically or facultatively in vitiligo melanocytes to amplify quinone-medicated oxidative stress correlating with their preferential apoptotic response.

Quinones are a ubiquitous class of compounds that can in turn undergo enzymatic and nonenzymatic redox cycling with their corresponding semiquinone radical and as a result generate superoxide anion radicals.[250–252] The subsequent enzymatic or spontaneous dismutation of these superoxide anion radicals gives rise to hydrogen peroxide, which reacts with trace amounts of iron or other transitional metals to form cellular hydroxyl radicals. The hydroxyl radicals are powerful oxidizing agents that are responsible for damage to essential protein, lipid, carbohydrate, and DNA macromolecules. For example, oxidation of cysteine residues in proteins leads to disulfide bond formation that can dramatically alter protein structure and function. Hydroxyl radicals also can catalyze oxidation of lipids, generating lipid hydroperoxides that can lead to formation of lipid peroxide–derived malondialdehyde DNA adducts.[253] Ultimately, the molecular and cellular damage caused by the aberrantly generated plethora of ROS results in programmed cell death, that is, apoptosis.[254] It is logical that the cytotoxicity induced by precipitating factors as 4-TBP is mediated via the generation of their related quinones.[269,270]

Phenols and catechols are compounds with oxygen-containing substituents that can be converted within cells to quinones by monooxygenase (e.g., tyrosinase or Tyrp1) or peroxidase enzymes, metal ions, and in some cases molecular oxygen.[250] Therefore, the cytotoxicity or apoptosis induced in melanocytes exposed to 4-TBP is a result of oxidative stress generated from the induction of ROS, putatively initiated via the conversion of 4-TBP to its related quinones, or increased melanin intermediates, respectively (Fig. 38.6).

Role of Melanocytes Within the Skin Immune System

In the late 1980s, Streilein and colleagues[271] developed the concept that lymphoid tissues outside the thymus and bone marrow may be involved in educating the immune system about self versus nonself, and danger versus no danger. The concept of skin-associated lymphoid tissue (SALT) emerged, highlighting the role of normal tissue cells in local immune responses.[271] Within the skin, keratinocytes receive much attention for their similarity to thymic epithelial cells and their ability to activate and educate T cells in vitro.[272,273] Less abundant melanocytes were long overlooked and were not described as part of the skin immune system until their malignant counterpart, the melanoma cell, displayed its relatively immunogenic nature and emerged in the 1990s as a model target type for antitumor vaccines.[274] Simultaneously it was

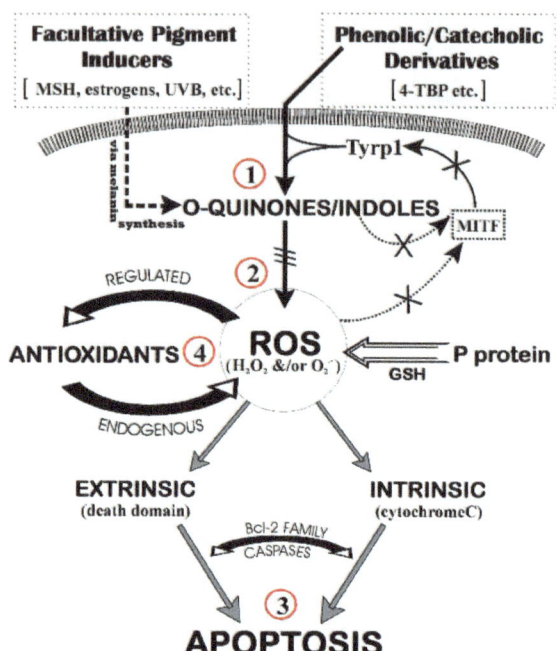

FIG. 38.6. Diagram of the proposed mechanism underlying the selective induction of apoptosis in vitiligo melanocytes. Exposure of melanocytes to facultative pigment inducers or 4-tert-butylphenol (4-TBP), via the action of tyrosinase related protein 1 (Tyrp1), results in the generation of intracellular quinones (1) that in turn produces reactive oxygen species (ROS) (2) and induces oxidative stress. Production of ROS stimulates the apoptotic pathway (3) that potentially could lead to cell death or interact with endogenous/regulated antioxidants (4) that could lead to cell survival, the balance of which is genetically determined. Therefore, the melanocyte's ability to survive these exogenous triggers of oxidative stress is dictated by the capacity to tolerate or combat ROS and prevent apoptosis—processes that may be genetically impaired in vitiligo melanocytes

acknowledged that melanocytes are well capable of generating primary cytokines, which are important in initiating a local immune response.[275,276]

Phagocytosis usually is considered a function of macrophages. However, it has been demonstrated that fibroblasts can ingest collagen during matrix remodeling and keratinocytes can phagocytose melanosomes and other particles.[277–279] Phagocytosis is followed by phagosome-lysosome fusion in macrophages. The digested content of the phagosome is presented to the immune system in the context of major histocompatibility complex (MHC) class II molecules to initiate an immune response.

Melanosomes are specialized lysosomes. It is likely that melanosomes are involved in immune-related functions.[280] Expression of HLA-DR by epidermal cells is generally restricted to Langerhans' cells and members of the dendritic cell family involved in detecting and clearing cutaneous assaults.[281] Under exceptional circumstances, apparently restricted to vitiligo and melanoma, melanocytic cells express MHC class II molecules.[222] The process of antigen presentation by melanocytes is of particular interest, as it may explain in part the immunogenicity of melanocytic cells.[282] Within melanocytes, melanin is synthesized in melanosomes. The synthetic pathway requires several enzymes including tyrosinase, TRP-1 and TRP-2, gp100, and MART-1. These same proteins are the primary targets of the immune response to melanoma.[283] Melanosomes like lysosomes in other cells fuse with incoming phagosomes visible by electron microscopy.[279] Thus it is likely that melanocytes, engaged in antigen processing and presentation in the context of MHC class II, present peptides derived from melanogenic compounds to the immune system that otherwise remain secluded within the melanosome.[284]

The importance of melanosomal localization for the immunogenicity of melanocytic proteins is supported by experiments in which a melanosomal target sequence tagged to an otherwise nonimmunogenic protein can render that protein increasingly immunogenic.[285] Indeed, it has been proposed that melanosomes are packages of tumor antigens that can be targeted in melanoma.[283] It is possible that melanocytes are preferentially targeted in autoimmune vitiligo as a consequence of (1) the immunogenicity of melanocytes expressing melanosome-associated proteins aberrantly perceived as nonself when presented in the context of class II; (2) the location of melanocytes within the epidermis, continuously exposed to signals from the environment and particularly vested in protection from radical uproar; and (3) a constellation of autoimmune-associated gene polymorphisms and mutations that may predispose to vitiligo rather than other autoimmune phenomena.

Vitiligo and the Innate Immune Response

The involvement of autoimmune responses in active vitiligo was overlooked. This is not surprising, given the dispersed distribution of melanocytes throughout the epidermis. Even in active disease, immune infiltrates are restricted to the narrow border of an advancing lesion. The infiltrates contain macrophages apparently clearing melanocytes in distress. Distress may be more pronounced in vitiligo patients than controls because of reduced expression of complement protective molecules DAF (decay acceleration factor), MCP (membrane cofactor protein), and CD59.[214] These studies are of particular interest given the finding that vitiligo is associated with a polymorphism in the C4 component of complement.[216] It is not immediately clear why these conditions predispose patients to the development of vitiligo, but leaving surrounding keratinocytes unharmed. Why does vitiligo target melanocytes, whereas psoriasis targets keratinocytes? The similarities of these two diseases targeting distinctly different cell types suggest the involvement of specific immunity in the form of humoral or cell-mediated immunity.

Humoral Immunity to Melanocytes

Melanocyte-reactive antibodies have been identified in the sera of patients with active vitiligo.[286] The majority of serum antibodies are either not specifically reactive with melanocytes or not reactive with cell-surface antigens. Whether melanocyte reactive antibodies play an etiologic role in vitiligo has been a point of discussion. In this respect, melanin concentrating hormone receptor (MCHR) is a membrane molecule among the antigens targeted by the humoral response,[287] and in experiments with xenografted human skin and vitiligo-derived serum transferred to mice it was observed that human antibodies targeted melanocytes within the xenografts.[288] Antibodies binding to melanocytes can cause melanocyte death through antibody-dependent cellular cytotoxicity (ADCC), or by the aforementioned complement activation.[289]

A Role for Skin-Infiltrating, Melanocyte-Reactive T Cells

Patients with active vitiligo have increased numbers of melanocyte-reactive cytotoxic T cells in the circulation, demonstrated with tetramer technology to identify antigen-specific T cells.[290] Additional properties have to be taken into account before assigning a causative role to CD8 T cells in progressive depigmentation. Melanocyte-reactive T cells must be destined for the skin, and should express high avidity for their targets to distinguish them from cytotoxic T cells reactive with melanocytes observed in control individuals. Evidence for such properties is found in CLA expression by circulating and skin infiltrating lymphocytes in both inflammatory and generalized vitiligo.[197,221,290] When propagated from blood or, more importantly, from skin biopsies of depigmenting vitiliginous skin, T cells express cytotoxic activity toward autologous melanocytes.[55,291,292] Reactivity to tyrosinase, MART-1, and gp100 has been detected among vitiligo skin–derived T cells.[292,293] Cytotoxic T cells from patients with vitiligo have superior avidity for their targets compared to T cells reactive with the same antigens in melanoma.[293,294] In part, superior reactivity of vitiligo-derived T cells may be explained by an environment conducive to immune reactivity in vitiligo, for example, through the absence of an effective regulatory response.[295] An additional factor appears to be the expression of high-affinity T-cell receptors (TCR). In fact, the analysis of *TCR* genes expressed by vitiligo skin–infiltrating T cells is supportive of a role for the α-subunit in defining T-cell affinity.[296]

A persisting enigma is why vitiligo T cells escape negative selection in the thymus and how these cells are allowed to enter the circulation. It is of interest that vitiligo is among autoimmune phenomena observed in patients with mutations in the *AIRE* gene, which helps define thymic selection.[297]

The progressive nature of depigmentation in vitiligo patients can be explained by T cells responding to alarm signals by stressed melanocytes. They induce a cytotoxic response, proliferate, and migrate centrifugally toward epidermal sites containing additional target cells.[198] In the absence of a regulatory response and in the presence of continuous stimulation, the activated T cells induce a progressive course of the disease.[298,299] Further insight into the autoimmune aspect of vitiligo can help to develop therapeutic measures to halt disease progression and prepare the skin for the intricate process of epidermal repigmentation.[300]

Genetic Basis for Vitiligo

Genes that are Involved in Vitiligo

Susceptibility for developing vitiligo has a genetic basis. The incidence of vitiligo globally is about 0.5% of the population at large.[301,302] However, siblings or other first-degree relatives of a patient with vitiligo have a relative risk of developing vitiligo of about 6% to 7%.[66,131,132,242] Even more indicative of the genetic basis of vitiligo is the observation that the concordance of vitiligo in monozygotic twins is elevated to 23%.[132] The genetic etiology of vitiligo appears to be multifactorial,[129,242,303,304] with a minimum of three di-allelic genes coordinately involved with the expression of vitiligo.[131] Recently both allelic association studies of candidate genes and genome-wide linkage analyses have facilitated the identification of some of these putative genes.[302]

A handful of genes have been identified by allelic association: (1) *VIT1* (i.e., *FBXO11*), which contains homologues with a G/T mismatch repair gene essential in recovery from DNA damage[305]; (2) catalase (i.e., *CAT*), an endogenous antioxidant; (3) tenascin, an adhesive integrin expressed by melanocytes[206]; (4) the estrogen receptor 1 (*ESR1*)[306]; (5) catechol-O-methyltransferase (*COMT*)[307]; and (6) angiotensin-converting enzyme (*ACE*).[308] Two other allelic associations have been reported between generalized vitiligo and the (7) *CTLA4*[309] and (8) *PTPN22*[310] genes, which have been broadly implicated in a number of other autoimmune diseases, and these genes may function as general autoimmunity/auto inflammatory susceptibility loci.[302]

Recently several other candidate genes have been identified by genetic linkage analysis. Most significant is embryonic transcription factor (9) *FOXD3*, which maps to an autoimmunity susceptibility locus.[311,312] However, mutations in *FOXD3* were originally found in one family with atypical vitiligo and are not expressed in most other patients with vitiligo.[302] Recently, Spritz's group,[304] using high-density single nucleotide polymorphism (SNP) genotyping and pedigree-based association, confirmed that vitiligo results from homozygosity at multiple recessive loci, one of which encodes (10) MALP1, a molecular component of the macrophage/neutrophil inflammasome responsible for activating inflammatory caspases.

Functions of Vitiligo-Associated Genes and Their Role in Melanocyte Destruction

There is ample clinical support for an hereditary component of the pigmentary disorder vitiligo. It has also become clear over time that several genes act in concert to confer susceptibility to vitiligo. The complexity of vitiligo inheritance patterns have posed a challenge for clinical geneticists and basic scientists wishing to identify the underlying genes involved in vitiligo etiology. Investigating vitiligo-associated gene function is thus of immediate importance to the vitiligo patient population.

Evidence of vitiligo as an inherited autoimmune disease can be found in several publications demonstrating an association between gradual depigmentation and HLA genotypes. Vitiligo has been associated most frequently with expression of specific MHC class II molecules, specifically with HLA-DRB1 in Mexican, Turkish, and U.S. populations.[313–315] HLA-DRB1 expression has been associated with several autoimmune diseases in the past as noted by Fain et al.[315] Expression of MHC class II molecules is generally restricted to professional antigen-presenting cells, and preferential expression of HLA-DRB1 suggests that this MHC class II can efficiently present melanocyte-derived antigens to the immune system, thus eliciting an immune response to melanocytes.

Fewer publications elude to an association between HLA class I haplotypes and vitiligo, and such associations are restricted to certain subpopulations. Most frequent associations include HLA-Cw6 in Northern Italians, Kuwaiti, and Saudis,[316–318] Bw6 in Saudi and Oman,i[318,319] A2 in Northern Germans and Slovaki,[320,321] and Cw7 in Saudis and Dutch.[318,322] Given the importance of MHC class I molecules for optimal presentation of antigens to cytotoxic T cells, when performed on a global scale these studies may clarify the most efficient means to present melanosomal antigens to the immune system. It will be of interest to learn whether the same HLA molecules confer resistance to the development of melanoma.

Besides antigen-presenting molecules that can affect antigen recognition by the immune system, the efficiency of antigen processing may also affect the probability that melanocyte self-antigens will be targeted by the immune system. In this respect, Casp et al. have demonstrated gene polymorphisms in LMP2, LMP7, and TAP-1.[323] At this point it is not clear how these polymorphisms will affect the function or longevity of the gene product.

Enhanced antigen processing and presentation will theoretically affect recognition of target cells other than melanocytes as well, and it is not surprising that vitiligo has been associated with other autoimmune disease, most notably with autoimmune thyroiditis.[324] Vitiligo is also a (late) manifestation of autoimmune polyendocrinopathy-candidiasis-ectodermal dystrophy syndrome (APCAPED) or autoimmune polyglandular syndrome (APS), a disease associated with mutations in the *AIRE* gene that defines presentation of autoantigens to T cells in primary lymphoid organs.[297,325,326] The *AIRE* gene is normally important in clonal deletion of autoreactive T cells with a high affinity for their targets. Indeed, vitiligo can be regarded as an autoimmune disease where T cells with high-affinity T-cell receptors reactive with melanocyte antigens escape clonal deletion and enter the circulation, contributing to destruction of melanocytes when these T cells find their way to the skin. Another indication for the involvement of autoimmunity in vitiligo is the definitive association between AIS-1 through AIS-4 mutations and vitiligo as described for large families with an increased prevalence of vitiligo by Spritz's group.[302,327]

Finally, in the effector phase, levels of intact *CTLA-4* expression are important to compete with B7 for its association with CD28 in order to prevent a self-perpetuating immune response.[328] In this respect, *CTLA-4* polymorphisms associated with vitiligo exist that may interfere with B7–CD28 effective intervention.[309,329,330] It is not clear how the described polymorphism will identify with altered function or longevity of the *CTLA-4* gene product. There is currently an interest in TNF-α and its role in autoimmunity. Vitiligo is associated with class I cytokine expression including TNF-α, and anti–TNF-α treatment has been proposed for vitiligo patients.[331] Whereas this treatment may prove effective, there does not appear to be a mutation in the promoter region of the gene associated with vitiligo.[332]

Vitiligo not only involves autoresponsiveness of the immune system, but is also believed to affect the efficiency by which the defining cell type, the melanocyte, can respond to conditions of skin stress and subsequent generation of radicals within the skin environment. Thus genes associated with vitiligo will likely be associated with melanocyte viability. The compound etiology of vitiligo, involving susceptibility genes, stress to the skin affecting melanocyte viability, and a progressive autoimmune response to melanocytes, is illustrated in Fig. 38.7. At a functional level, there has been discussion of the involvement of antiapoptotic proteins in vitiligo etiology. Elevated p53 expression has been demonstrated in vitiligo skin,[333,334] which is important in the (anti)apoptotic response.

To identify genes differentially expressed in vitiligo melanocytes compared to control melanocytes,

gene expression analysis has been performed which has led to the identification of a novel gene (*VIT1*). The *VIT1* transcript is largely complementary to a G/T mismatch repair gene, and reduced expression in vitiligo melanocytes likely signifies an increased need for G/T mismatch repair in vitiligo melanocytes.[305] Another gene that appears to confer selective sensitivity to environmental cues in vitiligo melanocytes is catechol-O-methyltransferase *(COMT)*. Significantly elevated expression of *COMT* in vitiligo skin again supports the need for neutralization of radicals generated within vitiligo skin.[335] More commonly associated with Parkinson's disease, it is interesting that polymor-

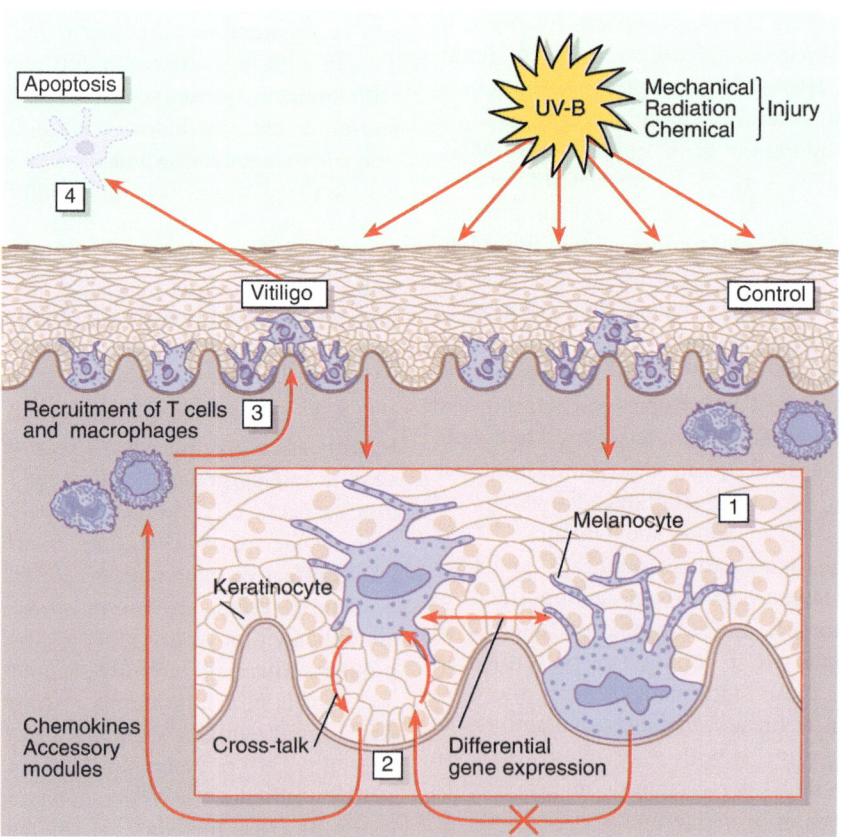

FIG. 38.7. Essentials of vitiligo etiology. Stress to the skin in the form of wounds or burns, excessive sun exposure, or contact with bleaching phenols will differentially affect melanocytes from vitiligo patients and control individuals (1). Differential gene expression among melanocytes and cross-talk with neighboring keratinocytes contribute to expression of chemokines and accessory molecules (2), recruiting an inflammatory infiltrate of T cells and macrophages (3) that further induce melanocyte apoptosis and selectively eliminate remaining melanocytes and melanocytic cell remnants from vitiligo epithelium (4)

phisms in the *COMT* gene have been described among vitiligo patients.[307]

Most research with respect to enhanced susceptibility of vitiligo melanocytes to environmental stress, however, has been performed in relation to catalase gene expression. Catalase function appears to be impaired in vitiligo, and pseudocatalase treatment for vitiligo patients is based on the principle that the oxidative stress balance may be relieved in vitiligo skin by this treatment[336,337] (see Medical Therapies, above). Thus several investigative groups have set out to identify alterations in the underlying catalase gene among vitiligo patients.[338–340] The relative abundance of specific allelic variants among vitiligo patients has been investigated, yet existing allelic variants are not known to affect catalase function. Other genes proposed to be associated with vitiligo include angiotensin-converting enzyme,[308,341] lymphoid tyrosine phosphatase,[310,342] vitamin D receptor Apa-I[343] and an estrogen receptor gene,[306] and finally transcription factor FoxD3,[312] all of which may selectively affect melanocyte physiology in ways not fully understood to date. Clearly, a further understanding of genes associated with vitiligo etiology can provide us with an understanding of the relative importance of melanocyte susceptibility and the immune system, and point to novel treatments for this disease.

Conclusion

Vitiligo vulgaris is defined as an idiopathic, acquired type of leukoderma manifested by depigmentation of the epidermis resulting from destruction of melanocytes. In vitiligo, certain sets of genes render the melanocyte fragile and susceptible to undergoing apoptosis. The genetic basis for vitiligo is multifactorial. Vitiligo usually affects interfollicular melanocytes and spares follicular melanocytes, but both types of cells can be destroyed in severe cases. Early vitiligo results in hypopigmentation, that is, tri- or pentachrome vitiligo, but advanced vitiligo causes depigmentation. Medical therapies for vitiligo involve ultraviolet radiation or topical medications, such as steroids or immunomodulators. Surgical treatment for vitiligo involves grafting of autologous skin.

Acknowledgments. The authors would like to acknowledge research funding by the National Vitiligo Foundation and by the National Institutes of Health (NIH)/National Institute of Skin and Musculoskeletal diseases (NIAMS)(RO3AR050137) and NIH/National Cancer Institute (NCI) (RO1CA128068) to I.C.L.P. and by NIH/NIAMS (R01AR46115) to R.E.B. for data described in this publication.

References

1. Kopera D. History and cultural aspects of vitiligo. In: Hann S-K, Nordlund J, eds. Vitiligo: A Monograph on the Basic and Clinical Science. Oxford: Blackwell Scientific, 2000:13–17.
2. Porter J. Psychosocial effects of skin disease. In: Medical and Health Annual. Chicago: Encyclopedia Britannica, 1989:388–90.
3. Porter J, Beuf A. Response of older people to impaired appearance: the effect of age on disturbance by vitiligo. J Aging Studies 1988;2:167–81.
4. Porter J, Beuf A, Nordlund JJ, Lerner AB. Personal responses of patients to vitiligo: the importance of the patient-physician interaction. Arch Dermatol 1978;114:1384–5.
5. Porter J, Beuf A, Lerner AB, Nordlund JJ. Response to cosmetic disfigurement: patients with vitiligo. Cutis 1987;39:493–4.
6. Porter JR, Beuf AH, Lerner A, Nordlund JJ. The psychosocial effect of vitiligo: a comparison of vitiligo patients with "normal" controls, with psoriasis patients, and with patients with other pigmentary disorders. J Am Acad Dermatol 1986;15:220–4.
7. Porter JR, Beuf AH, Lerner AB, Nordlund JJ. The effect of vitiligo on sexual relationship. J Am Acad Dermatol 1990;22:221–2.
8. Porter J. The psychological effects of vitiligo: response to impaired appearance. In: Hann SK, Nordlund JJ, eds. Vitiligo: A Monograph on the Basic and Clinical Science. Oxford: Blackwell Scientific, 2000:97–100.
9. el Mofty AM, Nada MM. On the treatment of vitiligo. Int J Dermatol 1971;10(4):262–6.
10. Mercurialis H. De Morbis Cutaneis et Omnibus Corporis Humani Excrementis Tractatus. Kansas City, MO: Lowell Press, 1572.
11. Im S, Nordlund JJ. Physiological alterations in the depigmented skin of patients with vitiligo. In: Hann S, Nordlund J, eds. Vitiligo: A Monograph on the Basic and Clinical Science. Oxford: Blackwell Scientific, 2000:254–69.

12. Nordlund JJ, Ortonne JP. Vitiligo vulgaris. In: Nordlund JJ, Boissy RE, Hearing VJ, King RA, Oetting WS, Ortonne JP, eds. The Pigmentary System: Physiology and Pathophysiology, 2nd ed. Oxford: Blackwell Scientific, 2006:591–8.

13. Nordlund JJ. The epidermal melanin unit: an expanded concept. Dermatol Clin 2007;25(3):271–81.

14. Lerner AB, Nordlund JJ. Vitiligo. What is it? Is it important? JAMA 1978;239:1183–7.

15. Nordlund JJ, Lerner AB. Vitiligo: It is important. Arch Dermatol 1982;118:5–8.

16. Nordlund JJ. The loss of melanocytes from the epidermis: the mechanism for depigmentation in vitiligo vulgaris. In: Hann SK, Nordlund JJ, eds. Vitiligo: Monograph on the Basic and Clinical Science. Oxford, London: Blackwell Science, 2000:7–12.

17. Concetta-Fargnoli M, Bolognia L. Pentachrome vitiligo. J Am Acad Dermatol 1995;33:853–6.

18. Dupre A, Christol B. Cockade-like vitiligo and linear vitiligo a variant of Fitzpatrick's trichrome vitiligo. Arch Dermatol Res 1978;262(2):197–203.

19. Nordlund JJ, Boissy RE, Hearing VJ, King RA, Oetting WS, Ortonne JP, eds. The Pigmentary System: Physiology and Pathophysiology, 2nd ed. Oxford: Blackwell Scientific, 2006.

20. Boissy RE, Hornyak TJ. Extracutaneous melanocytes. In: Nordlund JJ, Boissy RE, Hearing VJ, King RA, Oetting WS, Ortonne JP, eds. The Pigmentary System: Physiology and Pathophysiology, 2nd ed. Oxford: Blackwell Scientific, 2006:91–107.

21. Goldgeier MH, Klein LE, Klein-Angerer S, Moellmann G, Nordlund JJ. The distribution of melanocytes in the leptomeninges of the human brain. J Invest Dermatol 1984;82:235–8.

22. Albert DM, Sober AJ, Fitzpatrick TB. Iritis in patients with cutaneous melanoma and vitiligo. Arch Ophthalmol 1978;96(11):2081–4.

23. Barnes L. Vitiligo and the Vogt-Koyanagi-Harada syndrome. Dermatol Clin 1988;6(2):229–39.

24. Gass JD. Vitiliginous chorioretinitis. Arch Ophthalmol 1981;99(10):1778–87.

25. Nettleship E. Remarks on sympathetic ophthalmitis with whitening of the eyelashes. Trans Ophthalmol Soc UK 1884;4:83–4.

26. Boissy RE, Moellmann GE, Lerner AB. Morphology of melanocytes in hair bulbs and eyes of vitiligo mice. Am J Pathol 1987;127:380–8.

27. Lerner AB, Nordlund JJ. Vitiligo: Loss of pigment in skin, hair and eyes. Jpn J Dermatol 1978;5:1–8.

28. Nordlund JJ, Albert DM, Forget BM, Lerner AB. Halo nevi and the Vogt-Koyanagi-Harada syndrome: manifestations of vitiligo. Arch Dermatol 1980;116:690–2.

29. Nordlund JJ, Todes-Taylor N, Albert DM, Wagner MD, Lerner AB. Prevalence of vitiligo and polio-

sis in patients with uveitis. J Am Acad Dermatol 1981;4:528–36.

30. Park S, Albert DM, Bolognia JL. Ocular manifestations of pigmentary disorders. Dermatol Clin 1992;10(3):609–22.

31. Moorthy RS, Inomata H, Rao NA. Vogt-Koyanagi-Harada syndrome (review). Surv Ophthalmol 1995;39:265–92.

32. Beniz J, Forster DJ, Lean JS, Smith RE, Rao NA. Variations in clinical features of the Vogt-Koyanagi-Harada syndrome. Retina 1991;11:275–80.

33. Kumakiri M, Kimura T, Miura Y, Tagawa Y. Vitiligo with an inflammatory erythema in Vogt-Koyanagi-Harada disease: demonstration of filamentous masses and amyloid deposits. J Cutan Pathol 1982;9(4):258–66.

34. Ozdirim E, Renda Y, Baytok V. Vogt-Koyanagi-Harada syndrome in siblings (with a brief review of the literature). Eur J Pediatr 1980;135(2):217–9.

35. Catona A, Lanzer D. Monobenzone, Superfade, vitiligo and confetti-like depigmentation. Med J Aust 1987;146(6):320–1.

36. Cummings MP, Nordlund JJ. Chemical leukoderma: fact or fancy. Am J Contact Dermatitis 1995;6:122–7.

37. Mosher DB, Parrish JA, Fitzpatrick TB. Monobenzyl ether of hydroquinone: a retrospective study of treatment of 18 vitiligo patients and a review of the literature. Br J Dermatol 1977;97:669–79.

38. Huang CL, Nordlund JJ, Boissy R. Vitiligo: a manifestation of apoptosis? Am J Clin Dermatol 2002;3(5):301–8.

39. Brochez L, Boone B, Naeyert JM. Hypomelanoses associated with melanocytic neoplasia. In: Nordlund JJ, Boissy RE, Hearing VJ, King RA, Oetting WS, Ortonne JP, eds. The Pigmentary System: Physiology and Pathophysiology, 2nd ed. Oxford: Blackwell Scientific, 2006:705–10.

40. Lerner AB, Kirkwood JM. Vitiligo and melanoma: Can genetically abnormal melanocytes result in both vitiligo and melanoma within a single family? J Am Acad Dermatol 1984;11:696–701.

41. Nordlund JJ, Kirkwood JM, Forget BM, et al. A demographic study of clinically atypical (dysplastic) nevi in patients with melanoma and comparison subjects. Cancer Res 1985;45:1855–61.

42. Lerner AB. On the etiology of vitiligo and grey hair. Am J Med 1971;51:141–7.

43. Steingrinssom E, Copeland NG, Jenkins NA. Melanocytes stem cell maintenance and hair graying. Cell 2005;121:9–12.

44. Nishimura EK, Granter SR, Fisher DE. Mechanisms of hair graying: Incomplete melanocyte stem cell maintenance in the niche. Science 2005; 307:720–24.

45. Balabanov K, Andreev VC, Tchernozemski I. Malignant melanoma and vitiligo. Dermatologica 1969;139(3):211–9.

46. Duhra P, Ilchyshyn A. Prolonged survival in metastatic malignant melanoma associated with vitiligo. Clin Exp Dermatol 1991;16(4):303–5.

47. Fodor J, Bodrogi I. Vitiligo and malignant melanoma. Neoplasia 1975;22:445–8.

48. Koh HK, Sober AJ, Nakagawa H, Albert DM, Mihm MC, Fitzpatrick TB. Malignant melanoma and vitiligo-like leukoderma: An electron microscopic study. J Am Acad Dermatol 1983;9:696–708.

49. Milton GW, McCarthy WH, Carlon A. Malignant melanoma and vitiligo. Australas J Dermatol 1971;12:131–42.

50. Perrot H, Ortonne JP, Schmitt D. Vitiliginous achromia with malignant melanoma. Tyrosinase activity and ultrastructural study of achromic and normal skin. Arch Dermatol Res 1977;257:247–53.

51. Cavallari V, Cannavo SP, Ussia AF, Moretti G, Albanese A. Vitiligo associated with metastatic malignant melanoma. Int J Dermatol 1996;35(10):738–40.

52. Frenk E. Depigmentations vitiligineuses ches des patients atteints de melanommes malins. Dermatologica 1969;139:84–91.

53. Nordlund JJ, Kirkwood J, Forget BM, Milton G, Lerner AB. Vitiligo in patients with metastatic melanoma: A good prognostic sign. J Am Acad Dermatol 1983;9:689–95.

54. Rosenberg SA, White DE. Vitiligo in patients with melanoma: normal tissue antigens can be targets for cancer immunotherapy. J Immunother Emphasis Tumor Immunol 1996;19:81–4.

55. Yee C, Thompson JA, Roche P, et al. Melanocyte destruction after antigen-specific immunotherapy of melanoma: direct evidence of t cell-mediated vitiligo. J Exp Med 2000;192(11):1637–44.

56. Le Gal FA, Avril MF, Bosq J, et al. Direct evidence to support the role of antigen-specific CD8(+) T cells in melanoma-associated vitiligo. J Invest Dermatol 2001;117(6):1464–70.

57. Juranic ZD, Stanojevic-Bakic N, Zizak Z, et al. Antimelanoma immunity in vitiligo and melanoma patients. Neoplasma 2003;50(4):305–9.

58. Wankowicz-Kalinska A, Le Poole C, van den Wijngaard R, Storkus WJ, Das PK. Melanocyte-specific immune response in melanoma and vitiligo: two faces of the same coin? Pigment Cell Res 2003;16(3):254–60.

59. Kiniwa Y, Fujita T, Akada M, et al. Tumor antigens isolated from a patient with vitiligo and T-cell-infiltrated melanoma. Cancer Res 2001;61(21):7900–7.

60. Overwijk WW, Restifo NP. Autoimmunity and the immunotherapy of cancer: targeting the "self" to destroy the "other." Crit Rev Immunol 2000;20(6):433–50.

61. Osanto S, Schiphorst PP, Weijl NI, et al. Vaccination of melanoma patients with an allogeneic, genetically modified interleukin 2–producing melanoma cell line. Human Gene Ther 2000;11(5):739–50.

62. Das SK, Majumder PP, Chakraborty R, Majumdar TK, Haldar B. Studies on vitiligo I. Epidemiological profile in Calcutta, India. Genet Epidemiol 1985;2:71–8.

63. Das SK, Majumder PP, Majumdar TK, Haldar B. Studies on vitiligo II. Familial aggregation and genetics. Genet Epidemiol 1985;2:255–62.

64. Howitz J, Brodthagen H, Schwartz M, Thomsen K. Prevalence of vitiligo: Epidemiological survey on the Isle of Bornholm, Denmark. Arch Dermatol 1977;113:47–52.

65. Mehta NR, Shah KC, Theodore C, Vyas VP, Patel AB. Epidemiological study of vitiligo in Surat area, South Gujarat. Indian J Med Res 1973;61:145–54.

66. Nordlund JJ, Majumder PP. Recent investigations on vitiligo vulgaris. Dermatol Clin 1997;15:69–78.

67. Ortonne J. Special Features of Vitiligo. In: Hann S, Nordlund J, eds. Vitiligo: A Monograph on the Basic and Clinical Science. Oxford: Blackwell Scientific, 2000:70–5.

68. Arrunategui A, Arroyo C, Garcia L, et al. Melanocyte reservoir in vitiligo. Int J Dermatol 1994;33(7):484–7.

69. Cui J. The melanocyte reservoir and its necessity. In: Hann S-K, Nordlund JJ, eds. Vitiligo: Monograph on Basic and Clinical Science, 1st ed. Oxford, England: Blackwell Scientific, 2000:163–5.

70. Arata J, Abe-Matsuura Y. Generalized vitiligo preceded by a generalized figurate erythematosquamous eruption. J Dermatol 1994;21(6):438–41.

71. Falabella R. Repigmentation of stable leukoderma by autologous minigrafting. J Dermatol Surg Oncol 1986;12:172–9.

72. Hatchome N, Kato T, Tagami H. Therapeutic success of epidermal grafting in generalized vitiligo is limited by the Koebner phenomenon. J Am Acad Dermatol 1990;22:87–91.

73. Falabella R, Arrunategui A, Barona MI, Alzate A. The minigrafting test for vitiligo: detection of stable lesions for melanocyte transplantation. J Am Acad Dermatol 1995;32(2 pt 1):228–32.

74. Moellmann G, Klein-Angerer S, Scollay D, Nordlund JJ, Lerner AB. Extracellular granular material and degeneration of keratinocytes in the normally pigmented epidermis of patients with vitiligo. J Invest Dermatol 1982;79:321–30.

75. Hann SK, Koo SW, Kim JB, Park YK. Detection of antibodies to human melanoma cells in vitiligo and alopecia areata by Western blot analysis. J Dermatol 1996;23(2):100–3.

76. Hann SK. Clinical features of segmental vitiligo. In: Hann SK, Nordlund JJ, eds. Vitiligo: A Monograph on the Basic and Clinical Science. Oxford: Blackwell Scientific, 2000:49–60.

77. Grimes PE, Billips M. Childhood vitiligo: clinical spectrum and therapeutic approaches. In: Hann SK, Nordlund JJ, eds. Vitiligo: A Monograph on Basic and Clinical Science. Oxford: Blackwell Scientific, 2000:61–9.

78. Hann SK, Nordlund JJ. Clinical features of generalized vitiligo. In: Hann SK, Nordlund JJ, eds. Vitiligo: A Monograph on the Basic and Clinical Science. Oxford: Blackwell Scientific, 2000:35–48.

79. Seo SL, Kim IH. Squamous cell carcinoma in a patient with generalized vitiligo. J Am Acad Dermatol 2001;45(suppl 6):S227–S9.

80. Abdullah AN, Keczkes K. Cutaneous and ocular side-effects of PUVA photochemotherapy—a 10–year follow-up study [Review]. Clin Exp Dermatol 1989;14(6):421–4.

81. Schallreuter KU, Tobin DJ, Panske A. Decreased photodamage and low incidence of non-melanoma skin cancer in 136 sun-exposed Caucasian patients with vitiligo. Dermatology 2002;204(3):194–201.

82. Calanchini-Postizzi E, Frenk E. Long-term actinic damage in sun-exposed vitiligo and normally pigmented skin. Dermatologica 1987;174:266–71.

83. Wildfang IL, Jacobsen FK, Thestrup-Pedersen K. PUVA treatment of vitiligo: a retrospective study of 59 patients. Acta Derm Venereol 1992;72(4):305–6.

84. Yashiro K, Nakagawa T, Takaiwa T, Inai M. Actinic keratoses arising only on sun-exposed vitiligo skin. Clin Exp Dermatol 1999;24(3):199–201.

85. King RA. Albinism. In: Nordlund JJ, Boissy RE, Hearing VJ, King RA, Ortonne J-P, eds. The Pigmentary System Physiology and Pathophysiology. New York: Oxford University Press, 1998:553–75.

86. Kromberg JGR, Castle D, Zwane EM, Jenkins T. Albinism and skin cancer in Southern Africa. Clin Genet 1989;36:43–52.

87. Lookingbill DP, Lookingbill GL, Leppard B. Actinic damage and skin cancer in albinos in northern Tanzania: findings in 164 patients enrolled in an outreach skin care program. J Am Acad Dermatol 1995;32(4):653–8.

88. Lookingbill DP, Lookingbill GL, Leppard B. Actinic lentigines versus skin cancer risk in albinos in northern Tanzania. J Am Acad Dermatol 1995;33:299–300.

89. Yakubu A, Mabogunje OA. Skin cancer in African albinos. Acta Oncol 1993;32(6):621–2.

90. Luande J, Henschke CI, Mohammed N. The Tanzanian human albino skin. Natural history. Cancer 1985;55(8):1823–8.

91. Pehamberger H, Honigsmann H, Wolff K. Dysplastic nevus syndrome with multiple primary amelanotic melanomas in oculocutaneous albinism. J Am Acad Dermatol 1984;11:731–5.

92. Streutker CJ, McCready D, Jimbow K, From L. Malignant melanoma in a patient with oculocutaneous albinism. J Cutan Med Surg 2000;4(3):149–52.

93. van de Kerkhof PC, Fokkink HJ. Irritancy of dithranol in normally pigmented and depigmented skin of patients with vitiligo. Acta Derm Venereol 1989;69:236–8.

94. Westerhof W, Buehre Y, Pavel S, et al. Increased anthralin irritation response in vitiliginous skin. Arch Dermatol Res 1989;281:52–6.

95. Askenase PW, Van Loveren H, Kraeuter-Kops S, et al. Defective elicitation of delayed-type hypersensitivity in W/Wv and SI/SId mast cell-deficient mice. J Immunol 1983;131(6):2687–94.

96. Lerner AB, Shiohara T, Boissy RE, Jacobson KA, Lamoreux ML, Moellmann GE. A possible mouse model for vitiligo. J Invest Dermatol 1986;87:299–304.

97. Lamoreux ML, Boissy RE, Womack JE, Nordlund JJ. The vit gene maps to the Mi (Microphthalmia) locus of the laboratory mouse. J Hered 1992;83:435–9.

98. Palkowski MR, Nordlund ML, Rheins LA, Nordlund JJ. Langerhans' cells in hair follicles of the depigmenting C57Bl/Ler-vit.vit mouse. A model for human vitiligo. Arch Dermatol 1987;123(8):1022–8.

99. Rheins LA, Palkowski MR, Nordlund JJ. Alterations in cutaneous immune reactivity to dinitrofluorobenzene in graying C57BL/vi.vi mice. J Invest Dermatol 1986;86:539–42.

100. Nordlund JJ, Csato M, Babcock G, Takei F. Low ICAM-1 expression in the epidermis of depigmenting C57BL/6J-mi^{vit}/mi^{vit} mice: A possible cause of muted contact sensitization. Exp Dermatol 1995;3:20–9.

101. Nordlund JJ, Forget B, Kirkwood J, Lerner AB. Dermatitis produced by applications of monobenzone in patients with active vitiligo. Arch Dermatol 1985;121:1141–5.

102. Hatchome N, Aiba S, Kato T, Torinuki W, Tagami H. Possible functional impairment of Langerhans cells in vitiliginous skin: reduced ability to elicit dinitrochlorobenzene contact sensitivity reaction and decreased stimulatory effect in the allogeneic mixed skin cell lymphocyte culture reaction. Arch Dermatol 1987;123:51–4.

103. Uehara M, Miyauchi H, Tanaka S. Diminished contact sensitivity response in vitiliginous skin. Arch Dermatol 1984;120:195–8.

104. Anstey A, Marks R. Colocalization of lichen planus and vitiligo [letter]. Br J Dermatol 1993;128(1):103–4.

105. Brenner W, Diem E, Gschnait F. Coincidence of vitiligo, alopecia areata, onychodystrophy, localized scleroderma and lichen planus. Dermatologica 1979;159(4):356–60.

106. Cecchi R, Giomi A, Tuci F, Bartoli L, Seghieri G. Pityriasis rubra pilaris, lichen planus, alopecia universalis and vitiligo in a patient with chronic viral hepatitis C. Dermatology 1994;188(3): 239–40.

107. Chapman RS. Coincident vitiligo and psoriasis in the same individual. Arch Dermatol 1973;107(5):776.

108. Enhamre A, Ros AM, Nordlind K. Co-existing vitiligo and small-plaque parapsoriasis [letter]. Dermatologica 1986;173(2):103–4.

109. Iakovleva NI, Sen'kin VI. [Case of alopecia associated with vitiligo and psoriasis]. Vestn Dermatol Venerol 1984;10:70–1.

110. Koransky JS, Roenigk HH, Jr. Vitiligo and psoriasis. J Am Acad Dermatol 1982;7(2):183–9.

111. Menter A, Boyd AS, Silverman AK. Guttate psoriasis and vitiligo: anatomic cohabitation. J Am Acad Dermatol 1989;20(4):698–700.

112. de Moragas JM, Winkelmann RK. Psoriasis and vitiligo. Arch Dermatol 1970;101(2):235–7.

113. Julian CG, Bowers PW. Strict anatomical coexistence of vitiligo and psoriasis vulgaris—a Koebner phenomenon? [letter; comment]. Clin Exp Dermatol 1996;21(6):464.

114. Papadavid E, Yu RC, Munn S, Chu AC. Strict anatomical coexistence of vitiligo and psoriasis vulgaris—a Koebner phenomenon? [see comments]. Clin Exp Dermatol 1996;21(2):138–40.

115. Rubisz-Brzezinska J, Buchner SA, Itin P. Vitiligo associated with lichen planus. Is there a pathogenetic relationship? [see comments]. Dermatology 1996;192(2):176–8.

116. Dhar S, Malakar S. Colocalization of vitiligo and psoriasis in a 9-year-old boy [letter]. Pediatr Dermatol 1998;15(3):242–3.

117. Sardana K, Sharma RC, Koranne RV, Mahajan S. An interesting case of colocalization of segmental lichen planus and vitiligo in a 14-year-old boy. Int J Dermatol 2002;41(8):508–9.

118. Melato M, Gorji N, Rizzardi C, Maglione M. Associated localization of morphea and lichen planus of the lip in a patient with vitiligo. Minerva Stomatol 2000;49(11–12):549–54.

119. Porter SR, Scully C, Eveson JW. Coexistence of lichen planus and vitiligo is coincidental [letter]. Clin Exp Dermatol 1994;19(4):366.

120. Powell FC, Dicken CH. Psoriasis and vitiligo. Acta Derm Venereol 1983;63:246–9.

121. Powell FC, Dicken CH. Vitiligo and psoriasis [letter]. J Am Acad Dermatol 1983;8(1):136–7.

122. Tan RS. Ulcerative colitis, myasthenia gravis, atypical lichen planus, alopecia areata, vitiligo. Proc R Soc Med 1974;67(3):195–6.

123. Allende MF, Reed E. Dermatitis herpetiformis and vitiligo. Arch Dermatol 1964;89:156–8.

124. Hazelrigg DE. Dermatitis herpetiformis and vitiligo [letter]. Cutis 1987;39(3):232.

125. Hogan DJ, Lane PR. Dermatitis herpetiformis and vitiligo. Cutis 1986;38(3):195–7.

126. Olholm-Larsen P, Kavli G. Dermatitis herpetiformis and vitiligo. Dermatologica 1980;160(1):41–4.

127. Amato L, Gallerani I, Fuligni A, Mei S, Fabbri P. Dermatitis herpetiformis and vitiligo: report of a case and review of the literature. J Dermatol 2000;27(7):462–6.

128. Ortonne JP, Perrot H, Thivolet J. Clinical and statistical study of 100 patients with vitiligo. II. Associated lesions. Sem Hop 1976;52:679–86.

129. Hafez M, Sharaf L, El-Nabi SMA. The genetics of vitiligo. Acta Derm Venereol 1983;63:249–51.

130. Tripathi R, Fanders DJ, Young TL, et al. Evaluation of MITF locus linkage to human vitiligo and osteopetrosis. Presented to the Third Joint Clinical Genetics Meeting, 1995; abstract.

131. Majumder P, Nordlund JJ, Nath SK. Pattern of familial aggregation of vitiligo. Arch Dermatol 1993;129:994–8.

132. Alkhateeb A, Fain PR, Thody A, Bennett DC, Spritz RA. Epidemiology of vitiligo and associated autoimmune diseases in Caucasian probands and their families. Pigment Cell Res 2003;16(3):208–14.

133. Majumder PP, Das DK, Li CC. A genetical model for vitiligo. Am J Hum Genet 1988;43:119–25.

134. Cui J, Shan L, Wang G. Role of hair follicles in the repigmentation of vitiligo. J Invest Dermatol 1991;97:410–6.

135. Dourmishev AL, Aleksandrov II, Zlatkov NB, Trifonov SD. On the mechanism of perifollicular repigmentation in vitiligo. Doklady Bolgarskoi Academii Navk 1982;35:789–91.

136. Falabella R. Surgical Therapies for Vitiligo. In: Hann S-K, Nordlund J, eds. Vitiligo: Monograph on Basic and Clinical Science, 1st ed. Oxford, England: Blackwell Scientific, 2000:193–202.

137. Halder RM, Nordlund JJ. Surgical treatments of pigmentary disorders. In: Nordlund JJ, Boissy RE, Hearing VJ, King RA, Oetting WS, Ortonne JP, eds. The Pigmentary System: Physiology

and Pathophysiology, 2nd ed. Oxford: Blackwell Scientific, 2006:1191–7.

138. Falabella R. Repigmentation of segmental vitiligo by autologous minigrafting. J Am Acad Dermatol 1983;9:514–21.

139. Falabella R. Treatment of localized vitiligo by autologous minigrafting. Arch Dermatol 1988;124:1649–55.

140. Le Poole IC, Das PK, van den Wijngaard RM, Bos JD, Westerhof W. Review of the etiopatho-mechanism of vitiligo: a convergence theory. Exp Dermatol 1993;2(4):145–53.

141. El-Mofty AM, Nada MM. Vitiligo and its treatment. Australas J Dermatol 1974;15:15–22.

142. Gupta AK, Anderson TF. Psoralen photochemo-therapy. J Am Acad Dermatol 1987;17(5):703–34.

143. Tran D, Kwok YK, Goh CL. A retrospective review of PUVA therapy at the National Skin Centre of Singapore. Photodermatol Photoimmunol Photomed 2001;17(4):164–7.

144. Ortonne JP, MacDonald DM, Micoud A, Thivolet J. PUVA-induced repigmentation of vitiligo: a histo-chemical (split-DOPA) and ultrastructural study. Br J Dermatol 1979;101:1–12.

145. Ortonne JP, Schmitt D, Thivolet J. PUVA-induced repigmentation of vitiligo: scanning electron microscopy of hair follicles. J Invest Dermatol 1980;74:40–2.

146. Pathak MA, Fitzpatrick TB. The evolution of pho-tochemotherapy with psoralens and UVA (PUVA): 2000 BC to 1992 AD. J Photochem Photobiol B 1992;14(1–2):3–22.

147. Halder RM, Nordlund JJ. Chemophototherapy of pigmentary disorders. In: Nordlund JJ, Boissy RE, Hearing VJ, King RA, Oetting WS, Ortonne JP, eds. The Pigmentary System: Physiology and Pathophysiology, 2nd ed. Oxford: Blackwell Scientific, 2006:1175–82.

148. Harrist TJ, Pathak MA, Mosher DB, Fitzpatrick TB. Chronic cutaneous effects of long-term psoralen and ultraviolet radiation therapy in patients with vitiligo. Natl Cancer Inst Monogr 1984;66:191–6.

149. Basarab T, Millard TP, McGregor JM, Barker JN. Atypical pigmented lesions following extensive PUVA therapy. Clin Exp Dermatol 2000;25(2):135–7.

150. Lindelof B, Sigurgeirsson B, Tegner E, et al. PUVA and cancer risk: the Swedish follow-up study. Br J Dermatol 1999;141(1):108–12.

151. Tjioe M, Gerritsen MJ, Juhlin L, van de Kerkhof PC. Treatment of vitiligo vulgaris with narrow band UVB (311 nm) for one year and the effect of addition of folic acid and vitamin B12. Acta Derm Venereol 2002;82(5):369–72.

152. Spencer JM, Nossa R, Ajmeri J. Treatment of vitil-igo with the 308–nm excimer laser: a pilot study. J Am Acad Dermatol 2002;46(5):727–31.

153. Scherschun L, Kim JJ, Lim HW. Narrow-band ultraviolet B is a useful and well-tolerated treatment for vitiligo. J Am Acad Dermatol 2001;44(6):999–1003.

154. Menchini G, Tsoureli-Nikita E, Hercogova J. Narrow-band UV-B micro-phototherapy: a new treatment for vitiligo. J Eur Acad Dermatol Venereol 2003;17(2):171–7.

155. Dogra S, Parsad D. Combination of narrowband UV-B and topical calcipotriene in vitiligo. Arch Dermatol 2003;139(3):393.

156. Leone G, Iacovelli P, Paro Vidolin A, Picardo M. Monochromatic excimer light 308 nm in the treat-ment of vitiligo: a pilot study. J Eur Acad Dermatol Venereol 2003;17(5):531–7.

157. Samson Yashar S, Gielczyk R, Scherschun L, Lim HW. Narrow-band ultraviolet B treatment for vitiligo, pru-ritus, and inflammatory dermatoses. Photodermatol Photoimmunol Photomed 2003;19(4):164–8.

158. Taneja A, Trehan M, Taylor CR. 308–nm excimer laser for the treatment of localized vitiligo. Int J Dermatol 2003;42(8):658–62.

159. Passeron T, Ortonne JP. UVB Therapy for Pigmentary Disorders. In: Nordlund JJ RB, VJ Hearing, RA King, W Oetting, JP Ortonne, ed. The Pigmentary System: Physiology and Pathophysiology, 2nd ed. Oxford: Blackwell Scientific, 2006:1183–7.

160. Njoo MD, Bos JD, Westerhof W. Treatment of gen-eralized vitiligo in children with narrow-band (TL-01) UVB radiation therapy. J Am Acad Dermatol 2000;42(2 pt 1):245–53.

161. Schallreuter K, Moore J, Wood J. Pseudocatalase in the Treatment of Vitiligo. In: Hann S-K, Nordlund J, eds. Vitiligo: Monograph on Basic and Clinical Science, 1st ed. Oxford, England: Blackwell Scientific, 2000:182–92.

162. Patel DC, Evans AV, Hawk JL. Topical pseudocata-lase mouse and narrowband UVB phototherapy is not effective for vitiligo: an open, single-centre study. Clin Exp Dermatol 2002;27(8):641–4.

163. Hann SK. Steroid treatment for vitiligo. In: Hann SK, Nordlund JJ, eds. Vitiligo: A Monograph on the Basic and Clinical Science. Oxford: Blackwell Scientific, 2000:173–81.

164. Halder RM, Nordlund JJ. Topical treatment for pigmentary disorders. In: Nordlund JJ, Boissy RE, Hearing VJ, King RA, Oetting WS, Ortonne JP, eds. The Pigmentary System: Physiology and Pathophysiology, 2nd ed. Oxford: Blackwell Scientific, 2006:1165–74.

165. Grimes PE, Kelly AP, Cline DJ, et al. Management of vitiligo in children, Symposium. Pediatr Dermatol 1986;3(6):498–510.

166. Halder RM, Grimes PE, Cowan CA, Enterline JA, Chakrabarti SG, Kenney JA Jr. Childhood vitiligo. J Am Acad Dermatol 1987;16(5):948–54.

167. Kumari J. Vitiligo treated with topical clobetasol propionate. Arch Dermatol 1984;120:631–5.

168. Cockayne SE, Messenger AG, Gawkrodger DJ. Vitiligo treated with topical corticosteroids: children with head and neck involvement respond well. J Am Acad Dermatol 2002;46(6):964–5.

169. Grimes PE, Soriano T, Dytoc MT. Topical tacrolimus for repigmentation of vitiligo. J Am Acad Dermatol 2002;47(5):789–91.

170. Smith DA, Tofte SJ, Hanifin JM. Repigmentation of vitiligo with topical tacrolimus. Dermatology 2002;205(3):301–3.

171. Castanedo-Cazares JP, Lepe V, Moncada B. Repigmentation of chronic vitiligo lesions by following tacrolimus plus ultraviolet-B-narrow-band. Photodermatol Photoimmunol Photomed 2003;19(1):35–6.

172. Tanghetti EA. Tacrolimus ointment 0.1% produces repigmentation in patients with vitiligo: results of a prospective patient series. Cutis 2003;71(2):158–62.

173. Kanwar AJ, Dogra S, Parsad D. Topical tacrolimus for treatment of childhood vitiligo in Asians. Clin Exp Dermatol 2004;29(6):589–92.

174. Silverberg NB, Lin P, Travis L, et al. Tacrolimus ointment promotes repigmentation of vitiligo in children: a review of 57 cases. J Am Acad Dermatol 2004;51(5):760–6.

175. Grimes PE, Morris R, Avaniss-Aghajani E, Soriano T, Meraz M, Metzger A. Topical tacrolimus therapy for vitiligo: therapeutic responses and skin messenger RNA expression of proinflammatory cytokines. J Am Acad Dermatol 2004;51(1):52–61.

176. Kawalek AZ, Spencer JM, Phelps RG. Combined excimer laser and topical tacrolimus for the treatment of vitiligo: a pilot study. Dermatol Surg 2004;30(2 pt 1):130–5.

177. Travis LB, Weinberg JM, Silverberg NB. Successful treatment of vitiligo with 0.1% tacrolimus ointment. Arch Dermatol 2003;139(5):571–4; discussion 573.

178. Kose O, Riza Gur A, Kurumlu Z, Erol E. Calcipotriol ointment versus clobetasol ointment in localized vitiligo: an open, comparative clinical trial. Int J Dermatol 2002;41(9):616–8.

179. Chiaverini C, Passeron T, Ortonne JP. Treatment of vitiligo by topical calcipotriol. J Eur Acad Dermatol Venereol 2002;16(2):137–8.

180. Hann S-K, Nordlund JJ, eds. Vitiligo: A Monograph on the Basic and Clinical Science, 1st ed. Oxford, London: Blackwell Scientific, 2000.

181. Kenney JA Jr, Grimes PE. How we treat vitiligo. Cutis 1983;32(4):347–8.

182. Boersma BR, Westerhof W, Bos JD. Repigmentation in vitiligo vulgaris by autologous minigrafting: results in nineteen patients. J Am Acad Dermatol 1995;33(6):990–5.

183. Falabella R, Escobar C, Borrero I. Treatment of refractory and stable vitiligo by transplantation of in vitro cultured epidermal autografts bearing melanocytes. J Am Acad Dermatol 1992;26(2 pt 1):230–6.

184. Plott RT, Brysk MM, Newton R, Raimer SS, Rajaraman S. A surgical treatment for vitiligo: Transplantation of autologous cultured epithelial grafts. J Dermatol Surg Oncol 1989;15:1161–6.

185. Hann SK, Im S, Bong HW, Park YK. Treatment of stable vitiligo with autologous epidermal grafting and PUVA. J Am Acad Dermatol 1995;32(6):943–8.

186. Falabella R, Barona M, Escobar C, Borrero I, Arrunategui A. Surgical combination therapy for vitiligo and piebaldism. Dermatol Surg 1995;21(10):852–7.

187. Westerhof W, Boersma B. The minigrafting test for vitiligo: detection of stable lesions for melanocyte transplantation [letter]. J Am Acad Dermatol 1995;33(6):1061–2.

188. Bhawan J, Bhutani LK. Keratinocyte damage in vitiligo. J Cutan Pathol 1983;10:207–12.

189. Gokhale BB, Mehta LN. Histopathology of vitiliginous skin. Int J Dermatol 1983;22:477–80.

190. Lever WF, Schaumberg-Lever G. Histopathology of the Skin. Philadelphia: JB Lippincott, 1991.

191. Mishima Y, Kawasaki H, Pinkus H. Dendritic cell dynamics in progressive depigmentations. Distinctive cytokinetics of dendritic cells revealed by electron microscopy. Arch Dermatol Res 1972;243(2):67–87.

192. Mishima Y. Histopathology of functional pigmentary disorders. Cutis 1978;21(2):225–30.

193. Morohashi M, Hashimoto K, Goodman TF Jr, Newton DE, Rist T. Ultrastructural studies of vitiligo, Vogt-Koyanagi syndrome, and incontinentia pigmenti achromians. Arch Dermatol 1977;113:755–66.

194. Pinkus H, Mehregan AH. A Guide to Dermatohistopathology. New York: Appleton-Century-Crofts, 1981.

195. Takei M, Mishima Y, Uda H. Immunopathology of vitiligo vulgaris, Sutton's leukoderma and melanoma-associated vitiligo in relation to ster-

oid effects. I. Circulating antibodies for cultured melanoma cells. J Cutan Pathol 1984;11(2):107–13.

196. Uda H, Takei M, Mishima Y. Immunopathology of vitiligo vulgaris, Sutton's leukoderma and melanoma-associated vitiligo in relation to steroid effects. II. The IgG and C3 deposits in the skin. J Cutan Pathol 1984;11(2):114–24.

197. Le Poole IC, van den Wijngaard RMJGJ, Westerhof W, Das PK. Presence of T cells and macrophages in inflammatory vitiligo skin parallels melanocyte disappearance. Am J Pathol 1996;148:1219–28.

198. al Badri AM, Todd PM, Garioch JJ, Gudgeon JE, Stewart DG, Goudie RB. An immunohistological study of cutaneous lymphocytes in vitiligo. J Pathol 1993;170(2):149–55.

199. Boissy RE, Beato KE, Nordlund JJ. Dilated rough endoplasmic reticulum and premature cell death in melanocytes cultured from the vitiligo mouse. Am J Pathol 1991;138:1511–25.

200. Bose SK. Absence of Merkel cells in lesional skin of vitiligo. Int J Dermatol 1994;33(7):481–3.

201. Boissy RE. Histology of vitiliginous skin. In: Hann S-K, Nordlund JJ, eds. Vitiligo: Monograph on the Basic and Clinical Science, 1st ed. Oxford, England: Blackwell Scientific, 2000:23–34.

202. Medrano EE, Nordlund JJ. Successful culture of adult human melanocytes from normal and vitiligo donors. J Invest Dermatol 1990;95:441–5.

203. Le Poole IC, van den Wijngaard RMJGJ, Westerhof W, Dutrieux RP, Das PK. Presence or absence of melanocytes in vitiligo lesions: an immunohistochemical investigation. J Invest Dermatol 1993;100:816–22.

204. Tobin D, Swanson N, Pittelkow M, Peters E, Schallreuter K. Melanocytes are not absent in lesional skin of long duration vitiligo. J Pathol 2000;191:407–16.

205. Gauthier Y, Cario Andre M, Taieb A. A critical appraisal of vitiligo etiologic theories. Is melanocyte loss a melanocytorrhagy? Pigment Cell Res 2003;16(4):322–32.

206. Le Poole IC, van den Wijngaard RM, Westerhof W, Das PK. Tenascin is overexpressed in vitiligo lesional skin and inhibits melanocyte adhesion. Br J Dermatol 1997;137:171–8.

207. Iyengar B, Misra RS. Neural differentiation of melanocytes in vitiliginous skin. Acta Anat 1988;133:62–5.

208. Ivanova K, van den Wijngaard R, Gerzer R, Lamers WH, Das PK. Non-lesional vitiliginous melanocytes are not characterized by an increased proneness to nitric oxide-induced apoptosis. Exp Dermatol 2005;14(6):445–53.

209. Bose SK. Probable mechanisms of loss of Merkel cells in completely depigmented skin of stable vitiligo. J Dermatol 1994;21(10):725–8.

210. Montes LF, Abulafia J, Wilborn WH, Hyde BM, Montes CM. Value of histopathology in vitiligo. Int J Dermatol 2003;42(1):57–61.

211. Al'Abadie MSK, Warren MA, Bleehen SS, Gawkrodger DJ. Morphologic observations on the dermal nerves in vitiligo: an ultrastructural study. Int J Dermatol 1995;34:837–40.

212. Liu PY, Bondesson L, Loentz W, Tohansson O. The occurrence of cutaneous nerve endings and neuropeptides in vitiligo vulgaris: a case-control study. Arch Dermatol Res 1996;288:670–5.

213. Lazarova R, Hristakieva E, Lazarov N, Shani J. Vitiligo-related neuropeptides in nerve fibers of the skin. Arch Physiol Biochem 2000;108(3):262–7.

214. van den Wijngaard RM, Asghar SS, Pijnenborg AC, Tigges AJ, Westerhof W, Das PK. Aberrant expression of complement regulatory proteins, membrane cofactor protein and decay accelerating factor, in the involved epidermis of patients with vitiligo. Br J Dermatol 2002;146(1):80–7.

215. Venneker GT, Vodegel RM, Okada N, Westerhof W, Bos JD, Asghar SS. Relative contributions of decay accelerating factor (DAF), membrane cofactor protein (MCP) and CD59 in the protection of melanocytes from homologous complement. Immunobiology 1998;198(4):476–84.

216. Venneker GT, Westerhof W, de Vries IJ, et al. Molecular heterogeneity of the fourth component of complement (C4) and its genes in vitiligo. J Invest Dermatol 1992;99(6):853–8.

217. Le Poole IC, Das PK. Microscopic changes in vitiligo. Clin Dermatol 1997;15(6):863–73.

218. Kao C-H, Yu H-S. Depletion and repopulation of Langerhans cells in nonsegmental type vitiligo. J Dermatol 1990;17:287–96.

219. Kroll TM, Bommiasamy H, Boissy RE, Nickoloff BJ, Mestril R, Le Poole IC. 4–Tertiary butyl phenol exposure sensitizes melanocytes to dendritic cell mediated killing. J Invest Dermatol 2005;124:798–806.

220. Ahn SK, Choi EH, Lee SH, Won JH, Hann SK, Park YK. Immunohistochemical studies from vitiligo—comparison between active and inactive lesions. Yonsei Med J 1994;35(4):404–10.

221. van den Wijngaard R, Wankowicz-Kalinska A, Le Poole C, Tigges B, Westerhof W, Das P. Local immune response in skin of generalized vitiligo patients. Destruction of melanocytes is associated with the prominent presence of CLA+ T cells at the perilesional site. Lab Invest 2000;80(8):1299–309.

222. Das PK, van den Wijngaard RM, Wankowicz-Kalinska A, Le Poole IC. A symbiotic concept of autoimmunity and tumour immunity: lessons from vitiligo. Trends Immunol 2001;22(3):130–6.

223. al Badri AM, Foulis AK, Todd PM, et al. Abnormal expression of MHC class II and ICAM-1 by melanocytes in vitiligo. J Pathol 1993;169(2):203–6.

224. Le Poole IC, Stennett LS, Bonish BK, et al. Expansion of vitiligo lesions is associated with reduced epidermal CDw60 expression and increased expression of HLA-DR in perilesional skin. Br J Dermatol 2003;149(4):739–48.

225. Li YL, Yu CL, Yu HS. IgG anti-melanocyte antibodies purified from patients with active vitiligo induce HLA-DR and intercellular adhesion molecule-1 expression and an increase in interleukin-8 release by melanocytes. J Invest Dermatol 2000;115(6):969–73.

226. Abdallah M, Abdel-Naser MB, Moussa MH, Assaf C, Orfanos CE. Sequential immunohistochemical study of depigmenting and repigmenting minigrafts in vitiligo. Eur J Dermatol 2003;13(6):548–52.

227. Breathnach AS, Bor S, Wyllie LM. Electron microscopy of peripheral nerve terminals and marginal melanocytes in vitiligo. J Invest Dermatol 1966;47:125–40.

228. Ito K. [Ultrastructual observations of dendritic cells in the repigmented area of vitiligo: electron microscopic studies on dopa oxidase in melanocytes which are present between the epidermal basal cells in the repigmented area of vitiligo (author's transl)]. Nippon Hifuka Gakkai Zasshi 1975;85(6):333–49.

229. Bleehen SS. The treatment of vitiligo with topical corticosteroids. Light and electronmicroscopic studies. Br J Dermatol 1976;94(suppl 12):43–50.

230. Hu F, Fosnaugh RP, Lesney PF. In vitro studies on vitiligo. J Invest Dermatol 1959;33:267–80.

231. Abdel-Naser MB, Kruger-Krasagakes S, Krasagakis K, Gollnick H, Orfanos CE. Further evidence for involvement of both cell mediated and humoral immunity in generalized vitiligo. Pigment Cell Res 1994;7(1):1–8.

232. Savill J, Fadok V, Henson P, Haslett C. Phagocyte recognition of cells undergoing apoptosis. Immunol Today 1993;14:131–6.

233. Martins LM, Earnshaw WC. Apoptosis: alive and kicking in 1997. Trends Cell Biol 1997;7:111–4.

234. Blois MS. Phagocytosis of melanin particles by human epidermal cells in vitro. J Invest Dermatol 1968;50:336–7.

235. Wolff K, Konrad K. Melanin pigmentation: an in vivo model for studies of melanosome kinetics within keratinocytes. Science 1971;174:1034–5.

236. Boissy RE, Liu Y-Y, Medrano EE, Nordlund JJ. Structural aberration of the rough endoplasmic reticulum and melanosome compartmentalization in long-term cultures of melanocytes from vitiligo patients. J Invest Dermatol 1991;97:395–404.

237. Malmusi M, Ackerman A. A critical review of apoptosis in historical perspective. Am J Dermatopathol 2000;22:291–3.

238. Gogvadze V, Orrenius S, Zhivotovsky B. Multiple pathways of cytochrome c release from mitochondria in apoptosis. Biochim Biophys Acta 2006;1757(5–6):639–47.

239. Proskuryakov SY, Gabai VL, Konoplyannikov AG, Zamulaeva IA, Kolesnikova AI. Immunology of apoptosis and necrosis. Biochemistry (Mosc) 2005;70(12):1310–20.

240. Boissy RE, Nordlund JJ. Biology of vitiligo. In: Arndt KA, LeBoit PE, Robinson JK, Wintroub BU, eds. Cutaneous Medicine and Surgery: An Integrated Program in Dermatology. Philadelphia: WB Saunders, 1995:1210–8.

241. Ortonne J-P, Mosher DB, Fitzpatrick TB. Vitiligo and Other Hypomelanoses of Hair and Skin. New York: Plenum Medical, 1983.

242. Nath SK, Majumder PP, Nordlund JJ. Genetic epidemiology of vitiligo: multilocus recessivity cross validated. Am J Hum Genet 1994;55:981–90.

243. Abdel-Malek Z, Suzuki I, Tada A, Im S, Akcali C. The melanocortin-1 receptor and human pigmentation. Ann NY Acad Sci 1999;885:117–33.

244. Yaar M, Eller MS, DiBenedetto P, et al. The trk family of receptors mediates nerve growth factor and neurotrophin-3 effects in melanocytes. J Clin Invest 1994;94:1550–62.

245. Halaban R, Langdon R, Birchall N, et al. Basic fibroblast growth factor from human keratinocytes is a natural mitogen for melanocytes. J Cell Biol 1988;107:1611–9.

246. Imokawa G, Miyagishi M, Yada Y. Endothelin-1 as a new melanogen: Coordinated expression of its gene and the tyrosinase gene in UVB-exposed human epidermis. J Invest Dermatol 1995;105:32–7.

247. Slominski A, Tobin DJ, Shibahara S, Wortsman J. Melanin pigmentation in mammalian skin and its hormonal regulation. Physiol Rev 2004;84(4):1155–228.

248. Hochstein P, Cohen G. The cytotoxicity of melanin precursors. Ann NY Acad Sci 1963;100:876–81.

249. Riley PA. Mechanisms of inhibition of melanin pigmentation. In: Nordlund JJ, Boissy RE, Hearing VJ, King RA, Ortonne J-P, eds. The Pigmentary System Physiology and Pathophysiology. New York: Oxford University Press, 1998:401–21.

250. Monks TJ, Hanzlik RP, Cohen GM, Ross D, Graham DG. Contemporary issues in toxicology. Quinone chemistry and toxicity. Toxicol Appl Pharmacol 1992;112:2–16.

251. Powis G. Metabolism and reactions of quinoid anticancer agents. Pharmacol Ther 1987;35(1–2): 57–162.

252. O'Brien PJ. Molecular mechanisms of quinone cytotoxicity. Chem Biol Interact 1991;80(1):1–41.

253. Marnett LJ. Lipid peroxidation-DNA damage by malondialdehyde. Mutat Res 1999;424(1–2):83–95.

254. Takahashi A, Masuda A, Sun M, Centonze VE, Herman B. Oxidative stress-induced apoptosis is associated with alterations in mitochondrial caspase activity and Bcl-2–dependent alterations in mitochondrial pH (pHm). Brain Res Bull 2004;62(6):497–504.

255. Boissy RE, Manga P. On the etiology of contact/occupational vitiligo. Pigment Cell Res 2004;17(3):208–14.

256. Jimbow K, Obata H, Pathak MA, Fitzpatrick TB. Mechanism of depigmentation by hydroquinone. J Invest Dermatol 1974;62:436–49.

257. McGuire J, Hinders J. Biochemical basis for depigmentation of skin by phenol germicides. J Invest Dermatol 1971;57:256–61.

258. Gellin GA, Maibach HI, Misiaszek MH. Detection of environmental depigmenting substances. Contact Dermatitis 1979;5:201–13.

259. Nakagawa Y, Tayama S, Moore G, Moldeus P. Cytotoxic effects of biphenyl and hydroxybiphenyls on isolated rat hepatocytes. Biochem Pharmacol 1993;45:1959–65.

260. Mans DR, Lafleur MV, Westmijze EJ, et al. Reactions of glutathione with the catechol, the ortho-quinone and the semi-quinone free radical of etoposide. Consequences for DNA inactivation. Biochem Pharmacol 1992;43:1761–8.

261. Halliwell B, Chirico S. Lipid peroxidation: its mechanism, measurement, and significance. Am J Clin Nutr 1993;57(suppl 5):715S-25S.

262. Yang F, Sarangarajan R, Le Poole IC, Medrano EE, Boissy RE. The cytotoxicity and apoptosis induced by 4–tertiary butylphenol in human melanocytes is independent of tyrosinase activity. J Invest Dermatol 2000;114:157–64.

263. Manga P, Sheyn D, Yang F, Sarangarajan R, Boissy RE. A role for tyrosinase related-protein 1 in 4-tert-butyl-phenol-induced toxicity in melanocytes. Implications for vitiligo. Am J Pathol 2006;169(5):1652–62.

264. Vijayasaradhi S, Doskoch PM, Houghton AN. Biosynthesis and intracellular movement of the melanosomal membrane glycoprotein gp75, the human brown locus product. Exp Cell Res 1991;196:233–40.

265. Kobayashi T, Urabe K, Winder AJ, et al. Tyrosinase-related protein 1 (TRP1) functions as a DHICA oxidase in melanin biosynthesis. EMBO J 1994;13:5818–25.

266. Boissy RE, Sakai C, Zhao H, Kobayashi T, Hearing VJ. Human tyrosinase related protein-1 (TRP-1) does not function as a DHICA oxidase activity in contrast to murine TRP-1. Exp Dermatol 1998;7:198–204.

267. Jimenez M, Tsukamoto K, Hearing VJ. Tyrosinases from two different loci are expressed by normal and by transformed melanocytes. J Biol Chem 1991;266:1147–56.

268. Zhao H, Zhao Y, Nordlund JJ, Boissy RE. Human TRP-1 has tyrosine hydroxylase activity but no dopa oxidase activity. Pigment Cell Res 1994;7:131–40.

269. Bolton JL, Trush MA, Penning TM, Dryhurst G, Monks TJ. Role of quinones in toxicology. Chem Res Toxicol 2000;13(3):135–60.

270. Thorneby-Andersson K, Sterner O, Hansson C. Tyrosinase-mediated formation of a reactive quinone from the depigmenting agents, 4–tert-butyl-phenol and 4–tert-butylcatechol. Pigment Cell Res 2000;13:33–8.

271. Streilein JW. Skin-associated lymphoid tissues (SALT): origins and functions. J Invest Dermatol 1983;8(suppl):12s-6s.

272. Patel DD, Whichard LP, Radcliff G, Denning SM, Haynes BF. Characterization of human thymic epithelial cell surface antigens: phenotypic similarity of thymic epithelial cells to epidermal keratinocytes. J Clin Immunol 1995;15(2):80–92.

273. Sugita K, Kabashima K, Atarashi K, Shimauchi T, Kobayashi M, Tokura Y. Innate immunity mediated by epidermal keratinocytes promotes acquired immunity involving Langerhans cells and T cells in the skin. Clin Exp Immunol 2007;147(1):176–83.

274. Restifo NP, Rosenberg SA. Developing recombinant and synthetic vaccines for the treatment of melanoma. Curr Opin Oncol 1999;11(1):50–7.

275. Kruger-Krasagakes S, Krasagakis K, Garbe C, Diamantstein T. Production of cytokines by human melanoma cells and melanocytes. Recent Results Cancer Res 1995;139:155–68.

276. Swope VB, Sauder DN, McKenzie RC, et al. Synthesis of interleukin-1α and β by normal human melanocytes. J Invest Dermatol 1994;102:749–53.

277. Lee H, Overall CM, McCulloch CA, Sodek J. A critical role for the membrane-type 1 matrix metalloproteinase in collagen phagocytosis. Mol Biol Cell 2006;17(11):4812–26.

278. Van Den Bossche K, Naeyaert JM, Lambert J. The quest for the mechanism of melanin transfer. Traffic 2006;7(7):769–78.

279. Le Poole IC, van den Wijngaard RMJGJ, Westerhof W, et al. Phagocytosis by normal human melanocytes (in vitro). Exp Cell Res 1993;205:388–95.

280. Raposo G, Fevrier B, Stoorvogel W, Marks MS. Lysosome-related organelles: a view from

immunity and pigmentation. Cell Struct Funct 2002;27(6):443–56.

281. Berger CL, Vasquez JG, Shofner J, Mariwalla K, Edelson RL. Langerhans cells: mediators of immunity and tolerance. Int J Biochem Cell Biol 2006;38(10):1632–6.

282. Le Poole IC, Mutis T, van den Wijngaard RMJGJ, et al. A novel, antigen-presenting function of melanocytes and its possible relationship to hypopigmentary disorders. J Immunol 1993;151:7284–92.

283. Sakai C, Kawakami Y, Law LW, Furumura M, Hearing VJ Jr. Melanosomal proteins as melanoma-specific immune targets. Melanoma Res 1997;7(2):83–95.

284. Touloukian CE, Leitner WW, Topalian SL, et al. Identification of a MHC class II-restricted human gp100 epitope using DR4–IE transgenic mice. J Immunol 2000;164(7):3535–42.

285. Wang S, Bartido S, Yang G, et al. A role for a melanosome transport signal in accessing the MHC class II presentation pathway and in eliciting CD4+ T cell responses. J Immunol 1999;163(11):5820–6.

286. Harning R, Cui J, Bystryn JC. Relation between the incidence and level of pigment cell antibodies and disease activity in vitiligo. J Invest Dermatol 1991;97(6):1078–80.

287. Gottumukkala RV, Gavalas NG, Akhtar S, et al. Function-blocking autoantibodies to the melanin-concentrating hormone receptor in vitiligo patients. Lab Invest 2006;86(8):781–9.

288. Gilhar A, Zelickson B, Ulman Y, Etzioni A. In vivo destruction of melanocytes by the IgG fraction of serum from patients with vitiligo. J Invest Dermatol 1995;105:683–6.

289. Norris DA, Kissinger GM, Naughton GM, Bystryn J-C. Evidence for immunologic mechanisms in human vitiligo: Patients' sera induce damage to human melanocytes in vitro by complement-mediated damage and antibody-dependent cellular cytotoxicity. J Invest Dermatol 1988;90:783–9.

290. Ogg GS, Rod Dunbar P, Romero P, Chen JL, Cerundolo V. High frequency of skin-homing melanocyte-specific cytotoxic T lymphocytes in autoimmune vitiligo. J Exp Med 1998;188:1203–8.

291. Palermo B, Campanelli R, Garbelli S, et al. Specific cytotoxic T lymphocyte responses against Melan-A/MART1, tyrosinase and gp100 in vitiligo by the use of major histocompatibility complex/peptide tetramers: the role of cellular immunity in the etiopathogenesis of vitiligo. J Invest Dermatol 2001;117(2):326–32.

292. Wankowicz-Kalinska A, van den Wijngaard RM, Tigges BJ, et al. Immunopolarization of CD4+ and CD8+ T cells to Type-1–like is associated with melanocyte loss in human vitiligo. Lab Invest 2003;83(5):683–95.

293. Oyarbide-Valencia K, van den Boorn JG, Denman CJ, et al. Therapeutic implications of autoimmune vitiligo T cells. Autoimmun Rev 2006;5(7):486–92.

294. Palermo B, Garbelli S, Mantovani S, et al. Qualitative difference between the cytotoxic T lymphocyte responses to melanocyte antigens in melanoma and vitiligo. Eur J Immunol 2005;35(11):3153–62.

295. Levings MK, Allan S, d'Hennezel E, Piccirillo CA. Functional dynamics of naturally occurring regulatory T cells in health and autoimmunity. Adv Immunol 2006;92:119–55.

296. Mantovani S, Garbelli S, Palermo B, et al. Molecular and functional bases of self-antigen recognition in long-term persistent melanocyte-specific CD8+ T cells in one vitiligo patient. J Invest Dermatol 2003;121(2):308–14.

297. Collins SM, Dominguez M, Ilmarinen T, Costigan C, Irvine AD. Dermatological manifestations of autoimmune polyendocrinopathy-candidiasis-ectodermal dystrophy syndrome. Br J Dermatol 2006;154(6):1088–93.

298. Halder RM, Walters CS, Johnson BA, Chakrabarti SG, Kenney JA Jr. Aberrations in T lymphocytes and natural killer cells in vitiligo: a flow cytometric study. J Am Acad Dermatol 1986;14(5 pt 1):733–7.

299. Steitz J, Wenzel J, Gaffal E, Tuting T. Initiation and regulation of CD8+ T cells recognizing melanocytic antigens in the epidermis: implications for the pathophysiology of vitiligo. Eur J Cell Biol 2004;83(11–12):797–803.

300. Whitton ME, Ashcroft DM, Barrett CW, Gonzalez U. Interventions for vitiligo. Cochrane Database Syst Rev 2006;(1):CD003263.

301. Majumder PP. Genetics and prevalence of vitiligo vulgaris. In: Hann SK, Nordlund JJ, eds. Vitiligo: A Monograph on the Basic and Clinical Science. Oxford, UK: Blackwell Scientific, 2000:18–20.

302. Spritz RA. The genetics of generalized vitiligo and associated autoimmune diseases. J Dermatol Sci 2006;41(1):3–10.

303. Kim SM, Chung HS, Hann SK. The genetics of vitiligo in Korean patients. Int J Dermatol 1998;37:908–10.

304. Jin Y, Mailloux C, Bennett D, Dinarello C, Fain P, Spritz R. NALP1, a key regulator of the innate immune system, is a novel major gene for multiple autoimmune/autoinflammatory disease [abstract 160]. In. Presented at the annual meeting of The American Society of Human Genetics, October 9–13, 2006, New Orleans, LA. http://www.ashg.org/genetics/ashg06s/.

305. Le Poole IC, Sarangarajan R, Zhao Y, et al. "VIT1," a novel gene associated with vitiligo. Pigment Cell Res 2001;14(6):475–84.

306. Jin SY, Park HH, Li GZ, et al. Association of estrogen receptor 1 intron 1 C/T polymorphism in Korean vitiligo patients. J Dermatol Sci 2004;35(3):181–6.

307. Tursen U, Kaya TI, Erdal ME, Derici E, Gunduz O, Ikizoglu G. Association between catechol-O-methyltransferase polymorphism and vitiligo. Arch Dermatol Res 2002;294(3):143–6.

308. Jin SY, Park HH, Li GZ, et al. Association of angiotensin converting enzyme gene I/D polymorphism of vitiligo in Korean population. Pigment Cell Res 2004;17(1):84–6.

309. Blomhoff A, Kemp EH, Gawkrodger DJ, et al. CTLA4 polymorphisms are associated with vitiligo, in patients with concomitant autoimmune diseases. Pigment Cell Res 2005;18(1):55–8.

310. Canton I, Akhtar S, Gavalas NG, et al. A single-nucleotide polymorphism in the gene encoding lymphoid protein tyrosine phosphatase (PTPN22) confers susceptibility to generalised vitiligo. Genes Immun 2005;6(7):584–7.

311. Alkhateeb A, Stetler GL, Old W, et al. Mapping of an autoimmunity susceptibility locus (AIS1) to chromosome 1p31.3–p32.2. Hum Mol Genet 2002;11:661–7.

312. Alkhateeb A, Fain PR, Spritz RA. Candidate functional promoter variant in the FOXD3 melanoblast developmental regulator gene in autosomal dominant vitiligo. J Invest Dermatol 2005;125(2):388–91.

313. Tastan HB, Akar A, Orkunoglu FE, Arca E, Inal A. Association of HLA class I antigens and HLA class II alleles with vitiligo in a Turkish population. Pigment Cell Res 2004;17(2):181–4.

314. Orozco-Topete R, Cordova-Lopez J, Yamamoto-Furusho JK, Garcia-Benitez V, Lopez-Martinez A, Granados J. HLA-DRB1 *04 is associated with the genetic susceptibility to develop vitiligo in Mexican patients with autoimmune thyroid disease. J Am Acad Dermatol 2005;52(1):182–3.

315. Fain PR, Babu SR, Bennett DC, Spritz RA. HLA class II haplotype DRB1*04–DQB1*0301 contributes to risk of familial generalized vitiligo and early disease onset. Pigment Cell Res 2006;19(1):51–7.

316. al-Fouzan A, al-Arbash M, Fouad F, Kaaba SA, Mousa MA, al-Harbi SA. Study of HLA class I/IL and T lymphocyte subsets in Kuwaiti vitiligo patients. Eur J Immunogenet 1995;22(2):209–13.

317. Orecchia G, Perfetti L, Malagoli P, Borghini F, Kipervarg Y. Vitiligo is associated with a significant increase in HLA-A30, Cw6 and DQw3 and a decrease in C4AQ0 in northern Italian patients. Dermatology 1992;185(2):123–7.

318. Abanmi A, Harthi FA, Baqami RA, et al. Association of HLA loci alleles and antigens in Saudi patients with vitiligo. Arch Dermatol Res 2006;298(7):347–52.

319. Venkataram MN, White AG, Leeny WA, al Suwaid AR, Daar AS. HLA antigens in Omani patients with vitiligo. Clin Exp Dermatol 1995;20(1):35–7.

320. Schallreuter KU, Levenig C, Kuhnl P, Loliger C, Hohl-Tehari M, Berger J. Histocompatibility antigens in vitiligo: Hamburg study on 102 patients from northern Germany. Dermatology 1993;187(3):186–92.

321. Buc M, Busova B, Hegyi E, Kolibasova K. Vitiligo is associated with HLA-A2 and HLA-Dw7 in the Slovak populations. Folia Biol (Praha) 1996;42(1–2):23–5.

322. Venneker GT, de Waal LP, Westerhof W, D'Amaro J, Schreuder GM, Asghar SS. HLA associations in vitiligo patients in the Dutch population. Dis Markers 1993;11(4):187–90.

323. Casp CB, She JX, McCormack WT. Genes of the LMP/TAP cluster are associated with the human autoimmune disease vitiligo. Genes Immun 2003;4(7):492–9.

324. Laberge G, Mailloux CM, Gowan K, et al. Early disease onset and increased risk of other autoimmune diseases in familial generalized vitiligo. Pigment Cell Res 2005;18(4):300–5.

325. Gustafsson J, Alimohammadi M, Ekwall O, et al. [APS I–a severe autoimmune disease with endocrine and non-endocrine symptoms]. Lakartidningen 2004;101(24):2096–8, 101–3.

326. Dittmar M, Kahaly GJ. Polyglandular autoimmune syndromes: immunogenetics and long-term follow-up. J Clin Endocrinol Metab 2003;88(7):2983–92.

327. Fain PR, Gowan K, LaBerge GS, et al. A genome-wide screen for generalized vitiligo: Confirmation of AIS1 on chromosome 1p31 and evidence for additional susceptibility loci. Am J Hum Genet 2003;72:1560–4.

328. Kristiansen OP, Larsen ZM, Pociot F. CTLA-4 in autoimmune diseases—a general susceptibility gene to autoimmunity? Genes Immun 2000;1(3):170–84.

329. Kemp EH, Ajjan RA, Waterman EA, et al. Analysis of a microsatellite polymorphism of the cytotoxic T-lymphocyte antigen-4 gene in patients with vitiligo. Br J Dermatol 1999;140:73–8.

330. Itirli G, Pehlivan M, Alper S, et al. Exon-3 polymorphism of CTLA-4 gene in Turkish patients with vitiligo. J Dermatol Sci 2005;38(3):225–7.

331. Birol A, Kisa U, Kurtipek GS, et al. Increased tumor necrosis factor alpha (TNF-alpha) and inter-leukin 1 alpha (IL1–alpha) levels in the lesional skin of patients with nonsegmental vitiligo. Int J Dermatol 2006;45(8):992–3.

332. Yazici AC, Erdal ME, Kaya TI, et al. Lack of association with TNF-alpha-308 promoter poly-morphism in patients with vitiligo. Arch Dermatol Res 2006;298(1):46–9.

333. Van Den Wijngaard R, Aten J, Scheepmaker A, et al. Expression and modulation of apopto-sis regulatory molecules in human melano-cytes: significance in vitiligo. Br J Dermatol 2000;143:573–81.

334. Schallreuter KU, Behrens-Williams S, Khaliq TP, et al. Increased epidermal functioning wild-type p53 expression in vitiligo. Exp Dermatol 2003;12(3):268–77.

335. Le Poole IC, van den Wijngaard RM, Smit NP, Oosting J, Westerhof W, Pavel S. Catechol-O-methyltransferase in vitiligo. Arch Dermatol Res 1994;286(2):81–6.

336. Schallreuter KU. Effectiveness of pseudocata-lase formulations in vitiligo. Clin Exp Dermatol 2003;28(5):562–3; author reply 563.

337. Goth L, Rass P, Pay A. Catalase enzyme mutations and their association with diseases. Mol Diagn 2004;8(3):141–9.

338. Casp CB, She JX, McCormack WT. Genetic association of the catalase gene (CAT) with vitiligo susceptibility. Pigment Cell Res 2002;15:62–6.

339. Gavalas NG, Akhtar S, Gawkrodger DJ, Watson PF, Weetman AP, Kemp EH. Analysis of allelic variants in the catalase gene in patients with the skin depigmenting disorder vitiligo. Biochem Biophys Res Commun 2006;345(4):1586–91.

340. Park HH, Ha E, Uhm YK, et al. Association study between catalase gene polymorphisms and the susceptibility to vitiligo in Korean population. Exp Dermatol 2006;15(5):377–80.

341. Akhtar S, Gavalas NG, Gawkrodger DJ, Watson PF, Weetman AP, Kemp EH. An insertion/deletion polymorphism in the gene encoding angiotensin converting enzyme is not associated with gen-eralised vitiligo in an English population. Arch Dermatol Res 2005;297(2):94–8.

342. Vang T, Congia M, Macis MD, et al. Autoimmune-associated lymphoid tyrosine phos-phatase is a gain-of-function variant. Nat Genet 2005;37(12):1317–9.

343. Birlea S, Birlea M, Cimponeriu D, et al. Autoimmune diseases and vitamin D receptor Apa-I polymorphism are associated with vitiligo in a small inbred Romanian community. Acta Derm Venereol 2006;86(3):209–14.

39
Alopecia Areata

Richard S. Kalish and Amos Gilhar

Key Points

- Alopecia areata is an autoimmune disease of the hair follicle and nail matrix.
- Alopecia areata is associated with other autoimmune conditions, such as thyroid disease and vitiligo.
- There are no gender differences in the incidence of alopecia areata.
- Polymorphisms of interleukin-1 receptor antagonist, alleles of macrophage migration inhibitory factor, and Notch4 are associated with alopecia areata.
- The primary histology of alopecia areata is a perifollicular lymphocytic infiltrate, predominately CD4+ cells.
- The inflammatory T cells of alopecia areata are cytotoxic and possess both the Fas/Fas ligand and granzyme B cytotoxic mechanisms.
- The inflammatory T cells of alopecia areata have a T-helper-1 cytokine bias and express interferon-γ.
- During early alopecia areata, anagen arrest is followed by conversion of the hair follicle from anagen to catagen, followed by telogen.
- Neuroendocrine factors may result in loss of immune privilege that may mediate initiation of alopecia areata.
- Limited alopecia areata has a high rate of spontaneous resolution, but can be treated with steroids, anthralin, topical sensitizers, or topical minoxidil.

Alopecia areata is an autoimmune disease of the hair follicle and nail matrix. The two principal findings are hair loss and nail pitting. The hair loss is reversible with immunosuppression or immune modulation, and the disease is associated with other autoimmune conditions including thyroid disease and vitiligo. Hair loss can progress to alopecia totalis, which is the complete loss of scalp hair, or to alopecia universalis, which is the complete loss of all body hair. The social and psychological burden for affected patients is considerable.

Epidemiology

The best estimate for the incidence of alopecia areata in the United States was derived from a population-based study of Olmstead County Minnesota.[1] The incidence of alopecia was 20.2 per 100,000 person-years, with an estimated lifetime risk of 1.7%. There was no difference between the sexes. The strength of this study is that it was population based, but the limitation of this study is that Olmstead County is relatively homogeneous compared to the population of the U.S.

A family history of alopecia areata varies greatly between populations and is a function of the severity of the disease as well as the age of onset. A positive family history among first-degree relatives has been reported to be as high as 47% for patients with early onset, in contrast to 1.6% for all patients.[2] The first onset is usually prior to age 40, with no difference between the sexes. A study of childhood alopecia areata in Kuwait determined the mean age of onset to be 5.7 years, with a positive family history of 51%.[3] Eighty percent of patients had mild disease. The high rate of positive family history in this study may reflect the early onset of disease.

The role of stress and psychiatric factors in alopecia areata remains controversial. Many patients attribute the onset of their disease to stress.[4] However, population-based studies have found little evidence of a significant correlation between psychiatric factors and onset of disease.[5] However, patients with alopecia areata do have significantly higher levels of anxiety disorders and depression.[6,7]

Alopecia areata is also associated with thyroid disease and vitiligo. The rate of thyroid disease may vary greatly depending on population and other risk factors, such as age of onset and positive family history. Rates quoted for thyroid disease vary: 8.9% (Iran),[8] 2.3% (Singapore),[9] and 7.2% (Thailand).[10] Vitiligo has been reported to have an incidence of 4.1%.[9] Association with thyroid disease is a lifetime risk and is not limited to the onset of the episode of alopecia.

Clinical relevance of this population data includes prognostic factors, and screening. Poor prognostic factors are early age of onset, extent of disease, and Down syndrome.[9] Although the association with thyroid disease is variable, it is good practice to perform regular thyroid disease screening.

Genetics

Family studies demonstrate that alopecia areata has a genetic component. Multiple loci have been associated with increased risk of disease. As with most autoimmune conditions, alopecia areata has an association with major histocompatibility complex (MHC) antigens. Human leukocyte antigen (HLA)-DQ3 is associated with alopecia areata across multiple populations,[11,12] and the frequency of HLA-DQ3 is increased in patients with early onset, severe disease. DRB1*0401 (DR4) and DQB1*0301 (DQ7) are associated with alopecia totalis and universalis,[13] indicating that there is genetic heterogeneity between mild and severe disease. HLA-A*02, -A*03, -B*18, -B*27, -B*52, and -Cw*0704 are all increased in a Chinese population, demonstrating that MHC class I can be a involved in pathogenesis.[14]

Down syndrome is associated with alopecia areata,[15] and genes on chromosome 21 are implicated in disease risk. Autoimmune polyendocrinopathy–candidiasis–ectodermal dystrophy (APECED) is an autosomal recessive condition marked by mucocutaneous candidiasis with multiple autoimmune endocrine failure including hypothyroidism, hypogonadism, and type 1 diabetes mellitus. It is caused by mutations in the autoimmune regulator gene (AIRE), mapping to 21q22.3.[16] Up to 30% of patients with APECED have alopecia areata, which is generally severe.[17] However, AIRE mutations are not associated with alopecia areata in the general population.

Cytokine and cytokine receptor alleles are also associated with autoimmune disease. Polymorphisms of interleukin-1 (IL-1) receptor antagonist are associated with severe early-onset disease,[18] as are alleles of macrophage migration inhibitory factor (MIF),[19] and Notch4.[20] Lymphoid protein tyrosine phosphatase (PTPN22), a C1858T allele, is associated with susceptibility to autoimmune disorders including severe alopecia areata.[21]

With the exception of AIRE mutations, most of the known genetic risks for alopecia areata are common alleles resulting in a two- to eightfold increases in relative risk. The diversity of genes involved suggests there are multiple genetic pathways to alopecia areata. A genome-wide linkage analysis of alopecia areata risk in the C3H/HeJ mouse also found multiple regions of interest,[22] supporting a polygenetic inheritance. There is an alopecia areata registry in the U.S. devoted to further mapping and identifying genetic risks for alopecia areata.[23] Such studies can potentially shed light on the processes by which multiple genes with a variety of functions can interact to induce autoimmune disease.

Clinical Features and Evaluation

The classic presentation of mild alopecia areata is a round area of hair loss with no clinical signs of inflammation (Fig. 39.1). The hair loss tends to be nearly complete within the lesion. There is no clinical evidence of scarring or loss of hair follicles. Other features include "exclamation point" hairs, vellus hairs, and a positive hair-pull test. The latter is a clinical index of disease activity, and is an important part of the exam. Examination should include eyebrows, eyelashes, facial hair, and fingernails. The typical nail change is pitting, often in a linear array,[24] and may include trachyonychia and longitudinal ridging.[25] Nail pitting may be a function of disease activity. Alopecia areata may present as a solitary lesion, or as a multitude of

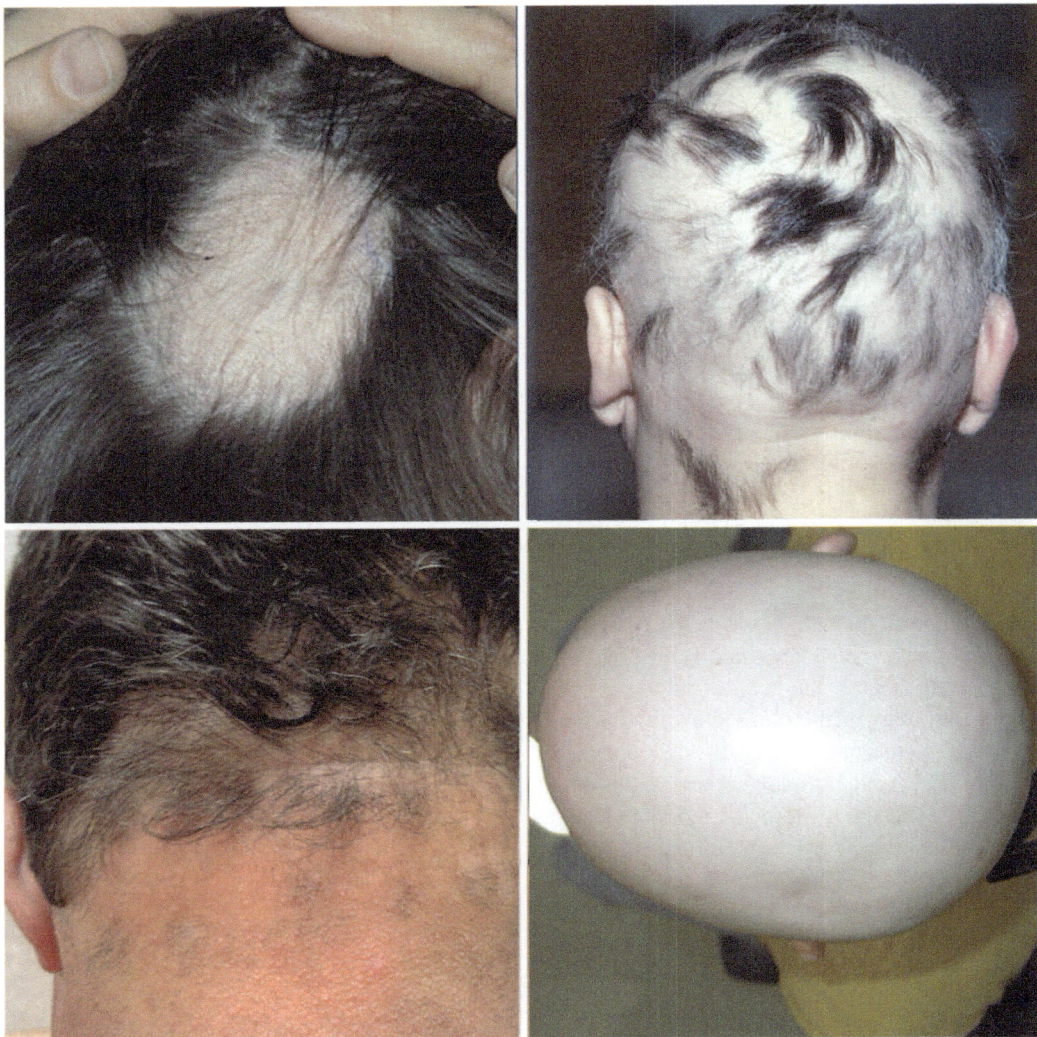

FIG. 39.1. Clinical presentations of alopecia areata. From left to right: limited alopecia areata, reticular diffuse alopecia areata, ophiasis pattern, and alopecia universalis

circular lesions, which may progress to widespread reticular alopecia areata. Alopecia areata of the occipital scalp, the ophiasis region, is common, and tends to be more recalcitrant to therapy. Eyebrows and eyelids are also commonly involved. Patients may report scalp symptoms with disease activity, including "tingling." Diffuse alopecia areata is an atypical presentation of rapid-onset alopecia involving the entire scalp. Other than a grossly positive hair-pull test, the typical findings may be absent, and diagnosis may require a biopsy. In patients with mixed gray and dark hairs, alopecia areata tends to spare white hairs, and the initial hair regrowth may be white. This has led to specula-

tion on the role of melanocyte antigens in alopecia areata. Alopecia areata may progress to alopecia totalis, involving the entire scalp, or alopecia universalis, involving all scalp and body hair including eyebrows and eyelids.

Evaluation of patients with alopecia areata should include a complete history, as well as examination of the scalp, facial hair, and nails. The history should include a personal history of atopy, and a family history of alopecia areata, thyroid disease, and vitiligo. Diseases to be excluded include inflammatory diseases of the scalp, such as lupus erythematosus, and lichen planopilaris. Alopecia areata should not exhibit erythema or scaling. Other conditions to be excluded include frontal fibrosing alopecia, which may mimic alopecia areata, but has histologic features of lichen planopilaris,[26] and trichotillomania. The hair-pull test is important both in diagnosis and clinical evaluation of alopecia areata. A positive hair pull is defined as the removal of five hairs with a gentle pull. The test is not diagnostic. Positive results may also be obtained with severe telogen effluvium.[27] However, the hair pull is the best clinical index of disease activity and should be performed both at the perimeter of existing lesions as well as diffusely throughout the scalp.

Laboratory evaluation should include a complete blood count and thyroid function tests. There is some evidence that patients with iron-deficiency anemia respond poorly to treatment, and serum ferritin determination may be appropriate in patients with a low mean cell volume (MCV) on a screening blood count.[28] Patients should be instructed to have thyroid function tests obtained yearly by their primary care provider.

An important part of the clinical evaluation is a determination of the patient's ability to cope with the condition, as well as interference with social functioning. A scoring system for alopecia areata has been published for use in clinical studies.[29] The percentage of hair loss is graded from S1 to S5 in 25% increments, with S1 indicating 0% and S5 indicating 100% hair loss. This scoring system is essential for clinical studies in that it provides standard comparisons. However, it remains primarily a research tool.

Histology of Alopecia Areata

The primary pathology of alopecia areata is a perifollicular lymphocytic infiltrate.[30] However, the pathologic changes vary with stage of disease.[31] Early active disease is associated with a lymphocytic infiltrate around the terminal hair bulb (Fig. 39.2). Anagen arrest follows, with conversion of the hair follicle from anagen to catagen, followed by telogen. The numbers of telogen hairs increase dramatically. The follicle attempts to cycle into anagen, which is aborted by inflammation, resulting in a miniaturized anagen or telogen hair. Terminal hairs are replaced by vellus hairs, or nanogen hairs, which are located in the mid-dermis and lack hair shafts. Quantitative changes in terminal, telogen, catagen, and vellus hairs are best observed in horizontal sections. Recovery is associated with resolution of inflammation and increase in terminal hairs.

Evidence of an Autoimmune Pathogenesis

Alopecia areata is associated with autoimmune thyroid disease and vitiligo. Risk factors include specific immune response genes. Histology is marked by perifollicular infiltrates of T lymphocytes. The perifollicular lymphocytes are predominantly CD4+ T cells, whereas the few intrafollicular lymphocytes tend to be CD8+ T cells. Further support for an autoimmune pathogenesis has been derived from human scalp graft/severe combined immunodeficiency disease (SCID) mouse studies, and animal models.[32,33]

Grafting of bald scalp from alopecia areata patients to nude mice results in hair regrowth, suggesting that hair growth is prevented by immunologic factors.[34] Autoantibodies to hair follicles are consistently found in alopecia areata.[35,36] However, the follicular structures labeled are variable and the role of antibodies in pathogenesis is uncertain. Furthermore, injection of patient serum into human skin grafts on nude mice does not induce hair loss.[37]

Hair Follicle Immune Privilege and Its Role in Alopecia Areata

Hair follicles have properties of an immune privileged site.[38] This is true of both mice and humans. During anagen, the proximal (lower) hair follicular epithelium of normal hair follicles does not express major histocompatibility complex (MHC) class I or class II molecules.[39,40] Absence of MHC during anagen is localized to keratinocytes of the matrix and inner root sheath. There is also a decrease of Langerhans' cell and dendritic cell density in the proximal hair follicle.[41] Other mechanisms of immune privilege in the anagen hair follicle include production of immunosuppressive cytokines melanocyte-stimulating hormone-α (MSH-α), transforming growth factor-β (TGF-β),

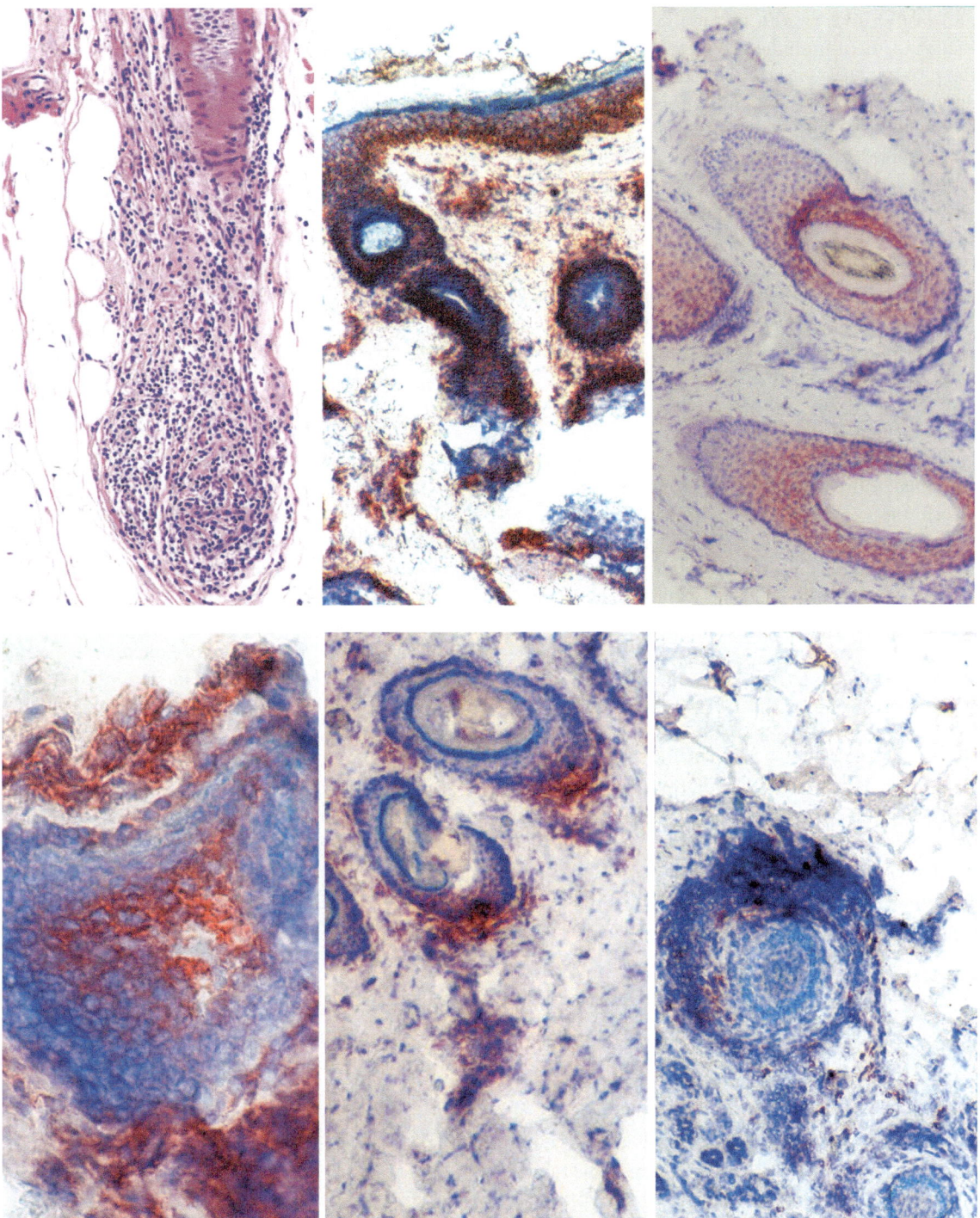

Fig. 39.2. Histology and immunohistochemistry of alopecia areata. (A) Histology demonstrating dense perifollicular lymphocytic infiltrate. (B) Human leukocyte antigen (HLA)-A,B,C expression on follicular epithelium as well as epidermis. (C) HLA-DR expression on follicular epithelium. (D) Intercellular adhesion molecule 1 (ICAM-1). (E) CD4+ T cells, perifollicular. (F) CD8+ T cells, intrafollicular

and insulin-like growth factor-I (IGF-I).[38] Similar mechanisms of immune privilege are also found in the proximal nail matrix, another target for alopecia areata.[42] The role of hair follicle immune privilege is uncertain. One obvious role would be to protect hair follicles from autoimmune attack, since loss of hair could be fatal to an animal. However, the bulge region containing hair follicle stem cells expresses MHC class I and is not subject to this protection.[38] It was proposed by Paus et al.[39] that loss of immune privilege allows for T-cell recognition of sequestered autoantigens, resulting in alopecia areata.

Alopecia areata is associated with loss of hair follicle immune privilege. Both humans and C3H/HeJ mice with alopecia areata express MHC classes I and II on proximal follicular epithelium (Fig. 39.2).[43] Such expression of MHC I and II on proximal follicular epithelium can be induced by interferon-γ (IFN-γ).[44] Induction of MHC class I on proximal hair follicles may initiate an autoaggressive response by melanocyte reactive CD8+ T cells.[39] These CD8+ cells may then induce HLA-DR on the affected hair follicles by production of IFN-γ, resulting in a second wave of CD4+ cells.

The immune privilege hypothesis for alopecia areata was tested in the C3H/HeJ mouse system. These mice develop spontaneous alopecia areata with age. Follicular expression of MHC classes I and II can be induced by intravenous injection of IFN-γ. Injection of C3H/HeJ female mice with IFN-γ resulted in a significant increase in the rate of development of alopecia areata associated with follicular expression of MHC class I and II.[45] Hair loss could only be induced in genetically susceptible C3H/HeJ mice.

Lessons from Animal Models

Alopecia areata develops spontaneously in 20% of female C3H/HeJ mice by 6 months of age.[46] The histology of these lesions is similar to that of the human disease, with a perifollicular inflammatory infiltrate of lymphocytes, as well as abnormal expression of HLA-DR, HLA-A,B,C, and intercellular adhesion molecule 1 (ICAM-1) by follicular epithelium. It is possible to transfer the alopecia areata to unaffected C3H/HeJ mice by grafting involved skin.[47] Transfer of the disease requires an intact immune system in the recipient animal. Both CD4+ and CD8+ T cells have a role in the alopecia,[48] in a direct parallel to the human condition.[49] The DEBR rat is a second similar model of spontaneous alopecia.[50] Alopecia areata in C3H/HeJ mice is dependent on IFN-γ, as IFN-γ–deficient mice are resistant to development of alopecia areata following skin grafting.[51] Deficiency in IL-2 also protects mice from the transfer of alopecia areata.[52] These data indicate that murine alopecia areata is mediated by cooperation between CD4+ and CD8+ lymphocytes and has a T-helper-1 (Th1) cytokine profile.

Direct Evidence of T Cells in the Pathogenesis of Alopecia Areata

T cells are capable of transferring alopecia areata in a human skin graft model.[53] Lesional (bald) human scalp plugs are grafted onto immunodeficient SCID mice. Following loss of passenger lymphocytes, the scalp hair regrows on the mouse. Additional scalp biopsies are obtained for isolation of lesional T cells. These T cells are cultured with homogenized hair follicles as a source of autoantigen, as well a autologous antigen presenting cells and IL-2. Following in vitro culture, the T cells are injected into the scalp grafts, resulting in loss of hair. T-cell injected grafts express HLA-A,B,C as well as HLA-DR and ICAM-1. Hair follicle homogenate is essential to activate the T cells to induce hair loss, and presumably functions as a source of autoantigen.

Optimal transfer of hair loss in this system requires both CD4+ and CD8+ T cells.[49] It is proposed that the CD4+ T cells provide help for the effector function of the CD8+ T cells. Inflammatory T cells of alopecia areata are cytotoxic and possess both the Fas/Fas ligand and granzyme B cytotoxic mechanisms.[54] Inflammatory T cells of alopecia areata have a Th1 cytokine bias and express IFN-γ.[55]

The clinical observation that alopecia areata tends to spare white hairs has led to the hypothesis that melanocyte antigens may have a role. This hypothesis was directly tested by using melanocyte antigens to stimulate lesional T cells in the human scalp graft system described above. Multiple melanocyte-associated HLA-A2 restricted peptides were found to stimulate lesional T cells to induce hair loss,[56] suggesting epitope spreading. This finding does not rule out other non–melanocyte-associated epitopes.

Neuropeptides and Alopecia Areata

Hair follicles are integrated into the neuroendocrine network. They are innervated, produce hormones, and express receptors for neuropeptides. Hair follicles even express a microcosm of the pituitary/adrenal axis, with production of corticotropin-releasing hormone, adrenocorticotropic hormone (ACTH), and cortisol.[57] Neurons innervating hair follicles express substance P, nerve growth factor (NGF), calcitonin gene–related peptide (CGRP), and vasoactive intestinal peptide (VIP). These neuropeptides are capable of inducing neurogenic inflammation, or immunosuppression in part through activation of mast cells.[58] Calcitonin gene–related peptide can be immunosuppressive,[59] and CGRP-containing neurons are deficient in alopecia areata lesions.[60] Substance P and NGF are both increased in mouse hair follicles following stress, and induce the hair follicles to enter catagen.[61] Stress also induces increases in perifollicular antigen presenting cells and activation of mast cells.[62] Potentially, neuroendocrine factors can result in loss of immune privilege that may mediate initiation of alopecia areata.

Treatment

Limited alopecia areata often responds well to treatment, and has a high rate of spontaneous resolution. However, extensive, long-standing disease has a poor prognosis and responds poorly to treatment. Common practice is to inject limited scalp lesions with intralesional triamcinolone (2.5 to 5 mg/mL). Response rates of 82%[4] to 63%[63] have been reported for excellent to complete response, with better responses in patients with limited disease of shorter duration. The hair-pull test can be used to determine areas of active disease for intralesional injection.

Betamethasone foam and liquid are both reported effective for mild to moderate disease[64]; however, this finding conflicts with the general clinical experience. The most impressive results with topical corticosteroids have been achieved with Clobetasol propionate 0.05% with plastic film occlusion.[65] Good regrowth was seen at 14 weeks in 28% of patients with alopecia totalis or universalis. This is impressive given the poor prognosis of patients with such extensive disease. Side effects included a follicular eruption secondary to occlusion.

Anthralin is used topically for alopecia areata as an alternative to corticosteroids. Use of anthralin is limited by irritation, and it has been proposed that irritation is required for efficacy.[66] Cosmetically significant or complete response rates have been reported of 25%[67] and 56%[68] for patchy alopecia areata after 23 or 20 weeks of treatment. Adverse effects that are intrinsic to the treatment are pruritus, erythema, and scale. The mechanism of action of anthralin is not established, but may involve counterirritation, analogous to the countersensitization described for topical sensitizers.

Topical sensitizers have established activity against alopecia totalis and universalis. Contact sensitizers such as dinitrochlorobenzene, diphenylcyclopropenone, or squaric acid dibutylester are first used to sensitize the patient. The agent is then painted on the scalp chronically at a minimal erythema concentration. Dinitrochlorobenzene was the first such compound in clinical use, but has fallen out of favor because it is positive in the Ames mutagenicity test. Squaric acid dibutyl ester has been reported to have success rates as high as 43%.[69,70] However, relapse is common. Diphenylcyclopropenone (diphencyprone, DPCP) initial sensitization is performed with 2%, and application starts with 0.001%, which is progressively increased to maintain erythema.[71] Cosmetically significant response rates in totalis/universalis patients are reported as 59%,[71] 71%,[72] and 48%.[73] Adverse effects include erythema, pigmentation, enlarged lymph nodes, bullous eczematous reactions, extension of contact dermatitis, and sleep disturbance. Unfortunately, the response tends to decrease over time such that only 60% of responders maintain response at 1 year, for an intent-to-treat analysis of 27% response at 1 year.[73] Other studies have reported good regrowth in 39% at 30-month follow-up.[74] Prognostic factors for response to diphenylcyclopropenone include the extent of disease, the age of onset, the duration, and atopy.[75]

Contact sensitizers are a hazard to all personnel who handle them, and precautions should be taken to avoid accidental contact. None of these sensitizing compounds is approved in the U.S. by the Food and Drug Administration (FDA) for application to humans. It is strongly recommended for this reason that all of these compounds be used in the U.S. only with approved human investigation protocols. Despite these problems and adverse effects, topical sensitizers warrant further investigation because of their ability to effectively treat the most severe disease. Some European experts consider contact sensitizers the preferred treatment for alopecia totalis or universalis.[76]

Systemic psoralen plus ultraviolet A (PUVA) phototherapy has shown efficacy in alopecia areata.[77,78] However, topical PUVA has given conflicting results. PUVA both eliminates lymphocytes in the papillary dermis, and has local and systemic immunosuppressive effects. The adverse effects of PUVA include burn, nausea, inconvenience, photoaging, and increased risk of skin cancer. PUVA should be used with great caution in children because of the high lifetime skin cancer risk.

Topical minoxidil (3% to 5%) may have modest efficacy for alopecia areata, and may have a role as an adjuvant therapy. Significant response has only been reported for patients with mild disease with response rates of 38%.[79,80] Other studies with 3% minoxidil showed no difference from vehicle control.[81] In combination with a 6-week taper of oral prednisone, patients receiving 2% minoxidil were more likely to maintain hair regrowth.[82]

Systemic corticosteroids are effective for alopecia areata and have been well studied. Use is limited by systemic adverse effects and relapse after treatment. In one study, 43 patients were randomized to oral prednisone 200 mg once per week vs. placebo for 3 months. After 6 months' observation, eight of 23 patients treated with prednisone had significant regrowth vs. none of 20 in placebo group. However, two of eight responders relapsed when they were taken off prednisone, resulting in six of 23 (26%) long-term responders.[83] Other protocols include oral prednisone 80 mg on 3 consecutive days every 3 months,[84] intramuscular triamcinolone acetonide 40 mg once a month for 6 months,[84] methylprednisolone (8 mg/kg) IV on 3 consecutive days at 4-week intervals for three courses (67% response),[85] dexamethasone 5 mg po on 2 consecutive days each week (63%

response),[86] and 300 mg prednisolone monthly oral pulse (60% response).[87] All the above protocols require significant corticosteroids with associated adverse effects. An alternative use of systemic corticosteroids is as a temporary bridge in patients with very active extensive disease, while treating with topical agents or intralesional corticosteroids.

Biologic response modifiers have not yet shown efficacy in alopecia areata. Agents that have been tested with negative results include etanercept[88] and efalizumab.[89] Lack of response to efalizumab was surprising, since this agent both inhibits lymphocyte homing and antigen presentation. Oral cyclosporine at high doses (6 mg/kg/day) is effective in alopecia areata.[90] However, both topical cyclosporine[91] and tacrolimus[92] are ineffective, presumably because of poor penetration.

Treatment would be incomplete without attention to the patient's ability to cope with the disease. It is the role of the physician to help, not necessarily to cure. Many patients with poor prognosis need to resort to wigs (scalp prosthesis). The physician can help by submitting the forms for insurance coverage for these expensive items. Patients should be monitored for signs of depression or anxiety and appropriately referred. It is also important to inform patients as to the nature of their disease. The best referral for additional information and patient support is the National Alopecia Areata Foundation (www. naaf.org).

Future Prospects

Although initial trials with biologic response modifiers have been disappointing, there are many pathways to be explored. Alopecia areata activity is associated with a Th1 T-cell response, and hair regrowth is associated with IL-10. It may be possible to deviate the immune response from Th1 to Th2 by treatment with IL-10 or anti–IL-12. Paus et al.[38] suggested that the ultimate treatment for alopecia areata and other organ-specific autoimmune diseases is to reestablish immune privilege. Theoretically, this may be achieved with immunosuppressive cytokines produced by the proximal hair follicle such as TGF-β and MSH-α.

Conclusion

Alopecia areata is an autoimmune disease of the hair follicle and nail matrix. It is associated with other autoimmune conditions, such as thyroid disease and vitiligo. Although alopecia areata has a genetic component, there are no gender differences in its incidence. Polymorphisms of IL-1 receptor antagonist, alleles of macrophage migration inhibitory factor, and Notch4 are associated with alopecia areata. The primary history of alopecia areata is a perifollicular lymphocytic infiltrate, predominately CD4+ cells. During early alopecia areata, anagen arrest is followed by conversion of the hair follicle from anagen to catagen, followed by telogen. The inflammatory T cells of alopecia areata are cytotoxic and possess both the Fas/Fas ligand and granzyme B cytotoxic mechanisms. In addition, these inflammatory cells have a Th1 cytokine bias and express IFN-γ. Neuroendocrine factors may result in loss of immune privilege that may mediate initiation of alopecia areata. Limited alopecia areata has a high rate of spontaneous resolution, but can be treated with a variety of interventions including steroids, anthralin, topical sensitizers, and topical minoxidil.

References

1. Safavi KH, Muller SA, Suman VJ, et al. Incidence of alopecia areata in Olmsted County, Minnesota, 1975 through 1989. Mayo Clin Proc 1995;70:628–33.

2. Yang S, Yang J, Liu JB,et al. The genetic epidemiology of alopecia areata in China. Br J Dermatol 2004;151:16–23.

3. Nanda A, Alsaleh QA, Al-Hasawi F, et al. Thyroid function, autoantibodies, and HLA tissue typing in children with alopecia areata. Pediatr Dermatol 2002;19:486–91.

4. Tan E, Tay YK, Goh CL, et al. The pattern and profile of alopecia areata in Singapore—a study of 219 Asians. Int J Dermatol 2002;41:748–53.

5. Picardi A, Pasquini P, Cattaruzza MS, et al. Psychosomatic factors in first-onset alopecia areata. Psychosomatics 2003;44:374–81.

6. Koo JY, Shellow WV, Hallman CP, et al. Alopecia areata and increased prevalence of psychiatric disorders. Int J Dermatol 1994;33:849–50.

7. Colon EA, Popkin MK, Callies AL, et al. Lifetime prevalence of psychiatric disorders in patients with alopecia areata. Compr Psychiatry 1991;32: 245–51.

8. Seyrafi H, Akhiani M, Abbasi H, et al. Evaluation of the profile of alopecia areata and the prevalence of thyroid function test abnormalities and serum autoantibodies in Iranian patients. BMC Dermatol 2005;5:11.

9. Tan E, Tay YK, Goh CL, et al. The pattern and profile of alopecia areata in Singapore—a study of 219 Asians. Int J Dermatol 2002;41:748–53.

10. Puavilai S, Puavilai G, Charuwichitratana S, et al. Prevalence of thyroid diseases in patients with alopecia areata. Int J Dermatol 1994;33:632–3.

11. Colombe BW, Price VH, Khoury EL, et al. HLA class II antigen associations help to define two types of alopecia areata. J Am Acad Dermatol 1995;33:757–64.

12. Akar A, Orkunoglu E, Sengul A, et al. HLA class II alleles in patients with alopecia areata. Eur J Dermatol 2002;12:236–9.

13. Colombe BW, Lou CD, Price VH. The genetic basis of alopecia areata: HLA associations with patchy alopecia areata versus alopecia totalis and alopecia universalis. J Invest Dermatol Symp Proc 1999;4:216–9.

14. Xiao FL, Ye DQ, Yang S, et al. Association of HLA haplotype with alopecia areata in Chinese Hans. J Eur Acad Dermatol Venereol 2006;20:1207–13.

15. Schepis C, Barone C, Siragusa M, et al. An updated survey on skin conditions in Down syndrome. Dermatology 2002;205:234–8.

16. Buzi F, Badolato R, Mazza C, Giliani S, et al. Autoimmune polyendocrinopathy-candidiasis-ectodermal dystrophy syndrome: time to review diagnostic criteria? J Clin Endocrinol Metab 2003;88:3146–8.

17. Tazi-Ahnini R, Cork MJ, Gawkrodger DJ, et al. Role of the autoimmune regulator (AIRE) gene in alopecia areata: strong association of a potentially functional AIRE polymorphism with alopecia universalis. Tissue Antigens 2002;60:489–95.

18. Tazi-Ahnini R, Cox A, McDonagh AJ, et al. Genetic analysis of the interleukin-1 receptor antagonist and its homologue IL-1L1 in alopecia areata: strong severity association and possible gene interaction. Eur J Immunogenet 2002;29:25–30.

19. Shimizu T, Hizawa N, Honda A, et al. Promoter region polymorphism of macrophage migration inhibitory factor is strong risk factor for young onset of extensive alopecia areata. Genes Immun 2005;6:285–9.

20. Tazi-Ahnini R, Cork MJ, Wengraf D, et al. Notch4, a non-HLA gene in the MHC is strongly associated with the most severe form of alopecia areata. Hum Genet 2003;112:400–3.

21. Kemp EH, McDonagh AJ, Wengraf DA, et al. The non-synonymous C1858T substitution in the PTPN22 gene is associated with susceptibility to

the severe forms of alopecia areata. Hum Immunol 2006;67:535–9.

22. Sundberg JP, Silva KA, Li R, et al. Adult-onset Alopecia areata is a complex polygenic trait in the C3H/HeJ mouse model. J Invest Dermatol 2004;123:294–7.

23. Duvic M, Norris D, Christiano A, et al. Alopecia areata registry: an overview. J Invest Dermatol Symp Proc 2003;8:219–21.

24. Tosti A, Morelli R, Bardazzi F, et al. Prevalence of nail abnormalities in children with alopecia areata. Pediatr Dermatol 1994;11:112–5.

25. Tan E, Tay YK, Goh CL, et al. The pattern and profile of alopecia areata in Singapore—a study of 219 Asians. Int J Dermatol 2002;41:748–53.

26. Tosti A, Piraccini BM, Iorizzo M, et al. Frontal fibrosing alopecia in postmenopausal women. J Am Acad Dermatol 2005;52:55–60.

27. Guarrera M, Semino MT, Rebora A. Quantitating hair loss in women: a critical approach. Dermatology 1997;194:12–6.

28. Trost LB, Bergfeld WF, Calogeras E. The diagnosis and treatment of iron deficiency and its potential relationship to hair loss. J Am Acad Dermatol 2006;54:824–44.

29. Olsen EA, Hordinsky MK, Price VH, et al. Alopecia areata investigational assessment guidelines—part II. J Am Acad Dermatol 2004;51:440–7.

30. Sperling LC, Lupton GP. Histopathology of nonscarring alopecia. J Cutan Pathol 1995;22:97–114.

31. Whiting DA. Histologic features of alopecia areata. Arch Dermatol 2003;139:1555–1559.

32. Kalish RS, Gilhar A. Alopecia areata: autoimmunity, the evidence is compelling. J Invest Dermatol Symp Proc 2003;8:164–167.

33. Gilhar A, Kalish RS. Alopecia areata: a tissue specific autoimmune disease of the hair follicle. Autoimmun Rev 2006;5:64–9.

34. Gilhar A, Krueger GG. Hair growth in scalp grafts from patients with alopecia areata and alopecia universalis grafted onto nude mice. Arch Dermatol 1987;123:44–50.

35. Okamoto M, Ogawa Y, Watanabe A, et al. Autoantibodies to DFS70/LEDGF are increased in alopecia areata patients. J Autoimmun 2004;23:257–66.

36. Tobin DJ, Hann SK, Song MS, et al. Hair follicle structures targeted by antibodies in patients with alopecia areata. Arch Dermatol 1997;133:57–61.

37. Gilhar A, Pillar T, Assy B, et al. Failure of passive transfer of serum from patients with alopecia areata and alopecia universalis to inhibit hair growth in transplants of human scalp skin grafted on to nude mice. Br J Dermatol 1992;126:166–171.

38. Paus R, Nickoloff BJ, Ito T. A "hairy" privilege. Trends Immunol 2005;26:32–40.

39. Paus R, Eichmuller S, Hofmann U, et al. Expression of classical and non-classical MHC class I antigens in murine hair follicles. Br J Dermatol 1994;131: 177–183.

40. Paus R, Christoph T, Muller-Rover S. Immunology of the hair follicle: a short journey into terra incognita. J Invest Dermatol Symp Proc 1999;4:226–234.

41. Christoph T, Muller-Rover S, Audring H, et al. The human hair follicle immune system: cellular composition and immune privilege. Br J Dermatol 2000;142:862–873.

42. Ito T, Ito N, Saathoff M, et al. Immunology of the human nail apparatus: the nail matrix is a site of relative immune privilege. J Invest Dermatol 2005;125:1139–48.

43. Messenger AG, Bleehen SS. Expression of HLA-DR by anagen hair follicles in alopecia areata. J Invest Dermatol 1985;85:569–572.

44. Gilhar A, Etzioni A, Assy B, et al. Response of grafts from patients with alopecia areata transplanted onto nude mice, to administration of interferon-gamma. Clin Immunol Immunopathol 1993;66:120–6.

45. Gilhar A, Kam Y, Assy B, et al. Alopecia areata induced in C3H/HeJ mice by interferon-gamma: evidence for loss of immune privilege. J Invest Dermatol 2005;124:288–9.

46. Sundberg JP, Cordy WR, King LE Jr. Alopecia areata in aging C3H/HeJ mice. J Invest Dermatol 1994;102:847–856.

47. McElwee KJ, Boggess D, King LE Jr, et al. Experimental induction of alopecia areata-like hair loss in C3H/HeJ mice using full-thickness skin grafts. J Invest Dermatol 1998;111:797–803.

48. McElwee KJ, Hoffmann R, Freyschmidt-Paul P, et al. Resistance to alopecia areata in C3H/HeJ mice is associated with increased expression of regulatory cytokines and a failure to recruit CD4+ and CD8+ cells. J Invest Dermatol 2002;119:1426–33.

49. Gilhar A, Landau M, Assy B, et al. Alopecia areata is mediated by cooperation between CD4+ and CD8+ T-lymphocytes: Transfer to human scalp explants on Prkdc[scid] mice. Arch Dermatol 2002;138:916–22.

50. Michie HJ, Jahoda CA, Oliver RF, et al. The DEBR rat: an animal model of human alopecia areata. Br J Dermatol 1991;125:94–100.

51. Freyschmidt-Paul P, McElwee KJ, Hoffmann R, et al. Interferon-gamma-deficient mice are resistant to the development of alopecia areata. Br J Dermatol 2006;155:515–21.

52. Freyschmidt-Paul P, McElwee KJ, Hoffmann R, et al. Reduced expression of interleukin-2 decreases the frequency of alopecia areata onset in C3H/HeJ mice. J Invest Dermatol 2005;125:945–51.

53. Gilhar A, Ullmann Y, Berkutzki T, et al. Alopecia areata transferred to human scalp explants on SCID mice with T-lymphocyte injections. J Clin Invest 1998;101:62–7.

54. Bodemer C, Peuchmaur M, Fraitaig S, et al. Role of cytotoxic T cells in chronic alopecia areata. J Invest Dermatol 2000;114:112–16.

55. Gilhar A, Landau M, Assy B, et al. Transfer of alopecia areata in the human scalp graft/Prkdc^scid (SCID) mouse system is characterized by a TH1 response. Clin Immunol 2003;106:181–7.

56. Gilhar A, Landau M, Assay B, et al. Melanocyte associated T-cell epitopes can function as autoantigens for transfer of alopecia areata to human scalp explants on Prkdcscid mice. J Invest Dermatol 2001;117:1357–62.

57. Arck PC, Slominski A, Theoharides TC, et al. Neuroimmunology of stress: skin takes center stage. J Invest Dermatol 2006;126:1697–704.

58. Streilein JW;Alard P;Niizeki H. Neural influences on induction of contact hypersensitivity. Ann NY Acad Sci 1999;885:196–208.

59. Niizeki H, Alard P, Streilein JW. Calcitonin gene-related peptide is necessary for ultraviolet B-impaired induction of contact hypersensitivity. J Immunol 1997;159:5183–6.

60. Rossi R, Del Bianco E, Isolani D, et al. Possible involvement of neuropeptidergic sensory nerves in alopecia areata. Neuroreport 1997;8:1135–8.

61. Peters EM, Arck PC, Paus R. Hair growth inhibition by psychoemotional stress: a mouse model for neural mechanisms in hair growth control. Exp Dermatol 2006;15:1–13.

62. Peters EM, Handjiski B, Kuhlmei A, et al. Neurogenic inflammation in stress-induced termination of murine hair growth is promoted by nerve growth factor. Am J Pathol 2004;165:259–71.

63. Kubeyinje EP. Intralesional triamcinolone acetonide in alopecia areata amongst 62 Saudi Arabs. East Afr Med J 1994;71:674–5.

64. Mancuso G, Balducci A, Casadio C, et al. Efficacy of betamethasone valerate foam formulation in comparison with betamethasone dipropionate lotion in the treatment of mild-to-moderate alopecia areata: a multicenter, prospective, randomized, controlled, investigator-blinded trial. Int J Dermatol 2003;42:572–5.

65. Tosti A, Piraccini BM, Pazzaglia M, et al. Clobetasol propionate 0.05% under occlusion in the treatment of alopecia totalis/universalis. J Am Acad Dermatol 2003;49:96–8.

66. Nelson DA, Spielvogel RL. Anthralin therapy for alopecia areata. Int J Dermatol 1985;24:606–7.

67. Fiedler-Weiss VC, Buys CM. Evaluation of anthralin in the treatment of alopecia areata. Arch Dermatol 1987;123:1491–3.

68. Sasmaz S, Arican O. Comparison of azelaic acid and anthralin for the therapy of patchy alopecia areata: a pilot study. Am J Clin Dermatol 2005;6:403–6.

69. Ajith C, Gupta S, Kanwar AJ. Efficacy and safety of the topical sensitizer squaric acid dibutyl ester in Alopecia areata and factors influencing the outcome. J Drugs Dermatol 2006;5:262–6.

70. Dall'oglio F, Nasca MR, Musumeci ML, et al. Topical immunomodulator therapy with squaric acid dibutylester (SADBE) is effective treatment for severe alopecia areata (AA): results of an open-label, paired-comparison, clinical trial. J Dermatol Treat 2005;16:10–4.

71. Aghaei S. Topical immunotherapy of severe alopecia areata with diphenylcyclopropenone (DPCP): experience in an Iranian population. BMC Dermatol 2005;26;5–6.

72. Galadari I, Rubaie S, Alkaabi J, et al. Diphenylcyclopropenone (diphencyprone, DPCP) in the treatment of chronic severe alopecia areata (AA). Allerg Immunol (Paris) 2003;35:397–401.

73. Cotellessa C, Peris K, Caracciolo E, et al. The use of topical diphenylcyclopropenone for the treatment of extensive alopecia areata. J Am Acad Dermatol 2001;44:73–6.

74. Gordon PM, Aldrige RD, McVittie E, et al. Topical diphencyprone for alopecia areata: evaluation of 48 cases after 30 months' follow-up. Br J Dermatol 1996;134:869–71.

75. Weise K, Kretzschmar L, John SM, et al. Topical immunotherapy in alopecia areata: anamnestic and clinical criteria of prognostic significance. Dermatology 1996;192:129–33.

76. MacDonald Hull SP, Wood ML, Hutchinson PE, et al. Guidelines for the management of alopecia areata. Br J Dermatol 2003;149:692–9.

77. Broniarczyk-Dyla G, Wawrzycka-Kaflik A, Dubla-Berner M, et al. Effects of psoralen-UV-A-Turban in alopecia areata. Skinmed 2006;5:64–8.

78. Mohamed Z, Bhouri A, Jallouli A, et al. Alopecia areata treatment with a phototoxic dose of UVA and topical 8–methoxypsoralen. J Eur Acad Dermatol Venereol 2005;19:552–5.

79. Fiedler-Weiss VC. Topical minoxidil solution (1% and 5%) in the treatment of alopecia areata. J Am Acad Dermatol 1987;16:745–8.

80. Shapiro J, Tan J, Ho V, et al. Treatment of chronic severe alopecia areata with topical diphenylcyclopropenone and 5% minoxidil: a clinical and immunopathologic evaluation. J Am Acad Dermatol 1993;29:729–35.

81. Ranchoff RE, Bergfeld WF, Steck WD, et al. Extensive alopecia areata. Results of treatment with 3% topical minoxidil. Cleve Clin J Med 1989;56:149–54.

82. Olsen EA, Carson SC, Turney EA. Systemic steroids with or without 2% topical minoxidil in the treatment of alopecia areata. Arch Dermatol 1992;128:1467–73.

83. Kar BR, Handa S, Dogra S, et al. Placebo-controlled oral pulse prednisolone therapy in alopecia areata. J Am Acad Dermatol 2005;52:287–90.

84. Kurosawa M, Nakagawa S, Mizuashi M, et al. A comparison of the efficacy, relapse rate and side effects among three modalities of systemic corticosteroid therapy for alopecia areata. Dermatology 2006;212:361–5.

85. Seiter S, Ugurel S, Tilgen W, et al. High-dose pulse corticosteroid therapy in the treatment of severe alopecia areata. Dermatology 2001;202:230–4.

86. Sharma VK, Gupta S. Twice weekly 5 mg dexamethasone oral pulse in the treatment of extensive alopecia areata. J Dermatol 1999;26:562–5.

87. Sharma VK, Muralidhar S. Treatment of widespread alopecia areata in young patients with monthly oral corticosteroid pulse. Pediatr Dermatol 1998;15:313–7.

88. Strober BE, Siu K, Alexis AF, et al. Etanercept does not effectively treat moderate to severe alopecia areata: an open-label study. J Am Acad Dermatol 2005;52:1082–4.

89. Price V, Hordinsky M, Leonardi C, et al. Safety and efficacy results of a clinical study of efalizumab in patients with alopecia areata. J Invest Dermatol 2006;126:105, 2006.

90. Gupta AK, Ellis CN, Cooper KD, et al. Oral cyclosporine for the treatment of alopecia areata. A clinical and immunohistochemical analysis. J Am Acad Dermatol 1990;22:242–50.

91. Gilhar A, Pillar T, Etzioni A. Topical cyclosporin A in alopecia areata. Acta Derm Venereol 1989;69:252–3.

92. Price VH, Willey A, Chen BK. Topical tacrolimus in alopecia areata. J Am Acad Dermatol 2005;52:138–9.

40
Cutaneous Lupus Erythematosus

David F. Fiorentino and Richard D. Sontheimer

Key Points

- *Cutaneous lupus erythematosus* is a term that describes a spectrum of skin disease that has a pathophysiology related to lupus erythematosus and is bound by common histopathologic or molecular criteria.
- Cutaneous lupus erythematosus may occur in the setting of systemic disease or in the absence of detectable disease.
- Cutaneous lupus erythematosus may be classified as acute, subacute, or chronic, based on the clinical presentation.
- In systemic lupus erythematosus, skin lesions are second only to joint disease as the most frequently affected organ.
- Other morphologic variants can occur in the skin, such as vesicular lesions (bullous lupus erythematosus), mucosal lesions (ulcers), and panniculitis.
- Specific laboratory abnormalities can occur in systemic lupus erythematosus, and may be associated with some clinical variants of cutaneous lupus erythematosus.
- The pathogenesis of systemic lupus erythematosus and cutaneous lupus erythematosus represent an autoimmune response targeted to various tissues. This occurs because of genetic susceptibility and environmental factors (such as UV light).
- There are a variety of treatments for cutaneous lupus erythematosus, ranging from photoprotection from UV light, to topical and systemic glucocorticosteroids, as well as nonsteroidal antiinflammatory agents (antimalarials).

Lupus erythematosus (LE) is a broad term referring to disease phenotypes that are characterized by a particular form of aberrant immune activation. Disease presentation is heterogeneous, ranging from a single-organ (i.e., skin) disorder to a multisystemic disease. As such, the term *lupus erythematosus* should be used with certain modifiers to more precisely specify the type of clinical illness that is being discussed. Systemic lupus erythematosus (SLE) refers to a unique medical diagnosis that is characterized by involvement of multiple organ systems and, although heterogeneous, is bound by certain commonalities of immune dysfunction. Cutaneous lupus erythematosus (CLE) refers to the spectrum of skin disease that has a pathophysiology that is related to LE and is bound by common histopathologic or molecular criteria (see below). After accepting this definition of CLE, it is important to understand that the same lesions can also be found as isolated cutaneous findings in an otherwise healthy individual.

When considering the patient with SLE, one must remember that CLE is not the only form of skin disease related to the underlying disease. It is useful to consider the classification scheme developed by Gilliam and Sontheimer[1] in which the skin findings in a patient with SLE are further characterized as either LE specific or LE nonspecific. LE-specific skin disease refers to CLE and generally has one or more of the following histologic features: lichenoid tissue reaction with or without basal keratinocyte vacuolar change, hyperkeratosis, thickening of the epidermal basement membrane, perivascular or perifollicular mononuclear cell infiltrate, and dermal mucin deposition.

In contrast, LE nonspecific disease refers to those cutaneous findings that, although driven by the underlying SLE, do not possess the typical histologic features of CLE and can also be seen in other disorders. LE nonspecific disease includes vascular abnormalities (e.g., vasculitis, vasculopathy, Raynaud's), mucosal ulceration, alopecia, and photosensitivity.[2] This chapter discusses only LE-specific skin disease (i.e., CLE). However, it should be noted that LE nonspecific skin disease is of paramount importance to the clinician, as its presence can be an indicator of systemic disease and can reflect SLE disease activity.

Classification

Lupus erythematosus (LE)-specific skin disease can be classified clinically, serologically, or histopathologically. We employ the scheme of Gilliam and Sontheimer,[1] which relies heavily on clinical manifestations, and divides lesions into acute (ACLE), subacute (SCLE), and chronic (CCLE). It should be noted that these terms refer to both the morphologies and the pace of the cutaneous lesions themselves. The fact that some forms of LE-specific skin disease such as ACLE are strongly associated with SLE disease activity is one reason why it is so vital to carefully categorize LE-specific disease, as this can give a clue to whether the findings are isolated or are occurring in the context of SLE. With any classification system, there are cases that do not fit neatly into a group; one example of this would be what has been designated "LE indeterminate" skin disease that has been described in African-American patients.[3] In addition, these categories are not mutually exclusive; that is, patients may have more than one type of LE-specific skin lesion either at the same time or during the course of their disease.

Epidemiology

There are few population-based data concerning the epidemiology of CLE, particularly isolated forms of CLE such as SCLE and classic discoid LE (DLE) that typically are not associated with clinically significant SLE. From a comprehensive review of the literature, Tebbe and Orfanos[4] have estimated that patients having isolated forms of CLE might outnumber patients having SLE by severalfold.

In the context of SLE, the skin appears to be second only to the joints as the most frequently affected organ.[5–7] For ACLE, the association is so strong with SLE that the epidemiology of ACLE would be expected to be similar to that of patients with SLE.[3] Assuming that ACLE is synonymous with "malar rash" as well as "maculopapular rash," facial ACLE appears to occur in 20% to 60% of large LE patient cohorts, while the "maculopapular rash" of SLE occurs in 35% of SLE patients.[6] Malar rash/ACLE is more common in whites than blacks, and in women and younger patients.[6,8,9]

Subacute CLE occurs predominantly in white females of all ages. The original cohort of Sontheimer et al.[10] showed that 70% were female and 85% were white, with a mean age of 43.3 years. These patients have been shown to comprise 7% to 27% of the total LE cohort in several studies.[3] A recent study using an anti-Ro/SSA registry followed by patient-reported photosensitive skin disease estimates an incidence and prevalence of 4.8 (per year) and 6.2 to 14 per 100,000 persons, respectively, for SCLE.[11]

Chronic CLE really has no reliable population-based data, as these patients are underrepresented in studies from rheumatologists and internists and overrepresented by dermatologists. Also, many of the studies were done before the creation of the updated American College of Rheumatology (ACR) clinical classification criteria and before the advent of certain serologic and laboratory tests that made classification of LE-specific disease more tenable. It appears that DLE lesions, the most common form of CCLE, can be found in 15% to 30% of SLE patients at some point in time during their disease course.[12] Approximately 5% to 10% of SLE patients present with DLE skin lesions.[13] The female/male ratio of DLE is between 3:2 and 3:1 (much lower than in SLE), and typical age of onset is between 20 and 40 years.[14] It is controversial whether whites are more commonly affected than blacks.[14,15]

Cutaneous Manifestations

Acute Cutaneous Lupus Erythematosus

Acute CLE can either be localized to the face or generalized. The classic "butterfly rash" consists of confluent or patchy macular erythema with or without papules, edema, and induration, scattered across the malar eminences and bridge of the nose. The forehead, chin, and V-area of the neck can be involved (Fig. 40.1A). The nasolabial folds are typically spared. Although it is usually symmetrical, this is not always the case. There can be some mild degree of hyperkeratosis.

Generalized ACLE is less common and presents as a widespread morbilliform eruption, often accentuated in a photodistributed pattern over the extensor aspects of the arms, forearms, and dorsal hands and fingers. Over the dorsal fingers during the early phase of the disease, the hair-bearing interphalangeal areas are especially targeted while the knuckles are spared. Some patients experience an extreme form of ACLE that simulates toxic epider-mal necrolysis (TEN), due to the intense lichenoid inflammation.[16] Of note this is one mechanism for the development of vesicular lesions in CLE.

Lupus erythematosus patients can experience several types of vesiculobullous skin disease. In bullous SLE, patients typically with active SLE can present with vesicles (which appear similar to dermatitis herpetiformis) or bullae on the face, arms, and trunk.[3] Histopathologic examination of the skin often reveals papillary dermal neutrophilic microabscesses as well as deposition of multiple immunoreactants at the dermal–epidermal junction. In some cases, these antibodies have been shown to bind type VII collagen, while in others the multiple immunoreactants are more consist-

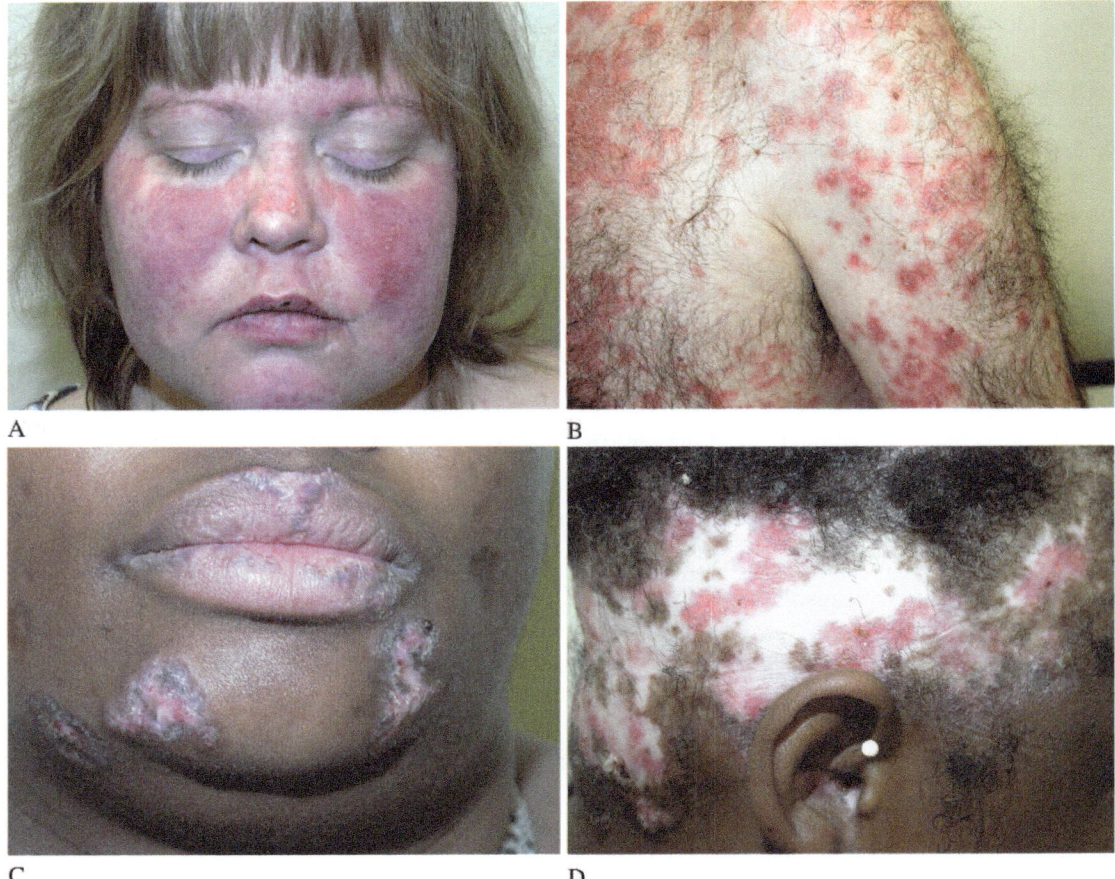

A B

C D

FIG. 40.1. Lupus-specific skin disease. (A) Acute cutaneous lupus erythematosus (LE). (B) Drug-induced subacute cutaneous LE secondary to rabeprazole (Aciphex; R. D. Sontheimer, personal unpublished observation). (C) Classic discoid LE affecting the chin and lips. (D) Classic discoid LE affecting the scalp and external ears with scarring alopecia and postinflammatory hypopigmentation

ent with nonspecific immune complex deposition. Thus, these lesions clinically and histologically simulate dermatitis herpetiformis or epidermolysis bullosa acquisita, but the clinical distribution and multiplicity of immunoreactants distinguish these cases. As "bullous SLE" does not share the histopathologic findings that are typical of CLE, it can be considered as a form of LE-nonspecific vesiculobullous skin disease. Vesiculobullous annular SCLE is an example of vesiculobullous LE-specific skin disease. Of note, vesiculation can also result from other blistering disorders, such as bullous pemphigoid, dermatitis herpetiformis, porphyria cutanea tarda, and pemphigus vulgaris that have rarely been reported to occur concordantly with LE.

In addition, superficial ulceration of the oral or nasal mucosa can occur in ACLE. These lesions are often asymptomatic, transient, and tend to occur on the hard palate (although virtually any area of the oral mucosa can be involved).[2,17]

The lesions of ACLE are typically photosensitive and transient, usually lasting several days or weeks. Patients can concurrently develop SCLE, or, less commonly, DLE lesions. The ACLE lesions do not scar but can result in predominate postinflammatory pigmentary alteration, especially in dark-skinned patients.

The differential diagnosis for ACLE includes any dermatosis that can produce a red face, with common diagnoses being acne rosacea, dermatomyositis, seborrheic dermatitis, contact dermatitis, polymorphous light eruption (PMLE), and drug eruptions. Special note should be made regarding PMLE, which can occur in up to 50% of patients with SLE, and can often be distinguished by a more rapid onset (i.e., hours) and resolution of the photosensitive lesions.[18]

Subacute Cutaneous Lupus Erythematosus

First described as a distinct entity by Gilliam in 1977, SCLE is the prototype of a LE-specific skin disease that is defined by clinical, serologic, and genetic features.[10] Clinically, these lesions present as either scaling papules or small plaques ("psoriasiform type") (Fig. 40.1B) or scaling, annular, or polycyclic plaques ("annular type"); these forms are equally prevalent.[14] In general, one individual

presents with one or the other type, though both forms can occur in a patient.

Lesions are characteristically photodistributed on the chest, back, extensor arms, and V-area of the neck; it is the experience of the authors and others that these lesions occur less commonly on the face compared to ACLE and DLE.[14,19] Eighty-five percent of all SCLE patients report photosensitivity.[20] The inactive central portion of the radially spreading annular lesions is often hypopigmented. Rarely, patients can present with erythema multiforme–like lesions, simulating Rowell syndrome (erythema multiforme–like lesions occurring in SLE patients with La/SS-B antibodies).[21] As in ACLE (see above), intense basovacuolar degeneration of epidermal keratinocytes can result in vesiculation or crusting, which usually occurs at the active edge of annular lesions. This can resemble TEN in its extreme form.[22] Lesions of SCLE typically heal without scarring, but permanent hypopigmentation or telangiectasias can occur. Subacute CLE patients can also develop the lesions of ACLE or classic DLE. Localized facial ACLE has been reported to occur in 20% of patients,[3] while various reports document DLE lesions in 0% to 30% of SCLE patients.[11,20] In contrast to SCLE, ACLE lesions tend to be more transient, less scaly, more edematous, and associated with less pigmentary change, and, as previously mentioned, more commonly affect the face. The absence of induration in SCLE lesions can serve as a clinical distinguisher from DLE and LE tumidus.

The differential diagnosis for SCLE includes psoriasis, dermatophyte infections, pityriasis rubra pilaris, polymorphous light eruption (PMLE), nummular eczema, dermatomyositis, and mycosis fungoides. Annular lesions can be confused with granuloma annulare, erythema multiforme, and gyrate erythemas. However, the inactive centers of SCLE lesions are typically hypopigmented while those of other annular disorders are typically pigmented normally or hyperpigmented.

Chronic Cutaneous Lupus Erythematosus

Classic DLE is the most common form of CCLE. These lesions begin as erythematous papules, which then develop scale and evolve into larger plaques covered by adherent scale that are usually associated with follicular plugging and peripheral hyperpigmentation. When the adherent scale is peeled back, follicle-sized keratotic spikes can be seen to project from the underside (the so-called "carpet tack sign"). The lesions expand slowly, leaving central atrophy, scarring, telangiectasia, and depigmentation (Fig. 40.1C). Hyperpigmentation is often seen at the active borders of lesions. The combination of peripheral hyperpigmentation and central depigmentation is especially prominent in African American DLE patients (Fig 40.1D). Some lesions of DLE can present only as macular hyperpigmentation, especially in Asian Indians.[23]

Discoid LE lesions occur most often on the face, ears (especially the conchae), scalp, V-area of the neck, and extensor aspect of the arms. Any facial structure can be involved, including eyebrows, eyelids, nose, and lips. Periocular lesions are often misdiagnosed and can present as blepharitis, conjunctivitis, or periorbital edema.[14] Lesions can occur in the malar distribution, but their chronicity, epidermal change, and scarring should distinguish them from the classic malar rash of ACLE. An acneiform pattern (often in the perioral area or the chin) that resolves with pitted scarring is rarely seen.[14,24] Compared with ACLE or SCLE, DLE is less commonly reported to be associated with ultraviolet (UV) exposure. Patients are often unaware of the time lag (up to 4 weeks) following sun exposure, and many lesions do not occur in sun-exposed areas (e.g., hairy-bearing scalp, conchal bowl of ears).[25,26]

Scalp involvement occurs in 60% of patients with DLE, with persistent activity resulting in permanent scarring (Fig. 40.1D). However, alopecia that is associated with DLE can be reversible when it is secondary to early inflammation of DLE, the telogen effluvium that represents an increase in underlying SLE activity, or alopecia areata that has been shown to be commonly associated with DLE.[27]

Discoid LE lesions are considered to be localized if they occur only on the head and neck, while lesions above and below the neck are referred to as generalized. Lesions can also occur on the palmar or plantar surfaces,[28,29] the nail unit,[14,30] in areas of trauma (the Koebner or isomorphic response).[31] Follicular DLE lesions have been described, often around the elbow, and may be more common in African-American and Asian patients.[31,32]

Hypertrophic DLE is a rare variant in which hyperkeratotic lesions occur (often on the extensor extremities, upper back, and face). Histopathology can reveal features of squamous cell carcinoma, which can lead to confusion regarding diagnosis.[33] Even if patients have classic DLE lesions elsewhere, the clinician should still be aware that squamous cell carcinoma can develop in long-standing, scarring DLE lesions.[34,35]

Well-developed lesions of DLE do not usually present a problem with differential diagnosis, although early lesions can be confused with PMLE, granuloma faciale, sarcoidosis, cutaneous lymphoid hyperplasia, lupus vulgaris, angiolymphoid hyperplasia with eosinophilia, and tertiary syphilis.

Mucosal DLE occurs in approximately 25% of CCLE patients.[17] Oral lesions tend to occur on the buccal mucosa, and less commonly on the palate, gums, and tongue. Lesions have a sharply marginated, scalloped white border with central erythema. Central areas can erode, although lesions are typically painless. The surfaces of well-developed plaques on the palate can have a meshwork of raised hyperkeratotic strands giving a "honeycomb" appearance.[17] Fixed mucosal DLE lesions can be distinguished clinically from the transient superficial mucosal ulcerations that are often seen in active SLE patients. The lips can be involved with well-defined plaques or a diffuse cheilitis.[3] Such lesions can degenerate into squamous cell carcinoma.[36] Involvement of the nasal, conjunctival, and genital mucosa can occur.[37]

Chilblain LE is characterized by red-purple patches or papules on the toes, fingers, or face that are precipitated by cold or damp climates. At the onset these lesions are clinically indistinguishable from simple chilblain (or pernio) lesions that occur in healthy individuals.[38,39] However, chilblain LE lesions tend to evolve into more classic acral DLE lesions, and it is postulated that this may be the result of a Koebner phenomenon in otherwise typical lesions of perniosis.[3] Differential diagnosis includes other cold-induced vasculopathies, such as cold agglutinin disease or cryoglobulinemia.

Lupus erythematosus profundus, also called LE panniculitis, is a form of CCLE characterized by inflammation in the lower dermis or subcutis. This lesion occurs more commonly in women and is seen in 1% to 3% of SLE patients.[3] Approximately 70% of patients have overlying DLE lesions.[40,41]

Some have used the term *LE profundus* to specify those lesions that have concurrent overlying DLE activity, and the term *LE panniculitis* to refer to lesions displaying only subcutaneous inflammation. However, this is not a universally accepted convention.

Lupus erythematosus profundus/panniculitis lesions are characterized by 1- to 3-cm firm, deep nodules with initially normal-appearing overlying skin. With time, the nodules resolve and draw the surface of the skin inward, leaving deep, saucerized depressions. Lesions tend to occur in the head, upper arms, buttocks, and thighs. Rarely, this entity can present as periorbital edema. Dystrophic calcification can occur in older lesions. Breast lesions ("lupus mastitis") can be confused with carcinoma.[14] Persistent, extensive LE profundus/panniculitis lesions of the breast can necessitate mastectomy. Early lesions can be confused with morphea, while other forms of panniculitis (subcutaneous panniculitic T-cell lymphoma, sarcoidosis, factitial or traumatic panniculitis, subcutaneous granuloma annulare), and lipoatrophy (partial lipodystrophy associated with autoimmune disease, drug-induced lipoatrophy, HIV-associated lipoatrophy) must be ruled out.

Typical lesions of lupus erythematosus tumidus (LET) are succulent, edematous papules, and plaques that arise due to accumulation of dermal mucin. These lesions are found with decreasing frequency on the face, back, arms, and chest.[42,43] In some individuals, large annular edematous plaques can be seen. The largest series reported resolution with no or mild topical treatment in nearly half of cases,[43] although it has since been questioned that this series may have included many patients with PMLE.[42] It is possible that this might account for the extreme photosensitivity that was reported in these patients.[43] Other authors report these lesions to be chronic and difficult to treat and such patients are typically antinuclear antibody (ANA)-negative. Most affected patients do not have SLE.[42–45] Lesions are characterized by perivascular and periappendiceal lymphocytic inflammation with dermal mucin deposition. Unlike other forms of LE-specific skin disease, there is absence of basal vacuolar changes in 80% to 100% of cases, with positive cases showing only focal and sparse keratinocyte necrosis.[42,46] The LET lesions must be differentiated from PMLE,

Jessner's lymphocytic infiltrate, atypical lymphoid infiltrates, mycosis fungoides, reticular erythematous mucinosis, DLE, SCLE, and figurate erythemas. Some have argued that LE tumidus and Jessner's lymphocytic infiltrate in reality cannot be clearly distinguished.[43]

Laboratory Abnormalities

Little data are available concerning laboratory assessment of patients with ACLE. It is assumed that they would closely parallel the data that are available for patients with SLE.

Approximately 60% to 80% of SCLE patients have detectable ANAs, with a speckled/particulate ANA pattern being most common.[47] This disease is characterized by positive anti-Ro/SSA antibodies, present in 40% to 100% of patients, depending on the assays used.[48,49] Anticardiolipin antibodies are present in 10% to 16%.[50] Rheumatoid factor is present in one third of SCLE patients,[48] and some patients initially present with rheumatoid arthritis long before a diagnosis of SCLE is made. Sm, double-stranded DNA (dsDNA), and U1 ribonucleoprotein (U1RNP) antibodies are present in 10% of SCLE patients.[48] Antithyroid antibodies were reported in 18%[51] and 44%[52] of SCLE patients. Depending on the presence of SLE disease activity, cytopenias, hypergammaglobulinemia, proteinuria, hematuria, and depressed complement levels can also be seen.

In DLE, low ANA titers/levels (e.g., ≤1:40) are present 30% to 40% of the time in assays that employ human tumor cells as substrates. However, higher titers that are typically seen in SLE (≥1:160) are rarely encountered in patients having isolated forms of DLE.[14] Anti-Ro/SSA antibodies are occasionally found, but the presence of anti-Sm, dsDNA, and La/SS-B antibodies is uncommon.[53] Fewer than 10% of patients have immunoglobulin G (IgG) anticardiolipin antibodies.[54] A small percentage of DLE patients have positive rheumatoid factor, slight depression in complement, and leukopenia (see below). Antinuclear antibodies are present in approximately 75% of patients with lupus profundus/panniculitis.[14] The frequency of ANAs in patients with chilblain lupus was reported as nine of 14 patients, with anti-dsDNA antibodies in four of

14 patients; these numbers might be an over-estimate.[39] Anti-Ro/SS-A antibodies have been variably found in these patients, and some authors have suggested that this is a marker for this disorder.[39,55]

Relationship to Systemic Disease

The rash of ACLE is generally presumed to always accompany SLE. One study suggests that the course of rash severity parallels SLE activity.[12] Interestingly, studies have failed to support an association with renal or central nervous system (CNS) disease, although this has not been studied adequately.[14] One small study indicated that SCLE and DLE patients with normal lymphocyte counts are unlikely to have SLE.[56]

Approximately 50% of patients with SCLE meet ACR criteria for SLE.[48,57] However, severe systemic disease (e.g., nephritis, CNS disease) develops in only 10% of SCLE patients.[48] Some data confirm that the papulosquamous form of SCLE is more associated with renal involvement.[14] As stated above, rheumatoid arthritis has been reported to precede as well as follow a diagnosis of SCLE. In addition, 3% to 12% of SCLE patients later develop Sjögren syndrome.[14] Finally, there are some reports that suggest that SCLE might be a paraneoplastic syndrome,[14] but due to the paucity of cases, a causal relationship has not been proven.

Approximately 5% to 10% of patients presenting only with DLE lesions eventually develop SLE.[14] Risk factors for progression include lesions above and below the neck, unexplained anemia, leukopenia, persistently positive high-titer ANA, hypergammaglobulinemia, and positive lupus band test of nonlesional skin.[58] Patients with evidence of nephropathy or arthralgias are also at increased risk of having SLE.[59] Similar to SCLE, patients with lupus panniculitis have a 50% chance of having SLE, although this is usually mild, with only 10% meeting strict ACR criteria for SLE.[14]

In patients with known SLE, the presence of CCLE lesions (namely DLE, lupus panniculitis, or chronic mucosal plaques), appears to be associated with less severe systemic disease.[14]

Histopathology

The histopathology of CLE will be mentioned only briefly as it has been described in detail elsewhere.[14] In general, ACLE, SCLE, and DLE have similar features, thus making it difficult to distinguish the subsets of CLE. Characteristic findings include liquefactive degeneration of the epidermal basal cell layer, variable hyperkeratosis, dermal edema and mucin deposition, and mononuclear cell infiltration around the dermal–epidermal junction and dermis. This infiltrate consists mainly of $CD3^+$ (both $CD4^+$ and $CD8^+$ cells, with other cell types including histiocytes and plasmacytoid dendritic cells (see below). In DLE, the dermal infiltrate is generally denser and can extend more deeply into the reticular dermis. In addition, DLE lesions can demonstrate follicular plugging and more pronounced basement membrane thickening.

Variable deposition of immunoglobulin (IgM, IgG, IgA in decreasing frequency) and complement components can also be detected at the basement membrane zone of lesional skin. The frequency and intensity with which this is detected vary among studies and by the anatomic location of skin biopsies and the type of CLE.[14]

Hypertrophic forms of DLE are characterized by a greater degree of epidermal acanthosis and hyperkeratosis. Notably, some areas can have features of squamous cell carcinoma or keratoacanthoma. Lupus panniculitis/profundus generally spares the dermal–epidermal junction (if overlying DLE is not present), and is characterized by a lobular panniculitis and perivascular mononuclear cell infiltrate.[14] The infiltrate in the fat is composed of histiocytes and lymphocytes (sometimes forming nodules) and can show variable hyaline-fat necrosis or calcification. LE tumidus shows a perivascular and periadnexal lymphocytic infiltrate with dermal mucin deposition. Studies show focal spotty keratinocyte necrosis in 0% to 20% of cases.[42,46] Chilblain LE shows basal vacuolar degeneration, superficial dermal edema, and a perivascular lymphocytic infiltrate. Some authors conclude that these entities can be distinguished by histopathology, with idiopathic chilblains being characterized by perieccrine inflammation and spongiosis.[60,61]

Pathogenesis

Most of the work pertaining to pathogenesis of cutaneous lupus relates to those forms of CLE that are characterized by interface dermatitis (i.e., ACLE, SCLE, and DLE). Thus, this section focuses on these manifestations of CLE. In addition, much of the discussion does not distinguish among the different types of CLE, except when otherwise noted.

Before considering the etiology of LE-specific skin disease, it is interesting to consider its relationship with disease mechanisms that are associated with SLE. Evidence of a pathogenic relationship between cutaneous and systemic disease includes the association of LE-specific skin disease with SLE as well as the fact that, even in skin-limited disease, certain characteristic T- and B-lymphocyte abnormalities can be found systemically that mirror those seen in SLE.[62,63] The general concept that genetic susceptibility (i.e., human leukocyte antigen [HLA] haplotypes) and environmental triggers (infection, medication, ultraviolet light) result in a loss of immunologic self-tolerance that then is manifested by the generation of autoantibodies and antigen-specific T lymphocytes that mediate tissue injury is likely operative in both cutaneous and systemic disease. However, it should be noted that there is no definitive evidence at present that demonstrates that the cutaneous inflammation of CLE is due to an autoimmune response to antigen(s) in the skin. However, studies showing an oligoclonal expansion of T cells in the CCLE lesions are suggestive of an antigen-driven reaction either in the skin or on the periphery.[64,65] Interestingly, there is no evidence for this in infiltrates of lupus panniculitis.[66]

Various genetic abnormalities are associated with different forms of LE-specific skin disease. Several HLA haplotypes have been associated with ACLE, SCLE, and DLE.[3] This implicates a role for T lymphocytes, which may specifically be their role in providing help for antigen-specific B-cell responses, as a particular HLA-B8-DR2 (DRB1*1501) DR3 (DRB1*0301) extended haplotype correlates with the anti-Ro/SS-A response.[14] A polymorphic variant in the tumor necrosis factor-α (TNF-α) promoter that is associated with increased TNF-α production is highly associated with SCLE

and neonatal LE.[67,68] Genetic deficiencies in complement components, such as C2, C3, C4, and C5 have been associated with SCLE or DLE.[14] The role of C1q seems important, as complete congenital genetic deficiencies of this protein are a strong risk factor for photosensitive SLE.[14] In addition, a polymorphism in the *C1QA* gene is associated with SCLE.[69]

Environmental factors play a role in the pathogenesis of CLE. The paramount role of UV irradiation is discussed below. Assuming that ACLE is triggered by the same mechanisms as for SLE, chemicals such as L-canavanine, which is present in alfalfa sprouts and induces SLE, may be important.[14] Infections, especially those caused by viruses, are also triggers for SLE. Multiple medications have been associated with the clinical induction of SCLE and less so with DLE[14] (Table 40.1). It has been proposed that these may do so via inducing photosensitivity, which might result in disease activity via UV-specific mechanisms or simply via the Koebner phenomenon that results from photodamage. Although numerous drugs can induce SLE (e.g., procainamide, hydralazine, isoniazid), drug-induced SLE is typically not associated with cutaneous findings. Similarly, trauma appears to induce a Koebner phenomenon, especially in DLE patients. Smoking has been implicated as a risk factor for the development of SCLE and DLE.[14] It is unclear if this reflects a primary role for smoking in the disease process or simply results from its known association with antimalarial resistance.

Any consideration of how the molecular pathogenesis of CLE must involve consideration of the role of UV light. Evidence of the role of UV light in CLE is strong. First, most CLE lesions are in photo-exposed regions of the body; second, 50% of patients with lupus report photosensitivity; third, 54% of patients with CLE demonstrate UV photoprovocation of their lesions in the lab[70]; and fourth, an immune response against UV-altered DNA has been shown to occur in both mouse models of lupus and patients with SLE. However, the relative importance of UV light in the pathogenesis of likely multiple genetic and phenotypic forms of CLE is not currently known. It is likely that other environmental triggers (e.g., infection, cellular injury, medications) can lead to CLE as well, although the mechanisms for this are not well worked out. Thus, although most of the data

TABLE 40.1. Drugs that have been implicated in triggering the clinical expression of subacute cutaneous lupus erythematosus (SCLE), listed alphabetically within groups.

Acid blockers
   Lansoprazole
   Omeprazole**
   Ranitidine*/**
   Rabeprazole*/**
Angiotensin-converting enzyme (ACE) inhibitors
   Captopril*
   Cilazapril
Anticonvulsants
   Phenytoin*
Antihistamines
   Cinnarazine/triethylperazine
Antimalarials
   Hydroxychloroquine*
Antimicrobials
   Griseofulvin*
   Terbinafine*
Beta-blockers
   Acebutolol
   Oxprenolol
Calcium channel blockers
   Diltiazem*
   Nifedipine*
   Nitrendipine
Chemotherapy
   Taxotere (Docetaxel)*
   Tamoxifen
Diuretics
   Hydrochlorothiazide*
   Spironolactone*
Lipid lowering
   Pravastatin*
   Simvastatin*
Nonsteroidal antiinflammatory agents
   Naproxen*
   Piroxicam*
Sulfonylureas
   Glyburide*
Others
   Bupropion*
   Etanercept/infliximab*
   Interferon-α*
   Insecticides
   d-Penicillamine**
   Procainamide
   Leflunomide*
   Tetracycline derivatives (COl-3)*
   Tiotropium (inhaled)
   Ticlopidine

*Drugs reported to be capable of producing photosensitivity skin reactions in individuals not having SCLE.
**Unpublished personal observation by one of the authors (R.D.S.).
Source: Table adapted from Sontheimer.[122]

presented related to how UV light induces CLE, other forms of keratinocyte damage or activation of the cutaneous immune system can be applied in the final model.

Although it is clear that UV light (UVA or UVB) can induce CLE lesions in susceptible patients, the mechanistic link between UV exposure and the cutaneous inflammation that is observed is still not clear; many of the proposed mechanisms may be operating simultaneously. Ultraviolet light can generate neoantigens, such as UV-modified DNA; when injected into mice, this altered DNA can cause lupus-like disease.[70] Another mechanism might be the ability of UV light to induce apoptosis of keratinocytes by multiple mechanisms, including oxidative damage to mitochondrial membranes, damage to DNA, induction of p53, activation of membrane death receptors (Fas), and sensitization to TNF-α (and TNF-related apoptosis-inducing ligand [TRAIL]). Normally, the immunologic clearance of apoptotic cells is a noninflammatory event. An increased rate of formation or decreased ability to "clear" these apoptotic cells, however, can lead to early necrosis of cells and result in their capacity to stimulate the immune system. This occurs via multiple mechanisms, including the ability of necrotic elements to induce maturation and activation of local antigen-presenting cells.[71] Necrotic cells can release proinflammatory mediators such as high mobility group 1 (HMG1) protein, which is found in high levels in the skin of CLE patients.[72] The C1QA and other complement deficiencies that are associated with CLE suggest that these patients might have a defect in removal of apoptotic cells. Is there evidence of defective clearance of apoptotic keratinocytes in CLE? Data are conflicting in this regard.[73,74] Whether or not CLE patients have an increased number of apoptotic cells, it is still possible that these cells could somehow lead to inflammatory sequelae in CLE patients. Indeed, a recent observation suggests that detectable inflammation correlates with the presence of apoptotic cells in the near vicinity in CLE patients.[74]

If one accepts that in CLE patients UV damages keratinocytes with an inflammatory response, then how might such a response be propagated? One theory is that the binding of circulating autoantibodies against cellular constituents of dying keratinocytes results in a local inflammatory response (via FcR-dependent or complement-dependent mechanisms).[70] Since the seminal observation by Casciola-Rosen and colleagues[75] that UV light induces translocation of intracellular keratinocyte antigens to the cell surface (in structures called blebs), and that these antigens include the SSA/Ro and SSB/La antigens that are the targets of commonly found autoantibodies in CLE (especially SCLE), the ability to definitively link this process with the clinical findings of CLE has eluded investigators. In fact, the frequency or titers of SSA/Ro antibodies do not always correlate with skin activity in CLE patients.[70] However, recently it has been suggested that SSA/Ro autoantibodies are capable of interfering with the clearance of apoptotic cells.[76] Still, it might be that the critical antibodies are not being measured, and that apoptotic-modified forms of these antigens are the critical targets.[70] In general, LE patients have antibodies that appear to be directed against antigens involved in the cellular-stress response and heat shock response. Whatever the answer, it seems unlikely that such autoantibodies play a role in initiating CLE disease, as the deposition of antibodies in CLE tends to follow, not precede, the cellular inflammation.[77]

Ultraviolet light can also promote inflammation by inducing the secretion of cytokines and chemokines, as well as upregulating the expression of adhesion molecules.[78] Ultraviolet B induces IL-1α and TNF-α in the epidermis. These cytokines induce release of IL-6, prostaglandin E$_2$ (PGE$_2$), IL-8, and granulocyte-monocyte colony-stimulating factor (GM-CSF) by keratinocytes.[70] The end result is activation of Langerhans' cells, chemotaxis of lymphocytes, and upregulation of adhesion molecules on keratinocytes (intercellular adhesion molecule 1 [ICAM-1]) and endothelial cells (ICAM-1, vascular cell adhesion molecule 1 [VCAM-1], E-selectin). UVB irradiation also induces expression of chemokines, such as CCL5, CCL27, and CXCL8[79]; these have all been found to be at high levels in CLE skin, and function to recruit memory T cells into the vicinity. Via production of oxygen-free radicals, UVA upregulates ICAM-1 in keratinocytes, but, because it can penetrate deeper into the skin, it is also able to upregulate vascular endothelial ICAM-1 and E-selectin, which allows leukocyte extravasation into the skin.[70] In addition, UVA is able to induce secretion of IL-12, a potent immunostimulant.[70]

T lymphocytes are likely to play a major pathologic role in CLE. Skin infiltrates consist primarily of CD3$^+$ T cells, both CD4$^+$ and CD8$^+$.[70] CD4$^+$ cells appear early in the skin, with CD8$^+$ appearing later. Recent data suggest that skin homing (CLA$^+$) CD8$^+$ cytotoxic cells might be responsible for the scarring that is seen in CCLE.[80] These cells are seen predominantly in the skin of DLE patients (as opposed to other CLE subsets), and an expanded population of circulating, CCR4$^+$, CLA$^+$ CD8$^+$ cells is associated exclusively with generalized DLE.[81] These cells secrete granzyme B, a serine protease that causes tissue death and could conceivably account for injury (and resulting scar) to adnexal and epidermal structures. Interferon-γ (IFN-γ) may also play a role in this process, as local IFN-γ activity was found to be correlated with CD8$^+$ cell infiltration. Further evidence for the role of activated T cells in CLE comes from the increased expression of HLA-DR and CD25 (both activation markers) on circulating CD4$^+$ and CD8$^+$ cells in patients with DLE and SCLE; furthermore, these levels correlated with cutaneous disease activity.[62,63]

The cytokine expression pattern found in DLE lesions is representative of a mixed Th1 and Th2 profile. Lesions are characterized by high levels of IL-1, IL-2, IFN-γ, TNF-α, IFN-α, IL-5, and IL-10.[70,82] Tumor necrosis factor-α is found in increased levels in the skin of DLE and SCLE patients, and serum levels correlate with disease.[82,83] TNF-α can promote many of the findings seen in CLE: translocation of SSA/Ro to the cell surface of keratinocytes, apoptosis of keratinocytes, hyperkeratosis, and increased expression of adhesion molecules that favor cutaneous leukocyte infiltration.[84] In addition to the effects mentioned above, IFN-γ has been shown to cause keratinocyte apoptosis[85]; a mouse strain that overexpresses IFN-γ in keratinocytes results in clinical features of SLE and cutaneous inflammation.[70] Interleukin-1 is generated by keratinocytes in response to UV light, and transgenic expression of IL-1 in mice results in hair loss, scaling, and focal inflammatory lesions.[70] Keratinocytes also express an antagonist of the IL-1 receptor, and null alleles of this protein have been reported in SLE patients with photosensitivity as well as in CCLE patients.[70]

The role of the innate immune system in CLE is beginning to be explored. It has recently been discovered that IFN-γ plays an important role in the pathogenesis of SLE[86]; evidence shows that the source of this IFN-γ is the plasmacytoid dendritic cell (pDC). High numbers of pDCs have been detected in the lesions of CLE,[87] with accompanying high levels of local IFN-γ activity.[81,87–89] Interferon-γ is known to induce the chemokines CXCL9, CXCL10, and CXCL11, which are also at high levels in CLE skin.[79] The ligand for these chemokines, CXCR3, is found on infiltrating T cells in CLE. Thus, local emigration of activated pDC to the skin of CLE patients might represent the mechanism whereby T cells initially migrate into cutaneous lupus lesions. At present it is unclear what the signals are that cause pDC migration to the skin; however, it is tempting to speculate that locally deposited immune complexes (i.e., the lupus band) might play a role in their ongoing local activation, since it is known that immune complexes containing nucleic acid (from apoptotic cells) activate pDC via Toll-like receptors (TLRs), resulting in the production of IFN-γ.[90]

Treatment

Due to the critical role of UV light in CLE pathogenesis, the mainstay of any treatment regimen is sun protection. Protection against UVB and UVA are critical, as both can induce CLE in the laboratory.[26,91] Patients should be counseled on the importance of avoiding direct sun exposure, as well as the benefits of tightly woven clothing. Broad-spectrum sunscreens are important, and there is evidence that the use of these agents inhibits experimentally induced CLE lesions in patients[92] as well as potentially decreasing the burden of systemic disease in SLE patients.[93]

Local therapy with corticosteroids or calcineurin inhibitors (tacrolimus or pimecrolimus) can be used in CLE.[14] The current strengths and formulations of calcineurin inhibitors available in the United States have limited efficacy on skin sites other than the face. However, higher concentrations of calcineurin inhibitors have been reported anecdotally to be of value in classic DLE.[94] Calcineurin inhibitors are presumed to act by inhibiting activation of infiltrating T cells that are known to be present in CLE.

Antimalarials (hydroxychloroquine, chloroquine, and quinacrine) are used as first-line systemic agents for SCLE or DLE lesions, with approximately 75%

of patients responding favorably.[3] Efficacy data are based mostly on anecdotal reports, although one controlled trial with hydroxychloroquine suggested 50% efficacy for DLE or SCLE,[95] while another with chloroquine showed 82% efficacy for ACLE, SCLE, or DLE.[96] More common side effects include gastrointestinal disturbance, and blue-black pigmentation of skin or mucosa. Rarer side effects include retina, muscle, nerve, and hepatic toxicity. Potential mechanisms of action include inhibition of antigen presentation (via their known ability to disrupt lysosomal acidification), inhibition of cytokine secretion, interference with activation of extracellular signal-regulated kinases (ERKs), inhibition of prostaglandins, stabilization of membranes, and photoprotection.[97] Recent evidence suggests that they might operate via interference with intracellular TLR signaling,[98] which is tantalizing given the mounting evidence for a role of the innate immune system (i.e., pDCs) in LE and its dependence on TLR signaling.

Diaminodiphenylsulfone (Dapsone) is also used for CLE, especially when treating the patient with LE-nonspecific vesiculobullous lesions related to SLE.[2] Others have reported efficacy in SCLE.[99] Hematologic, renal, and hepatic toxicity can occur with this drug. Dapsone is known to affect neutrophil function at many levels (chemotaxis, cd11b-mediated epidermal adherence, enzyme production, generation of reactive oxygen intermediates),[100] and this may be relevant in light of the variable cutaneous infiltrate of neutrophils that is seen in CLE.

Retinoids (acitretin and isotretinoin) are advocated for SCLE and hypertrophic DLE lesions,[14] although disease usually returns following discontinuation of the drug. The mechanism of action is unclear, although inhibition of cutaneous T lymphocyte infiltration has been demonstrated in humans and animal models.[101,102]

Thalidomide can be especially effective for SCLE and DLE,[14] with a response seen in 75% of antimalarial-resistant patients.[103] Efficacy is seen as early as 2 weeks and peaks at 3 months, although relapses following cessation of therapy are common. The most common side effect is sedation. Besides its teratogenicity, it can produce a sensory neuropathy in 50% to 70% of patients, with no correlation between cumulative dose and duration of treatment.[103] Recent reports of thromboembolic events occurring in thalidomide-treated patients should prompt caution with its use in high-risk patients, including those with antiphospholipid antibodies. Thalidomide has a wide range of immunosuppressive effects, including inhibition of cytokine (notably TNF-α) production, inhibition of leukocyte chemotaxis, and inhibition of nuclear factor κB (NF-κB) effects.[104] The inhibition of NF-κB might be quite important, as this signaling pathway is important for both TNF-α– and TLR-mediated inflammatory effects, which are suspected to be instrumental in CLE.

Traditional immunosuppressive agents are sometimes used for CLE. These include methotrexate, mycophenolate mofetil, azathioprine, and cyclophosphamide.[14] Methotrexate has perhaps the most data to support its use, with a recent retrospective study of 43 CLE patients (including ACLE, SCLE, and DLE) showing improvement in 98% of patients.[105] Mounting evidence suggests that, in contrast to the traditional thinking that it acts as an antiproliferative agent, the immunomodulatory effects of methotrexate likely result from an increase in signaling via adenosine receptors.[106] This results in inhibition of neutrophil migration and decreased production of reactive oxygen metabolites and leukotriene B_4, decreased expression of cutaneous lymphocyte antigen on mononuclear cells in blood, downregulation of endothelial E-selectin on endothelial cells, inhibition of lymphocyte proliferation, and a variable decrease in TNF-α and IL-1 synthesis.[106]

Intravenous immunoglobulin (IVIG) has been used in some cases of CLE, the largest being an open label prospective study of 12 patients with SCLE or DLE in which five of 12 had virtual clearing of disease.[107] Some investigators, however, have not observed a beneficial effect.[108] Possible mechanisms of action have been reviewed elsewhere.[109]

One intriguing and somewhat counterintuitive therapy for LE is that of UV light, namely low-dose UVA1 (340 to 400 nm). This may not be so unexpected, as the wavelengths responsible for inducing SLE flares are thought to be within the UVB (280 to 320 nm) and UVA2 (320 to 340 nm) wavebands,[26,110] and "pure" (not contaminated in UVC or longer wavelengths) UVA1 and UVB do not induce (and may improve) CLE.[111] Several small trials using low-dose UVA1 (6 to 12 J/cm^2) have demonstrated benefit in systemic symptoms of SLE (including a decrease in autoantibodies). As for the skin, one of the trials noted "improvement of rash,"[112] and this was also reported separately in

two patients DLE.[113] Caution should be taken, as exacerbation of skin disease has been noted in some patients.[114,115] The mechanism of action is unclear, but might involve immunodeviation to Th1 patterns, apoptosis of resident T cells, inhibition of antigen presentation, or inhibition of TNF-α production.[116]

Future Directions

An increased understanding of the immune dysregulation seen in CLE will lead to more effective therapies for this disease. Many of these therapies will parallel the development of treatments for SLE.[117] Novel treatments might include agents targeted at T lymphocytes, such as anti-CD4 antibodies or CTLA4-Ig (which blocks T-cell co-stimulation). Although clearly important in SLE, the role of B lymphocytes is unclear in CLE, and it will be interesting to evaluate the current application of B-cell–directed therapies (such as Rituximab) for efficacy in LE-related skin disease. The known increase in ICAM-1 in lesions of CLE suggests that interference with its ligand (lymphocyte function–associated antigen 1 [LFA-1]) might be effective. Efalizumab, an antibody directed against LFA-1, has indeed shown some promise in a small open-label trial of patients with DLE.[118] There is anecdotal evidence for efficacy of TNF-α inhibitors such as etanercept in some forms of CLE.[119–121] However, the tendency for this class of biologics to induce lupus serologic changes (ANA, double-stranded DNA antibodies) and, at times, clinical changes of cutaneous and SLE limits their value in this regard. The increasing role of innate immunity, pDCs, and TLR signaling suggests that agents specifically designed to inhibit TLR signaling or pDC infiltration/maturation might be very effective for CLE. The compelling role of IFN-γ, along with studies showing that interference with type I interferon receptor signaling improves lupus-like disease in mice, make this an attractive target.

Conclusion

Cutaneous LE is a tissue-based autoimmune reaction that is unmasked by environmental factors such as ultraviolet light. Many morphologic variants may occur in the skin. Current therapies are conventional antiinflammatory agents such as glucocorticosteroids and antimalarial agents. Ongoing research into the pathophysiology of this disease suggests that targeted therapies (biologic-based treatments) that block effector cells or molecules may play an important role in the management of this disease.

Acknowledgments. Dr. Fiorentino is partially supported by a career development award from the Dermatology Foundation. Dr. Sontheimer's efforts on this project were supported by the Richard and Adeline Fleischaker Chair in Dermatology Research.

References

1. Gilliam JN, Sontheimer RD. Distinctive cutaneous subsets in the spectrum of lupus erythematosus. J Am Acad Dermatol 1981;4(4):471–475.
2. Costner MI, Sonthalmer RD, Lupus erythematosus-nonspecific skin disease. In: Hahn B and Wallace DP, eds. Dubols' Lupus Erythematosus (Chapter 31); Seventh edition, Lippincott, William and Wilkins, Philadelphia, PA, 2007.
3. Costner MI, Sontheimer RD, Provost TT. Lupus erythematosus. In: Sontheimer RD, Provost TT, eds. Cutaneous Manifestations of Rheumatic Diseases, 2nd ed. Philadelphia: Lippincott Williams & Wilkins, 2004:15–64.
4. Tebbe B, Orfanos CE. Epidemiology and socioeconomic impact of skin disease in lupus erythematosus. Lupus 1997;6(2):96–104.
5. Dubois EL, Wallace DJ. Clinical and laboratory manifestations of systemic lupus erythematosus. In: Wallace DJ, Dubois EL, eds. Lupus erythematosus, 3rd ed. Philadelphia: Lea & Febiger, 1987:317.
6. Cervera R, Khamashta MA, Font J, et al. Systemic lupus erythematosus: clinical and immunologic patterns of disease expression in a cohort of 1,000 patients. The European Working Party on Systemic Lupus Erythematosus. Medicine (Baltimore) 1993;72(2):113–124.
7. Pistiner M, Wallace DJ, Nessim S, Metzger AL, Klinenberg JR. Lupus erythematosus in the 1980s: a survey of 570 patients. Semin Arthritis Rheum 1991;21(1):55–64.
8. Jonsson H, Nived O, Sturfelt G. The effect of age on clinical and serological manifestations in unselected patients with systemic lupus erythematosus. J Rheumatol 1988;15(3):505–509.
9. Font J, Cervera R, Navarro M, et al. Systemic lupus erythematosus in men: clinical and immunological characteristics. Ann Rheum Dis 1992;51(9):1050–1052.
10. Sontheimer RD, Thomas JR, Gilliam JN. Subacute cutaneous lupus erythematosus: a cutaneous marker for a distinct lupus erythematosus subset. Arch Dermatol 1979;115(12):1409–1415.
11. Popovic K, Nyberg F, Wahren-Herlenius M. A serology-based approach combined with clinical examination of 125 Ro/SSA-positive patients to define incidence and prevalence of subacute cutaneous lupus erythematosus. Arthritis Rheum 2006;56(1):255–264.
12. Vlachoyiannopoulos PG, Karassa FB, Karakostas KX, Drosos AA, Moutsopoulos HM. Systemic lupus erythematosus in Greece. Clinical features, evolution and outcome: a descriptive analysis of 292 patients. Lupus 1993;2(5):303–312.
13. Dubois EL, Tuffanelli DL. Clinical manifestations of systemic lupus erythematosus. Computer analysis of 520 cases. JAMA 1964;190:104–111.
14. McCauliffe DP, Sontheimer RD: Lupus erythematosus-specific skin disease. In: Hahn B and Wallace DP, eds: Dubols' Lupus Erythematosus (Chapter 30), Seventh edition, Lippincott, William and Wilkins, Philadelphine, PA, 2007.
15. Hochberg MC, Boyd RE, Ahearn JM, et al. Systemic lupus erythematosus: a review of clinico-laboratory features and immunogenetic markers in 150 patients with emphasis on demographic subsets. Medicine (Baltimore) 1985;64(5):285–295.
16. Gilliam JN, Sontheimer RD. Subacute cutaneous lupus erythematosus. Clin Rheum Dis 1982;8(2):343–352.
17. Urman JD, Lowenstein MB, Abeles M, Weinstein A. Oral mucosal ulceration in systemic lupus erythematosus. Arthritis Rheum 1978;21(1):58–61.
18. Nyberg F, Hasan T, Puska P, et al. Occurrence of polymorphous light eruption in lupus erythematosus. Br J Dermatol 1997;136(2):217–221.
19. David-Bajar KM, Bennion SD, DeSpain JD, Golitz LE, Lee LA. Clinical, histologic, and immunofluorescent distinctions between subacute cutaneous lupus erythematosus and discoid lupus erythematosus. J Invest Dermatol 1992;99(3):251–257.
20. Hymes SR, Russell TJ, Jordon RE. The anti-Ro antibody system. Int J Dermatol 1986;25(1):1–7.
21. Rowell NR, Beck JS, Anderson JR. Lupus erythematosus and erythema multiforme-like lesions. A syndrome with characteristic immunological abnormalities. Arch Dermatol 1963;88:176–180.
22. Scheinman PL. Acral subacute cutaneous lupus erythematosus: an unusual variant. J Am Acad Dermatol 1994;30(5 pt 1):800–801.
23. George R, Mathai R, Kurian S. Cutaneous lupus erythematosus in India: immunofluorescence profile. Int J Dermatol 1992;31(4):265–269.
24. Kouba DJ, Owens NM, Mimouni D, Klein W, Nousari CH. Milia en plaque: a novel manifestation of chronic cutaneous lupus erythematosus. Br J Dermatol 2003;149(2):424–426.

25. Sanders CJ, Van Weelden H, Kazzaz GA, Sigurdsson V, Toonstra J, Bruijnzeel-Koomen CA. Photosensitivity in patients with lupus erythematosus: a clinical and photobiological study of 100 patients using a prolonged phototest protocol. Br J Dermatol 2003;149(1):131–137.

26. Lehmann P, Holzle E, Kind P, Goerz G, Plewig G. Experimental reproduction of skin lesions in lupus erythematosus by UVA and UVB radiation. J Am Acad Dermatol 1990;22(2 pt 1):181–187.

27. Werth VP, White WL, Sanchez MR, Franks AG. Incidence of alopecia areata in lupus erythematosus. Arch Dermatol 1992;128(3):368–371.

28. Wong KO. Systemic lupus erythematosus: a report of forty-five cases with unusual clinical and immunological features. Br J Dermatol 1969;81(3):186–190.

29. Parish LC, Kennedy RJ, Hurley J. Palmar lesions in lupus erythematosus. Arch Dermatol 1967;96(3):273–276.

30. Romero RW, Nesbitt LT Jr, Reed RJ. Unusual variant of lupus erythematosus or lichen planus. Clinical, histopathologic, and immunofluorescent studies. Arch Dermatol 1977;113(6):741–748.

31. Lodin A. Discoid lupus erythematosus and trauma. Acta Derm Venereol 1963;43:142–148.

32. Morihara K, Kishimoto S, Shibagaki R, Takenaka H, Yasuno H. Follicular lupus erythematosus: a new cutaneous manifestation of systemic lupus erythematosus. Br J Dermatol 2002;147(1):157–159.

33. Daldon PE, Macedo de Souza E, Cintra ML. Hypertrophic lupus erythematosus: a clinicopathological study of 14 cases. J Cutan Pathol 2003;30(7):443–448.

34. Velthuis PJ, van Weelden H, van Wichen D, Baart de la Faille H. Immunohistopathology of light-induced skin lesions in lupus erythematosus. Acta Derm Venereol. 1990;70(2):93–98.

35. Wolska H, Blaszczyk M, Jablonska S. Phototests in patients with various forms of lupus erythematosus. Int J Dermatol 1989;28(2):98–103.

36. Andreasen JO. Oral Manifestations in Discoid and Systemic Lupus Erythematosus. I. Clinical Investigation. Acta Odontol Scand 1964;22:295–310.

37. Burge SM, Frith PA, Juniper RP, Wojnarowska F. Mucosal involvement in systemic and chronic cutaneous lupus erythematosus. Br J Dermatol 1989;121(6):727–741.

38. Doutre MS, Beylot C, Beylot J, Pompougnac E, Royer P. Chilblain lupus erythematosus: report of 15 cases. Dermatology 1992;184(1):26–28.

39. Viguier M, Pinquier L, Cavelier-Balloy B, et al. Clinical and histopathologic features and immunologic variables in patients with severe chilblains. A study of the relationship to lupus erythematosus. Medicine (Baltimore) 2001;80(3):180–188.

40. Ng PP, Tan SH, Tan T. Lupus erythematosus panniculitis: a clinicopathologic study. Int J Dermatol 2002;41(8):488–490.

41. Tuffanelli DL. Lupus erythematosus panniculitis (profundus). Arch Dermatol 1971;103(3):231–242.

42. Alexiades-Armenakas MR, Baldassano M, Bince B, et al. Tumid lupus erythematosus: criteria for classification with immunohistochemical analysis. Arthritis Rheum 2003;49(4):494–500.

43. Kuhn A, Richter-Hintz D, Oslislo C, Ruzicka T, Megahed M, Lehmann P. Lupus erythematosus tumidus—a neglected subset of cutaneous Lupus erythematosus: report of 40 cases. Arch Dermatol 2000;136(8):1033–1041.

44. Makhoul E, Abadjian G, Bendaly-Halaby E, Hourany N, Hobeika P. [Tuberculous lupusopos of a case of tuberculous lupus tumidus]. J Med Liban 1997;45(1):43–45.

45. Choonhakarn C, Poonsriaram A, Chaivoramukul J. Lupus erythematosus tumidus. Int J Dermatol 2004;43(11):815–818.

46. Kuhn A, Sonntag M, Ruzicka T, Lehmann P, Megahed M. Histopathologic findings in lupus erythematosus tumidus: review of 80 patients. J Am Acad Dermatol 2003;48(6):901–908.

47. Callen JP, Klein J. Subacute cutaneous lupus erythematosus. Clinical, serologic, immunogenetic, and therapeutic considerations in seventy-two patients. Arthritis Rheum 1988;31(8):1007–1013.

48. Sontheimer RD. Subacute cutaneous lupus erythematosus: a decade's perspective. Med Clin North Am 1989;73(5):1073–1090.

49. Lee LA, Roberts CM, Frank MB, McCubbin VR, Reichlin M. The autoantibody response to Ro/SSA in cutaneous lupus erythematosus. Arch Dermatol 1994;130(10):1262–1268.

50. Fonseca E, Alvarez R, Gonzalez MR, Pascual D. Prevalence of anticardiolipin antibodies in subacute cutaneous lupus erythematosus. Lupus 1992;1(4):265–268.

51. Callen JP, Kulick KB, Stelzer G, Fowler JF. Subacute cutaneous lupus erythematosus. Clinical, serologic, and immunogenetic studies of forty-nine patients seen in a nonreferral setting. J Am Acad Dermatol 1986;15(6):1227–1237.

52. Konstadoulakis MM, Kroubouzos G, Tosca A, et al. Thyroid autoantibodies in the subsets of lupus erythematosus: correlation with other autoantibodies and thyroid function. Thyroidology 1993;5(1):1–7.

53. Callen JP, Fowler JF, Kulick KB. Serologic and clinical features of patients with discoid lupus erythematosus: relationship of antibodies to single-stranded deoxyribonucleic acid and of other antinuclear antibody subsets to clinical manifestations. J Am Acad Dermatol 1985;13(5 pt 1):748–755.

54. Mayou SC, Wojnarowska F, Lovell CR, Asherson RA, Leigh IM. Anticardiolipin and antinuclear antibodies in discoid lupus erythematosus—their clinical significance. Clin Exp Dermatol 1988;13(6):389–392.

55. Franceschini F, Calzavara-Pinton P, Quinzanini M, et al. Chilblain lupus erythematosus is associated with antibodies to SSA/Ro. Lupus 1999;8(3):215–219.

56. Wenzel J, Bauer R, Uerlich M, Bieber T, Boehm I. The value of lymphocytopenia as a marker of systemic involvement in cutaneous lupus erythematosus. Br J Dermatol 2002;146(5):869–871.

57. Tan EM, Cohen AS, Fries JF, et al. The 1982 revised criteria for the classification of systemic lupus erythematosus. Arthritis Rheum 1982;25(11):1271–1277.

58. Callen JP. Chronic cutaneous lupus erythematosus. Clinical, laboratory, therapeutic, and prognostic examination of 62 patients. Arch Dermatol 1982;118(6):412–416.

59. Tebbe B, Mansmann U, Wollina U, et al. Markers in cutaneous lupus erythematosus indicating systemic involvement. A multicenter study on 296 patients. Acta Derm Venereol 1997;77(4):305–308.

60. Crowson AN, Magro CM. Idiopathic perniosis and its mimics: a clinical and histological study of 38 cases. Hum Pathol 1997;28(4):478–484.

61. Cribier B, Djeridi N, Peltre B, Grosshans E. A histologic and immunohistochemical study of chilblains. J Am Acad Dermatol 2001;45(6):924–929.

62. Wenzel J, Henze S, Brahler S, Bieber T, Tuting T. The expression of human leukocyte antigen-DR and CD25 on circulating T cells in cutaneous lupus erythematosus and correlation with disease activity. Exp Dermatol 2005;14(6):454–459.

63. Wouters CH, Diegenant C, Ceuppens JL, Degreef H, Stevens EA. The circulating lymphocyte profiles in patients with discoid lupus erythematosus and systemic lupus erythematosus suggest a pathogenetic relationship. Br J Dermatol 2004;150(4):693–700.

64. Kita Y, Kuroda K, Mimori T, et al. T cell receptor clonotypes in skin lesions from patients with systemic lupus erythematosus. J Invest Dermatol 1998;110(1):41–46.

65. Volc-Platzer B, Anegg B, Milota S, Pickl W, Fischer G. Accumulation of gamma delta T cells in chronic cutaneous lupus erythematosus. J Invest Dermatol 1993;100(1):84S–91S.

66. Massone C, Kodama K, Salmhofer W, et al. Lupus erythematosus panniculitis (lupus profundus): clinical, histopathological, and molecular analysis of nine cases. J Cutan Pathol 2005;32(6):396–404.

67. Clancy RM, Backer CB, Yin X, et al. Genetic association of cutaneous neonatal lupus with HLA class II and tumor necrosis factor alpha: implications for pathogenesis. Arthritis Rheum 2004;50(8):2598–2603.

68. Werth VP, Zhang W, Dortzbach K, Sullivan K. Association of a promoter polymorphism of tumor necrosis factor-alpha with subacute cutaneous lupus erythematosus and distinct photoregulation of transcription. J Invest Dermatol 2000;115(4):726–730.

69. Racila DM, Sontheimer CJ, Sheffield A, Wisnieski JJ, Racila E, Sontheimer RD. Homozygous single nucleotide polymorphism of the complement C1QA gene is associated with decreased levels of C1q in patients with subacute cutaneous lupus erythematosus. Lupus 2003;12(2):124–132.

70. Dutz J, Sontheimer RD, Werth V. Pathomechanisms of cutaneous lupus erythematosus; 2007:550–573.

71. Rovere P, Vallinoto C, Bondanza A, et al. Bystander apoptosis triggers dendritic cell maturation and antigen-presenting function. J Immunol 1998;161(9):4467–4471.

72. Popovic K, Ek M, Espinosa A, et al. Increased expression of the novel proinflammatory cytokine high mobility group box chromosomal protein 1 in skin lesions of patients with lupus erythematosus. Arthritis Rheum 2005;52(11):3639–3645.

73. Kuhn A, Herrmann M, Kleber S, et al. Accumulation of apoptotic cells in the epidermis of patients with cutaneous lupus erythematosus after ultraviolet irradiation. Arthritis Rheum 2006;54(3):939–950.

74. Reefman E, de Jong MC, Kuiper H, et al. Is disturbed clearance of apoptotic keratinocytes responsible for UVB-induced inflammatory skin lesions in systemic lupus erythematosus? Arthritis Res Ther 2006;8(6):R156.

75. Casciola-Rosen LA, Anhalt G, Rosen A. Autoantigens targeted in systemic lupus erythematosus are clustered in two populations of surface structures on apoptotic keratinocytes. J Exp Med 1994;179(4):1317–1330.

76. Clancy RM, Neufing PJ, Zheng P, et al. Impaired clearance of apoptotic cardiocytes is linked to anti-SSA/Ro and -SSB/La antibodies in the pathogenesis of congenital heart block. J Clin Invest 2006;116(9):2413–2422.

77. Angotti C. Immunology of cutaneous lupus erythematosus. Clin Dermatol-Apr 2004;22(2):105–112.

78. Bennion SD, Norris DA. Ultraviolet light modulation of autoantigens, epidermal cytokines and adhesion molecules as contributing factors of the pathogenesis of cutaneous LE. Lupus 1997;6(2):181–192.

79. Meller S, Winterberg F, Gilliet M, et al. Ultraviolet radiation-induced injury, chemokines, and leukocyte recruitment: An amplification cycle triggering cutaneous lupus erythematosus. Arthritis Rheum 2005;52(5):1504–1516.

80. Wenzel J, Uerlich M, Worrenkamper E, Freutel S, Bieber T, Tuting T. Scarring skin lesions of discoid lupus erythematosus are characterized by high numbers of skin-homing cytotoxic lymphocytes

associated with strong expression of the type I interferon-induced protein MxA. Br J Dermatol 2005;153(5):1011–1015.

81. Wenzel J, Henze S, Worenkamper E, et al. Role of the chemokine receptor CCR4 and its ligand thymus- and activation-regulated chemokine/CCL17 for lymphocyte recruitment in cutaneous lupus erythematosus. J Invest Dermatol 2005;124(6): 1241–1248.

82. Toro JR, Finlay D, Dou X, Zheng SC, LeBoit PE, Connolly MK. Detection of type 1 cytokines in discoid lupus erythematosus. Arch Dermatol 2000;136(12):1497–1501.

83. Zampieri S, Alaibac M, Iaccarino L, et al. Tumour necrosis factor alpha is expressed in refractory skin lesions from patients with subacute cutaneous lupus erythematosus. Ann Rheum Dis 2006;65(4):545–548.

84. Gerl V, Hostmann B, Johnen C, et al. The intracellular 52–kd Ro/SSA autoantigen in keratinocytes is up-regulated by tumor necrosis factor alpha via tumor necrosis factor receptor I. Arthritis Rheum 2005;52(2):531–538.

85. Trautmann A, Akdis M, Kleemann D, et al. T cell-mediated Fas-induced keratinocyte apoptosis plays a key pathogenetic role in eczematous dermatitis. J Clin Invest 2000;106(1):25–35.

86. Ronnblom L, Eloranta ML, Alm GV. The type I interferon system in systemic lupus erythematosus. Arthritis Rheum 2006;54(2):408–420.

87. Farkas L, Beiske K, Lund-Johansen F, Brandtzaeg P, Jahnsen FL. Plasmacytoid dendritic cells (natural interferon- alpha/beta-producing cells) accumulate in cutaneous lupus erythematosus lesions. Am J Pathol 2001;159(1):237–243.

88. Chow S, Chen C, Xiang Z, Sinha A. Interferon-inducible signatures in the skin and peripheral blood of patients with cutaneous lupus. J Invest Dermatol 2005;124(S4):A89.

89. Blomberg S, Eloranta ML, Cederblad B, Nordlin K, Alm GV, Ronnblom L. Presence of cutaneous interferon-alpha producing cells in patients with systemic lupus erythematosus. Lupus 2001;10(7):484–490.

90. Lovgren T, Eloranta ML, Bave U, Alm GV, Ronnblom L. Induction of interferon-alpha production in plasmacytoid dendritic cells by immune complexes containing nucleic acid released by necrotic or late apoptotic cells and lupus IgG. Arthritis Rheum 2004;50(6):1861–1872.

91. Nived O, Johansen PB, Sturfelt G. Standardized ultraviolet-A exposure provokes skin reaction in systemic lupus erythematosus. Lupus 1993;2(4):247–250.

92. Stege H, Budde MA, Grether-Beck S, Krutmann J. Evaluation of the capacity of sunscreens to photoprotect lupus erythematosus patients by employing the photoprovocation test. Photodermatol Photoimmunol Photomed 2000;16(6):256–259.

93. Vila LM, Mayor AM, Valentin AH, et al. Association of sunlight exposure and photoprotection measures with clinical outcome in systemic lupus erythematosus. P R Health Sci J 1999;18(2):89–94.

94. Walker SL, Kirby B, Chalmers RJ. The effect of topical tacrolimus on severe recalcitrant chronic discoid lupus erythematosus. Br J Dermatol 2002;147(2):405–406.

95. Ruzicka T, Sommerburg C, Goerz G, Kind P, Mensing H. Treatment of cutaneous lupus erythematosus with acitretin and hydroxychloroquine. Br J Dermatol 1992;127(5):513–518.

96. Bezerra EL, Vilar MJ, da Trindade Neto PB, Sato EI. Double-blind, randomized, controlled clinical trial of clofazimine compared with chloroquine in patients with systemic lupus erythematosus. Arthritis Rheum 2005;52(10):3073–3078.

97. Van Beek MJ, Piette WW. Antimalarials. Dermatol Clin 2001;19(1):147–160, ix.

98. Kyburz D, Brentano F, Gay S. Mode of action of hydroxychloroquine in RA-evidence of an inhibitory effect on toll-like receptor signaling. Natl Clin Pract Rheumatol 2006;2(9):458–459.

99. Holtman JH, Neustadt DH, Klein J, Callen JP. Dapsone is an effective therapy for the skin lesions of subacute cutaneous lupus erythematosus and urticarial vasculitis in a patient with C2 deficiency. J Rheumatol 1990;17(9):1222–1225.

100. Modschiedler K, Weller M, Worl P, von den Driesch P. Dapsone and colchicine inhibit adhesion of neutrophilic granulocytes to epidermal sections. Arch Dermatol Res 2000;292(1):32–36.

101. Jimenez-Balderas FJ, Tapia-Serrano R, Fonseca ME, et al. High frequency of association of rheumatic/autoimmune diseases and untreated male hypogonadism with severe testicular dysfunction. Arthritis Res 2001;3(6):362–367.

102. Ikeda T, Nishide T, Ohtani T, Furukawa F. The effects of vitamin A derivative etretinate on the skin of MRL mice. Lupus 2005;14(7):510–516.

103. Pelle MT, Werth VP. Thalidomide in cutaneous lupus erythematosus. Am J Clin Dermatol 2003;4(6):379–387.

104. Wu JJ, Huang DB, Pang KR, Hsu S, Tyring SK. Thalidomide: dermatological indications, mechanisms of action and side-effects. Br J Dermatol 2005;153(2):254–273.

105. Wenzel J, Brahler S, Bauer R, Bieber T, Tuting T. Efficacy and safety of methotrexate in recalcitrant cutaneous lupus erythematosus: results of a retrospective study in 43 patients. Br J Dermatol 2005;153(1):157–162.

106. Cronstein BN. The mechanism of action of methotrexate. Rheum Dis Clin North Am 1997;23(4): 739–755.

107. Goodfield M, Davison K, Bowden K. Intravenous immunoglobulin (IVIg) for therapy-resistant cutaneous lupus erythematosus (LE). J Dermatol Treat 2004;15(1):46–50.

108. De Pita O, Bellucci AM, Ruffelli M, Girardelli CR, Puddu P. Intravenous immunoglobulin therapy is not able to efficiently control cutaneous manifestations in patients with lupus erythematosus. Lupus 1997;6(4):415–417.

109. Colsky AS. Intravenous immunoglobulin in autoimmune and inflammatory dermatoses. A review of proposed mechanisms of action and therapeutic applications. Dermatol Clin 2000;18(3):447–457, ix.

110. Hasan T, Nyberg F, Stephansson E, et al. Photosensitivity in lupus erythematosus, UV photoprovocation results compared with history of photosensitivity and clinical findings. Br J Dermatol 1997;136(5):699–705.

111. Lokitz ML, Billet S, Patel P, et al. Failure of physiologic doses of pure UVA or UVB to induce lesions in photosensitive cutaneous lupus erythematosus: implications for phototesting. Photodermatol Photoimmunol Photomed 2006;22(6):290–296.

112. Polderman MC, Huizinga TW, Le Cessie S, Pavel S. UVA-1 cold light treatment of SLE: a double blind, placebo controlled crossover trial. Ann Rheum Dis 2001;60(2):112–115.

113. Mitra A, Yung A, Goulden V, Goodfield MD. A trial of low-dose UVA1 phototherapy for two patients with recalcitrant discoid lupus erythematosus. Clin Exp Dermatol 2006;31(2):299–300.

114. McGrath H, Martinez-Osuna P, Lee FA. Ultraviolet-A1 (340–400 nm) irradiation therapy in systemic lupus erythematosus. Lupus 1996;5(4):269–274.

115. Polderman MC, le Cessie S, Huizinga TW, Pavel S. Efficacy of UVA-1 cold light as an adjuvant therapy for systemic lupus erythematosus. Rheumatology (Oxford) 2004;43(11):1402–1404.

116. Pavel S. Light therapy (with UVA-1) for SLE patients: is it a good or bad idea? Rheumatology (Oxford) 2006;45(6):653–655.

117. Schattner A, Naparstek Y. The future of the treatment of systemic lupus erythematosus. Clin Exp Rheumatol 2005;23(2):254–260.

118. Usmani N, Goodfield MD. Efalizumab in the treatment of patients with discoid lupus erythematosus. Br J Dermatol 2006;155(suppl 1):2.

119. Fautrel B, Foltz V, Frances C, Bourgeois P, Rozenberg S. Regression of subacute cutaneous lupus erythematosus in a patient with rheumatoid arthritis treated with a biologic tumor necrosis factor alpha-blocking agent: comment on the article by Pisetsky and the letter from Aringer et al. Arthritis Rheum 2002;46(5):1408–1409; author reply 1409.

120. Drosou A, Kirsner RS, Welsh E, Sullivan TP, Kerdel FA. Use of infliximab, an anti-tumor necrosis alpha antibody, for inflammatory dermatoses. J Cutan Med Surg 2003;7(5):382–386.

121. Norman R, Greenberg RG, Jackson JM. Case reports of etanercept in inflammatory dermatoses. J Am Acad Dermatol 2006;54(3 suppl 2):S139–142.

122. Sontheimer RD. Subacute cutaneous lupus erythematosus: 25-year evolution of a prototypic subset (subphenotype) of lupus erythematosus defined by characteristic cutaneous, pathological, immunological, and genetic findings. Autoimmun Rev 2005;4(5):253–263.

41
Fibrotic Skin Diseases

Irina G. Luzina and Sergei P. Atamas

Key Points

- Dermal fibrosis is excessive scarring of the skin, and is a result of a pathologic wound healing response.
- There is a wide spectrum of fibrotic skin diseases: scleroderma, nephrogenic fibrosing dermopathy, mixed connective tissue disease, scleromyxedema, scleredema, and eosinophilic fasciitis. Exposures to chemicals or physical agents are also potential causes of fibrotic skin disease.
- Dermal fibrosis may be driven by immune, autoimmune, and inflammatory mechanisms.
- The balance of collagen production and degradation by fibroblasts plays a critical role in the pathophysiology of fibrotic processes in the skin.
- Certain cytokines promote would healing and fibrosis, such as transforming growth factor-β (TGF-β) and interleukin-4 (IL-4), whereas others are antifibrotic, such as interferon-γ (IFN-γ) and transforming growth factor-α (TNF-α).

Dermal fibrosis, or excessive scarring of the skin, is a consequence of exaggerated healing response, particularly disproportionate fibroblast proliferation and extracellular matrix (ECM) production in the dermis. Clinically, skin fibrosis manifests as thickened, tightened, and hardened areas of skin. Ultimately, skin fibrosis may lead to dermal contractures that affect the ability to flex and extend the joints.

The spectrum of fibrotic skin diseases is wide and includes scleroderma in both localized (morphea, linear scleroderma) and systemic forms, graft-versus-host disease (GVHD), nephrogenic fibrosing dermopathy (NFD), and mixed connective tissue disease. Collagen accumulation also occurs in scleredema, scleromyxedema, and eosinophilic fasciitis. Cicatricial pemphigoid is an autoimmune process associated with scarring, in which dermal fibroblasts may produce excessive amounts of collagen, a collagen-folding chaperone heat shock protein 47 (HSP47), and transforming growth factor-β (TGF-β).[1] Excessive scarring may also occur in chromoblastomycosis.[2] Dermal fibroses may result from environmental or professional exposures to various chemicals (e.g., in eosinophilia-myalgia syndrome induced by L-tryptophan) or from metabolic disorders. Ionizing radiation-induced and post-burn trauma skin fibroses, hypertrophic scars and keloids, lipodermatosclerosis, and collagenomas are often placed in this group of diseases as well.

Despite this variety of causes and disease-specific pathophysiologic processes leading to skin fibrosis, the cellular and molecular mechanisms of excessive extracellular matrix accumulation in the skin are fairly universal. Extensive research in the mechanisms of dermal, pulmonary, hepatic, and renal fibrosis revealed profound similarities between the molecular and cellular mechanisms of fibrosis and wound healing. Tissue fibrosis is often viewed as abnormal, exaggerated wound healing process. Normally, an injury to the skin tissues causes a rapid (within hours) early acute inflammatory response, followed by the late-phase inflammation (within days since the injury), and finally followed by a healing response (within weeks). It is during this latter phase that fibroblasts become

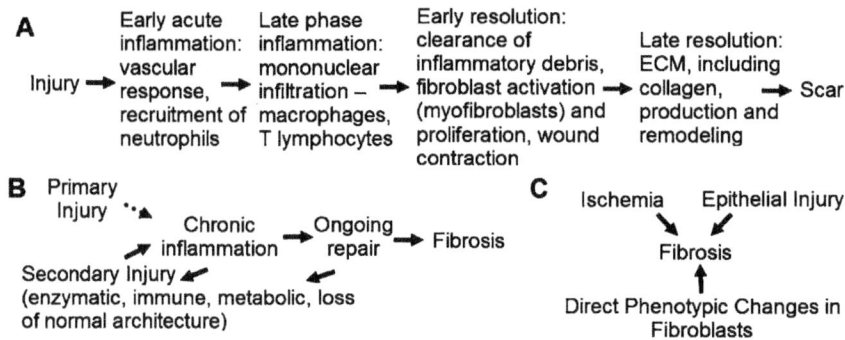

FIG. 41.1. Simplified staging of normal wound healing resolving with formation of scar tissue (A), as opposed to chronic inflammation (B) and inflammation-independent factors (C) that lead to excessive scarring and fibrosis. Each of the phases in these processes is complex and involves processes at the molecular, cellular, tissue, and organismal levels (even though the injury may be local). Numerous cytokines appear to be critical regulators of each phase. Despite the extreme pleiotropy and functional redundancy of the multiple cytokines involved, these processes are precisely regulated. An oversimplified but useful generalization related to panel A is that the cytokines of the early inflammation phase (e.g., tumor necrosis factor-α [TNF-α], interferon-γ [IFN-γ]) are directly antifibrotic, whereas the cytokines of late inflammation and repair phases (transforming growth factor-β [TGF-β], connective tissue growth factor [CTGF], and Th2/Tc2) are directly profibrotic

activated, undergo phenotypic transformation into myofibroblasts (by expressing not only collagen but also α-smooth muscle actin), and cause wound contraction. These myofibroblasts also proliferate, and accelerate production of the extracellular matrix components, particularly collagen, normally leading to formation of a scar (Fig. 41.1A).

If the primary injury is persistent or is followed by a secondary injury from excessive inflammation or immune activation (e.g., autoimmunity), then the inflammatory process becomes chronic, with tissue injury, inflammation, and repair ongoing simultaneously (Fig. 41.1B). In the latter case, tissue fibrosis is likely to develop as a result of

ongoing repair that becomes excessive and disorganized. Since fibrosis is often preceded and accompanied by chronic inflammation, it has been assumed for a long time that inflammation is a necessary contributor to fibrosis (Table 41.1). The timing and intensity of the processes in the sequence that is outlined schematically in Figure 41.1A is controlled by cytokines, many of which have direct stimulatory or inhibitory effect on the proliferation of, or collagen production in, fibroblasts. The disturbances of this regulation in dermal fibrosis is reviewed below. Our understanding of the immune and inflammatory mechanisms leading to fibrosis is far from complete; we do know,

TABLE 41.1. Mechanisms of tissue fibrosis.

Causes of tissue fibrosis	Characteristics
Chronic inflammation	Caused by an ongoing primary or secondary injury to the tissues and infiltration with monocytic inflammatory cells (macrophages, T cells); often associated with immune/autoimmune activation and damage; antiinflammatory and immunosuppressive therapies effective
Inflammation-unrelated mechanisms: epithelial injury and activation, vascular insufficiency	Antiinflammatory and immunosuppressive therapies ineffective
Intrinsic profibrotic phenotypic changes in fibroblasts: accelerated proliferation and production of ECM in vivo and in cell culture, slowed ECM turnover	Likely a consequence of the mechanisms above, becomes an independent contributor to fibrosis later in the disease, when these phenotypic changes become irreversible

ECM, extracellular matrix.

however, that such mechanisms are complex and involve numerous cells types and dozens or even hundreds of genes.[3-5]

Recent considerations suggested that not all cases of tissue fibrosis are inflammation-dependent. For example, limited inflammation is seen in the lungs of patients with a deadly fibrotic lung disease, idiopathic pulmonary fibrosis, and it is believed to be an epiphenomenon rather than the driving force of the disease; the antiinflammatory therapies are ineffective in attenuating the rapid decline in pulmonary function, resulting in the death of the patient within 3 to 5 years after the diagnosis. It is believed that instead of chronic inflammation, multiple cycles of epithelial cell injury and activation drive the fibrosis through a variety of inflammation-independent fibrotic mechanisms. Similarly, dermal fibrosis may develop in association with limited, if any, inflammation. For example, the chronic venous insufficiency rather than inflammatory changes is a likely driving force of dermal fibrosis in the affected skin of patients with lipodermatosclerosis (hardening and hyperpigmentation of lower leg skin associated with chronic venous insufficiency).[6] Nevertheless, the fibrotic mechanisms seem to be similar to those observed in an inflammation-driven fibrosis, such as increased levels and activity of matrix metalloproteinases (MMPs)[7] and abnormal spatial distribution of the profibrotic cytokines.[8]

In addition to the inflammation-related, epithelial injury–related, or systemic (e.g., chronic ischemia) mechanisms, the genuine phenotypic disturbances in dermal fibroblasts (Table 41.1) are thought to be the manifestation, and simultaneously a driving force, of tissue fibrosis. Such changes include persistent accelerated proliferation and ECM production, slow ECM turnover (degradation by MMPs), increased resistance to apoptosis, and disturbed interactions with the components of the ECM.[9-11] These may be genuine phenotypic changes in the majority of fibroblasts or a result of clonal selection of activated fibroblast subpopulations during the course of the disease.[12] Recent gene array studies suggested that such phenotypic changes in fibroblasts are rather complex, but failed to clarify any causal relationships between changes in the expression of individual genes.[3-5]

Dermal fibrosis is usually driven by inflammatory and immune, including autoimmune, mechanisms.

Such mechanisms are considered in this chapter. The mostly nonimmune mechanisms of lipodermatosclerosis or collagen-producing tumors such as dermatofibromas, dermatofibrosarcomas, and collagenomas are not discussed here, although they may develop in association with autoimmunity and under control of the same inflammatory cells and profibrotic factor as those involved in the immune- and inflammation-driven collagen accumulation. The exact timing of response to injury is critical to normal repair process (Fig. 41.1); when the normal timing and levels of cytokine production become disturbed, dermal fibrosis ensues.

It is important to differentiate the direct and indirect regulation of fibroblast proliferation and collagen production. The cells and cytokines of early inflammation are either directly antifibrotic (tumor necrosis factor-α [TNF-α] and interferon-γ [IFN-γ]) or have no direct effect on fibroblasts (interleukin-1 [IL-1], IL-6). Yet, dysregulated inflammation may lead to an exaggerated healing response, with excessive production of directly profibrotic cytokines (TGF-β, IL-4, CCL2), overly active collagen production and overly suppressed collagen turnover, and finally fibrosis. Thus, the immediate effect of early inflammation is antifibrotic, yet its long-term effect may be profibrotic.

Selected Fibrotic Skin Diseases and Animal Models

Scleroderma

Although rare, scleroderma is a prototypic fibrotic disease. A better understanding of the mechanisms of fibrosis in scleroderma, particularly the contribution of autoimmune processes, would have major implications for fibrotic complications in other diseases. The pathophysiology of progressive systemic sclerosis (SSc) is characterized by a triad of (1) immune system activation and autoimmunity, (2) proliferative and obliterative small vessel vasculopathy, and (3) fibrosis. This is a true systemic disease, with numerous organs and systems of organs involved, but dermal manifestations of the disease are most obvious. There are two major categories of cutaneous scleroderma: limited (skin involvement distal to the elbows and knees, with possible face and neck involvement), and diffuse (skin involvement on the trunk and proximal parts of the limbs). A subset of patients with limited cutaneous scleroderma present with the so-called CREST syndrome (*c*alcinosis, *R*aynaud's phenomenon, *e*sophageal dysmotility, *s*clerodactyly, and *t*elangiectasia). Both categories of patients are at risk for internal organ involvement, although life-threatening end-organ damage of the lungs, heart, gut, and kidneys is more common in diffuse scleroderma. Such involvement of internal organs does not occur in localized scleroderma (morphea, linear scleroderma).

Although determination of autoantibodies against characteristic targets is helpful in assessing the prognosis, monitoring, and treatment of scleroderma patients, the pathophysiologic roles of such antibodies remains unclear. For example, autoantibodies to the ECM protein fibrillin-1 are present in the sera of scleroderma patients, and appear to be highly disease-specific.[13] However, there are striking ethnic differences in the occurrence of these antibodies and their antigenic epitope specificity, and there is no correlation with major clinical features, the presence of other autoantibodies, or human leukocyte antigen (HLA) class II alleles.[13] These observations raise the question of whether these antibodies are a mere epiphenomenon of the disease rather than a pathophysiologic contributor. Although one recent study implicated anti–fibrillin-1 autoantibodies in the direct activation of normal dermal fibroblasts into a profibrotic phenotype,[14] the role of this mechanism in the disease remains unclear as less than 50% of Caucasians with scleroderma show seroreactivity with recombinant fibrillin-1.[13] Similarly, anti-DNA topoisomerase I (anti-Scl-70) antibodies, the major autoantibodies in the sera of patients with systemic sclerosis, react with the immunodominant domains that are heterogeneous, influenced by ethnic background,[15] and are highly variable over time.[16] These autoantibodies may play a specific, autoantigen-driven, pathogenic role or, as a nonexclusive alternative, they may be a secondary by-product of other processes, such as excessive activation of innate, antigen-nonspecific mechanisms.

Self-reactive T cells may play a more profound pathogenic role in scleroderma. Such cells target autologous type I collagen[17] and topoisomerase I,[18] and are clonally expanded,[19,20] suggesting a variety of self-antigens involved in the activation of these cells. The pathogenic contribution of these cells to the disease is that they produce a variety of cytokines and express abnormal patterns of cell-surface molecules that are thought to contribute to excessive collagen accumulation.[11]

Chronic Cutaneous Graft-Versus-Host Disease

Chronic graft-versus-host disease (GVHD) is the most common serious long-term complication of allogeneic hematopoietic stem cell transplantation, and a major cause of late morbidity and mortality in these patients. The skin is the major target organ in GVHD; the 5-year cumulative incidence of sclerodermatous GVHD is 11.5% in all transplanted patients and 15.5% in patients with chronic GVHD.[21] Patients with chronic cutaneous GVHD present with either the lichenoid or sclerodermoid form of the disease, with the latter form often manifesting initially as morpheaform plaques but later progressing to diffuse areas of sclerosis. Also, lichen sclerosus and eosinophilic fasciitis are possible in sclerodermatous GVHD, as the most superficial and the deepest manifestations, respectively.[22] Chronic GVHD may or may not be preceded by acute GVHD. The sclerodermatous GVHD clinically resembles scleroderma, and the implied immune mechanisms of these two diseases are so similar that a murine GVHD is used as a model of human scleroderma.[23] Studies in animal models suggested that a specific disease phenotype depends on particular immunodominant antigens targeted by the engrafted immune cells.[24]

Nephrogenic Fibrosing Dermopathy

This very recently recognized uncommon scleroderma-like disorder of unclear etiology and pathophysiologic mechanism develops in patients with end-stage renal disease who undergo long-term hemo- or peritoneal dialysis. In some instances, it can also develop in patients with acute renal failure never requiring dialysis. Although nephrogenic fibrosing dermopathy (NFD) has been originally described as a purely cutaneous scleroderma-like disease, the fibrotic changes are truly systemic, involving fibrosis of the lung and cardiac tissues, fascia, and muscles.[25,26]

Dermal Fibroses Following Traumas

Excessive scarring may develop following wounding, burns, and ionizing radiation injuries to the skin. Although immune involvement is not primary to the dermal fibrotic processes initiated by such traumas, the primary injury initiates an inflammatory cascade that significantly contributes to fibrosis in a manner seen in (auto)immune-associated fibrotic processes. Mechanical trauma, surgery, or burns may lead to hypertrophic scars, keloids, and contractures, whereas ionizing radiation injury often leads to delayed accumulation of collagen in the dermis and subcutaneous tissues.

Unlike other fibrotic disorders of the skin in which collagen accumulation is the dominant mechanism and fibroblast proliferation is a secondary contributor to scarring, hypertrophic scars and keloids are primarily fibroproliferative disorders, although accompanied by excessive collagen deposition. They are characterized by accumulation of inflammatory cells, particularly macrophages and T cells, and a polarized profibrotic T-helper-2 (Th2) pattern of cytokine production.[27] Similarly, inflammation seems to play a crucial role in the development of ionizing radiation–induced dermal fibrosis, which is a major morbidity factor limiting therapeutic benefits of radiotherapy in cancer patients or develops following severe environmental exposures (e.g., after the Chernobyl power plant accident). A proinflammatory cytokine, IL-1β, is directly upregulated by radiation in keratinocytes, and is central to the development of late radiation fibrosis[28]—a perfect example of an indirectly profibrotic, inflammation-mediated effect (Fig. 41.1). Radiation injury to the skin and subsequent inflammation ultimately drive the excessive production of TGF-β, a potent activator of collagen production[29]; decreased production of MMPs, the enzymes mediating collagen turnover; and excessive production of tissue inhibitor of matrix metalloproteinases (TIMP).[30] In the absence of Smad3, a key intracellular mediator of TGF-β effects, ionizing radiation induces significantly lesser inflammatory and fibrotic response.[31]

Animal Models of Skin Fibrosis

Animal models recapitulate many features of dermal fibrosis in humans and have proven to be valuable for better mechanistic understanding of the pathogenesis of dermal fibrosis. Among spontaneous animal models are tight skin (Tsk) mice, including Tsk1 and Tsk2 variants, and avian scleroderma in University of California, Davis line 200 white leghorn chickens. The induced models include bleomycin- or ionizing radiation injury–induced, sclerodermatous GVHD models, and genetically manipulated (knock-in, or transgenic, and knockout) models.

Tight-Skin (Tsk) Mouse Models

There are two tight-skin models, Tsk1, or simply Tsk, and Tsk2. The homozygote mutants Tsk/Tsk are not viable in either model; therefore, the heterozygote Tsk/+ model is commonly studied. The Tsk1/+ model has a spontaneous genetic defect (tsk-Fbn1) on chromosome 2, a large in-frame duplication in the fibrillin-1 (Fbn1) gene, manifesting in a phenotype that resembles scleroderma. These mice overproduce collagen in their skin, heart, and other internal organs, and develop characteristic defects in pulmonary architecture. They also develop characteristic autoantibodies against topo I, fibrillin-1 (Fbn-1), RNA polymerase I, collagen type I, and Fcγ receptors.[32,33] However, Tsk/+ mice do not develop mononuclear infiltration in the dermis, although they have increased mast cell density in the skin in association with the increased levels of TGF-β1.[34] Since fibrosis in humans is often associated with inflammatory infiltration, this model may be only partially relevant to the mechanism of human disease. Nevertheless, the Tsk/+ model has been instrumental in revealing a pathogenic role of and a close crosstalk between important profibrotic cytokines TGF-β and IL-4.[35–37]

The tight skin-2 (Tsk2/+) mouse has a different genetic defect resulting from a mutation localized on the proximal arm of mouse chromosome 1. This appears to be a more suitable animal model of SSc, as not only do these animals produce and accumulate excess collagen type I and III,[38] but they also develop mononuclear cellular infiltrates in the dermis.[39] They also have numerous autoantibodies similar to those in patients with SSc, such as anti-Scl70, anti-CENP-B (centromere protein B), and anti–double-stranded DNA (dsDNA).[39,40] T lymphocytes appear to be involved in the pathogenesis of the disease, with restricted T-cell populations participating in the inflammatory cell infiltrates.[41,42]

Graft-Versus-Host Disease Model

A murine Scl GVHD model developed by Gilliam's group[23] recapitulates many features of human scleroderma, such as prominent skin thickening, upregulation of cutaneous collagen messenger RNA (mRNA) cutaneous immune cell infiltrates, TGF-β1 overproduction, and lung fibrosis. In this model, lethally irradiated BALB/c (H-2^d) mice are transplanted with the major histocompatibility complex (MHC) matched B10.D2 (H-2^d) bone marrow and spleen cells. The development of fibrosis in this model is associated with the increased expression of a host of chemokines and cell-surface molecules in a pattern similar to that in human scleroderma.[3,43] This is also an excellent model for studies of the cell types that drive fibrosis, such as CD4+ and CD8+ T cells, natural killers, mast cells, and cells of myeloid origin.

Bleomycin Model

In the bleomycin-induced model, repeated injections of bleomycin cause fibrosis, with some noticeable variations in the intensity and time required for this effect to develop in various strains of mice. The dermal infiltrates in the bleomycin model are composed predominantly of macrophages, T cells, and mast cells, as well as fibroblasts. Excessive apoptosis, which is mediated by Fas/Fas ligand pathway and caspase-3 activation, contributes to fibrosis, possibly by playing an inflammatory role.[44] Profibrotic cytokines, specifically TGF-β, IL-4, and monocyte chemoattractant protein 1 (MCP-1), that are produced by the inflammatory cells activate their respective receptors and intracellular signaling and mediate collagen accumulation in the dermis.[45–47]

Roles of Cells and Cytokines in Dermal Fibrosis

The ECM synthesis and turnover is regulated by the systemic stimuli, interactions with the extracellular matrix, and with numerous cell types (Fig. 41.2). Activation of the immune and late inflammatory mechanisms, particularly in association with dermal

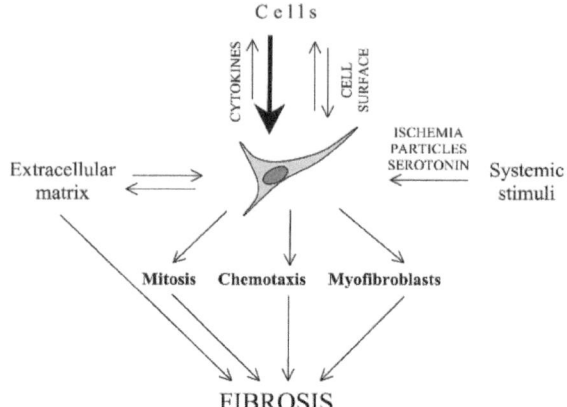

FIG. 41.2. The overall complexity of fibroblast interaction with the environment. Fibroblasts (in the middle of the diagram) are subject to systemic stimuli; they also interact with extracellular matrix and with other cells. Any of these interactions can lead to fibrosis. Interaction with other cells takes place through soluble factors (cytokines) and cell-surface molecules. The bold arrow from other cells to fibroblasts symbolizes the emphasis of this review on the role of cytokines in fibrosis. (From Atamas,[11] with permission.)

infiltration of inflammatory cells, is the predominant driving force of dermal fibrosis. The vastness and complexity of these mechanisms goes beyond the scope of a single review. We focus here on the immune- and inflammation-related aspects of pro- and antifibrotic regulation, particularly its molecular and cellular aspects, with an emphasis on cytokines, as these seem to play the central role in such regulation. A host of cytokines is involved in the complex processes that ultimately lead to dermal fibrosis in humans and in experimental animals.

Cytokines are small hormone-like proteins secreted by various cell types. Because of the great variety of their functional effects and enormous diversity of the secreting and responding cells, the systemic phenomena of the cytokine network are very difficult to understand in their entirety.[9–11] The situation is further complicated by the cytokines' redundancy (different cytokines having similar functional effects), functional pleiotropy (a single cytokine having diverse effects), and intricate functional differences between alternative splice variants.[48] In many cases, the effects of cytokines acting alone are different from the effects of the same cytokines acting in combination or at different times or in a different order. Moreover, a cell activated by a cytokine or cytokines in many cases becomes a source of cytokines itself. The cytokine-mediated activation involves other regulatory factors such as nonprotein mediators, cell-surface molecules, antibodies, fibronectin, and many others. Despite this complexity, some important common themes and general rules have been developed as a result of intensive research in the field. In this section we focus on the cytokines that are known to directly regulate fibroblast proliferation, collagen production, and turnover in primary fibroblast cell culture. In a simplified, teleologic view, numerous cytokines can be assigned to either those promoting acute inflammation and simultaneously inhibiting fibrosis, and those inhibiting acute inflammation and promoting fibrosis (the most potent selected representatives of both groups are listed in Fig. 41.3).

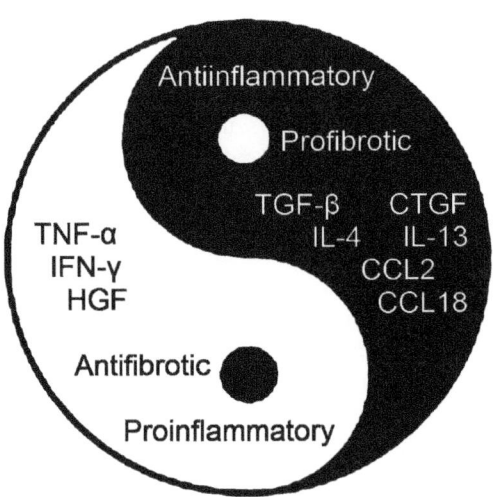

FIG. 41.3. Main profibrotic/antiinflammatory and antifibrotic/proinflammatory cytokines presented as a yin and yang duality. This symbolism is surprisingly complete. The dots of the opposite force within each semicircle represent the fact that the generally antifibrotic cytokines can act indirectly profibrotically in some in vivo situations (e.g., by stimulating production of profibrotic factors late in inflammation following injury), and, conversely, the generally profibrotic cytokines can exert indirect antifibrotic action in vivo (e.g., by promoting inflammation when they are expressed in a disturbed spatiotemporal pattern following injury)

Cellular Players of Skin Fibrosis

Resident Fibroblasts and Fibrocytes

Fibrosis is a direct result of accelerated collagen production by resident tissue fibroblasts, slowed collagen turnover, and accelerated fibroblast proliferation. Recently, an additional mechanism has been demonstrated—the transdifferentiation into fibroblasts of other cell types, such as local epithelial cells (epithelial-mesenchymal transition), monocytes, and so-called fibrocytes.[49] The latter cells are represented by a minor circulating population of CD45+ leukocytes with precursor features (CD34+) that display fibroblast-like properties (collagen+), and are, in fact, fibroblastic precursors in transit from bone marrow to the sites of tissue damage. They contribute to normal and abnormal wound healing by homing to injured tissues, phenotypically transitioning to mature myofibroblasts, and producing collagen.[50–52]

Two additional factors have to be considered regarding the role of fibroblasts in fibrosis. First, not only do fibroblasts deposit collagen, but they also participate in the inflammatory and repair processes by secreting cytokines of their own, expressing cell-surface molecules, and interacting with numerous other cell types. For example, unlike normal dermal fibroblasts, scleroderma fibroblasts spontaneously express CCL2 (MCP-1), which promotes dermal infiltration by attracting monocytes to the skin; moreover, CCL2 stimulates the producing fibroblasts to express more of the same factor, thus creating a self-perpetuating vicious circle.[53] Second, in virtually all cases of fibrosis, fibroblasts become phenotypically changed, to the extent that they can drive excessive collagen production on their own, by creating regulatory "vicious circles" of autocrine and paracrine cytokines. For example, the same excessive autocrine CCL2 loop also maintains excessive MMPs, TIMPs, and collagen production by scleroderma fibroblasts.[45,54] The fibroblasts make and activate excess TGF-β,[55,56] which further stimulates them in an autocrine fashion through an abnormally enhanced, profibrotic signaling cascade.[57] They also become resistant to the induction of apoptosis.[58,59] At those later stages of fibrosis, the involvement of immune and inflammatory cells in the fibrotic regulation seems almost unnecessary, as fibroblasts become capable of sustaining the abnormal self-propelling profibrotic networks.

T Lymphocytes

Despite the early enthusiasm about the implied mechanistic role of T lymphocytes in (auto)immune fibrosis, there has been little progress in the systematic understanding of this issue. It seems that new research brings more and more confusion to the subject, yet it suggests that T cells have a central role in the mechanism of fibrosis.[60–65] A variety of secreted molecules, including cytokines, and direct cell-surface contacts through Fas-FasL, CD40–CD40L, and surface-bound cytokines are involved in the profibrotic T-cell–fibroblast interactions. Depending on the phenotypic polarization of the T cells involved, the outcome of such interaction can be either pro- or antifibrotic, or have no effect on collagen accumulation. Th2/Tc2 cells are profibrotic,[62–65] although this effect can be overridden by the antifibrotic effect of cell-surface–bound TNF-α or IFN-γ.[60,61] In contrast, Th1/Tc1 cells are antifibrotic.[66] Importantly, the disturbed regulation between T cells and fibroblasts is mutual, with T cells regulating fibroblast activities and fibroblasts regulating T-cell expansion, for example in scleroderma.[67]

B Lymphocytes

In addition to producing numerous autoantibodies in association with fibrosis (see Scleroderma, above), B cells are hyperresponsive to transmembrane signals and spontaneously produce autoantibodies in Tsk mice.[32] Depletion of B cells in Tsk mice during disease onset normalizes the Th1/Th2 balance in the skin and attenuates autoantibody production and collagen accumulation.[68] However, depletion of B cells in the adult Tsk mice with established disease has little if any effect on autoantibody levels and collagen accumulation, suggesting that B cells are required for the initiation, but not for the maintenance, of the disease.[32,68] Expression of CD19 appears to be critical for the B cells' involvement in autoimmune processes.[69]

Other Cell Types

Other inflammatory and structural cells contribute to fibrosis. *Activated macrophages* are involved in dermal infiltrates in association with collagen deposits and may release profibrotic factors TGF-β and platelet-derived growth factor (PDGF), and

reactive oxygen species. *Mast cells* are involved in dermal infiltrates in scleroderma, hypertrophic scars, and skin in animal models. They have been associated with the elevated levels of cytokines, particularly TGF-β, IL-4, and MCP-1, and the development of skin fibrosis.[34,70,71] The mast cell–related neutral proteases also act profibrotically.[72,73] During normal wound healing, *keratinocytes* are actively engaged in the regulation of myofibroblastic differentiation and ECM production by fibroblasts, a process that is enhanced by TGF-β and inhibited by IL-1.[74] Epidermis contributes to collagen accumulation in hypertrophic scars,[75] keloids,[76,77] and radiation-induced fibrosis.[78] A disturbed interaction between keratinocytes and fibroblasts also involves connective tissue growth factor (CTGF) as a key player contributing to keloid pathogenesis.[77] There is evidence of the profibrotic roles of endotheliocytes and granulocytes in dermal fibrosis.

Profibrotic and Antifibrotic Cytokines

Many of the factors that drive fibrosis are truly systemic and have a broad spectrum of functional properties. These factors include ischemia, serotonin, heparin, retinoic acid, histamine, adenosine, endothelin, thrombin, leptin, relaxin, angiotensin, so-called matricellular proteins such as thrombospondins and SPARC, and components of the extracellular matrix such as collagens, fibronectin, and tenascins. These regulators are not discussed here either because their involvement in immune- or inflammation-mediated fibrosis has not been systematically understood or because it is difficult to differentiate their effect on fibroblasts from the effects on a variety of other cell types and processes.

Other factors, mostly cytokines, have only a modulating effect on fibroblasts, meaning that they have been implicated in inflammation, immune activation, and associated fibrosis in vivo, but have a mild, variable, or no direct effect on fibroblasts in cell culture. These cytokines likely regulate fibrosis indirectly, through their effects on epithelial or endothelial cells, macrophages, T cells, or keratinocytes, all of which in turn produce direct regulators of fibroblasts. These indirect factors can also synergize with or antagonize the effects of the direct regulators reviewed below. In some cases (e.g., Oncostatin M), the profibrotic effect of a cytokine on fibroblast proliferation or collagen production may be direct, but the exact mechanism of its action remains obscure. Such indirect factors or those with obscure mechanisms of action are the cytokines fibroblast growth factors (FGFs), granulocyte colony-stimulating factor (G-CSF), granulocyte-macrophage colony-stimulating factor (GM-CSF), hepatocyte growth factor (HGF), insulin-like growth factor (IGF), IL-1, IL-6, IL-11, Oncostatin M, platelet-derived growth factor (PDGF), SCF, and vascular endothelial growth factor (VEGF); the chemokines macrophage inflammatory protein 1α (MIP-1α), MCP-3, RANTES (regulated on activation, normal T-cell expressed and secreted), IL-8, cell-surface interactions Fas-FasL, CD40–CD40L or integrin-mediated, and others.[9–11,63,79] It is important to remember that although they are not discussed here because of their mechanistically indirect or unclear involvement, many of these factors are potent regulators associated with either profibrotic (notably PDGF) or antifibrotic (notably HGF) effects. One or more of these factors may be the key to resolving the problem of tissue fibrosis, a possibility that will be clarified by future research. Below we focus on direct regulators of fibrosis that have proven to be active on collagen production and fibroblast proliferation in vivo and in cell culture, that have been investigated in a relatively detailed fashion, and that have been extensively implicated in fibrotic diseases of the skin.

Transforming Growth Factor-β and Connective Tissue Growth Factor

Transforming growth factor-β is the most potent known profibrotic cytokine. There are at least five highly homologous isoforms (TGF-β1 to TGF-β5), of which TGF-β1 has been most extensively studied. Inflammatory cells, such as macrophages and lymphocytes, produce TGF-β, as do fibroblasts, epithelial and endothelial cells, platelets, and other cell types. This cytokine is secreted in a latent form and has to be activated by removal of the so-called latency-associated peptide (LAP) in order to exert its profibrotic action. The mechanisms or TGF-β activation are numerous and their regulation is

complex. Such activation can be mediated by proteolytic enzymes (plasmin, MMP-2, MMP-9), a matricellular protein thrombospondin-1, reactive oxygen species, acidic environment, and αV-containing integrins such as integrins αVβ6, αVβ8, αVβ5, and αVβ3.[55,56]

The profibrotic function of TGF-β has been extensively studied, and it is now clear that the involvement of TGF-β is central to fibrosis in the skin as well as every other organ investigated (e.g., the lung, liver, kidney, and esophagus). This cytokine is also intimately involved in a variety of other physiologic and pathologic processes such as various aspects of embryonic development, regulation of inflammation and immune response, and wound healing. Elevated levels of TGF-β mRNA and total and active protein have been found in virtually all fibrotic diseases in every organ, including the skin, and in virtually all animal models of skin fibrosis and of immune response, and in the scarring models of other organs. Despite obvious beneficial effects of TGF-β neutralization in fibrosis,[80–82] its functional pluripotency might limit the possibility of the systemic targeting of TGF-β in humans, because of the implied severe systemic side effects of such therapy. Instead, local TGF-β activating mechanisms may be a better target of future antifibrotic therapies.

Based on the well-known involvement of TGF-β in normal wound healing and in tissue fibrosis in various organs, it would be intuitive to expect that excess TGF-β accelerates wound healing. However, the timing of TGF-β expression in the skin is of essence, as it is elevated in the damaged skin only in a narrow window of time after the injury, whereas constitutive overexpression of this cytokine by keratinocytes in transgenic mice unexpectedly leads to profound inflammation and delayed wound healing.[83] Similarly, transgenic mice that overexpress a well-known TGF-β activator integrin αVβ6 in the epithelium, develop, as expected, a significant elevation in the active TGF-β levels in the skin, but, instead of generalized skin fibrosis, they develop spontaneous, progressing fibrotic chronic ulcers.[84]

Despite this complexity of systemic TGF-β effects, the specific intracellular signaling of TGF-β in fibroblasts is a target of numerous attempts to abrogate the profibrotic effect of this cytokine. These key intracellular signaling molecules of the TGF-β signaling pathway are Smad2, Smad3, Smad4,[46,47,85,86] c-Abl,[87] and Egr-1.[88] It has been also suggested that the function of an inhibitory intracellular factor of the TGF-β pathway, Smad7, is attenuated in scleroderma fibroblasts, thus making the fibroblasts less resistant to the profibrotic effect of TGF-β[57,89]; restoration of the inhibitory function of Smad7 may be another valuable therapeutic approach.

The profibrotic action of TGF-β is often associated with CTGF, which is also known as CCN2. This is one of matricellular proteins, a family that regulate cell adhesion, migration, proliferation, survival, and differentiation. Transforming growth factor-β is a potent inducer of CTGF in quiescent fibroblasts, but in scleroderma and other dermal fibroses CTGF is constitutively overexpressed,[90,91] contributing to fibrosis. Transforming growth factor-β and CTGF acting together exert a more severe profibrotic effect than each factor alone.[92]

Interleukin-4 and Interleukin-13

Interleukin-4 and IL-13 define a cell phenotype and a pattern of cytokine production that are commonly referred to as type 2, as opposed to type 1 that is defined by IFN-γ and IL-12. The helper T cells (CD3+CD4+) that produce IL-4 or IL-13 (type 2) are designated as Th2 (as opposed to the IFN-γ–producing Th1), whereas the corresponding cytotoxic T cells (CD3+CD8+) are designated Tc2 and Tc1. Generally, type 2 cytokines are directly profibrotic, whereas type 1 cytokines are directly antifibrotic. In the complexity of the in vivo situation, however, the prolonged expression of the type 1 pattern, although directly antifibrotic, may facilitate the secondary activation of type 2 cytokine production, and ultimately lead to tissue fibrosis. Both IL-4 and IL-13 share the cell-surface receptor and the intracellular signaling pathway that involves factors Jak1, Jak2, Jak3, STAT6, and phosphatidylinositol-3-kinase (PI3K), yet there are some fine differences in the functional effects of these two cytokines.

Studies by Bona's group[36,37] demonstrated that the expression of IL-4 receptor is elevated in Tsk/+ fibroblasts in comparison with normal fibroblasts, and that the former cells were hyperresponsive to IL-4, showing higher intensity of IL-4–induced intracellular signaling and more

accelerated IL-4–stimulated collagen production. Administration of neutralizing anti-IL-4 antibodies to Tsk/+ mice prevented the development of dermal fibrosis,[62] as did deletion of IL-4 receptor by a targeted mutation.[37] There is substantial crosstalk between IL-4 and TGF-β pathways that appears to be important in the fibrotic process in vivo.[35–37] Interleukin-13 is also directly profibrotic[93] and appears to be involved in the murine bleomycin model of fibrosis and in the pathogenesis of scleroderma.[94]

CC Chemokine Ligands (CCL) 2 and 18

Chemokines are a group of cytokines that attract leukocytes (their name is a hybrid of the words *chemoattractant* and *cytokine*), and have other functions such as regulation of cell proliferation and expression of intracellular, secreted, and cell-surface molecules in various cell types. The only two known chemokines that are directly profibrotic are CCL2 and CCL18, although numerous other chemokines are involved in inflammation and repair and thus indirectly regulate accumulation of ECM in the skin. CCL2, also known as monocyte chemoattractant protein 1 (MCP-1), stimulates collagen production by fibroblasts.[45,54,70] Whether this is a direct or indirect autocrine TGF-β–mediated effect on fibroblasts remains a subject of controversy.[95] The expression of the receptor for CCL2, CCR2, is upregulated on various cell types in patients with diffuse cutaneous SSc.[96] Contradicting these findings, a study found no difference between SSc and normal fibroblasts in the expression of CCR2,[97] and no effect of CCL2 on collagen production by fibroblasts,[97,98] yet this chemokine appeared to promote fibrosis by inducing the differentiation of Th2 cells. Despite these mechanistic controversies, the involvement of CCL2 in facilitating tissue fibrosis appears to be universally accepted. An abrogation of either CCL2 or its receptor reduces fibrosis in animal models.[45] Similar to CCL2, CCL18 (also known as PARC) is involved in the pathogenesis of scleroderma,[99] and directly stimulates collagen production in fibroblasts by activating an intracellular signaling cascade that leads to the transcriptional upregulation of the collagen gene promoter.[100–102] However, it is important to mention that compared with TGF-β and IL-4/IL-13, dramatically higher (100- to 1000-fold) concentrations of CCL2 or

CCL18 are needed for the direct activation of collagen production in fibroblasts. It is likely that in the in vivo situation these two chemokines act profibrotically by attracting late inflammatory cells, such as T cells and macrophages, to the sites of injury and inflammation.[103]

Tumor Necrosis Factor-α

Tumor necrosis factor-α is secreted by a variety of inflammatory and structural cell types during inflammation. In a sense, TNF-α is a functional counterpart of TGF-β: the former is proinflammatory and antifibrotic, whereas the latter is antiinflammatory and profibrotic. In other words, TNF-α drives inflammation, whereas TGF-β drives repair. Consistent with such generalization, mice deficient in TNF receptor p55 show less infiltration of the wound sites with leukocytes and their wounds heal in an accelerated fashion.[104] In another study, inhibition of TNF-α with continued systemic administration of TNF-binding protein attenuated the wound breaking strength in rats.[105] The cell-surface membrane–bound TNF-α on T cells renders these lymphocytes antifibrotic, despite their Th2 phenotype, which is usually profibrotic.[61] Exposure to TNF-α induces NIK- and TRAF2–independent nuclear factor κB (NF-κB)-mediated intracellular signaling[106] in human dermal fibroblasts. Such exposure also causes downregulation of TGF-βRII on fibroblasts, with subsequent dramatic downregulation of collagen and TIMP-1 production.[107] Tumor necrosis factor-α prevents TGF-β–induced Smad-specific gene transactivation in human dermal fibroblasts by blocking the Smad3-mediated gene transcription.[108] Tumor necrosis factor-α also suppresses the induction of CTGF by TGF-β.[109] Thus, TNF-α is not only a directly antifibrotic cytokine, but it also desensitizes fibroblasts to the profibrotic signals.

Interferon-γ

Interferon-γ (IFN-γ) is a strongly proinflammatory type 1 cytokine and a powerful inhibitor of fibroblast proliferation and collagen production, signaling in fibroblasts through STAT1, C/EBPβ, p300/CBP, and YB-1 pathways.[110–113] In response to skin wounding, the expression of mRNA and protein for IFN-γ, as well as for its inducers IL-12 and IL-18, is detectable at day 1 after injury, peaks at day 3, and then gradually declines. Macrophages and T lymphocytes are the main sources of IFN-γ in the wound.[113] Mice that have been genetically manipulated to eliminate expression of IFN-γ (knockout mice) exhibited accelerated wound healing with a concomitant reduction in leukocyte infiltration, and enhanced angiogenesis and collagen deposition at the wound sites.[113] Simultaneously, there was a significant increase in the levels of mature TGF-β1 protein as well as elevation in Smad2 phosphorylation at the wound sites of IFN-γ knockout mice,[113] further supporting the concept of functional antagonism between IFN-γ and TGF-β. This antagonism suggested initially that IFN-γ might be used as for antifibrotic therapies. There have been sporadic reports on the beneficial use of the IFN-γ therapy. Unfortunately, IFN-γ failed to antagonize TGF-β–mediated fibrotic response in keloid-derived dermal fibroblasts,[114] and was ineffective in the treatment of localized scleroderma in a double-blind, randomized, placebo-controlled, multicenter study.[115] Similarly, IFN-γ therapy was ineffective in a large, randomized, multinational, double-blind, placebo-controlled trial in a well-defined population of patients with idiopathic pulmonary fibrosis.[116] It is important to consider that the half-life of the injected recombinant IFN-γ is short,[117] and its bioavailability in the dermis is not known.

Conclusion

How can one decipher the complexity discussed in this chapter? More importantly, how can one affect it pharmacologically to the patients' benefit? Past experience suggests that successful therapeutic, particularly pharmacologic, targeting of complex pathophysiologic networks is clearly possible. Modern understanding of complex networks indicates that due to pleiotropic interactions and vast functional redundancy of their elements, these networks are very robust and resistant to random interventions, yet they remain vulnerable to effects on the key elements of the system.[118] Such key elements in complex networks are those that lack redundancy but are functionally connected to numerous other elements.

In a pathophysiologic network, nonredundant but pleiotropic cytokines and cell-surface and signaling molecules can be pharmacologically targeted in order to effectively disrupt the disease process. A purpose of the mechanistic biomedical research, therefore, is identifying such key elements of pathophysiologic networks and developing tools for their selective targeting. A striking example of the successful identification of a key pathophysiologic player and its successful targeting is the recent astounding success of anti–TNF-α therapies in rheumatoid arthritis. This factor (TNF-α) not only is increased along with a host of other proinflammatory molecules in chronic inflammatory diseases, but also is an irreplaceable cause of the increase in the levels of the molecules.[119] Thus, by neutralizing TNF-α, production of other proinflammatory factors and the entire inflammatory process can be abrogated.

Unfortunately, similar systemic targeting of TGF-β is likely to produce severe systemic effects due to its broad pleiotropic key functions beyond the connective tissue homeostasis. Also, the complexity of the TGF-β–driven network may require a combined targeting of several factors. For example, imatinib mesylate, a small molecule that selectively inhibits a tyrosine kinase c-Abl, has potent antifibrotic effects in vitro and in vivo due to its selective dual inhibition of TGF-β and PDGF pathways.[87] However, anti–TGF-β antibody therapy had no efficacy in scleroderma patients.[120]

Nevertheless, the new information about the cells and molecular regulators of fibrosis already propels the vigorous clinical trials and implementation of new antifibrotic therapies. Since the mechanisms of dermal fibrosis are largely driven by immune activation and inflammation, and are mediated by the cytokines, the traditional and new therapies aim at immune suppression, resetting the entire immunity through stem cell transplantation with or without immune ablation, and molecular targeting of individual cytokines or their signaling pathways. The new information about the molecular pathways contributing to tissue fibrosis has formed the basis for the ongoing clinical trials of more specific pharmacologic agents, such as imatinib (Gleevec), which targets c-Abl, a critical enzyme of the TGF-β and PDGF signaling pathways; bosentan (Tracleer), an endothelin receptor antagonist that besides its efficacy in pulmonary arterial hypertension may have a beneficial effect on skin fibrosis; and imiquimod, a small molecule

that induces production of IFN-γ. We should expect a further acceleration of research leading to the broadening of potential cellular and molecular targets in dermal fibrosis.

Acknowledgments. We thank Drs. Anthony Gaspari and David Kouba for their invaluable suggestions and comments. The authors' research has been supported in part by grants from the National Institutes of Health (R01HL074067, R03AR47110), Department of Veterans Affairs (Merit Review Type I Award), Arthritis Foundation, Scleroderma Foundation, Baltimore Research and Education Foundation, and University of Maryland Intramural Awards. We are indebted to those researchers whose hard work and important results have not been mentioned here but are crucially important for creating the basis for future antifibrotic therapies.

References

1. Razzaque MS, Ahmed AR. Collagens, collagen-binding heat shock protein 47 and transforming growth factor-beta 1 are induced in cicatricial pemphigoid: possible role(s) in dermal fibrosis. Cytokine 2002;17:311–6.
2. Ricard-Blum S, Hartmann DJ, Esterre P. Monitoring of extracellular matrix metabolism and cross-linking in tissue, serum and urine of patients with chromoblastomycosis, a chronic skin fibrosis. Eur J Clin Invest 1998;28:748–54.
3. Zhou L, Askew D, Wu C, Gilliam AC. Cutaneous gene expression by DNA microarray in murine sclerodermatous graft-versus-host disease, a model for human scleroderma. J Invest Dermatol 2007;127:281–92.
4. Zhou X, Tan FK, Xiong M, et al. Systemic sclerosis (scleroderma): specific autoantigen genes are selectively overexpressed in scleroderma fibroblasts. J Immunol 2001;167:7126–33.
5. Whitfield ML, Finlay DR, Murray JI, Troyanskaya, et al. Systemic and cell type-specific gene expression patterns in scleroderma skin. Proc Natl Acad Sci USA 2003;100:12319–24.
6. Degiorgio-Miller AM, Treharne LJ, McAnulty RJ, et al. Procollagen type I gene expression and cell proliferation are increased in lipodermatosclerosis. Br J Dermatol 2005;152:242–9.
7. Herouy Y, May AE, Pornschlegel G, et al. Lipodermatosclerosis is characterized by elevated

expression and activation of matrix metallopro-teinases: implications for venous ulcer formation. J Invest Dermatol 1998;111:822–7.

8. Quatresooz P, Henry F, Paquet P, et al. Deciphering the impaired cytokine cascades in chronic leg ulcers (review). Int J Mol Med 2003;11:411–8.

9. Atamas SP, White B. The role of chemokines in the pathogenesis of scleroderma. Curr Opin Rheumatol 2003;15:772–7.

10. Atamas SP, White B. Cytokine regulation of pul-monary fibrosis in scleroderma. Cytokine Growth Factor Rev 2003;14:537–50.

11. Atamas SP. Complex cytokine regulation of tissue fibrosis. Life Sci 2002;72:631–43.

12. Jelaska A, Strehlow D, Korn JH. Fibroblast heteroge-neity in physiological conditions and fibrotic disease. Springer Semin Immunopathol 1999;21:385–95.

13. Tan FK, Arnett FC, Reveille JD, et al. Autoantibodies to fibrillin 1 in systemic sclerosis: ethnic differences in antigen recognition and lack of correlation with specific clinical features or HLA alleles. Arthritis Rheum 2000;43:2464–71.

14. Zhou X, Tan FK, Milewicz DM, et al. Autoantibodies to fibrillin-1 activate normal human fibroblasts in culture through the TGF-beta pathway to recapitulate the "scle-roderma phenotype." J Immunol 2005;175:4555–60.

15. Kuwana M, Kaburaki J, Medsger TA Jr, et al. An immunodominant epitope on DNA topoisomerase I is conformational in nature: heterogeneity in its rec-ognition by systemic sclerosis sera. Arthritis Rheum 1999;42:1179–88.

16. Henry PA, Atamas SP, Yurovsky VV, et al. Diversity and plasticity of the anti-DNA topoisomerase I autoan-tibody response in scleroderma. Arthritis Rheum 2000;43:2733–42.

17. Warrington KJ, Nair U, Carbone LD, et al. Characterisation of the immune response to type I col-lagen in scleroderma. Arthritis Res Ther 2006;8:R136.

18. Hu PQ, Oppenheim JJ, Medsger TA Jr, et al. T cell lines from systemic sclerosis patients and healthy controls recognize multiple epitopes on DNA topoi-somerase I. J Autoimmun 2006;26:258–67.

19. Marie I, Cordel N, Lenormand B, et al. Clonal T cells in the blood of patients with systemic sclerosis. Arch Dermatol 2005;141:88–9.

20. Sakkas LI, Xu B, Artlett CM, et al. Oligoclonal T cell expansion in the skin of patients with systemic sclerosis. J Immunol 2002;168:3649–59.

21. Skert C, Patriarca F, Sperotto A, et al. Sclerodermatous chronic graft-versus-host disease after allogeneic hemat-opoietic stem cell transplantation: incidence, predictors and outcome. Haematologica 2006;91:258–61.

22. Schaffer JV, McNiff JM, Seropian S, et al. Lichen sclerosus and eosinophilic fasciitis as manifesta-

tions of chronic graft-versus-host disease: expanding the sclerodermoid spectrum. J Am Acad Dermatol 2005;53:591–601.

23. Zhang Y, McCormick LL, Desai SR, et al. Murine sclerodermatous graft-versus-host disease, a model for human scleroderma: cutaneous cytokines, chemokines, and immune cell activation. J Immunol 2002;168:3088–98.

24. Kaplan DH, Anderson BE, McNiff JM, et al. Target antigens determine graft-versus-host disease pheno-type. J Immunol 2004;173:5467–75.

25. Jimenez SA, Artlett CM, Sandorfi N, et al. Dialysis-associated systemic fibrosis (nephrogenic fibrosing dermopathy): study of inflammatory cells and trans-forming growth factor beta1 expression in affected skin. Arthritis Rheum 2004;50:2660–6.

26. Levine JM, Taylor RA, Elman LB, et al. Involvement of skeletal muscle in dialysis-associated systemic fibrosis (nephrogenic fibrosing dermopathy). Muscle Nerve 2004;30:569–77.

27. Tredget EE, Yang L, Delehanty M, et al. Polarized Th2 cytokine production in patients with hyper-trophic scar following thermal injury. J Interferon Cytokine Res 2006;26:179–89.

28. Liu W, Ding I, Chen K, et al. Interleukin 1beta (IL1B) signaling is a critical component of radiation-induced skin fibrosis. Radiat Res 2006;165:181–91.

29. Martin M, Lefaix JL, Pinton P, et al. Temporal modu-lation of TGF-beta 1 and beta-actin gene expression in pig skin and muscular fibrosis after ionizing radia-tion. Radiat Res 1993;134:63–70.

30. Lafuma C, El Nabout RA, Crechet F, et al. Expression of 72–kDa gelatinase (MMP-2), collagenase (MMP-1), and tissue metalloproteinase inhibitor (TIMP) in primary pig skin fibroblast cultures derived from radiation-induced skin fibrosis. J Invest Dermatol 1994;102:945–50.

31. Flanders KC, Sullivan CD, Fujii M, et al. Mice lacking Smad3 are protected against cutaneous injury induced by ionizing radiation. Am J Pathol 2002;160:1057–68.

32. Saito E, Fujimoto M, Hasegawa M, et al. CD19-dependent B lymphocyte signaling thresholds influ-ence skin fibrosis and autoimmunity in the tight-skin mouse. J Clin Invest 2002;109:1453–62.

33. Muryoi T, Kasturi KN, Kafina MJ, et al. Antitopoisomerase I monoclonal autoantibodies from scleroderma patients and tight skin mouse interact with similar epitopes. J Exp Med 1992;175:1103–9.

34. Wang HW, Tedla N, Hunt JE, et al. Mast cell accumulation and cytokine expression in the tight skin mouse model of scleroderma. Exp Dermatol 2005;14:295–302.

35. Kodera T, McGaha TL, Phelps R, et al. Disrupting the IL-4 gene rescues mice homozygous for the tight-

skin mutation from embryonic death and diminishes TGF-beta production by fibroblasts. Proc Natl Acad Sci USA 2002;99:3800–5.

36. McGaha TL, Le M, Kodera T, et al. Molecular mechanisms of interleukin-4–induced up-regulation of type I collagen gene expression in murine fibroblasts. Arthritis Rheum 2003;48:2275–84.

37. McGaha T, Saito S, Phelps RG, et al. Lack of skin fibrosis in tight skin (TSK) mice with targeted mutation in the interleukin-4R alpha and transforming growth factor-beta genes. J Invest Dermatol 2001;116:136–43.

38. Christner PJ, Hitraya EG, Peters J, et al. Transcriptional activation of the alpha1(I) procollagen gene and up-regulation of alpha1(I) and alpha1(III) procollagen messenger RNA in dermal fibroblasts from tight skin 2 mice. Arthritis Rheum 1998;41:2132–42.

39. Christner PJ, Peters J, Hawkins D, et al. The tight skin 2 mouse. An animal model of scleroderma displaying cutaneous fibrosis and mononuclear cell infiltration Arthritis Rheum 1995;38:1791–8.

40. Gentiletti J, McCloskey LJ, Artlett CM, et al. Demonstration of autoimmunity in the tight skin-2 mouse: a model for scleroderma. J Immunol 2005;175:2418–26.

41. Wallace VA, Kondo S, Kono T, et al. A role for CD4+ T cells in the pathogenesis of skin fibrosis in tight skin mice. Eur J Immunol 1994;24:1463–6.

42. Wooley PH, Sud S, Langendorfer A, et al. T cells infiltrating the skin of Tsk2 scleroderma-like mice exhibit T cell receptor bias. Autoimmunity 1998;27:91–8.

43. Sugerman PB, Faber SB, Willis LM, et al. Kinetics of gene expression in murine cutaneous graft-versus-host disease. Am J Pathol 2004;164:2189–202.

44. Yamamoto T, Nishioka K. Possible role of apoptosis in the pathogenesis of bleomycin-induced scleroderma. J Invest Dermatol 2004;122:44–50.

45. Yamamoto T, Nishioka K. Role of monocyte chemoattractant protein-1 and its receptor, CCR-2, in the pathogenesis of bleomycin-induced scleroderma. J Invest Dermatol 2003;121:510–6.

46. Takagawa S, Lakos G, Mori Y, et al. Sustained activation of fibroblast transforming growth factor-beta/Smad signaling in a murine model of scleroderma. J Invest Dermatol 2003;121:41–50.

47. Lakos G, Takagawa S, Chen SJ, et al. Targeted disruption of TGF-beta/Smad3 signaling modulates skin fibrosis in a mouse model of scleroderma. Am J Pathol 2004;165:203–17.

48. Atamas SP. Alternative splice variants of cytokines: making a list. Life Sci 1997;61:1105–12.

49. Postlethwaite AE, Shigemitsu H, Kanangat S. Cellular origins of fibroblasts: possible implications for organ fibrosis in systemic sclerosis. Curr Opin Rheumatol 2004;16:733–8.

50. Chesney J, Metz C, Stavitsky AB, et al. Regulated production of type I collagen and inflammatory cytokines by peripheral blood fibrocytes. J Immunol 1998;160:419–25.

51. Yang L, Scott PG, Dodd C, et al. Identification of fibrocytes in postburn hypertrophic scar. Wound Repair Regen 2005;13:398–404.

52. Ishii G, Sangai T, Sugiyama K, et al. In vivo characterization of bone marrow-derived fibroblasts recruited into fibrotic lesions. Stem Cells 2005;23:699–706.

53. Yamamoto T, Eckes B, Krieg T. High expression and autoinduction of monocyte chemoattractant protein-1 in scleroderma fibroblasts. Eur J Immunol 2001;31:2936–41.

54. Yamamoto T, Eckes B, Mauch C, et al. Monocyte chemoattractant protein-1 enhances gene expression and synthesis of matrix metalloproteinase-1 in human fibroblasts by an autocrine IL-1 alpha loop. J Immunol 2000;164:6174–9.

55. Asano Y, Ihn H, Yamane K, et al. Increased expression of integrin alphavbeta5 induces the myofibroblastic differentiation of dermal fibroblasts. Am J Pathol 2006;168:499–510.

56. Asano Y, Ihn H, Yamane K, et al. Increased expression of integrin alpha(v)beta3 contributes to the establishment of autocrine TGF-beta signaling in scleroderma fibroblasts. J Immunol 2005;175:7708–18.

57. Asano Y, Ihn H, Yamane K, et al. Impaired Smad7–Smurf-mediated negative regulation of TGF-beta signaling in scleroderma fibroblasts. J Clin Invest 2004;113:253–64.

58. Jelaska A, Korn JH. Role of apoptosis and transforming growth factor beta1 in fibroblast selection and activation in systemic sclerosis. Arthritis Rheum 2000;4310:2230–9.

59. Moulin V, Larochelle S, Langlois C, et al. Normal skin wound and hypertrophic scar myofibroblasts have differential responses to apoptotic inductors. J Cell Physiol 2004;198:350–8.

60. Chizzolini C, Rezzonico R, Ribbens C, et al. Inhibition of type I collagen production by dermal fibroblasts upon contact with activated T cells: different sensitivity to inhibition between systemic sclerosis and control fibroblasts. Arthritis Rheum 1998;41:2039–47.

61. Chizzolini C, Parel Y, De Luca C, et al. Systemic sclerosis Th2 cells inhibit collagen production by dermal fibroblasts via membrane-associated tumor necrosis factor alpha. Arthritis Rheum 2003;48:2593–604.

62. Ong C, Wong C, Roberts CR, et al. Anti-IL-4 treatment prevents dermal collagen deposition in the tight-skin mouse model of scleroderma. Eur J Immunol 1998;28:2619–29.

63. Atamas SP. FCP (http://fibro.biobitfield.com/fcp. php): a bioinformatic tool assisting in PubMed

searches for literature on fibrosis-related cytokines. Arthritis Rheum 2003;48:2083–4.

64. Atamas SP, Luzina IG, Dai H, et al. Synergy between CD40 ligation and IL-4 on fibroblast proliferation involves IL-4 receptor signaling. J Immunol 2002;168:1139–45.

65. Atamas SP, Yurovsky VV, Wise R, et al. Production of type 2 cytokines by CD8+ lung cells is associated with greater decline in pulmonary function in patients with systemic sclerosis. Arthritis Rheum 1999;42:1168–78.

66. Rezzonico R, Burger D, Dayer JM. Direct contact between T lymphocytes and human dermal fibroblasts or synoviocytes down-regulates types I and III collagen production via cell-associated cytokines. J Biol Chem 1998;273:18720–8.

67. De Palma R, Del Galdo F, Lupoli S, et al. Peripheral T lymphocytes from patients with early systemic sclerosis co-cultured with autologous fibroblasts undergo an oligoclonal expansion similar to that occurring in the skin. Clin Exp Immunol 2006;144:169–76.

68. Hasegawa M, Hamaguchi Y, Yanaba K, et al. B-lymphocyte depletion reduces skin fibrosis and autoimmunity in the tight-skin mouse model for systemic sclerosis. Am J Pathol 2006;169:954–66.

69. Sato S, Hasegawa M, Fujimoto M, et al. Quantitative genetic variation in CD19 expression correlates with autoimmunity. J Immunol 2000;165:6635–43.

70. Yamamoto T, Hartmann K, Eckes B, et al. Role of stem cell factor and monocyte chemoattractant protein-1 in the interaction between fibroblasts and mast cells in fibrosis. J Dermatol Sci 2001;26:106–11.

71. Trautmann A, Krohne G, Brocker EB, et al. Human mast cells augment fibroblast proliferation by heterotypic cell-cell adhesion and action of IL-4. J Immunol 1998;160:5053–7.

72. Kakizoe E, Shiota N, Tanabe Y, et al. Isoform-selective upregulation of mast cell chymase in the development of skin fibrosis in scleroderma model mice. J Invest Dermatol 2001;116:118–23.

73. Abe M, Kurosawa M, Ishikawa O, et al. Effect of mast cell-derived mediators and mast cell-related neutral proteases on human dermal fibroblast proliferation and type I collagen production. J Allergy Clin Immunol 2000;106:S78–84.

74. Shephard P, Martin G, Smola-Hess S, et al. Myofibroblast differentiation is induced in keratinocyte-fibroblast co-cultures and is antagonistically regulated by endogenous transforming growth factor-beta and interleukin-1. Am J Pathol 2004;164:2055–66.

75. Bellemare J, Roberge CJ, Bergeron D, et al. Epidermis promotes dermal fibrosis: role in the pathogenesis of hypertrophic scars. J Pathol 2005;206:1–8.

76. Funayama E, Chodon T, Oyama A, et al. Keratinocytes promote proliferation and inhibit apoptosis of the underlying fibroblasts: an important role in the pathogenesis of keloid. J Invest Dermatol 2003;121:1326–31.

77. Khoo YT, Ong CT, Mukhopadhyay A, et al. Upregulation of secretory connective tissue growth factor (CTGF) in keratinocyte-fibroblast coculture contributes to keloid pathogenesis. J Cell Physiol 2006;208:336–43.

78. Sivan V, Vozenin-Brotons MC, Tricaud Y, et al. Altered proliferation and differentiation of human epidermis in cases of skin fibrosis after radiotherapy. Int J Radiat Oncol Biol Phys 2002;53:385–93.

79. Gharaee-Kermani M, Phan SH. Role of cytokines and cytokine therapy in wound healing and fibrotic diseases. Curr Pharm Des 2001;7:1083–103.

80. McCormick LL, Zhang Y, Tootell E, et al. Anti-TGF-beta treatment prevents skin and lung fibrosis in murine sclerodermatous graft-versus-host disease: a model for human scleroderma. J Immunol 1999;163:5693–9.

81. Zhang Y, McCormick LL, Gilliam AC. Latency-associated peptide prevents skin fibrosis in murine sclerodermatous graft-versus-host disease, a model for human scleroderma. J Invest Dermatol 2003;21:713–9.

82. Santiago B, Gutierrez-Canas I, Dotor J, et al. Topical application of a peptide inhibitor of transforming growth factor-beta1 ameliorates bleomycin-induced skin fibrosis. J Invest Dermatol 2005;125:450–5.

83. Wang XJ, Han G, Owens P, et al. Role of TGFbeta-mediated inflammation in cutaneous wound healing. J Invest Dermatol 2006;126:112–7.

84. Hakkinen L, Koivisto L, Gardner H, et al. Increased expression of beta6–integrin in skin leads to spontaneous development of chronic wounds. Am J Pathol 2004;164:229–42.

85. Mori Y, Chen SJ, Varga J. Expression and regulation of intracellular SMAD signaling in scleroderma skin fibroblasts. Arthritis Rheum 2003;48:1964–78.

86. Gao Z, Wang Z, Shi Y, et al. Modulation of collagen synthesis in keloid fibroblasts by silencing Smad2 with siRNA. Plast Reconstr Surg 2006;118:1328–37.

87. Distler JH, Jungel A, Huber LC, et al. Imatinib mesylate reduces production of extracellular matrix and prevents development of experimental dermal fibrosis. Arthritis Rheum 2007;56:311–22.

88. Chen SJ, Ning H, Ishida W, et al. The early-immediate gene EGR-1 is induced by transforming growth factor-beta and mediates stimulation of collagen gene expression. J Biol Chem 2006;281:21183–97.

89. Dong C, Zhu S, Wang T, et al. Deficient Smad7 expression: a putative molecular defect in scleroderma. Proc Natl Acad Sci USA 2002;99:3908–13.

90. Leask A, Denton CP, Abraham DJ. Insights into the molecular mechanism of chronic fibrosis: the role of connective tissue growth factor in scleroderma. J Invest Dermatol 2004;122:1–6.

91. Holmes A, Abraham DJ, Chen Y, et al. Constitutive connective tissue growth factor expression in scleroderma fibroblasts is dependent on Sp1. J Biol Chem 2003;278:41728–33.

92. Mori T, Kawara S, Shinozaki M, et al. J Role and interaction of connective tissue growth factor with transforming growth factor-beta in persistent fibrosis: A mouse fibrosis model. Cell Physiol 1999;181:153–9.

93. Jinnin M, Ihn H, Yamane K, et al. Interleukin-13 stimulates the transcription of the human alpha2(I) collagen gene in human dermal fibroblasts. J Biol Chem 2004;279:41783–91.

94. Granel B, Chevillard C, Allanore Y, et al. Evaluation of interleukin 13 polymorphisms in systemic sclerosis. Immunogenetics 2006;58:693–9.

95. Gharaee-Kermani M, Denholm EM, Phan SH. Costimulation of fibroblast collagen and transforming growth factor beta1 gene expression by monocyte chemoattractant protein-1 via specific receptors. J Biol Chem 1996;271:17779–84.

96. Carulli MT, Ong VH, Ponticos M, et al. Chemokine receptor CCR2 expression by systemic sclerosis fibroblasts: evidence for autocrine regulation of myofibroblast differentiation. Arthritis Rheum 2005;52:3772–82.

97. Distler JH, Jungel A, Caretto D, et al. Monocyte chemoattractant protein 1 released from glycosaminoglycans mediates its profibrotic effects in systemic sclerosis via the release of interleukin-4 from T cells. Arthritis Rheum 2006;54:214–25.

98. Distler O, Pap T, Kowal-Bielecka O, et al. Overexpression of monocyte chemoattractant protein 1 in systemic sclerosis: role of platelet-derived growth factor and effects on monocyte chemotaxis and collagen synthesis. Arthritis Rheum 2001;44:2665–78.

99. Luzina IG, Atamas SP, Wise R, et al. Gene expression in bronchoalveolar lavage cells from scleroderma patients. Am J Respir Cell Mol Biol 2002;26:549–57.

100. Luzina IG, Highsmith K, Pochetuhen K, et al. PKCalpha mediates CCL18–stimulated collagen production in pulmonary fibroblasts. Am J Respir Cell Mol Biol 2006;35:298–305.

101. Luzina IG, Tsymbalyuk N, Choi J, et al. CCL18–stimulated upregulation of collagen production in lung fibroblasts requires Sp1 signaling and basal Smad3 activity. J Cell Physiol 2006;206:221–8.

102. Atamas SP, Luzina IG, Choi J, et al. Pulmonary and activation-regulated chemokine stimulates collagen production in lung fibroblasts. Am J Respir Cell Mol Biol 2003;29:743–9.

103. Luzina IG, Papadimitriou JC, Anderson R, et al. Induction of prolonged infiltration of T lymphocytes and transient T lymphocyte-dependent collagen deposition in mouse lungs following adenoviral gene transfer of CCL18. Arthritis Rheum 2006;54:2643–55.

104. Mori R, Kondo T, Ohshima T, et al. Accelerated wound healing in tumor necrosis factor receptor p55–deficient mice with reduced leukocyte infiltration. FASEB J 2002;16:963–74.

105. Lee RH, Efron DT, Tantry U, et al. Inhibition of tumor necrosis factor-alpha attenuates wound breaking strength in rats. Wound Repair Regen 2000;8:547–53.

106. Kouba DJ, Nakano H, Nishiyama T, et al. Tumor necrosis factor-alpha induces distinctive NF-kappa B signaling within human dermal fibroblasts. J Biol Chem 2001;276:6214–24.

107. Yamane K, Ihn H, Asano Y, et al. Antagonistic effects of TNF-alpha on TGF-beta signaling through down-regulation of TGF-beta receptor type II in human dermal fibroblasts. J Immunol 2003;171:3855–62.

108. Verrecchia F, Pessah M, Atfi A, et al. Tumor necrosis factor-alpha inhibits transforming growth factor-beta /Smad signaling in human dermal fibroblasts via AP-1 activation. J Biol Chem 2000;275:30226–31.

109. Abraham DJ, Shiwen X, Black CM, et al. Tumor necrosis factor alpha suppresses the induction of connective tissue growth factor by transforming growth factor-beta in normal and scleroderma fibroblasts. J Biol Chem 2000;275:15220–5.

110. Ghosh AK, Bhattacharyya S, Mori Y, et al. Inhibition of collagen gene expression by interferon-gamma: novel role of the CCAAT/enhancer binding protein beta (C/EBPbeta). J Cell Physiol 2006;207:251–60.

111. Ghosh AK, Yuan W, Mori Y, et al. Antagonistic regulation of type I collagen gene expression by interferon-gamma and transforming growth factor-beta. Integration at the level of p300/CBP transcriptional coactivators. J Biol Chem 2001;276:11041–8.

112. Higashi K, Inagaki Y, Fujimori K, et al. Interferon-gamma interferes with transforming growth factor-beta signaling through direct interaction of YB-1 with Smad3. J Biol Chem 2003;278:43470–9.

113. Ishida Y, Kondo T, Takayasu T, et al. The essential involvement of cross-talk between IFN-gamma and TGF-beta in the skin wound-healing process. J Immunol 2004;172:1848–55.

114. Hasegawa T, Nakao A, Sumiyoshi K, et al. IFN-gamma fails to antagonize fibrotic effect of TGF-beta on keloid-derived dermal fibroblasts. J Dermatol Sci 2003;32:19–24.

115. Hunzelmann N, Anders S, Fierlbeck G, et al. Double-blind, placebo-controlled study of intralesional

interferon gamma for the treatment of localized scleroderma. J Am Acad Dermatol 1997;36:433–5.

116. Raghu G, Brown KK, Bradford WZ, et al. A placebo-controlled trial of interferon gamma-1b in patients with idiopathic pulmonary fibrosis. N Engl J Med 2004;350:125–33.

117. Bolinger AM, Taeubel MA. Recombinant interferon gamma for treatment of chronic granulomatous disease and other disorders. Clin Pharm 1992;11:834–50.

118. Virtual Round Table on ten leading questions for network research. Eur Phys J [B] 2004;38:143–5.

119. Feldmann M, Bondeson J, Brennan FM, et al. The rationale for the current boom in anti-TNFalpha treatment. Is there an effective means to define therapeutic targets for drugs that provide all the benefits of anti-TNFalpha and minimise hazards? Ann Rheum Dis 1999;58:I27–31.

120. Denton CP, Merkel PA, Furst DE, et al. Recombinant human anti-transforming growth factor beta1 antibody therapy in systemic sclerosis: A multicenter, randomized, placebo-controlled phase I/II trial of CAT-192. Arthritis Rheum 2007;56:323–33.

42
Pemphigus Family of Diseases

Masayuki Amagai

Key Points

- Pemphigus is a group of autoimmune blistering diseases of the skin and mucous membranes, which are mediated by immunoglobulin G (IgG) autoantibodies against the cadherin type of cell–cell adhesion molecules in desmosomes, desmogleins.
- Pemphigus is histologically characterized by acantholysis, that is, intraepidermal blisters due to the loss of cell–cell adhesion of keratinocytes, and immunopathologically by the finding of in-vivo–bound and circulating IgG autoantibodies directed against the cell surface of keratinocytes.
- Pemphigus has three major forms: pemphigus vulgaris, pemphigus foliaceus, and paraneoplastic pemphigus. Pemphigus vegetans is a variant of pemphigus vulgaris. Pemphigus erythematosus is a localized variant of pemphigus foliaceus, and fogo selvagem is an endemic variant of pemphigus foliaceus.
- Patients with pemphigus vulgaris and pemphigus foliaceus have IgG autoantibodies against desmoglein 3 and desmoglein 1, respectively, while patients with paraneoplastic pemphigus have IgG autoantibodies against plakin molecules in addition to desmogleins.
- Systemic corticosteroids are the mainstay of therapy for pemphigus, and adjuvant therapies, including immunosuppressive agents, plasmapheresis, and high-dose intravenous immunoglobulin, are used for severe cases.

Historical Background

The term *pemphigus* stems from the Greek *pemphix*, meaning blister or bubble, and it describes a group of chronic blistering skin diseases in which autoantibodies are directed against the cell surface of keratinocytes, resulting in the loss of cell–cell adhesion of keratinocytes through a process called acantholysis (Table 42.1). The modern history of pemphigus began with the discovery by Beutner and Jordon[1] in 1964 of circulating antibodies directed against the cell surface of keratinocytes in the sera of pemphigus vulgaris patients. In the late 1970s to early 1980s, pemphigus autoantibodies were shown to have a pathogenic activity in induction of blister formation in skin organ-culture systems as well as by passive transfer of patients' immunoglobulin G (IgG) to neonatal mice.[2,3] In the mid- and late 1980s, the target antigens of pemphigus were characterized by immunochemical methods, such as immunoprecipitation and immunoblotting.[4,5] In the early 1990s, the isolation of complementary DNA (cDNA) for pemphigus antigens demonstrated that the target antigens in pemphigus are desmogleins.[6,7]

Pathogenesis

Pemphigus Target Antigens are Desmogleins

The hallmark of pemphigus is the finding of IgG autoantibodies against the cell surface of keratinocytes. The pemphigus autoantibodies found in

TABLE 42.1. Classification of pemphigus.

Pemphigus vulgaris
    Pemphigus vegetans
Pemphigus foliaceus
    Pemphigus erythematosus: localized
    Fogo selvagem: endemic
Paraneoplastic pemphigus
Drug-induced pemphigus
IgA pemphigus

patients' sera play a primary pathogenic role in inducing blisters. When the IgG fraction from patients is passively transferred to neonatal mice, the mice develop blisters with typical histologic findings.[3] Even monovalent Fab' fragments of IgG from patients are sufficient to cause blisters in neonatal mice, indicating that complement activation and surface cross-linking may not be relevant in keratinocyte detachment.[8]

Immunoelectron microscopy localized both pemphigus vulgaris and pemphigus foliaceus antigens to the desmosomes, the most prominent cell–cell adhesion junctions in stratified squamous epithelia.[9] Immunochemical characterization of pemphigus antigens by immunoprecipitation or immunoblotting with extracts from cultured keratinocytes or epidermis demonstrated that the pemphigus vulgaris and foliaceus antigens were 130-kd and 160-kd transmembrane glycoproteins, respectively.[4,5,10] The 160-kd protein recognized by pemphigus foliaceus sera was subsequently shown to be identical to desmoglein 1 (Dsg1) by comparative immunochemical studies.[11]

Molecular cloning of cDNA encoding Dsg1 and pemphigus vulgaris antigens indicated that both molecules were desmogleins, which are the members of the cadherin supergene family[6,7] (Fig. 42.1). Thus, pemphigus was discovered to be an

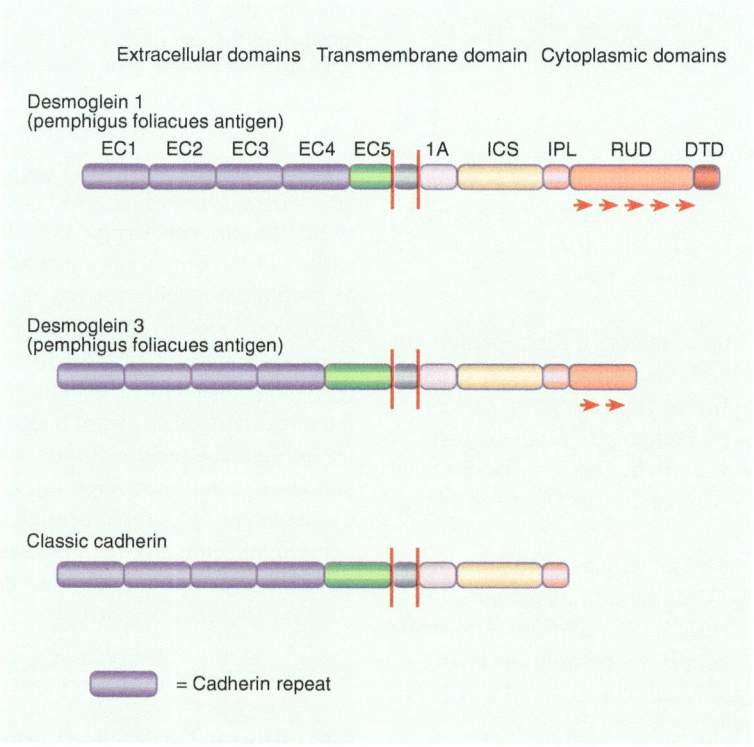

FIG. 42.1. Molecular structure of the pemphigus antigens. Cadherin is a single span transmembrane protein with unique structure. The extracellular (EC) region of each cadherin member has four cadherin repeats of about 110 amino acid residues with calcium-binding motifs. Boxes with the same color have similarities in their amino acid sequences. Desmogleins have their own unique sequences of 29 ± 1 residues (repeating unit domain or RUD). ICS, intracellular cadherin-specific domain; IA, intracellular anchor domain; IPL, intracellular proline-rich linker; DTD, desmoglein-specific terminal domain

anti-desmoglein autoimmune disease. The pemphigus vulgaris antigen was termed desmoglein 3 (Dsg3).

Desmosomes are intercellular adhesive junctions in the epidermis and mucous membranes and contain two major transmembrane components, desmogleins and desmocollins, both of which are cadherin-type cell adhesion molecules. Desmogleins have four isoforms (Dsg1 to Dsg4). Expression of Dsg1 and Dsg3 is basically restricted to stratified squamous epithelia, where blisters are formed in pemphigus, while Dsg2 is expressed in all desmosome-possessing tissues, including simple epithelia and myocardium.[12] Dsg4 plays an important adhesive role mainly in hair follicles because mutations in the *DSG4* gene cause abnormal hair development.[13] The molecular structure of desmogleins are unique and they have four cadherin repeats in their extracellular domains, as do classic cadherins, and have an extra carboxyl-terminal domain containing repeats of 29 ± 1 residues (Fig. 42.1).

Compelling evidence has accumulated that IgG autoantibodies against Dsg1 and Dsg3 are pathogenic and play a primary role in inducing the blister formation in pemphigus. Essentially, all patients with pemphigus have IgG autoantibodies against Dsg1 or Dsg3, depending on the subtype of pemphigus.[14,15] When anti-desmoglein IgG autoantibodies are removed from patients' sera of pemphigus vulgaris, pemphigus foliaceus, or paraneoplastic pemphigus by immunoadsorption with recombinant desmoglein proteins, the sera are no longer pathogenic in blister formation.[16,17] Furthermore, anti-desmoglein IgG autoantibodies that were affinity-purified from pemphigus sera on the desmoglein recombinant proteins can cause blisters when injected in neonatal mice.[17,18] Some pemphigus sera react with Dsg4 due to cross-reactivity of a subset of anti-Dsg1 IgG, although Dsg4/Dsg1 cross-reacting IgG has no demonstrable pathogenic effect.[19] IgG autoantibodies against acetylcholine receptors or annexin-like molecules are reported, but their pathogenic relevance in pemphigus remains to be determined.[20–22]

Thus, the basic pathophysiology of pemphigus is that IgG autoantibodies raised against Dsg1 or Dsg3 inhibit their adhesive function and lead to the loss of the cell–cell adhesion of keratinocytes, resulting in blister formation.

Desmoglein Compensation Theory as Explanation for Localization of Blisters

Although the disruption of desmoglein-dependent cell adhesion by autoantibodies is the basic pathophysiology underlying blister formation in pemphigus, the clinical spectrum is more complex. This complex clinical features of pemphigus are explained logically by the desmoglein compensation theory: Dsg1 and Dsg3 compensate for each other when they are coexpressed in the same cell.[23–25]

The intraepithelial expression pattern of Dsg1 and Dsg3 is different between the skin and mucous membranes. In the skin, Dsg1 is expressed throughout the epidermis, but more intensely in the superficial layers, while Dsg3 is expressed in the lower portion of the epidermis, primarily in the basal and parabasal layers. In contrast, Dsg1 and Dsg3 are expressed throughout the squamous layers of mucosa, but Dsg1 is expressed at a much lower level than Dsg3.

Patients with pemphigus foliaceus have only anti-Dsg1 IgG autoantibodies (Table 42.2). Patients with the mucosal dominant type of pemphigus vulgaris have only anti-Dsg3 IgG autoantibodies, whereas those with the mucocutaneous type of pemphigus vulgaris have both anti-Dsg3 and anti-Dsg1 IgG autoantibodies.[26,27]

For example, when sera contain only anti-Dsg1 IgG, which interferes with the function of Dsg1, the presence of Dsg3 compensates for the loss of function of Dsg1 in the lower epidermis. In contrast, in upper epidermis, there is no compensation by Dsg3. Therefore, blisters only appear in the superficial epidermis of the skin because that is the only area in which Dsg1 is present without coexpression of Dsg3. Although the anti-Dsg1 IgG binds to mucosa, no blisters are formed because of the coexpression of Dsg 3. Thus, sera containing only anti-Dsg1 IgG cause superficial blisters in the skin without mucosal involvement, as is seen in patients with pemphigus foliaceus.

The desmoglein compensation theory also explains the clinical and histologic phenotype of bullous impetigo and staphylococcal scalded skin syndrome (SSSS).[25] The blisters of bullous impetigo and SSSS are caused by exfoliative toxin (ET), which is produced by *Staphylococcus aureus*. ET

TABLE 42.2. Target antigens in pemphigus.

Diseases	Autoantibodies	Antigens
Pemphigus vulgaris		
Mucosal dominant type	IgG	Desmoglein 3
Mucocutaneous type	IgG	Desmoglein 3
		Desmoglein 1
Pemphigus foliaceus	IgG	Desmoglein 1
Paraneoplastic pemphigus	IgG	Desmoglein 3
		Desmoglein 1
		Plectin
		Desmoplakin I
		Desmoplakin II
		BPAG1
		Envoplakin
		Periplakin
		170-kd antigen
Drug-induced pemphigus	IgG	Desmoglein 3
		Desmoglein 1
IgA pemphigus		
SPD type	IgA	Desmocollin 1
IEN type	IgA	?

BPAG, bullous pemphigoid antigen; IEN, intraepidermal neutrophilic; Ig, immunoglobulin; SPD, subcorneal pustular dermatosis.

was recently discovered to bind specifically to Dsg1 and cleave only the site after glutamic acid residue 381 between extracellular domains 3 and 4.[28–30] When ET reaches the skin and digests Dsg1 in the lower layers of the epidermis, Dsg3 compensates for the loss of function of Dsg1 and manages to maintain cell–cell adhesion, while no compensation by Dsg3 occurs in the superficial layers of the epidermis. Therefore, ET induces superficial blisters on the skin. In mucous membranes, the Dsg3 expressed throughout the squamous layers of the mucosa compensates for the impaired Dsg1 and maintains cell–cell adhesion with no mucosal involvement.

Paraneoplastic Pemphigus has More Complex Autoimmune Reaction Than Classic Pemphigus

In addition to IgG autoantibodies against Dsg3 or Dsg1, patients with paraneoplastic pemphigus (PNP) develop characteristic IgG autoantibodies against multiple antigens with molecular weights of 500, 250, 230, 210, 190, and 170 kd[17,31] (Table 42.2). By immunochemical studies and cDNA cloning, most of these antigens were identified. The 500-kd antigen is plectin. The 250- and 210-kd antigens are desmoplakins I and II, respectively. The 230-kd antigen is bullous pemphigoid antigen 1, the major plaque protein of the epidermal hemidesmosome and also a target antigen in bullous pemphigoid. The 210-kd band also contains envoplakin. The 190-kd antigen is periplakin, while the 170-kd antigen is a transmembrane cell-surface protein that has yet to be identified.[32]

Anti-desmoglein antibodies play a role in inducing the loss of cellular adhesion of keratinocytes and initiate blister formation, while the pathophysiologic relevance of the anti-plakin autoantibodies is unclear. The intracellular location of plakin proteins makes it unlikely that anti-plakin autoantibodies initiate pathology in PNP because IgG cannot penetrate cell membranes. It is also important to bear in mind that not only humoral immunity but also cell-mediated cytotoxicity is involved in the pathogenesis of PNP, in which more severe and refractory oral erosions and stomatitis as well as more polymorphic skin eruptions are seen compared with classic forms of pemphigus.

Clinical Features

Pemphigus Vulgaris

Pemphigus vulgaris has two clinical subtypes: mucosal dominant type and mucocutaneous type. Patients with the mucosal dominant type show mucosal erosions mainly in the oral cavity with minimal or limited skin involvement. Patients with the mucocutaneous type show extensive flaccid blisters and erosions on the skin in addition to the mucosal erosions. Any stratified squamous epithelia where Dsg1 or Dsg3 are expressed can be involved in pemphigus vulgaris.

Mucous membrane lesions are usually seen as painful erosions (Fig. 42.2). Intact blisters are rare, probably because they are fragile and break easily. Scattered and often extensive erosions may be seen on any part of the oral cavity. Extensive erosions and painful lesions in the mouth may result in decreased food and drink intake. Involvement of throat may

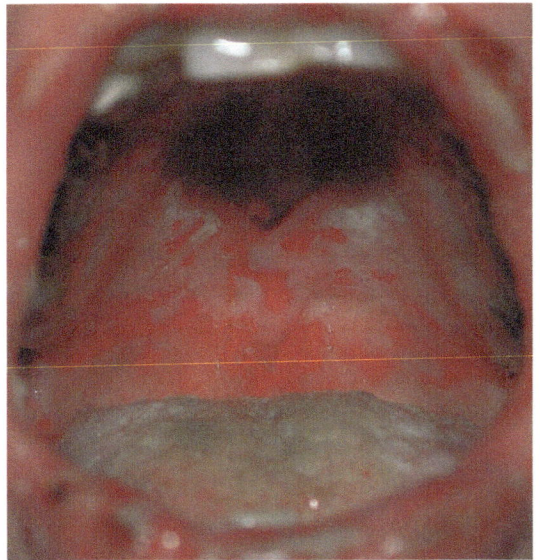

FIG. 42.2. Pemphigus vulgaris. Essentially all patients develop painful oral mucous membrane erosions

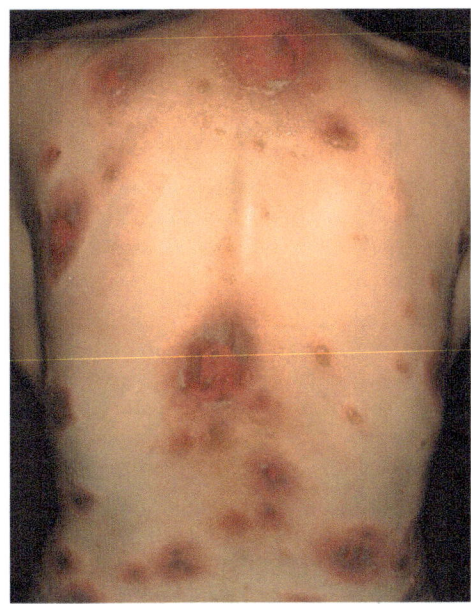

FIG. 42.3. Pemphigus vulgaris. Skin lesions are flaccid blisters that are fragile and soon rupture to form painful erosions that ooze and bleed easily

produce hoarseness and difficulty in swallowing. The esophagus, conjunctiva, nasal mucosa, vagina, penis, anus, and labia may also be involved. The diagnosis of pemphigus vulgaris tends to be delayed in patients presenting with only oral involvement, as compared to patients with skin lesions.

The primary skin lesions of pemphigus vulgaris are flaccid, thin-walled, easily ruptured blisters that appear anywhere on the skin surface (Fig. 42.3). The blisters arise on normal-appearing skin or erythematous bases. The blisters are fragile and soon rupture to form painful erosions that ooze and bleed easily. The erosions soon become partially covered with crusts that have little or no tendency to heal. Without appropriate treatment, pemphigus vulgaris can be fatal because a large area of the skin loses epidermal barrier function, leading to loss of body fluids or secondary bacterial infection. Because of the absence of cohesion in the epidermis, the upper layers are easily made to slip laterally by slight pressure or rubbing in active patients with pemphigus (Nikolsky sign).

Pemphigus Foliaceus

Patients with pemphigus foliaceus develop scaly, crusted erosions, often on an erythematous base in the skin, but do not have apparent mucous mem-

brane involvement even with widespread disease (Fig. 42.4). The absence of oral involvement may be a clue to clinically differentiate pemphigus foliaceus from pemphigus vulgaris.

The onset of disease is often subtle, with a few scattered crusted lesions that come and go, and are frequently mistaken for impetigo. These lesions are usually well demarcated and scattered in a sebor-

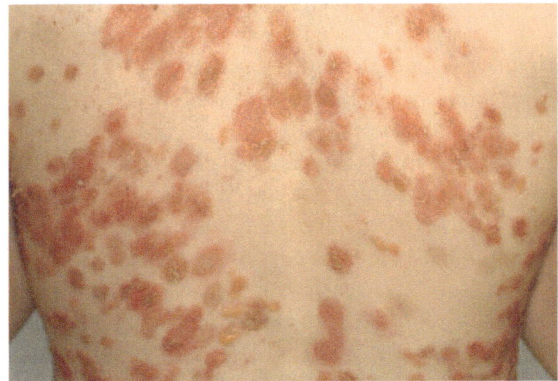

FIG. 42.4. Pemphigus foliaceus. Skin lesions are scaly crusted erosions and vesicles that are fragile and easily ruptured

rheic distribution, including face, scalp, and upper trunk. Because the vesicle is so superficial and fragile, often only the crust and scale that result from ruptured vesicles are seen. Disease may stay localized for years or may rapidly progress, in some cases, to generalized involvement resulting in an erythrodermic exfoliative dermatitis. Nikolsky sign is present. Generally patients with pemphigus foliaceus are not severely ill.

Paraneoplastic Pemphigus

Paraneoplastic pemphigus is a recently described form of pemphigus that occurs in association with underlying neoplasms.[31,32] It is unique and distinct from the classic forms of pemphigus vulgaris and foliaceus by clinical, histologic, and immunopathologic criteria. The associated neoplasms are non-Hodgkin's lymphoma (42%), chronic lymphocytic leukemia (29%), Castleman's tumor (10%), malignant and benign thymoma (6%), spindle cell neoplasms (reticulum cell sarcoma)(6%), and Waldenström's macroglobulinemia (6%). The combination of non-Hodgkin's lymphoma and chronic lymphocytic leukemia represents almost two thirds of cases. Castleman's disease, which is a very rare lymphoproliferative lesion, is the third most commonly associated neoplasm. The absence of common tumors, such as adenocarcinoma of breast or bowel and squamous cell carcinomas, is notable.

The most constant clinical feature of paraneoplastic pemphigus is the presence of intractable stomatitis (Fig. 42.5). The severe stomatitis is usually the earliest presenting sign, and after treatment it is the one that persists and is extremely resistant to therapy. This stomatitis consists of erosions and ulcerations that affect all surfaces of the oropharynx and characteristically extend onto the vermillion of the lip. Most patients also have a severe pseudomembranous conjunctivitis with scarring. Esophageal, nasopharyngeal, vaginal, labial, and penile mucosal lesions may also be affected.

The cutaneous lesions are quite polymorphic and may appear as erythematous macules, flaccid blisters and erosions resembling pemphigus vulgaris, tense blisters resembling bullous pemphigoid, erythema multiforme-like lesions, and lichenoid eruptions. Extensive cases show clinical resemblance with toxic epidermal necrolysis

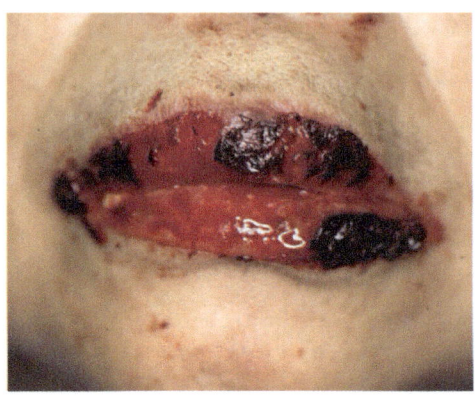

FIG. 42.5. Paraneoplastic pemphigus. The characteristic clinical feature is severe intractable stomatitis that extends onto the vermillion of the lip

(TEN). The occurrence of blisters and erythema multiforme–like lesions on the palms and soles can be used to clinically differentiate paraneoplastic pemphigus from pemphigus vulgaris. Cutaneous lichenoid eruptions are very common together with severe stomatitis. In the chronic form of the disease lichenoid eruption may predominate over blistering lesions.

Paraneoplastic pemphigus is the only form of pemphigus that has involvement of nonstratified squamous epithelia. Approximately, 30% to 40% of patients develop pulmonary symptom.[33,34] The earliest symptoms are progressive dyspnea, and pulmonary function studies show airflow obstruction, involving large and small airways, as seen in bronchiolitis obliterans, which can be fatal through respiratory failure.

Other Forms of Pemphigus

Pemphigus Vegetans

Pemphigus vegetans is a rare vegetative variant of pemphigus vulgaris and considered to be one reactive pattern of the skin to autoimmune insult of pemphigus vulgaris. Pemphigus vegetans is characterized by flaccid blisters that become erosions and form fungoid vegetations or papillomatous proliferations, especially in the intertriginous area and in the scalp or on the face. Pustules rather than vesicles characterize early lesions but these soon progress to vegetative plaques.

Pemphigus Erythematosus (Senear-Usher Syndrome)

Pemphigus erythematosus is simply a localized variant of pemphigus foliaceus. Typical scaly and crusted lesions of pemphigus foliaceus occur across the malar area of the face and in other seborrheic areas. Originally, pemphigus erythematosus was introduced for patients with immunologic features of both lupus erythematosus and pemphigus, such as in vivo IgG and C3 deposition on keratinocyte cell surfaces as well as basement membrane zone and circulating antinuclear antibodies.[35] However, only a few patients have been reported to actually have the two diseases concurrently.[36]

Drug-Induced Pemphigus

There are sporadic cases of pemphigus in association with the use of drugs, such as penicillamine and captopril.[37] Pemphigus foliaceus is more common than pemphigus vulgaris in penicillamine-treated patients. Although most patients with drug-induced pemphigus are shown to have autoantibodies against Dsg1 or Dsg3,[38] evidence suggests that some drugs may induce acantholysis without production of antibodies. Both penicillamine and captopril contain sulfhydryl groups that are speculated to interact with the sulfhydryl groups in desmoglein 1 and 3. Most, but not all, patients with drug-induced pemphigus go into remission after the offending drug is stopped.

Immunoglobulin A Pemphigus

Immunoglobulin A (IgA) pemphigus is a newly characterized group of autoimmune intraepidermal blistering diseases presenting with a vesiculopustular eruption, neutrophilic infiltration, and in-vivo–bound and circulating IgA autoantibodies against keratinocyte cell surfaces, but no IgG autoantibodies.[39–41] IgA deposition on cell surfaces of the epidermis is present in all cases by direct immunofluorescence, and many patients have detectable circulating IgA autoantibodies by indirect immunofluorescence. There have been two distinct types of IgA pemphigus: subcorneal pustular dermatosis (SPD) type and intraepidermal neutrophilic (IEN) type. IgA autoantibodies

in the SPD type react with desmocollin 1.[40] while autoimmune targets of the IEN type remains to be identified (Table 42.2). A subset of IgA pemphigus patients have IgA autoantibodies against Dsg1 or Dsg3, making the autoimmune target of IgA pemphigus more heterogeneous. The exact pathogenic role of IgA autoantibodies in pustular formation in IgA pemphigus remains to be elucidated.

The patients with both types of IgA pemphigus clinically present with flaccid vesicles or pustules both on erythematous or normal skin. In the both types the pustules tend to coalesce to form an annular or circinate pattern with crusts in the central area, although a sunflower-like configuration of pustules is a characteristic sign of the IEN type. The predilection sites are the axillary and groin areas, but the trunk, proximal extremities, and lower aspect of the abdomen are commonly involved. Mucous membrane involvement is rare. Pruritus is often a significant symptom. Because the SPD type of IgA pemphigus is clinically and histologically indistinguishable from classic subcorneal pustular dermatosis (Sneddon-Wilkinson disease), immunologic characterization is essential to differentiate the two diseases.

Histology

Pemphigus Vulgaris

The characteristic histologic finding of the classic form of pemphigus is intraepidermal blister formation due to loss of cell–cell adhesion (acantholysis) of keratinocytes without keratinocyte necrosis. In pemphigus vulgaris, acantholysis usually occurs just above the basal cell layer (suprabasilar acantholysis) (Fig. 42.6). A few rounded-up (acantholytic) keratinocytes as well as clusters of epidermal cells are often seen in the blister cavity. Although the basal cells lose the contact with their neighbors, they maintain their attachment to the basement membrane, thus giving the appearance of a "row of tombstones." Eosinophilic spongiosis can be also seen in very early lesions of pemphigus.

Pemphigus Foliaceus

In pemphigus foliaceus, acantholysis is found in the upper epidermis, within or adjacent to the

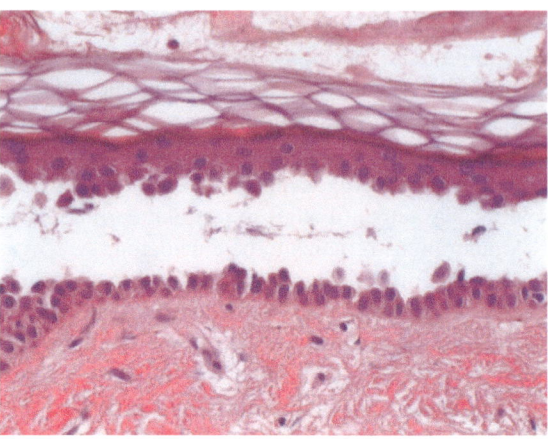

FIG. 42.6. Histology of pemphigus vulgaris. The characteristic histologic finding of pemphigus is intraepidermal blister formation due to loss of cell–cell adhesion of keratinocytes without keratinocyte necrosis. In pemphigus vulgaris, blisters usually occur just above the basal cell layer (suprabasilar acantholysis)

granular layer. As the blisters are superficial, it is often very difficult to obtain an intact lesion for diagnosis. These histologic findings of superficial blisters are indistinguishable from those seen in staphylococcal scalded skin syndrome or bullous impetigo, because desmoglein 1 is targeted in both diseases. Sometimes the blister contains numerous acute inflammatory cells, particularly neutrophils.

Paraneoplastic Pemphigus

In paraneoplastic pemphigus, the histologic findings of lesions show considerable variability, reflecting the polymorphism of the clinical lesions. The lesions show a unique combination of pemphigus vulgaris–like histology and erythema multiform–like or lichen planus–like histology. Intact cutaneous blisters may show suprabasilar acantholysis and individual keratinocyte necrosis with lymphocytic infiltration in the epidermis. In addition, basal cell liquefactive degeneration or band-like dense lymphocytic infiltration in the upper dermis can be seen.

Diagnosis

Once the diagnosis of pemphigus is suspected from clinical findings, it is important to take a biopsy for histology and direct immunofluorescence as well

as perform serum tests to look for IgG autoantibodies against cell surfaces of keratinocytes or desmogleins. The definitive diagnosis of pemphigus requires the demonstration of the IgG autoantibodies. Methods to demonstrate pemphigus autoantibodies include direct immunofluorescence, indirect immunofluorescence, immunoprecipitation, immunoblot, and enzyme-linked immunosorbent assay (ELISA).

Direct immunofluorescence examines patients' skin or mucous membranes to demonstrate in-vivo–bound IgG deposition on the keratinocyte cell surfaces (Fig. 42.7). Direct immunofluorescence is a most reliable and sensitive diagnostic test for all forms of pemphigus. If the direct immunofluorescence is negative, the diagnosis of pemphigus should be seriously questioned. The biopsy specimen should be taken from perilesional normal skin or mucous membrane, because blister sites may yield false negatives. IgM deposition is not seen, but occasionally IgA deposition may be seen in addition. Complement (C3) deposition is not necessarily demonstrated, probably because the dominant subclass of IgG is IgG4, which does not fix complement. In IgA pemphigus, IgA deposition, but not IgG deposition, is detected on keratinocyte cell surfaces.

Indirect immunofluorescence examines patients' sera to demonstrate circulating IgG autoantibodies, which react with epithelial cell surfaces. The

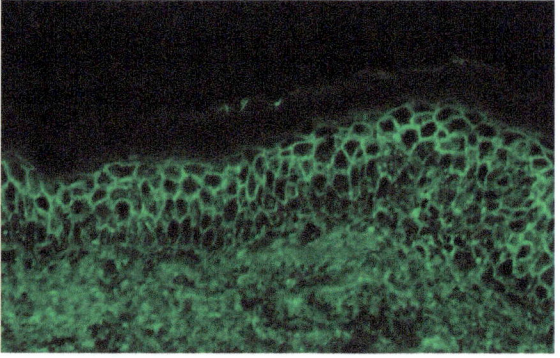

FIG. 42.7. Direct immunofluorescence of pemphigus foliaceus. Direct immunofluorescence using patients' skin as a substrate show in-vivo–bound immunoglobulin G (IgG) deposition on the keratinocyte cell surfaces, indicating IgG autoantibodies bind to the native target antigen, desmoglein1 or desmoglein3, as an initial step of blister formation in pemphigus

expression level of Dsg1 and Dsg3 varies among different epithelial cells. As a substrate of indirect immunofluorescence staining, monkey esophagus is more suitable for detecting anti-Dsg3 IgG autoantibodies, and normal human skin or guinea pig esophagus is better for anti-Dsg1 IgG autoantibodies. Rat bladder is used for paraneoplastic pemphigus or anti-plakin autoantibodies. Despite the different antigens involved in pemphigus vulgaris and foliaceus, the staining pattern using direct or indirect immunofluorescence is similar, which makes it difficult to serologically distinguish the two diseases.

Enzyme-linked immunosorbent assay provides a specific, sensitive, and quantitative assay to detect and measure circulating IgG autoantibodies in the diagnosis of pemphigus.[14,15] The patient's serum is tested on ELISA plates that are precoated with recombinant proteins of Dsg1 or Dsg3. Enzyme-linked immunosorbent assay enables us to serologically distinguish subtypes of pemphigus vulgaris and foliaceus. In general, if a serum is positive against Dsg1 but negative against Dsg3, it suggests a diagnosis of pemphigus foliaceus. If negative against Dsg1 but positive against Dsg3, it suggests a diagnosis of the mucosal dominant type of pemphigus foliaceus. If positive against both Dsg1 and Dsg3, it suggests a diagnosis of the mucocutaneous type of pemphigus vulgaris. Furthermore, ELISA scores show parallel fluctuation with the disease activity. Thus ELISA is also useful to monitor the disease activity to plan tapering schedules of corticosteroids and to predict flares or relapses before clinical evidence of disease flares is noticed.

Treatment

The introduction of systemic glucocorticoids and immunosuppressive agents has greatly improved the prognosis of pemphigus; however, the morbidity and mortality are still significant because death sometimes occurs from the complications of therapy. Systemic glucocorticoids are the mainstay of therapy for pemphigus, and immunosuppressive reagents are often used for a steroid-sparing effect to reduce the side effects of steroids. The goal of therapy is to control the disease at the lowest possible dose of glucocorticoids.

Prednisone at 1.0 mg/kg/day (usually 60 mg/day) is a typical initial treatment. The therapeutic effects are clinically estimated by the number of new blisters per day or the rate of healing of the new lesions, and prednisone is planned to be gradually tapered. However, once clinical remission is obtained, changes in the titers of circulating autoantibodies as determined by ELISA are helpful in gauging the dose of prednisone.[15,42–44]

Immunosuppressive agents, such as azathioprine (2 to 4 mg/kg/day) and cyclophosphamide (1 to 3 mg/kg/day), when combined with corticosteroids, are beneficial to gain early control of the disease and increased numbers of remissions.[45–47] If complete clinical remission is achieved with the combined therapy, the dosage of the immunosuppressive drug is maintained while the prednisone is gradually tapered to 5 mg/day. In young patients the potential increase in malignancies that might be associated with the use of these drugs must be taken into account. Mycophenolate mofetil (2 to 3 g/day) is another choice for an effective immunosuppressive agent of the combination therapy with glucocorticoids.[48]

Plasmapheresis is useful to quickly reduce the titers of circulating autoantibodies and should be considered for severe pemphigus if the disease is unresponsive to a combination of prednisone and immunosuppressives.[49] Concomitant immunosuppression with glucocorticoids and cyclophosphamide prevents a rebound increase in the production of autoantibody.

High-dose intravenous immunoglobulin is another option for resistant disease.[50] Intravenous immunoglobulin has immunomodulatory effects when used in a high dose, although their exact mechanisms remains to be elucidated. Recently, anti-CD20 monoclonal antibody (rituximab) was reported to be effective in patients with refractory pemphigus.[51–53]

Conclusion

Pemphigus is a group of autoimmune blistering diseases in which the pathogenic autoantibodies have been well characterized, as well as the targets of the autoimmune response, desmogleins 1 and 3. Glucorticoids, immunosuppressive drugs, and biologic agents are effective in treating this disease because they interfere with either the effector cascades that disrupt the epidermis, or the autoantibody synthesis or circulating half-life of the pathogenic antibody.

References

1. Beutner EH, Jordon RE. Demonstration of skin antibodies in sera of pemphigus vulgaris patients by indirect immunofluorescent staining. Proc Soc Exp Biol Med 1964;117(505):505–510.

2. Schiltz JR, Michel B. Production of epidermal acantholysis in normal human skin in vitro by the IgG fraction from pemphigus serum. J Invest Dermatol 1976;67(254):254–260.

3. Anhalt GJ, Labib RS, Voorhees JJ, Beals TF, Diaz LA. Induction of pemphigus in neonatal mice by passive transfer of IgG from patients with the disease. N Engl J Med 1982;306(1189):1189–1196.

4. Stanley JR, Yaar M, Hawley NP, Katz SI. Pemphigus antibodies identify a cell surface glycoprotein synthesized by human and mouse keratinocytes. J Clin Invest 1982;70(281):281–288.

5. Hashimoto T, Ogawa MM, Konohana A, Nishikawa T. Detection of pemphigus vulgaris and pemphigus foliaceus antigens by immunoblot analysis using different antigen sources. J Invest Dermatol 1990;94(3):327–331.

6. Koch PJ, Walsh MJ, Schmelz M, Goldschmidt MD, Zimbelmann R, Franke WW. Identification of desmoglein, a constitutive desmosomal glycoprotein, as a member of the cadherin family of cell adhesion molecules. Eur J Cell Biol 1990;53(1):1–12.

7. Amagai M, Klaus-Kovtun V, Stanley JR. Autoantibodies against a novel epithelial cadherin in pemphigus vulgaris, a disease of cell adhesion. Cell 1991;67(5):869–877.

8. Rock B, Labib RS, Diaz LA. Monovalent Fab' immunoglobulin fragments from endemic pemphigus foliaceus autoantibodies reproduce the human disease in neonatal Balb/c mice. J Clin Invest 1990;85(296):296–299.

9. Karpati S, Amagai M, Prussick R, Cehrs K, Stanley JR. Pemphigus vulgaris antigen, a desmoglein type of cadherin, is located within keratinocyte desmosomes. J Cell Biol 1993;122(2):409–415.

10. Stanley JR, Koulu L, Thivolet C. Distinction between epidermal antigens binding pemphigus vulgaris and pemphigus foliaceus autoantibodies. J Clin Invest 1984;74(313):313–320.

11. Koulu L, Kusumi A, Steinberg MS, Klaus-Kovtun V, Stanley JR. Human autoantibodies against a desmosomal core protein in pemphigus foliaceus. J Exp Med 1984;160(1509):1509–1518.

12. Schafer S, Koch PJ, Franke WW. Identification of the ubiquitous human desmoglein, Dsg2, and the expression catalogue of the desmoglein subfamily of desmosomal cadherins. Exp Cell Res 1994;211(2):391–9.

13. Kljuic A, Bazzi H, Sundberg JP, et al. Desmoglein 4 in hair follicle differentiation and epidermal adhesion: evidence from inherited hypotrichosis and acquired pemphigus vulgaris. Cell 2003;113(2):249–60.

14. Ishii K, Amagai M, Hall RP, et al. Characterization of autoantibodies in pemphigus using antigen-specific ELISAs with baculovirus expressed recombinant desmogleins. J Immunol 1997;159:2010–2017.

15. Amagai M, Komai A, Hashimoto T, et al. Usefulness of enzyme-linked immunosorbent assay (ELISA) using recombinant desmogleins 1 and 3 for serodiagnosis of pemphigus. Br J Dermatol 1999;140:351–357.

16. Amagai M, Hashimoto T, Shimizu N, Nishikawa T. Absorption of pathogenic autoantibodies by the extracellular domain of pemphigus vulgaris antigen (Dsg3) produced by baculovirus. J Clin Invest 1994;94:59–67.

17. Amagai M, Nishikawa T, Nousari HC, Anhalt GJ, Hashimoto T. Antibodies against desmoglein 3 (pemphigus vulgaris antigen) are present in sera from patients with paraneoplastic pemphigus and cause acantholysis in vivo in neonatal mice. J Clin Invest 1998;102:775–782.

18. Amagai M, Hashimoto T, Green KJ, Shimizu N, Nishikawa T. Antigen-specific immunoadsorption of pathogenic autoantibodies in pemphigus foliaceus. J Invest Dermatol 1995;104:895–901.

19. Nagasaka T, Nishifuji K, Ota T, Whittock NV, Amagai M. Defining the pathogenic involvement of desmoglein 4 in pemphigus and staphylococcal scalded skin syndrome. J Clin Invest 2004;114(10):1484–92.

20. Nguyen VT, Ndoye A, Grando SA. Pemphigus vulgaris antibody identifies pemphaxin. A novel keratinocyte annexin-like molecule binding acetylcholine. J Biol Chem 2000;275(38):29466–76.

21. Grando SA. Autoimmunity to keratinocyte acetylcholine receptors in pemphigus. Dermatology 2000;201(4):290–5.

22. Nguyen VT, Ndoye A, Shultz LD, Pittelkow MR, Grando SA. Antibodies against keratinocyte antigens other than desmogleins 1 and 3 can induce pemphigus vulgaris-like lesions. J Clin Invest 2000;106(12):1467–79.

23. Mahoney MG, Wang Z, Rothenberger KL, Koch PJ, Amagai M, Stanley JR. Explanation for the clinical and microscopic localization of lesions in pemphigus foliaceus and vulgaris. J Clin Invest 1999;103:461–468.

24. Udey MC, Stanley JR, Pemphigus—diseases of antidesmosomal autoimmunity. JAMA 1999;282(6):572–576.

25. Stanley JR, Amagai M. Pemphigus, bullous impetigo, and the staphylococcal scalded-skin syndrome. N Engl J Med 2006;355(17):1800–10.

26. Ding X, Aoki V, Mascaro JM, Lopez-Swiderski A, Diaz LA, Fairley JA. Mucosal and mucocutaneous (generalized) pemphigus vulgaris show dis-

tinct autoantibody profiles. J Invest Dermatol 1997;109:592–596.

27. Amagai M, Tsunoda K, Zillikens D, Nagai T, Nishikawa T. The clinical phenotype of pemphigus is defined by the anti-desmoglein autoantibody profile. J Am Acad Dermatol 1999;40:167–170.

28. Amagai M, Matsuyoshi N, Wang ZH, Andl C, Stanley JR. Toxin in bullous impetigo and staphylococcal scalded skin syndrome targets desmoglein 1. Nature Medicine 2000;6(11):1275–1277.

29. Hanakawa Y, Schechter NM, Lin C, et al. Molecular mechanisms of blister formation in bullous impetigo and staphylococcal scalded skin syndrome. J Clin Invest 2002;110(1):53–60.

30. Hanakawa Y, Schechter NM, Lin C, Nishifuji K, Amagai M, Stanley JR. Enzymatic and molecular characteristics of the efficiency and specificity of exfoliative toxin cleavage of desmoglein 1. J Biol Chem 2004;279(7):5268–5277.

31. Anhalt GJ, Kim S, Stanley JR, et al. Paraneoplastic pemphigus. An autoimmune mucocutaneous disease associated with neoplasia. N Engl J Med 1990;323(1729):1729–1735.

32. Anhalt GJ. Paraneoplastic pemphigus. Adv Dermatol 1997;12:77–97.

33. Fullerton SH, Woodley DT, Smoller BR, Anhalt GJ. Paraneoplastic pemphigus with autoantibody deposition in bronchial epithelium after autologous bone marrow transplantation. JAMA 1992;267(11):1500–2.

34. Nousari HC, Deterding R, Wojtczack H, et al. The mechanism of respiratory failure in paraneoplastic pemphigus. N Engl J Med 1999;340(18):1406–10.

35. Senear FE, Usher B. An unusual type of pemphigus combining features of lupus erythematosus. Arch Dermatol Syphilol 1926;13:761–781.

36. Gomi H, Kawada A, Amagai M, Matsuo I. A case of classic pemphigus erythematosus: detection of anti-desmoglein 1 antibody by ELISA. Dermatology 1999;199(2):188–189.

37. Brenner S, Bialy-Golan A, Ruocco V. Drug-induced pemphigus. Clin Dermatol 1998;16:393–397.

38. Brenner S, Bialy-Golan A, Anhalt GJ. Recognition of pemphigus antigens in drug-induced pemphigus vulgaris and pemphigus foliaceus. J Am Acad Dermatol 1997;36:919–23.

39. Robinson ND, Hashimoto T, Amagai M, Chan LS. The new pemphigus variants. J Am Acad Dermatol 1999;40(5):649–671.

40. Hashimoto T, Kiyokawa C, Mori O, et al. Human desmocollin 1 (Dsc1) is an autoantigen for the sub-corneal pustular dermatosis type of IgA pemphigus. J Invest Dermatol 1997;109:127–131.

41. Nishikawa T, Hashimoto T. Dermatoses with intraepidermal IgA deposits. Clin Dermatol 2000;18:315–318.

42. Harman KE, Seed PT, Gratian MJ, Bhogal BS, Challacombe SJ, Black MM. The severity of cutaneous and oral pemphigus is related to desmoglein 1 and 3 antibody levels. Br J Dermatol 2001;144(4):775–80.

43. Cheng SW, Kobayashi M, Tanikawa A, Kinoshita-Kuroda K, Amagai M, Nishikawa T. Monitoring disease activity in pemphigus with enzyme-linked immunosorbent assay using recombinant desmoglein 1 and 3. Br J Dermatol 2002;147(2):261–265.

44. Herzog S, Schmidt E, Goebeler M, Brocker EB, Zillikens D. Serum levels of autoantibodies to desmoglein 3 in patients with therapy-resistant pemphigus vulgaris successfully treated with adjuvant intravenous immunoglobulins. Acta Derm Venereol 2004;84(1):48–52.

45. Aberer W, Wolff SE, Stingl G, Wolff K. Azathioprine in the treatment of pemphigus vulgaris. A long-term follow-up. J Am Acad Dermatol 1987,16(527):527–533.

46. Fellner MJ, Katz JM, McCabe JB. Successful use of cyclophosphamide and prednisone for initial treatment of pemphigus vulgaris. Arch Dermatol 1978;114(889):889–894.

47. Fine JD. Management of acquired bullous skin diseases. N Eng J Med 1995;333(22):1475–1484.

48. Enk AH, Knop J. Mycophenolate is effective in the treatment of pemphigus vulgaris. Arch Dermatol 1999;135(1):54–56.

49. Bystryn JC, Steinman NM, The adjuvant therapy of pemphigus. An update. Arch Dermatol 1996;132(2):203–12.

50. Jolles S. A review of high-dose intravenous immunoglobulin (hdIVIg) in the treatment of the autoimmune blistering disorders. Clin Exp Dermatol 2001;26(2):127–31.

51. Ahmed AR, Spigelman Z, Cavacini LA, Posner MR. Treatment of pemphigus vulgaris with rituximab and intravenous immune globulin. N Engl J Med 2006;355(17):1772–9.

52. Schmidt E, Seitz CS, Benoit S, Brocker EB, Goebeler M. Rituximab in autoimmune bullous diseases: mixed responses and adverse effects. Br J Dermatol 2007;156(2):352–6.

53. Joly P, Mouquet H, Roujeau JC, et al. A single cycle of riboximab for the treatment of severe pemphigus. N Engl J Med 2007;357(6):545–552.

43
The Pemphigoid Spectrum

Kelly Nelson, Ning Li, Zhi Liu, and Luis A. Diaz

Key Points

- Bullous pemphigoid (BP) is a subepidermal autoimmune blistering skin disease, and is predominantly a disease of the elderly in its classic presentation.
- There are distinct clinical variants of this disease: bullous pemphigoid, cicatricial pemphigoid, and pemphigoid gestationis.
- The autoimmune response in BP is directed against two hemidesmosomal antigens, BP180 (BPantigen2 or collagen XVII) and BP230 (BPantigen1). In CP, autoantibodies recognize multiple autoantigens, including BP180, BP230, laminin-5, laminin-6, and integrin B4 subunit. Autoantibodies in pemphigoid gestations are maily reative with BP180.
- The diagnosis of this condition is based on clinical findings, histology, and the demonstration of tissue bound immunoreactants (direct immunofluorescence).
- Therapy can range from topical glucocorticosteroids for mild disease, to oral antibiotics, to systemic glucocorticosteroids alone or with cytotoxic drugs or intravenous immunoglobulin (IVIG).

Bullous Pemphigoid

Overview

Bullous pemphigoid (BP) is a subepidermal autoimmune bullous disorder that commonly occurs in elderly patients and is the most common adult bullous disorder. The patient typically presents with generalized pruritic tense bullae, with rare involvement of the mucous membranes. The pathogenesis of BP has been clarified by advances in the field of immunodermatology, which have also aided in diagnosis of atypical cases. Therapy focuses on immunosuppression to attenuate the autoimmune response.

Historical Background

Bullous pemphigoid was first described by Lever[1] in 1953 as a subepidermal bullous dermatosis seen in elderly individuals (Fig. 43.1). Based on histologic evaluation, BP was characterized by detachment of the epidermis and an intense inflammatory cell infiltrate in the upper dermis. Jordon and Beutner et al.[2] discovered anti-skin autoantibodies in BP patients, which are present in the serum and bound to the dermal–epidermal junction in a linear fashion. Further specification of the anti-skin autoantibodies was provided by Stanley et al.,[3] with the characterization of antibodies against a 230-kd epidermal protein within the sera of BP patients. Mutasim et al.[4] observed that BP autoantibodies recognized hemidesmosomes, and Labib et al.[5] described the binding of BP autoantibodies to an 180-kd epidermal protein.

Further molecular characterization of the BP 180 antigen has been performed by Diaz et al.[6] Specifically, the BP180 antigen is a transmembrane hemidesmosomal glycoprotein with both an extracellular C-terminus projecting into the lamina lucida, and an intracellular N-terminus. Development of a passive transfer murine model, and progress toward an active immunization murine model by Liu et al.[7] have provided further clarification of the pathogenesis of BP.

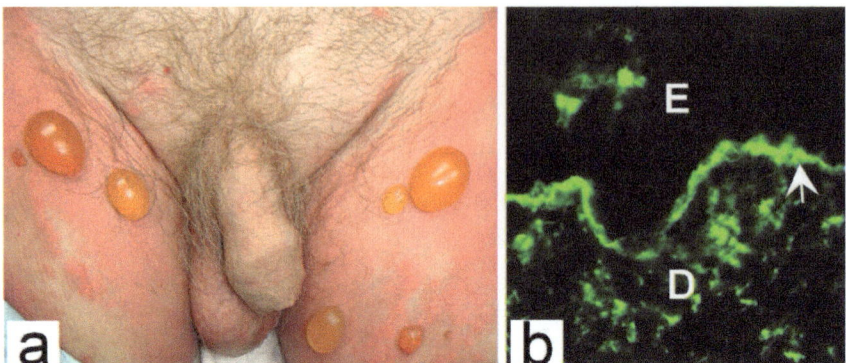

FIG. 43.1. Bullous pemphigoid (BP). (A) Large, tense blisters and erosions are seen in a BP patient. (B) Direct immunofluorescence shows in situ deposition of immunoglobulin G (IgG) and C3 at the cutaneous basement membrane zone (arrow). D, dermis; E, epidermis

Epidemiology

With onset typically occurring after the sixth decade, BP is classically considered a disease of the elderly. Indeed, in comparing patients older than 90 years of age to those less than 60 years of age, the relative risk of developing BP is approximately 300.[8] Given the age of most patients with BP, assessing survival in this patient population has provided variable figures, with 1-year mortality ranging from 25% to 40%.[9–15] However, both increased patient age and poor general health condition have been associated with increased mortality in BP.[9,16] Correlation of the extent of the bullous lesions, patient gender, and dosing of oral steroids with patient mortality have been variable.[8,9,16]

Various human leukocyte antigen (HLA) classes have been associated with BP, specifically in regard to patient race. In Caucasians, HLA-DQB1*0301, has been associated with not only BP, but also ocular and mucous membrane involvement.[17,18] Among patients of Japanese descent with BP, increased incidence of the HLA-DRB1*04, DRB1*1101, and DQB1*0302 alleles have been noted.[19] Focusing on the geographic region of northern China, comparison of patients with BP to controls revealed decreased frequency of HLA-DRB1*08 and HLA-DQB1*06 in patients afflicted with BP.[20]

Pathogenesis

The autoimmune response in BP is directed against two hemidesmosomal antigens, BP180 (BP antigen 2 or collagen XVII), and BP230 (BP antigen 1). BP180 has been characterized at the molecular level as possessing both an intracellular N-terminus, and an extracellular C-terminus, which projects into the lamina lucida.[6] In contrast, BP230 is a cytoplasmic protein with structural similarity to plectin and desmoplakins I and II.[21,22] As part of

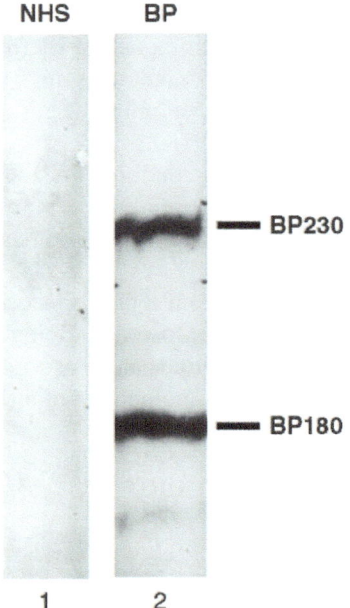

FIG. 43.2. Bullous pemphigoid autoantigens. By immunoblotting analysis, sera of patients with BP recognize BP180 and BP230 in skin protein extracts (lane 2). Normal human serum (NHS) controls show no immune reactivity with skin protein extracts (lane 1)

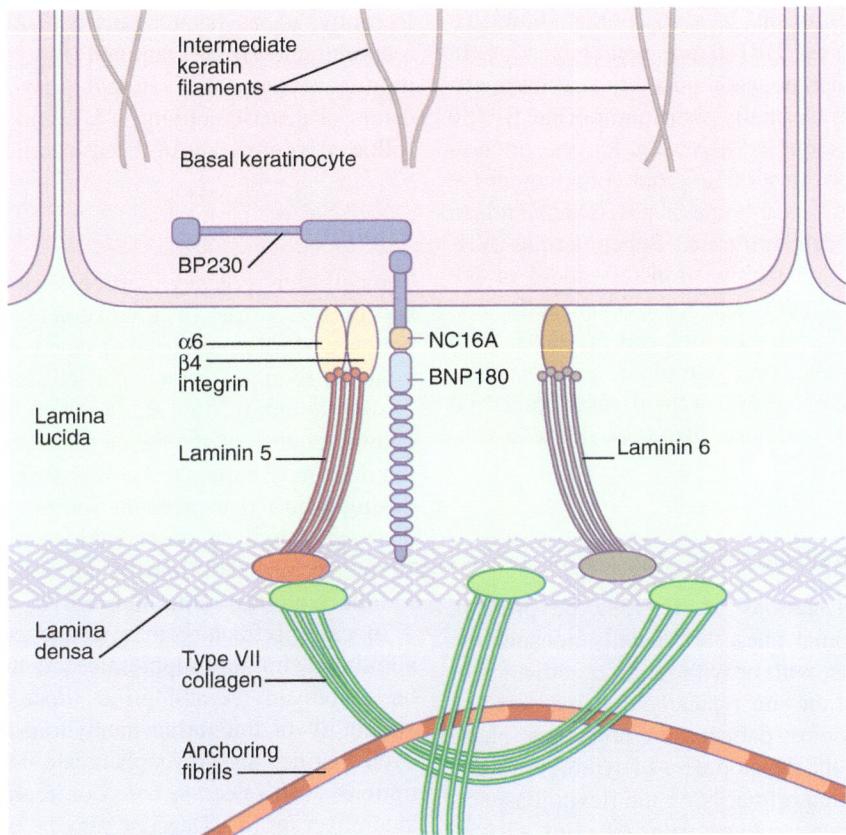

Fig. 43.3. A diagram of hemidesmosomal antigens and their interactive extracellular matrix proteins at the dermal-epidermal junction. BK, basal keratinocyte; IKF, intermediate keratin filaments; LL, lamina lucida; LD, lamina densa

the hemidesmosome, BP180 and BP230 promote adhesion of the basement membrane to the basal layer of keratinocytes (Figs. 43.2 and 43.3).

Characterization of autoantibodies reveals a polyclonal response, with the majority of antibodies recognizing a cluster of epitopes about the largest noncollagen domain (referred to as NC16A) of the BP180 antigen.[23,24] The BP180NC16A-specific autoantibodies are predominantly immunoglobulin E (IgE), IgG1, and IgG4.[25–27] Titers of the BP180NC16A autoantibodies have been correlated with the degree of clinical severity.[26–28]

B-cell production of pathogenic autoantibodies likely begins with development of autoreactive T cells. Most patients with BP demonstrate circulating autoreactive BP180-specific CD4 T cells.[29] T-helper-2 (Th2) and Th1 responses against the BP180 ectodomain were identified in the majority of the studied BP patients.[30,31] BP180-reactive Th cells

and IgG autoantibodies recognized similar or identical epitopes clustered in distinct regions of the BP180 ectodomain; the majority of autoreactive Th2 and Th1 cells and B cells recognized epitopes within the NC16A, followed by reactivity against the COOH-terminal and central regions.[31–34] More significantly, T- and B-cell reactivity against the BP180NC16A ectodomain was associated with severe BP, with widespread blisters and erosions, while the central portion was more frequently recognized in limited BP, with few blisters and erosions.[33] BP patients (less than 50%) also showed a combined T- and B-cell response against the COOH- and NH_2-terminal globular domains of BP230.[34]

The characteristic histologic and clinical features of BP are a result of the inflammatory cascade triggered by the binding of pathogenic autoantibodies to the antigen targets within the hemidesmosome structure. In vitro and in vivo studies show that antibodies against BP180 are pathogenic.[35,36] In the in vivo model, neonatal mice injected intraperitoneally or intradermally with antimurine BP180 antibodies develop BP-like skin lesions, including in situ deposition of IgG and complement C3 at the basement membrane zone (BMZ) and an inflammatory cell infiltrate. Subepidermal blistering in this IgG passive transfer model of BP requires complement activation, mast cells, and neutrophils.[37–40] Inflammatory cell products, such as neutrophil elastase, gelatinase, and plasmin, result in tissue destruction at the dermal–epidermal junction, which manifests histologically as a subepidermal split.[41–45]

Clinical Features

Clinical manifestations of BP may be protean, and the prodromal phase is typically nonspecific. Intense pruritus, with or without an eczematous or urticarial eruption, are typically the first signs of the disease. In most patients, the prodromal phase is followed by the development of symmetric tense bullae, distributed primarily on the flexural aspects of the extremities and lower trunk (see Fig. 43.1A). The bullae are symptomatically pruritic, and may be filled with clear or hemorrhagic fluid. Rupture of the bullae results in shallow crusted erosions. Involvement of intertriginous areas may produce vegetative moist plaques. The mucous membranes are involved in approximately a third of patients.

Diagnosis

Once the suspicion of BP is raised on the basis of clinical and historical patient information, definitive diagnosis is based not only on histologic evaluation, but also on further characterization of the autoantibody response through direct and indirect immunofluorescence (IF) microscopy. Standard histologic evaluation via light microscopy reveals a subepidermal split, with a sparse inflammatory infiltrate composed mainly of eosinophils. Direct IF (from perilesional, uninvolved skin) demonstrates a fine linear band at the dermal–epidermal junction of IgG or C3 (see Fig. 43.1B). Indirect IF (from patient's serum) demonstrates in most patients the presence of autoantibodies that bind the dermal–epidermal junction in a linear fashion.

Recently, it has been reported that titers against recombinant BP180 antigen by enzyme-linked immunosorbent assay (ELISA) may be good indicators of disease activity in BP, and titers may be followed as a marker of disease activity.[46]

Therapy

Topical high potency corticosteroids are useful for limited areas of involvement in motivated patients. More generalized or severe manifestations typically require systemic corticosteroids, in initial dosing ranging from 0.5 to 1 mg/kg/day. After gaining control of the development of new bullae, the dose may be tapered over 6 to 8 months, with dosing adjusted to account for the recurrence of disease. A study suggests that high-potency topical steroids (clobetasol) may be an excellent approach to induce clinical remission in BP.[47]

In cases refractory to systemic corticosteroids, additional immunosuppressive medications may be employed. Azathioprine (dose adjusted for variability in thiopurine methyltransferase levels), cyclosporine, and mycophenolate mofetil are all options, with selection based on each medication's side-effect profile. Dapsone may be useful in some cases where systemic steroids or immunosuppressive drugs are not indicated. Plasmapheresis and intravenous immunoglobulin (IVIG) have been used successfully to induce remission in BP.[48–50] While other dermatologists have found tetracycline and nicotinamide useful in the control of BP, in our hands it has had a limited effect in some rare patients.

Cicatricial Pemphigoid

Overview

Cicatricial pemphigoid (CP), also known as mucous membrane pemphigoid, is a rare chronic autoimmune blistering disorder, characterized by mucosal involvement, with high risk of scarring occurring within the affected areas. Any or all mucous membranes may be involved in any individual patient. Patients demonstrate linear deposition of autoantibodies against various basement membrane zone components. The clinical course tends to be chronic, and best managed with a multidisciplinary approach to avoid major sequelae occurring secondary to scarring.[51]

Historical Background

Chronic blistering conditions with both skin and eye involvement were described throughout the 1800s.[52,53] Up to the mid-1900s, CP was considered a variant of pemphigus, until Civatte[54] and Lever[55] separated the disorder based on histopathologic criteria. Lever suggested changing the name from "benign mucous membrane pemphigoid" to "cicatricial pemphigoid" based on the tendency for scar formation.[56,57] Tissue-bound immunoglobulins and complement components along the basement membrane zone were identified in the 1970s.[58,59] Circulating autoantibodies were demonstrated by Dantzig[60] and Bean[61] shortly thereafter.

Epidemiology

Cicatricial pemphigoid has been documented to occur at any age, and is one of the most rare subepidermal bullous diseases, with an estimated annual incidence of approximately 0.25 per million.[62] In a recent review of patients with circulating antibodies recognizing laminin-5, over 30% of patients demonstrated internal malignancy.[63]

Clinical Features

While any mucosal surface may be affected in CP, the oral site is most commonly involved, followed by, in decreasing order of involvement, the ocular, nasal, nasopharyngeal, anogenital, laryngeal, and esophageal sites.[64–66] Oral disease may present as erosive or desquamative gingivitis; intact blisters are rarely observed. Chronic erosions on the palate and lateral tongue are commonly seen, as well. Once healed, the areas may resemble lesions of lichen planus, with white reticulated striations.

Conjunctival involvement is also commonly seen, and, if not appropriately addressed, may result in blindness. Conjunctival inflammation, erosions, symblepharon, and entropion may be present. Similar to the appearance of lesions in the oral mucosa, intact bullae are very rarely observed.[65]

Nasopharyngeal involvement may be associated with lesions of the upper aerodigestive tract.[66] Symptoms suggestive of nasopharyngeal involvement include nasal crusting, recurrent epistaxis, and nasal airway obstruction. A history of persistent pharyngalgia, dysphagia, odynophagia, dysphonia, or dyspepsia, may sug-gest pharyngeal and laryngeal involvement.[67] Development of strictures or stenosis of the pharynx or larynx may prove life-threatening, if not identified at an early stage.

Genital and anal involvement is relatively rare. Progressive disease may lead to narrowing of the introitus in women, or to phimosis in men. Anal involvement may lead to scarring, and potentially to stricture. The skin is involved in approximately a quarter of patients with CP. Erythematous plaques develop recurrent blisters, and heal with atrophic scarring.

Pathogenesis and Diagnosis

Diagnosis of CP relies on immunofluorescent (IF) evaluation. Direct IF performed on perilesional mucosa or skin reveals IgG, IgA, or C3 in a continuous fine linear pattern along the basement membrane zone.[51,64–73] Direct IF is most likely to provide conclusive information when performed on an area of mucosa adjacent to an area of inflammation.[51] To minimize the risk of conjunctival scarring, other anatomic areas of involvement should be biopsied preferentially, as injury to the conjunctiva may increase disease activity.[51] Indirect IF reveals anti-BMZ antibodies in 20% to 30% of patients with clinical disease. Localization of autoantibodies, when performed on human salt-split skin substrate, is variable, depending on the diversity of each patient's autoantibody milieu.[74–79] Commonly recognized target antigens in CP include BP180, BP230, laminin-5, laminin-6, and integrin β_4 subunit.[80,81]

Therapy

In patients with mild, low-risk disease (defined as oral mucosa involvement, with or without skin involvement), potent topical corticosteroids may be sufficient. However, in patients with high-risk disease (defined as involvement of ocular, genital, laryngeal, nasopharyngeal, esophageal sites), initial therapy should involve systemic corticosteroids, with consideration of the addition of cyclophosphamide or azathioprine.[51] Dapsone is also a consideration for stable or mild disease. Case reports document the use of various other modalities, including intravenous immunoglobulin, etanercept, and mycophenolate mofetil.[82–84]

Herpes Gestationis (Gestational Pemphigoid)

Overview

Herpes gestationis (HG) is a rare dermatosis of pregnancy and the immediate postpartum period characterized by grouped intensely pruritic urticarial lesions. Most patients demonstrate autoantibodies to the BP180 antigen, with generation of a subepidermal separation on histologic evaluation. In pregnancies affected with HG, there is increased risk of prematurity and small-for-gestational-age birth. The clinical course tends to be quite variable, and most cases resolve following delivery.

Historical Background

The term *herpes gestationis* was first cited by Milton in 1872, with demonstration of complement deposition along the basement membrane zone first documented by Provost and Tomasi[85] in 1973. In 1976, Jordon et al.[86] and Katz et al.[87] characterized the "HG" factor as an IgG antibody that activates the complement pathway. Guidice et al.[88,89] identified the structural antigen for the HG factor as BP180, and provided further structural analysis of the antigen.

Epidemiology

Herpes gestationis is a rare disorder exclusively found in during pregnancy and the immediate postpartum period. Even more rare is its association with trophoblastic malignancy or molar pregnancy.[90,91] Estimates of incidence for HG range from 1 in 10,000 to 1 in 50,000 pregnancies.[92,93] It often recurs in subsequent pregnancies, and may occur earlier and in a more severe form.[94] Also, with subsequent pregnancies, the time to resolution in the postpartum period may become progressively prolonged.[95]

Pathogenesis

Generation of autoreactive T cells stimulates production of autoantibodies against the NC16A region of the BP180 antigen, prompting histopathologic and clinical manifestations of HG. Characterization of the autoreactive T cells has revealed expression of a Th1 cytokine profile, supporting the production of IgG1 autoantibodies against BP180.[96,97]

Deposition of the autoantibodies prompts complement activation, primarily through the classic pathway, followed by mast cell recruitment, degranulation, recruitment of inflammatory cells (primarily eosinophils), and production of destructive products.[98-100] The resultant damage at the dermal–epidermal junction manifests as a subepidermal separation on histologic examination.

Herpes gestationis has been associated with HLA-DR3 or HLA-DR4 or both alleles.[101-104] Correspondingly, patients with HG are at increased risk for the development of other autoimmune disorders, such as Graves' disease.[104]

Clinical Features

Typically, abdominal urticarial lesions appear abruptly during the second or third trimester, followed by the appearance of a generalized bullous reaction sparing the face, mucous membranes, palms, and soles.[93,105-107] However, initial onset in the immediate postpartum period has been described in 20% of cases.[108] Most patients experience a flare with delivery, which spontaneously resolves over weeks to months following delivery. Flares with subsequent pregnancies, menstruation, or initiation of oral contraceptive use are common.[106,109]

Neonatal vesicles are present in approximately 10% of cases, presumably secondary to passive transfer of pathogenic antibodies.[106,110,111] While the lesions are transient and typically mild, they are at increased risk of superinfection secondary to the infant's relatively immunocompromised status. Although associations have been reported in regard to preterm delivery and small-for-gestational-age infants, there have been no reports of increased fetal morbidity or mortality.[112,113]

Diagnosis

Standard light microscopy of involved skin reveals a subepidermal vesicle with a lymphocytic and eosinophilic perivascular infiltrate. Direct IF of perilesional skin demonstrates linear C3 along the BMZ; occasionally, IgG is also present, but to a lesser degree than C3.[98,114] While standard indirect IF is rarely positive, complement-added indirect IF is almost universally positive for pathogenic IgG antibodies.[114,115]

Therapy

For limited disease, high-potency topical corticos-teroids along with oral antihistamines may provide sufficient control. However, more severe erup-tions may require oral corticosteroids for adequate response. More therapeutic options are feasible during the postpartum period, such as cyclophos-phamide and methotrexate, although only sporadic reports of variable efficacy are available.[116,117]

Conclusion

Bullous pemphigoid is a blistering skin disease in which skin-specific autoantibodies are responsible for a subepidermal split. It is likely that this autoim-mune disease is common in the elderly because of a progressive loss of immune self-tolerance that occurs with the senescence of the immune system. It is possible to induce remissions in this disease with systemic glucocorticosteroids alone or when combined with glucocorticosteroid-sparing agents such as cytotoxic drugs. Certain clinical variants are very difficult to treat, such as ocular pemphig-oid and mucosal pemphigoid.

References

1. Lever W. Pemphigus. Medicine 1953;32:1–123.
2. Jordon R, Beutner E, Witebsky E, et al. Basement zone antibodies in bullous pemphigoid. JAMA 1967;200:751–758.
3. Stanley J, Hawley-Nelson P, Yuspa S, et al. Characterization of bullous pemphigoid antigen: a unique basement membrane protein of stratified epi-thelia. Cell 1981;24:897–903.
4. Mutasim D, Takahaski Y, Labib R, et al. A pool of bullous pemphigoid antigen(s) is intracellular and associated with the basal cell cytoskeleton-hemidesmosome complex. J Invest Dermatol 1985;84:47–53.
5. Labib R, Anhalt G, Patel H, et al. Molecular hetero-geneity of bullous pemphigoid antigens as detected by immunoblotting. J Immunol 1986;136:1231–1235.
6. Diaz L, Ratrie III H, Saunders W, et al. Isolation of a human epidermal cDNA corresponding to the 180-kD autoantigen recognized by bullous pemphig-oid and herpes gestationis sera. Immunolocalization of this protein to the hemidesmosome. J Clin Invest 1990;86:1088–1094.

7. Liu Z, Diaz L, Troy J, et al. A passive transfer model of the organ-specific autoimmune disease, bullous pemphigoid, using antibodies generated against the hemidesmosomal antigen, BP 180. J Clin Invest 1993;92:2480–2488.
8. Rzany B, Weller N. Epidemiology of autoimmune skin disorders. In: Hertl M, ed. Autoimmune Diseases of the Skin. New York: Springer-Verlag, 2001:21–38.
9. Roujeau J, Lok C, Bastuji-Garin S, et al. High risk of death in elderly patients with extensive bullous pemphigoid. Arch Dermatol 1998;134:465–469.
10. Bernard P, Bedane C, Bonnetblanc J. Anti-BP180 autoantibodies as a marker of poor prognosis in bullous pemphigoid: a cohort analysis of 94 elderly patients. Br J Dermatol 1997;136:694–698.
11. Bernard P, Enginger V, Venot J, et al. Survival prog-nosis in pemphigoid: a cohort analysis of 78 patients. Ann Dermatol Venereol 1995;122:751–757.
12. Venning V, Wojnarowska F. Lack of predictive fac-tors for the clinical course of bullous pemphigoid. J Am Acad Dermatol 1992;26:585–589.
13. Savin J. The events leading to the death of patients with pemphigus and pemphigoid. Br J Dermatol 1979;101:521–534.
14. Joly P, Roujeau J, Benichou J, et al. A comparison of oral and topical corticosteroids in patients with bul-lous pemphigoid. N Engl J Med 2002;346:321–327.
15. Rzany B, Partscht K, Jung M, et al. Risk factors for lethal outcome in patients with bullous pemphigoid. Arch Dermatol 2002;138:903–908.
16. Joly P, Benichou J, Lok C, et al. Prediction of sur-vival for patients with bullous pemphigoid: a pro-spective study. Arch Dermatol 2005;141:691–8.
17. Delgado J, Turbay D, Yunis E, et al. A common major histocompatibility complex class II allele HLA-DQB1*0301 is present in clinical variants of pemphigoid. Proc Natl Acad Sci USA 1996;93: 8569–8571.
18. Oyama N, Setterfield J, Powell A et al. Bullous pemphigoid antigen II (BP180) and its soluble extra-cellular domains are major autoantigens in mucous membrane pemphigoid: the pathogenic relevance to HLA class II alleles and disease severity. Br J Dermatol 2005;154:90–98.
19. Okazaki A, Miyagawa S, Yamashina Y, et al. Polymorphisms of HLA-DR and -DQ genes in Japanese patients with bullous pemphigoid. J Dermatol 2000;27:149–56.
20. Gao X, Winsey S, Li G, et al. HLA-DR and -DQ polymorphisms in bullous pemphigoid from northern China. Clin Exp Dermatol 2002;27:319–21.
21. Fontao L, Favre B, Riou S, et al. Interaction of the bullous pemphigoid antigen 1 (BP230) and desmo-plakin with intermediate filaments is mediated by

distinct sequences within their COOH terminus. Mol Biol Cell 2003;14:1978–92.

22. Sawamura D, Li K, Nomura K, et al. Bullous pemphigoid antigen: cDNA cloning, cellular expression, and evidence for polymorphism of the human gene. J Invest Dermatol 1991;96:908–15.

23. Giudice G, Emery D, Zelickson B, et al. Bullous pemphigoid and herpes gestationis autoantibodies recognize a common non-collagenous site on the BP180 ectodomain. J Immunol 1993;151:5742–5750.

24. Zillikens D, Rose P, Balding S, et al. Tight clustering of extracellular BP180 epitopes recognized by bullous pemphigoid autoantibodies. J Invest Dermatol 1997;109:573–579.

25. Bernard P, Aucouturier P, Denis F, et al. Immunoblot analysis of IgG subclasses of circulating antibodies in bullous pemphigoid. Clin Immunol Immunopathol 1990;54:484–494.

26. Dopp R, Schmidt E, Chimanovitch I, et al. IgG4 and IgE are the major immunoglobulins targeting the NC16A domain of BP180 in bullous pemphigoid: serum levels of these immunoglobulins reflect disease activity. J Am Acad Dermatol 2000;42: 577–583.

27. Laffitte E, Skaria M, Jaunin F, et al. Autoantibodies to the extracellular and intracellular domain of bullous pemphigoid 180, the putative key autoantigen in bullous pemphigoid, belong predominantly to the IgG1 and IgG4 subclasses. Br J Dermatol 2001;144:760–768.

28. Haase C, Budinger L, Borradori L, et al. Detection of IgG autoantibodies in the sera of patients with bullous and gestational pemphigoid: ELISA studies utilizing a baculovirus-encoded form of bullous pemphigoid antigen 2. J Invest Dermatol 1998;110:282–286.

29. Budinger L, Borradori L, Yee C, et al. Identification and characterization of autoreactive CD4+ T cell responses to the extracellular domain of bullous pemphigoid antigen 2 in patients with bullous pemphigoid and normals. J Clin Invest 1998;102: 2082–2089.

30. Büdinger L, BorradoriL, Yee C, et al. Identification and characterization of autoreactive T cell responses to bullous pemphigoid antigen 2 in patients and healthy controls. J Clin Invest 1998;102:2082–2089.

31. Lin M, Fu C, Giudice G, et al. Epitopes targeted by bullous pemphigoid T lymphocytes and autoantibodies map to the same sites on the bullous pemphigoid 180 ectodomain. J Invest Dermatol 2000;115:955–961.

32. Hofmann S, Thoma-Uszynski S, Hunziker T, et al. Severity and phenotype of bullous pemphigoid relate to autoantibody profile against the NH2- and COOH-terminal regions of the BP180 ectodomain. J Invest Dermatol 2002;119:1065–1073.

33. Thoma-Uszynski S, Uter W, Schwietzke S, et al. BP230- and BP180-specific auto-antibodies in bullous pemphigoid. J Invest Dermatol 2004;122:1413–1422.

34. Thoma-Uszynski S, Uter W, Schwietzke S, et al. Autoreactive T and B cells from bullous pemphigoid (BP) patients recognized epitopes clustered in distinct regions of BP180 and BP230. J Immunol 2006;176:2015–2023.

35. Liu Z, Diaz L, Troy J, et al. A passive transfer model of the organ-specific autoimmune disease, bullous pemphigoid, using antibodies generated against the hemidesmosomal antigen, BP180. J Clin Invest 1993;92:2480–2488.

36. Sitaru C, Schmidt E, Petermann S, et al. Autoantibodies to bullous pemphigoid antigen 180 induce dermal-epidermal separation in cryosections of human skin. J Invest Dermatol 2002;118:664–671.

37. Jordon R, Kawana S, Fritz K. Immunopathogenic mechanisms in pemphigus and bullous pemphigoid. J Invest Dermatol 1985;85(1 suppl):72s–78s.

38. Nelson K, Zhao M, Schroeder P, et al. Role of different pathways of the complement cascade in experimental bullous pemphigoid. J Clin Invest 2006;116:2892–900.

39. Chen R, Zhou X, Diaz L, et al. Mast cells play a key role in neutrophil recruitment in experimental bullous pemphigoid. J Clin Invest 2001;108:1151–1158.

40. Liu Z, Giudice G, Zhou X, et al. A major role for neutrophils in experimental bullous pemphigoid. J Clin Invest 1997;100:1256–1263.

41. Stahle-Backdahl M, Inoue M, Giudice G, et al. 92–kD gelatinase is produce by eosinophils at the site of blister formation in bullous pemphigoid and cleaves the extracellular domain of recombinant 180kD in bullous pemphigoid autoantigen. J Clin Invest 1994;93:2022–230.

42. Liu Z, Shapiro S, Zhou X, et al. Neutrophil elastase plays a direct role in dermal-epidermal junction separation in experimental bullous pemphigoid. J Clin Invest 2000;105:113–123.

43. Liu Z, Shipley J, Vu T, et al. Gelatinase B-deficient mice are resistant to experimental BP. J Exp Med 1998;188:475–482.

44. Verraes S, Hornebeck W, Polette M, et al. Proteinase/proteinase inhibitor balance in the capacity of 92kDa gelatinase and neutrophil elastase to degrade BP180 (collagen XVII) in bullous pemphigoid. J Invest Dermatol 2001;117:1091–6.

45. Liu Z, Li N, Diaz L, et al. Synergy between a plasminogen cascade and MMP-9 in autoimmune disease. J Clin Invest 2005;115:879–887.

46. Kobayashi M, Amagai M, Kuroda-Kinoshita K, et al. BP180 ELISA using bacterial recombinant NC16a

protein as a diagnostic and monitoring tool for bullous pemphigoid. J Dermatol Sci 2002;30:224–32.

47. Joly P, Roujeau J, Benichou J, et al. A comparison of oral and topical corticosteroids in patients with bullous pemphigoid. N Engl J Med 2002;346:321–7.

48. Lee J, Fumimori T, Kurose K, et al. A case of bullous pemphigoid successfully treated by plasmapheresis: assessment of the change in titers of circulating antibodies by immunoblotting and enzyme-linked immunosorbent assay. J Dermatol 2003;30:326–31.

49. Hatano Y, Katagiri K, Arawaka S, et al. Successful treatment by double-filtration plasmapheresis of a patient with bullous pemphigoid: effects in vivo on transcripts of several genes for chemokines and cytokines in peripheral blood mononuclear cells. Br J Dermatol 2003;148:573–9.

50. Harman KE, Black MM. High-dose intravenous immune globulin for the treatment of autoimmune blistering diseases: an evaluation of its use in 14 cases. Br J Dermatol 1999;140: 865–74.

51. Chan I, Ahmed A, Anhalt G, et al. The first international consensus on mucous membrane pemphigoid: definition, diagnostic criteria, pathogenic factors, medical treatment, and prognostic indicators. Arch Dermatol 2002;138:370–9.

52. Cooper W. Pemphigus of the conjunctiva. Opthal Hosp Rep 1858;1:155–7.

53. Morris M, Roberts H. Pemphigus of the skin and mucous membranes of the mount, associated with "essential shrinking" and pemphigus of the conjunctivae. Br J Dermatol 1889;1:175–81.

54. Civatte A. Le diagnostic des dermatoses bulleuses an laboratorie. Arch Belg Dermatol Syphiligr 1949;5: 273–5.

55. Lever W. Pemphigus: a histopathologic study. Arch Dermatol Syphilol 1951;64:727–53.

56. Lever W. Pemphigus. Medicine 1953;32:1–123.

57. Lever W. Commentary on Brunsting LA, Perry HO. Benign pemphigoid? A report of seven cases with chronic, scarring, herpetiform plaques about the head and neck. Arch Dermatol 1957;75:489–501.

58. Bean S, Waisman M, Michel B, et al. Cicatricial pemphigoid: immunofluorescent studies. Arch Dermatol 1972;105:195–9.

59. Heydenreich G, From E, Diederichsen H. Some unusual findings obtained by the immunofluorescence method in bullous pemphigoid and benign mucous membrane pemphigoid. Acta Derm Venereol 1972;52:201–4.

60. Dantzig P. Circulating antibodies in cicatricial pemphigoid. Arch Deramtol 1973;108:264–6.

61. Bean S. Cicatricial pemphigoid: immunofluorescent studies. Arch Dermatol 1974;110:552–5.

62. Bernard P, Vaillant L, Labeille B, et al. Incidence and distribution of subepidermal autoimmune bullous skin disease in three French regions. Bullous Diseases French Study Group. Arch Dermatol 1995;131:48–52.

63. Matsushima S, Horiguchi Y, Honda T, et al. A case of anti-epiligrin cicatricial pemphigoid associated with lung carcinoma and severe laryngeal stenosis: review of Japanese cases and evaluation of risk for internal malignancy. J Dermatol 2004;31:10–5.

64. Hardy K, Parry H, Pingree G, et al. Benign mucous membrane pemphigoid. Arch Dermatol 1971;104:467–475.

65. Chan L, Yancey K, Hammerberg C, et al. Immune mediated subepithelial blistering diseases of mucous membranes: pure ocular cicatricial pemphigoid is a unique clinical and immunopathological entity distinct from bullous pemphigoid and other subsets identified by antigen specificity of autoantibodies. Arch Dermatol 1993;129:448–455.

66. Hanson R, Olsen K, Rogers R III. Upper aerodigestive tract manifestations of cicatricial pemphigoid. Br J Dermatol 1988;118:209–217.

67. Alexandre M, Brette M, Pascal F, et al. A prospective study of upper aerodigestive tract manifestations of mucous membrane pemphigoid. Medicine 2006;85:239–252.

68. Rogers R III, Perry H, Bean S, et al. Immunopathology of cicatricial pemphigoid: studies of complement deposition. J Invest Dermatol 1977;68:39–43.

69. Mondino B, Ross A, Rabin B, et al. Autoimmune phenomena in ocular cicatricial pemphigoid. Am J Ophthalmol 1977;83:443–450.

70. Rogers R III, Sheridan P, Nightingdale S. Desquamative gingivitis: clinical, histopathologic, immunopathologic, and therapeutic observations. J Am Acad Dermatol 1982;7:729–735.

71. Fine J, Gabrielle R, Neises B, et al. Immunofluorescence and immuno-electron microscopic studies in cicatricial pemphigoid. J Invest Dermatol 1984;82:39–43.

72. Foster C. Cicatricial pemphigoid. Trans Am Opthalmol Soc 1986;84:527–663.

73. Silverman S, Gorsky M, Lozada-Nur F, et al. Oral mucous membrane pemphigoid: a study of 65 patients. Oral Surg Oral Med Oral Pathol 1986;61:233–237.

74. Setterfield J, Shirlaw P, Bhogal B, et al. Cicatricial pemphigoid: serial titers of circulating IgG and IgA antibasement membrane antibodies correlate with disease activity. Br J Dermatol 1999;140:645–650.

75. Setterfield J, Shirlaw P, Karr-Muir M, et al. Mucous membrane pemphigoid: a dual circulating antibody response with IgG and IgA signifies a more severe and persistent disease. Br J Dermatol 1998;138:602–610.

76. Gammon W, Briggaman R, Inman A, et al. Differentiating anti-lamina lucida and anti-sublamina densa anti-BMZ antibodies by indirect immunofluorescence on 1.0M sodium chloride-separated skin. J Invest Dermatol 1984;82:139–144.

77. Kelly S, Wojnarowska F. The use of chemically split tissue in the detection of circulating anti-basement membrane zone antibodies in bullous pemphigoid and cicatricial pemphigoid. Br J Dermaol 1991;24:952–958.

78. Sarrett Y, Hall R, Cobo M, et al. Salt-split human skin substrate for the immunofluorescent screening of serum from patients with cicatricial pemphigoid and a new method of immunoprecipitation with IgA antibodies. J Am Acad Dermatol 1991;24:952–958.

79. Shimizu H, Masunaga T, Ishiko A, et al. Autoantibodies from patients with cicatricial pemphigoid target different sites in epidermal basement membrane. J Invest Dermatol 1995;104:370–373.

80. Egan C, Yancey K. The clinical and immunopathological manifestations of anti-epiligrin cicatricial pemphigoid, a recently defined subepithelial autoimmune blistering disease. Eur J Dermatol 2000;10:585–9.

81. Lazarova Z, Yee C, Darling T, et al. Passive transfer of anti-laminin 5 antibodies induces subepidermal blisters in neonatal mice. J Clin Invest 1996;98:1509–18.

82. Sami N, Bhol K, Razzaque Ahmed A. Intravenous immunoglobulin therapy in patients with multiple mucosal involvement in mucous membrane pemphigoid. Clin Immunol 2002;102:59–67.

83. Canizares M, Smith D, Conners M, et al. Successful treatment of mucous membrane pemphigoid with etanercept in 3 patients. Arch Dermatol 2006;11:1457–61.

84. Thorne J, Jabs D, Qazi F, et al. Mycophenolate mofetil therapy for inflammatory eye disease. Ophthalmology 2005;112:1472–7.

85. Provost T, Tomasi T. Evidence for complement activation via the alternate pathway in skin diseases. I. Herpes gestationis, systemic lupus erythematosus and bullous pemphigoid. J Clin Invest 1973;52:1779–87.

86. Jordon R, Heine K, Tappeiner G, et al. The immunopathology of herpes gestationis. Immunofluorescence studies and characterization of "HG factor." J Clin Invest 1976;57:1426–31.

87. Katz S, Hertz K, Yaoita H. Herpes gestationis. Immunopathology and characterization of the HG factor. J Clin Invest 1976;57:1434–41.

88. Guidice G, Emery D, Diaz L. Cloning and primary structural analysis of the bullous pemphigoid antigen. J Invest Dermatol 1992;99:234–50.

89. Guidice G, Emery D, Zelickson B, et al. Bullous pemphigoid and herpes gestationis autoantibodies recognize a common non-collagenous site on the BP180 ectodomain. J Immunol 1993;151:5742–50.

90. do Valle Chiossi M, Costa R, Ferreira Roselino A. Titration of herpes gestationis factor fixing to C3 in pemphigoid herpes gestationis associated with choriocarcinoma. Arch Dermatol 2000;136:129–30.

91. Tindall J, Rea T, Shulman I, et al. Herpes gestationis in association with a hydatidiform mole: immunopathologic studies. Arch Dermatol 1981;117:510–2.

92. Engineer L, Bhol K, Ahmed A. Pemphigoid gestationis: a review. Am J Obstet Gynecol 2000;183:483–91.

93. Yancey K. Herpes gestationis. Dermatol Clin 1990;8:727–34.

94. Shornik J. Herpes gestationis. J Am Acad Dermatol 1987;17:539–56.

95. Holmes R, Williamson D, Black M. Herpes gestationis persisting for 12 years post partum letter. Arch Dermatol 1986;122:375–6.

96. Lin M, Gharia M, Fu C, et al. Molecular mapping of the major epitopes of BP180 recognized by herpes gestationis autoantibodies. Clin Immunol 1999;92:285–92.

97. Lin M, Gharia M, Swartz S, et al. Identification and characterization of epitopes recognized by T lymphocytes and autoantibodies from patients with herpes gestationis. J Immunol 1999;162:4991–7.

98. Shornick J. Dermatoses of pregnancy. Semin Cutan Med Surg 1998;17:172–81.

99. Carruthers J, Ewins A. Herpes gestationis: studies on the binding characteristics, activity and pathogenetic significance of the complement-fixing factor. Clin Exp Dermatol 1978;31:38–44.

100. Scheman A, Hordinsky M, Groth D, et al. Evidence for eosinophil degranulation in the pathogenesis of herpes gestationis. Arch Dermatol 1989;125:1079–83.

101. Garcia-Gonzales E, Castro-Llamas J, Karchmer S, et al. Class II histocompatibility complex typing across the ethnic barrier in pemphigoid gestationis: a study in Mexicans. Int J Dermatol 1999;38:46–51.

102. Schornick J, Stastny P, Gilliam J. High frequency of histocompatibility antigens HLA-DR3 and DR4 in herpes gestationis. J Clin Invest 1981;68:553–5.

103. Shornick J, Stastny P, Gilliam J. Paternal histocompatibility (HLA) antigens and maternal anti-HLA antibodies in herpes gestationis. J Invest Dermatol 1983;81:407–9.

104. Shornik J, Black M. Secondary autoimmune diseases in herpes gestationis (pemphigoid gestationis). J Am Acad Dermatol 1992;26:563–6.

105. Shornik J, Bangert J, Freeman R, et al. Herpes gestationis in blacks. Arch Dermatol 1984;120:511–3.

106. Shornik J, Bangert J, Freeman R, et al. Herpes gestationis: clinical and histologic features in twenty-eight cases. J Am Acad Dermatol 1983;8:214–24.

107. Shornik J. Herpes gestationis. J Am Acad Dermatol 1987;17:539–56.

108. Kolodny R. Herpes gestationis: a new assessment of incidence and foetal prognosis. Am J Obstet Gynecol 1969;104:39–45.

109. Holmes R, Black M, Jurecka W, et al. Clues to the etiology and pathogenesis of herpes gestationis. Br J Dermatol 1983;109:131–9.

110. Karna P, Broecker A. Neonatal herpes gestationis. J Pediatr 1991;119:299–301.

111. Chen S, Chopra K, Evans T, et al. Herpes gestationis in a mother and child. J Am Acad Dermatol 1999;40:847–9.

112. Lawley T, Stingl G, Katz S. Fetal and maternal risk factors in herpes gestationis. Arch Dermatol 1978;114:552–5.

113. Shornick J, Black M. Fetal risks in herpes gestationis. J Am Acad Dermatol 1992;26:63–8.

114. Morrison L, Anhalt G. Herpes gestationis. J Autoimmun 1991;4:37–45.

115. Anhalt G, Morrison L. Pemphigoid: bullous, gestational and cicatricial. In: Provost T, Weston W, eds. Bullous Diseases. St. Louis: Mosby, 1993:63–113.

116. Castle S, Mather-Mondrey M, Bennion S, et al. Chronic herpes gestationis and antiphospholipid antibody syndrome successfully treated with cyclophosphamide. J Am Acad Dermatol 1996;34:333–6.

117. Fine J, Omura E. Herpes gestationis: persistent disease activity 11 years post partum. Arch Dermatol 1985;121:924–6.

44
Epidermolysis Bullosa Acquisita

Julie Burnett, Jennifer Remington, Mei Chen, and David T. Woodley

Key Points

- Epidermolysis bullosa acquisita is an autoimmune, blistering skin condition, in which there is an autoantibody to type VII collagen, a component of the anchoring fibril complex of the basement membrane zone.
- There are a number of clinical presentations of this disease: the classic porphyria cutanea tarda (PCT)-like, noninflammatory mechanobullous disease; the bullous pemphigoid presentation of widespread inflammatory blisters; the cicatricial pemphigoid–like presentation with mucous membrane involvement; the Brunsting-Perry–like presentation (disease localized to the head and neck area); the immunoglobulin A (IgA) bullous dermatosis–like presentation (inflammatory presentation with a neutrophil-rich infiltrate).
- There are associated complications of this disease, such as esophageal strictures, loss of nails, scarring, and contractures of the hands.
- Epidermolysis bullosa acquisita may be associated with underlying diseases such as inflammatory bowel disease, systemic lupus erythematosus, amyloidosis, and other inflammatory and autoimmune conditions.
- Direct immunofluorescence, along with histology and clinical findings, is used to confirm this diagnosis. Indirect immunofluorescence for mapping studies on NaCl split skin can facilitate distinguishing EBA from bullous pemphigoid. Western blotting confirms that the sera from EBA patients bind to a 290-kd autoantigen (type VII collagen).

- Epidermolysis bullosa acquisita can be challenging to treat. Colchicines and systemic glucocorticosteroids alone or with cytotoxic drugs or cyclosporine have been used to treat severe disease.

Two cases of a blistering disease with adult onset and features highly reminiscent of hereditary dystrophic EB were reported by Elliott in 1895. These clinical features included skin fragility, erosions, blisters, and a healing response characterized by scarring and the formation of milia cysts.

In the early 1970s, Roenigk et al.[1] summarized the epidermolysis bullosa acquisita (EBA) world literature, reported three new cases, and suggested the first diagnostic criteria: (1) a negative family and personal history for a previous blistering disorder, (2) an adult onset of the eruption, (3) spontaneous or trauma-induced blisters that resemble those of hereditary dystrophic epidermolysis bullosa (EB), and (4) the exclusion of all other bullous diseases.

Kushniruk,[2] Gibbs and Minus,[3] and Nieboer et al.[4] showed that patients with EBA had immunoglobulin G (IgG) deposits at the dermal–epidermal junction just like patients with bullous pemphigoid (BP). Nieboer et al. and Yaoita et al.[5] showed that the IgG deposits in EBA were within and below the lamina densa area of the basement membrane zone (BMZ), whereas BP immune deposits are within hemidesmosomes and high in the lamina lucida. Distinguishing EBA from the BP group is important because the clinical, pathologic, and immunologic presentations of EBA may be identical with BP and cicatricial pemphigoid (CP)[6–11] (see below).

Clinical Findings

As noted above the cutaneous lesions of EBA can be quite varied and can mimic other type of acquired autoimmune bullous diseases. The common denominator for patients with EBA is autoimmunity to type VII (anchoring fibril) collagen.[10-13] Although the clinical spectrum of EBA is still being defined, there are at least five clinical presentations: (1) a classic presentation, (2) a BP-like presentation, (3) a CP-like presentation, (4) a presentation reminiscent of Brunsting-Perry pemphigoid with scarring lesions and a predominant head and neck distribution, and (5) a presentation reminiscent of linear IgA bullous dermatosis or chronic bullous disease of childhood.

Classic Presentation

The classic presentation is of a noninflammatory bullous disease with an acral distribution that heals with scarring and milia formation. This presentation is reminiscent of porphyria cutanea tarda (PCT) when it is mild and of the hereditary form of recessive dystrophic EB when it is severe. The classic form of EBA is thus a mechanobullous disease marked by skin fragility. These patients have erosions, tense blisters within noninflamed skin, and scars over trauma-prone surfaces such as the backs of the hands, knuckles, elbows, knees, sacral area, and toes. Some blisters may be hemorrhagic or develop scales, crusts, or erosions. The lesions heal with scarring and frequently with the formation of pearl-like milia cysts within the scarred areas. Although this presentation may be reminiscent of PCT, these patients do not have other hallmarks of PCT, such as hirsutism, a photodistribution of the eruption, or scleroderma-like changes, and their urinary porphyrins are within normal limits. A scarring alopecia and some degree of nail dystrophy may be seen.

Although the disease is usually not as severe as that of patients with hereditary forms of recessive dystrophic EB, EBA patients with the classic form of the disease may have many of the same sequelae, such as scarring, loss of scalp hair, loss of nails, fibrosis of the hands and fingers, and esophageal stenosis.[14-27]

Bullous Pemphigoid–Like Presentation

A second clinical presentation of EBA is of a widespread, inflammatory vesiculobullous eruption involving the trunk, central body, and skin folds in addition to the extremities.[6] The bullous lesions are tense and surrounded by inflamed or even urticarial skin. Large areas of inflamed skin may be seen without any blisters, and only erythema or urticarial plaques. These patients often complain of pruritus and do not demonstrate prominent skin fragility, scarring, or milia formation. This clinical constellation is more reminiscent of BP than of a mechanobullous disorder. Like BP, the distribution of the lesions may show an accentuation within flexural areas and skin folds. About 25% of patients with EBA may present with a BP-like clinical appearance.

Cicatricial Pemphigoid–Like Presentation

Both the classic and BP-like forms of EBA may have involvement of mucosal surfaces. However, EBA also may present with such predominant mucosal involvement that the clinical appearance is reminiscent of CP.[7] These patients usually have erosions and scars on the mucosal surfaces of the mouth, upper esophagus, conjunctiva, anus, or vagina with or without similar lesions on the glabrous skin. The clinical phenotype of EBA that is reminiscent of pure CP occurs in fewer than 10% of all EBA cases.

Brunsting-Perry Pemphigoid–Like Presentation

Brunsting-Perry cicatricial bullous pemphigoid is a chronic recurrent vesiculobullous eruption localized to the head and neck and characterized by residual scars, subepidermal bullae, IgG deposits at the dermal–epidermal junction, and minimal or no mucosal involvement. The antigenic target for the IgG autoantibodies, however, has not been defined. Nevertheless, a patient reported with this constellation of findings had IgG autoantibodies directed to anchoring fibrils below the lamina densa.[11] Therefore, it appears that EBA patients may present with a clinical phenotype of Brunsting-Perry pemphigoid.

Immunoglobulin A Bullous Dermatosis–Like Presentation

This form of EBA is manifested by a subepidermal bullous eruption, a neutrophilic infiltrate, and linear IgA deposits at the BMZ when viewed by direct immunofluorescence (DIF). It may resemble linear IgA bullous dermatosis (LABD), dermatitis herpetiformis, or chronic bullous disease of childhood (CBDC), and may feature tense vesicles arranged in an annular fashion and involvement of mucous membranes.[28–33] The autoantibodies are usually IgA, IgG, or both. Some clinicians regard these patients as having purely LABD,[30] whereas others regard them as having a subset of EBA.[31]

Childhood EBA is a rare disease. It has a variable presentation, with five of 14 patients reviewed presenting with an LABD-like disease, five with BP-like disease, and four with the classic type.[33] Mucosal involvement is frequent in childhood EBA, but the overall prognosis is more favorable than for adults with EBA.[29,33]

In addition to the protean clinical manifestations of EBA, the EBA patient may suffer a number of associated clinical problems that add to the morbidity of the disease. These include oral erosions, esophageal strictures, nail loss, milia formation, scarring, and a degree fibrosis of the hands. These are all associated clinical conditions that are shared (albeit usually milder) with hereditary dystropic EB.

Epidermolysis bullosa acquisita has been linked to some systemic diseases. Inflammatory bowel disease occurs in 20% to 30% of all EBA patients. In addition, anecdotal reports suggest that EBA may have other associated systemic diseases including systemic lupus erythematosus (SLE), amyloidosis, thyroiditis, multiple endocrinopathy syndrome, rheumatoid arthritis, pulmonary fibrosis, chronic lymphocytic leukemia, thymoma, diabetes, and other diseases in which an autoimmune pathogenesis has been implicated.[34,35]

Pathology

Pathology of an EBA lesion shows a subepidermal blister. In the classic mechanobullous presentation of EBA, there is an overall paucity of dermal inflammatory cells. Since EBA lesions tend to occur over and over in the same trauma-prone sites, one frequently observes fibrosis and scarring. In the BP-like EBA presentation, the pathology shows a significant dermal inflammatory infiltrate of lymphocytes, macrophages, monocytes, neutrophils, histiocytes, and eosinophils. In the bullous pemphigoid-like forms and in the IgA EBA form, there is often a predominance of neutrophils.

Direct Immunofluorescence

Krushnick et al.,[2] Gibbs and Minor[3] Nieboer et al.,[4] and Yaoita et al.[5] have shown that a positive DIF is necessary for the diagnosis of EBA. Immunoglobulin G deposits are present at the dermal–epidermal junction by DIF from a perilesional biopsy. One problem with the routine DIF is that it may look exactly like that of bullous pemphigoid in any of the varieties of inflammatory EBA. Performing salt-split skin DIF and indirect immunofluorescence (IIF) are necessary to distinguish EBA from the pemphigoid group of disorders. Perilesional skin is incubated in 1 mol/L cold NaCl for 72 hours, which fractures the dermal–epidermal junction through the lamina lucida of the dermal–epidermal junction. This places the bullous pemphigoid autoantigens associated with the hemidesmosome (i.e., BPAg 1 and BPAg 2, also known as type XVII collagen) on the epidermal roof of the separation.[36–43] The EBA antigen, which is type VII collagen, remains with the dermal floor.[44] If the patient has EBA, the immune deposits are detected on the dermal side of the separation.

Indirect Immunofluorescence

Many, but not all, EBA patients have an anti–BMZ IgG autoantibody circulating in their blood that can be detected by IIF. The EBA serum autoantibodies label frozen sections of human skin or monkey esophagus, producing a crisp linear fluorescent staining at the dermal–epidermal junction of the frozen sections. As with the routine DIF procedure, one cannot distinguish EBA from the pemphigoid group of diseases without doing salt-split IIF, which is always done on human skin substrate. Human skin is incubated in 1 mol/L NaCl, and the dermal–epidermal junction fractures cleanly through the lamina lucida zone, placing the BP antigens on the epidermal roof and the EBA antigen (type VII anchoring fibril collagen) on the dermal floor.[38] Salt-split skin substrate can be used to distinguish EBA and BP sera.[39] If the serum antibody is IgG and labels the epidermal roof, the patient does not have EBA, and BP should be considered. If, on the other hand, the antibody labels the dermal side of the separation, the patient usually has either EBA or bullous SLE. The latter can be ruled out by other serology and by clinical criteria.

Rare Diseases that Give Dermal Staining by Salt-Split Immunofluorescence

It was thought that only EBA and bullous SLE show dermal staining of the salt-split skin on IIF or DIF. In recent years, other very rare autoimmune diseases have been shown to have IgG deposits in the lower lamina lucida space that stay down with the dermis when the skin substrate is fractured by salt. These diseases include anti-laminin 5 cicatricial pemphigoid,[40] a BP-like disease in which the patients have autoantibodies to a 105-kd lamina lucida glycoprotein that is unrelated to laminin-5,[41] a newly discovered disease reported by Ghohestani and colleagues,[43] with IgG autoantibodies directed against the α5 chain of type IV (lamina densa) collagen in association with renal failure, and another BP-like disease called protein 200 pemphigoid in which the autoantigen is a 200-kd glycoprotein in the lower part of the lamina lucida.

Pathogenesis

Although EBA does not have a mendelian pattern of inheritance, African-American EBA patients in the Southeastern part of the United States have a high incidence of the human leukocyte antigen (HLA)-DR2 phenotype. The calculated relative risk for EBA in HLA-DR2+ individuals is 13.1 in these patients.[26] It is thought that although it is not the primary cause, these patients have an immune profile that makes them susceptible to the disease.

While the etiology of EBA is unknown, it appears that when IgG autoantibodies bind to the patient's anchoring fibrils, a paucity of normal anchoring fibrils at the BMZ develops, and this is associated with poor dermal–epidermal adherence. This is exactly the same problem as hereditary dystrophic forms of EB due to a gene defect in the gene that encodes for type VII collagen.

Epidermolysis bullosa acquisita likely has an autoimmune etiology. Direct immunofluorescence of perilesional skin biopsies from EBA patients reveals IgG deposits at the dermal–epidermal junction.[2-5] The EBA antibodies bind to type VII collagen within anchoring fibrils,[12,13] structures that emanate perpendicularly from the BMZ and attached to the papillary dermis. Anchoring fibrils anchor the BMZ to the papillary dermis. In EBA, the IgG autoantibodies binding to the type VII collagen α-chains result in decreased anchoring fibrils, but the pathway leading to this reduction is unknown. Type VII collagen has affinity for fibronectin, a large glycoprotein in the papillary dermis.[21] The interaction between fibronectin and type VII collagen may play a role in adhering the basement membrane beneath the epidermis onto the dermis. It is conceivable that EBA autoantibodies binding to type VII collagen interrupt the interaction between type VII collagen and fibronectin and a separation ensues.

Electron Microscopy

Electron microscopy (EM) shows that the dermal–epidermal separation in an EBA lesion is associated with a paucity of normal anchoring fibrils and an amorphous, electron dense band beneath the lamina densa due to the IgG deposits over the anchoring fibrils.[8] Despite the sublamina densa deposits, EBA blisters frequently separate above the immune deposits within the lamina lucida.[36]

Immunoelectron Microscopy

Immunoelectron microscopy (IEM) localizes the EBA IgG autoantibody deposits in the BMZ to within and below the lamina densa, the location of the anchoring fibrils. Immunoelectron microscopy showing these sublamina densa IgG deposits is the gold standard for the diagnosis, as first demonstrated by Nieboer et al.[4] and Yaoita et al.[5] This localization is distinct from BP IgG deposits, which are localized to the hemidesmosomes of the basal keratinocytes and the IgG autoantibody deposits in CP, which are confined to the lower lamina lucida.

Western Immunoblotting

Antibodies in EBA sera bind to a 290-kd band in Western blots of human skin basement membrane proteins containing type VII collagen, whereas sera from all other primary blistering diseases do not.[12] This band is the α-chain of type VII collagen. Often a second band of 145 kd will be labeled with EBA antibodies. This band is the amino-terminal globular NC1 domain of the type VII collagen α-chain, which is rich in carbohydrate and contains the antigenic epitopes of EBA autoantibodies, bullous SLE autoantibodies, and monoclonal antibodies against type VII collagen.[12,45]

Enzyme-Linked Immunosorbent Assay

Now that unlimited quantities of purified, recombinant, human, type VII collagen are available, an enzyme-linked immunosorbent assay (ELISA) for the diagnosis of EBA was developed by Chen et al.[23,46] It has proven to be more sensitive for detecting EBA autoantibodies in the sera of patients than either IIF or Western blotting analysis.

Diagnosis

The diagnostic criteria for EBA developed by Yaoita et al.[5] still stand. These criteria, with slightly updated modifications, are as follows:

- A bullous disorder within the clinical spectrum outlined earlier
- No family history of a bullous disorder
- Histology showing a subepidermal blister
- Deposition of IgG deposits within the dermal–epidermal junction, that is, a positive DIF of perilesional skin
- IgG deposits localized to the lower lamina densa or sublamina densa zone of the dermal–epidermal junction when perilesional skin is examined by IEM

Alternatives for the last item are indirect or direct salt-split skin immunofluorescence, Western blotting, and ELISA.

Treatment

Epidermolysis bullosa acquisita can be very refractory to most therapies. Probably the least risky form of treatment is colchicine at fairly high doses. The side effects of colchicine are relatively benign compared with other therapeutic choices. Diarrhea is a common side effect of colchicine, especially at higher doses. We do not use colchicine in EBA patients who also have inflammatory bowel disease. Colchicine is a well-known microtubule inhibitor, but it also inhibits antigen presentation to T cells and downregulates autoimmunity.[47,48]

The noninflammatory, mechanobullous type of EBA is notoriously resistant to systemic steroids. Other immunosuppressants such as mycophenolic acid, azathioprine, methotrexate, cyclosporin A, and cyclophosphamide may be somewhat helpful in controlling EBA when it appears as an inflammatory BP-like disease. When using cyclosporin A, relatively high doses are needed in the range of 6 mg/kg, and the nephrotoxicity of this drug sometimes limits its use.[49,50] Some EBA patients improve on dapsone, especially when neutrophils are present in their dermal infiltrate.

Supportive therapy is warranted in all patients with EBA. This includes instruction in open wound care and strategies for avoiding trauma. Patients should be warned not to overwash or overuse hot water or harsh soaps, and to avoid prolonged or vigorous rubbing of their skin with a washcloth or towel. In some patients it appears that prolonged sun exposure may aggravate or promote new lesions on the dorsal hands and knuckles. Avoidance of prolonged sun exposure and the use of sunscreens may be helpful. The patient should be educated to recognize localized skin infections and to seek medical care and antibiotic therapy promptly when they occur.

Photophoresis has been used with success anecdotally in various autoimmune bullous diseases. One reported case of life-threatening EBA had a remarkable recovery when treated with photophoresis.[51] In a small trial of three EBA patients, photophoresis lowered the circulating anti–type VII collagen antibodies in the patients' sera, increased the suctioning blistering times of the patients, and improved the clinical disease.[52]

Intravenous immunoglobulin has been reported to be effective in some patients with EBA.[53] The mechanism by which gamma globulin may invoke a positive response in EBA is unknown.

The anti–tumor necrosis factor-α (TNF-α) biologics have been tried in EBA with some success in limited open trials.

Conclusion

Epidermolysis bullosa acquisita is an example of skin specific autoimmune response, in which there is a type VII collagen autoantibody that is presumed to be pathogenic, and the cause of blistering in the skin. There are a number of clinical variants that can be diagnosed with clinical findings, histology and direct immunofluorescence, and indirect immunofluorescence. When this disease is diagnosed, it is imperative to consider complications of the disease, as well as the associated autoimmune and inflammatory conditions that are frequently associated with EBA. Immunosuppressive therapy is usually required.

References

1. Roenigk HH, et al. Epidermolysis bullosa acquisita: Report of three cases and review of all published cases. Arch Dermatol 1971;103:10.
2. Kushniruk W. The immunopathology of epidermolysis bullosa acquisita. Can Med Assoc J 1973;108:1143.
3. Gibbs RB, Minus HR. Epidermolysis bullosa acquisita with electron microscopical studies. Arch Dermatol 1975;111:215.
4. Nieboer C, et al. Epidermolysis bullosa acquisita: Immunofluorescence, electron microscopic and immunoelectron microscopic studies in four patients. Br J Dermatol 1980;102:383.
5. Yaoita H, et al. Epidermolysis bullosa acquisita: Ultrastructural and immunological studies. J Invest Dermatol 1981;76:288.
6. Gammon WR, et al. Epidermolysis bullosa acquisita: a pemphigoid-like disease. J Am Acad Dermatol 1984;11:820.
7. Dahl MGC. Epidermolysis bullosa acquisita: a sign of cicatricial pemphigoid? Br J Dermatol 1979;101:475.
8. Richter BJ, McNutt NS. The spectrum of epidermolysis bullosa acquisita. Arch Dermatol 1979;115:1325.
9. Provost TT, et al. Unusual sub-epidermal bullous diseases presenting as an inflammatory bullous disease. Arch Dermatol 1979;115:156.
10. Woodley DT. Epidermolysis bullosa acquisita. Prog Dermatol 1988;22:1.
11. Kurzhals G, et al. Acquired epidermolysis bullosa with the clinical features of Brunsting-Perry cicatricial bullous pemphigoid. Arch Dermatol 1991;127:391.
12. Woodley DT, et al. Identification of the skin basement membrane autoantigen in epidermolysis bullosa acquisita. N Engl J Med 1984;310:1007.
13. Woodley DT, et al. The epidermolysis bullosa acquisita antigen is the globular carboxyl terminus of type VII procollagen. J Clin Invest 1988;81:683.
14. Ray TL, et al. Epidermolysis bullosa acquisita and inflammatory bowel disease. J Am Acad Dermatol 1982;6:242.
15. Christiano AM, et al. A common insertion mutation in COLA1 in two Italian families with recessive dystrophic epidermolysis bullosa. J Invest Dermatol 1996;106:679.
16. Parente MG, et al. Human type VII collagen: cDNA cloning and chromosomal mapping of the gene. Proc Natl Acad Sci USA 1991;88:6931.
17. Shimizu H. Molecular basis of recessive dystrophic epidermolysis bullosa: Genotype/phenotype correlation in a case of moderate clinical severity. J Invest Dermatol 1996;106:119.
18. Woodley DT, et al. Burn wounds resurfaced by cultured epidermal autografts show abnormal reconstitution of anchoring fibrils. JAMA 1988;259:2566.
19. Lapiere J-C, et al. Epitope mapping of type VII collagen: Identification of discrete peptide sequences recognized by sera from patients with acquired epidermolysis bullosa. J Clin Invest 1993;92:1831.
20. Jones DA, et al. Immunodominant autoepitopes of type VII collagen are short, paired peptide sequences within the fibronectin type III homology region of the non-collagenous (NC1) domain. J Invest Dermatol 1995;104:231.
21. Woodley DT, et al. Specific affinity between fibronectin and the epidermolysis bullosa acquisita antigen. J Clin Invest 1987;179:1826.
22. Lapiere J-C, et al. Type VII collagen specifically binds fibronectin via a unique subdomain within the collagenous triple helix. J Invest Dermatol 1994;103:637.
23. Chen M, et al. Interactions of the amino-terminal noncollagenous (NC1) domain of type VII collagen with extracellular matrix components. J Biol Chem 1997;272:14516.
24. Gammon WR, et al. Evidence that antibasement membrane zone antibodies in bullous eruption of systemic lupus erythematosus recognize epidermolysis bullosa acquisita autoantigens. J Invest Dermatol 1985;84:472.
25. Barradori L, et al. Passive transfer of autoantibodies from a patient with mutilating epidermolysis bullosa acquisita induces specific alterations in the skin of neonatal mice. Arch Dermatol 1995;131:590.
26. Gammon WR, et al. Increased frequency of HLA DR2 in patients with autoantibodies to EBA antigen: Evidence that the expression of autoimmunity to

type VII collagen is HLA class II allele associated. J Invest Dermatol 1988;91:228.

27. Stewart MI, Woodley DT. Acquired epidermolysis bullosa and associated symptomatic esophageal webs. Arch Dermatol 1991;127:373.

28. Park SB, et al. Epidermolysis bullosa acquisita in childhood: a case mimicking chronic bullous dermatosis of childhood. Clin Exp Dermatol 1997;22:220.

29. Callot-Mellot C, et al. Epidermolysis bullosa acquisita in childhood. Arch Dermatol 1997;133:1122.

30. Hashimoto T, et al. A case of linear IgA bullous dermatosis with IgA anti-type VII collagen autoantibodies. Br J Dermatol 1996;134:336.

31. Bauer JW, et al. Ocular involvement in IgA-epidermolysis bullosa acquisita. Br J Dermatol 1999;141:887.

32. Lee CW. Serum IgA autoantibodies in patients with epidermolysis bullosa acquisita: a high frequency of detection. Dermatology 2000;200:83.

33. Edwards S, et al. Bullous pemphigoid and epidermolysis bullosa acquisita: presentation, prognosis and immunopathology in 11 children. Pediatr Dermatol 1998;15:184.

34. Burke WA, et al. Epidermolysis bullosa acquisita in a patient with multiple endocrinopathies syndrome. Arch Dermatol 1986;122:187.

35. Chan L, Woodley DT. Pemphigoid: bullous and cicatricial. In: Lichtenstein LM, Fauci AS, eds. Current Therapy in Allergy, Immunology and Rheumatology, 5th ed. St. Louis: Mosby, 1996:93.

36. Fine JD, et al. The presence of intra-lamina lucida blister formation in epidermolysis bullosa acquisita: possible role of leukocytes. J Invest Dermatol 1989;92:27.

37. Briggaman RA, et al. Degradation of the epidermal-dermal junction by proteolytic enzymes from human skin and human polymorphonuclear leukocytes. J Exp Med 1984;160:1027.

38. Woodley DT, et al. Localization of basement membrane components after dermal-epidermal junction separation. J Invest Dermatol 1983;81:149.

39. Gammon WR, et al. Differentiating anti-lamina lucida and antisublamina dense anti-BMZ antibodies by direct immunofluorescence on 1.0 M sodium chloride separated skin. J Invest Dermatol 1983;84:215.

40. Domloge-Hultsch N, et al. Antiepiligrin cicatricial pemphigoid: a subepithelial bullous disorder. Arch Dermatol 1994;130:1521.

41. Chan LS, et al. A newly identified 105-kDa lower lamina lucida autoantigen is an acidic protein distinct from the 105-kDa gamma 2 chain of laminin 5. J Invest Dermatol 1995;105:75.

42. Ceilley E, et al. Labeling of fractured human skin with antibodies to BM 600/nicein, epiligrin, kalinin and other matrix components. J Dermatol Sci 1993;5:97.

43. Ghohestani RF, et al. The a5 chain of type IV collagen is the target of IgG autoantibodies in a novel autoimmune disease with subepidermal blisters and renal insufficiency. J Biol Chem 2000;275:16002.

44. Gammon WR, et al. Direct immunofluorescence studies of sodium chloride–separated skin in the differential diagnosis of bullous pemphigoid and epidermolysis bullosa acquisita. J Am Acad Dermatol 1990;22:664.

45. Woodley DT, et al. Epidermolysis bullosa acquisita antigen, a new major component of cutaneous basement membrane, is a glycoprotein with collagenous domains. J Invest Dermatol 1986;86:668.

46. Chen M, et al. Development of an ELISA for rapid detection of anti–type VII collagen autoantibodies in epidermolysis bullosa acquisita. J Invest Dermatol 1997;108:68.

47. Cunningham BB, et al. Colchicine for epidermolysis bullosa (EBA). J Am Acad Dermatol 1996;34:781.

48. Mekori YA, et al. Inhibition of delayed hypersensitivity reaction by colchicine: Colchicine inhibits interferon-gamma-induced expression of HLA-DR on an epithelial cell line. Clin Exp Immunol 1989;78:230.

49. Connolly SM, Sander HM. Treatment of epidermolysis bullosa acquisita with cyclosporin. J Am Acad Dermatol 1987;16:890.

50. Crow LL, et al. Clearing of epidermolysis bullosa acquisita on cyclosporin A. J Am Acad Dermatol 1988;19:937.

51. Miller JL, et al. Remission of severe epidermolysis bullosa acquisita induced by extracorporeal photochemotherapy. Br J Dermatol 1995;133:467.

52. Gordon K, et al. Treatment of refractory epidermolysis bullosa acquisita with extracorporeal photochemotherapy. Br J Dermatol 1997;136:415.

53. Meier F, et al. Epidermolysis bullosa acquisita: efficacy of high dose intravenous immunoglobulins. J Am Acad Dermatol 1993;29:334.

45
Immunoglobulin A Dermatoses

Todd V. Cartee and Robert A. Swerlick

Key Points

- Immunoglobulin A (IgA) dermatoses are a diverse group of conditions in which the disease process occurs directly from IgA in the lesional or perilesional skin.
- This group of diseases has in common the presence of a neutrophil-rich inflammatory infiltrate and pharmacologic responsiveness to dapsone therapy.
- The cellular receptor for IgA (FcαR1) are of limited distribution (predominantly neutrophils), which may, in part, explain the neutrophil-rich infiltrates observed in these disorders. Engagement of the IgA receptor can activate neutrophils to degranulate, mediate cytotoxicity, develop a respiratory burst, and activate endocytosis. All of these activation processes are likely to play a role in the tissue damage that is observed in the IgA dermatoses.
- This group of diseases includes dermatitis herpetiformis, linear IgA bullous dermatosis, IgA pemphigus (both subcorneal and intraepidermal types), and Henoch-Schönlein purpura.

The diseases reviewed in this chapter all share one common immunohistologic feature. In each, the cutaneous deposition of immunoglobulin A (IgA) is demonstrable by direct immunofluorescence. It is presumed, though not proven, that the cutaneous eruptions manifest in these diseases stem directly from immunologic responses to this IgA. All these dermatoses typically possess two characteristics: (1) a neutrophil predominant infiltrate, and (2) a pharmacologic sensitivity to dapsone.

These commonalities aside, however, it is important to note that these diseases are also linked by a relatively poor understanding of their respective pathophysiologies, especially when compared to IgG-mediated dermatoses, rendering proper categorization based on a common biologic mechanism difficult. Therefore, the adopted grouping of IgA dermatoses in this chapter has its limitations. Furthermore, in addition to the accepted IgA dermatoses, IgA deposition is not infrequently detected in skin biopsies from connective tissue and autoimmune diseases, where IgG or IgM is generally considered the predominant immunoreactant (e.g., cutaneous lupus erythematosus and bullous pemphigoid). Whether the presence of IgA in these disorders is incidental or possesses pathologic, diagnostic, or prognostic significance is not known. In our experience, the clinical presentation of diseases discussed in this chapter may resemble their IgG-mediated counterparts more closely than they resemble each other.

Immunoglobulin A

Of the five antibody classes (IgA, IgD, IgG, IgE, and IgM), IgA is by far the predominant antibody in mucosal secretions, where it assumes its well-characterized role in neutralizing respiratory, gastrointestinal, and genitourinary pathogens. Perhaps less well appreciated, IgA is also the second most prevalent antibody in human serum at a concentration of 2 to 3 mg/mL (compared to 12 mg/mL IgG), and, given a serum half-life of one-fifth that of IgG, this implies the rate of production of serum IgA equals or exceeds that of IgG. The large energy expenditure in producing this tremendous quantity of nonsecretory IgA would suggest critical immunologic functions outside of mucosal defense, but this role for IgA remains mysterious.[1]

Two subclasses of IgA exist: IgA1 and IgA2. Except for the colon, IgA1 is the predominant isoform, both in serum and in bodily secretions, though IgA2 is relatively more abundant in the latter. Approximately 90% of serum IgA consists of monomeric IgA1 that is produced by the bone marrow with no apparent relationship to mucosally derived IgA. Secretory IgA (S-IgA) generally exists as a dimer with the Fc regions covalently linked by a protein known as the J-chain, which also forms the hub of the IgM pentamer. Secretory IgA is further adorned with a polypeptide, the secretory component that is enzymatically cleaved from the epithelial cell-surface receptor, the polymeric immunoglobulin receptor (pIgR). PIgR coordinates the transport of IgA from mucosal lymphoid tissue, where it is synthesized, to the apical epithelial border, where it is secreted.[2]

Secretory IgA protects the mucosa from a constant barrage of pathogens, toxins, and foreign antigens. By physically coating critical epitopes, S-IgA impairs microbial adherence and function and shields the body from toxins or, potentially worse, from innocuous antigens that might otherwise stimulate undesirable or unnecessary immune responses.[1] More recently, interactions between IgA and immune cells have been elucidated, which mediate important immunologic events in various extramucosal tissues including the skin. Immunoglobulin A is a relatively weak activator of complement and does not readily opsonize microbes. However, a receptor for IgA, FcαR1, is expressed on neutrophils, primarily, and also on eosinophils, monocytes, and some macrophages. Whereas IgG receptors (FcγRs) are present on all immune cells, FcαR1 has a more limited distribution, which may explain why the infiltrate typically observed in IgA-mediated dermatoses is so consistently neutrophil predominant. Engagement of FcαRI by IgA immune complexes can trigger numerous biologic responses, including endocytosis, antigen presentation, antibody-dependent cell-mediated cytotoxicity (ADCC), respiratory burst, and degranulation. Presumably, these processes provide the mechanism for the clinical sequelae

of cutaneous IgA deposition. Furthermore, given this distinct biologic activity, differences in clinical presentations and biologic behavior between IgA dermatoses and those mediated by antibodies that are more efficient fixers of complement (IgG and IgM) should not be surprising.

General Features of Immunoglobulin A Dermatoses

Immunoglobulin A dermatoses are defined as cutaneous diseases that demonstrate IgA deposition in involved or perilesional skin. While their proper diagnosis is contingent on positive immunofluorescence studies, there are some general similarities among these diseases that stem from the unique characteristics of the IgA antibody class. Because the IgA initiated immunologic responses detailed above are all cell-mediated, the pathogenesis of IgA-mediated disease requires the presence of immune cells, which can interact with antigen-bound IgA. Thus, IgA dermatoses tend to exhibit a marked neutrophilic infiltrate with varied numbers of eosinophils and macrophages. This group of diseases also responds to drugs that antagonize neutrophil function. The chief example is dapsone, which has been shown to inhibit neutrophil myeloperoxidase, the key enzyme responsible for the respiratory burst, and the secretion of proteases, such as elastase.[3] Dapsone also clearly interferes with neutrophil chemotaxis. Dapsone inhibits integrin-mediated neutrophilic adhesion and attenu-

TABLE 45.1. Immunoglobulin A (IgA) dermatoses and their IgG counterparts.

IgA dermatoses	IgG counterpart
Dermatitis herpetiformis	None
Linear IgA bullous dermatoses/chronic bullous disease of childhood	Bullous pemphigoid
IgA pemphigus: subcorneal pustular dermatosis type	Pemphigus foliaceus
IgA pemphigus: intraepidermal type	Pemphigus vulgaris
IgA vasculitis (Henoch-Schönlein purpura)	Cutaneous leukocytoclastic vasculitis (LCV)*

*IgtM immune complex deposition is more common than IgG in cutaneous LCV.

ates intracellular signaling induced by a number of neutrophil chemoattractants—leukotriene B_4 (LTB_4), interleukin-8 (IL-8), and C5a—in vitro.[4]

The diseases selected for discussion in this chapter are listed in Table 45.1 along with the IgG-mediated disease, when one exists, which demonstrates a similar pattern of antibody deposition.

Dermatitis Herpetiformis

Dermatitis herpetiformis (DH) is a chronic, severely pruritic subepidermal blistering disease mainly affecting the extensor skin surfaces. It is also known as Duhring's disease, named after the University of Pennsylvania physician, Dr. Louis Duhring, who first described DH in 1884. The cutaneous manifestations are thought to be secondary to an immune response engendered by IgA immune complex deposition in the dermal papillae. The disease is strongly if not uniformly associated with gluten-sensitive enteropathy (celiac disease), which is characteristically, though not always, subclinical.

Epidemiology

Dermatitis herpetiformis predominantly afflicts individuals of Northern European descent, with few reported cases in other ethnic groups. Most studies demonstrate a male/female ratio of 1.5:1 to 2:1. Onset of disease generally occurs between ages 20 and 45, but DH does occur in children, in whom a female preponderance was observed in one published series. The only U.S. prevalence study was conducted in a relatively homogeneous Northern European population in Utah with a reported prevalence of 11.2 per 100,000.[5]

A remarkably strong association with a few specific major histocompatibility complex (MHC) class II molecules within the human leukocyte antigen (HLA) DQ2 serotype has been reported in DH patients. Each human haplotype possesses three loci on chromosome 6 coding for three MHC class II heterodimers: HLA-DP, -DQ, and –DR. HLA-DQ is composed of immensely polymorphic α (A1) and β (B1) chains. One unique A1 gene product of the HLA-DQA1*0501 allele combined with any one of four nearly identical B1 gene products from alleles sharing the HLA-DQB1*02

designation has been shown in 86% of DH patients compared to 25% of healthy controls. The majority of the remaining patients express an HLA-DQ8 antigen, genotype (A1*03, B1*0302).[6] Previous reported associations with the class II HLA-DR3 and class I HLA-B8 serotypes are now thought to result from linkage disequilibrium, that is, a nonrandom association between the alleles coding for these antigens and those coding for the DQ2 antigen, the class II heterodimer correlating most strongly with DH.

Pathogenesis

A revolution in our understanding of DH occurred in 1967 with the proposal of a link between DH and celiac disease (CD).[7] It has now been well established that virtually all patients with DH show histologic changes in the jejunal mucosa that are indistinguishable from those in CD, including intraepithelial lymphocytes, increased lymphocytes and plasma cells in the lamina propria, and variable degrees of villous atrophy. However, cardinal gastrointestinal symptoms of CD (foul-smelling diarrhea, steatorrhea, flatulence, abdominal cramps, and bloating) are quite uncommon in DH, as are the extraintestinal effects of malabsorption (anemia, osteopenia, vitamin deficiencies). Only 20% of DH patients have clearly demonstrable sequelae of CD by history or laboratory examination, and these are almost always mild.

Because the manifestations of both CD and DH are so exquisitely dependent on its ingestion, gluten has long been implicated as the inciting factor in the pathogenesis of both diseases. Gluten is a mixture of proteins present in wheat, barley, and rye. Gliadin is the alcohol soluble fraction of gluten and it possesses the immunogenic proteins. Antigliadin antibodies are very common in patients with gluten-sensitive disorders but do not appear to be pathogenic. Gliadin has never been identified in the skin of patients with DH. However, resolution of both CD and DH is almost invariable when patients remove gluten from their diets, underscoring a critical if seemingly indirect role.

In contrast to other immunobullous disease such as bullous pemphigoid or pemphigus, patients with DH do not have circulating antibodies that bind to any component of the dermis or epidermis when examined using indirect immunofluorescence (IIF) techniques. Patients with DH frequently have circulating antibodies that react with esophageal smooth muscle termed anti–endomysial antibodies (EMAs), which are specific for both DH and CD. The target antigen for EMA has been identified as tissue transglutaminase (TGc), which is now the accepted autoantigen of CD.[8] TGc is present both in the gut and in the skin, where it catalyzes the cross-linking of polypeptides. Gliadin forms irreversible complexes with TGc, which enzymatically alters gliadin, creating antigenic epitopes. In genetically susceptible people, there seems to be progression over time from gliadin reactive T cells to TGc-reactive T cells by epitope spreading. Anti-TGc antibodies may be responsible for the enteropathy, but TGc is not present in dermal papillae of patients with DH. Furthermore, it has never been clear why only a small portion of CD patients exhibit DH despite the shared autoantibodies.

An important clue to resolving this quandary emerged in 2002 when Sardy et al.[9] proposed that epidermal transglutaminase (TGe) was the autoantigen of DH. They presented evidence that, while both DH and CD patients have circulating anti-TGc antibodies, only DH patients have specific, high-avidity antibodies against TGe. In addition, TGe, which is normally present exclusively in the epidermis, was shown to colocalize with IgA in the granular deposits within dermal papillae of DH patients. TGe may covalently cross-link IgA to dermal proteins, potentially explaining the remarkable persistence of dermal IgA deposits in DH, which have been observed even after a decade of gluten-free dietary restriction. Covalent linkage would also account for the inability to extract IgA complexes from DH skin, a phenomenon that had thwarted previous efforts to characterize the DH autoantigen.

The identification of a unique population of autoantibodies in DH represents an important advance in our understanding of its pathogenesis. Sardy et al.'s[9] results support the widely held contention that DH is an immune-complex–mediated disease. Where the TGe-IgA complexes form and why they preferentially deposit in the dermis remain areas of active investigation.

As in the other IgA dermatoses, the clinical manifestations of DH are secondary to the destructive effects of activated neutrophils. IgA complexes are certainly capable of activating neutrophils via FcαR1 engagement, but the factors that mediate the immigration of neutrophils into the dermis have never been identified. In DH, patients' IgA deposits are present in unaffected, perilesional skin, and IgA deposits persist in the dermis long after complete clinical resolution on a gluten-free diet. Obviously, other pathogenic factors beyond IgA-TGe deposition must be involved in actual skin lesion formation, but their identification has been elusive.

A promising new development in DH research came fortuitously when researchers, in an attempt to generate a mouse model of CD, observed the emergence of a blistering disorder that histologically and clinically was remarkably similar to DH.[10] Fifteen of 90 nonobese diabetic (NOD) mice, which have an increased susceptibility to autoimmune disease, expressing human HLA-DQ8 and challenged with gluten, both intraperitoneally and orally, developed subepidermal blistering of their ears. Histology showed IgA deposits in the dermal papillae with neutrophilic infiltrate. Blistering resolved on a gluten-free diet. However, the mice did not exhibit any enteropathy, and no EMA, anti-TGc, or anti-TGe antibodies were detectable. Although the model is an imperfect reproduction of DH, studying the gluten-sensitive bullous disease evoked in these mice may provide some answers to the many perplexing, unanswered questions regarding the pathophysiology of DH.

Clinical Features

Dermatitis herpetiformis is characterized by a symmetric polymorphic eruption along extensor surfaces. The forearms, elbows, back, buttocks, and knees are favored sites. In contrast to the other immunobullous diseases with which DH is frequently grouped in textbooks, it rarely presents with bullae. The pruritus of DH is so intense that lesions seldom evolve beyond small vesicles before being mechanically ruptured by the suffering patient. Thus, grouped herpetiform, papules, and vesicles on an erythematous base with excoriations and hemorrhagic crusting is the most common clinical picture (Fig. 45.1A). Lesions may coalesce into urticarial plaques (Fig. 45.1B). Often patients experience localized burning, stinging, or itching 12 to 24 hours prior to the emergence of skin lesions. Dermatitis

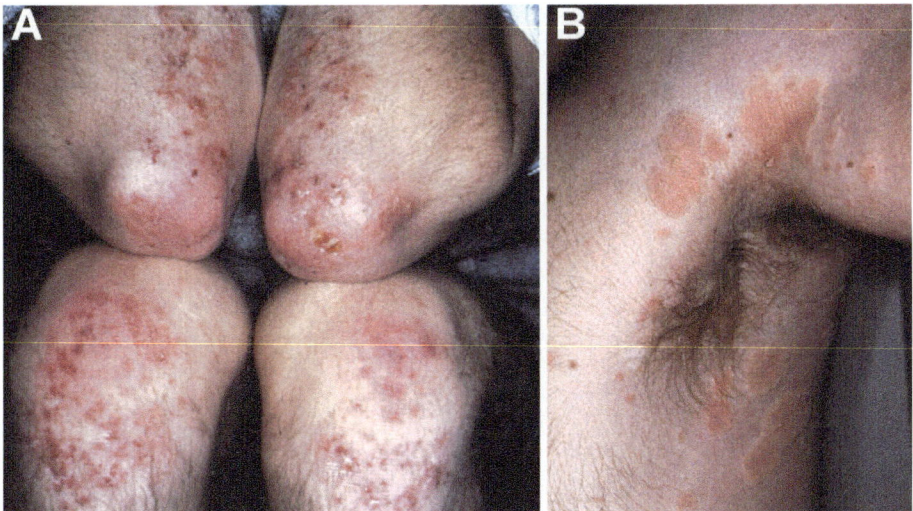

F<small>IG</small>. 45.1. Dermatitis herpetiformis. (A) Typical presentation demonstrating symmetric erythematous papules and vesicles with hemorrhagic crusting and excoriations on elbows and knees. (B) Urticarial plaques are a common clinical variant

herpetiformis tends to have a chronic remitting and relapsing course. Intense flares may be associated with a particularly robust gluten challenge. Mucous membrane involvement is uncommon.

An association with autoimmune thyroiditis is well established, with 32% of DH patients exhibiting hypo- or hyperthyroidism in one series, and should prompt thyroid function tests in all newly diagnosed patients.[11] Other autoimmune disorders have also been associated with DH. Non-Hodgkin's lymphoma, chiefly enteropathy type T-cell lymphoma of the small intestine, occurs at a rate of about 1% in DH patients with men being at higher risk.[12] Dapsone and related drugs suppress cutaneous disease, but only a gluten-free diet results in a reduction in lymphoma risk, providing the primary rationale for adherence to a difficult to manage diet when other gastrointestinal (GI) symptoms are absent.

Histology

Biopsies of nonexcoriated early lesions provide the most useful information for conventional histology. Early primary lesions exhibit dermal edema and a prominent neutrophilic infiltrate with variable numbers of eosinophils. The changes may be concentrated in the dermal papillae where

neutrophilic microabscesses are seen (Fig. 45.2A). While highly suggestive of a diagnosis of DH, none of these features is pathognomonic. One cannot overemphasize that routine histology is inadequate to distinguish DH from other subepidermal blistering disorders consistently and reliably.

As in all the diseases in this chapter, immunofluorescent studies are essential for definitive diagnosis. Unaffected skin should be obtained for direct immunofluorescence (DIF). One small study suggested that biopsies obtained 3 to 5 mm from noninflamed, perilesional skin demonstrate the most robust IgA deposits,[13] although these authors have not observed significantly better diagnostic yields from perilesional specimens. Instead, we routinely biopsy photoprotected skin from the upper arm or buttock. Nonuniform IgA distribution in affected patients may require more than a single biopsy to demonstrate the characteristic IgA deposits. Unquestionably biopsy of involved skin may yield false negatives, as the epidermis may be missing, and deposited IgA is frequently destroyed by the exuberant neutrophilic response in DH. Granular deposits of IgA in the dermal papillae or along the basement membrane zone are diagnostic (Fig. 45.2B). Less commonly, IgA deposits may be seen decorating the fibrillar network of proteins extensively through the papillary dermis. Indirect

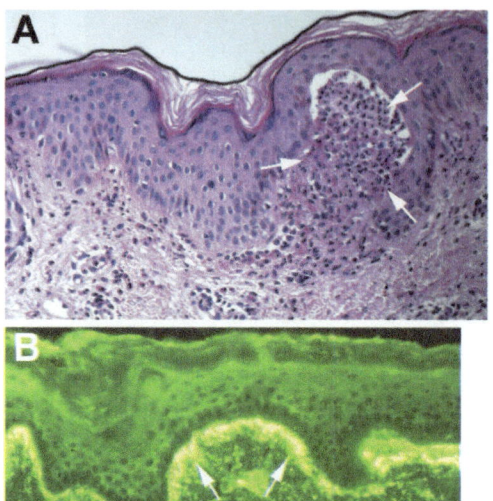

Fig. 45.2. Dermatitis herpetiformis. (A) Intense neutrophilic infiltrate localized in a papillary microabscess (arrows). (B) Direct immunofluorescence reveals dense granular deposits of immunoglobulin A (IgA) along the basement membrane that is most intense in the dermal papillae (arrows)

immunofluorescence using skin substrates should be negative, but IIF studies looking for EMA may provide additional information supportive of a diagnosis of DH.

Treatment

Pharmacologic approaches to DH are heavily reliant on the sulfone antibiotic dapsone (diaminodiphenyl sulfone). Sulfapyridine, a sulfonamide antibiotic, may also be effective for DH, with the potential trade-off of better tolerability for modestly less efficacy. However, this medication is no longer available in the United States. Either agent effects a rapid cessation of new lesion formation and resolution of pruritus. Prior to the widespread availability of immunofluorescence studies, a positive therapeutic trial of dapsone was believed to represent solid diagnostic evidence of DH. However, subsequent follow-up revealed misdiagnosis in almost half of patients diagnosed on this basis.[14]

Dapsone is widely used throughout the world to treat leprosy, prevent malaria, and provide prophylaxis for patients at risk for *Pneumocystis* pneumonia. It is generally well tolerated at modest doses but can cause problems in genetically predisposed individuals in both a dose-dependent and idiosyncratic fashion (Table 45.2). All patients who take dapsone in sufficient doses suffer some degree of red blood cell hemolysis, with greater effects seen at greater doses. Patients with DH can be started at 50 mg daily, which may result in a transient 1- to 2-g drop in hemoglobin due to the lysis of older red blood cells. Hemoglobin levels generally rebound quickly.

The dose should be increased by 25 to 50 mg every 2 to 4 weeks until adequate suppression of symptoms is achieved. Most patients respond to 100 mg of dapsone daily or less. Since the most common side effects are dose dependent, the minimal effective dose should be sought. Patients generally tolerate dosages up to 200 mg daily. Intractable cases may be approached with dosages as high as 400 mg qd, but side effects typically prohibit prolonged therapy at this level. Once the skin rash is controlled, the daily dapsone dose should be tapered at a rate of 25 mg every 2 to 4 weeks with the goal of establishing a stable maintenance regimen at 25 or 50 mg qd.

Patients who are genetically deficient in glucose-6-phosphate dehydrogenase (G6PD) may suffer from severe hemolysis after taking even modest doses of dapsone. While G6PD deficiency

TABLE 45.2. Adverse effects of dapsone therapy.

Dose dependent (Rarely significant at doses ≤100 mg/d)	Hemolytic anemia
	Methemoglobinemia
	Headache
	Nausea
	Lethargy
	Cyanosis
Idiosyncratic	Agranulocytosis
	Gastrointestinal irritation
	Cholestasis
	Psychosis
	Peripheral neuropathy (distal motor)
	Dapsone hypersensitivity syndrome
	Mononucleosis-like illness with fever, polymorphic skin eruption, and lymphadenopathy
	Toxic hepatitis and hepatosplenomegaly

occurs most frequently in those of African and Mediterranean descent, it has been reported in most ethnic groups. In addition, although G6PD deficiency is an X-linked recessive disorder, carriers may experience hemolytic crises. Therefore, a prudent approach is to screen all patients to be treated with dapsone for G6PD deficiency.

Methemoglobinemia is another invariable consequence of dapsone therapy but is uncommonly symptomatic at doses below 150 mg daily in otherwise healthy individuals. Methemoglobin is an oxidized form of hemoglobin that lacks oxygen-carrying capacity. Thus, the symptoms of methemoglobinemia are those of anemia or hypoxia and include headache, lethargy, cyanosis, and dyspnea. Patients with compromised cardiovascular function are more sensitive to the conversion of relatively small amounts of their hemoglobin to methemoglobin. Both vitamin E (800 IU/day) and cimetidine (400 mg t.i.d.) confer some protection against methemoglobinemia and hemolysis, with the latter probably the more efficacious agent. Intravenous or oral methylene blue may be used acutely in severe methemoglobinemia.

Dapsone may also cause a variety of adverse reactions on an idiosyncratic or allergic basis (Table 45.2), of which potentially fatal agranulocytosis is the most worrisome. Interestingly, DH patients appear to be at markedly higher risk for dapsone-induced agranulocytosis than patients on dapsone for leprosy or malaria prophylaxis. The risk among a series of DH patients in Sweden was measured at 1:240 to 1:425.[15] Cases present an average of 7 weeks after initiation of therapy and are rare after 12 weeks. Fever and sore throat must immediately evoke suspicion for this uncommon but serious reaction.

A second notable idiosyncratic reaction is the "dapsone hypersensitivity syndrome," which presents with the triad of fever, rash, and internal organ involvement (typically hepatitis). A mononucleosis-like illness with a polymorphic but most often morbilliform rash presenting 1 to 6 weeks after starting dapsone is characteristic. Elevated erythrocyte sedimentation rate and liver transaminases occur in all patients.

A prior allergic reaction to sulfonamide antibiotics modestly increases the risk of dapsone allergy over that in the general population, and dapsone is not strictly contraindicated in patients with a history of mild sulfonamide hypersensitivity reactions.[16] Administration of sulfones in this setting can be considered, but close observation and education of such patients are mandatory.

Dapsone therapy requires vigilant laboratory monitoring. A complete blood cell count with differential and a comprehensive metabolic panel including liver function tests should be obtained before starting therapy. As mentioned earlier, thyroid function and G6PD activity should also be assessed at this time. Complete blood cell counts should be checked twice monthly for the first 2 months of dapsone therapy followed by monthly checks for the next 2 months. In addition, liver function tests should be checked monthly for the first 4 months. Thereafter, complete blood parameters should be obtained every 3 to 6 months depending on the clinical context. Patients without confounding medical problems on long-term therapy with moderate doses without evidence of dapsone toxicity require less laboratory scrutiny and may need only annual studies.

The chief alternative therapeutic strategy to dapsone is a gluten-free diet (GFD). The strict avoidance of gluten leads to resolution of skin lesions and is the only effective therapy for gluten-sensitive enteropathy. However, control of the skin eruption may take months to years on GFD alone, so concomitant administration of dapsone is customary. After several months of combined dietary and pharmacologic treatment, dapsone may be tapered and often discontinued. Although the lifelong avoidance of gluten is a considerable challenge, it should be offered to all patients. A GFD may be especially attractive to patients with bothersome gastrointestinal symptoms or those desirous of nonpharmacologic therapy. Clearly, in patients unable to tolerate sulfones or with significant G6PD deficiency or hemoglobinopathies, GFD is the treatment of choice. Copious information and support for patients are available from the Celiac Sprue Association (http://www.csaceliacs.org/).

There is also an important role for medium- and high-potency topical steroids in DH. Topical corticosteroids can alleviate symptoms and expedite the healing of skin lesions. They are appropriate for patients who experience occasional localized disease flairs and are otherwise well controlled on GFD or dapsone therapy.

Linear Immunoglobulin A Bullous Dermatosis

Linear IgA bullous dermatosis (LABD) is an acquired, autoimmune, subepidermal blistering disorder that affects both children and adults. When presenting in children, it is commonly referred to as chronic bullous disease of childhood (CBDC), but the almost complete identity in pathophysiology argues against classification of CBDC as a separate entity. The label LABD encompasses dermatoses that are heterogeneous in distribution and morphology but are unified by the presence of a linear deposition of IgA at the basement membrane of perilesional skin. In its two most common presentations, LABD can either resemble DH or have an appearance reminiscent of bullous pemphigoid (BP).

Epidemiology

The disease is sufficiently rare to make any detailed epidemiologic data difficult to obtain. Age of onset exhibits a bimodal distribution, affecting either the elderly or children between 1 and 10 years of age. However, LABD can occur at any age. No racial or consistent gender predilections have been reported. Incidence is at least 20-fold less than DH.

The HLA associations have not been as extensively studied as in DH, and a precise association with a specific genotype has yet to emerge. The largest series demonstrated that LABD patients were more than twice as likely to carry the HLA-Cw7, -DR3, or -B8 serotypes as ethnically matched controls.[17]

Pathogenesis

Unlike DH, selected patients with LABD have circulating IgA class antibodies whose target antigens are present in normal skin; that is, IIF is frequently positive. One consensus basement membrane autoantigen for all of the dermatoses that meet the current immunofluorescent criterion for a diagnosis of LABD does not exist. The antigenic profile of LABD is as heterogeneous as its clinical presentations. Studies examining generally small numbers of LABD patient sera have yielded discordant results, with rare agreement on the most prevalent autoantigen, highlighting the complexity of the immune response in LABD.

A recent analysis of a large series of LABD patients, using a more sensitive immunoblotting technique in concert with IIF, found 10 different autoantigens among the 76% of patients with identifiable epidermal antigens and the 61% with dermal antigens.[18,19] The significant overlap between the two groups casts doubt on the utility of dividing LABD into subtypes based on autoantigen location, which has been proposed by others (e.g., LABD-sublamina densa type). The authors did not explicitly state if any patients had antibodies solely against a dermal antigen, but the vast majority, if not all, of the patients with identifiable autoantigens had epidermal antigens. 94% of these patients had antibodies against BP180, a keratinocyte transmembrane protein and critical hemidesmosomal component, which is the target for the pathogenic antibodies in bullous pemphigoid. Of the dermal antigens detected by patient sera, LAD285 was the most common (58%), followed closely by BP180. Other antigens commonly identified were BP230 and LABD97; the latter is a proteolytic product of the extracellular domain of BP180. Reactivity to multiple antigens was common (42%). The authors speculate that the multiplicity of antigens within individuals results from inter- and intramolecular epitope spreading over time from BP180, the presumed initial focus of the autoimmune response. Circulating IgG antibodies against a more limited spectrum of autoantigens (primarily BP180 with a few positive for BP230) were present in 47% of patients. The pathophysiologic significance of IgG in these patients is not clear.

Regardless of the target antigen, once IgA is deposited in the skin, the pathophysiology of LABD follows the general theme of IgA dermatoses. Unlike its IgG-mediated cousin BP, where cell-poor variants have been described, a pronounced neutrophilic infiltrate is a sine qua non of LABD. The epidermal–dermal separation is thus deemed secondary to the elaboration of proteases and potent oxidants by the invading neutrophils. The dependence of the manifestations of LABD on neutrophilic function rather than direct antibody effects is consistent with the lack of specificity in the autoantibodies detected among groups of patients with this disease. The presence of IgA at the BMZ is necessary, but the particular target of that IgA is perhaps less significant.

As in DH, an animal model has been developed. A mouse monoclonal IgA antibody directed against the LABD97 fragment of BP180 was injected into severe combined immunodeficiency (SCID) mice bearing human skin grafts. Although no macroscopic disease was elicited, basement membrane IgA deposition was demonstrable in all mice, and an enhanced neutrophilic infiltrate was observed in half of the injected animals. Five of 12 mice showed histologic evidence of blistering.

Clinical Features

The eruption of LABD is heterogeneous in appearance and may consist of erythematous grouped papulovesicles and urticarial plaques as seen in DH (Fig. 45.3A) or tense bullae similar to the lesions of

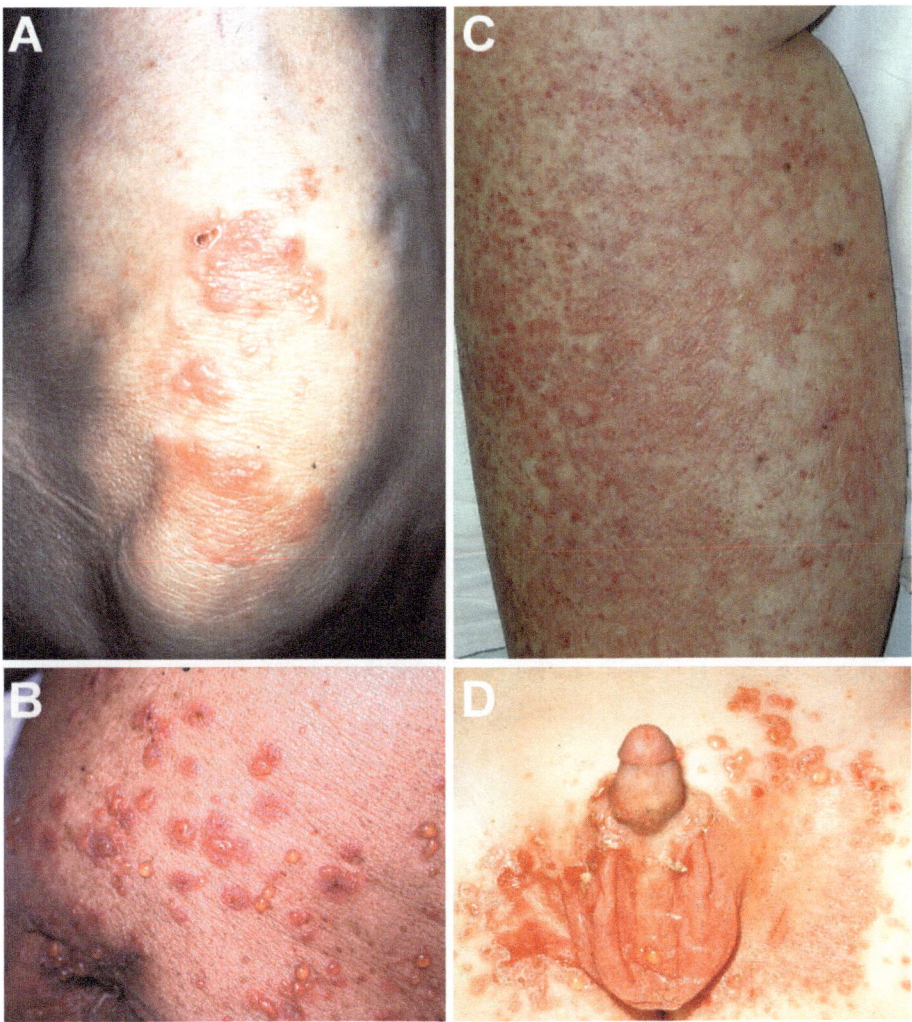

FIG. 45.3. Linear IgA bullous dermatosis (LABD). (A) Erythematous papulovesicles on the elbow of an adult suggestive of dermatitis herpetiformis (DH). (B) This adult's periumbilical eruption emphasizes the polymorphic nature of LABD. Tense bullae on a nonerythematous base are seen characteristic of cell-poor bullous pemphigoid in combination with deeply erythematous papulovesicular and urticarial lesions. (C) The leg of a patient with vancomycin-induced LABD. There is diffuse erythema and superficial blistering indicative of toxic epidermal necrolysis. (D) Typical inguinal and scrotal blistering of childhood LABD

BP (Fig. 45.3B). The bullae often are arranged in linear or arciform patterns. Annular erythematous bullae, the so-called crown of jewels, are a classic finding in childhood LABD. Less commonly, patients may present with erythema multiforme–like lesions. The trunk is most often involved, but LABD can arise on the extremities, face, and scalp. In children, facial, inguinal, and perineal involvement is characteristic, with subsequent spread to the trunk and extremities. Mucosal involvement is extremely common, perhaps as high as 70% in adults.[20] On occasion, LABD initially presents as predominant or exclusive and severe mucosal disease with scarring, compatible with a clinical diagnosis of cicatricial pemphigoid. Pruritus is a nearly universal complaint.

Linear IgA bullous dermatosis is frequently drug-induced. Over 20 different agents have been associated with LABD, but by far the most frequent inciting drug is vancomycin. Other agents appearing in several case reports include β-lactam and cephalosporin antibiotics, nonsteroidal antiinflammatory drugs (NSAIDs), and captopril (Table 45.3). The clinical picture of drug-induced LABD does not deviate significantly from the idiopathic form, although mucosal involvement is somewhat less common in the former. The eruption presents within 1 to 2 weeks from initiation of an offending drug and resolves 2 to 6 weeks after the agent is withdrawn. Of note, seven cases of especially severe drug-induced LABD have been reported

TABLE 45.3. Drugs associated with linear IgA bullous dermatosis.

Common	Vancomycin
Multiple reports	Captopril
	β-lactams
	Cephalosporins
	NSAIDs
	Phenytoin
Isolated reports	Acetaminophen
	Amiodarone
	Atorvastatin
	Benazepril
	Candesartan/eprosartan
	Carbamazepine
	Furosemide
	Gemcitabine
	Interleukin-2
	Lithium
	Somatostatin
	Trimethoprim/sulfamethoxazole

that clinically mimicked toxic epidermal necrolysis (TEN), of which five were secondary to vancomycin. Two succumbed to comorbidities, but the remainder enjoyed a resolution of their cutaneous disease upon discontinuation of the offending drug. It is therefore important to consider drug-induced LABD in the evaluation of any patient with suspected TEN (Fig. 45.3C).

Patients with LABD may have an increased incidence of lymphoproliferative malignancies of B-cell origin (three of 70 adults in one series[21]). Scattered reports of other coexistent malignancies in LABD patients are probably serendipitous. Associations with disparate autoimmune disorders, including connective tissue diseases and thyroiditis, have also been proposed, but a compelling link has only been established with inflammatory bowel disease, primarily ulcerative colitis, which is seen in up to 7% of patients.[22]

Histology

Routine histology of lesional skin in LABD follows a similar pattern as the clinical presentation. Histologic findings may be essentially indistinguishable from DH, exhibiting subepidermal blistering with a neutrophilic infiltrate (Fig. 45.4A). The infiltrate tends to be more diffuse than in DH, but papillary microabscesses may still be observed. However, roughly an equivalent percentage will display histologic features that are indistinguishable from bullous pemphigoid, although the density of eosinophils in the inflammatory infiltrate is on average less than that observed in typical pemphigoid.

The accurate diagnosis of LABD is contingent on immunofluorescence studies of perilesional skin. Direct immunofluorescence reveals a homogeneous linear deposition of IgA along the basement membrane and is pathognomonic for LABD (Fig. 45.4B). Patients with homogeneous linear deposition of IgA have a disorder that is distinct from the disorder in patients with linear deposits of granular IgA. Virtually all patients with granular IgA deposition in either a linear or dermal papillary pattern have dermatitis herpetiformis.

Immunoglobulin G co-deposition is seen in a minority of patients and may complicate differentiation from BP. Initial investigations

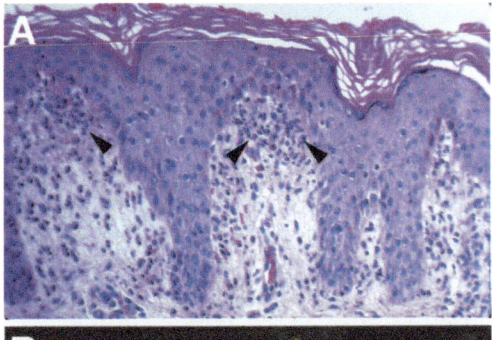

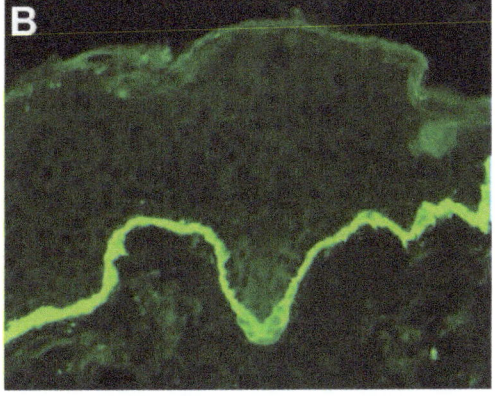

FIG. 45.4. Linear IgA bullous dermatosis. (A) Biopsy of the patient pictured in Figure 45.3A with DH-like LABD showed a dermal papillary neutrophilic infiltrate (arrowheads). (B) Homogeneous linear IgA deposition along the basement membrane is diagnostic

looking for circulating autoantibodies in LABD patients with IIF using intact skin as substrate were largely negative. Incubation of human skin with 1 mol/L NaCl results in epidermal separation at the level of the lamina lucida. The use of salt-split skin (SSK) greatly enhances the sensitivity of IIF in IgA dermatoses in general because of its increased capacity to detect the relatively low titers of autoantibodies common in these disorders. With SSK, >60% of LABD patients demonstrate positive IIF in selected studies.[18] Researchers studying LABD often draw a distinction between the majority of patients who possess epidermal antigens (positive IIF along the roof of SSK) and the minority with dermal antigens (positive along the base), but as discussed previously this dichotomy may have limited clinical or pathophysiologic significance.

Treatment

Despite the clinical and histologic heterogeneity that mark LABD, most patients respond dramatically to sulfone therapy at doses that are comparable to patients affected with DH. However, one third to one half of patients with LABD may require low to modest doses of oral corticosteroids to achieve adequate control of disease, although corticosteroid requirements have not been studied in any systematic way.[23] Concurrent deposition of immunoreactants in addition to IgA does not appear to predict differences in sulfone responsiveness.

Subsets of patients with LABD may present with much more extensive and difficult to treat disease marked by partial and inadequate responses to sulfone treatment. Furthermore, while the cutaneous disease is generally quite sulfone responsive, predominant mucosal disease tends to be substantially more resistant.[24] In difficult cases, a therapeutic approach borrowed from experience in the treatment of bullous pemphigoid or cicatricial pemphigoid appears to be promising. A variety of isolated reports have identified patients who ultimately responded to more aggressive treatments including azathioprine, mycophenolate mofetil, cyclophosphamide, and intravenous immunoglobulin (IVIG).

Immunoglobulin A Pemphigus

Immunoglobulin A pemphigus is the most popular term applied to a newly characterized and extremely rare group of disorders defined by the presence of intercellular, epidermal deposits of IgA. In the literature, this entity has been alternatively labeled intraepidermal neutrophilic IgA dermatosis, intraepidermal IgA pustulosis, and intercellular IgA (vesiculopustular) dermatosis. Although no agreement on nomenclature has been reached, we prefer the laconic designation IgA pemphigus, which emphasizes its immunologic and histologic parallels with the well-characterized pemphigus family of diseases. In concordance with its IgG-mediated counterpart, desmosomal components are the targets of the pathogenic antibodies in the cases of IgA pemphigus where an antigen has been identified.

Two subtypes of IgA pemphigus are recognized. The subcorneal pustular dermatosis (SPD) type exhibits upper epidermal IgA staining on DIF and resembles Sneddon-Wilkinson disease clinically. The intraepidermal neutrophilic (IEN) type shows intercellular IgA spanning the entire epidermis with consequent deeper appearing pustular lesions.

Epidemiology

Approximately 70 cases of IgA pemphigus have been reported, with most cases occurring in the U.S., Europe, and Japan. A review of 49 of these cases revealed a slight predominance of the SPD type and an overall female/male ratio of 1.45:1.[25] Most patients were in their fifth or later decade of life.

Pathogenesis

Sera obtained from patients with IgA pemphigus have consistently failed to react to any proteins on immunoblots, presumably because the tertiary structure of the antigen must be preserved for antibody binding. By expressing desmosomal proteins in mammalian cells, where they assume their native conformation, and assaying for autoantibodies by living cell immunofluorescence, Hashimoto et al.[26] demonstrated that desmocollin 1, a member of the cadherin superfamily, is an autoantigen in the SPD type of IgA pemphigus.[26] The transmembrane cell-adhesion proteins within desmosomes, which through their heterophilic (and possibly also homophilic) interactions provide tight interepithelial binding, belong to one of two groups of cadherins: desmocollins and desmogleins. The latter are the target antigens in classic pemphigus. Except for a few isolated cases where a desmoglein has been implicated, an autoantigen in IgA pemphigus-IEN type has not been established.

In classic pemphigus, IgG impairs its target cadherins directly, disrupting intercellular adhesion and resulting in acantholysis. The process can proceed without the assistance of complement fixation or immune cells. Indeed, monovalent antigen binding fragments (Fab) isolated from pathogenic pemphigus antibodies, which lack the Fc portion of the antibody necessary for interactions with complement and effector cells, are sufficient to elicit bullae in experimental models. In contrast, the presence of neutrophils is essential

for the evolution of skin lesions in IgA pemphigus. Acantholysis, though often present, is not a cardinal feature of IgA pemphigus, which is instead most notable for the interepithelial abscesses that develop. Thus, clinically, IgA pemphigus exhibits a more pustular phenotype distinct from the vesiculobullous nature of the early lesions in its IgG-mediated counterparts.

Clinical Features

Immunoglobulin A pemphigus presents with vesiculopustular lesions often arising within thin erythematous plaques. The trunk and proximal extremities are affected with extensive involvement of intertriginous areas commonplace. The postauricular skin and scalp may also be involved. Pruritus can be pronounced. Pustules in the SPD type often assume annular and serpiginous arrangements with central crusting similar to classic SPD (Sneddon-Wilkinson disease). The IEN type may have a similar appearance, although a distinguishing "sunflower-like" lesion has been described, consisting of vesiculopustules fringing a deeply erythematous plaque. Erosions and desquamation may be observed in both types. The mucous membranes are usually spared. No disease associations have been established.

Histology

Intraepidermal pustules with microabscesses and a dermal and epidermal neutrophilic infiltrate are seen in affected skin of both subtypes. The pustules are in the superficial epidermis in the SPD type and are located throughout the epidermis in the IEN type. Acantholysis and acantholytic cells are occasionally seen but are not typical and are especially rare in the IEN type. Direct immunofluorescence demonstrates fairly uniform intercellular IgA encircling the keratinocytes within the upper epidermal layers in the SPD type and throughout the epidermis in the IEN type. Similar patterns are seen with IIF, which is positive in approximately 50% of patients.

Treatment

Immunoglobulin A pemphigus is a chronic condition but is relatively indolent, with considerably less morbidity than classic pemphigus. Dapsone is the initial therapy of choice in both subtypes of IgA pemphigus. A dosage of 75 to 100 mg daily is often effective. Long-term maintenance therapy at a lower dosage is usually required after disease control is achieved. In general, the SPD subtype is less responsive to treatment than the IEN type. If the response to dapsone is inadequate, the patient may be switched to an oral retinoid or, more typically, the two used in combination. Several cases of the SPD type appearing in the literature have resolved with etretinate treatment, but this drug is no longer available in the United States, leaving either Soriatane or isotretinoin as the preferred second-line agent. Oral corticosteroids have been used extensively because of their efficacy in classic pemphigus. Dapsone in conjunction with corticosteroids have achieved disease remission in several cases of IEN-type IgA pemphigus, and this regimen is an appropriate secondary option in patients with this subtype who fail dapsone monotherapy. Rarely, recalcitrant cases of IgA pemphigus (usually of the SPD type) have required more aggressive immunosuppressive therapy.

Immunoglobulin A Vasculitis (Henoch-Schönlein Purpura)

Immunoglobulin A–mediated dermal small-vessel vasculitis is most commonly associated with, and in many clinicians' minds equated with, the clinical syndrome of Henoch-Schönlein purpura (HSP), which is characterized by the tetrad of palpable purpura, arthralgias, gastrointestinal symptoms, and glomerulonephritis. Immunoglobulin A class antibodies have been frequently observed within vessel walls in cases of isolated cutaneous leukocytoclastic vasculitis (LCV).[27] Immunoglobulin A deposits are also commonly identified in secondary cutaneous vasculitides associated with connective tissue diseases such as lupus erythematosus, Sjögren's syndrome, and rheumatoid arthritis, or in larger vessel systemic necrotizing vasculitides such as polyarteritis nodosa.[28,29] Furthermore, IgA antineutrophilic cytoplasmic antibodies (ANCAs) have been identified in erythema elevatum diutinum and other cases of LCV. The pathogenicity and significance of IgA in all of these settings remains unclear and may very well be incidental. Henoch-Schönlein purpura represents the only

distinct entity for which IgA antibodies are broadly imputed a central role in diagnosis and in pathophysiology and therefore will be the focus of this section. A full discussion of the wide range of vasculitic syndromes where IgA has been detected by DIF is beyond the scope of this chapter.

While adults are also affected, HSP is predominantly a childhood disease and is the most common pediatric vasculitis. It represents an immunologic response to a precipitating infection or drug and is usually self-limited. However, recurrences are common, and a minority of patients develop a persistent nephropathy.

Epidemiology

The peak age of onset of HSP is between 2 and 10 years. Girls are affected about 50% more often than boys, but there is no gender differential among adults. Approximately 70% of children[30,31] and 40% of adults[29] have a history of a recent upper respiratory infection, viral or streptococcal. Pharmaceuticals, foods, and hematologic malignancies have also been implicated as precipitating agents. No convincing association with any MHC molecules has been reported.

Pathogenesis

The classification schemes and general pathophysiologies of the numerous vasculitides are reviewed in detail in Chapter 19. The majority of vasculitic syndromes can be classified by their central pathogenesis according to the operative class of hypersensitivity reaction as described by Coombs and Gell. As a neutrophil-predominant, DIF-positive vasculitis, HSP best fits into the category of type III hypersensitivity reactions; that is, immune complex deposition is directly culpable, along with cutaneous LCV from which HSP is histologically indistinguishable. A few studies from three decades ago demonstrated circulating IgA immune complexes in HSP,[32,33] but most evidence implicating immune complexes in pathogenesis is indirect. Clearly IgA is present in the vessel walls, but whether it is bound to an in-situ antigen or represents a deposited immune complex has never been definitively established. No antigen has ever been associated with the vascular IgA in HSP. There are numerous conflicting reports of IgA ANCA in the serum of adults and children with HSP. About as many studies have reported the absence of IgA ANCA as have its presence. The most recent series revealed a high prevalence of IgA ANCA in children with HSP and a strong correlation with disease activity but not with disease severity.[34] Concerns linger, though, over the possible technical issues with these studies. The high concentrations of (potentially physiologically abnormal) IgA in HSP patients' sera may facilitate weak, nonspecific interactions with components of neutrophilic extracts, yielding false-positive results.

For now, the consensus holds that IgA immune complexes are pathogenic in HSP. Presumably, an immunologic response to a microbial or tumoral antigen or drug hapten in susceptible individuals generates circulating IgA immune complexes. The immune complexes tend to deposit in the glomeruli and in the walls of the small blood vessels within the dermis of the lower extremities. These represent general predilection areas in immune complex-mediated vasculitis. Immune complex deposition occurs in the vascular beds of the other target organs, namely the joints and the gastrointestinal tract. The IgA immune complexes engender an exuberant neutrophilic response leading to a necrotizing vasculitis, enzymatic and ischemic destruction of surrounding tissues, and erythrocyte extravasation.

As in the other diseases in this chapter, IgA1 appears to be the primary subclass involved. Some studies have demonstrated abnormal glycosylation of IgA1 in HSP patients relative to normal controls.[35] This structural variation may confer on IgA1 some unusual properties, which are of theoretical importance in HSP pathogenesis, such as increased half-life, increased ability to complex in plasma, increased tendency to deposit in target organs, and the capacity to fix complement more efficiently. Further research on the potentially distinct biochemical properties of IgA in HSP is necessary to substantiate any of these intriguing hypotheses.

Clinical Features

Palpable purpura represents the predominant cutaneous manifestations of HSP and is essentially universal (Fig. 45.5A). It usually develops in dependent areas: the lower extremities, buttocks,

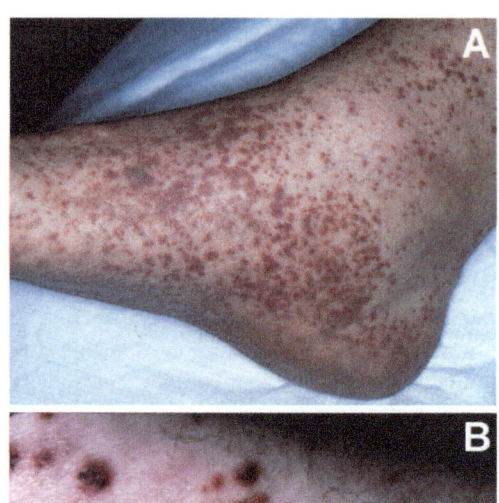
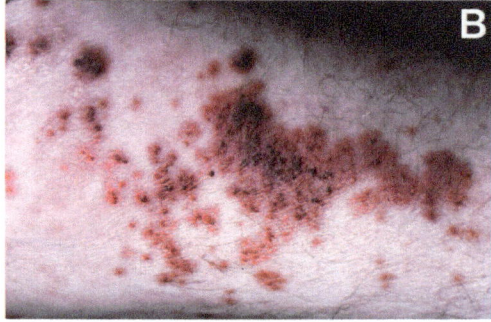

FIG. 45.5. Henoch-Schönlein purpura. (A) The foot of an adult displaying punctate purpura and coalescent purpuric plaques consistent with a leukocytoclastic vasculitis. (B) This adult demonstrated the characteristic irregular plaques containing a retiform pattern of hemorrhage

and scrotum. The upper extremities and trunk are less commonly involved. Macular, petechial, and urticarial lesions may also be observed, but they typically evolve into purpura over 24 to 48 hours. Acral and scalp edema is a frequent finding and may confuse the diagnosis with acute hemorrhagic edema of infancy in the very young. Bullous, necrotic, and ulcerative lesions are rare in children but occur in up to 60% of adults,[29] suggesting involvement of larger dermal or subcutaneous arteries. In adults, irregular purpuric plaques containing a "retiform" pattern of hemorrhage or superficial necrosis has been proposed as a distinctive lesion in IgA-mediated vasculitis by one group[36] (Fig. 45.5B), but the uniqueness of this finding has not been corroborated in other series.

Arthralgias and abdominal pain may precede purpura by up to 2 weeks in 30% to 40% of patients, but renal manifestations almost always follow the characteristic rash. Arthritis occurs in approximately 80% of patients and abdominal pain in 60%. Colicky abdominal pain may be accompanied by emesis. Gastrointestinal bleeding, mostly occult, occurs in approximately 30% of patients.[37,38] Rarely, more serious gastrointestinal involvement can arise, and the clinician must maintain concern for ischemic bowel or intussusception in patients with worrisome abdominal exams.

Immunoglobulin A glomerulopathy is the only potential source of long-term morbidity in HSP and should be ruled out in any vasculitis with significant IgA on DIF. The other manifestations of HSP usually resolve in an average of 4 weeks and only occasionally persist beyond 8 weeks.[30] As with any glomerulonephritis, hematuria is a defining feature of HSP nephritis and occurs in about 34% of children with HSP according to a recent meta-analysis.[39] The majority of patients (98%) with isolated hematuria with or without proteinuria do not suffer from long-term renal impairment. The incidence of nephrotic or nephritic syndrome is about 7% at presentation, and less than 2% of children have a persistent nephropathy. Overall, the prognosis of HSP nephritis in the child is therefore good; however, several studies have reported more severe renal involvement in adults.[40]

The natural history of HSP is surprisingly chronic with frequent relapses, which is reminiscent of secondary vasculitides in the setting of connective tissue diseases. This contrasts with primary LCV associated with a drug or microbial trigger, which typically presents as a single, self-limited episode. The perplexing multi-episodic nature of HSP has never been explained. But it is this unique natural history that creates some dissatisfaction with the simple drug- or bug-induced immune-complex etiology outlined previously. A search for an autoimmune component in the pathogenesis of HSP (e.g., ANCA or antiendothelial antibodies) is therefore an important ongoing pursuit.

Histology

Conventional histology shows a superficial necrotizing small-vessel vasculitis with perivascular neutrophilic infiltrate that cannot be differentiated from typical LCV (see Chapter 19). In patients with bullous and ulcerative lesions, involvement of deep dermal vessels may also be seen. Direct immunofluorescence reveals predominant IgA deposits and variable amounts of C3 in the walls of both involved and uninvolved vessels. Although all cases of HSP exhibit IgA deposition, the converse is not true. As mentioned previously, vascular IgA deposits may be observed in numerous settings. Other vasculitic syndromes must be ruled out on clinical or histologic grounds.

Treatment

Because of the self-limited nature of HSP, treatment is mostly supportive. A urinalysis, measures of renal function, and blood pressure should be obtained in all patients upon diagnosis and the beginning of each recurrent episode. If results are normal, urinalysis and blood pressure should be rechecked for 6 months after which point the risk of new-onset renal involvement is negligible. Children with isolated hematuria or proteinuria (i.e., normal creatinine, blood pressure, and urine output) typically enjoy a full resolution of their nephritis, and long-term follow-up is probably unnecessary. Children presenting with nephritic or nephrotic syndrome are at high risk (20%) of chronic renal insufficiency and should be referred to a nephrologist. A similar degree of vigilance is prudent in all adults with evidence of nephritis.

Corticosteroids have been used extensively for decades in the treatment of HSP. They seem to be the most effective agents for alleviating abdominal and joint symptoms but, in usual doses, have never been shown to alter the natural history of any element of the disease. The most important goal of therapy is prevention of chronic renal insufficiency. In a prospective but uncontrolled trial, children with severe glomerulonephritis experienced promising improvement in acute renal pathology and limited disease progression when high-dose pulse methylprednisolone followed by oral corticosteroids was initiated early in the course of the disease.[41] Oral or IV corticosteroids in combination with azathioprine is another common regimen for HSP nephritis that has yielded good long-term outcomes in retrospective reviews.[42]

Purpura and other cutaneous manifestations, if severe enough to warrant treatment, often respond well to dapsone.[43] Dapsone does not seem to ameliorate the vasculitis in other target organs.

Conclusion

Immunoglobulin A dermatosis are a diverse group of dermatologic diseases that share IgA deposition in tissue, which more importantly plays an important role in the pathophysiologic process. Neutrophils are one of the few cell types that express IgA receptors (FcαR1), and hence are a major component of the cellular infiltrate, as well as important effector cells that mediate tissue damage. Because neutrophils are important in the IgA dermatoses (dermatitis herpetiformis, linear IgA bullous dermatosis, IgA pemphigus and Henoch-Schönlein purpura), this group of diseases exhibits pharmacologic responsiveness to sulfone therapy (dapsone and related compounds).

References

1. Woof JM, Kerr MA. The function of immunoglobulin A in immunity. J Pathol 2006;208(2):270–82.
2. Wines BD, Hogarth PM. IgA receptors in health and disease. Tissue Antigens 2006;68(2):103–14.
3. Suda T, Suzuki Y, Matsui T, et al. Dapsone suppresses human neutrophil superoxide production and elastase release in a calcium-dependent manner. Br J Dermatol 2005;152(5):887–95.
4. Debol SM, Herron MJ, Nelson RD. Anti-inflammatory action of dapsone: inhibition of neutrophil adherence is associated with inhibition of chemoattractant-induced signal transduction. J Leukoc Biol 1997;62(6):827–36.
5. Smith JB, Tulloch JE, Meyer LJ, et al. The incidence and prevalence of dermatitis herpetiformis in Utah. Arch Dermatol 1992;128(12):1608–10.
6. Spurkland A, Ingvarsson G, Falk ES, et al. Dermatitis herpetiformis and celiac disease are both primarily associated with the HLA-DQ (alpha 1*0501, beta 1*02) or the HLA-DQ (alpha 1*03, beta 1*0302) heterodimers. Tissue Antigens 1997;49(1):29–34.
7. Fry L, Keir P, McMinn RM, et al. Small-intestinal structure and function and haematological changes in dermatitis herpetiformis. Lancet 1967;2(7519):729–33.
8. Dieterich W, Ehnis T, Bauer M, et al. Identification of tissue transglutaminase as the autoantigen of celiac disease.[see comment]. Nature Med 1997;3(7):797–801.
9. Sardy M, Karpati S, Merkl B, et al. Epidermal transglutaminase (TGase 3) is the autoantigen of dermatitis herpetiformis. J Exp Med 2002;195(6):747–57.
10. Marietta E, Black K, Camilleri M, et al. A new model for dermatitis herpetiformis that uses HLA-DQ8 transgenic NOD mice. J Clin Invest 2004;114(8):1090–7.
11. Gaspari AA, Huang CM, Davey RJ, et al. Prevalence of thyroid abnormalities in patients with dermatitis herpetiformis and in control subjects with HLA-B8/-DR3. Am J Med 1990;88(2):145–50.
12. Sigurgeisson B, Agnarsson BA, Lindelof B. Risk of lymphoma in patients with dermatitis herpetiformis. BMJ 1994;308(6920):13–.
13. Zone JJ, Meyer LJ, Petersen MJ. Deposition of granular IgA relative to clinical lesions in dermatitis herpetiformis. Arch Dermatol 1996;132(8):912–8.
14. Fry L, Walkden V, Wojnarowska F, et al. A comparison of IgA positive and IgA negative dapsone responsive dermatoses. Br J Dermatol 1980;102(4):371–82.
16. Holtzer CD, Flaherty JF Jr, Coleman RL. Cross-reactivity in HIV-infected patients switched from trimethoprim-sulfamethoxazole to dapsone. Pharmacotherapy 1998;18(4):831–5.
17. Collier PM, Wojnarowska F, Welsh K, et al. Adult linear IgA disease and chronic bullous disease of childhood: the association with human lymphocyte antigens Cw7, B8, DR3 and tumour necrosis factor influences disease expression. Br J Dermatol 1999;141(5):867–75.
18. Allen J, Wojnarowska F. Linear IgA disease: the IgA and IgG response to the epidermal antigens demonstrates that intermolecular epitope spreading is associated with IgA rather than IgG antibodies, and is more common in adults. Br J Dermatol 2003;149(5):977–85.
19. Allen J, Wojnarowska F. Linear IgA disease: the IgA and IgG response to dermal antigens demonstrates a chiefly IgA response to LAD285 and a dermal 180–kDa protein. Br J Dermatol 2003;149(5):1055–8.
20. Peters MS, Rogers RS. Clinical correlations of linear IgA deposition at the cutaneous basement membrane zone. J Am Acad Dermatol 1989;20(5 pt 1):761–70.
21. Godfrey K, Wojnarowska F, Leonard J. Linear IgA disease of adults: association with lymphoproliferative malignancy and possible role of other triggering factors.[see comment]. Br J Dermatol 1990;123(4):447–52.
22. Paige DG, Leonard JN, Wojnarowska F, et al. Linear IgA disease and ulcerative colitis. Br J Dermatol 1997;136(5):779–82.
23. Leonard JN, Haffenden GP, Ring NP, et al. Linear IgA disease in adults. Br J Dermatol 1982;107(3):301–16.
24. Wojnarowska F, Marsden RA, Bhogal B, et al. Chronic bullous disease of childhood, childhood cicatricial pemphigoid, and linear IgA disease of adults.

A comparative study demonstrating clinical and immunopathologic overlap. J Am Acad Dermatol 1988;19(5 pt 1):792–805.

25. Yasuda H, Kobayashi H, Hashimoto T, et al. Subcorneal pustular dermatosis type of IgA pemphigus: demonstration of autoantibodies to desmocollin-1 and clinical review. Br J Dermatol 2000;143(1):144–8.

26. Hashimoto T, Kiyokawa C, Mori O, et al. Human desmocollin 1 (Dsc1) is an autoantigen for the subcorneal pustular dermatosis type of IgA pemphigus. J Invest Dermatol 1997;109(2):127–31.

27. Barnadas MA, Perez E, Gich I, et al. Diagnostic, prognostic and pathogenic value of the direct immunofluorescence test in cutaneous leukocytoclastic vasculitis.[see comment]. Int J Dermatol 2004;43(1):19–26.

28. Magro CM, Crowson AN. A clinical and histologic study of 37 cases of immunoglobulin A-associated vasculitis. Am J Dermatopathol 1999;21(3):234–40.

29. Tancrede-Bohin E, Ochonisky S, Vignon-Pennamen MD, et al. Schonlein-Henoch purpura in adult patients. Predictive factors for IgA glomerulonephritis in a retrospective study of 57 cases.[see comment]. Arch Dermatol 1997;133(4):438–42.

30. Allen DM, Diamond LK, Howell DA. Anaphylactoid purpura in children (Schonlein-Henoch syndrome): review with a follow-up of the renal complications. Am J Dis Child 1960;99:833–54.

31. Sterky G, Thilen A. A study on the onset and prognosis of acute vascular purpura (the Schoenlein-Henoch syndrome) in children. Acta Paediatr 1960;49:217–29.

32. Kauffmann RH, Herrmann WA, Meyer CJ, et al. Circulating IgA-immune complexes in Henoch-Schonlein purpura. A longitudinal study of their relationship to disease activity and vascular deposition of IgA. Am J Med 1980;69(6):859–66.

33. Levinsky RJ, Barratt TM. IgA immune complexes in Henoch-Schonlein purpura. Lancet 1979;2(8152):1100–3.

34. Ozaltin F, Bakkaloglu A, Ozen S, et al. The significance of IgA class of antineutrophil cytoplasmic antibodies (ANCA) in childhood Henoch-Schonlein purpura. Clin Rheumatol 2004;23(5):426–9.

35. Saulsbury FT. Alterations in the O-linked glycosylation of IgA1 in children with Henoch-Schonlein purpura. J Rheumatol 1997;24(11):2246–9.

36. Piette WW, Stone MS. A cutaneous sign of IgA-associated small dermal vessel leukocytoclastic vasculitis in adults (Henoch-Schonlein purpura). Arch Dermatol 1989;125(1):53–6.

37. Saulsbury FT. Henoch-Schonlein purpura in children. Report of 100 patients and review of the literature. Medicine 1999;78(6):395–409.

38. Calvino MC, Llorca J, Garcia-Porrua C, et al. Henoch-Schonlein purpura in children from northwestern Spain: a 20–year epidemiologic and clinical study. Medicine 2001;80(5):279–90.

39. Narchi H. Risk of long term renal impairment and duration of follow up recommended for Henoch-Schonlein purpura with normal or minimal urinary findings: a systematic review. Arch Dis Child 2005;90(9):916–20.

40. Pillebout E, Thervet E, Hill G, et al. Henoch-Schonlein Purpura in Adults: Outcome and Prognostic Factors. J Am Soc Nephrol 2002;13(5):1271–8.

41. Niaudet P, Habib R. Methylprednisolone pulse therapy in the treatment of severe forms of Schonlein-Henoch purpura nephritis. Pediatr Nephrol 1998; 12(3):238–43.

42. Foster BJ, Bernard C, Drummond KN, et al. Effective therapy for severe Henoch-Schonlein purpura nephritis with prednisone and azathioprine: a clinical and histopathologic study. J Pediatr 2000;136(3):370–5.

43. Iqbal H, Evans A. Dapsone therapy for Henoch-Schonlein purpura: a case series. Arch Dis Child 2005;90(9):985–a-6.

Index